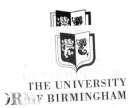

Cell Biology

CELL BIOLOGY

Thomas D. Pollard, M.D.
Higgins Professor of Molecular, Cellular and Developmental Biology
Yale University
New Haven, Connecticut

William C. Earnshaw, Ph.D., FRSE
Professor and Wellcome Trust Principal Research Fellow
University of Edinburgh
Scotland, United Kingdom

Illustrated by Graham T. Johnson

SAUNDERS
An Imprint of Elsevier Science
Philadelphia London New York St. Louis Sydney Toronto

SAUNDERS
An Imprint of Elsevier Science

The Curtis Center
Independence Square West
Philadelphia, Pennsylvania 19106

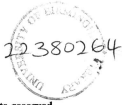

CELL BIOLOGY

ISBN 0-7216-3997-6

Notice

Medicine is an ever-changing field. Standard safety precautions must be followed, but as new research and clinical experience broaden our knowledge, changes in treatment and drug therapy may become necessary or appropriate. Readers are advised to check the most current product information provided by the manufacturer of each drug to be administered to verify the recommended dose, the method and duration of administration, and contraindications. It is the responsibility of the treating physician, relying on experience and knowledge of the patient, to determine dosages and the best treatment for each individual patient. Neither the Publisher nor the author assume any liability for any injury and/or damage to persons or property arising from this publication.

The Publisher

Library of Congress Cataloging-in-Publication Data

Pollard, Thomas D.
　　Cell biology / Thomas D. Pollard, William C. Earnshaw; illustrated by Graham T. Johnson.—1st ed.
　　　　p.　cm
　　Includes bibliographical references and index.
　　ISBN 0-7216-3997-6
　　　　1. Cytology.　I. Earnshaw, William C.　II. Title.

QH581.2.P65 2002
571.6—dc21

2002021189

Acquisitions Editor: William R. Schmitt
Senior Developmental Editor: Hazel N. Hacker
Production Manager: Donna Morrissey

PIT/QWK

Printed in the United States of America

Last digit is the print number:　9　8　7　6　5　4　3　2　1

To Patty and Margarete and our families

In memory of Keith Porter, Bernie Gilula, Thomas Kreis, and Paul Sigler

We would like to remember four friends who left us during the writing of this first edition: Keith Porter, the father of modern cell biology; Norton B. Gilula, who shaped the development of modern cell biology through his outstanding research and his insightful, compassionate, and critical leadership of the *Journal of Cell Biology;* Thomas Kreis, one of the rising stars of the field of molecular cell biology, whose career was cruelly cut short; Paul Sigler, x-ray crystallographer extraordinaire, who showed us how many important macromolecular complexes actually work.

PREFACE

To understand the chain of life from molecules through cells to tissues and organisms is the ultimate goal of cell biologists. To understand how cells work, we need to know a good deal about the identities and structures of molecules, how they fit together, and what they do. It is therefore tempting to compare cells to a complex piece of machinery, like a jet airliner, whose complexity may rival certain aspects of the cell. However, cells are much more complex than jet airliners. First, cells are enormously adaptable—unlike a simple assembly of mechanical parts, they can profoundly change their structure, physiology, and functions in response to environmental changes. Second, in multicellular organisms, cells provide only an intermediate level of complexity. Groups of specialized cells organize themselves into communities called tissues, and these tissues are further organized into organs that function in coordinated ways to produce life as we experience it. Finally, cells differ from complex machines in that there exists as yet no blueprint that completely describes how cells work. However, biologists who study a wide range of different aspects of cellular structure and function are beginning to compile such a blueprint. This has elucidated not only the molecular details of fundamental processes such as oxidative phosphorylation and protein synthesis but also many ways in which defects in individual molecular components can disrupt cell function and cause diseases.

Because the blueprint does not yet exist, this book necessarily represents a collection of vignettes from the lives and functions of cells. To some extent, these stories have been selected to demonstrate the general principles that we see as important. However, to a very real extent, they have also been selected by chance. This is the nature of scientific exploration and discovery: the scientist may set out on an investigation with a particular goal in mind only to discover that he or she has landed somewhere entirely different. Ultimately, our intent is to provide the student with a working knowledge of the major macromolecular systems of the cell, together with an understanding of how these principles were discovered and how the processes are coordinated to enable cells to function both autonomously and in tissues. The latter is important because most genetic diseases result from a single mutated molecule but manifest themselves by disrupting function in tissues. Cancer, which originates as a disease of single cells and can result from many different molecular lesions, is the exception.

This book's guiding theme is that cellular structure and function ultimately result from specific macromolecular interactions. In addition to water, salts, and small metabolites, cells are composed mainly of proteins, nucleic acids, lipids, and polysaccharides. Nucleic acids store genetic information required for reproduction and specify the sequences of thousands of RNAs and proteins. Both proteins and RNA serve as enzymes for the biosynthesis of all cellular constituents. Many RNAs have structural roles, but proteins—which are able to form the specific protein-protein, protein–nucleic acid, protein-lipid, and protein-polysaccharide bonds that hold the cell together—are the predominant structural elements of cells. A remarkable feature of these vital interactions between macromolecules is that few covalent bonds are involved. The striking conclusion is that the structure and function of the cell (and therefore the existence of life on earth) depends on highly specific, but often relatively tenuous, interactions between complementary surfaces of macromolecules.

The specificity of these interactions relies to a great extent on the structure of protein molecules. Molecular biologists discovered how the information for the primary structure (the amino acid sequence) of proteins is stored in the genes, and they continue to search for the mechanisms that cells use to control the expression of the thousands of genes whose products define the properties of each cell. Biochemists and biophysicists established that the three-dimensional structure of each protein is determined solely by its amino acid sequence: once synthesized, polypeptides fold either spontaneously or with the assistance of chaperones into specific three-dimensional structures. A folded protein may be biologically active, catalyzing a reaction, binding oxygen, or carrying out a myriad of other functions. However, in many cases it is inactive, waiting for the products of other genes to convert it to an active form. The ability of cells to regulate the expression of banks of genes and to fine-tune the activities of proteins after they have been made exemplifies the plasticity that enables cells to succeed in an ever-changing world.

Seeking to take the story a step farther, cell biologists ask this question: Do simple self-associations among the molecules account for the properties of the living cell? Is life, that is, merely a very complex molecular jigsaw puzzle? The answer developed in this book is both yes and no. To a large extent, cell structure and function clearly result from macromolecular interactions. However, living cells do not spontaneously self-assemble from mixtures of all their cellular constituents. The assembly reactions required for life reach completion only inside preexisting living cells; therefore, the existence of each cell depends on its historical continuity with past cells. This special historical feature sets biology apart from chemistry and physics. A cell can be viewed as the temporary repository of the genes of the species and the only microenvironment that allows macromolecular self-assembly reactions to continue the processes of life.

In our view, the field of cell biology is emerging from a Linnaean phase, where genetic and biochemical methods have been used to gather an inventory of many of the cell's molecules, into a more mechanistic phase, where new insights will come from detailed biophysical studies of these molecules at atomic resolution and of their dynamics in living cells. The molecular inventory of genes and gene products is massive, almost overwhelming, in its detail. But this genetic inventory is far from the complete story, especially at the interface of basic cell biology with medicine. On a weekly basis, investigators continue to track down the genes for defective proteins that predispose people to human disease. In addition to revealing the many genes that cause the spectrum of diseases known as cancer, this work has revealed the molecules responsible for muscular dystrophy, cystic fibrosis, hypertrophic cardiomyopathy, and blistering skin diseases, among many others, and will continue to grow as

scientists seek the causes of more complex multifactorial diseases. Because virtually every gene expressed in the human body is subject to mutation, it is quite possible that eventually a great many genes will be directly or indirectly implicated in the predisposition to disease.

For both the basic scientist who seeks general principles about cellular function, often in "model" organisms, and the physician who applies knowledge of the molecular mechanisms of normal cellular function to the understanding of cellular dysfunction in human disease, the future lies in insights about how the cellular repertoire of macromolecules interact with one another. Understanding at this level requires not only the knowledge of atomic structures and rates of molecular interactions but also the development of molecular probes to follow these interactions in living cells. With respect to this area of recent explosive progress, this book presents both current technological advances and lessons already learned.

Given the complexity of the molecular inventory (about 35,000 different genes in humans), gaining an understanding of the details of molecular interactions might, in principle, be equivalent to the daunting task of learning a set of 35,000 Chinese characters and all the rules of spelling and grammar that govern their use. However, it is already clear that the origin of complex life forms by evolution has simplified the task. For example, although the genome encodes about 800 protein kinases (enzymes that transfer a phosphate from ATP to a protein), each kinase has much in common with all other kinases because of their evolution from a common ancestor. The same is true of membrane receptors with seven α-helices traversing the lipid bilayer. Detailed knowledge about any one of these kinases or receptors provides informative general principles about how the whole family of related molecules works. Thus, although there are more than a few names, structures, binding partners, and reaction rates to learn, we are confident that many general concepts have already emerged and will continue to emerge. These will enable us to develop a set of "first principles" that we can use to deduce how novel pathways are put together and function when we are confronted with new genes and structures.

Although we feel that the time is right to take a molecular approach to cellular structure and function, this is not a biochemistry book. Readers who are interested in a fuller understanding of metabolism, the biosynthesis of cellular building blocks, enzymology, and other purely biochemical topics should consult one of the many excellent biochemistry texts. Similarly, although we consider herein some of the specialized manifestations of cells found in specific tissues and how these tissues are formed, this is not a histology or developmental biology book. We focus instead on the general properties of eukaryotic cells that are common to their successful function.

We have written this book with the busy student in mind. Carefully limiting the text's size and illustrating all the main points with original drawings, we anticipate that, in a single course, an undergraduate, medical, or graduate student will be able to read through the entire book. In our effort to keep the book concise, however, we have been careful to maintain appropriate depth. Most chapters contain a few complex figures that show either how some important points were discovered or how multiple processes are integrated with one another. A few of these figures may initially present a challenge; however, an understanding of these figures will ultimately provide insight into the integrated network of cellular life. Throughout this book, we have presented the very latest discoveries in cell biology, and in each section we have defined as closely as possible the frontiers of our knowledge. We hope that upon completion of the study of this text, our readers will share not only a comprehensive, up-to-date knowledge of how cells work but also our personal excitement about these basic insights into life itself. It is our sincerest hope that the questions raised herein will inspire some of our readers to experience the challenges and rewards of cell biology research for themselves and to contribute to the ongoing challenge of completing the blueprint of the life of the cell.

Organization of the Book

We anticipate that our readers will find many ways to use this book, which covers the structure and function of all parts of the cell and all major cellular processes. We have aimed to maintain uniform depth of coverage of each topic, including up-to-date descriptions of general principles and of the structures of the major molecules and an explanation of how the system works. The emphasis is on animal cells, but we have included many examples from fungi. Our inclusion of plants and prokaryotes distinguishes their special aspects, such as rotary flagella, two-component signal transduction pathways, and photosynthesis.

We divide the material into many highly focused stories that deal with particular molecules and mechanisms. Whereas an in-depth course in cell biology might cover the whole book, a variety of shorter courses might easily be fashioned by picking a subset of topics. Our 49 short chapters are clustered into 8 sections that discuss the major aspects of cellular structure and function: (1) molecules, self-assembly, and research strategies; (2) membranes; (3) genomes, gene expression, and nuclear organization; (4) organelle biogenesis and membrane traffic; (5) signal transduction; (6) adhesion and the extracellular matrix; (7)

cytoskeleton and cell motility; and (8) the cell cycle. Many of the chapters can be read in a single sitting.

We use molecular structures as the starting point for explaining how each cellular system is constructed and how it operates. Most of the eight major sections begin with one or more chapters that cover the key molecules that run the systems under consideration. For example, the section on signaling (Reception and Transduction of Environmental Information) begins with separate chapters on receptors, cytoplasmic signal transduction proteins, and second messengers. Noting the concentrations of key molecules and the rates of their reactions should help the student to appreciate the rapidly moving molecular environment inside cells.

We explain the evolutionary history and molecular diversity of each class of molecules as a basis for understanding how each system works. And we ask and answer two questions: How many varieties of this type of molecule exist in animals? Where did they come from in the evolutionary process? Thus, readers have the opportunity to see the big picture rather than just a mass of details. For example, a single original figure in Chapter 9 shows the evolution of all types of membrane ion channels followed by text that spells out the properties of each of these families.

After introducing the molecular hardware, each section finishes with one or more chapters that illustrate how these molecules function together in physiological process. This organization allows for a clearer exposition regarding the general principles of each class of molecules, since they are treated as a group rather than specific examples. More important still, the operation of complex processes, such as signaling pathways, is presented as an integrated whole, without the diversions that arise when it is necessary to introduce the various components as they arise along the pathway. Teachers of short courses may choose to concentrate on a subset of the examples in these systems chapters, or they may choose to use parts of the hardware chapters as reference material.

The seven chapters on the cell cycle that conclude the book clearly illustrate our approach. Having now covered the previous sections on nuclear structure and function, gene expression, membrane physiology, signal transduction and the cytoskeleton, and cell motility, the reader is prepared to appreciate the coordination of all cellular systems as step by step the cell transverses the cell cycle. This final section begins with a chapter that deals with general principles of cell cycle control and proceeds with chapters on each aspect of cell growth and death (including apoptosis), each integrating the contribution of all the cellular systems.

The chapters on cellular functions integrate material on specialized cells and tissues. Epithelia, for example, are covered under membrane physiology and junctions, excitable membranes of neurons and muscle under membrane physiology, connective tissues under the extracellular matrix, the immune system under connective tissue cells and signal transduction, muscle under the cytoskeleton and cell motility, and cancer under the cell cycle and signal transduction. We use clinical examples to illustrate physiological functions throughout the book. This is possible, since connections have now been made between most cellular systems and disease. These medical "experiments of nature" are woven into the text along with laboratory experiments on model organisms.

Most of the experimental evidence is presented in figures that include numerous micrographs, molecular structures, and key graphs that emphasize the results rather than the experimental details. Original references are given for many of the experiments. Many of the methods used will be new to our readers. The chapter on experimental methods in cell biology introduces how and why particular approaches (such as microscopy, classical genetics, genomics and reverse genetics, and biochemical methods) are used to identify new molecules, map molecular pathways, or verify physiological functions.

Most of the papers that are cited in the chapters' Selected Readings sections are reviews of the primary literature taken from major review journals, such as the *Annual Reviews* (*of Biochemistry, Cell Biology, Biophysics*), *Trends* (*in Cell Biology, Biochemical Sci-*

ences), and *Current Opinion* (*in Cell Biology, Structural Biology*), or from the review sections of major journals in the field, such as *Current Biology, Journal of Cell Biology, Nature, Proceedings of the National Academy of Sciences,* and *Science*. These references, although helpful to us in writing this book, will rapidly become dated. With very little effort, readers can update the reference lists on-line. Pubmed (http://www.ncbi.nlm.nih.gov/entrez/query.fcgi), the wonderful tool provided by the National Institutes of Health, is an invaluable resource. Simply type in the name of the molecule or the process of interest followed by a space and the word "review" (no quotation marks). In no time, you will access an up-to-date reference list. The abstracts given in Pubmed will help you choose the best articles for your purposes. Many institutions have electronic versions of the major journals in the field, so you can find and display a new review in a matter of seconds. Although the same route can be used to access the original research literature, the number of web site hits will be much greater than if the "review" restriction is used, so be prepared to spend more time searching. The Pubmed site also allows searches for atomic structures, genes, genomes, and proteins. Each of the numerous molecular structures displayed in our figures comes with a Protein Data Base (PDB) accession number. Anyone with an Internet connection to Pubmed or PDB can thus find the original data, display an animated molecule, and directly search links to the original literature.

ACKNOWLEDGMENTS

The days are long gone when an in-depth cell biology textbook can be written by one or two people—the field has simply been too successful, and the weight of knowledge is now too great. Thus, although the core team of TDP, WCE, and GJ account for much of this effort, completion of this book depended on essential contributions from many others. TDP based the framework for Chapters 7 to 10 on lectures given by Peter Maloney and Bill Agnew at Johns Hopkins Medical School. Bill Agnew, in turn, thanks Fred Sigworth of Yale Medical School for lecture material on ion channels. Jeff Corden wrote Chapter 14. Barbara Sollner-Webb wrote Chapter 15, with Christine Smith providing essential help with the design of a number of the figures. Ann Hubbard, David Castle, and Pat Shipman wrote the original versions of Chapters 17 to 24 on protein synthesis, organelle biogenesis, membrane traffic, and degradation mechanisms. Sandy Schmid rewrote Chapters 17 and 22 to 24. Bill Balch and TDP revised and updated Chapters 18 to 21. And WCE and Maria del Mar Carmena wrote Chapter 48. We thank one and all for contributing very considerable insights to the project. TDP and WCE edited all of the chapters and bear the responsibility for any errors that crept in during the process.

Many of us have written scientific review articles and remember the challenge of trying to encapsulate an entire field fairly and correctly. Having now completed the present exercise, we authors have experienced the humbling effort of trying to produce a text where comprehensive reviews represent only small subheadings or a single phrase within much larger chapters. We could not do this alone, and we have relied on many critics and advisors to keep us on track. The book is a much closer approximation to the truth than it would have been without the painstaking time that they spent in reading various drafts and suggesting improvements. These include (in alphabetical order) Bill Agnew, Peter Agre, James Allen, James Anderson, Denis Baylor, Philip Beachy, Jean Beggs, Jeremy Berg, Magdalena Bezanilla, Adrian Bird, Julian Blow, Henry Bourne, David Bredt, Gerta Breitwieser, Mike Caplow, Sherwood Casjens, Don Caspar, Senyon Choe, Don Cleveland, John A. Cooper, Pierre Coulombe, Gerry Crabtree, Enrique De La Cruz, John Diffley, Russ Doolittle, John Dowling, Barbara Ehrlich, Beverley Emerson, Harold Erickson, John Exton, Justin Fallon, Susan Forsburg, Joachim Frank, Elaine Fuchs, Tony Gallione, David Garbers, Ian Gibbons, Susan Gilbert, Bernie Gilula, Mark Ginsberg, Pete Godlewski, Bob Goldman, Joe Goldstein, Larry Goldstein, Dan Goodenough, Holly Goodson, Steve Gould, Kathleen Green, Barry Gumbiner, Barbara Hamkalo, Heidi Hamm, Vince Hascall, Ron Hay, Margarete Heck, Steve Heinemann, Silke Heinisch, Harry Higgs, Beth Holleran, Rick Horwitz, Rick Huganier, Maj Hulten, Tim Hunt, Tony Hunter, Richard Hynes, Ken Jacobson, Erick Jakobsson, Rob Jensen, David Jones, Jonathan Jones, Kristine Kamm, Scott Kaufmann, Kenneth Keegstra, Joe Kelleher, Dave Kovar, Jeff Kuhn, Ned Landau, David Leach, Dan Leahy, Bob Lefkowitz, Sam Lehrer, David Levy, Richard Linck, David Luck, Laura Machesky, David MacLennon, Stuart MacNeill, Peter Maloney, Dyche Mullins, Doug Murphy, Shigekazu Nagata, James Nelson, Alexandra Newton, Joe Noel, Joanna Olmsted, Bjorn Olsen, Charlotte Omoto, Leslie Orgel, Mike Ostap, Jonathon Pines, Dan Pollard, Katie Pollard, Mary Porter, Steve Quirk, Dan Raben, Rajini Rao, Tom Rappaport, Ivan Rayment, Randy Reed, Tom Roberts, Jon Sachs, Ted Salmon, Peter Satir, Immo Scheffler, Ron Schnaar, Danny Schnell, David Shortle, Tom Silhavy, Volodia Sirotkin, Ahna Skop, Paul Slesinger, Greenfield Sluder, Sol Snyder, Mitch Sogin, Tim Springer, Tom Steitz, Gail Stetten, Murray

Stewart, Sriram Subramanian, Lee Sweeney, Susan Taylor, David Thanassi, David Tollervey, Kirsi Turbedsky, Ron Vale, Kevin Vaughn, Jeff Wahl, Michael Way, Michael Welsh, Sarah Wheelan, Ian Wilson, Cynthia Wohlberger, Mark Yeager. We thank all for their helpful suggestions and apologize for any errors, which remain our own.

Now that the book is in circulation, we hope to hear from many readers about errors that have crept through in the process. We would like to use these suggestions, which can be posted on the book's web site (http://www.harcourthealth.com/SIMON/Pollard/) to improve future editions.

TDP and WCE thank and acknowledge our third author, artist Graham Johnson, who entered the project as an employee but over time assumed his rightful place as an equal contributor. Not only did he transform well over 1300 sketches into highly polished figures; he also acquired enough knowledge of the science behind each figure to contribute to its concept and design and ensured that all the molecules in each figure were drawn to the same scale. He downloaded the coordinates for the molecular structures from PDB files and chose the view that best illustrates each message. No other book has ever succeeded in presenting such realistic molecules to scale. Graham, we salute you for these efforts.

Graham thanks Witek Kwiatkowski, Max Nano, and Kirsi Turbedsky for introducing him to UNIX and molecular modeling software and Magdalena Bezanilla for answering many science questions and for providing input on the figures. Joanne Haderer assisted with the organization of the photo collection from contributing authors and created a few of the illustrations for Chapter 42. Her ideas for the first cover are still visible in the final cover and in the background graphics in the text. Emiko Koike and Quade Paul generously contributed endless artistic input for the figures and helped to finalize some sketches when time was short.

Individuals too numerous to list (consult the credits in each figure legend) provided original micrographs and figures. We must, however, single out Don Fawcett, Professor of Anatomy Emeritus at Harvard Medical School, as deserving special thanks. Don eagerly returned to the darkroom to print many beautiful electron micrographs especially for this book. The generosity of all the contributors helped us set a new standard for artwork in cell biology texts. Many thanks for these contributions. All unattributed figures were drawn by GJ or came from the collections of TDP and WCE.

A special note of thanks is due to Bill Schmitt at Saunders for believing in the project over the (many) years of its gestation and for allowing us an uncommon degree of editorial and design freedom. We also thank Andrew Stevenson for his involvement in bringing all to a successful culmination. Carol Vartanian skillfully edited early versions of many chapters. The production team, including Hazel Hacker, Donna Morrisey, and Joan Vidal, skillfully edited and assembled the book.

Personal Thanks

We thank our wives, Patty and Margarete (and the Earnshaw children, Charles and Irina), for never complaining when "The Book" meant that yet again they were left to fend for themselves. Finally, WCE thanks the members of his lab, past and present, and his longtime collaborator and friend Scott Kaufmann for similarly making allowances during those many times when the door was shut, the e-mails were unanswered, and deadlines were kept by the smallest of margins.

CONTENTS

chapter 1

GENERAL PRINCIPLES OF CELLULAR ORGANIZATION

▌ Historical Prologue

Biology is based on the fundamental laws of nature embodied in chemistry and physics, but the origin and evolution of life on earth was an historical event. This makes biology more like astronomy than like chemistry and physics. Neither the organization of the universe nor life as we know it had to evolve as it did. Chance played a central role. Throughout history and continuing today, the genes of some organisms sustain chemical changes that are inherited by their progeny. Many of the changes reduce the fitness of the organism, but some improve fitness. Over the long term, competition between sister organisms with random differences in their genes determines which survive in various environments. Although these genetic differences assure survival, they do not necessarily optimize each chemical life process. The variants that survive merely have a selective advantage over the alternatives. Thus, the molecular strategy of life processes works well, but is often illogical. Readers would likely be able to suggest simpler or more elegant mechanisms for many cellular processes. This historical prologue sets the stage for all that follows. Recent research has redrawn the tree of life (Fig. 1–1), providing a sound basis for understanding how life evolved and how contemporary organisms are related to each other.

The Unity of Biology at the Molecular Level

As the molecular mechanisms of life have become clearer, the underlying similarities are more impressive than the differences. Humans share with baker's yeast similar mechanisms to control our cell cycles, to guide protein secretion, and to segregate chromosomes at mitosis. Human versions of essential proteins can of-

ten substitute for their yeast counterparts. Biologists are confident that a limited number of general principles, summarizing common molecular mechanisms, will eventually explain even the most complex life processes in terms of straightforward chemistry and physics.

These general principles apply to all forms of life, because 3 or 4 billion years ago, all living things had a common ancestor (Box 1–1; see also Fig. 1–1). This organism no longer exists, but it must have utilized biochemical mechanisms similar to those that sustain contemporary cells. This retention of common molecular mechanisms in all parts of the **phylogenetic tree** is remarkable, given that the major phylogenetic groups have been separated for vast times and subjected to different selective pressures. The biochemical mechanisms in the branches of the phylogenetic tree could have diverged radically from each other, but they did not. To be sure, living things differ in size and complexity and are adapted to life in environments as extreme as deep sea hydrothermal vents at temperatures of 113°C or pockets of water at 0°C in frozen Antarctic lakes. They also differ in strategies to extract energy from their environments. Plants and some bacteria use sunlight for photosynthesis. Some bacteria and Archaea oxidize reduced inorganic compounds, such as hydrogen, hydrogen sulfide, or iron. Many organisms in all parts of the tree, including ourselves, extract energy from reduced organic compounds. Nevertheless, all organisms share a common genetic code, store genetic information in nucleic acids (usually **DNA**), transfer genetic information from DNA to **RNA** to protein, employ proteins (and occasionally, RNAs) to catalyze chemical reactions, synthesize proteins on **ribosomes,** derive energy by breaking down simple sugars, use adenosine triphosphate (**ATP**) as energy currency, and separate their cyto-

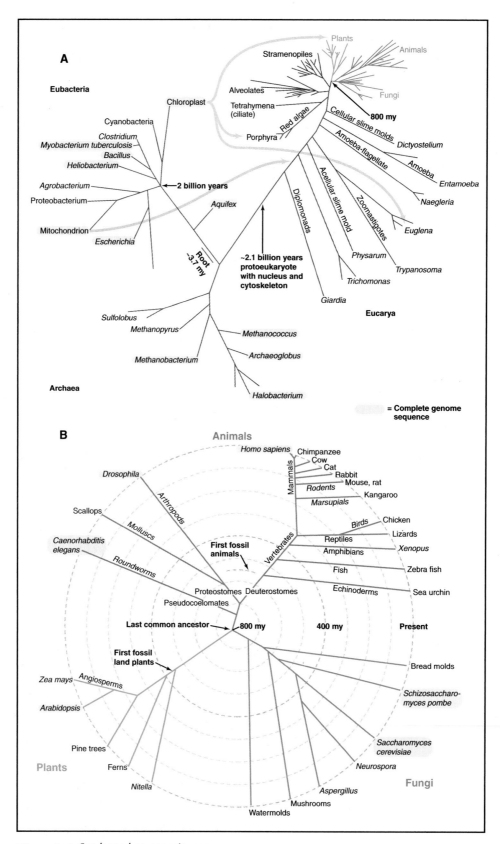

Figure 1-1 *See legend on opposite page*

plasm from their environment by means of phospholipid **membranes** containing **pumps, carriers,** and **channels.** These ancient biochemical strategies are so well adapted for survival that they have been protected from change during natural selection of the surviving species.

The common evolutionary origin of contemporary forms of life explains the underlying similarity of biochemical mechanisms across the phylogenetic tree. A practical consequence of the common ground provided by evolution is that the general principles of cellular function can be learned by studying any cell that is favorable for experimentation. This text will cite many examples where research on bacteria, insects, protozoa, or fungi has revealed fundamental mechanisms shared by human cells.

Not all cells are the same (Fig. 1–2). In particular, all eukaryotes (protists, plants, fungi, and animals) differ in important ways from the two extensive groups of prokaryotes (Eubacteria and Archaea). All eukaryotic cells have a compartmentalized cytoplasm (consisting of organelles including a nucleus) and a cytoskeleton. The basic features of eukaryotic organelles and the cytoskeleton were refined more than 1.5 billion years ago, before the major groups of eukaryotes diverged. To put human life in perspective, note that multicellular eukaryotes (green, blue, red in Fig. 1–1) evolved relatively recently, hundreds of millions of years after earlier, single-celled eukaryotes. Also note

that plants branched off before fungi, our nearest relatives on the tree of life.

Many interesting creatures have been lost to extinction during evolution. Extinction is irreversible because the cell is the only place where the entire range of life-sustaining biochemical reactions, including gene replication, molecular biosynthesis, targeting, and assembly, can go to completion. Thus, cells are such a special environment that the chain of life has required an unbroken lineage of cells stretching from each contemporary organism back to the earliest forms of life.

Introduction to Cells

This text focuses on the underlying molecular mechanisms of biological function at the cellular level. This chapter starts with a brief description of the main features that set eukaryotes apart from prokaryotes and then covers the general principles that apply equally well to eukaryotes and prokaryotes. It closes with a preview of the major components of eukaryotic cells.

Two Features That Distinguish Eukaryotic and Prokaryotic Cells

1. *Eukaryotic cells are compartmentalized.* A plasma membrane surrounds all cells, and additional in-

Figure 1-1 The tree of life. *A,* Universal tree based on comparisons of ribosomal RNA sequences. The tree has its root deep in the Eubacterial lineage 3 to 4 billion years ago. All current organisms, arrayed at the ends of branches, fall into three domains: Bacteria, Archaea and Eucarya (eukaryotes). The lengths of the segments and branches are based solely on differences in RNA sequences. Because the rate of random changes in the genes for rRNA has not been constant, the lengths of the lines leading to all contemporary organisms are not equal. Fossil records provide the estimated times of a few key events. Complete sequences of a few genomes (*orange,* see ⟨tigr.org/tdbv/ mdb.html⟩) verify this tree, but also show that genes moved laterally between Eubacteria and Archaea and within each of these domains. Genes also moved from Eubacteria to Eucarya when proteobacteria gave rise to mitochondria (transferring many of their genes to the eukaryotic nucleus) and when cyanobacteria gave rise to chloroplasts by a similar mechanism. Protozoa branched near the bottom of the eukaryotic lineage and relatively recently gave rise to other eukaryotic kingdoms: plants, fungi, and animals (*enlarged in Fig. 1–1*B). Analysis of rRNA sequences shows that organisms formerly classified as algae, as well as organisms formerly classified elsewhere, actually belong to four large branches near the top of the tree: alveolates (including dinoflagellates, ciliates, and sporozoans), stramenopiles (including diatoms and brown algae), rhodophytes (red algae), and plants (including the green alga *Chlamydomonas*). Molecular analysis also established that cellular slime molds (e.g., *Dictyostelium*) and acellular slime molds (e.g., *Physarum*) are not fungi and arose at different times. Unicellular amoeboid organisms arose multiple times during evolution and do not form a coherent group. *B,* Time line for the divergence of animals, plants, and fungi. In contrast to *A,* this tree has a radial time scale originating about 800 million years (my) ago with the last common ancestor. Contemporary organisms and time are at the circumference. Lengths of branches are arbitrary. With one exception, the order of branching is firmly established, based on comparisons of gene sequences. The exception is the branching of nematode round worms, shown here as an early event. New work suggests that nematodes are more closely related to arthropods. The times of branching of the oldest common ancestor of each pair of diverging lineages are only estimates, since the calibration of the molecular clocks is uncertain and the early fossil records are sparse. (*A,* Original drawing, adapted from the branching pattern from Sogin M, Marine Biological Laboratory, Pace N: A molecular view of microbial diversity and the biosphere. Science 276:734–740, 1997. *B,* Original drawing, based on timing for animals, adapted from Kuman S, Hedges SB: A molecular timescale for vertebrate evolution. Nature 392:917–920, 1998; based on timing for plants, adapted from ⟨ucjeps.herb.berkeley.edu/bryolab/ greenplantpage.html⟩; based on timing for fungi, adapted from ⟨phylogeny.arizona.edu/tree/eukaryotes/fungi/ ascomycota/axcomycota.html⟩.)

box 1–1

ORIGIN AND EVOLUTION OF LIFE

All living things belong to one of three great divisions: Eubacteria, Archaea, or Eucarya (see Fig. 1–1). Archaea and Eubacteria were considered as one kingdom until the 1970s when ribosomal RNA sequences revealed that they were different divisions of the tree of life, having branched from each other almost as long ago as they branched from eukaryotes.

No one is certain how life began, but the ancestor of all living things populated the earth nearly 4 billion years ago, not long after the earth formed 4.6 billion years ago. Common biochemical features of all succeeding cells suggest that this primitive microscopic cell had about a thousand genes. These genes diversified in later cells by the process of duplication and random mutations in their sequences. Where these modified genes provided a selective advantage, they were retained in future generations. This mechanism accounts for the huge families of related but specialized proteins, such as pumps and carriers found in the cell membranes of all forms of life. Where conditions did not require a gene, it was lost. For example, the simple pathogenic bacteria, *Mycoplasma genitalium,* has but 470 genes, since it can rely on its animal host for most nutrients, rather than making them de novo. Similarly, the slimmed down genome of budding yeast, with only 6144 genes, lost nearly 400 genes common to lower organisms. Vertebrates also lost many genes that had been maintained for 3 billion years in earlier forms of life. For instance, humans lack the enzymes to synthesize certain essential amino acids, which must be supplied in our diets.

The Eubacteria and Archaea that branched nearest the base of the tree of life mainly live at high temperatures and use hydrogen as their energy source. The common ancestor may have shared these features. Archaea and Eucarya briefly shared a common lineage. This is reflected in similarities in their apparatus for copying DNA into messenger RNA, but Archaea are closer to bacteria than Eucarya in most other ways.

Since the beginning, microorganisms dominated the earth in terms of numbers, variety of species, and range of habitats. Eubacteria and Archaea remain the most abundant organisms in the seas and in the earth. Less than 1% of Eubacteria and Archaea can be grown in the laboratory, so most varieties have escaped detection by traditional means. Now, new species can be identified by amplifying and sequencing characteristic genes from minute samples. Remarkably, only a very small proportion of Eubacterial species and no Archaea cause human disease. Chlorophyll-based photosynthesis originated in Eubacteria. More recently, the form of photosynthesis that produces reduced carbon compounds and oxygen from carbon dioxide and water was perfected in cyanobacteria. This raised the oxygen concentration in the earth's atmosphere to current levels and generated the organic compounds that many other forms of life depend upon for energy.

We know little about the earliest Eucarya other than the fact that their genomes may be nearly as old as those of Eubacteria and Archaea. The most primitive-appearing contemporary **eukaryote** is an amoeba lacking mitochondria called *Pelomyxa palustris.* Throughout evolution, the most numerous and heterogeneous eukaryotes have been microscopic single-celled protists. Symbiotic bacteria similar to proteobacteria (see Fig. 1–1*A*) brought respiration to early eukaryotes. Over time, most of the bacterial genes moved to the host **nucleus,** leaving behind a small number of genes in the organelle that we call a **mitochondrion.** Organisms that branched first from the eukaryotic lineage, such as *Giardia* (the cause of "hiker's diarrhea"), lack mitochondria, but the presence of a few bacterial genes in their nuclei may be evidence of transient associations with bacteria. Relatively late during evolution, cyanobacterial symbionts brought photosynthesis to red algae, brown algae, and green algae/plants. As the bacteria evolved into **chloroplasts,** most of the bacterial genes moved to the nucleus of the host.

The multicellular lifestyle emerged multiple times more than a billion years ago in colonial bacteria, cellular slime molds, and red, brown, and green algae. Some of these organisms, such as kelp, a tree-size brown alga found along many seashores, are huge. According to analysis of ribosomal RNA, animals, plants, and fungi arose from algae-like organisms some time between 670 and 1200 million years ago, well before the first fossils of these types. The existence of fossils about 570 million years old that are strikingly similar to contemporary animal embryos supports a hypothesis that early multicellular animals were small creatures similar to contemporary invertebrate larvae or embryos. Similar, tiny, early animals may have existed much earlier. If the major branches of the animal tree diverged before macroscopic animals developed, this might account for the disagreement between the molecular data and the fossil record, which suggests a much more recent divergence of animals.

tracellular membranes divide eukaryotes into compartments, each with a characteristic structure, biochemical composition, and function (see Fig. 1–2). The **nuclear envelope** separates the two major compartments: nucleoplasm and cytoplasm. The **chromosomes** carrying the cell's genes and the machinery to express these **genes** reside inside the nucleus; they are in the cytoplasm of prokaryotes. Most eukaryotic cells have **endoplasmic reticulum** (the site of protein and phospholipid synthesis), a **Golgi apparatus** (an organelle that adds sugars to membrane proteins,

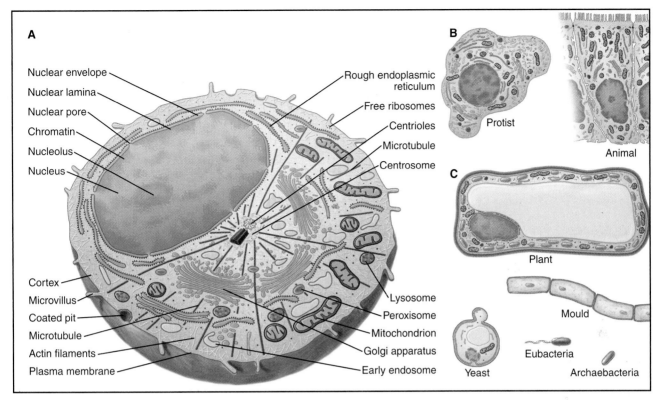

Figure 1-2 Basic cellular architecture. *A,* Drawing of a section through a eukaryotic cell showing the internal components. *B and C,* Drawings comparing cells from the major branches of the phylogenetic tree with color-coded components.

lysosomal proteins, and secretory proteins), **lyso-somes** (a compartment for digestive enzymes), **peroxisomes** (containers for enzymes involved in oxidative reactions), and **mitochondria** (structures that convert energy stored in the chemical bonds of nutrients into ATP). Table 1–1 lists the major cellular components and some of their functions.

Compartments give eukaryotic cells a number of advantages. The membranes provide a barrier that allows each type of organelle to maintain novel ionic and enzymatic interior environments. Each of these special environments favors a subset of the biochemical reactions required for life. The following three examples demonstrate this concept.

- Segregation of digestive enzymes in lysosomes prevents them from destroying other cellular components.
- ATP synthesis depends on the impermeable membrane around mitochondria; energy-releasing reactions produce a proton gradient across the membrane that enzymes in the membrane use to drive ATP synthesis.
- The nuclear envelope provides a compartment where the synthesis and editing of RNA copies of the genes can be completed before the ma-

ture messenger RNAs exit to the cytoplasm where they direct protein synthesis.

2. *Eukaryotic cells have a cytoskeleton.* Three protein polymers—**actin filaments, microtubules,** and **intermediate filaments**—form a viscous and elastic cytoplasmic matrix to provide mechanical support for the cell. In addition, actin filaments and microtubules are tracks for a variety of motor proteins that move the whole cell and the organelles within the cytoplasm. The actin filament and microtubule **cytoskeletons** are essential for life even in fungi and plants, which have rigid cell walls that provide mechanical support and prevent locomotion of the whole cell. Although encased in their cell walls, these cells depend on the cytoskeleton and its associated motors to transport organelles in the cytoplasm and to segregate the chromosomes.

Some Universal Principles of Living Cells

1. *Genetic information stored in one-dimensional chemical sequences in DNA (occasionally RNA) is duplicated and passed on to daughter cells* (Fig. 1–3). The information required for cellular growth, multiplication, and function is stored in long polymers of DNA called chromosomes. Each

table 1–1

INVENTORY OF CELLULAR COMPONENTS*

Cellular Component	Description
Plasma membrane	A lipid bilayer, 7 nm thick, with integral and peripheral proteins; the membrane surrounds cells and contains channels and pumps for ions and nutrients, receptors for growth factors, hormones and (in nerves and muscles) neurotransmitters, plus the molecular machinery to transduce these stimuli into intracellular signals
Adherens junction	A punctate or belt-like link between cells with actin filaments attached on the cytoplasmic surface
Desmosome	A punctate link between cells associated with intermediate filaments on the cytoplasmic surface
Gap junction	A localized region where the plasma membranes of two adjacent cells join to form minute intercellular channels for small molecules to move from the cytoplasm of one cell to the other
Tight junction	An annular junction sealing the gap between epithelial cells
Actin filament	"Microfilaments," 8 nm wide; form a viscoelastic network in the cytoplasm and act as tracks for myosin-powered movements
Intermediate filament	Filaments, 10 nm wide, composed of keratin-like proteins that act as inextensible "tendons" in the cytoplasm
Microtubule	A tubular polymer of tubulin, 25 nm in diameter, that is the main structural component of cilia, flagella, and the mitotic spindle; microtubules provide tracks for organelle movements powered by dynein and kinesin
Centriole	A short cylinder of 9 microtubule triplets located in the cell center (centrosome) and at the base of cilia and flagella; pericentrosomal material nucleates and anchors microtubules
Microvillus (or filopodium)	A thin, cylindrical projection of the plasma membrane supported internally by a bundle of actin filaments
Cilia/flagella	Motile organelles projecting from the cell surface and surrounded by plasma membrane; their bending motions are powered by an axoneme consisting of 9 doublet and 2 singlet microtubules with the energy-transducing enzyme, dynein
Glycogen particle	Storage form of polysaccharide
Ribosome	RNA/protein particle that catalyzes protein synthesis
Rough endoplasmic reticulum	Flattened, intracellular bags of membrane with associated ribosomes that synthesize secreted and integral membrane proteins
Smooth endoplasmic reticulum	Flattened, intracellular bags of membrane without ribosomes involved in lipid synthesis, drug metabolism, and sequestration of Ca^{2+}
Golgi apparatus	A stack of flattened membrane bags and vesicles that packages secretory proteins and participates in protein glycosylation
Nuclear envelope	A pair of membranes connected to the endoplasmic reticulum that limits the nucleus
Nuclear pore	Large, gated channels across the nuclear envelope that control all traffic of proteins and RNA in and out of the nucleus
Euchromatin	Dispersed, active form of interphase chromosomes
Heterochromatin	Condensed, inactive chromatin
Nucleolus	Intranuclear site of ribosomal RNA synthesis and processing; ribosome assembly
Lysosome	Impermeable, membrane-bound bags of hydrolytic enzymes
Peroxisome	Membrane-bound bags containing catalase and various oxidases
Mitochondria	Organelles surrounded by a smooth outer membrane and a convoluted inner membrane folded into cristae; they contain enzymes for fatty acid oxidation and oxidative phosphorylation of ADP

*See Figure 1–2.

DNA molecule is composed of a covalently linked linear sequence of four different nucleotides (adenine [A], cytosine [C], guanine [G], and thymine [T]). In the double-helix DNA molecule, each nucleotide base preferentially forms a specific complex with a complementary base on the other strand. Specific noncovalent interactions stabilize the pairing between complementary nucleotide bases, A with T and C with G. During DNA replication, the two DNA strands are separated, each serving as a template for the synthesis of a new complementary strand. The enzymes that carry

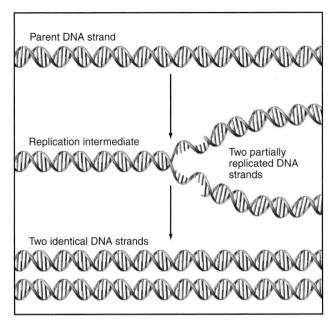

Parent DNA strand

Replication intermediate

Two partially replicated DNA strands

Two identical DNA strands

Figure 1-3 DNA structure and replication. The genes stored as the sequence of bases in DNA are replicated enzymatically, forming two identical copies from one double-stranded original.

complicated ensemble of trillions of specialized cells that function harmoniously for decades in an ever-changing environment.

3. *Macromolecular structures assemble from subunits* (Fig. 1–5). Many cellular components form by **self-assembly** of their constituent molecules without the aid of templates or enzymes. The protein, nucleic acid, and lipid molecules themselves contain the information required to assemble complex structures. Diffusion usually brings the molecules together during these assembly processes. Exclusion of water from their complementary surfaces ("lock and key" packing), as well as electrostatic and hydrogen bonds, provide the energy to hold the subunits together. In some cases, protein chaperones assist with assembly by preventing the precipitation of partially or incorrectly folded intermediates. Examples of important macromolecular assemblies include the packaging of DNA by proteins to form **chromatin,** the co-

out DNA synthesis recognize the structure of complementary base pairs and insert only the correct complementary nucleotide at each position, thereby producing two identical copies of the DNA. Precise segregation of one, newly duplicated, double helix to each daughter cell then guarantees the transmission of intact genetic information to the next generation.

2. *One-dimensional chemical sequences are stored in DNA code for both the linear sequences and three-dimensional structures of RNAs and proteins* (Fig. 1–4). Enzymes called polymerases copy the information stored in genes into linear sequences of nucleotides of RNA molecules. Some genes specify RNAs with structural roles or enzymatic activity, but most genes produce **messenger RNA** (mRNA) molecules that act as templates for protein synthesis specifying the sequence of amino acids during the synthesis of **polypeptides** by ribosomes. The amino acid sequence of most polypeptides contains sufficient information to determine how to fold into a unique three-dimensional structure with biological activity. Genetically encoded control circuits, which are modified by environmental stimuli, control the production and processing of RNA and protein from tens of thousands of genes. The basic plan for the cell contained in the genome, together with ongoing regulatory mechanisms (see points 7 and 8 below), work so well that each human develops with few defects from a single fertilized egg into a

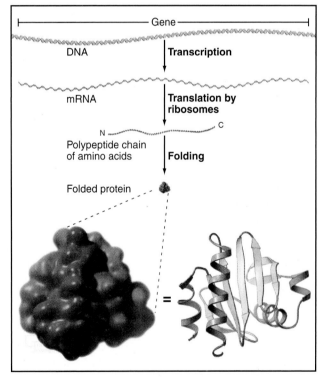

Gene

DNA — Transcription

mRNA — Translation by ribosomes

N — C

Polypeptide chain of amino acids — Folding

Folded protein

=

Figure 1-4 Scale drawings showing how genetic information contained in the base sequence of DNA determines the amino acid sequence of a protein and its three-dimensional structure. Enzymes copy (transcribe) the sequence of bases in a gene to make a messenger RNA (mRNA). Ribosomes use the sequence of bases in the mRNA as a template to synthesize (translate) a corresponding linear polymer of amino acids. This polypeptide folds spontaneously to form a three-dimensional protein molecule, in this example, the actin-binding protein profilin. (Protein data base [PDB] file: 1ACF.)

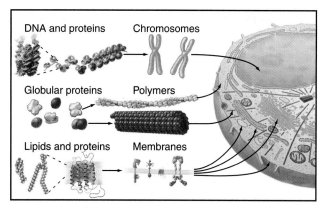

Figure 1-5 Macromolecular assembly. Many macromolecular components of cells assemble spontaneously from the constituent molecules without the guidance of templates. Proteins and DNA assemble chromatin. Globular proteins assemble cytoskeletal filaments. Proteins and lipids assemble membranes that grow by lateral expansion of preexisting membranes. The endoplasmic reticulum is the site of most lipid biosynthesis and also the site where new proteins are inserted into the growing membrane.

assembly of RNA and proteins to form ribosomes, the polymerization of proteins to form cytoskeletal polymers, and the assembly of lipids and proteins to form membranes.

4. *Membranes grow by expansion of preexisting membranes* (see Figs. 1–5 and 1–6). Biological membranes composed of phospholipids and proteins do not form de novo in cells; instead, they grow only by expansion of preexisting lipid bilayers. As a consequence, organelles, such as mitochondria and endoplasmic reticulum, form only by growth and division of preexisting organelles and are inherited maternally starting from the egg. The endoplasmic reticulum (ER) plays a central role in membrane biogenesis as the site of phospholipid synthesis. Through a series of budding and fusion events, membrane made in the ER provides material for the Golgi apparatus, which, in turn, provides lipids and proteins for lysosomes and the plasma membrane.

5. *Signal-receptor interactions target cellular constituents to their correct locations* (see Fig. 1–6). Specific recognition signals incorporated into the structures of proteins and nucleic acids route these molecules to their proper cellular compartments. Receptors recognize these signals and guide each molecule to its correct compartment. For example, most proteins destined for the nucleus contain short sequences of amino acids that bind receptors that facilitate their passage through nuclear pores into the nucleus. Similarly, a peptide signal sequence first targets lysosomal proteins into the lumen of the ER. Subsequently, the

Golgi apparatus adds a sugar-phosphate group recognized by receptors that target these proteins to lysosomes.

6. *Cellular constituents move by diffusion, pumps, and motors* (Fig. 1–7). Most small molecules move through the cell or across membrane channels by diffusion. Movements of small molecules across membranes against concentration gradients and movements of larger objects, like organelles, through cytoplasm, require the expenditure of energy. Electrochemical gradients or ATP hydrolysis provide energy for molecular pumps to drive molecules across membranes against concentration gradients. ATP-burning **motor proteins** move organelles and other cargo along microtubules or

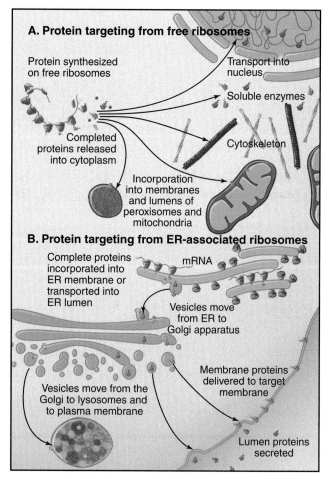

Figure 1-6 Protein targeting. Signals built into the amino acid sequence of proteins target them to all compartments of the eukaryotic cell. *A,* Proteins synthesized on free ribosomes can be used locally in the cytoplasm or guided by different signals to the nucleus, mitochondria, or peroxisomes. *B,* Other signals target proteins for insertion into the membrane or lumen of the endoplasmic reticulum (ER). From there, a series of vesicular budding and fusion reactions carry the membrane proteins and lumen proteins to the Golgi apparatus, lysosomes, or plasma membrane.

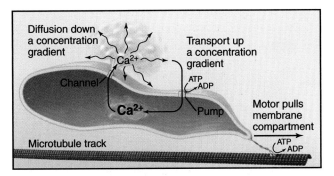

Figure 1-7 Molecular movements by diffusion, pumps, and motors. *Diffusion*: Molecules up to the size of globular proteins diffuse in the cytoplasm. Concentration gradients can provide a direction to diffusion, such as the diffusion of Ca^{++} from a region of high concentration inside the endoplasmic reticulum through a membrane channel to a region of low concentration in the cytoplasm. *Pumps*: ATP-driven protein pumps can transport ions up concentration gradients. *Motors*: ATP-driven motors move organelles and other large cargo along microtubules and actin filaments.

actin filaments. In a more complicated example, protein molecules destined for mitochondria diffuse from their site of synthesis in the cytoplasm to a mitochondrion (see Fig. 1–6) where they bind to a receptor. An energy-requiring reaction then transports the protein into the mitochondria.

7. *Receptors and signaling mechanisms allow cells to adapt to environmental conditions* (Fig. 1–8). Environmental stimuli modify cellular behavior and biochemistry. Faced with an unpredictable environment, cells must decide which genes to express, which way to move, and whether to proliferate, differentiate into a specialized cell, or die. Some of these choices are programmed genetically, but minute-to-minute decisions generally in-

volve the reception of chemical or physical stimuli from outside the cell and the processing of these stimuli to change the behavior of the cell. Cells have an elaborate repertoire of **receptors** for a multitude of stimuli, including nutrients, growth factors, hormones, neurotransmitters, and toxins. Stimulation of these receptors activates signal-transducing mechanisms that produce chemical signals to generate a wide range of cellular responses. These responses regulate the electrical potential of the plasma membrane, gene expression, enzyme activity, cytoskeletal motors, and many other systems. Basic **signal transduction** mechanisms are very ancient, but many specific receptors and output systems have arisen during evolution. Thus, humans typically have a greater number of variations on the general themes than simpler organisms.

8. *Molecular feedback mechanisms control molecular composition, growth, and differentiation* (Fig. 1–9). Living cells are dynamic, constantly undergoing changes in composition or activity in response to external stimuli, nutrient availability, and internal signals. Change is constant, but through well-orchestrated recycling and renewal, the cell and its constituents remain relatively stable. Each cell regulates the balanced production and degradation of its constituent molecules to function optimally. Some "housekeeping" molecules are used by most cells for basic functions, such as intermediary metabolism. Other molecules are unique and are required for specialized functions of differentiated cells. The supply of each of thousands of proteins is controlled by a hierarchy of mechanisms: by regulatory proteins that turn specific genes on and off; by the rate of transla-

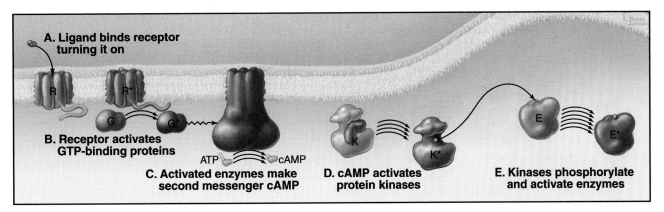

Figure 1-8 Receptors and signals. Activation of cellular metabolism by an extracellular ligand, such as a hormone. In this example, binding of the hormone (*A*) triggers a series of linked biochemical reactions (*B* to *E*), leading through a second messenger molecule (cyclic adenosine monophosphate, or cAMP) and a cascade of three activated proteins to a metabolic enzyme. The response to a single ligand is multiplied at steps *B*, *C*, and *E*, leading to thousands of activated enzymes. GTP, guanosine triphosphate.

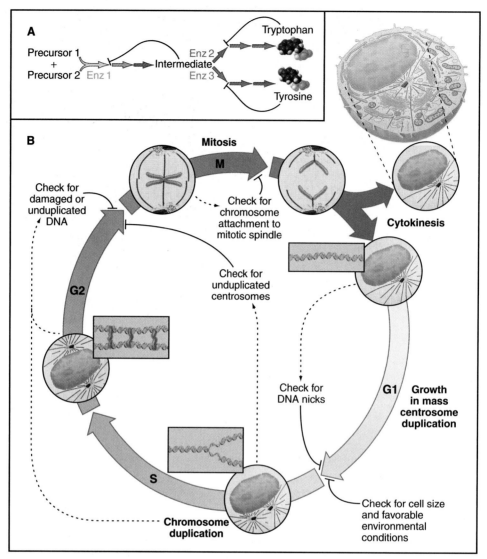

Figure 1-9 Molecular feedback loops. *A,* Control of the synthesis of aromatic amino acids. An intermediate and the final products of this biochemical pathway inhibit three of nine enzymes (enz) in a concentration-dependent fashion, automatically turning down the reactions that produced them. This maintains constant levels of the final products, two amino acids that are essential for protein synthesis. *B,* Control of the cell cycle. The cycle consists of four stages. During the G1 phase, the cell grows in size. During the S phase, the cell duplicates the DNA of its chromosomes. During the G2 phase, the cell checks for completion of DNA replication. In M phase, chromosomes condense and attach to the mitotic spindle, which separates the duplicated pairs in preparation for the division of the cell at cytokinesis. Biochemical feedback loops called checkpoints halt the cycle (*blunt bars*) at several points until the successful completion of key preceding events.

tion of messenger RNAs into protein; by the rate of degradation of specific RNAs and proteins; and by regulation of the distribution of each molecule within the cell. Some proteins are enzymes that determine the rate of synthesis or degradation of other proteins, nucleic acids, sugars, and lipids. Molecular feedback loops regulate all of these processes to ensure the proper levels of each cellular constituent.

Overview of Eukaryotic Cellular Organization and Functions

This section provides a brief preview of the major constituents and processes of eukaryotic cells. It is hoped that this will alleviate a practical problem with texts such as this, namely that all cellular components are interdependent. Thus, each chapter on a particular topic cross-references material covered in detail in

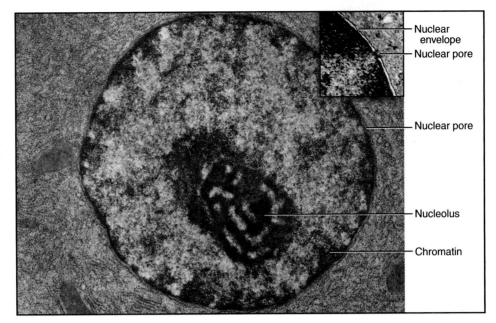

Nuclear envelope

Nuclear pore

Nuclear pore

Nucleolus

Chromatin

Figure 1-10 Electron micrograph of a thin section of a nucleus. (Courtesy of Don Fawcett, Harvard Medical School.)

other chapters. This overview provides enough of a refresher on concepts first encountered in basic biology courses to appreciate references to material in later chapters.

Nucleus

The nucleus (Fig. 1–10) stores genetic information in extraordinarily long DNA molecules called chromosomes. Surprisingly, genes make up only a small fraction (5%) of the 3 billion nucleotide pairs in human DNA, but more than 50% of the 97 million nucleotide pairs in a nematode worm. Most of the remaining DNA has no known function, although regions called telomeres stabilize the ends of chromosomes and centromeres ensure the distribution of chromosomes to daughter cells when cells divide. The DNA and its associated proteins are called chromatin. Interactions with histones and other proteins fold each chromosome compactly enough to fit inside the nucleus. During **mitosis,** chromosomes condense further into separate structural units that one can observe by light microscopy. Between cell divisions, chromatin becomes increasingly dispersed within the nucleus.

Proteins of the transcriptional machinery turn specific genes on and off in response to genetic, developmental, and environmental signals. Enzymes called polymerases make RNA copies of active genes. Messenger RNAs specify the amino acid sequences of proteins. Other RNAs have structural or catalytic functions. Most newly synthesized RNAs must be processed extensively before they are ready for use. Processing involves removal of intervening sequences or addition of specific structures at either end. For cytoplasmic RNAs, this processing occurs before RNA

molecules are exported from the nucleus through **nuclear pores.** The **nucleolus** assembles ribosomes from more than 40 different proteins and 3 RNA molecules. Genetic errors resulting in altered RNA and protein products cause or predispose individuals to many inherited human diseases.

The nuclear envelope is a double membrane that separates the nucleus from the cytoplasm. All traffic into and out of the nucleus passes through nuclear pores that bridge the double membranes. Inbound traffic includes all nuclear proteins, such as transcription factors and ribosomal proteins. Outbound traffic includes messenger RNAs and ribosomal subunits. Some macromolecules shuttle back and forth between the nucleus and cytoplasm.

Cell Cycle

Cellular growth and division are regulated by an integrated molecular network consisting of protein kinases (enzymes that add phosphate to the side chains of proteins), specific kinase inhibitors, transcription factors, and highly specific proteases. When conditions inside and outside a cell are appropriate for cell division (see Fig. 1–9B), changes in the stability of key proteins allow specific protein kinases to escape from negative regulators and to trigger a chain of events leading to DNA replication and cell division. Once DNA replication is initiated, the specific destruction of components of these kinases allows cells to complete the process. Once DNA replication is complete, activation of the cell cycle kinase Cdk1 pushes the cell into mitosis, the process that separates chromosomes into two daughter cells. Three controls sequentially activate Cdk1: (1) synthesis of a regulatory subunit; (2) trans-

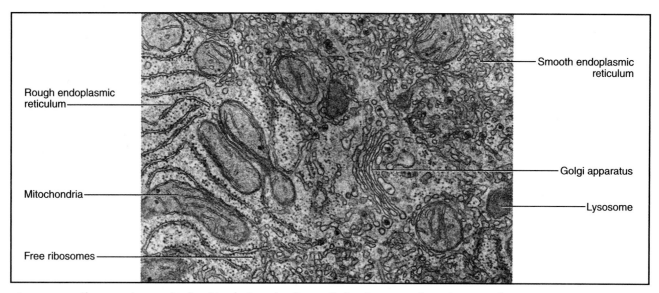

Rough endoplasmic reticulum

Mitochondria

Free ribosomes

Smooth endoplasmic reticulum

Golgi apparatus

Lysosome

Figure 1–11 Electron micrograph of a thin section of a liver cell showing organelles. (Courtesy of Don Fawcett, Harvard Medical School.)

port into the nucleus; and (3) removal of inhibitory phosphate groups.

Phosphorylation of proteins by Cdk1 leads directly or indirectly to disassembly of the nuclear envelope (in most but not all cells), condensation of mitotic chromosomes, and assembly of the **mitotic spindle.** Selective proteolysis of Cdk1 regulatory subunits and key chromosomal proteins then leads to segregation of identical copies of each chromosome to each daughter cell and division of the two cells. At the end of mitosis, the nuclear envelope reassembles on the surface of the clustered chromosomes.

A key feature of the cell cycle is built-in quality controls, called **checkpoints** (see Fig. 1–9), that ensure that each stage of the cycle is completed successfully before allowing the process to continue. These checkpoints also detect damage to cellular constituents and block cell cycle progression until the damage is repaired. Misregulation of checkpoints and other cell cycle controls is a common cause of cancer. Remarkably, the entire cycle of DNA replication, chromosomal condensation, nuclear envelope breakdown, and reformation, including the modulation of these events by checkpoints, can be carried out in cell-free extracts in a test tube.

Ribosomes and Protein Synthesis

Ribosomes catalyze the synthesis of proteins using the nucleotide sequences of messenger RNA molecules to specify the sequence of amino acids (see Figs. 1–4, 1–6, and 1–11). If the protein being synthesized has a signal sequence for ER receptors, the ribosome is bound to the ER, so that the protein can be inserted into the ER membrane bilayer or into the lumen of the

ER. Otherwise, ribosomes are free in cytoplasm and the newly synthesized protein enters the cytoplasm.

Endoplasmic Reticulum

The endoplasmic reticulum is a continuous system of flattened membrane sacks and tubules (see Fig. 1–11) that is specialized for protein processing and lipid biosynthesis. Motor proteins move along microtubules to pull the ER membranes into a branching network spread throughout the cytoplasm. ER also forms the outer half of the nuclear envelope. ER pumps and channels regulate the cytoplasmic Ca^{++} concentration, and ER enzymes metabolize drugs.

Ribosomes synthesizing proteins for insertion into cellular membranes or for export from the cell associate with specialized regions of the ER, called rough ER owing to the attached ribosomes (see Fig. 1–6). These proteins carry **signal sequences** of amino acids that guide their ribosomes to ER receptors. As a polypeptide chain grows, its sequence determines whether the protein folds up in the lipid bilayer or translocates into the lumen of the ER. Some of these proteins are retained in the ER, but most move on to other parts of the cell.

Endoplasmic reticulum is very dynamic. Continuous bidirectional traffic moves small vesicles between the ER and the Golgi apparatus. These vesicles carry soluble proteins in their lumens, in addition to membrane lipids and proteins. Proteins on the cytoplasmic surface of the membranes catalyze each membrane budding and fusion event. The use of specialized proteins for budding and fusion of membranes at different sites in the cell prevents the membrane components from getting mixed up.

Golgi Apparatus

The Golgi apparatus processes the sugar side chains of secreted and membrane glycoproteins and sorts the proteins for transport to other parts of the cell (see Figs. 1–6 and 1–11). The Golgi apparatus is a stack of flattened, membrane-bound sacks with many associated vesicles. Membrane vesicles come from the ER and fuse with the Golgi apparatus. As a result of a series of vesicle budding and fusion events, the membrane molecules and soluble proteins in the lumen pass through the stacks of Golgi apparatus from one side to the other. During this passage, Golgi enzymes, retained in specific layers of the Golgi apparatus by transmembrane anchors, modify the sugar side chains of secretory and membrane proteins. On the downstream side of the Golgi apparatus, the processed proteins segregate into different vesicles destined for lysosomes or the plasma membrane. The Golgi apparatus is characteristically located in the middle of the cell near the nucleus and the centrosome.

Lysosomes

An impermeable membrane separates degradative enzymes inside lysosomes from other cellular compo-

nents. Lysosomal proteins are synthesized by rough ER and transported to the Golgi apparatus where enzymes recognize a three-dimensional site on the proteins' surface that targets them for addition of a modified sugar, phosphorylated mannose (see Fig. 1–6). Vesicular transport, guided by phosphomannose receptors, delivers the lysosomal proteins to the lumen of the lysosome.

Membrane vesicles, called **endosomes** and **phagosomes,** deliver ingested microorganisms and other materials destined for destruction to lysosomes. Fusion of these vesicles with lysosomes exposes these substrates to lysosomal enzymes in the lumen. Deficiencies of lysosomal enzymes cause many congenital diseases. In each of these diseases, a deficiency in the ability to degrade a particular biomolecule leads to its accumulation in quantities that can impair the function of the brain, liver, or other organs.

Plasma Membrane

The plasma membrane is the interface of the cell with its environment (Fig. 1–12). Owing to the hydrophobic interior of its lipid bilayer, the plasma membrane is impermeable to ions and most water-soluble

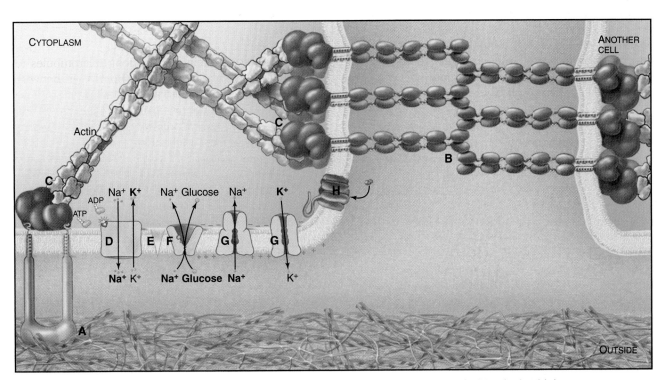

Figure 1–12 Drawing illustrating the structure and functions of an animal cell plasma membrane. The lipid bilayer forms a permeability barrier between the cytoplasm and the extracellular environment. Transmembrane adhesion proteins anchor the membrane to the extracellular matrix (A) or to like receptors on other cells (B) and transmit forces to the cytoskeleton (C). ATP-driven enzymes (D) pump Na^+ out and K^+ into the cell against concentration gradients (E) to establish an electrical potential across the lipid bilayer. Other transmembrane carrier proteins (F) use these ion concentration gradients to drive the transport of nutrients into the cell. Selective ion channels (G) open and shut transiently to regulate the electrical potential across the membrane. A large variety of receptors (H) bind specific extracellular ligands and send signals across the membrane to the cytoplasm.

molecules. Consequently, they only cross the membrane through transmembrane channels, carriers, and pumps, which provide the cell with nutrients, control internal ion concentrations, and establish a transmembrane electrical potential. A single amino acid change in one plasma membrane pump and Cl⁻ channel causes cystic fibrosis.

Other plasma membrane proteins mediate the interaction of the cell with its immediate environment. Transmembrane receptors bind extracellular signaling molecules, such as hormones and growth factors, and transduce their presence into chemical or electrical signals that influence the activity of the cell. Genetic defects in signaling proteins, which turn on signals for growth in the absence of appropriate extracellular stimuli, cause some human cancers.

Adhesive glycoproteins of the plasma membrane allow cells to bind specifically to each other or to the **extracellular matrix.** These selective interactions allow cells to form multicellular structures, like epithelia. Similar interactions allow white blood cells to bind bacteria, so that they can be ingested and digested in lysosomes. In cells subjected to mechanical forces, like muscle and epithelia, the adhesive proteins of the plasma membrane are reinforced by association with cytoskeletal filaments inside the cell. In skin, defects in these attachments cause blistering diseases.

ER synthesizes phospholipids and proteins for the plasma membrane (see Fig. 1–6). After insertion into the lipid bilayer of the ER, proteins move through the Golgi apparatus by vesicular transport to the plasma membrane. Many components of the plasma membrane are not permanent residents; receptors for extracellular molecules, including nutrients and some hormones, can recycle from the plasma membrane to endosomes and back to the cell surface many times before they are degraded. Defects in the receptor for low-density lipoproteins cause arteriosclerosis.

Mitochondria

Mitochondrial enzymes convert most of the energy released from the breakdown of nutrients into the synthesis of ATP, the common currency for most energy-requiring reactions in cells (see Fig. 1–11). This efficient mitochondrial system uses molecular oxygen to complete the oxidation of fats, proteins, and sugars to carbon dioxide and water. A less efficient glycolytic system in the cytoplasm extracts energy from the partial breakdown of glucose to make ATP. Mitochondria cluster near sites of ATP utilization, such as sperm tails, membranes engaged in active transport, nerve terminals, and the contractile apparatus of muscle cells.

Mitochondria also have a key role in cellular responses to toxic stimuli from the environment. In response to drugs such as many used in cancer chemotherapy, mitochondria release into the cytoplasm a toxic cocktail of enzymes and other proteins that brings about the death of the cell. Defects in this form of cellular suicide, known as **apoptosis,** lead to autoimmunity, cancer, and some neurodegenerative diseases.

Mitochondria form in a fundamentally different way from the ER, Golgi apparatus, and lysosomes (see Fig. 1–6). Free ribosomes synthesize most of the mitochondrial proteins, which are released into the cytoplasm. Receptors on the surface of mitochondria recognize and bind signal sequences on mitochondrial proteins. Energy-requiring processes transport these proteins into the lumen or insert them into the outer or inner mitochondrial membranes.

DNA, ribosomes, and messenger RNAs located inside mitochondria produce a small number of the proteins that contribute to the assembly of the organelle. This machinery is left over from an earlier stage of evolution when mitochondria arose from symbiotic Eubacteria (see Fig. 1–1). Defects in the maternally inherited mitochondrial genome cause several diseases, including deafness, diabetes, and ocular myopathy.

Peroxisomes

Peroxisomes are membrane-bound organelles containing enzymes that participate in oxidative reactions (see Fig. 1–11). Like mitochondria, peroxisomal enzymes oxidize fatty acids, but the energy is not used to synthesize ATP. Peroxisomes are particularly abundant in plants, as well as some animal cells. Peroxisomal proteins are synthesized in the cytoplasm and imported using the same strategy, but different targeting sequences and transport machinery, as mitochondria (see Fig. 1–6). Genetic defects in peroxisomal biogenesis cause several forms of mental retardation.

Cytoskeleton and Motility Apparatus

A cytoplasmic network of three protein polymers—actin filaments, intermediate filaments, and microtubules (Fig. 1–13)—maintains the shape of a cell. Each polymer has distinctive properties and dynamics. The ability of skin cells to resist mechanical forces illustrates the cytoskeletal function of these polymers.

Actin filaments and microtubules also provide tracks for the ATP-powered motor proteins that produce most cellular movements (Fig. 1–14), including cellular locomotion, muscle contraction, transport of organelles through the cytoplasm, mitosis, and the beating of **cilia** and **flagella.** The specialized forms of motility exhibited by muscle and sperm are exaggerated, highly organized versions of the motile processes used by most other eukaryotic cells.

Networks of cross-linked actin filaments anchored to the plasma membrane reinforce the surface of the

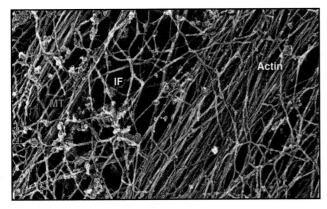

Figure 1-13 Electron micrograph of the cytoplasmic matrix of a fibroblast prepared by detergent extraction of soluble components, rapid freezing, sublimation of ice, and coating with metal. IF, intermediate filaments. (Courtesy of J. Heuser, Washington University.)

Microtubules are rigid cylindrical polymers with two main functions. They serve as (1) mechanical reinforcing rods for the cytoskeleton and (2) as the tracks for two classes of motor proteins. They are the only cytoskeletal polymer that can resist compression. The polymer has a molecular polarity that determines the rate of growth at the two ends and the direction of movement of motor proteins. Virtually all microtubules in cells have the same polarity relative to the

cell (Fig. 1–13). In many cells, tightly packed bundles of actin filaments support finger-like projections of the plasma membrane. These filopodia or microvilli increase the surface area of the plasma membrane for transporting nutrients and other processes, including sensory transduction in the ear. Genetic defects in a membrane-associated, actin-binding protein called dystrophin cause the most common form of muscular dystrophy.

Actin filaments participate in movements in two ways. Assembly of actin filaments produces some movements, like the extension of pseudopods. Other movements result from force produced by the motor protein, **myosin,** moving along actin filaments (see Fig. 1–14). A family of different types of myosin uses the energy from ATP hydrolysis to produce movements. Muscles use a highly organized assembly of actin and myosin filaments to produce forceful, rapid, one-dimensional contractions. Myosin also drives the contraction of the cleavage furrow during cell division. External signals, such as chemotactic molecules, can influence both actin filament organization and the direction of motility. Genetic defects in myosin cause enlargement of the heart and sudden death.

Intermediate filaments are flexible but strong intracellular tendons used to reinforce the epithelial cells of the skin and other cells subjected to substantial physical stresses. All intermediate filament proteins are related to the keratin molecules found in hair. Intermediate filaments characteristically form bundles that link the plasma membrane to the nucleus. Other intermediate filaments reinforce the nuclear envelope. Reversible phosphorylation regulates rearrangements of intermediate filaments during mitosis and cell movements. Genetic defects in keratin intermediate filaments cause blistering diseases of the skin.

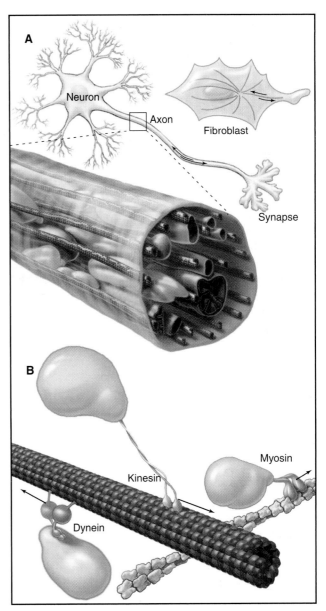

Figure 1-14 Transport of cytoplasmic particles along actin filaments and microtubules by motor proteins. *A,* Overview of organelle movements in a neuron and fibroblast. *B,* Details of the molecular motors. The microtubule-based motors—dynein and kinesin—move in opposite directions. The actin-based motor—myosin—moves in one direction along actin filaments. (Original drawing, adapted from Atkinson SJ, Doberstein SK, Pollard TD: Moving off the beaten track. Curr Biol 2:326–328, 1992. Copyright 1992, with permission from Elsevier Science.)

organizing centers that initiate their growth (e.g., the **centrosome**) (see Fig. 1–2). Their rapidly growing ends are oriented toward the periphery of the cell. Individual cytoplasmic microtubules are remarkably dynamic, growing and shrinking on a time scale of minutes.

Two classes of motor proteins use the energy liberated by ATP hydrolysis to move along the microtubules. **Kinesin** moves its associated cargo (vesicles and RNA protein particles) out along the microtubule network radiating from the centrosome, whereas **dynein** moves its cargo towards the cell center. Together, they form a two-way transport system in the cell that is particularly well developed in the axons and dendrites of nerve cells. Toxins can impair this transport system and cause nerve malfunctions.

During mitosis, the cell assembles a mitotic apparatus of highly dynamic microtubules and uses microtubule motor proteins to separate the chromosomes into the daughter cells. The motile apparatus of cilia and flagella is built from a complex array of stable microtubules that bends when dynein slides the microtubules past each other. A genetic absence of dynein immobilizes these appendages, causing male infertility and lung infections (Kartagener's syndrome).

Microtubules, intermediate filaments, and actin filaments each provide mechanical support for the cytoplasm that is enhanced by interactions between these polymers. Associations of microtubules with intermediate filaments and actin filaments unify the cytoskeleton into a continuous mechanical structure that resists forces applied to cells. These polymers also maintain the organization of the cell by providing a scaffolding for some cellular enzyme systems and a matrix between the membrane-bound organelles.

▌ Selected Readings

Doolittle RF: Microbial genomes opened up. Nature 392:339–342, 1998.

Doolittle WF: A paradigm gets shifty. (Origins of eukaryotes). Nature 392:15–16, 1998.

Kuman S, Hedges SB: A molecular timescale for vertebrate evolution. Science 392:917–920, 1998.

Margulis L, Schwartz KV: Five Kingdoms: An Illustrated Guide to the Phyla of Life on Earth. New York: W. H. Freeman, 1998, p. 520.

Orgel LE: The origin of life—A review of facts and speculations. Trends Biochem Sci 23:491–494, 1998.

Pace NR: A molecular view of microbial diversity and the biosphere. Science 276:734–740, 1997.

Pennisi E, Roush W: Developing a new view of evolution. Science 277:34–37, 1997.

Tatusov RL, Koonin EV, Lipman DJ: A genomic view on protein families. Science 278:631–637, 1997.

Xiao S, Zhang Y, Knoll AH: Three-dimensional preservation of algae and animal embryos in a Neoproterozoic phosphorite. Nature 391:553–558, 1998.

BASIC CHEMICAL AND PHYSICAL CONCEPTS

chapter 2

MOLECULAR STRUCTURES

This chapter describes the essential properties of water, proteins, nucleic acids, and carbohydrates as they pertain to cell biology. Chapter 6 covers lipids in the context of biological membranes.

Water

Water is the most abundant and important molecule in cells and tissues. Humans are about two thirds water. Water is not only the solvent for virtually all other compounds in the cell, but it is a reactant or product in thousands of different biochemical reactions catalyzed by enzymes, including the synthesis and degradation of proteins and nucleic acids and the synthesis and hydrolysis of adenosine triphosphate (ATP), to name a few examples. Water is also an important determinant of biological structure, as lipid bilayers, folded proteins, and macromolecular assemblies are all stabilized by the hydrophobic effect derived from the exclusion of water from nonpolar surfaces (see Chapter 3). Additionally, water forms hydrogen bonds with polar groups of many cellular constituents ranging in size from small metabolites to large proteins. It also associates with small inorganic ions.

Water is so familiar that one tends to neglect its role in cell biology and its fascinating properties. Despite years of research, a completely satisfactory understanding of the physical chemistry of water has not yet been achieved, largely because it is one of the most complex of all liquids. However, a few essential features of water relevant to its role in cell biology have been elucidated.

The water molecule is roughly tetrahedral in shape (Fig. 2–1) with two hydrogen bond donors and two hydrogen bond acceptors. The more electronegative oxygen withdraws the electrons from the O—H covalent bonds, leaving a partial positive charge on the hydrogens and a partial negative charge on the oxygen. These properties give hydrogen bonds between water molecules a special character. They are partly electrostatic because of the charge separation (induced dipole), but they also have some covalent character owing to overlap of the electron orbitals. Thus, the strength of hydrogen bonds is dependent on their orientation, being strongest along the lines of tetrahedral orbitals. One can think of oxygens from two water molecules sharing a hydrogen-bonded hydrogen.

Given two hydrogen bond donors and acceptors, water can be fully hydrogen-bonded as it is in ice (Fig. 2–2). Crystalline water in ice has a well-defined structure with a complete set of tetragonal hydrogen bonds and a remarkable amount (35%) of unoccupied space.

Neither theoretical calculations nor physical observations of liquid water have revealed a consistent picture of its organization. When ice melts, the volume decreases by only about 10%, so liquid water has considerable empty space too. The heat required to melt ice is a small fraction (15%) of the heat required to convert ice to a gas, where all the hydrogen bonds are lost. Because the heat of melting reflects the number of bonds broken, liquid water must retain most of the hydrogen bonds that stabilize ice. These hydrogen bonds create a continuous, three-dimensional network of water molecules connected at their tetrahedral vertices, allowing water to remain a liquid at a higher temperature than a similar molecule, ammonia. On the other hand, because liquid water does not have a well-defined, long-range structure, it must be very heterogeneous and dynamic, with rapidly fluctuating regions of local order and disorder (see Fig. 2–1C). This incomplete picture of water structure limits our

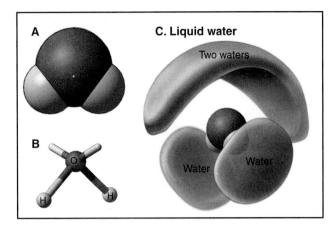

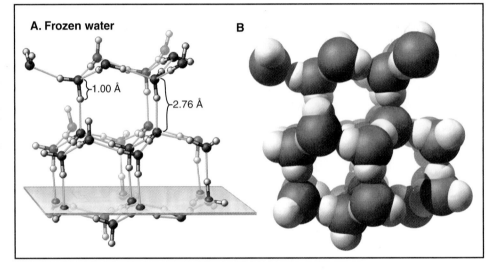

Figure 2-1 *A* and *B,* Water molecules. *A,* Space-filling model. *B,* Orientation of the tetrahedral electron orbitals that define the directions of the hydrogen bonds. *C,* Computer representation of approximately tetrahedral local order in liquid water. The three-dimensional map shows regions around the central water molecule where the local density of oxygen is at least 40% higher than average. Two adjacent water oxygens are centered near the two hydrogen bond donors, and two other waters are positioned in an elongated cap so that their protons can hydrogen-bond with the central water oxygen.

Figure 2-2 Crystal structure of ice. *A,* Stick figure showing the tetrahedral network of hydrogen bonds. *B,* A space-filling model showing the large amount of unoccupied space. (From ice.pdb; waterbox.pdb from <www.nyu.edu/pages/math mol/library/water), Project Math-Mol Scientific Visualization Lab, New York University.)

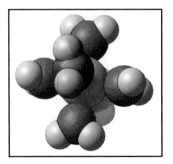

Figure 2-3 Shells of water molecules travel with solute ions. Diagram of a potassium ion and its shell of waters. Small ions, such as Li^+, Na^+, and F^-, bind water more tightly than do larger ions, such as K^+, Cl^-, and I^-.

ability to understand macromolecular interactions in an aqueous environment.

The properties of water have profound effects on all other molecules in the cell. For example, ions organize shells of water around themselves that compete effectively with other ions with which they might interact electrostatically (Fig. 2–3). This shell of water travels with the ions, governing the size of pores that they can penetrate. Similarly, hydrogen bonding with water strongly competes with the hydrogen bonding that occurs between solutes, including macromolecules. By contrast, water does not interact as favorably with nonpolar molecules as it does with itself, so the solubility of nonpolar molecules in water is low, and they tend to aggregate to reduce their surface area in contact with water. These interactions of nonpolar groups are energetically favorable because they minimize the unfavorable interactions of water with the nonpolar groups and increase the favorable interactions of water molecules with each other—the hydrophobic effect (see Chapter 3). Collectively, these interactions of water dominate the behavior of solute molecules in an aqueous environment. They strongly influence the assembly of proteins, lipids, and nucleic acids into the structures that they assume in the cell, as well as the interactions of these molecules. On the other hand, strategically placed water molecules can bridge two macromolecules in functional assemblies.

Proteins

Proteins are major components of all cellular systems. This section presents some basic concepts about protein structure that explain how proteins function in cells. More extensive coverage of this topic is available in biochemistry books and specialized books on protein chemistry.

Proteins consist of one or more linear polymers called **polypeptides,** which consist of various combinations of 20 different **amino acids** (Figs. 2–4 and 2–5) linked together by **peptide bonds** (Fig. 2–6). When linked in polypeptides, amino acids are referred to as residues. The sequence of amino acids in each type of polypeptide is unique. It is specified by the gene encoding the protein and is read out precisely during protein synthesis (see Chapter 18). The polypeptides of proteins with more than one chain are usually synthesized separately. However, in some cases, a single chain is divided into pieces by cleavage after synthesis.

Polypeptides have a wide range of lengths. Small peptide hormones, such as oxytocin, consist of as few as nine residues. By contrast, some giant structural proteins—titin, for example (see Chapter 42)—have more than 25,000 residues. Most cellular proteins fall in the range of 100 to 1000 residues. In the absence of stabilization by disulfide bonds or bound metal ions, a minimum of 40 residues seems to be required for a polypeptide to adopt a stable three-dimensional structure in water.

The sequence of amino acids in a polypeptide can be determined chemically by removing one amino acid at a time from the amino terminus and identifying the product. This procedure, called **Edman degradation,** can be repeated about 50 times before declining yields limit progress. Longer polypeptides can be divided into fragments of less than 50 amino acids by chemical or enzymatic cleavage, after which they are purified and sequenced separately. Even easier, one can sequence the gene or a complementary DNA **(cDNA)** copy of the messenger RNA for the protein (see Fig. 2–18) and use the genetic code to infer the amino acid sequence. Analysis of protein fragments by mass spectrometry can be used to sequence even tiny quantities of proteins.

Properties of the Amino Acids

Every student of cell biology should know the chemical structures of the amino acids used in proteins (see Fig. 2–4). Without these structures in mind, reading the literature and this book would be like spelling without knowledge of the alphabet. In addition to their full names, amino acids are frequently designated by three-letter or single-letter abbreviations.

All but one of the 20 amino acids commonly used in proteins consist of an **amino group,** linked to the **α-carbon,** linked to a **carboxyl group.** The exception is proline, which has a cyclic side chain bonded back to the nitrogen to form an imino group. Both the amino group (pK ~7) and carboxyl group (pK ~4) are partially ionized under physiological conditions. All amino acids, with the exception of glycine, have a β-carbon and a proton bonded to the α-carbon. (Glycine has a second proton instead.) This makes the α-carbon an asymmetrical center with two possible configurations. The L-isomers are used almost exclusively in living systems. (Compared with natural proteins, proteins constructed artificially from D-amino acids have mirror-image structures and properties. In addition to the β-carbon, each amino acid has a distinctive **side chain,** or R group, that determines its unique chemical and physical properties.

The amino acids are conveniently grouped in small families according to their R groups (Figure 2–4 denotes the special features of each group of amino acids). These side chains are distinguished by the presence of ionized groups, polar groups capable of

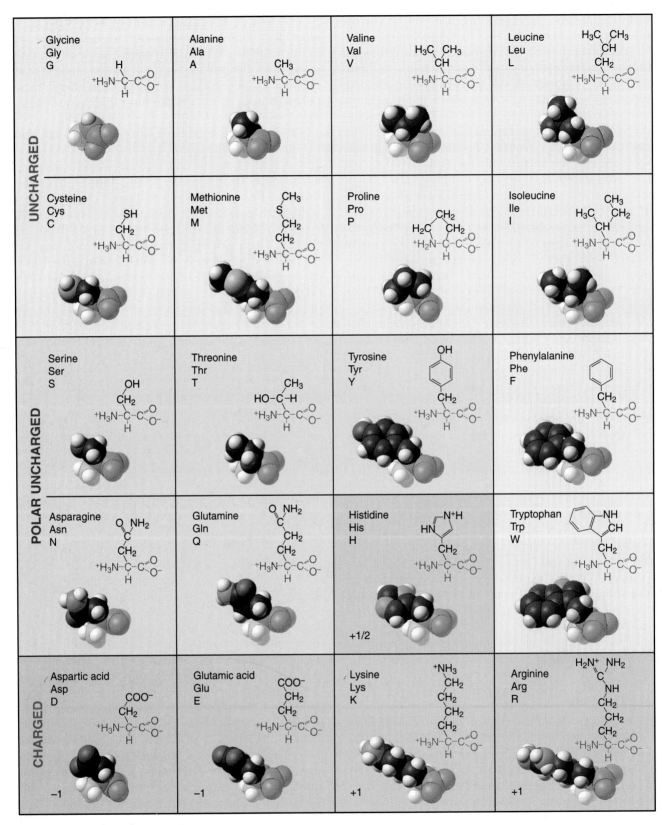

Figure 2-4 *See legend on opposite page*

Figure 2-4 The 20 L-amino acids specified by the genetic code. For each is shown the full name, the three-letter abbreviation, the single-letter abbreviation, a stick figure of the atoms, and a space-filling model of the atoms where hydrogen is white, carbon is black, oxygen is red, nitrogen is blue, and sulfur is yellow. For all, the amino group is protonated and carries a +1 charge, whereas the carboxyl group is ionized and carries a −1 charge. The amino acids are grouped according to the side chains attached to the α-carbon. *Uncharged amino acids:* These side chains fall into three subgroups. The aliphatic (G, A, V, L, I, C, M, P) and aromatic (Y, F, W) side chains partition into nonpolar environments, as they interact poorly with water. The uncharged side chains with polar hydrogen bond donors, or acceptors (S, T, N, Q, Y) can hydrogen-bond with water. *Charged amino acids:* At neutral pH, the basic amino acids K and R are fully protonated and carry a charge of +1, the acidic amino acids (D, E) are fully ionized and carry a charge of −1, and histidine (pK ~6.0) carries a partial positive charge. All the charged residues interact favorably with water, although the aliphatic chains of R and K also give them significant nonpolar character.

forming hydrogen bonds, chemically reactive groups, and their apolar surface area, which interacts poorly with water. Glycine and proline are special cases owing to their unique effects on the polymer backbone (see later section).

This repertoire of amino acids is sufficient to construct tens of thousands of different proteins, each with different capacities for interacting with other cellular constituents. This is possible because each protein has a unique three-dimensional structure (Fig. 2–7), each displaying the relatively modest variety of functional groups in a different way on its surface.

Enzymes modify many amino acids after their incorporation into polypeptides. These **posttranslational modifications** can have both structural and regulatory functions. Figure 2–5 illustrates some of the major modifications. These modifications will be referred to many times in this book, especially the reversible phosphorylation of amino acid side chains, the most common regulatory reaction in biochemistry (see Chapter 27).

Architecture of Proteins

Our knowledge of protein structure is based largely on x-ray diffraction studies of protein crystals or nuclear magnetic resonance (NMR) spectroscopy studies of small proteins in solution. These methods provide us with pictures showing the arrangement of the atoms in space. X-ray diffraction requires three-dimensional crystals of the protein and yields a three-dimensional contour map showing the density of electrons

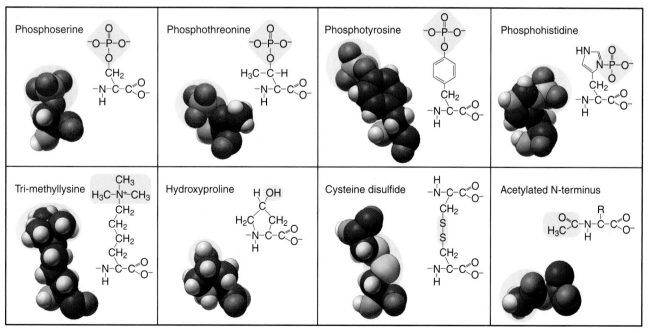

Figure 2-5 Modified amino acids. Protein kinases add a phosphate group to serine, threonine, tyrosine, histidine, and aspartic acid (not shown). Other enzymes add one or more methyl groups to lysine or histidine (not shown), a hydroxyl group to proline, or an acetate to the N-terminus of many proteins. The reducing environment of the cytoplasm minimizes the formation of disulfide bonds, but under oxidizing conditions within the membrane compartments of the secretory pathway (see Chapters 20 to 22), intramolecular or intermolecular disulfide (S—S) bonds form between adjacent cysteine residues.

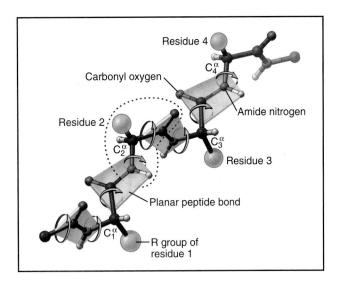

Residue 4

Carbonyl oxygen

C_4^α

Amide nitrogen

Residue 2

C_2^α C_3^α

Residue 3

Planar peptide bond

C_1^α

R group of residue 1

Figure 2–6 The polypeptide backbone. This perspective drawing shows three planar peptide bonds, the four participating α-carbons (labeled 1 to 4), the R groups represented by the β-carbons, amide protons, carbonyl oxygens, and the two rotatable backbone bonds (ϕ and φ). (Adapted from Creighton TE: Proteins: Structure and Molecular Principles. New York: W.H. Freeman and Co., 1983.)

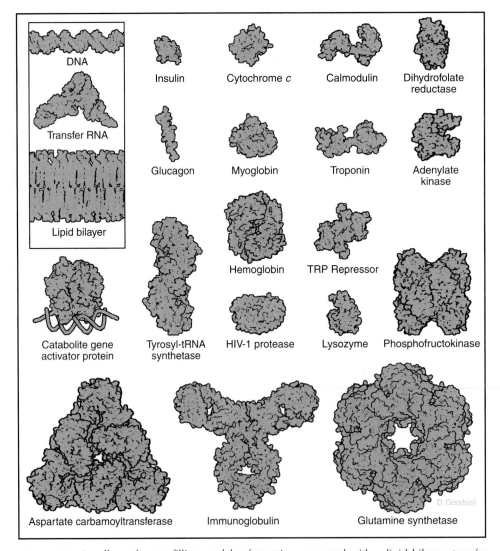

DNA

Transfer RNA

Lipid bilayer

Insulin

Cytochrome *c*

Calmodulin

Dihydrofolate reductase

Glucagon

Myoglobin

Troponin

Adenylate kinase

Catabolite gene activator protein

Tyrosyl-tRNA synthetase

Hemoglobin

TRP Repressor

HIV-1 protease

Lysozyme

Phosphofructokinase

Aspartate carbamoyltransferase

Immunoglobulin

Glutamine synthetase

D. Goodsell

Figure 2–7 A gallery of space-filling models of proteins compared with a lipid bilayer, transfer RNA, and DNA, all on the same scale. (Modified from, and reproduced with permission from Goodsell D, Olsen AJ: Soluble proteins: Size, shape, and function. Trends Biochem Sci 18:65–68, 1993. Copyright 1993, with permission from Elsevier Science.)

around each atom (Fig. 2–8). In the best cases, all the atoms except the hydrogens are clearly resolved, along with the water molecules occupying fixed positions in and around the protein. By contrast, NMR spectroscopy requires concentrated solutions of protein and reveals the distances between identified protons. Given enough distance constraints, it is possible to calculate the unique fold of the protein that is consistent with these spacings of the protons. In a few cases, electron microscopy of two-dimensional crystals has also revealed atomic structures (see Chapters 5, 6, and 37).

Each amino acid residue contributes three atoms to the polypeptide backbone: the nitrogen from the amino group, the α-carbon, and the carbonyl carbon from the carboxyl group (see Fig. 2–6). The peptide bond linking the amino acids together is formed by dehydration synthesis (see Chapter 18), a common chemical reaction in biological systems. Water is removed in the form of a hydroxyl from the carboxyl group of one amino acid and a proton from the amino group of the next amino acid in the polymer. Ribosomes catalyze this reaction in cells. Chemical synthesis can achieve the same result in the laboratory. The peptide bond nitrogen has an **(amide) proton,** and the carbon has a double-bonded **(carbonyl) oxygen.** The amide proton is an excellent hydrogen bond donor, whereas the carbonyl oxygen is an excellent hydrogen bond acceptor.

The end of a polypeptide with the free amino group is called the **amino terminus** or **N-terminus.** The numbering of the residues in the polymer starts with the N-terminal amino acid, as the biosynthesis of the polymer begins there. The other end of a polypeptide has a free carboxyl group and is called the **carboxyl terminus** or **C-terminus.**

The peptide bond has some characteristics of a double bond owing to resonance of the electrons, and it is relatively rigid and planar. The bonds on either side of the α-carbon can rotate through 360 degrees, although a relatively narrow range of bond angles is highly favored. Steric hindrance between the β-carbon (on all the amino acids but glycine) and the α-carbon of the adjacent residue favors a *trans* configuration in which the side chains alternate from one side of the polymer to the other (see Fig. 2–6). Folded proteins generally use a limited range of rotational angles to avoid steric collisions of atoms along the backbone. Glycine without a β-carbon is free to assume a wider range of configurations and is useful for making tight turns in folded proteins.

Folding of Polypeptides

The three-dimensional structure of a protein is determined solely by the sequence of the amino acids in the polypeptide chain. This was established by reversi-

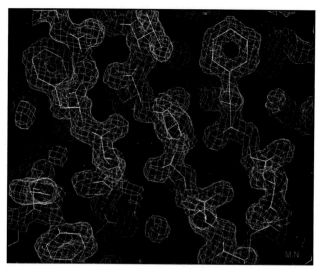

Figure 2–8 Protein structure determination by x-ray crystallography. A small part of an electron density map at 1.5 Å resolution of the cytoplasmic T1 domain of the shaker potassium channel from *Aplysia*. The chicken-wire map shows the electron density. The stick figure shows the superimposed atomic model. (Based on original data from M. Nanao and S. Choe, Salk Institute for Biological Studies.)

bly unfolding and refolding proteins in a test tube. Many, but not all, proteins unfolded by harsh treatments (high concentrations of urea or extremes of pH), will refold to regain full activity when returned to physiological conditions. Although proteins may be flexible enough to undergo conformational changes (see later discussion), polypeptides rarely fold into more than one final stable structure.

A major unfulfilled goal in biology is to predict the three-dimensional structure of proteins from the sequence of amino acids. This ability would have profound practical consequences. Presently, the number of known protein sequences (>200,000) far exceeds the number of established protein structures (about 4000), and the disparity widens as the complete genomes of various organisms are sequenced. Some of the factors that dominate the folding process are known, but the rules derived to date fall short of enabling prediction of whole folded structures. Some of the parameters responsible for folding are as follows:

1. Hydrophobic side chains pack very tightly in the core of proteins to minimize their exposure to water. Little free space exists inside proteins; the hydrophobic core is more like a hydrocarbon crystal than like an oil droplet (Fig. 2–9). Accordingly, the most conserved residues in families of proteins are found in the interior. Nevertheless, the internal packing is malleable enough to tolerate mutations that change the size of buried side chains, as the neighboring chains can rearrange without changing the overall shape of the protein.

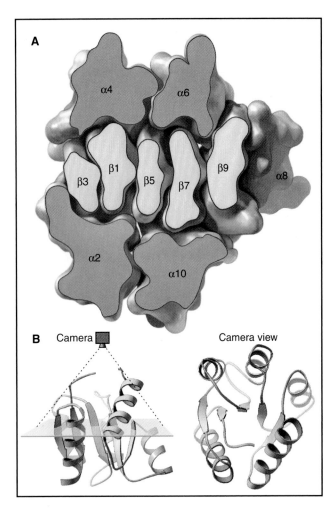

Figure 2-9 Space-filling *(A)* and ribbon *(B)* models of a cross section of the bacterial chemotaxis protein CheY illustrate some of the factors that contribute to protein folding. α-Helices pack on both sides of the central, parallel β-sheet. Most of the polar and charged residues are on the surface. The tightly packed interior of largely apolar residues excludes water. The buried backbone amides and carbonyls are fully hydrogen-bonded to other backbone atoms in both the α-helices and β-sheet. (From protein data base [PDB] file: 2chf.)

Although many hydrophobic residues are inside, roughly half the residues exposed to solvent on the outer surface are also hydrophobic.

2. Most charged and polar side chains are exposed on the surface, where they interact favorably with water. Amino acid residues on the surface typically appear to play a minor role in protein folding. Experimentally, one can substitute many residues on the surface of a protein with any other residue without changing the stability or three-dimensional structure. Interior charged or polar residues frequently form hydrogen bonds or salt bridges to neutralize their charge.

3. The polar amide protons and carbonyl oxygens of the polypeptide backbone maximize their potential to form hydrogen bonds with other backbone atoms, side chain atoms, or water. In the hydrophobic core of proteins, this is commonly achieved by hydrogen bonds with other backbone atoms in the two major types of **secondary structures: α-helices** and **β-sheets** (Fig. 2–10).

4. Elements of secondary structure usually extend

Figure 2-10 Models of secondary structures and turns of proteins. *A,* α-Helix. The stick figure *(left)* shows a right-handed α-helix with the N-terminus at the bottom and side chains R represented by the β-carbon. The backbone hydrogen bonds are indicated by cyan dashed lines. In this orientation, the carbonyl oxygens point up, the amide protons point down, and the R groups trail toward the N-terminus. Space-filling models *(middle)* show a polyalanine α-helix. The end-on views show how the backbone atoms fill the center of the helix. A space-filling model *(right)* of α-helix 5 from bacterial rhodopsin shows the side chains. *B,* Stick figure and space-filling models of an antiparallel β-sheet. The arrows indicate the polarity of each chain. With the polypeptide extended in this way, the amide protons and carbonyl oxygens lie in the plane of the sheet, where they make hydrogen bonds with the neighboring strands. The amino acid side chains alternate pointing up and down from the plane of the sheet. *C,* Stick figure and space-filling models of a parallel β-sheet. All strands have the same orientation *(arrows).* The orientations of the hydrogen bonds are somewhat less favorable than in an antiparallel sheet. *D* and *E,* Stick figures of two types of reverse turns found between strands of antiparallel β-sheets. *F,* Stick figure of an omega loop. (*A,* From PDB file: 1BAD: *B,* From PDB file: 1SLK: *D* and *E,* From PDB file: 1IMM: *F,* From PDB file: 1LNC.)

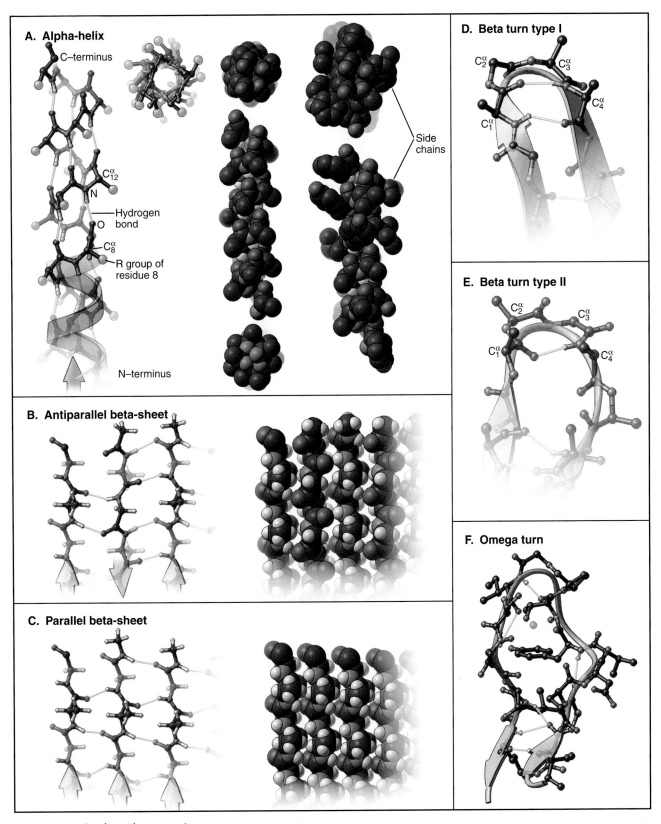

A. Alpha-helix

C–terminus

C_{12}^{α}

N

Hydrogen bond

O

C_8^{α}

R group of residue 8

N–terminus

Side chains

B. Antiparallel beta-sheet

C. Parallel beta-sheet

D. Beta turn type I

C_2^{α} C_3^{α}

C_1^{α} C_4^{α}

E. Beta turn type II

C_2^{α} C_3^{α}

C_1^{α} C_4^{α}

F. Omega turn

Figure 2–10 *See legend on opposite page*

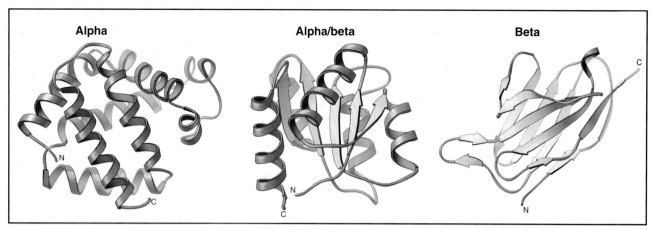

Figure 2-11 Ribbon diagrams of protein structures showing β-strands as flattened arrows, α-helices as coils, and other parts of the polypeptide chains as ropes. *Left,* The β-subunit of hemoglobin consists entirely of tightly packed α-helices. *Middle,* CheY is a mixed α/β structure, with a central parallel β-sheet flanked by α-helices. Note the right-handed twist of the sheet (defined by the sheet turning away from the viewer at the upper right) and right-handed pattern of helices (defined by the helices angled toward the upper right corner of the sheet) looping across the β-strands. (Compare the cross section in Figure 2–9). *Right,* The immunoglobulin V$_L$ domain consists of a sandwich of two antiparallel β-sheets. (*Left,* From PDB file: 1MBA. *Middle,* From PDB file: 2CHf. *Right,* From PDB file: 2IMM.)

completely across compact domains. Consequently, loops connecting α-helices and β-strands are on the surface, not in the interior of proteins (Fig. 2–11).

All these features tend to maximize the stability of the folded protein, but folded proteins are relatively unstable. The standard free energy difference (see Chapter 3) between a folded and unfolded protein is only about 40 kJ mol^{-1}, much less than that of a single covalent bond! This allows proteins to make conformational changes as part of their biological function. On the other hand, minor changes in structure can destabilize a protein. This explains why subtle mutations almost anywhere in a protein can occasionally have global effects on protein structure and function, even causing a disease.

Secondary Structure

Much of the polypeptide backbone of proteins folds into stereotyped elements of secondary structure, especially α-helices and β-sheets (see Fig. 2–10). They are shown as spirals and polarized ribbons in the ribbon diagrams of protein organization used throughout this book. Both α-helices and β-strands are linear, so that globular proteins can be thought of as compact bundles of straight or gently curving rods, laced together by surface turns.

α-Helices provide a way for a polypeptide to maximize hydrogen bonding of backbone polar groups while using highly favored rotational angles around the α-carbons and tight packing of atoms in the core of the helix (see Figs. 2–10 and 2–11). All these features stabilize the α-helix. Viewed with the

amino terminus at the bottom, the amide protons all point down and the carbonyl oxygens all point up. The side chains project radially around the helix, tilted toward its N-terminus. Given 3.6 residues in each right-handed turn of the helix, the carbonyl oxygen of residue number one is positioned perfectly to form a linear hydrogen bond with the amide proton of residue number five. This n to n+4 pattern of hydrogen bonds repeats along the whole α-helix.

The orientation of the backbone hydrogen bonds in α-helices has two important consequences. First, the whole helix has an electrical dipole moment, negative at the C-terminus. Second, the ends of the helices are less stable than the middle, as four potential hydrogen bonds are not completed by backbone interactions at each end. These unmet backbone hydrogen bonds can be completed by interaction with appropriate donors or acceptors on the side chains of the terminal residues. Interactions with serine and asparagine are favored as "caps" at the N-termini of helices because their side chains can complete the hydrogen bonding of the backbone amide nitrogens. Lysine, histidine, and glutamine are favored hydrogen bonding caps for the C-terminus of helices.

All the amino acids are found in naturally occurring α-helices, but glycine and proline are uncommon, as they tend to destabilize the configuration of the backbone of the helix. In fact, proline is favored to initiate helices and glycine to complete helices because they allow backbone conformations found in bends.

A second strategy used to stabilize the backbone structure of polypeptides is hydrogen bonding (see Chapter 3) of β-strands laterally to neighboring β-strands (see Figs. 2–10 and 2–11). A group of hydrogen-bonded β-strands is called a **β-sheet.** The peptide chain in the individual β-strands is extended in a configuration close to *all-trans* with side chains alternating on the top and bottom and the amide protons and carbonyl oxygens alternating to the right and left. β-Strands can form a complete set of hydrogen bonds, with neighboring strands running in the same or opposite directions in any combination. However, the hydrogen bond donors and acceptors are more favorably oriented to form linear hydrogen bonds in a β-sheet with antiparallel strands, compared with parallel strands. Largely parallel β-sheets are usually extensive and completely buried in proteins. β-Sheets have a natural right-handed twist in the direction along the strands. Antiparallel β-sheets are stable even if the strands are short and extensively distorted by twisting. Antiparallel sheets can wrap around completely to form a **β-barrel** with as few as five strands, but the natural twist of the strands and the need to fill the core of the barrel with hydrophobic residues favors eight strands.

Up to 25% of the residues in globular proteins are present in bends at the surface (see Fig. 2–10D to F). The residues that constitute the bends are generally hydrophilic. The presence of glycine or proline in a turn allows the backbone to deviate from the usual geometry in tight turns, but the composition of bends is highly variable and not a strong determinant of folding or stability. The turns of the polypeptide backbone between linear elements of secondary structure are called **reverse turns,** as they reverse the direction of the polypeptide chain. Those between β-strands have a few characteristic conformations and are called β-bends.

Many parts of polypeptide chains in proteins do not have a regular structure (see Fig. 2–11). At one extreme, small segments of polypeptide, frequently at the N- or C-terminus of the chain, are truly disordered in the sense that they are mobile. On the other hand, many irregular segments of polypeptide are tightly packed into the protein structure and should not be referred to as random coil. **Omega loops** are compact structures consisting of 6 to 16 residues, generally on the protein surface, that connect adjacent elements of secondary structure (see Fig. 2–10F). They lack regular structure but typically have the side chains packed in the middle of the loop. Some are mobile, but many are rigid. Omega loops form the antigen-binding sites of antibodies. In other proteins, they bind metal ions or participate in the active sites of enzymes.

Packing of Secondary Structure in Proteins

The elements of secondary structure can pack together in almost any way (see Fig. 2–11), but a few themes are favored enough to be found in many proteins. For example, two β-sheets tend to pack face to face at an angle of about 40 degrees with nonpolar residues packed tightly, knobs into holes, in between. α-Helices tend to pack at an angle of about 30 degrees across β-sheets, always in a right-handed arrangement (see Fig. 2–11). Adjacent α-helices tend to pack together at an angle of either +20 degrees or −50 degrees owing to packing of side chains from one helix into grooves between side chains on the other helix.

Coiled-coils are an extreme example of regular superstructure (Fig. 2–12). Two α-helices pair to form a fibrous structure that is widely used to create stable polypeptide dimers in structural proteins (see Chapter 39) and transcription factors (see Chapter 14). Typically two identical α-helices wrap around each other in register in a left-handed super helix that is stabilized by hydrophobic interactions at the interface of the two helices. Intermolecular ionic bonds between the side chains of the two polypeptides also stabilize coiled-coils. Given 3.6 residues per turn, the sequence of a coiled-coil has hydrophobic residues regularly spaced at positions 1 and 4 of a **"heptad repeat."** This pattern allows one to predict the tendency of a polypeptide to form coiled-coils from its amino acid sequence.

Interaction of Proteins with Solvent

The surface of proteins is almost entirely covered with protons (Fig. 2–13). Some are potential hydrogen bond donors, but many are inert, being bonded to backbone or side chain aliphatic carbons. Although most charged side chains are exposed on the surface, so are many nonpolar side chains. Many water molecules are ordered on the surface of proteins by virtue of hydrogen bonds to polar groups. These water molecules appear in electron density maps of crystalline proteins, but they exchange rapidly, on a picosecond (10^{-12} second) time scale. Waters in contact with nonpolar atoms maximize hydrogen bonding with each other, forming a dynamic layer of water with reduced translational diffusion compared with the bulk water. This lowers the entropy of the water and provides a thermodynamic impetus to protein folding pathways that minimize the number of hydrophobic atoms displayed on the surface (see Chapter 3).

Protein Dynamics

Pictures of proteins tend to give the wrong impression that they are rigid and static. On the contrary, even when packed in crystals, the atoms of proteins vibrate around their mean positions on a picosecond (10^{-12} sec) time scale with amplitudes up to 0.2 nm and velocities of 200 m per second. This motion is an inevitable consequence of the kinetic energy of each

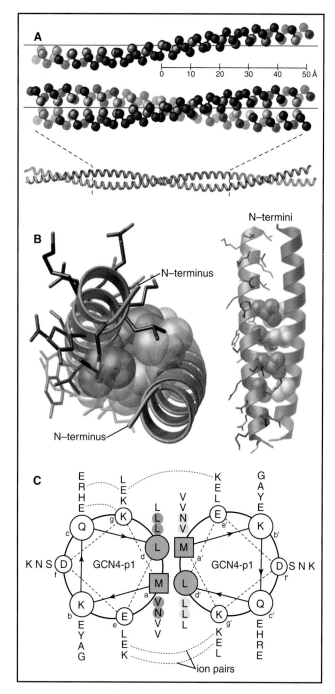

Figure 2-12 Coiled-coils. *A,* Comparison of a single α-helix, represented by spheres centered on the α-carbons, and a two-stranded, left-handed coiled-coil. Two identical α-helices make continuous contact along their lengths by the interaction of the first and fourth residue in every two turns (seven residues) of the helix. *B,* Atomic structure of the GCN4 coiled-coil, viewed end-on. The coiled-coil holds together two identical peptides of this transcription factor dimer (see Chapter 14 for information on its function). Hydrophobic side chains fit together like knobs into holes along the interface between the two helices. *C,* Helical wheel representation of the GCN4 coiled-coil. Following the arrows around the backbone of the polypeptides, one can read the sequences from the single-letter code, starting with the boxed residues and proceeding to the most distal residue. Note that hydrophobic residues in the first (*a*) and fourth (*d*) positions of each two turns of the helices make hydrophobic contacts that hold the two chains together. Electrostatic interactions *(dashed lines)* between side chains at positions *e* and *g* stabilize the interaction. (*A,* From PDB file: 2TMA. *B,* From PDB file: GCN4. *C,* Redrawn from O'Shea E, et al: X-ray structure of the GCN4 leucine zipper, a two-stranded, parallel coiled-coil. Science 254:539–544, 1991.)

atom, about 2.5 kJ mol⁻¹ at 25°C. This allows the protein as a whole to explore a variety of subtly different conformations on a fast time scale. Binding to a ligand or a change in conditions may favor one of these conformations.

In addition to relatively small, local variations in structure, many proteins can undergo large conformational changes. These changes in structure are often reflected by a change of activity or physical properties. **Conformational changes** are believed to play a role in many biological processes ranging from opening and closing of ion channels (see Chapter 9) to cell motility

(see Chapter 39). Many conformational changes have been observed indirectly by spectroscopy or hydrodynamic methods, and a few have been documented at atomic resolution. The best examples (Fig. 2–14) are enzymes that change their shape when they bind substrate (e.g., hexokinase, elongation factor EF-Tu), when they bind a regulatory molecule (e.g., phosphofructokinase), or when they are phosphorylated (e.g., glycogen phosphorylase). When the substrate, glucose, binds to the enzyme, hexokinase, the two lobes of the protein rotate 12 degrees about a hinge consisting of two polypeptide strands. When guanosine triphos-

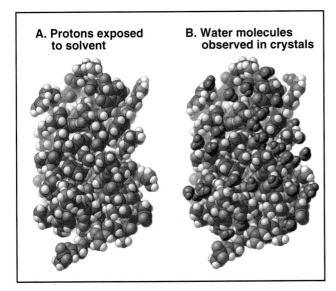

Figure 2-13 Water associated with the surface of a protein. *A,* Protein protons exposed to solvent *(white)* on the surface of a small protein, bovine pancreatic trypsin inhibitor. *B,* Water molecules observed on the surface of the protein in crystal structures. (From PDB file: 5bti.)

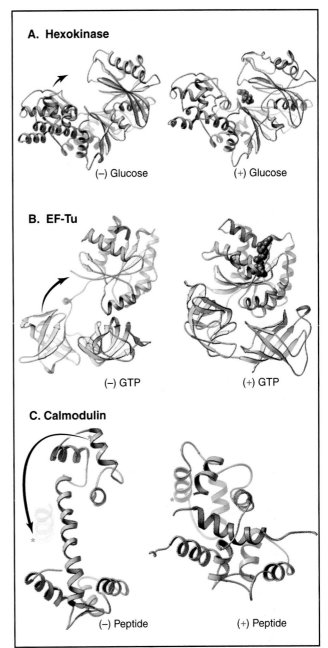

Figure 2-14 Conformational changes of proteins. *A,* The glycolytic enzyme hexokinase. The two domains of the protein hinge together to surround the substrate, glucose. *B,* EF-Tu, a cofactor in protein synthesis (see Chapter 18), folds more compactly when it binds GTP. *C,* Calmodulin (see Chapter 28) binds Ca^{2+} and wraps itself around an α-helix *(red)* in target proteins. Note the large change in position of the helix marked with an asterisk. *(A,* From PDB files: 2YHX and 1HKg. *B,* From PDB files: 1EFU and 1EFT. *C,* From PDB files: CLN and 2bbm.)

phate (GTP) binds the elongation factor EF-Tu, rotation about two glycine residues shifts a domain of the protein 90 degrees relative to the rest of the molecule! Similarly, phosphorylation of glycogen phosphorylase causes a local rearrangement of the N-terminus that transmits a structural change of more than 2 nm to the active site (see Chapter 29). A dramatic conformational change occurs when the Ca^{2+} binding regulatory protein, calmodulin, binds to its target proteins (see Fig. 2–14*C* and Chapter 28). The dumbbell-shaped calmodulin wraps itself tightly around the helical peptide it binds.

Modular Domains in Proteins

Many large polypeptides consist of linear arrays of independently folded, globular regions, or **domains,** connected in a modular fashion. Figure 2–15 provides a small sample of domains and their use. Later chapters introduce many other multi-use domains. Most of the modules consist of 40 to 100 residues, but kinase domains and motor domains can be much larger. Although homologous domains in different proteins usually differ significantly in their amino acid sequences, most domains can be recognized from their characteristic patterns of amino acids. For example, the cysteine residues of immunoglobulin G (Ig) domains are spaced in a characteristic pattern. Despite sequence differences, homologous domains have similar three-dimensional structures. This is extremely important, as it facilitates predictions of protein structure (and some functions) from amino acid sequences alone.

Each family of modular domains is thought to have arisen from a common ancestor. In this sense, the members of a family are said to be **homologous.** Through the processes of **gene duplication, transposition,** and **divergent evolution,** the most widely used domains (e.g., the immunoglobulin domain)

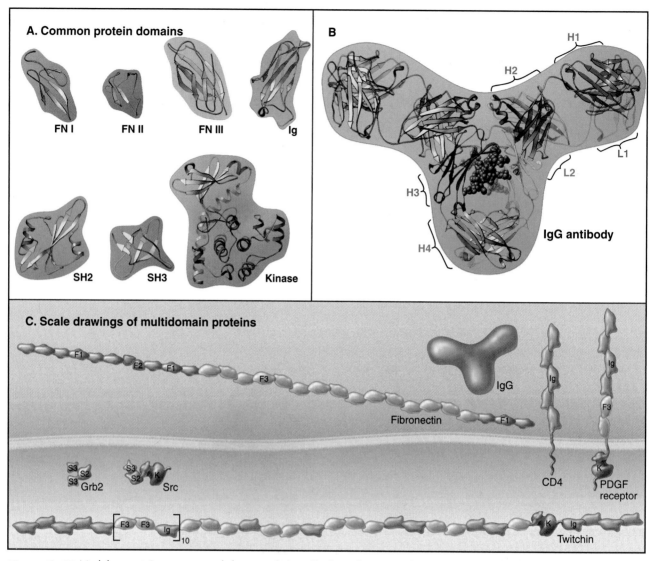

Figure 2-15 Modular proteins constructed from evolutionarily homologous, independently folded domains. *A,* Examples of protein domains used in many proteins: fibronectin 1 (FN I), fibronectin 2 (FN II), fibronectin 3 (FN III), immunoglobulin (Ig), Src homology 2 (SH2), Src homology 3 (SH3), kinase (SH1). *B,* Immunoglobulin G (IgG), a protein composed of 12 Ig domains on four polypeptide chains. Two identical heavy chains (H) consist of four Ig domains and two identical light chains (L) consist of two Ig domains. The sequences of these six Ig domains differ, but all of the domains are folded similarly. The two antigen-binding sites are located at the ends of the two arms of the Y-shaped molecule composed of highly variable loops contributed by domains H1 and L1. *C,* Examples of proteins constructed from the domains shown in *A:* fibronectin (see Chapter 31), CD4 (see Chapters 29 and 30), PDGF-receptor (see Chapter 26), Grb2 (see Chapter 27), Src (see Chapter 27) and twitchin (see Chapter 42). Each of the 31 FN3 domains in twitchin has a different sequence. F1 is FI, F2 is FII, F3 is FIII. (*A,* From PDB files: FN7, 1PDC, 1FNA, 1IG2, 1HCS, 1PRM, 1CTP. *B,* From PDB file: 1IG2.)

have become incorporated into dozens of different proteins where they serve unique functions. This theme recurs frequently. Much less commonly, some protein domains with related structures may have arisen independently during evolution and converged during functional selection toward a particularly favorable conformation, as postulated to explain the similarity of immunoglobulin, and fibronectin-III domains.

■ **Nucleic Acids**

Nucleic acids, polymers of a few simple building blocks called **nucleotides,** store and transfer all genetic information. This is not the limit of their functions, however, as nucleic acids contribute to the structures and enzyme activities of major cellular components, such as ribosomes (see Chapter 18) and spliceosomes (see Chapter 15). Furthermore, RNAs catalyze a number of biochemical reactions. In addition, nucleotides themselves transfer chemical energy between cellular systems and information in signal transduction pathways. Each of these topics is elaborated upon in other chapters. The following discussion gives the basic structures of these vital molecules.

Building Blocks of Nucleic Acids

Nucleotides consist of three parts: (1) a **base** built of one or two cyclic rings containing carbon and a few nitrogen atoms, (2) a five-carbon sugar, and (3) one or more phosphate groups (Fig. 2–16). **DNA** uses four main bases: the purines **adenine** (A) and **guanosine** (G) and the pyrimidines **cytosine** (C) and **thymine** (T). In **RNA, uracil** (U) is found in place of thymine. Some RNAs contain bases that are chemically modified after synthesis of the polymer. The RNA sugar is **ribose,** which has the aldehyde oxygen of carbon 4 cyclized to carbon 1. The DNA sugar is deoxyribose, which is similar to ribose but lacks the hydroxyl on carbon 2. In both RNA and DNA, carbon 1 of the sugar is conjugated with nitrogen 1 of a pyrimidine base or with nitrogen 9 of a purine base. The hydroxyl of sugar carbon 5 can be esterified to a chain of one or more phosphates, forming the **nucleotides** such as adenosine monophosphate **(AMP),** adenosine diphosphate **(ADP),** and ATP.

Covalent Structure of Nucleic Acids

DNA and RNA are polymers of nucleotides joined by **phosphodiester bonds** (Fig. 2–17). The backbone links a chain of six atoms (two oxygens and four carbons) from one phosphorous to the next. Unlike the backbone of proteins, in which the planar peptide bond greatly limits rotation, all six bonds along the polynucleotide backbone have some freedom to rotate, even that in the sugar ring. This feature gives nucleic acids much greater conformational flexibility than polypeptides, which have only two variable torsional angles per residue. The backbone phosphate group has a single negative charge at neutral pH. The N—C bond linking the base to the sugar is also free to rotate on a picosecond time scale, but rotation away from the backbone is strongly favored. The bases have a strong tendency to stack upon each other owing to favorable van der Waals interactions (see Chapter 3) between these planar rings.

Each type of nucleic acid has a unique sequence of nucleotides. Simple laboratory procedures employing the enzymatic synthesis of DNA allow the se-

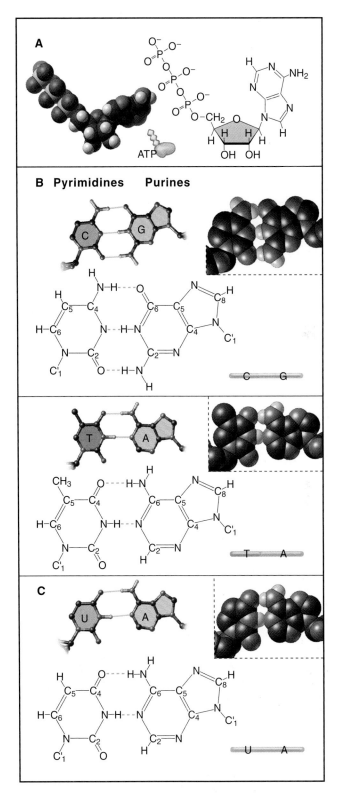

Figure 2–16 ATP and nucleotide bases. *A,* Stick figure and space-filling model of ATP. *B,* Four bases used in DNA. Stick figures show the hydrogen bonds used to form base pairs between thymine (T) and adenine (A) and between cytosine (C) and guanine (G). *C,* Uridine (U) replaces thymine in RNA. C_1' refers to carbon 1 of ribose and deoxyribose.

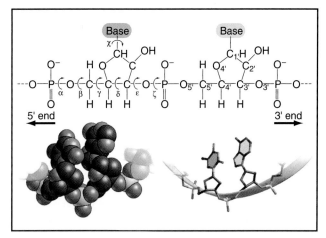

Figure 2–17 Rotational freedom of the backbone of a polynucleotide, RNA in this case. The stick figure of two residues shows that all six of the backbone bonds are rotatable, even the C'_4—C'_3 bond that is constrained by the ribose ring. This gives polynucleotides more conformational freedom than polypeptides. Note the phosphodiester bonds between the residues and the definition of the 3' and 5' ends. Space-filling and stick figures at the bottom show a uridine (U) and adenine (A) from part of Figure 2–19. (Redrawn from Jaeger JA, SantaLucia J, Tinoco I: Determination of RNA structure and thermodynamics. Annu Rev Biochem 62:255–287, 1993, with permission, from the *Annual Review of Biochemistry*, Vol. 62, © 1993 by Annual Reviews www.AnnualReviews.org.)

quence to be determined rapidly (Fig. 2–18). All DNA and RNA molecules are synthesized in the same direction (see Chapters 14 and 45) by adding a nucleoside triphosphate to the 3' sugar hydroxyl of the growing strand. The loss of the two terminal phosphates from the new subunit provides the energy for the extension of the polymer in the 5' to 3' direction. Newly synthesized DNA and RNA molecules have a phosphate at the 5' end and a 3' hydroxyl at the other end. In certain types of RNA (e.g., messenger RNA [mRNA]), the 5' nucleotide is modified by the addition of a specialized cap structure (see Chapter 15).

Secondary Structure of DNA

A few viruses have chromosomes consisting of single-stranded DNA molecules, but most DNA molecules are paired with a complementary strand to form a right-handed **double helix,** as originally proposed by Watson and Crick (Fig. 2–19). The essential features of the double helix are two strands running in opposite directions with the sugar-phosphate backbone on the outside and pairs of bases hydrogen-bonded to each other on the inside (see Fig. 2–16). These pairs of

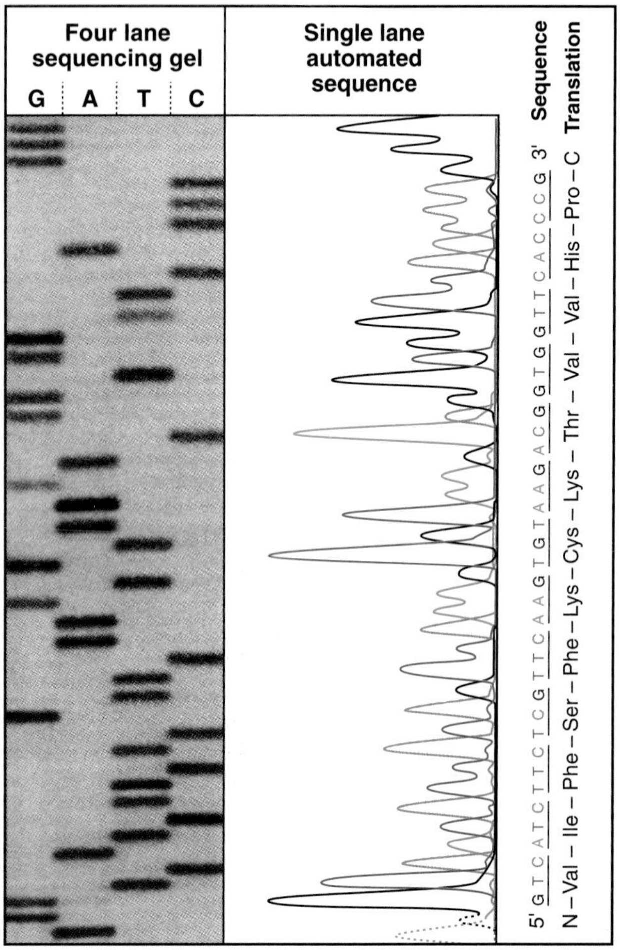

Four lane sequencing gel	Single lane automated sequence	Sequence Translation
G A T C		

5' G T C A T C T T C T C G T T C A A G T G T A A G A C G T G G T T C A C C C G 3'

N – Val – Ile – Phe – Ser – Phe – Lys – Cys – Lys – Thr – Val – Val – His – Pro – C

Figure 2–18 The sequence of a purified fragment of DNA is rapidly determined by in vitro synthesis (see Chapter 45) using the four deoxynucleoside triphosphates plus a small fraction of one dideoxynucleoside triphosphate. The random incorporation of the dideoxy residue terminates a few of the growing DNA molecules every time that base appears in the sequence. The reaction is run separately with each dideoxynucleotide, and fragments are separated according to size by gel electrophoresis (see Chapter 5), with the shortest fragments at the bottom. A radioactive label makes the fragments visible when exposed to an x-ray film. The sequence is read from the bottom as indicated. An automated method uses four different fluorescent dideoxynucleotides to mark the end of the fragments and electronic detectors to read the sequence. (Based on original data from W-L. Lee, Salk Institute for Biological Studies.)

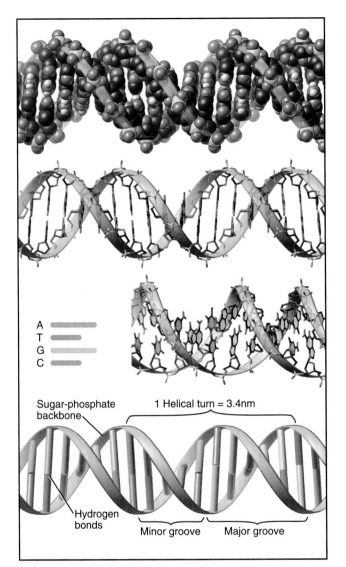

A
T
G
C

Sugar-phosphate backbone

1 Helical turn = 3.4nm

Hydrogen bonds

Minor groove   Major groove

Figure 2-19 Models of B-form DNA. The molecule consists of two complementary antiparallel strands arranged in a right-handed double helix with the backbone (see Fig. 2-17) on the outside and stacked pairs of hydrogen-bonded bases (see Fig. 2-16) on the inside. *Top,* Space-filling model. *Middle,* Stick figures, with the lower figure rotated slightly to reveal the faces of the bases. *Bottom,* Ribbon representation. (Idealized 24-base pair model built by Robert Tan, University of Alabama, Birmingham.)

bases are stacked 0.34 nm apart, nearly perpendicular to the long axis of the polymer. This regular structure is referred to as **B-DNA,** but real DNA is not completely regular. On average, in solution, B-DNA has 10.5 base pairs per turn and a diameter of 1.9 nm. Hydrogen bonds between adenine and thymine and between guanine and cytosine span nearly the same distance between the backbones, so the helix has a regular structure that, to a first approximation, is independent of the unique sequence of bases. One exception is a run of As that tend to bend adjoining parts of the helix. Because the bonds between the bases and

the sugars are asymmetrical, the helix is asymmetrical. Consequently, the major groove on one side of the helix is broader than the other, minor groove. Most cellular DNA is approximately in the B-DNA conformation, but proteins that regulate gene expression can distort the DNA significantly (see Chapter 14).

Under some laboratory conditions, DNA forms stable helical structures that differ from classic B-form DNA. All these variants have the phosphate-sugar backbone on the outside, and most have the usual complementary base pairs on the inside. A-form DNA has 11 base pairs per turn and an average diameter of 2.3 nm. DNA-RNA hybrids and double-stranded RNA also have A-form structure. Z-DNA is the most extreme variant, as it is a left-handed helix with 12 base pairs per turn. There is some circumstantial evidence for Z-DNA in cells.

DNA molecules are either linear or circular. Human chromosomes are single linear DNA molecules (see Chapter 12). Many, but not all, viral and bacterial chromosomes are circular. Eukaryotic mitochondria and chloroplasts also have circular DNA molecules.

When circular DNAs or linear DNAs with both ends anchored (as in chromosomes; see Chapter 13) are twisted about their long axis, the strain is relieved by the development of long-range bends and twists called **supercoils** or **superhelices** (Fig. 2-20). This supercoiling can be either positive or negative depending on whether the DNA helix is wound more tightly or somewhat unwound. Supercoiling is biologically important as it can influence the expression of genes. Under some circumstances, supercoiling favors the unwinding of the double helix, thus promoting

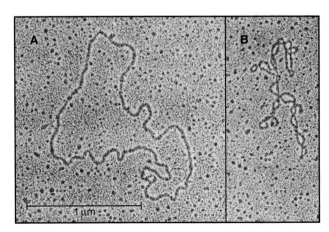

Figure 2-20 DNA supercoiling. Electron micrographs of a circular mitochondrial DNA molecule in a relaxed configuration *(A)* and a supercoiled configuration *(B).* (Reproduced, with permission, from David Clayton, Stanford University; originally in Stryer L: Biochemistry. 4th ed. New York: W.H. Freeman and Co., 1995.)

access of proteins involved in the regulation of transcription from DNA (see Chapter 14).

The degree of supercoiling can be regulated locally by enzymes called **topoisomerases.** Type I topoisomerases nick one strand of the DNA and cause the molecule to unwind by rotation about a backbone bond. Type II topoisomerases cut both strands of the DNA and use an ATP-driven conformational change (called gating) to pass an uncut DNA strand through the cut prior to rejoining the ends of the DNA. To avoid free DNA ends during this reaction, cleavage of the DNA is accomplished by a covalent linkage to tyrosine residues in the enzyme. The chemical bond energy is conserved throughout, so that ATP is not required for the re-ligation of the DNA at the end of the reaction.

Secondary and Tertiary Structure of RNAs

RNAs range in size from 76 nucleotides in transfer RNA (tRNA) to greater than 80,000 nucleotides in the mRNA for the giant muscle protein, titin (see Chapter 42). Because each nucleotide is about six times as massive as an amino acid, RNAs with a modest number of nucleotides are bigger than most proteins. The 16S RNA of the small ribosomal subunit of bacteria

consists of 1542 bases and has a mass of about 1 million D, much larger than any of the 21 proteins with which it interacts (see Chapter 18).

With the exception of a few viruses, RNAs do not

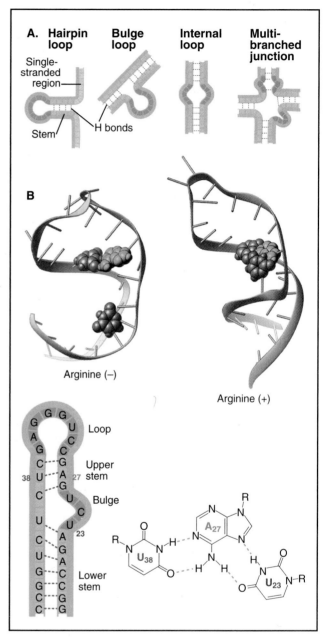

Figure 2–22 RNA secondary structure. A, Diagrams of an antiparallel base-paired stem which is part of a hairpin loop, a hairpin loop, a bulge loop, an internal loop, and a multibranched junction. B, Molecular models of NMR structures of a stem-loop structure, called TAR coded by HIV. In the presence of arginine (or a protein called TAT), TAR undergoes a major conformational change: two bases twist out of the helix into the solvent (top). U23 forms a base triplet with U38 and A27 (space-filling model), and the stem straightens. This conformational change promotes the transcription of the rest of the mRNA. (A, Redrawn from Jaeger JA, SantaLucia J, Tinoco I: Annu Rev Biochem 62:255–287, 1993, with permission, from the *Annual Review of Biochemistry*, Vol. 62, © 1993 by Annual Reviews www.AnnualReviews.org. B, From PDB files: 1ANR and 1AKX.)

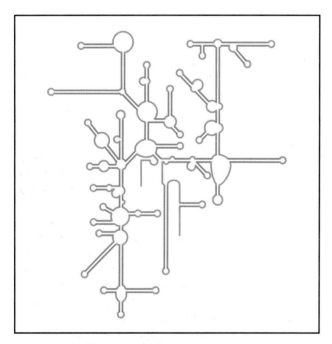

Figure 2–21 RNA secondary structure. Base pairing of *Escherichia coli* 16S ribosomal RNA determined by covariant analysis of nucleotide sequences of many different 16S ribosomal RNAs. The small circles represent the nucleotides. Note the numerous bulges and turns within and between segments of antiparallel, base-paired strands. (Redrawn from Huysmans E, DeWachter R: Compilation of small ribosomal subunit RNA sequences. Nucleic Acids Research 14Suppl:73–118, 1987.)

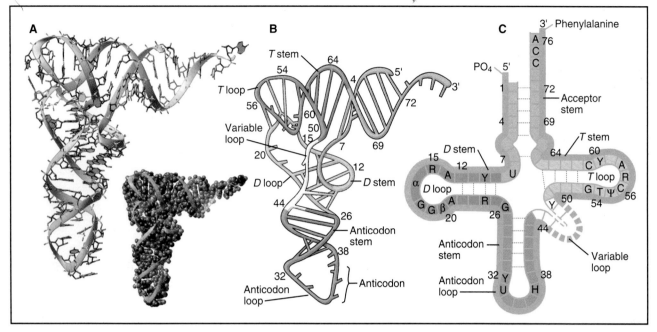

Figure 2-23 Atomic structure of phenylalanine transfer RNA (phe-tRNA) determined by x-ray crystallography. The conformation (*A* and *B*) is much freer than implied by the flat base-pairing scheme (*C*), including the base-paired segments that are much less regular than B-form DNA. In *A*, a ribbon is superimposed on the RNA backbone to trace its path. (From PDB file: 6TNA; redrawn from an original by Alex Rich, MIT.)

have a complementary strand to pair with each base, but they form specific secondary structures by optimizing *intramolecular* base pairing (Figs. 2–21 and 2–22). Comparison of homologous RNA sequences provides much of what is known about this intramolecular base pairing. The approach is to identify pairs of nucleotides that vary together across the phylogenetic tree. For example, if an A and a U at discontinuous positions in one RNA are changed together to C and G in other homologous RNAs, it is concluded that they are probably hydrogen-bonded together. This **co-variant method** works remarkably well, because hundreds to thousands of homologous sequences for the major classes of RNA are available from evolutionary studies. Conclusions about base pairing from covariant analysis have been confirmed often by experimental mutagenesis of RNAs or, more recently, by direct structure determination using x-ray diffraction or NMR spectroscopy.

The simplest type of RNA secondary structure is an antiparallel helix stabilized by hydrogen bonding of complementary bases (see Figs. 2–22 and 2–23). As in DNA, U pairs with A and G pairs with C. Unlike in DNA, G also frequently pairs with U in RNA. Helical base pairing occurs between both contiguous and discontiguous sequences. When contiguous sequences form a helix, the strand is often reversed by a tight turn, forming an antiparallel **stem-loop** structure. These hairpin turns frequently consist of just four

bases. A few sequences are highly favored owing to their compact, stable structures. Bulges secondary to extra bases or noncomplementary bases frequently interrupt base-paired helices of RNA.

The atomic structures of RNA—beginning with **tRNAs** (see Fig. 2–23 and Chapter 15) and a hammerhead **ribozyme** (Fig. 2–24)—established that RNAs have novel, specific, three-dimensional structures. The atomic structure of the ribosome (see Chapter 18) confirmed that larger RNAs also fold into specific structures using similar principles. Crystallization of RNAs is challenging, and NMR provides much less information on RNA than on proteins of the same size, so much is yet to be learned about RNA structures.

Like proteins, many residues in RNAs are in conventional secondary structures, especially stems consisting of base-paired double helices; however, the backbone also makes sharp turns that allow bases to make unconventional hydrogen bonds with each other, ribose hydroxyls, and backbone phosphates. Generally, the phosphodiester backbone is exposed on the surface, and most of the hydrophobic bases are stacked internally. Some bases are hydrogen-bonded together in triplets (see Fig. 2–22) rather than in pairs. Four or five Mg^{2+} ions stabilize regions of tRNA with high densities of negative charge. A variety of evidence suggests that RNAs are more flexible than proteins.

Like proteins, RNAs can change conformation. The

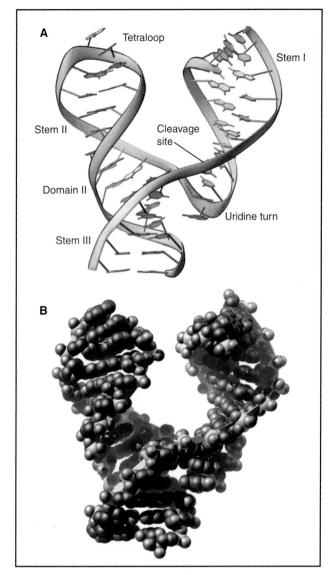

Figure 2–24 The x-ray structure of a hammerhead ribozyme, a self-cleaving RNA sequence found in plant virus RNAs. *A*, Stick figure. *B*, Space-filling model. The structure consists of an RNA strand of 34 nucleotides complexed to a DNA strand of 13 nucleotides (in vivo this is a 13-nucleotide stretch of RNA, which would be cleaved by the ribozyme). The RNA forms a central stem–loop structure (stem II) and base-pairs with the substrate DNA to form stems I and III. Interactions of the substrate strand with the sharp uridine turn distort the backbone and promote its cleavage. (*A*, Redrawn from Pley HW, Flaherty KM, McKay DB: Three-dimensional structure of a hammerhead ribozyme. Nature 372:68–74, 1994. *B*, From PDB file: 1HMH.)

TAR RNA is a stem-loop structure with a bulge formed by three unpaired nucleotides (see Fig. 2–22). It is located at the 5′ end of all RNA transcripts of the human immunodeficiency virus (HIV) that causes AIDS. Binding of a regulatory protein called TAT to TAR changes its conformation and promotes the elongation of the RNA. Binding arginine also changes the conformation of TAR.

Carbohydrates

Carbohydrates are a large family of biologically essential molecules made up of one or more sugar molecules. Sugar polymers differ from proteins and nucleic acids by having branches. Compared with proteins, which are generally compact, hydrophilic sugar polymers tend to spread out in aqueous solutions to maximize the hydrogen bonds with water. On a weight basis, carbohydrates may occupy 5 to 10 times the volume of a protein. The nomenclature for sugar polymers is in flux. The terms **glycoconjugate** or **complex carbohydrate** are currently preferred to polysaccharide.

Carbohydrates serve four main functions:

1. Chemical energy stored in covalent bonds of sugar molecules is a primary source of energy for cells.
2. Polymers of sugar molecules are the most abundant structural components on earth. Examples are the cellulose that forms the cell walls of plants, chitin that forms the exoskeletons of insects, and glycosaminoglycans that are found in the connective tissues of animals.
3. Sugars are essential components of the nucleotides that form the backbone of nucleic acids and participate in many metabolic reactions (see earlier discussion).
4. Single sugars and groupings of sugars form side chains on lipids (see Chapter 6) and proteins (see Chapters 20 and 21). These modifications provide molecular diversity beyond that inherent in the proteins and lipids themselves, changing their physical properties and vastly expanding the potential of these glycoproteins and glycolipids to interact with other cellular components in specific receptor-ligand interactions (see Chapters 32 and 34). On the other hand, the function of some glycoconjugates is to block inappropriate cellular interactions.

The vast array of different complex carbohydrates is constructed of a modest number of simple sugars (Fig. 2–25). They consist of three to seven carbons with one aldehyde or ketone group and multiple hydroxyl groups. In water, the common five-carbon **(pentose)** and six-carbon **(hexose)** sugars cyclize by reaction of the aldehyde or ketone group with one of the hydroxyl carbons. This forms a compact structure used in all the glycoconjugates considered in this book. Given several asymmetrical carbons in each sugar, a great many **stereochemical isomers** exist. For example, the hydroxyl on carbon 1 can either be above (β-isomer) or below (α-isomer) the plane of the ring. Proteins (enzymes, lectins, and receptors) that interact with sugars distinguish these stereoisomers.

Sugars are coupled to other molecules by highly

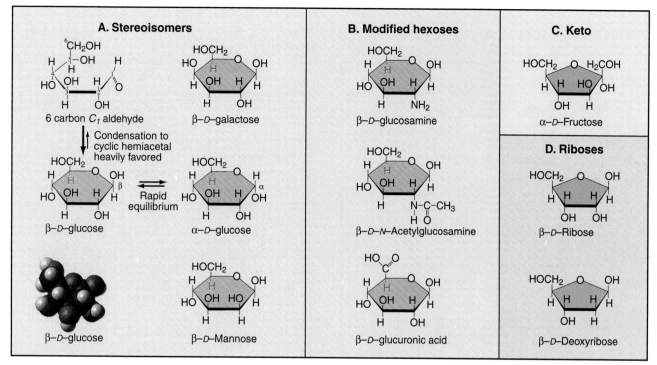

Figure 2-25 *A to C,* Simple sugar molecules. Stick figures and space-filling model of D-glucose showing the highly favored condensation of the carbon 5 hydroxyl with carbon 1 to form a hemiacetal. The resulting hydroxyl group on carbon 1 is in a rapid equilibrium between the α (down) or β (up) configurations. The space-filling model of β-D-glucose illustrates the stereochemistry of the ring; the stick figures are drawn as unrealistic planar rings to simplify comparisons. Stick figures show three stereoisomers of the 6-carbon glucose, three modifications of glucose, a 6-carbon keto sugar condensed into a five-membered ring, and two 5-carbon riboses.

specific enzymes, using a modest repertoire of intermolecular bonds (Fig. 2–26). The common *O*-glycosidic (carbon-oxygen-carbon) bond is formed by removal of water from two hydroxyls—the hydroxyl of the carbon bonded to the ring oxygen of a sugar and a hydroxyl oxygen of another sugar or the amino acids serine and threonine. A similar reaction couples a sugar to an amine, as in the bond between a sugar and a nucleoside base. Sugar phosphates with one or more phosphates esterified to a sugar hydroxyl are components of nucleotides, as well as of many intermediates in metabolic pathways.

Glycoconjugates—polymers of one or more types of sugar molecules—are present in massive amounts

Figure 2-26 Glycosidic bonds. Stick figures show the formation of *O*- and *N*-glycosidic bonds and a common example of each—the disaccharide sucrose and the nucleoside cytidine. Enzymes catalyze the formation of glycosidic bonds in cells. The chemical name of sucrose [glucose-α(1→2)fructose] illustrates the convention for naming the bonds of glycoconjugates.

Hemiacetal sugars	react with	to form	Examples
Glucose	Alcohols	*O*-glycosidic bond	Sucrose Glucose–α(1→2)–fructose
Ribose	Amines	*N*-glycosidic bond	Cytidine

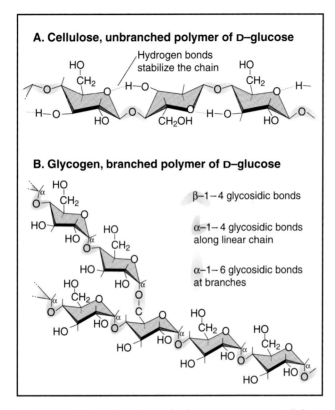

A. Cellulose, unbranched polymer of D–glucose

Hydrogen bonds stabilize the chain

B. Glycogen, branched polymer of D–glucose

β–1–4 glycosidic bonds

α–1–4 glycosidic bonds along linear chain

α–1–6 glycosidic bonds at branches

Figure 2–27 Examples of simple glycoconjugates. *A,* Cellulose, an unbranched homopolymer of glucose used to construct plant cell walls. *B,* Glycogen, a branched homopolymer of glucose used by animal cells to store sugar. Many glycoconjugates consist of several different types of sugar subunits (see Chapters 21 and 31).

in nature and are used as both energy stores and structural components (Fig. 2–27). Cellulose (unbranched β-1,4 polyglucose), which forms the cell walls of plants, and chitin (unbranched β-1,4 poly *N*-acetylglucosamine), which forms the exoskeletons of many invertebrates, are the first and second most abundant biological polymers found on earth. In animals, giant complex carbohydrates are essential components of the extracellular matrix of cartilage and other connective tissues (see Chapters 31 and 34). Glycogen, a branched α-1,4 polymer of glucose, is the major energy store in animal cells. Starch—polymers of glucose with or without a modest level of branching—performs the same function for plants.

Glycoconjugates differ from proteins and nucleic acids in that they have a broader range of conformations owing to the flexible glycosidic linkages between the sugar subunits. Although sugar polymers may be stabilized by extensive intramolecular hydrogen bonds, and some glycosidic linkages are relatively rigid, NMR studies have revealed that many glycosidic bonds rotate freely, allowing the polymer to change its conformation on a submillisecond time scale. This dynamic behavior limits efforts to determine glycoconjugate structures. They are reluctant to crystallize, and the multitude of conformations does not lend itself to NMR analysis. Structural details are best revealed by x-ray crystallography of a glycoconjugate bound to a protein, such as a lectin or a glycosidase (a degradative enzyme).

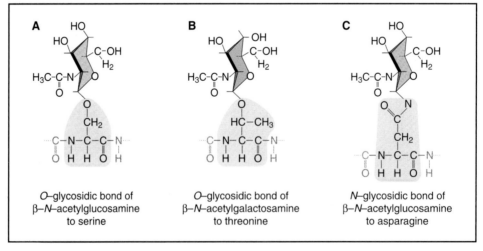

A O–glycosidic bond of β–*N*–acetylglucosamine to serine

B O–glycosidic bond of β–*N*–acetylgalactosamine to threonine

C N–glycosidic bond of β–*N*–acetylglucosamine to asparagine

Figure 2–28 Three types of glycosidic bonds link glycoconjugates to proteins. *A,* An *O*-glycosidic bond links *N*-acetylglucosamine to serine residues of many intracellular proteins. *B,* An *O*-glycosidic bond links *N*-acetylgalactosamine to serine or threonine residues of core proteins, initiating long glycoconjugate polymers called glycosaminoglycans on extracellular proteoglycans (see Chapter 31). *C,* An *N*-glycosidic bond links *N*-acetylglucosamine to asparagine residues of secreted and membrane glycoproteins (see Chapter 21). A wide variety of glycoconjugates extend the sugar polymer from the *N*-acetylglucosamine. These stick figures illustrate the conformations of the sugar rings.

Sugars are linked to proteins in three different ways (Fig. 2–28). The formation of each type of linkage is catalyzed by specific enzymes that recognize unique protein conformations. Glycoprotein side chains vary in size from one sugar to polymers of hundreds of sugars. These sugar side chains can exceed the mass of the protein to which they are attached. Glycoprotein biosynthesis is considered in Chapters 21 and 31.

Compared with the nearly invariant proteins and nucleic acids, glycoconjugates are heterogeneous because enzymes assemble these sugar polymers without the aid of a genetic template. These glycosyltransferases link high-energy sugar-nucleosides to acceptor sugars. These enzymes are specific for the donor sugar-nucleoside and selective, but not completely specific, for the acceptor sugars. Thus, cells require many different glycosyltransferases to generate the hundreds of types of sugar-sugar bonds found in glycoconjugates. Particular cells consistently produce the same range of specific glycoconjugate structures. This reproducible heterogeneity arises from the repertoire of glycosyltransferases expressed, their localization in specific cellular compartments, and the availability of suitable acceptors. The glycosyltransferases compete with each other for acceptors, yielding a variety of products at many steps in the synthesis of glycoconjugates. For example, the probability of encountering a particular glycosyltransferase depends upon the part of the Golgi apparatus (see Chapter 21) in which a particular acceptor finds itself.

The Aqueous Phase of Cytoplasm

The aqueous phase of cells contains a wide variety of solutes, including inorganic ions, the building blocks of the major organic constituents, the intermediates in metabolic pathways, carbohydrate and lipid energy stores, and high concentrations of proteins and RNA; in addition, eukaryotic cells have a dense network of cytoskeletal fibers (Fig. 2–29). Cells control the concentrations of solutes in each cellular compartment, because many (e.g., pH, Na^+, K^+, Ca^{2+}, and cyclic AMP) have essential regulatory or functional significance in particular compartments.

The high concentration of macromolecules and the network of cytoskeletal polymers make the cytoplasm a very different environment from the dilute salt solutions usually employed in biochemical experiments on cellular constituents. The presence of 300 mg/mL of protein and RNA causes the cytoplasm to be crowded. The concentration of bulk water in cytoplasm is less than the 55 M in dilute solutions, but the microscopic viscosity of the aqueous phase in live cells is remarkably close to that of pure water. Crowding lowers the diffusion coefficient of the molecules

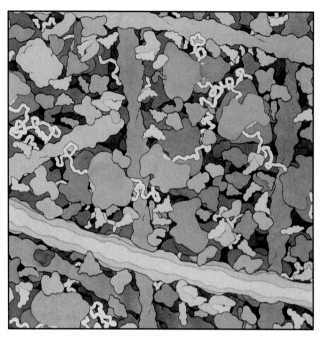

Figure 2–29 Crowded cytoplasm. Scale drawing of eukaryotic cell cytoplasm emphasizing the high concentrations of ribosomes *(shades of red)*, proteins *(shades of tan, blue, and green)*, and nucleic acids *(white)* among cytoskeletal polymers. (Original drawing from D. Goodsell, Scripps Research Institute.)

by a factor of about three, but it also enhances macromolecular associations by raising the chemical potential of the diffusing molecules through an "excluded volume" effect. The macromolecules take up space in the solvent, so the concentration of each molecule is higher relative to the available solvent. At cellular concentrations of macromolecules, the chemical potential of a molecule (see Chapter 3) may be one or more orders of magnitude higher than its concentration. (It is actually the chemical potential, rather than the concentration, that determines the rate of reactions.) Therefore, crowding favors protein-protein, protein–nucleic acid, and other macromolecular assembly reactions that depend on the chemical potential of the reactants. Crowding also changes the rates and equilibria of enzymatic reactions, usually increasing the activity as compared with values in dilute solutions. These striking effects are rarely considered in biochemical experiments.

Selected Readings

Baldwin RL, Rose GD: Is protein folding hierarchic? I. Local structure and peptide folding. Trends Biochem Sci 24: 26–33, 1999.

Brandon C, Tooze J: Introduction to Protein Structure. New York: Garland Publishing, 1999, p. 350.

Bryant RG: The dynamics of water-protein interactions. Annu Rev Biophys Biomol Struct 25:29–53, 1996.

Chothia C, Hubbard T, Brenner S, et al.: Protein folds in the all-β and all-α classes. Annu Rev Biophys Biomol Struct 26:597–627, 1997.

Creighton TE: Proteins: Structure and Molecular Principles. 2nd ed. New York: W.H. Freeman and Co., 1993, p. 507.

Drickamer K, Taylor M: Evolving views of protein glycosylation. Trends Biochem Sci 23:321–323, 1998.

Hagerman PJ: Flexibility of RNA. Annu Rev Biophys Biomol Struct 26:139–156, 1997.

Kuriyan J, Cowburn D: Modular peptide recognition domains in eukaryotic signaling. Annu Rev Biophys Biomol Struct 26:259–288, 1997.

Levitt M, Gerstein M, Huang E, et al.: Protein folding: The endgame. Annu Rev Biochem 66:549–580, 1997.

Lupas A: Coiled-coils: New structures and new functions. Trends Biochem Sci 21:375–382, 1996.

Murthy VL, Srinivasan R, Draper DE, Rose GD: A complete conformational map for RNA. J Mol Biol 291:313–327, 1999.

Narlikar GJ, Hershlag D: Mechanistic aspects of enzyme catalysis: Lessons from comparisons of RNA and protein enzymes. Annu Rev Biochem 66:19–60, 1997.

Rebecchi MJ, Scarlata RS: Pleckstrin homology domains: A common fold with diverse functions. Annu Rev Biophys Biomol Struct 27:503–528, 1998.

Scott WG, Klug A: Ribozymes: Structure and mechanism in RNA catalysis. Trends Biochem Sci 21:220–223, 1996.

Wedekind JE, McKay DR: Crystallographic structures of the hammerhead ribozyme: Relationship to ribozyme folding and catalysis. Annu Rev Biophys Biomol Struct 27:475–502, 1998.

chapter 3

BASIC BIOPHYSICAL CONCEPTS

The concepts in this chapter form the basis for understanding all the molecular interactions in chemistry and biology. Most molecular interactions are driven by the diffusion of reactants that simply collide with each other on a random basis. Similarly, the dissociation of molecular complexes is a random process occurring with a probability determined by the strength of the chemical bonds holding the molecules together. Many other reactions occur within molecules or molecular complexes. The aim of biophysical chemistry is to explain life processes in terms of these kinds of molecular interactions.

The extent of such reactions is characterized by the **equilibrium constant**; the rates of these reactions are described by **rate constants**. This chapter reviews the physical basis for rate constants and how they are related to the thermodynamic parameter, the equilibrium constant. These simple but powerful principles permit a deeper appreciation of the molecular interactions in cells. Based on the many examples presented in this book, it will become clear to the reader that rate constants are at least as important as equilibrium constants, since the rates of reactions govern the dynamics of the cell. The end of the chapter presents a discussion of the chemical bonds important in biochemistry. Box 3–1 lists key terms used in this chapter.

▌ First-Order Reactions

First-order reactions have one reactant (R) and produce a product (P). The general case is simply

$$R \longrightarrow P$$

Chapter adapted in part from Wachsstock DH, Pollard TD: Transient state kinetics tutorial using KINSIM. Biophys J 67:1260–1273, 1994.

Some common examples of first-order reactions (Fig. 3–1) include conformational changes, such as a change in shape of protein A to shape A*

$$A \longrightarrow A^*$$

and the dissociation of complexes, such as

$$AB \longrightarrow A + B$$

The rate of a first-order reaction is directly proportional to the concentration of the reactant (R, A, or AB in these examples). The rate of a first-order reaction, expressed as a differential equation (rate of change of reactant or product as a function of time [t]), is simply the concentration of the reactant times a constant, the rate constant k, with units of s^{-1}.

$$Rate = -d[R]/dt = d[P]/dt = k[R]$$

The rate of the reaction has units of M s^{-1}, where M is moles per liter and s is seconds (molar per second). As the reactant is depleted, the rate slows proportionally.

A first-order rate constant can be viewed as a **probability** per unit of time. For the conformational change, it is the probability that any A will change to A* in a unit of time. For the dissociation of complex AB, the first-order rate constant is determined by the strength of the bonds holding the complex together. This "dissociation rate constant" can be viewed as the probability that the complex will fall apart in a unit of time. The probability of the conformational change of any particular A to A* or of the dissociation of any particular AB is independent of its concentration. *The concentrations of A and AB are important only in determining the rate of the reaction observed in a bulk sample* (Box 3–2).

To review, the rate of a first-order reaction is sim-

KEY TERMS

Rate constants, designated by lowercase k's, relate the concentrations of reactants to the rate of a reaction.

Equilibrium constants are designated by uppercase K's. One important and useful concept to remember is that the *equilibrium constant for a reaction is related directly to the rate constants for the forward and reverse reactions, as well as the equilibrium concentrations of reactants and products.*

The **rate of a reaction** is usually measured as the rate of change of **concentration** of a reactant (R) or product (P). As reactants disappear, products are formed so that the rate of reactant loss is directly related to the rate of product formation in a manner determined by the stoichiometry of the mechanism. In all the reaction mechanisms in this book, the arrows indicate the direction of a reaction. In the general case, the reaction mechanism is expressed as

$$R \rightleftharpoons P$$

Reaction rates are expressed as follows:

$$\text{Forward rate} = k_+ [R]$$

$$\text{Reverse rate} = k_- [P]$$

$$\text{Net rate} = k_+ [R] - k_- [P]$$

At equilibrium, the forward rate equals the reverse rate:

$$k_+ [R_{eq}] = k_- [P_{eq}]$$

and concentrations of reactants R_{eq} and products P_{eq} do not change with time.

The equilibrium constant K is defined as the ratio of the concentrations of products and reactants at equilibrium:

$$K_{eq} = \frac{[P_{eq}]}{[R_{eq}]}$$

so it follows that

$$K_{eq} = \frac{k_+}{k_-}$$

In specific cases, these relationships depend on the reaction mechanism, particularly on whether one or more than one chemical species constitutes the reactants and products. The equilibrium constant will be derived from a consideration of the reaction rates, beginning with the simplest case where there is one reactant.

---

ply the product of a constant that is characteristic of the reaction and the concentration of the single reactant. The constant can be calculated from the half-time of a reaction (see Box 3–2).

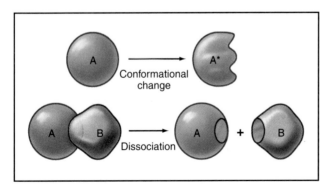

Figure 3-1 First-order reactions. In first-order reactions, a single reactant undergoes a change. In these examples, molecule A changes conformation to A* and the bimolecular complex AB dissociates to A and B. The rate constant for a first-order reaction (*arrow*) is a simple probability.

Second-Order Reactions

Second-order reactions have two reactants (Fig. 3–2). The general case is

$$R_1 + R_2 \longrightarrow \text{product}$$

A common example in biology is a bimolecular association reaction, such as

$$A + B \longrightarrow AB$$

where A and B are two molecules that bind together. Some examples are the binding of substrates to enzymes, the binding of ligands to receptors, and the binding of proteins to other proteins or nucleic acids.

The rate of a second-order reaction is the product of the concentrations of the two reactants, R_1 and R_2, and the second-order rate constant, k.

$$\text{Reaction rate} = d[P]/dt = k[R_1][R_2]$$

The second-order rate constant, k, has units of $M^{-1}\,s^{-1}$. The units for the reaction rate are

$$[R_1] \cdot [R_2] \cdot k = M \cdot M \cdot M^{-1}\,s^{-1} \text{ or } M\,s^{-1}$$

the same as a first-order reaction.

The value of a second-order "association" rate constant, k_+, is determined mainly by the rate at

box 3-2

RELATIONSHIP OF THE HALF-TIME TO A FIRST-ORDER RATE CONSTANT

When thinking about a first-order reaction, it is sometimes useful to refer to the half-time of the reaction. The half-time, $t_{1/2}$, is the time required for half of the existing reactant to be converted to product. For a first-order reaction, this time depends *only on the rate constant* and, therefore, is the same regardless of the starting concentration of the reactant. The relationship is derived as follows:

$$\frac{d[R]}{dt} = -k[R]$$

so

$$\frac{d[R]}{[R]} = -k\,dt$$

Thus, integrating,

$$\ln[R_t] - \ln[R_o] = -k\,t$$

where R_o is the initial concentration and R_t is the concentration at time t. Rearranging,

$$\ln[R_t] = \ln[R_o] - k\,t$$

or

$$[R_t] = [R_o]\,e^{-k\,t}$$

When the initial concentration R_o is reduced by half,

$$[R_t] = \tfrac{1}{2}[R_o]$$

so

$$\tfrac{1}{2}[R_o] = [R_o]\,e^{-k\,t_{1/2}}$$

$$\tfrac{1}{2} = e^{-k\,t_{1/2}}$$

or

$$2 = e^{k\,t_{1/2}}$$

Thus,

$$\ln 2 = k\,t_{1/2}$$

so, rearranging,

$$t_{1/2} = 0.693\,/\,k$$

or

$$k = 0.693\,/\,t_{1/2}$$

Therefore, a first-order rate constant can be estimated simply by dividing 0.7 by the half-time. Clearly, an analogous calculation yields the half-time from a first-order rate constant. This relationship is handy, as one frequently can estimate the extent of a reaction without knowing the absolute concentrations, and this relationship is independent of the extent of the reaction at the outset of the observations.

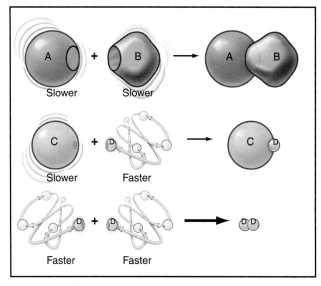

Figure 3-2 Second-order reactions. In second-order reactions, two molecules must collide with each other. The rate of these collisions is determined by their concentrations and by a collision rate constant (*arrows*). The collision rate constant depends on the sum of the diffusion coefficients of the reactants and the size of their interaction sites. The rate of diffusion in a given medium depends on the size and shape of the molecule. Large molecules, such as proteins, move slower than small molecules, such as adenosine triphosphate (ATP). The rate constants (*arrows*) are about the same for A + B and C + D, because the large diffusion coefficient of D offsets the small size of its interaction site on C. Despite the small interaction size, D + D is faster because both reactants diffuse rapidly.

which the molecules collide. This collision rate depends on the rate of diffusion of the molecules (see Fig. 3–2), which is determined by the size and shape of the molecule, the viscosity of the medium, and the temperature. These factors are summarized in a parameter called the **diffusion coefficient,** D, with units of $cm^2\ s^{-1}$. D is a measure of how fast a molecule moves in a given medium. The rate constant for collisions is described by the Debeye-Smoluchowski equation, a relationship that depends only on the diffusion coefficients and the area of interaction between the molecules:

$$k = 4\pi b(D_A + D_B)N_o\,10^{-3}$$

where b is the interaction radius of the two particles (in centimeters), the D's are the diffusion coefficients of the reactants, and N_o is Avogadro's number. The factor of 10^{-3} converts the value into units of $M^{-1}\ s^{-1}$.

For particles the size of proteins, D is approximately $10^{-7}\ cm^2\ s^{-1}$ and b is approximately 2×10^{-7} cm, so the rate constants for collisions of two proteins are in the range of $3 \times 10^8\ M^{-1}\ s^{-1}$. For small molecules such as sugars, D is approximately $10^{-5}\ cm^2\ s^{-1}$ and b is approximately 10^{-7} cm, so the rate constants for collisions of a protein and a small molecule are about 20 times larger than collisions of two proteins, in the range of 7×10^9 M^{-1} s^{-1}. On the other hand, the experimentally observed rate constants for the association of proteins are 20 to 1000 times smaller than the collision rate constant, on the order of 10^6 to 10^7 $M^{-1}s^{-1}$. The difference is attributed to a steric factor that accounts for the fact that macromolecules must be correctly oriented relative to each other in order to bind together when they collide. Thus, the complementary binding sites are aligned correctly only 0.1% to 5% of the times that the molecules collide.

Many binding reactions between two proteins, between enzymes and substrates, and between proteins and larger molecules (e.g., DNA) are said to be "diffusion limited" in the sense that the rate constant is determined by diffusion-driven collisions between the reactants. Thus, many association rate constants are in the range of 10^6 to 10^7 M^{-1} s^{-1}.

To review, the rate of a second-order reaction is simply the product of a constant that is characteristic of the reaction and the concentrations of the two reactants. In biology, the rates of many bimolecular association reactions are determined by the rates of diffusion-limited collisions between the reactants.

■ Reversible Reactions

Most reactions are reversible, so the net rate of a reaction will be equal to the difference between the forward and reverse reaction rates. The forward and reverse reactions can be any combination of first- or second-order reactions. A reversible conformational change of a protein from A to A* is an example of a pair of simple first-order reactions:

$$A \rightleftharpoons A^*$$

The forward reaction rate is k_+A with units of M s^{-1}, and the reverse reaction rate is k_-A^* with the same units. At equilibrium, at which point the net concentrations of A and A* no longer change,

$$k_+ [A] = k_- [A^*]$$

and

$$K_{eq} = k_+ / k_- = [A^*] / [A]$$

This equilibrium constant is unitless, since the units of concentration and the rate constants cancel out.

The same reasoning with respect to the equilibrium constant applies to a simple bimolecular binding reaction:

$$A + B \rightleftharpoons AB$$

where A and B are any molecule (e.g., enzyme, receptor, substrate, cofactor, or drug). The forward (binding) reaction is a second-order reaction, whereas the reverse (dissociation) reaction is a first-order one. The opposing reactions are

Rate of association $= k_+$ [A] [B]   units: M s^{-1}

Rate of dissociation $= k_-$ [AB]   units: M s^{-1}

The overall rate of the reaction is the forward rate minus the reverse rate:

Net rate = association rate − dissociation rate

$$= k_+ [A] [B] - k_- [AB]$$

Depending on the values of the rate constants and the concentrations of A, B, and AB, the reaction can go forward, backward, or nowhere.

At equilibrium, the forward and reverse rates are (by definition) the same:

$$k_+ [A] [B] = k_- [AB]$$

The equilibrium constant for such a bimolecular reaction can be written in two ways:

Association equilibrium constant

$$K_a = [AB] / [A] [B] = k_+/k_-$$

units: $M^{-1} = M / M \times M$

This is the classical equilibrium constant used in chemistry, where the strength of the reaction is proportional to the numerical value. For bimolecular reactions, the units of reciprocal molar are difficult to relate to, so biochemists frequently use the reciprocal relationship:

Dissociation equilibrium constant

$$K_d = [A] [B] / [AB] = k_-/k_+$$

units: $M = M \times M / M$

When half of the total A is bound to B, the concentration of free B is simply equal to the dissociation equilibrium constant.

■ Thermodynamic Considerations

The driving force for chemical reactions is the lowering of the free energy of the system when reactants are converted into products. The larger the reduction in free energy, the more completely reactants will be converted to products at equilibrium. A thorough consideration of thermodynamics is beyond the scope of this text, but an overview of this subject is presented to allow the reader to gain a basic understanding of its power and simplicity.

The change in Gibbs free energy, ΔG, is simply

the difference in the chemical potential, μ, of the reactants (R) and products (P):

$$\Delta G = \mu^P - \mu^R$$

The chemical potential of a particular chemical species depends on its intrinsic properties and its concentration, expressed as the equation

$$\mu = \mu^0 + RT \ln C$$

where μ^0 is the chemical potential in the standard state (1 M in biochemistry), R is the gas constant (8.3 J mol^{-1} degree^{-1}), T is the absolute temperature in degrees Kelvin, and C is the ratio of the concentration of the chemical species to the standard concentration. Because the standard state is defined as 1 M, the parameter C has the same numerical value as the molar concentration, but is, in fact, unitless. The term RT ln C adjusts for the concentration. When $C = 1$, $\mu = \mu^0$.

Under standard conditions where one mole of reactant is converted to one mole of product, the standard free energy change, ΔG^0, is

$$\Delta G^0 = \mu^{0P} - \mu^{0R}$$

However, because most reactions do not take place under these standard conditions, the chemical potential must be adjusted for the actual concentrations. This can be done by including the concentration term from the definition of the chemical potential. An equation for the free energy change that takes concentrations into account is

$$\Delta G = \mu^{0P} + RT \ln [P] - \mu^{0R} - RT \ln [R]$$

Substituting the definition of ΔG^0,

$$\Delta G = \Delta G^0 + RT \ln [P] - RT \ln [R]$$
$$= \Delta G^0 + RT \ln [P]/[R]$$

This relationship tells us that the free energy change for the conversion of reactants to products is simply the free energy change under standard conditions corrected for the actual concentrations of reactant and products.

At equilibrium, the concentrations of reactants and products do not change and the free energy change is zero, so

$$0 = \Delta G^0 - RT \ln [P_{eq}]/[R_{eq}]$$

or

$$\Delta G^0 = RT \ln [P_{eq}]/[R_{eq}]$$

The reader is already familiar with the fact that the equilibrium constant for a reaction is the ratio of the equilibrium concentrations of products and reactants.

Thus, that relationship can be substituted in this thermodynamic equation:

$$\Delta G^0 = RT \ln K$$

or

$$K = e^{-\Delta G^0/RT} = k_+/k_- = [P_{eq}] / [R_{eq}]$$

This profound relationship shows how the free energy change is related to the equilibrium constant. The change in the standard Gibbs free energy, ΔG^0, specifies the ratio of products and reactants when the reaction reaches equilibrium, *regardless of the rate or path of the reaction*. The free energy change provides no information about whether or not a given reaction will proceed on a time scale relevant to cellular activities. Nevertheless, because the equilibrium constant depends on the ratio of the rate constants, knowledge of the rate constants reveals the equilibrium constant and the free energy change for a reaction. Consider the consequences of various values of ΔG^0:

- If ΔG^0 equals 0, $e^{-\Delta G^0/RT}$ equals 1, and at equilibrium, the concentration of products will equal the concentration of reactants (or in the case of a bimolecular reaction, the product of the concentrations of the reactants).
- If ΔG^0 is less than 0, $e^{-\Delta G^0/RT}$ is greater than 1, and at equilibrium, the concentration of products will be greater than the concentration of reactants. Larger, negative, free energy changes will drive the reaction farther toward products. Favorable reactions have large negative ΔG^0 values.
- If ΔG^0 is greater than 0, $e^{-\Delta G^0/RT}$ is less than 1, and at equilibrium, the concentrations of reactants will exceed the concentration of products.

It is sometimes said that a reaction with a positive ΔG^0 will not proceed spontaneously. This is not strictly true. Reactants will still be converted to products, although relative to the concentration of reactants, the concentration of products will be small. The size and sign of the free energy change tell nothing about the rate of a reaction. For example, the oxidation of sucrose by oxygen is highly favored with a ΔG^0 of -5693 kJ/mol, but "a flash fire in a sugar bowl is an event rarely, if ever, seen."[*]

The free energy change is additionally related to two thermodynamic parameters that are important to the subsequent discussion of molecular interactions. The Gibbs-Helmholtz equation is the key relationship:

$$\Delta G = \Delta H - T\Delta S$$

where ΔH is the change in **enthalpy**, an approximation (with a small correction for pressure-volume work) of the bond energies of the molecules. Thus,

[*]Eisenberg D, Crothers D: Physical Chemistry with Applications to the Life Sciences. Menlo Park, CA: Benjamin Cummings Publishing Co., 1979.

ΔH is the heat given off when a bond is made, or the heat taken up when a bond is broken. The change in enthalpy is simply the difference in enthalpy of reactants and products. In biochemical reactions, the enthalpy term principally reflects energies of the strong covalent bonds and of the weaker hydrogen and electrostatic bonds. If no covalent bonds change, as in a binding reaction or a conformational change, ΔH is determined by the difference in the energy of the weak bonds of the products and reactants.

The change in **entropy**, expressed as ΔS, is a measure of the change in the order of the products and reactants. The value of the entropy is a function of the number of microscopic arrangements of the system, including the solvent molecules. Note the minus sign in front of the $T\Delta S$ term. Reactions are favored if the change in entropy is positive, that is, if the products are less well ordered than the reactants. Increases in entropy drive reactions by increasing the negative free energy change. For example, the hydrophobic effect, which is discussed later in this chapter, depends on an increase in entropy. Increases in entropy provide the free energy change for many biologic reactions, especially macromolecular folding (see Chapter 2) and assembly (see Chapter 4).

As emphasized in the case of ΔG, neither the rate of the reaction nor the path between reactants and products is relevant to the difference in enthalpy or entropy of reactants and products. The reader may consult a physical chemistry book for a fuller explanation of these basic principles of thermodynamics.

Linked Reactions

Many important processes in the cell consist of a single reaction, but most of cellular biochemistry involves a series of linked reactions (Fig. 3–3). For example, when two macromolecules bind together, the complex often undergoes some type of internal rearrangement or conformational change, linking a first-order reaction to a second-order reaction.

$$A + B \rightleftharpoons AB$$
$$AB \rightleftharpoons AB^*$$

One of thousands of such examples is GTP binding to a G protein, causing it to undergo a conformational change from the inactive to the active state (see Chapter 27).

Similarly, the basic enzyme reaction considered in most biochemistry books is simply a series of reversible second- and first-order reactions:

$$E + S \rightleftharpoons ES$$
$$ES \rightleftharpoons EP$$
$$EP \rightleftharpoons E + P$$

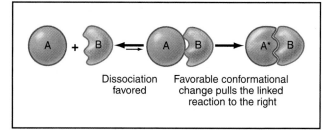

Figure 3–3 Linked reactions. Two molecules, A and B, bind together weakly and then undergo a favorable conformational change. The binding reaction is unfavorable owing to the high rate of dissociation of AB, but the favorable conformational change pulls the overall reaction far to the right.

where E is enzyme, S is substrate, and P is products. These and much more complicated reactions can be described rigorously by a series of rate equations like those explained earlier. For example, enzyme reactions nearly always involve one or more additional intermediates between ES and EP, coupled by first-order reactions, where the molecules undergo conformational changes.

Linking reactions together is the secret of how the cell carries out unfavorable reactions. All that matters is that the total free energy change for all coupled reactions is negative. An unfavorable reaction is driven forward by a favorable reaction upstream or downstream. For example, the unfavorable reaction producing adenosine triphosphate (ATP) from adenosine diphosphate (ADP) and inorganic phosphate is driven by being coupled to an energy source in the form of a proton gradient across the mitochondrial membrane (see Chapter 10). This proton gradient is derived, in turn, from the oxidation of chemical bonds of nutrients. To use a macroscopic analogy, a siphon can initially move a liquid uphill against gravity provided the outflow is placed below the inflow, so that the overall change in energy is favorable.

An appreciation of linked reactions makes it possible to understand how catalysts, including biochemical catalysts—protein enzymes and ribozymes—influence reactions. They do not alter the free energy change for reactions, but they enhance the rates of reactions by speeding up the forward and reverse rates of unfavorable intermediate reactions along pathways of coupled reactions. Given that the rates of both first- and second-order reactions depend on the concentration of the reactants, the overall reaction is commonly limited by the concentration of the least favored, highest energy intermediate, called a transition state. This might be a strained conformation of substrate in a biochemical pathway. Interaction of this transition state with an enzyme can lower its free energy, increasing its probability (concentration) and, thus, the rate of the limiting reaction. The acceleration of biochemical reactions by enzymes is impressive. Enhancement of reaction rates by 10 orders of magnitude is common.

A Strategy for Understanding Cellular Functions

One strategy for understanding the mechanism of any molecular process—including binding reactions, self-assembly reactions, and enzyme reactions—is to determine the existence of the various reactants, intermediates, and products along the reaction pathway and then to measure the rate constants for each step. Such an analysis yields additional information about the thermodynamics of each step, as the ratio of the rate constants reveals the equilibrium constant and the free energy change, even for transient intermediates that may be difficult or impossible to analyze separately.

In earlier times, biochemists lacked methods to evaluate the internal reactions along most pathways, but they could measure the overall rate of reactions, such as the steady-state rate of conversion of reactants to products by an enzyme. To analyze these data, they simplified complex mechanisms using relationships such as the Michaelis-Menten equation (described in virtually any biochemistry textbook). Now, abundant supplies of proteins, convenient methods for measuring rapid reaction rates, and computer programs that can be used to analyze complex reaction mechanisms generally make such simplifications unnecessary.

Chemical Bonds

Covalent bonds are responsible for the stable architecture of the organic molecules in cells (Fig. 3–4). They are very strong. C—C and C—H bonds have energies of about 400 kJ mol^{-1}. Bonds this strong do not dissociate spontaneously at body temperatures and pressures, nor are the reactive intermediates required to form these bonds present in finite concentrations in cells. To overcome this problem, living systems use enzymes, which stabilize high-energy transition states, to catalyze the formation and dissolution of covalent bonds. The energy for making strong covalent bonds

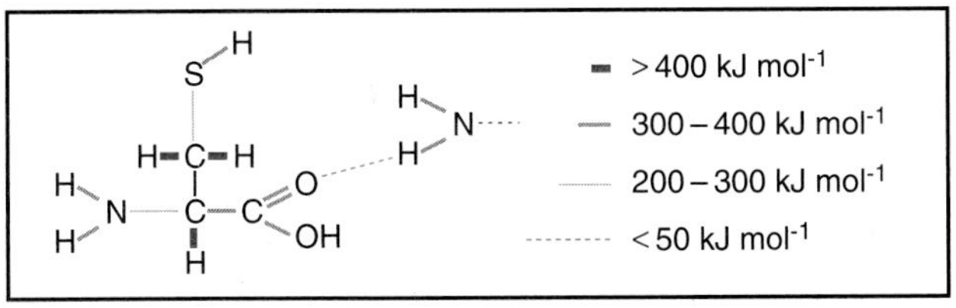

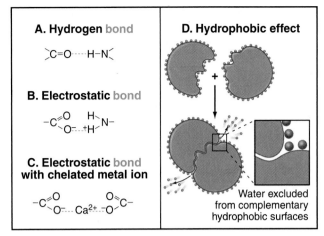

Figure 3–5 Weak interactions. *A,* Hydrogen bond. Opposite partial charges in the oxygen and hydrogen provide the attractive force. *B,* Electrostatic bond. Atoms with opposite charges are attracted to each other. *C,* Ca^{2+} chelated between two negatively charged oxygens. *D,* The hydrophobic effect arises when two complementary, apolar surfaces make contact, excluding water molecules that formerly were associated with the surfaces. The increased disorder of the water increases the entropy and provides the decrease in free energy to drive the association. van der Waals interactions between closely packed atoms on complementary surfaces also stabilize interactions.

is obtained indirectly by coupling to energy-yielding reactions. For example, metabolic enzymes convert energy released by breaking covalent bonds of nutrients, such as carbohydrates, lipids, and proteins, into ATP (see Chapter 10), which supplies the energy required to form new covalent bonds during the synthesis of polypeptides. The metabolic pathways relating the covalent chemistry of the molecules of life are covered in depth in many excellent biochemistry books.

For cell biologists, four types of relatively weak interactions (Fig. 3–5) are as important as covalent bonds because they are responsible for folding macromolecules into their active conformations and for holding molecules together in the structures of the cell. These weak interactions are (1) **hydrogen bonds,** (2) **electrostatic interactions,** (3) the **hydrophobic effect,** and (4) **van der Waals interactions.** None of these interactions is particularly strong on its own. The stable bonding between subunits of many macromolecular structures, between ligands and receptors, and between substrates and enzymes is a result of the additive effect of many weak interactions working in concert.

Hydrogen and Electrostatic Bonds

Hydrogen bonds (see Fig. 3–5) occur between a covalently bound donor H atom with a partial positive charge, $\delta+$ (due to electron withdrawal by a covalently bonded O or N), and an acceptor atom (usually

Figure 3–4 Covalent bonds. Bond energies for the amino acid cysteine.

O or N) with a partial negative charge, $\delta-$. These bonds are highly directional, with optimal bond energy (12 to 29 kJ mol^{-1}) when the H atom points directly at the acceptor atom. Hydrogen bonds are extremely important in the stabilization of secondary structures of proteins, such as α-helices and β-sheets and in the base pairing of DNA and RNA (see Chapter 2).

Electrostatic (or ionic) bonds occur between charged groups that have either lost or gained a proton (e.g., —COO$^-$ and —NH$_3^+$). Although these bonds are potentially about as strong as an average hydrogen bond (20 kJ mol^{-1}), it has been argued that they contribute little to biological structure. This is because a charged group is usually neutralized by an inorganic counter-ion (such as Na$^+$ or Cl$^-$) that is itself surrounded by a cloud of water molecules. The effect of having the cloud of water molecules is that the counter-ion does not occupy a single position with respect to the charged group on the macromolecule; thus, these interactions lack structural specificity.

The Hydrophobic Effect

Self-assembly and other association reactions that involve the joining together of separate molecules to form more ordered structures may seem unlikely when examined from the point of view of thermodynamics. Nonetheless, many binding reactions are highly favored, and when such processes are monitored in the laboratory, it can be shown that ΔS actually increases.

How can association of molecules lead to increased disorder? The answer is that the entropy of the system—including the macromolecules and the solvent—increases owing to the loss of order in the *water* surrounding the macromolecules (see Fig. 3–5). This increase in the entropy of the water more than offsets the increased order and decreased entropy of the associated macromolecules. Bulk water is a semi-structured solvent maintained by a loose network of hydrogen bonds (see Chapter 2). Water cannot form hydrogen bonds with nonpolar (hydrophobic) parts of lipids and proteins. Instead, water molecules form "cages" or "clathrates" of extensively H-bonded water molecules near these hydrophobic surfaces. These clathrates are more ordered than bulk water or water interacting with charged or polar amino acids.

When proteins fold (see Chapter 2), macromolecules bind together (see Chapter 4), and phospholipids associate to form bilayers (see Chapter 6), hydrophobic groups are buried in pockets or between interfaces that exclude the water. The highly ordered water formerly associated with these surfaces disperses into the less ordered bulk phase, and the entropy of the system increases.

The increase in the disorder of water that results when hydrophobic regions of macromolecules are buried is called the **hydrophobic effect**. Hydrophobic interactions are a major driving force, but they would not confer specificity on an intermolecular interaction except for the fact that the molecular surfaces must be complementary in order to exclude water. The hydrophobic effect is not a bond per se, but a thermodynamic factor that favors macromolecular interactions.

van der Waals Interactions

van der Waals interactions occur when adjacent atoms come close enough so that their outer electron clouds barely touch. This action induces charge fluctuations that result in a nonspecific, nondirectional attraction. These interactions are highly distance dependent, decreasing in proportion to the sixth power of the separation. The energy of each interaction is only about 4 kJ mol^{-1} (very weak when compared with the average kinetic energy of a molecule in solution, which is approximately 2.5 kJ mol^{-1}) and is significant only when many interactions are combined (as when surfaces have complementary shapes). Under optimal circumstances, van der Waals interactions can achieve bonding energies as high as 40 kJ mol^{-1}.

When two atoms get too close, they strongly repel each other. Consequently, imperfect fits between interacting molecules are energetically very expensive, preventing association if surface groups interfere sterically with each other. As a determinant of specificity of macromolecular interactions, this van der Waals repulsion is even more important than the favorable bonds discussed earlier, because it precludes many nonspecific interactions.

■ Selected Readings

Berg OG, von Hippel PH: Diffusion controlled macromolecular interactions. Ann Rev Biophys 14:131–160, 1985.

Eisenberg D, Crothers D: Physical Chemistry with Applications to the Life Sciences. Menlo Park, CA: Benjamin Cummings Publishing Co., 1979.

Johnson KA: Transient-state kinetic analysis of enzyme reaction pathways. Enzymes 20:1–61, 1992.

Northrup SH, Erickson HP: Kinetics of protein-protein association explained by Brownian dynamics computer simulation. Proc Natl Acad Sci USA 89:3338–3342, 1992.

Wachsstock DH, Pollard TD: Transient state kinetics tutorial using KINSIM. Biophys J 67:1260–1273, 1994.

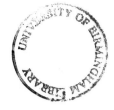

chapter 4

MACROMOLECULAR ASSEMBLY

The discovery that dissociated parts of viruses can assemble in a test tube led to the concept of **self-assembly,** one of the central principles in biology. In vitro analysis of true self-assembly from purified components of viruses, bacterial flagella, ribosomes, and cytoskeletal filaments has revealed the general properties of these processes. For example, large biological structures, such as the mitotic spindle (Fig. 4–1), are constructed from molecules that assemble by defined pathways without the aid of templates. The properties of the constituents determine the assembly mechanism and architecture of the final structure. Weak but highly specific noncovalent interactions hold together the building blocks, which include proteins, nucleic acids, and lipids. Even large cellular components, such as chromosomes, nuclear pores, transcription initiation complexes, vesicle fusion machinery, and intercellular junctions, assemble by the same strategy.

The ability of **subunit molecules** to assemble spontaneously into the complicated structures required for cellular function greatly increases the amount of information stored in the genome. The primary structure of a protein or nucleic acid specifies not only the folding of the individual protein or nucleic acid subunit, but also the bonds that it can make in a larger assembly.

Assembly of macromolecular structures differs fundamentally from the template-specified, enzymatic mechanisms with which cells replicate genes (see Chapter 45) and translate genes into RNAs and proteins (see Chapters 14 and 18). Macromolecular assembly does not require templates and rarely involves enzymatic formation or dissolution of covalent bonds. When enzymatic processing occurs during the assembly of some viruses (see Example 7 later in chapter), collagen (see Chapter 31), and elastin (see Chapter 31), it usually precludes reassembly of the dissociated parts.

This chapter presents five concepts that explain most assembly processes. Also included are descriptions of a series of model systems that illustrate these principles. Subsequent chapters return repeatedly to these ideas, as they help explain the structure, biogenesis, and function of most cellular components.

Assembly of Macromolecular Structures from Subunits

The use of subunits provides multiple advantages for assembly processes, as originally pointed out by Crane (Box 4–1). These advantages include the following:

- *Assembly of large structures from subunits conserves the genome.* The assembly of macromolecular structures from identical subunits, like bricks in a wall, obviates the need to specify separate parts. For example, a plant virus, the **tobacco mosaic virus** (TMV) (see Example 4 in this chapter), consists of 2130 protein subunits of 158 amino acids and a single-stranded RNA molecule of 6390 nucleotides. Having a separate gene for each viral coat protein would require 1,009,620 nucleotides of RNA, which would be about 160-fold longer than the entire viral RNA! The virus conserves its genome by using a single copy of the coat protein gene (474 nucleotides; 7.4% of the genome) to make 2130 identical copies of protein that assemble into the virus coat.
- *Using small subunits improves the chance of synthesizing error-free building blocks.* All biological processes are susceptible to error, and protein synthesis by ribosomes is no exception (see Chap-

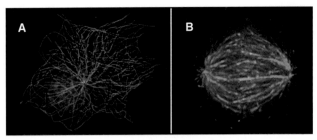

Figure 4-1 Microtubules (*green*) use recycled subunits to reorganize completely during the cell cycle. *A*, Interphase. Microtubules form a cytoplasmic network radiating from the microtubule organizing center at the centrosome, stained red. The nuclear DNA is blue. *B*, Mitosis. Duplicated centrosomes become the poles of the bipolar mitotic apparatus. Microtubules radiate from the poles to contact chromosomes (*blue*) at centromeres (*red*), pulling the chromosomes to the poles. After mitosis, the interphase arrangement of microtubules reassembles. (*A*, Courtesy of A. Khodjakov, Wadsworth Center Albany, N.Y. *B*, Courtesy of D. Cleveland, University of California, San Diego.)

ter 18). The error rate of translation is about 1 in 3000 amino acid residues. Therefore, the odds that any given amino acid residue is correct are 0.99967. With these odds, the chance that a TMV subunit will be translated correctly are 0.99967^{158}, or 0.949. Thus, about 95% of all TMV coat proteins in an infected cell are perfect, providing an ample supply of subunits with which to construct an infectious virus. Of the 5% of subunits with a mistake, some will be functional and others will not, depending on the nature and position of the amino acid substitution. Some amino acid substitutions pass unnoticed, whereas others result in loss of function. By contrast, the chance of correctly synthesizing the viral coat, if TMV coated its RNA with one huge polypeptide with 336,540 residues, is only 0.99967^{336540}, or 1.87×10^{-49}.

- *Construction from subunits provides a mechanism for eliminating faulty components.* Given that a significant fraction of all proteins have minor errors, good and bad subunits can be segregated on the basis of their ability to form correct bonds with their neighbors at the time of assembly. Many faulty subunits will not bond and thus are simply excluded from the final structure.
- *Subunits can be recycled.* Many macromolecular structures assemble reversibly, and because they are built of subunits, the subunits can be reused later. For example, the subunits of the mitotic spindle microtubules reassemble into the interphase array of microtubules (see Fig. 4–1 and Chapter 47). Subunits in actin (see Example 1 in this chapter) and myosin (see Example 2) filaments are also recycled.
- *Assembly from subunits provides multiple opportunities for regulation.* Simple modifications of subunits can regulate the state of assembly. For exam-

ple, many intermediate filaments disassemble during mitosis when their subunits are phosphorylated by protein kinases (see Chapters 38 and 47).

■ Specificity by Multiple Weak Bonds on Complementary Surfaces

Stable macromolecular assemblies require intermolecular interactions stronger than the forces tending to dissociate the subunits. Subunits diffusing independently in an aqueous milieu have a kinetic energy of about 2.5 kJ mol^{-1} at 25°C. Interactions in macromolecular assemblies must be strong enough to overcome this thermal energy, which tends to pull them apart. Forces holding subunits together can be estimated from analysis of atomic structures (see Examples 1, 4–6) and the effects of solution conditions on the stability of assemblies (see Example 2).

Subunits of macromolecular assemblies are usually held together by the same four weak interactions (see Chapter 3) that stabilize folded proteins: the hydrophobic effect, hydrogen bonds, electrostatic interactions, and van der Waals interactions. Although none of these interactions is particularly strong on its own, stable association of macromolecular subunits is achieved by combining the effects of multiple weak interactions. This is possible because the free energy changes contributed by each weak interaction are added together. With a small correction for entropy changes, the overall binding constant for the association of subunits is the product of the equilibrium constants for each weak interaction [$K_A = (K_1)(K_2)(K_3)(\ldots\ldots)(K_n)$].

Far from being a liability, multiple weak interactions provide assembly systems with the ability to achieve exquisite specificity that is derived from the "fit" between **complementary surfaces** of interacting molecules (illustrated by the viruses presented in Examples 4 and 5 in this chapter). Complementary surfaces are important for three reasons. First, atoms having the potential to form hydrogen bonds or electrostatic bonds must be placed in a complementary arrangement for the bonds to form. Second, complementary surfaces can exclude water between subunits, as required for the hydrophobic effect. Third and most important, repulsive forces arising from collisions between even a few atoms on imperfectly matching surfaces are strong enough to effectively cancel interaction between two potential bonding partners.

To use a macroscopic analogy, the interactions between subunits of macromolecular assemblies have much more in common with Velcro fasteners than with snaps. Snaps provide an easy way to attach components to one another, and they can attach compo-

box 4–1

CRANE'S HYPOTHESIS

In 1950, the physicist H. R. Crane predicted in *Scientific Monthly* that all macromolecular structures in biology are assembled from multiple subunits and according to the laws of **symmetry.** A symmetric structure is composed of numerous identical **subunits,** all in equivalent environments (i.e., making identical contacts with their neighbors). For example, Figure 4–2*A* shows a plane hexagonal array, with each subunit making identical contacts with the six surrounding subunits. This is the most efficient way to fill a flat surface with globular subunits.

Crane also predicted that elongated tubular structures are assembled with symmetry. This type of symmetry is known as a **helix.** One way of constructing a helix is to take a plane hexagonal array, cut it along one of its lattice lines, and roll it up into a tube (Fig. 4–2*B*). The bonds between adjacent subunits are nearly identical in the plane array and the helical tube, save for the fact that each bond is distorted just enough to roll the sheet into a tube. Introduction of five-fold vertices into a hexagonal array allows it to fold up into a closed polygon (see Fig. 4–2*D–F*).

Crane argued further that biological structures could avoid the problem of poisoning by defective subunits if such subunits were recognized and discarded. Crane's thinking about this problem was stimulated by a visit to a factory producing complex parts for vacuum tubes during World War II. When he asked the factory manager how much training the workers needed to assemble such a complex product, he was surprised to learn that the average was only 4 hours. The supervisor explained that they worked on an assembly line where each worker made only one small component (a subunit). If that component was defective, it was simply discarded, so that the final product was built only from perfect components. Crane suggested that cells use the same strategy.

Crane's theories led to the hypothesis that cellular structures "build" themselves by self-assembly. Thus, the design of the final structure is somehow incorporated into the shape of the individual subunits. Remarkably, all of Crane's predictions about subunits and assembly were correct.

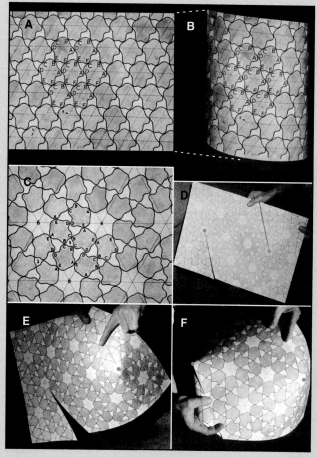

Figure 4–2 Folding of paper models of hexagonal arrays of identical particles into a helix or a closed polygon. *A,* A hexagonal array of particles similar to the arrangement of subunits in the tobacco mosaic virus. *B,* The sheet is rolled around onto itself to make a helix similar to the virus. *C,* A hexagonal array of particles with three identical subunits in each triangular unit. The subunits around one six-fold axis are colored pink. *D* to *F,* The sheet is cut along two lattice lines and folded, creating two five-fold vertices (*green dot*). Introduction of 12 such five-fold vertices creates an icosahedron. (From Caspar D, Klug A: Physical principles in the construction of regular viruses. Cold Spring Harbor Symp Quant Biol 27:1–24, 1962.)

nents whose surfaces touch only at the snaps. A single snap is often enough to hold two items together. By contrast, Velcro fasteners work because many tiny hooks become entrapped in a mesh of fibrous loops. The strength provided by each hook is minuscule, but when hundreds or thousands of hooks work together, bonding is strong. Velcro works best when the two bonding surfaces are smoothed against one another; in the case of rigid objects, a Velcro-like bond is tightest when the surfaces have complementary shapes. In molecular assemblies, tens of thousands of specific macromolecular associations are achieved by combining a small repertoire of weak bonds on complex, three-dimensional surfaces.

Many assembly reactions take advantage of flexibility in the protein subunits. In viral capsids (see Examples 5 and 6 in this chapter), hinges between the domains of the protein subunits provide the necessary flexibility to allow them to fit into more than one geometrical position. In some assemblies, flexible polypeptide strands knit subunits together (see Examples 1, 5, and 6). In other cases, assembly is coupled to the folding of the subunit proteins (see Examples 3, 4, and 6).

Symmetrical Structures Constructed from Identical Subunits with Equivalent (or Quasi-Equivalent) Bonds

Studies of relatively simple systems composed of identical subunits, such as viruses and bacterial flagella, have provided most of what is known about assembly processes. The symmetry of these structures makes them ideal for analysis by x-ray crystallography and electron microscopy, and their biochemical simplicity facilitates analysis of assembly mechanisms. Subunits in asymmetric assemblies, such as transcription factor complexes (see Chapter 14), are likely to interact in the same way. Continuing progress in determining their atomic structures will allow more detailed analysis of their assembly processes.

The subunits in a symmetrical macromolecular structure make identical bonds with one another. In practice, biologic assemblies use only three fundamental types of symmetry. Proteins that assemble into flat structures, such as membranes, typically have plane hexagonal symmetry; filaments have helical symmetry; and closed structures have polygonal symmetry.

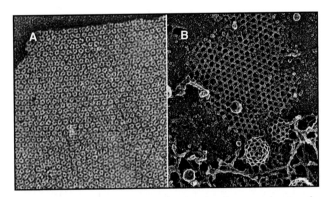

Figure 4-3 Electron micrographs showing hexagonal networks of membrane proteins. *A,* Integral membrane protein. Gap junction subunits called connexons span the lipid bilayer. An isolated junction was prepared by negative staining. *B,* Peripheral membrane proteins. Clathrin coats on the surface of a membrane in a hexagonal array. Introduction of five-fold vertices allows this sheet to fold up around a coated vesicle, shown at the bottom of the figure. This is a replica of the inner surface of the plasma membrane. (*A,* Courtesy of N. B. Gilula, Scripps Research Institute, La Jolla, CA. *B,* Courtesy of J. Heuser, Washington University.)

Subunits Arranged in Hexagonal Arrays in Plane Sheets

The simplest way to pack globular subunits in a plane is to form a hexagonal array with each subunit surrounded by six neighbors. This happens if one puts a layer of marbles in the bottom of a box and then tilts the box. A hexagonal array maximizes contacts between the surfaces of adjacent subunits. Membranes are the only flat surfaces in cells, and a number of membrane proteins crowd together in hexagonal arrays on or within the lipid bilayers. Connexons of gap junctions (Fig. 4–3), bacteriorhodopsin of purple membranes (see Fig. 6–8), and porin channels of bacterial membranes (see Fig. 6–8) all form regular hexagonal arrays in the plane of the lipid bilayer. Clathrin coats form hexagonal nets on the surface of membranes (see Fig. 4–3).

Helical Filaments Produced by Polymerization of Identical Subunits with Like Bonds

Helical arrays of identical subunits form cytoskeletal filaments (see Examples 1 and 2 in this chapter), bacterial flagella (see Example 3), and some viruses (see Example 4). Subunits are positioned like steps of a spiral staircase. Each subunit is located a fixed distance along the axis and rotated by a fixed angle relative to the previous subunit. Helices can have one or more strands. TMV has one strand of subunits (see Example 4), whereas bacterial flagella have 11 strands (see Example 3). Helices can be either solid, like actin filaments (see Example 1), or hollow, like bacterial flagella (see Example 2) and TMV (see Example 4).

The asymmetry of protein subunits gives most helical polymers in biology a polarity (see Examples 1, 3, and 4). Different bonding properties at the two ends of the polymer have important consequences for their assembly and functions. Myosin filaments (see Example 2) have a bipolar helix, a rare form of symmetry. (The DNA double helix [see Fig. 2–19] is geometrically symmetric, with one strand running in each direction, but the order of its nucleotide subunits gives each strand a polarity.)

Spherical Assemblies Formed by Regular Polygons of Subunits

Geometric constraints limit the ways that identical subunits can be arranged on a closed spherical surface with equivalent or nearly equivalent contacts between the subunits. By far, the most favored arrangement is based on a net of equilateral triangles. On a plane surface, these triangles will pack hexagonally with six-fold vertices (see Fig. 4–2). Since the time of Plato, it has been appreciated that introducing vertices sur-

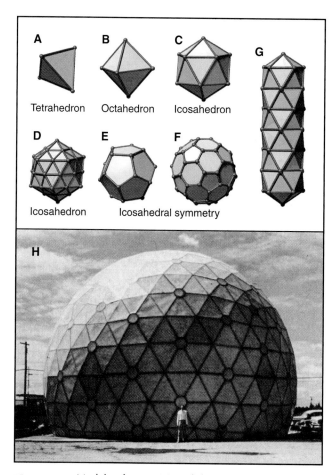

Figure 4-4 Models of geometric solids. *A,* A tetrahedron with four three-fold vertices and four triangular faces. *B,* An octahedron with six four-fold vertices and eight triangular faces. *C* to *H,* Various icosahedral solids with 12 five-fold vertices. Many other arrangements of subunits are possible. *C,* One triangle on each face. *D,* Four triangles on each face. *E,* A dodecahedron with 20 vertices and 12 faces. *F,* An intermediate polyhedron with 60 vertices and 32 faces (12 pentagons and 20 hexagons). *G,* An extended structure made by including rings of hexagons between two icosahedral hemispheres. *H,* A geodesic dome designed by R. Buckminster Fuller. (From Caspar D, Klug A: Physical principles in the construction of regular viruses. Cold Spring Harbor Symp Quant Biol 27:1–24, 1962.)

Most closed macromolecular assemblies in biology are polygons with five-fold vertices (see Examples 5 to 7). (The cubic iron-carrying protein, ferritin, is an exception.) An important reason for this is that most structures require some six-fold vertices to provide sufficient internal volume. This favors five-fold vertices for the puckers, as they require much less distortion of the subunits located on the triangular faces of the hexagonal plane sheet than three- or four-fold vertices. Further, the distortion in the contacts between the triangles is minimized if the five-fold vertices are in equivalent positions. Closed icosahedral shells can be assembled from any type of asymmetrical subunit given two provisions: (1) the subunit must be able to form bonds with like subunits in a triangular network; and (2) these subunits must be able to accommodate the distortion required to form both five- and six-fold vertices. Both fibrous (see Fig. 4–3) and globular subunits (see Examples 5 to 7) can fulfill these criteria.

These considerations indicate that subunits in a closed macromolecular assembly must be arranged in rings of five or six. A simple variation has three like protein subunits on each face, but three different protein subunits, or more than three like subunits, can be used on each face to construct icosahedrons. Closest packing is achieved if the protein subunits form pentamers and hexamers, but other arrangements on the 20 faces of an icosahedron are possible (see Example 6 in this chapter).

New Properties from Sequential Assembly Pathways

To fully understand any assembly mechanism, it is necessary to determine the order in which the subunits bind together and the rates of these reactions. For most assembly reactions, more is known about the pathways from genetic or biochemical identification of intermediates than about the reaction rates. The following section describes some general principles about pathways.

All self-assembly processes depend on diffusion-driven, random, reversible collisions between the subunits. As described in Chapter 3, the rate equation for such a second-order reaction is

$$\text{Rate} = k_{+}(A)(B) - k_{-}(AB)$$

where k_{+} is the association rate constant; k_{-} is the dissociation rate constant; and (A), (B), (AB) are the concentrations of the reactants and products. Elongation of actin filaments (see Example 1) illustrates this mechanism.

The association rate is directly proportional to the concentration of subunits and a rate constant (k_{+}).

rounded by three, four, or five triangles will cause such a network of triangles to pucker and, given an appropriate number of puckers, to close up into a complete shell (Fig. 4–4). Four three-fold vertices make a tetrahedron, six four-fold vertices an octahedron, and 12 five-fold vertices an **icosahedron.** Remarkably, no other ways of arranging triangles will complete a shell. In addition to three-, four-, or five-fold vertices that introduce puckers, a closed polygon can contain additional triangular faces and six-fold vertices to expand the volume. The six-fold vertices can be placed symmetrically with respect to the five-fold vertices to produce a spherical shell, or asymmetrically to form an elongated structure (see Fig. 4–4G).

This rate constant takes into account the rates of **diffusion** of the subunits, the size of their complementary surfaces, and the degree of tolerance in orientation permitted for binding. In general, association rate constants are limited by diffusion and are in the range of 10^5 to 10^7 $M^{-1}s^{-1}$ for most protein association reactions.

The rate of dissociation (k_-) determines which complexes formed by random collisions are stable enough to participate in an assembly pathway. Specificity is achieved by rapid dissociation of nonspecific complexes. The sequence of random collisions, each followed by separation or bonding, can be viewed as a scanning process that allows each molecule to sample a variety of interactions. At cellular concentrations (see Fig. 2–29), intermolecular collisions between macromolecules are extremely frequent but usually involve irrelevant molecules or molecules that could assemble but that collide in the wrong orientation. Given these frequent random collisions, it is extremely important that proteins not be intrinsically "sticky." Dissociation of unrelated molecules that have collided by chance is just as important as for specific associations to form. Because interactions of individual atoms on the surfaces of proteins are relatively weak, random collisions are very brief unless two complementary surfaces collide in an orientation close enough to allow a large number of simultaneous weak interactions or to allow flexible strands to intertwine two subunits. Molecules with poorly aligned or uncomplementary surfaces rapidly dissociate by diffusing away from each other. This is how specific associations are achieved by random collisions.

The stability of macromolecular complexes varies considerably owing to two factors. First, collision complexes have a wide spectrum of dissociation rate constants ranging from greater than 1000 s^{-1} for very unstable complexes to less than 0.00001 s^{-1} for very stable complexes. (The former complexes have a half-life of 0.7 ms, whereas the half-life of the latter is 16 h.) Second, conformational changes often follow formation of a collision complex between subunits. These reactions are difficult to observe, but assembly of bacterial flagella provides one clear example (see Example 3). Because the equilibrium constants for all of the coupled reactions are multiplied, such conformational changes can provide the major change in free energy holding a structure together (see Fig. 3–3). The weakly associated conformation characteristic of a free subunit can be thought of as an *unsociable* state, whereas the strongly associated conformation found in a completed structure is considered an *associable* state.

Although all assembly reactions occur by chance encounters, large structures usually assemble by specific pathways in which new properties emerge at most
steps. A new binding site for the next subunit may emerge from a conformational change in a newly incorporated subunit or by juxtaposition of two parts of a binding site on adjacent subunits. Such emergent properties favor addition of subunits in an orderly fashion until the process is completed. The assembly of myosin (see Example 2), tomato bushy stunt virus (see Example 5), and bacteriophage T4 (see Example 7) illustrates control of assembly by emergent properties.

Initiation of assembly is frequently much less favorable than its propagation. Free subunits associating randomly cannot participate in all the stabilizing interactions enjoyed by a subunit joining a preexisting structure. Consequently, assembly of the first few subunits to form a "nucleus" for further growth may be thousands of times less favorable than the steps that follow during the growth of the assembly (see Example 1). The chance of dissociation from the assembly is reduced once subunits can engage in the full complement of bonds made possible by conformational changes that stabilize the structure. Cells often solve the **nucleation** problem by constructing specialized structures to nucleate the formation of macromolecular assemblies (see Examples 3 and 6; Figs. 36–18 and 37–9). Nucleation is not always the slowest step; in the case of myosin minifilaments, the initial step is the fastest (see Example 2).

Regulation at Multiple Steps on Sequential Assembly Pathways

Many assembly reactions proceed spontaneously in vitro, but all seem to be tightly regulated in vivo. For example, at the time of mitosis, cells disassemble their entire microtubule network and reassemble the mitotic spindle with the same subunits (see Fig. 4–1). The following are some examples of the mechanisms that cells use to control assembly processes.

Regulation by Subunit Biosynthesis and Degradation

Cells regulate the supply of building blocks for assembly reactions. For example, a feedback mechanism controls the concentration of tubulin subunits available to form microtubules. The concentration of unpolymerized tubulin regulates the stability of tubulin mRNA. Experimental release of tubulin subunits in the cytoplasm results in degradation of tubulin mRNA and a decline in the rate of tubulin synthesis. On the other hand, red blood cells regulate the assembly of their membrane skeleton (see Fig. 6–10) by synthesizing a limiting amount of one subunit of the spectrin heterodimer. Following assembly of the membrane skeleton, proteolysis destroys the excess of the other subunit.

Regulation of Nucleation

Regulation of a rate-limiting nucleation step is particularly striking in the case of microtubules. Microtubule nucleation from subunits is so unfavorable that it rarely, if ever, occurs in a cell. Instead, all the microtubules grow from a discrete microtubule organizing center (see Fig. 4–1). In animal cells, the principal microtubule organizing center is the centrosome, a cloud of amorphous material surrounding the centrioles (see Fig. 37–9). Varying the number, position, and activity of microtubule organizing centers helps cells produce completely different microtubule arrays during interphase and mitosis.

Regulation by Changes in Environmental Conditions

Weak bonds between subunits allow cells to regulate assembly processes with relatively mild changes in conditions, such as in pH or ion concentrations. For example, when TMV infects a plant cell, the low concentration of Ca^{2+} in cytoplasm promotes disassembly of the virus because Ca^{2+} links the protein subunits together (see Example 4). Uncoating the RNA genome begins a new cycle of replication.

Regulation by Covalent Modification of Subunits

Phosphorylation of specific serine, threonine, or tyrosine residues (see Chapter 27) can regulate interactions of protein subunits in macromolecular assemblies. This is an excellent strategy because cell cycle and extracellular signals can control the activities of the kinases that add phosphate and the enzymes, called protein phosphatases, that reverse the modification. Given the uniform bonding between subunits of symmetrical macromolecular structures, the same phosphorylation of each subunit can cause the whole structure to disassemble.

Reversible phosphorylation regulates the assembly of the nuclear lamina, the filamentous network that supports the nuclear envelope (see Chapter 16). At the onset of mitosis, a protein kinase adds several phosphate groups to the lamina subunits (see Chapter 47). The network of filaments falls apart when negatively charged phosphate groups overcome the weak interactions between the protein subunits. Removing these phosphates at the end of mitosis is one step in the reassembly of the nucleus. Similarly, phosphorylation of centrosomal proteins may be responsible for changes in their microtubule nucleation properties during mitosis (see Fig. 4–1).

Several other chemical modifications regulate assembly reactions. Proteolysis is a drastic and irreversible modification used in the assembly of the bacterio-phage T4 head (see Example 7) and collagen (see Chapter 31). Collagen is an extreme example, since its assembly also requires hydroxylation of prolines and lysines, glycosylation, disulfide bond formation, oxidation of lysines, and chemical cross-linking. Subunits in other assemblies are modified by methylation, acetylation, glycosylation, fatty acylation, tyrosination, poly-glutamylation, or ubiquitination.

Regulation by Accessory Proteins

Self-assembly processes were originally thought to require only the components found in the final structure, but many assembly reactions either require or are facilitated by auxiliary factors. The **molecular chaperones** that promote protein folding (see Chapter 18) also promote assembly reactions. In fact, bacterial mutations that compromised assembly of bacteriophages led to the discovery of the original chaperonin-60, GroEL. This class of chaperones also facilitates assembly of oligomeric proteins, such as the chloroplast enzyme RUBISCO. These effects of chaperones may simply be due to their role in preventing aggregation during the folding of subunit proteins prior to their assembly. They may also participate directly in macromolecular assembly reactions, but this has not been proven.

Bacteriophage assembly also requires accessory proteins coded by the virus. T4 uses accessory proteins to assemble its head. Often proteolysis destroys these accessory proteins prior to insertion of the viral DNA (see Example 7). Bacteriophage P22 uses an accessory **"scaffolding protein"** to guide assembly of its icosahedral capsid protein. The building blocks are apparently heterodimers or small oligomers of the two proteins. Scaffolding protein forms an internal shell inside the capsid. Before the DNA is inserted, the scaffolding proteins exit intact from the head (by an unknown mechanism) and recycle to promote the assembly of another virus.

Accessory molecules can specify the size of assemblies. The length of the RNA genome precisely regulates the size of TMV (see Example 4). A giant α-helical polypeptide called nebulin runs from end to end of skeletal muscle actin filaments, determining their length (see Chapter 42). By contrast, a kinetic mechanism determines the length of skeletal muscle myosin filaments (see Example 2).

Numerous proteins regulate assembly of the cytoskeleton, and some are incorporated into the polymer network. Taking actin as an example, different classes of proteins regulate nucleotide exchange, determine the concentration of monomers available for assembly, nucleate and cap the ends of filaments, sever filaments, and cross-link filaments into bundles or random networks (see Chapter 36). Similar regulatory proteins likely are involved in other macromolecular assemblies, such as microtubules, intermediate filaments, myosin filaments, and coated vesicles.

The following examples will demonstrate how the principles discussed previously govern the assembly of real biological structures.

example 1
Actin Filaments: Rate-Limiting Nucleation and the Concept of Critical Concentration

Actin filaments consist of two strands of subunits wound helically around one another (Fig. 4–5). (Another description is a single, short-pitch helix including all of the subunits repeating every 5.5 nm.) Subunits all point in the same direction, so the polymer is polar. Each subunit contacts two subunits laterally and two other subunits longitudinally. Hydrogen bonds, electrostatic bonds, and hydrophobic interactions stabilize contacts between subunits. In addition, a hydrophobic polypeptide loop is thought to extend from each subunit into a hydrophobic pocket between neighboring subunits. This loop folds onto the surface of free monomers. The appearance of actin filaments with bound myosin (see Fig. 35–9) originally revealed the **polarity** now apparent at atomic resolution. The decorated filament looks like a line of arrowheads with points at one end and barbs at the other.

Actin binds adenosine diphosphate (ADP) or adenosine triphosphate (ATP) in a deep cleft. Irreversible hydrolysis of bound ATP during polymerization complicates the assembly process in a number of important ways (considered in Chapter 36). Here, assem-

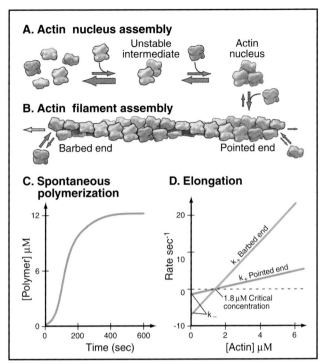

Figure 4–6 Actin filament assembly. *A*, Formation of a trimeric nucleus from monomers. *B*, Elongation of the two ends of a filament by association and dissociation of monomers. *C*, Time course of spontaneous polymerization of purified ADP-actin under physiological conditions. *D*, Dependence of the rates of elongation at the two ends of actin filaments on the concentration of ADP–actin monomers. (Reference: Pollard TD: Rate constants for the reactions of ATP- and ADP-actin with the ends of actin filaments. J Cell Biol 103:2747–2754, 1986, by copyright permission of the Rockefeller University Press.)

bly of ADP-actin, a relatively simple, reversible reaction, illustrates the concepts of nucleation and critical concentration.

Initiation of polymerization by pure actin monomers, also called **nucleation**, is so unfavorable that polymer accumulates only after a long lag (Fig. 4–6C). This time is required to form enough filaments to yield a detectable rate of polymerization. Initiation of each new filament is slow because small actin oligomers are exceedingly unstable. Actin dimers dissociate on a microsecond time scale, so their concentration is low, making addition of a third subunit rare. Actin trimers are the nucleus for filament growth (see Fig. 4–6A) because they are more stable than dimers and can add monomers rapidly. A trimer is a reasonable nucleus, since it is the smallest oligomer with a complete set of intermolecular bonds. Unfavorable nucleation reduces the chance that new filaments form spontaneously. This enables the cell to control this reaction with specific nucleating proteins (see Chapter 36).

Elongation of actin filaments is a bimolecular reaction between monomers and a single site on each end of the filament (see Fig. 4–6B and D). The growth

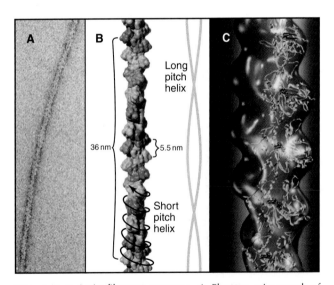

Figure 4–5 Actin filament structure. *A*, Electron micrograph of a negatively stained actin filament. *B*, Atomic model showing two ways to describe the helix: (1) two long pitch helices (*orange/yellow* and *blue/green*) or (2) a one start short pitch helix including all of the subunits, (*yellow* to *green* to *orange* to *blue*). *C*, Ribbon model of actin, including a space-filling model of ADP superimposed on a reconstruction of the filament from electron micrographs. (Courtesy of U. Aebi, University of Basel.)

rate of each filament is directly proportional to the concentration of subunits. (In a bulk sample, the rate of change in polymer concentration by elongation is proportional to both the concentrations of filament ends and subunits.) If the rate of assembly is graphed as a function of the concentration of actin monomer, the slope is the association rate constant, k_+. The y-intercept is the dissociation rate constant, k_-. The elongation rate is zero where the plot crosses the x-axis. This monomer concentration is called the **critical concentration**. Above this concentration, polymers grow longer. Below this concentration, polymers shrink. In vitro, polymers grow until the monomer concentration falls to the critical concentration. At the critical concentration, subunits bind and dissociate at the same rate. The rates of association and dissociation are somewhat different at the two ends of the polar filament. The rapidly growing end is called the barbed end and the slowly growing end the pointed end.

example 2
Myosin Filaments: New Properties Emerge as the Filaments Grow

Myosin-II forms bipolar filaments held together by interactions of the α-helical, coiled-coil tails of the molecules (Fig. 4–7). Antiparallel overlap of tails forms a central bare zone. On either side of the bare zone, parallel interactions extend the filament. The simplest myosin-II minifilaments from nonmuscle cells consist of just eight molecules (see Fig. 4–7B). Muscle myosin filaments are much larger, but are built on the same plan (see Fig. 4–7A and Chapter 42). Molecules are staggered at 14.3 nm intervals in these filaments. This arrangement maximizes the ionic bonds between

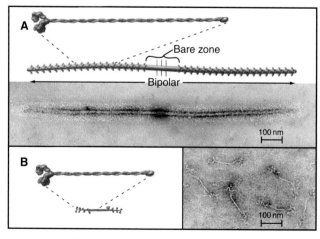

Figure 4–7 Structure of myosin filaments. *A*, Skeletal muscle myosin filament. Drawing and electron micrograph of a negatively stained filament. *B*, *Acanthamoeba* myosin-II minifilament. Drawing and electron micrograph of a negatively stained filaments. (*A*, Courtesy of J. Trinick, Bristol University, United Kingdom.)

zones of positive and negative charge that alternate along the tail. Hydrophobic interactions are also important; 170 water molecules dissociate from every molecule incorporated into a muscle myosin filament.

Minifilaments form in milliseconds by three successive dimerization reactions (Fig. 4–8). Under experimental conditions where filaments are partially assembled, antiparallel dimer and antiparallel tetramer intermediates can be detected by electron microscopy, light scattering, and analytical ultracentrifugation. Computer modeling of the time course of assembly provides limits on the rate constants for each transition. The association rate constants for formation of dimers and tetramers are larger than those predicted by diffusional collisions. Perhaps the long tails of the subunits form a variety of weakly bound complexes that rearrange rapidly to stable intermediates without dissociating.

This simple mechanism shows how new properties can emerge during an assembly process. The parallel interactions of tails seen in tetramers and octamers are not favored until the myosin has formed antiparallel dimers in the first step.

The elongation of muscle myosin filaments from the central bare zone provides a second example of how assembly properties can change as a structure forms. Muscle myosin forms stable dimers by side-by-side association of the tails. These are called parallel dimers because both pairs of heads are at the same end. Parallel dimers add to the ends of filaments in a diffusion-limited, bimolecular reaction. The reaction is unusual in that the dissociation rate constant increases with the length of the filament, eventually limiting the length of the polymer at the point where the dissociation rate equals the association rate.

example 3
Bacterial Flagella: Assembly with a Rate-Limiting Folding Reaction

Bacterial flagella are helical polymers of a protein called flagellin (Fig. 4–9). Eleven strands of subunits surround a narrow central channel. Each subunit has four domains: an outer globular domain that varies in size among bacterial species, a constant middle domain, and two constant inner domains. The inner domains are bundles of α-helices that run parallel to the long axis of the flagellum.

Nucleation of a flagellar filament is even less favorable than for an actin filament, so assembly in vitro depends absolutely on the presence of preexisting flagellar ends. Bacteria use structures called the base plate and hook assembly to initiate flagellar growth and to anchor the flagellum to the rotary motor that turns it (see Chapter 41).

Amazingly, flagella grow only at the end located farthest from the cell. Flagellin subunits synthesized in the cytoplasm diffuse through the narrow central

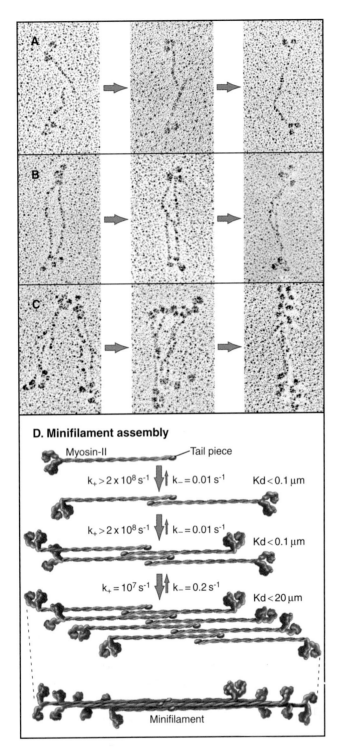

D. Minifilament assembly

Myosin-II — Tail piece

$k_+ > 2 \times 10^8\,s^{-1}$ $k_- = 0.01\,s^{-1}$ $Kd < 0.1\,\mu m$

$k_+ > 2 \times 10^8\,s^{-1}$ $k_- = 0.01\,s^{-1}$ $Kd < 0.1\,\mu m$

$k_+ = 10^7\,s^{-1}$ $k_- = 0.2\,s^{-1}$ $Kd < 20\,\mu m$

Minifilament

Figure 4-8 Assembly of amoeba myosin-II mini-filaments. *A* to *C*, Electron micrographs showing the successive assembly of dimers, tetramers, and octamers. *D*, Diagram of the assembly pathway with rate and equilibrium constants. A nonhelical tailpiece at the tip of the tail engages another myosin tail to form an antiparallel dimer with a 15-nm overlap. Two dimers form a tetramer, and two tetramers form an octamer. The second and third steps depend on completion of the first step. (*A* to *C*, Courtesy of J. Sinard, Yale Medical School. *D*, Reference: Sinard JH, Pollard TD: *Acanthamoeba* myosin-II minifilaments assemble on a millisecond time scale. J Biol Chem 265: 3654–3660, 1990.)

channel of the flagellum (see Fig. 4–9) out to the distal tip, where a cap consisting of an accessory protein prevents their escape before assembly.

Flagellar assembly in vitro is expected to be a bimolecular reaction dependent on the concentrations of flagellin monomers and polymer ends. This behavior is observed at low concentrations of flagellin, where the rate of elongation is proportional to the concentrations of flagellin and nuclei (Fig. 4–10).

Unexpectedly, the rate of elongation plateaus at a maximum of about three monomers per second at high subunit concentrations. This plateau can be explained if a relatively slow (first-order, concentration-independent) conformational change is required in the newly bound subunit before the next subunit can bind. This reaction limits growth at high rates of subunit binding. The parts of the flagellin monomer that form the core of the polymer are disordered in solu-

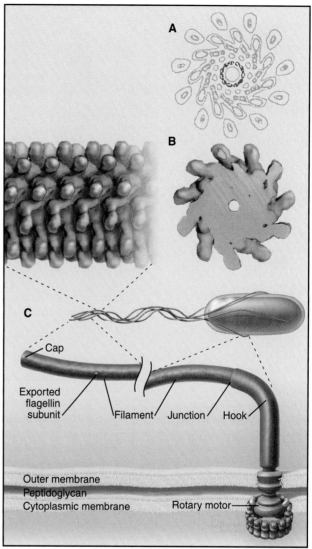

Figure 4-9 Structure of bacterial flagella. *A,* Cross section of a flagellum from *Salmonella typhimurium,* determined by image processing of electron micrographs, showing some internal details, including cross sections of the longitudinal helices *(red)* contributed by each of the 11 subunits lining the central channel. *B,* Surface view and cross section determined by image processing of electron micrographs. *C,* Drawing of a bacterium and a flagellar filament attached to the basal body, the rotary motor that turns the flagellum. (From Mimori-Kiyosue Y, Yamashita I, Fujiyoshi Y, et al: Role of the outermost subdomain of *Salmonella* flagellin in the filament structure revealed by electron cryomicroscopy. J Mol Biol 284:521–530, 1998; Morgan D, Owen C, Melanson L, DeRosier D: Structure of bacterial flagellar filaments at 11Å resolution. J Mol Biol 249:88–110, 1995.)

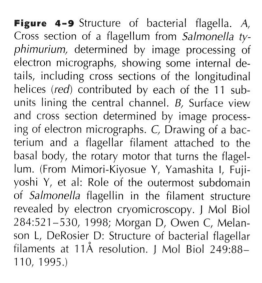

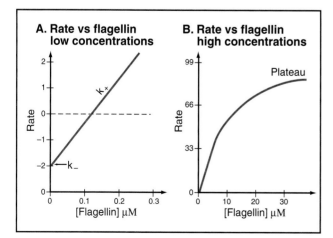

Figure 4-10 Elongation of flagellar filaments from seeds (fragments of flagella) in vitro. The plots show the dependence of the elongation rate on subunit concentration. *A,* Low concentrations. *B,* High concentrations. (Redrawn from Asakura S: A kinetic study of in vitro polymerization of flagellin. J Mol Biol 35: 237–239, 1968.)

tion, so the slow step may involve the folding of these disordered peptides into α-helices that interact to form the two concentric cylinders inside the flagellum. Slow folding converts an unsociable monomer into an associable subunit of the flagella and allows further growth.

example 4
Tobacco Mosaic Virus (TMV): A Helical Polymer Assembled with a Molecular Ruler of RNA

TMV was the first biological structure recognized to be a helical array of identical subunits, and it was the first helical protein structure to be determined at atomic resolution (Fig. 4–11). The virus is a cylindrical copolymer of one RNA molecule (the viral genome) and the 2130 protein subunits. The protein subunits are constructed from a bundle of four α-helices, shaped somewhat like a bowling pin. These subunits pack tightly in the virus and are held together by hydrophobic interactions, hydrogen bonds, and salt bridges, some of which use Ca^{2+} to link protein subunits. The

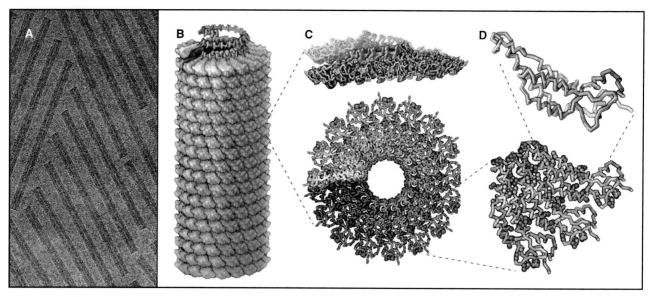

Figure 4–11 Structure of tobacco mosaic virus (TMV). *A*, Electron micrograph of TMV frozen in amorphous ice. *B*, Atomic structure showing the protein subunits in grey and the individual nucleotides of RNA in red. *C* and *D*, Details of the atomic structure of one turn of the helix and of subunits. Basic residues are blue; note the basic residues in the groove that binds the RNA. Acidic residues are red. (PDB file: 2tmv.) (*A*, Courtesy of R. Milligan, Scripps Research Institute, La Jolla, CA. *B*, *C*, and *D*, Courtesy of D. Caspar, Florida State University; Tallahassee. Reference: Namba K, Caspar D, Stubbs G: Enhancement and simplification of macromolecular images. Biophysical J 53:469–475, 1988.)

RNA follows the protein helix in a spiral from one end of the virus to the other, nestling in a groove in the protein subunits lined with arginine residues to neutralize the negative charges along the RNA backbone (see Fig. 4–11*C–D*). Each protein subunit also makes hydrophobic and electrostatic interactions with three of the RNA bases.

Production of infectious TMV from RNA and protein subunits was the first self-assembly reaction reproduced in vitro. At the time, during the 1950s, newspapers proclaimed, "Scientists create life in a test tube!"

RNA regulates assembly of the protein subunits in two ways. First, RNA allows the protein to polymerize at a physiological pH. Protein alone forms helical polymers of varying lengths at nonphysiological acidic pH, but at physiological pH, it forms only unstable oligomers of 30 to 40 protein subunits, slightly more than two turns of the helix (Fig. 4–12). Monomers and small oligomers of coat protein exchange rapidly with these oligomers, but disorder in the polypeptide loops lining the central channel limits growth beyond 40 subunits. RNA promotes folding of these disordered loops, acting as a switch to drive propagation of the helix by the incorporation of additional protein subunits. Second, RNA is the molecular ruler that determines the precise length of the assembled virus. Only after interacting with RNA at the growing end of the polymer can subunits fold into a structure compatible with a stable virus.

example 5
Tomato Bushy Stunt Virus: Flexibility within Protein Subunits Accommodates Quasi-Equivalent Bonding

The first atomic structure of a virus (tomato bushy stunt virus, TBSV) revealed that the flexibility required to form both five- and six-fold icosahedral vertices lies within the protein subunit rather than in the bonds between subunits. The 180 identical subunits associate in pairs in two different ways, distinguished in Figure 4–13 by the green-blue and red colors. The blue subunit of the green-blue pairs is used exclusively for five-fold vertices. Three red subunits and three green subunits form six-fold vertices. External contacts of both green-blue and red pairs with their neighbors are similar, but the contacts between pairs of red subunits differ from pairs of green-blue subunits. The difference is achieved by changing the position of the amino-terminal portion of the coat protein polypeptide chain. Two subunits in green-blue pairs pack tightly against each other, providing the sharp curvature required at five-fold vertices. In red dimers, the amino-terminal peptide acts as a wedge to pry the inner domains of the subunits apart and flatten the surface, as is appropriate for six-fold vertices. The flexible arm acts like a switch to determine the local curvature. This subunit flexibility accommodates the 12-degree difference in packing at five- and six-fold vertices. Other spherical viruses use a similar strategy to achieve **quasi-equivalent** packing of identical subunits.

forces the next three dimers to take the green-blue conformation, since no intermolecular binding sites are available for their arms. The greater curvature of the green-blue dimers dictates that five-fold vertices form at regular positions around the nucleating six-fold vertex. Additional five-fold vertices form appropriately as positions for this more favored association become available around the growing shell. The beauty of this idea is that local information (the availability of intermolecular binding sites for strands) auto-

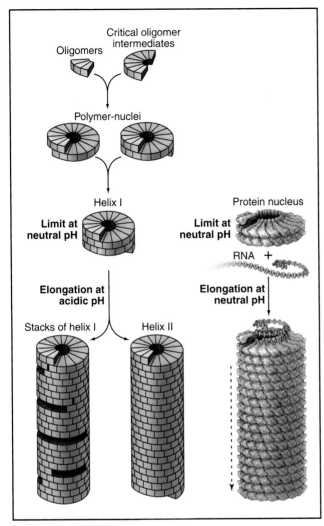

Figure 4-12 Assembly pathway of tobacco mosaic virus. The subunit protein forms small oligomers of two plus turns at neutral pH that can elongate in the presence of RNA. On their own, the protein oligomers can form imperfect protein helices at acid pH. (Redrawn from Potschka M, Koch M, Adams M, Schuster T: Time resolved solution x-ray scattering of tobacco mosaic virus coat protein, kinetics and structure of intermediates. Biochemistry 27:8481–8491, 1988. Copyright 1988 American Chemical Society.)

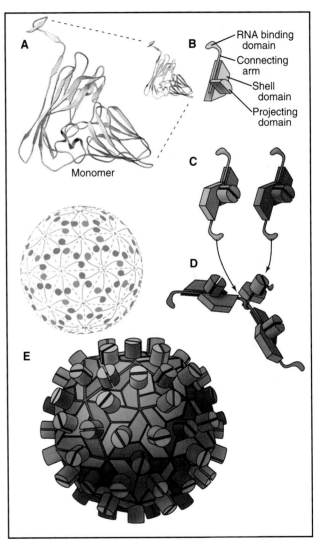

Figure 4-13 Tomato bushy stunt virus structure and assembly pathway. *A*, Ribbon diagram of a coat protein subunit. *B*, Block diagram of one subunit. *C*, Block diagrams of dimers of coat protein subunits. *D*, Proposed nucleus for a six-fold vertex with three dimers color-coded red. Three additional dimers (color-coded green-blue) are proposed to add to complete a six-fold vertex. Five blue subunits associate to make a five-fold vertex. *E*, Two different surface representations of the viral capsid showing the quasi-equivalent positions occupied by red, blue, and green subunits. (*A*, PDB file: 2tbv. *C* and *D* redrawn from Olsen A, Bricogne G, Harrison S: Structure of tomato bushy stunt virus IV. The virus particle at 2.9 Å resolution. J Mol Biol 171:61–93, 1983.)

TBSV provided the first of many examples of flexible arms that lace subunits together. Amino-terminal extensions of three red subunits intertwine at six-fold vertices. As if holding hands, these arms form a continuous network on the inner surface, reinforcing the coat.

Icosahedral plant viruses like TBSV assemble in vitro from pure protein and RNA. An attractive hypothesis is that local information built into the growing shell specifies the pathway, as follows. Building blocks are dimers of coat protein. To initiate assembly, three dimers in the red conformation bind a specific viral RNA sequence, forming a structure similar to a six-fold vertex. Folding of the arms in this nucleus

sheath subunits assemble inefficiently into a shorter and fatter helix.

The three assembly lines converge, joining heads to tails and then adding the six long, independently assembled tail fibers that give the completed virus its spider-like appearance. Attachment of tail fibers to the base plate somehow removes the "safety" that held the base plate in its hexagonal form. The finished bacteriophage is hardy enough to survive for 20 years at 4°C in a metastable state, poised to infect its bacterial host.

When tail fibers contact a susceptible bacterium, dramatic structural changes in the sheath force the tail core through both bacterial membranes in a syringe-like fashion (see Fig. 4–15B). The base plate changes from a hexagon into a six-pointed star that cuts loose the central plug with its attached tail core. Weak contacts between sheath and core allow the sheath to "recrystallize" into its preferred short, fat, helical form. Because the sheath is firmly attached at both the base plate and the top of the tail core, this spring-like contraction drives the core through the base plate into the bacterium. This action also unplugs the head, allowing the DNA to exit through the channel in the core into the bacterium. Thus, the linear assembly reactions produce a machine that can, when triggered, do physical work.

Selected Readings

Caspar DLD: Virus structure puzzle solved. Curr Biol 2:169–171, 1992.

Caspar DLD, Klug A: Physical principles in the construction of regular viruses. Cold Spring Harbor Symp Quant Biol 27:1–24, 1962.

Harrison SC: What do viruses look like? Harvey Lect 85:127–152, 1991.

Liddington RC, Yan Y, Moulai J, et al.: Structure of simian virus 40 at 3.8 Å resolution. Nature 354:278–284, 1991.

Namba K, Stubbs G: Structure of tobacco mosaic virus at 3.6 Å resolution: Implications for assembly. Science 231:1401–1406, 1986.

Oosawa F, Asakura S: Thermodynamics of the Polymerization of Protein. New York: Academic Press, 1975.

Pollard TD: Actin. Curr Opin Cell Biol 2:33–40, 1990.

Pollard TD, Blanchoin L, Mullins RD: Biophysics of actin filament dynamics in nonmuscle cells. Ann Rev Biophys Biomolec Struct 29:545–576, 2000.

Simpson AA, Tao Y, Leiman PG et al: Structure of the bacteriophage phi29 DNA packaging motor. Nature 408:745–750, 2000.

Sinard JH, Pollard TD: *Acanthamoeba* myosin-II minifilaments assemble on a millisecond time scale with rate constants greater than those expected for a diffusion limited reaction. J Biol Chem 265:3654–3660, 1990.

Wood WB: Genetic control of bacteriophage T4 morphogenesis. Symp Soc Dev Biol 31:29–46, 1973.

chapter 5

RESEARCH STRATEGIES

Research in cell biology aims to discover how cells work at the molecular level. Powerful tools are now available to achieve this goal. To understand how these methods contribute to the broad effort to explain cellular function, this chapter begins with a brief account of the synthetic approach used in cell biology. This strategy is based on the premise that one can understand a complex cellular process by reducing the system to its constituent parts and characterizing their properties. This approach, also called **reductionism,** has dominated cell biology research since the middle of the 20th century and has succeeded time after time. For example, most of what we understand about protein synthesis has come from isolating and characterizing ribosomes, messenger RNAs (mRNAs), transfer RNAs (tRNAs), and accessory factors. In this and many other cases, proof of function has been established by reconstituting a process from isolated parts of the molecular machine and verifying these conclusions with genetic experiments.

This reductionist approach involves much more than simply identifying the molecular parts of a cellular machine. Essential tasks include the following:

1. Conducting a complete inventory of molecular constituents
2. Determining atomic structures of the molecular components
3. Identifying molecular partners (and pathways)
4. Measuring rate and equilibrium constants
5. Testing for physiological function
6. Formulating a mathematical model of system behavior

This agenda is complete for remarkably few biological processes. Bacterial chemotaxis is one example (see Chapter 29). Often, much is known about some aspects of a process, such as a partial list of participating

molecules, the localization of these molecules in a cell, or a test for function by removing the genes for one or more molecules from an experimental organism. Rarely is enough information available about molecular concentrations and reaction rates to formulate a mathematical model of the process in order to verify that the system actually works as anticipated. Thus, much work remains to be done.

This chapter begins with imaging, one extremely valuable method for studying cells. Microscopy of live and fixed cells often provides initial hypotheses about the mechanisms of cellular process; it is also a valuable tool for genetic analysis and mechanism testing. The chapter then covers a selection of other methods used for the various tasks of the reductionist agenda.

The following list is a guide to experimental methods discussed throughout this book:

Method	Pages
1. Light microscopy	68–71
2. Electron microscopy	69–73
3. Gene and protein identification by classical genetics	73–76
4. Gene and protein identification by genomics and reverse genetics	76
5. Protein purification	76–80
6. Gel electrophoresis	77–78
7. Column chromatography	78–79
8. Organelle purification	78–80
9. Isolation of genes and cDNAs (PCR, cloning)	80–82
10. Molecular structure (hydrodynamics, x-ray crystallography, NMR)	23–25 82–83
11. Identification of binding partners by biochemistry	83
12. Identification of binding partners by genetics and genomics	83–85

Imaging

Microscopy is possible owing to fortunate coinci-dences within the electromagnetic spectrum. First, the wavelength of visible light is suitable for imaging whole cells, and the wavelength of electrons is right for imaging macromolecular assemblies and cellular organelles. Second, glass lenses may be used to focus visible light, and electromagnetic lenses can focus electrons. Resolution, the ability to discriminate two points, is directly related to the wavelength of the light. The limit of resolution with visible light and glass lenses is normally about 0.2 μm. Although short wavelength x-rays are not useful for imaging because there is no convenient way to focus them, analysis of their diffraction by molecular crystals is still the chief method for determining structures of cellular macro-molecules at atomic resolution.

Microscopes carry out two functions. The first is to enlarge an image of the specimen so that it can be seen with the eye or a camera. Everyone is familiar with the concept that a magnifying lens can enlarge an image. Just as important, but less appreciated, mi-croscopes must produce **contrast,** so that details of the enlarged image stand out from each other.

Light Microscopy

A half dozen optical tricks are used to produce con-trast in light micrographs of biological specimens (Ta-ble 5–1 and Fig. 5–1). These are called wide-field methods, as a broad beam of illuminating light is fo-cused on the specimen by a condenser lens.

The classic light microscopic method is **bright field,** whereby the specimen is illuminated with pure white light. Most cells absorb very little visible light and thus show little contrast with bright-field illumina-tion (Fig. 5–2A). For this reason, staining must be used to increase light absorption and contrast. Be-cause staining makes it difficult to see through thick tissues, specimens must also be relatively thin, about 1μm for critical work. Slides for histological and path-ological study are produced by fixing cells with cross-linking chemicals, embedding them in paraffin or plas-tic, making sections with a microtome (a device that cuts a series of thin slices from the surface of a speci-men), and staining with a variety of dyes (see Figs. 30–2, 30–3, 30–5, 30–7; 31–3, 31–8; 34–1 and 34–2). Alternatively, thin slices may be taken from frozen tissue and then stained. In either case, the cells are killed by fixation or sectioning prior to observation.

Observations of live cells require other methods to produce contrast. In every case, these methods are also useful for fixed cells. **Phase-contrast** microscopy generates contrast by interference between light scat-tered by the specimen and a slightly delayed reference beam of light. Small variations in either thickness or refractive index (speed of light) can be seen, even within specimens that absorb little or no light (Fig.

---

table 5–1

METHODS FOR PRODUCING CONTRAST IN LIGHT MICROSCOPY

Type	Principle	Requirements	Live Cells	Fixed Cells
Bright field	Absorption of visible light	Light-absorbing stains on a thin specimen	No	Yes
Fluorescence	Emission of light by fluorescent molecule	Cellular molecules labeled with fluorescent dyes or expression of fluores-cent proteins	Yes	Yes
Phase contrast	Variations in thickness and re-fractive index within specimen	Relatively flat cells	Yes	Yes
Differential interference contrast (DIC)	Gradient of refractive index across the specimen	None; may be used on thick, unstained speci-mens	Yes	Yes
Dark field	Scattering of light	Relatively thin, simple specimen	Yes	Yes
Polarization	Differences in refractive index for perpendicular beams of polarized light	Birefringent (highly ordered along a linear axis) ele-ments in specimen	Yes	Yes

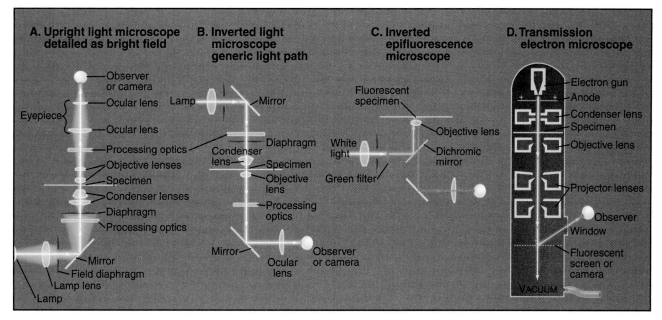

Figure 5-1 Light paths through various microscopes. *A,* Basic optical path in an upright light microscope set up for bright-field illumination. A condenser lens focuses light on the specimen. Light interacts with the specimen. An objective lens collects and recombines the altered beam. An ocular lens projects the enlarged image onto the eye or a camera. *B,* Optical path in an inverted light microscope. Processing optics produce contrast by phase contrast, differential interference, or polarization. *C,* Epi-illumination for fluorescence microscopy. The objective lens is used to focus the exciting, short-wavelength light (green, in this example) on the specimen. Fluorescent molecules in the specimen absorb exciting light and emit longer-wavelength light (red, in this example). The same objective lens collects emitted long-wavelength light. A dichroic mirror in the light path reflects exciting light and transmits emitted light. An additional filter blocks any short-wavelength light from reaching the viewer. *D,* Optical path in a transmission electron microscope. Electromagnetic lenses carry out the same functions as glass lenses in a light microscope. For visual observations, the electrons produce visible light from a fluorescent screen.

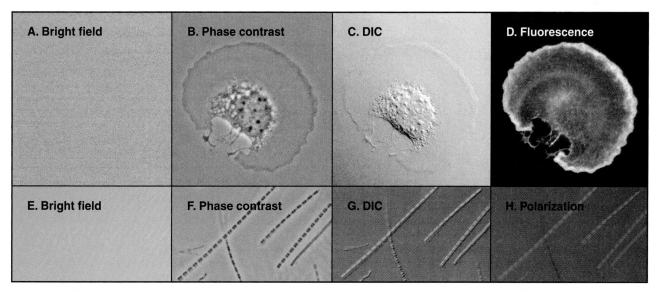

Figure 5-2 Comparison of methods to produce contrast. *A* to *D,* Micrographs of a spread mouse 3T3 cell grown in tissue culture on a microscope slide, then fixed and stained with rhodamine-phalloidin, a fluorescent peptide that binds actin filaments. Contrast methods include bright field (*A*), phase contrast (*B*), differential interference contrast (DIC) (*C*), and fluorescence (*D*). *E* to *H,* Micrographs of myofibrils isolated from skeletal muscle. Contrast methods include bright field (*E*), phase contrast (*F*), differential interference contrast (*G*), and polarization (*H*). The A-bands, consisting of parallel thick filaments of myosin, appear as dark bands with phase contrast and are birefringent (either bright or dark, depending on the orientation) with polarization. See Chapter 42 for further details on muscle structure. (*A* to *D,* Courtesy of R. Mahaffy, Yale University.)

5–2*B*). **Differential interference contrast** (DIC) produces an image that looks like it is illuminated by an oblique shaft of light (Fig. 5–2*C*). What actually happens is that two nearby beams interfere with each other, producing contrast in proportion to local differences (gradient) in the refractive index across the specimen. Thus, a vesicle with a high refractive index (slow speed of light) in cytoplasm will appear light on one side (where the index of refraction is increasing with respect to the cytoplasm) and dark on the other (where the index of refraction is decreasing).

Fluorescence microscopy requires a fluorescent dye or protein in the specimen. Remarkable sensitivity makes fluorescence microscopy a powerful tool. Under favorable conditions, single fluorescent dyes or fluorescent protein molecules can be imaged. When a fluorescent molecule absorbs a photon of light, an electron is excited into a higher state. Nanoseconds later, a longer-wavelength (lower-energy) photon is emitted when the electron falls back to the ground state. For example, the fluorescent dye rhodamine absorbs green light (shorter wavelength) and emits red light (longer wavelength). Fluorescence microscopes use filters and selectively reflective dichroic mirrors to illuminate fluorescent specimens with the exciting wavelength and to image the longer-emission wavelength. Because the emission filters remove the exciting light reflected by the specimen, only the fluorescent regions of the specimen appear bright. To provide fluorescence, a purified lipid, protein, or nucleic acid can be labeled with a fluorescent dye and injected into a live cell, where it will seek its natural location (see Fig. 40–8). Molecules labeled with a fluorescent dye can also be used to locate a target in a fixed and permeabilized cell. A powerful version of this strategy is to localize molecules in fixed cells with a fluorescent dye attached to an antibody (see Chapter 30); this then reacts with a single molecular target (Fig. 5–3*C*). Another is to label an oligonucleotide with a fluorescent dye to probe for nucleic acids with complementary sequences in fixed cells (see Fig. 13–10). Yet another approach is to localize actin filaments with a fluorescent dye attached to a small peptide that binds tightly to these filaments (see Fig. 5–2*D*).

The discovery of proteins whose amino acid sequence renders them naturally fluorescent, such as **green fluorescent protein** (GFP) found in jellyfish, has made fluorescence microscopy immensely valuable for observation of particular proteins in live cells. Typically, DNA-encoding GFP is joined to one end of the coding sequence for a cellular protein and introduced into live cells, which then produce a fusion protein consisting of GFP linked to the protein of interest. GFP fluorescence marks wherever the protein goes in the cell (see Fig. 5–3). Ideally, genetic experiments are done to confirm that the GFP fusion protein substitutes functionally for the endogenous protein.

Mutations in GFP can change its fluorescence properties, providing probes in a range of colors.

Dark-field and **polarization microscopy** have found specialized uses in biology. In dark-field microscopy the specimen is illuminated at an oblique angle, so that only light scattered by the specimen is collected by the objective lens. Recall how easy it is to detect small dust particles in a beam of light in a dark room. The contrast is so great that single microtubules stand out brightly from the dark background. However, for the images to be interpretable, the specimen must be very simple, much simpler than a cell. An image of something as complicated as cytoplasm is very confusing owing to multiple overlapping objects that scatter light. Like dark-field microscopy, polarization microscopy produces a bright image on a dark background. When a specimen is viewed between two crossed polarizing filters, only light whose polarization state is modified by the specimen will pass through the second polarizer to the image. Polarization microscopy relies on a specimen's crystalline order, or birefringence, to provide contrast. Birefringent specimens, such as filaments in striated muscle (see Fig. 5–2*D*) or microtubules in a mitotic spindle, are aligned just enough so that polarized light, oriented so that it vibrates along the length of the molecules, passes through more slowly than light vibrating perpendicular to the molecules (much as a knife cuts through meat faster when cutting with the grain than across it). Most cells do not have sufficient birefringence to produce a useful image with a conventional polarization microscope. New methods will make this approach more applicable in the future.

Computer processing can greatly enhance contrast and remove optical artifacts from images. For example, computer-enhanced DIC can image single microtubules (see Fig. 37–8). New methods of **image processing** can even improve the resolution beyond the classical limit determined by the wavelength of light (about 0.2 μm with green light). A processing method called **deconvolution** produces clear fluorescence images of thin optical sections by moving out of focus blur from overlapping regions of the specimen in traditional wide-field images (see Fig. 5–3*C*) back to the image plane where it belongs by means of an iterative computational process. Combining a series of deconvolved optical sections from the top to the bottom of a specimen produces remarkably detailed three-dimensional images.

Confocal microscopy is an alternative method for producing thin optical sections of fluorescent specimens. With this method, rather than illuminating with a wide beam of light, the fluorescent specimen is excited with a point of laser light sharply focused in all three directions: *x*, *y*, and *z*. A strategically placed pinhole next to the detector removes any emitted light that does not come directly from this focal point. The

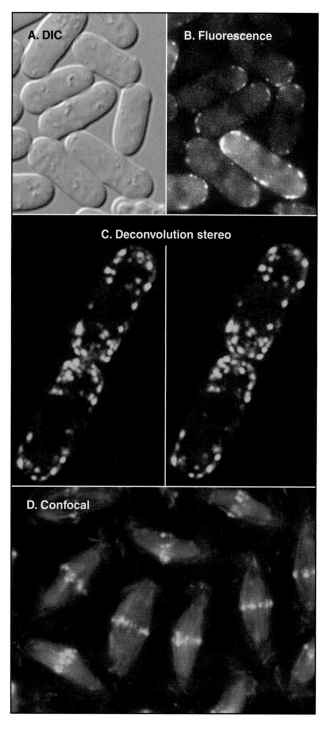

Figure 5-3 *A* to *C,* Light micrographs of live fission yeast expressing GFP fused to myosin-I. *A,* Differential interference contrast (DIC). *B,* Standard wide-field fluorescence of the same cells. *C,* Stereo pair of a three-dimensional reconstruction of a stack of optical sections made by deconvolution of wide-field images. Removal of out-of-focus blur improves the resolution and contrast of small patches enriched in myosin-I. A stereo view may be obtained by focusing your left eye on the left image and right eye on the right image. This can be achieved by holding the micrographs close to your eyes and then gradually withdrawing the page about 12 inches. *D,* Confocal fluorescence micrograph of mitotic spindles in a *Drosophila* embryo stained with a green fluorescent antibody to microtubules, a red fluorescent anticentromere antibody, and a blue dye (DAPI) for DNA. This is a thin optical section of a very thick specimen. (*A* to *C,* Reference: Lee W-L, Bezanilla M, Pollard TD: Fission yeast myosin-I, Myo1p, stimulates actin assembly by Arp2/3 complex and shares functions with WASp. J Cell Biol 151:789–800, 2000, by copyright permission of the Rockefeller University Press.)

exciting point of light is scanned across the specimen in a raster pattern (checkerboard pattern, like the electron beam in a TV) and the light emitted at each point is collected (see Fig. 5–3*D*). A computer reassembles the image from the fluorescence at each point in this checkerboard of fluorescence signals. A series of confocal images taken at different planes can be used for three-dimensional reconstructions.

Electron Microscopy

Transmission electron microscopes (TEMs; see Fig. 5–1 for optical path) can resolve points below 0.3 nm, but the practical resolution is usually limited by damage to the specimens from the electron beam and the methods used to prepare the specimens. Historically, the most common method used to prepare cells for

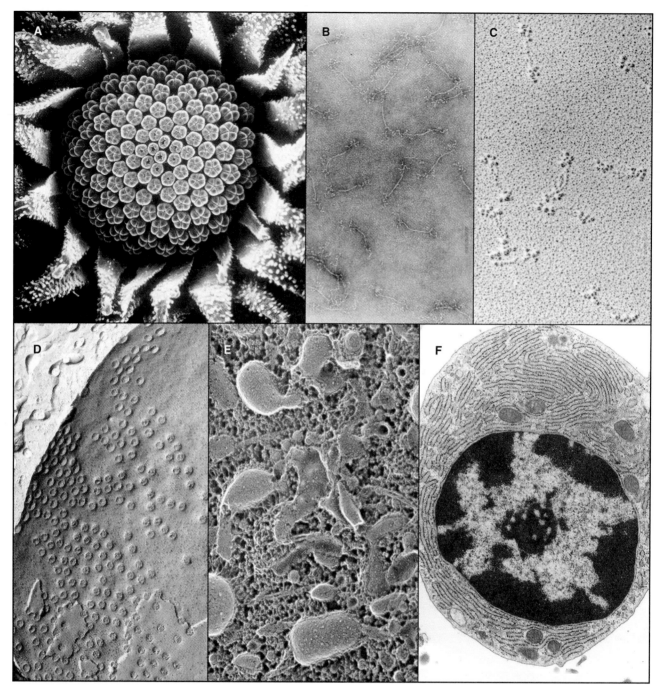

Figure 5–4 Electron micrographs. *A,* Scanning electron micrograph of developing flowers of the Western mountain aster. *B* to *F,* Transmission electron micrographs. *B,* Myosin-II minifilaments on a thin carbon film prepared by negative staining with uranyl acetate. *C,* Myosin-II minifilaments on a mica surface prepared by rotary shadowing with platinum. *D,* Freeze-fracturing. The cleavage plane passed through the cytoplasm and then split apart the two halves of the bilayer of the nuclear envelope. This fractured surface was then shadowed with platinum. The cytoplasm is in the upper left. Nuclear pores are prominent in the nuclear envelope. *E,* A cultured cell prepared by rapid freezing, fracturing, deep etching, and rotary shadowing with platinum. Membranes of the endoplasmic reticulum stand out against the porous cytoplasmic matrix. *F,* Thin section of a plasma cell, an immune cell specialized to synthesize and secrete antibodies. (*A,* Courtesy of J. L. Bowman, University of California, Davis. *C,* Courtesy of J. Sinard, Yale University. *E,* Courtesy of John Heuser, Washington University. *D* and *F,* Courtesy of Don W. Fawcett, Harvard Medical School.)

electron microscopy has been to fix the specimen with chemicals, embed it in plastic, cut the specimen into **thin sections,** and stain the sections with heavy metals (see Fig. 5–4F). With this technique, the resolution is limited to about 3 nm, but that is sufficient to bridge the gap between light microscopy and molecular structures. During the heyday of electron microscopy in cell biology, between 1950 and 1970, thin sections revealed most of what is known about the organization of organelles in cells.

The highest resolution is attained with regular specimens, such as two-dimensional protein crystals rapidly frozen and viewed while embedded in a thin film of vitreous (i.e., amorphous, noncrystalline) ice (see Fig. 4–11A). This is called **cryoelectron microscopy** because the stage holding the frozen specimen is cooled to liquid nitrogen temperatures. Electron micrographs and electron diffraction of frozen crystals have produced structures of bacteriorhodopsin (see Fig. 6–8), aquaporin water channels (see Fig. 9–12) and tubulin (see Fig. 37–5) at resolutions of 3 to 4 nm. Computational image processing methods are used to calculate the three-dimensional structure of proteins in these regular specimens. These methods are similar to those used to calculate electron density maps from x-ray diffraction patterns (see Fig. 2–8). Although the resolution is limited and data collection is tedious in electron crystallography, electron microscopic images have the advantage of containing the phase information that is often difficult to ascertain with x-ray diffraction.

Electron microscopy is extremely valuable for studying protein polymers and other large macromolecular specimens at less-than-atomic resolution. Diverse methods are used to prepare specimens and impart contrast. One way is to freeze filaments or macromolecular assemblies in vitreous ice, as described earlier (see Figs. 37–8 and 39–5A). A second is negative staining, whereby specimens are dried from aqueous solutions of heavy metal salts (Fig. 5–4B). A shell of dense stain encases particles in the specimen and can preserve structural details at a resolution of about 1 nm. Alternatively, macromolecules dried on a smooth surface can be sprayed with a thin coat of metal evaporated from an electrode (see Fig. 5–4C). A variation of this approach that improves preservation is to freeze specimens rapidly, evaporate the ice surrounding the molecules, and then apply a coat of platinum (see Figs. 32–4 and 37–10).

Computer image processing of micrographs of certain types of structures can yield an average three-dimensional reconstruction of a molecular structure. Particles with helical symmetry, such as actin filaments (see Fig. 36–8) and microtubules (Fig. 37–6), can be analyzed by an image-processing method called deconvolution to reconstruct the three-dimensional struc-

ture. Single particles may also be reconstructed by first classifying images of thousands of randomly oriented particles into categories corresponding to different views. Then, an average three-dimensional structure is calculated computationally from this ensemble. One example is the Sec61p translocon associated with a ribosome (see Fig. 20–4).

Cells and tissues can also be frozen rapidly and prepared for electron microscopy without chemical fixation. In the **freeze-fracture method,** the frozen specimen is cleaved to expose the inside of the cells, and exposed surfaces are rotary-shadowed with a thin coat of platinum. This surface coat is then viewed using the electron microscope (see Fig. 5–4D). Frequently, the cleavage plane splits lipid bilayers in half to reveal proteins embedded in the membrane. Also, if some of the frozen water in the specimen is evaporated from the surface before shadowing, three-dimensional details of deeper parts of the cytoplasm can be revealed. A variation of this method involves extracting soluble molecules and membranes with mild detergents before freezing, fracturing, evaporating frozen water, and rotary-shadowing (see Fig. 5–4E).

Scanning electron microscopes (SEMs) can be used on thicker specimens, such as whole cells or tissues that have been fixed, dried, and coated with a thin metal film. Here, an electron beam scans a raster pattern over the surface of specimens, and secondary electrons emitted from the surface at each point are collected and used to reconstruct an image (see Fig. 5–4A). The resolution of conventional SEM is limited, but nonetheless valuable, for studying surface features of cells and their three-dimensional relationships in tissues. SEMs that use special (field emission) guns to produce the electron beam have improved resolution, and these have been very useful for studying cellular substructures, such as nuclear pores (see Fig. 16–6B).

▌ Inventory: Gene and Protein Discovery

Classical Genetics

Communities of scientists invested years of hard work to develop both genetic and molecular genetic methods to study prokaryotes and eukaryotes (Table 5–2). Ideal **model organisms** have completely sequenced **genomes,** and facile methods have been developed to manipulate the genes, including the replacement of a gene with a modified gene, by the process of homologous recombination. **Haploid** organisms with one copy of each chromosome after mitotic division are particularly favorable for detecting the effects of changes in genes, called mutations (Box 5–1). However, it is useful for a haploid organism to have a

table 5–2

MODEL GENETIC ORGANISMS

Organism	Genome Size and Ploidy	Genome Sequenced	Number of Genes	Homologous Recombination	Meiotic Recombination	Biochemistry
Gram-negative bacterium, *Escherichia coli*	4.6 Mb, haploid	Yes	4288	Yes	No	Excellent
Cellular slime mold, *Dictyostelium discoideum*	? Mb, haploid	No	?	Yes	No	Excellent
Budding yeast, *Saccharomyces cerevisiae*	12.1 Mb, haploid	Yes	~6144	Yes	Yes	Good
Fission yeast, *Schizosaccharomyces pombe*	14 Mb, haploid	Yes	~4900	Yes	Yes	Good
Nematode worm, *Caenorhabditis elegans*	97 Mb, diploid	Yes	~18,266	Difficult	Yes	Poor
Fruit fly, *Drosophila melanogaster*	180 Mb, diploid	Yes	~13,338	Difficult	Yes	Fair
Mustard weed, *Arabidopsis thaliana*	100 Mb, diploid	Yes	~25,706	No	Yes	Poor
Mouse, *Mus musculus*	3000 Mb, diploid	Yes	?	Yes	Yes	Good
Human, *Homo sapiens*	3000 Mb, diploid	Yes	~35,000	Yes, cultured cells	Yes	Good

diploid stage with two copies of each chromosome and a sexual phase, during which **recombination** can occur between the chromosomes from the two parents. (See Chapter 48 and Figure 48–7 for details on recombination.) This allows one to construct strains with a variety of **mutations** and facilitates mapping a mutation to a particular gene.

Budding yeast and **fission yeast** meet all of these criteria, so they are widely used to study basic cellular functions. These free-living haploid organisms have a tractable diploid stage in their life cycles. Moving between haploid and diploid stages greatly simplifies the process of creating and analyzing recessive mutations. This is important because most loss-of-function mutations are recessive. Even before their genomes were sequenced, the availability of yeast for

box 5–1

KEY GENETIC TERMS

Allele: A version of a gene

Complementation: Providing gene function in *trans* (i.e., by another copy of a gene)

Conditional mutation: A mutation that gives an altered phenotype only under certain conditions, such as temperature, medium composition, etc.

Diploid: A genome with two copies of each chromosome, one from each parent

Dominant mutation: A mutation that gives an altered phenotype, even in the presence of a copy of the wild-type gene

Essential gene: A gene whose function is required for viability

Gene: The nucleotide sequence required to make a protein or RNA product, including the coding sequence, flanking regulatory sequences, and introns, if present

Genome: The entire genetic endowment of an organism

Genotype: The genetic complement, including particular mutations

Haploid: A genome with single copies of each chromosome

Mutant: An organism containing a mutation of interest

Mutation: A change in the chemical composition of a gene, including changes in nucleotide sequence, insertion, deletions, etc.

Pedigree: Family history of a genetic trait

Phenotype: (From the Greek term for "shining" or "showing") Appearance of the organism as dictated by its genotype

Plasmid: A circular DNA molecule that self-replicates in the cytoplasm of a bacterium or nucleus of a eukaryote

Recessive mutation: A mutation that gives an altered phenotype only when no wild-type version is present

Recombination: Physical exchange of regions of the genome between homologous chromosomes or between a plasmid and a chromosome

Wild type: The naturally occurring allele of a gene; the phenotype of the naturally occurring organism

genetic, biochemical, and microscopic analysis revolutionized research in cell biology. However, yeast are single cells with specialized lifestyles.

Multicellular organisms are required to study the development and function of tissues and organs. **Flies, nematode worms, mice,** and **humans** share many ancient, conserved genes that control their cellular and developmental systems, so flies and worms are popular for basic studies of animal development and tissue function. However, vertebrates have evolved a substantial number of new gene families (roughly 7% of total genes) and a large number of new proteins by rearranging ancient domains in new ways. Therefore, mice are used for experiments on many specialized vertebrate functions, especially those of the nervous system, despite being more difficult to work with than flies and worms. Although not an experimental organism, humans are included on this list because much can be learned by analysis of human genetic variation and its relation to disease. Humans are, of course, much more eloquent than the model organisms when it comes to describing their medical problems, many of which have a genetic basis that can be documented by analysis of **pedigrees** and DNA samples. **Arabidopsis** is the most popular plant for genetics because its genome is small, reproduction is rapid, and methods for genetic analysis are well developed. Its genome was the first of a plant to be completely sequenced. One drawback is the lack of methods to replace genes by homologous recombination (see later section).

Identification of Genes through Mutations

The approach in classical genetics is to damage genes (i.e., make mutations) for the purpose of identifying those mutations that compromise a particular cellular function, and then to find the responsible gene(s). This approach is extremely powerful, especially when little or nothing is known about a process, or when the gene product (usually a protein) is present at very low concentrations. Yeast genetic studies have been spectacularly successful in mapping out complex pathways, including identification of the proteins that regulate the cell cycle (see Chapters 43 to 47) and the proteins that operate the secretory pathway (see Chapters 17 to 23).

Because one generally does not know the relevant genes in advance, it is important that mutations are introduced randomly into the genome and, ideally, limited to one in each organism tested. A prerequisite for such a genetic screen is a good assay for the biological function of interest. Simplicity and specificity are essential, as interesting mutations may be rare and much effort may be expended characterizing each mutation. The assay may test the ability to grow under

certain conditions, drug resistance, morphologic changes, cell cycle arrest, or abnormal behavior. Mutations arise spontaneously at low rates, but usually, a chemical (e.g., ethyl methyl sulfonate or nitrosoguanidine) or radiation is used to increase the frequency of damage. Another approach is to insert an identifiable segment of DNA randomly into the genome. This disrupts genes and marks them for subsequent analysis. Because the damage is random, the trick is to find the particular damage that changes the physiology of the organism in an interesting way.

Haploid organisms are favorable for detecting mutations because damage to the single copy of a relevant gene will alter function, and either a loss of function or a gain of function can be detected with suitable test conditions (i.e., the ability to grow under certain conditions), biochemical assay, or morphologic assay. A disadvantage is that haploid organisms are not viable following the loss of function of an essential gene. Selecting for **conditional mutant** alleles allows the haploid organism to survive mutation of an essential gene under **permissive conditions** (e.g., low temperatures) but not under **restrictive conditions** (e.g., high temperatures). A further advantage of haploid organisms is that one can usually identify the mutated gene by a **complementation** experiment. Mutant cells are induced to take up a plasmid library containing fragments of the wild-type genome or cDNAs. **Plasmids** are circular DNA molecules that can be propagated readily in bacteria and, if suitably designed, in eukaryotes as well. Plasmids carrying the wild-type gene will correct loss-of-function mutations, allowing colonies of cells to grow normally. Plasmids complementing the mutation are isolated and sequenced to reveal the wild-type gene. Then the mutant gene can be isolated and sequenced to determine the nature of the damage. This complementation test can also be used to discover genes from other species that correct the mutation in the model organism. For example, genes for human cell cycle proteins can complement many cell cycle mutations in yeast (see Chapter 43). For gain-of-function mutations, a gene library from the mutant cell is inserted into plasmids, which are then tested for their ability to cause the altered phenotype in wild-type cells.

Genetics in diploid organisms is more complicated. Many mutations will appear to have no effect, provided the same gene on the other chromosome functions normally. These **recessive mutations** produce a phenotype only after crossing two mutant organisms, yielding 25% of offspring with two copies of the mutant gene. (Consult a genetics textbook for details.) Other mutations will yield an altered phenotype even when only one of the two genes is affected. These **dominant mutations** include simple loss of function when two wild-type genes are required to make sufficient product for normal function (called **haplo-insufficiency**); production of an altered protein that compromises the formation of a large assembly by normal protein subunits produced by the wild-type gene (called **dominant negative**); and production of an unregulated protein that cannot be controlled by partners in the cell (another type of dominant negative).

The classic method for identifying a mutated gene is **genetic mapping.** One observes the frequency of recombination between known markers and the mutation of interest in genetic crosses. With a complete genome sequence available, the mutated gene may first be mapped by performing genetic crosses. Then the database of sequenced genes in the area highlighted by mapping is examined to look for sensible candidate genes. These candidates can then be studied to establish which one carries the mutation. Another approach is to make the mutation by inserting a piece of DNA (called a transposable element) randomly into the genome. If one of these insertions causes a mutant phenotype, the transposable element with some of the surrounding gene may be excised and sequenced to identify the disrupted gene.

Once a gene required for the function of interest is sequenced, the primary structure of the protein (or RNA) is deduced from translating the coding sequence in a computer. Much can be learned by identifying RNAs or proteins with similar sequences or domains in the same or other species, particularly if something is known about the function of the corresponding gene product. Protein can often be expressed artificially from a cDNA copy of the mRNA, tested for activity and binding partners, and (when fused to GFP or when used to make an antibody) localized in cells.

Further insights regarding function are often obtained by disruption of a gene. Genomic DNA can be used to construct a plasmid containing two substantial "targeting" regions (usually several thousand base pairs) of a gene flanking a selectable marker gene. If introduced into cells under conditions where the targeting regions recombine into the chromosome, the region of the gene between them will be replaced by the selectable marker. This can produce a **null mutation,** in which that copy of the gene is completely removed. Creating such a null mutation is readily accomplished in yeast and, with somewhat more difficulty, in vertebrate cells, but is more complicated in flies where this gene-targeting technology is less well developed. Fortunately, an alternative method called RNAi (for **RNA interference**) can remove particular mRNAs from worms and cultured cells of flies and humans. When cells are induced to take up double-stranded RNA, a defense mechanism destroys the corresponding mRNA, preventing the expression of the gene.

Genomics and Reverse Genetics

Thanks to large-scale DNA sequencing projects, nearly complete sequences of the coding regions of the most popular experimental organism are now· available. When fully annotated (i.e., all sequences coding for genes identified and catalogued), these genome sequences will be the definitive inventory of genes. This is easier said than done, as accurate and complete identification of genes in raw sequence data is challenging. The task has been aided by millions of sequences of cDNA copies of expressed genes (**expressed sequence tags,** or ESTs), which help to document the diversity of products created by transcription and RNA processing (Chapter 15).

Nevertheless, even before genome annotation is complete, these sequences make possible a new approach for relating genes to biological function. First, one identifies as many genes as possible and uses the translated sequences to predict what each protein might do. Given the sequence of a gene of interest, the initial strategy is to search computer data bases for proteins with similar sequences and known functions. This is surprisingly fruitful as many genes occur as extended families. In addition, conserved sequence motifs of a few to several hundred amino acids can provide clues to function if the motifs have been characterized in other proteins. For example, this sort of analysis can readily identify a novel protein as a protein kinase (see Chapter 27). Once predicted sequences have been analyzed, one can check when and where the gene is expressed in the organism, test the consequences of deleting the gene, or test for interactions of the protein with other proteins (see later section). These tests can be done one gene at a time or on a genome-wide scale. For example, investigators have created strains of budding yeast lacking each of the 6000 genes and have tested for interaction of the products of each of these genes with the products of all other genes. These preliminary screening tests will often yield some information about function. Ultimately, however, function will only be understood when representatives of each family of protein are studied in detail by the biophysical, biochemical, and cellular methods described in the following sections.

Biochemical Fractionation

The biochemical approach (to the inventory) is to purify active molecules for analysis of structure and function. This requires a sensitive, quantitative assay to detect the component of interest in crude fractions, an assay to assess purity, and a battery of methods to separate it from the rest of the cellular constituents. Assays are as diverse as the processes of life. Enzymes are particularly easy to measure. Many molecules are

box 5–2

GEL ELECTROPHORESIS

An electrical field draws molecules in a sample through a gel matrix. **Agarose gels** (see Fig. 5–5A) are used commonly for nucleic acids, whereas **polyacrylamide gels** are used for both nucleic acids (see Fig. 2–18) and proteins (see Fig. 5–5B). Most often, buffers are employed to dissociate the components of the sample and to make their rate of migration through the gel depend on their size. The ionic detergent sodium dodecylsulfate **(SDS)** serves this purpose for proteins. SDS-binding unfolds polypeptide chains and gives them a uniform negative charge per unit length. Small molecules move rapidly and separate from slowly moving large molecules, which are more impeded by the matrix. By the time small molecules reach the end of the gel, all of the components in the sample are spread out according to size. Buffers containing the nonionic, denaturing agent urea also dissociate and unfold protein molecules. Electrophoresis in urea separates the proteins depending on both their charge and size. Negatively charged proteins move toward the positive electrode, whereas positively charged proteins move in the other direction. Another approach, called **isoelectric focusing,** uses a buffer containing molecules called ampholines, which have both positive and negative charges. In an electrical field across a gel, ampholines set up a pH gradient. Proteins (usually dissociated in urea) migrate to the pH where they have a net charge of zero, their isoelectric point. This is a sensitive approach to detect charge differences in proteins, such as those introduced by phosphorylation. Iso-electric focusing in one gel followed by SDS–

gel electrophoresis in a second dimension can resolve hundreds of individual proteins in complex samples (see Fig. 41–11A).

Many methods are available to detect molecules separated by gel electrophoresis. Proteins are detected by binding colored dyes or more sensitive metal reduction techniques. A single stained band on a heavily loaded SDS gel is the goal of those purifying proteins. Of course, some pure proteins consist of multiple polypeptide chains (see Fig. 5–5C); in such cases, multiple bands in some definite proportions are seen. Specific proteins are often detected with antibodies. Typically, the proteins are transferred electrophoretically from the polyacrylamide gel to a sheet of nitrocellulose or nylon before reaction with antibodies. This transfer step is called **blotting.** Antibodies labeled with radioactivity are detected by exposing a sheet of x-ray film. Antibodies are also detected by reaction with a second antibody conjugated to an enzyme that catalyzes a light-emitting reaction **(chemiluminescence),** which exposes a sheet of x-ray film. Some proteins can be detected by reaction with naturally occurring binding partners. Fluorescent dyes, such as ethidium bromide, bind to nucleic acids (see Fig. 5–5A). Following blotting of the separated nucleic acids from the gel onto nitrocellulose or nylon films, specific sequences are detected with complementary oligonucleotides or longer sequences of cloned DNA (probes) labeled with radioactivity or fluorescent dyes.

---

detected by binding a partner molecule. For example, nucleic acids bind complementary nucleotide sequences and sequence-specific regulatory proteins; receptors bind ligands; antibodies bind their antigens; and particular proteins bind partner proteins. More difficult assays reconstitute a cellular process, such as vesicle fusion, nuclear transport, or molecular motility. Devising such a sensitive and specific assay is one of the most creative parts of this approach. A second prerequisite for purification is a simple method for assessing purity. Various types of **gel electrophoresis** often work brilliantly (Box 5–2; Fig. 5–5).

With a functional assay and a method to assess purity, one can then set about purifying the molecule of interest. Highly abundant constituents, such as actin or tubulin, may require purification of only 20- to 100-fold, but many interesting and important molecules, such as signaling proteins and transcription factors, constitute less than 0.1% of the cell protein, so extensive purification is required.

First, the cell is disrupted gently to avoid damage to the molecule of interest. This may be accomplished physically by mechanical shearing with various types of **homogenizers** or, where appropriate, chemically, with mild detergents that extract lipids from cellular membranes. Next, the homogenate is **centrifuged** to separate particulate and soluble constituents. If the molecule of interest is soluble, it can be purified by sophisticated **chromatography** methods (Box 5–3, Fig. 5–6) given sufficient starting material.

If a cDNA copy of the mRNA for a protein of interest is available, rare proteins or modified proteins can often be expressed in large quantities in bacteria, yeast, or insect cells. An advantage of this approach is that mutations can be made at will, including substitution of one or more amino acids, deletion of parts of the protein, or addition of domains that are useful for characterizing the protein. Examples include the addition of short amino acid sequences corresponding to the binding site (epitope) for particular antibodies.

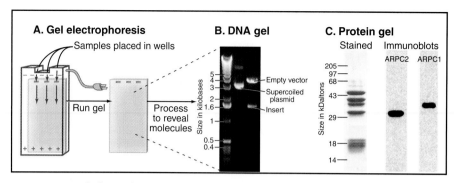

Figure 5-5 Gel electrophoresis. *A,* Schematic diagram showing a (generic) gel with three sample wells and an electric field. *B,* Agarose gel electrophoresis of DNA samples stained with ethidium bromide. The lane on the left shows size standards. The middle lane has a bacterial plasmid, a supercoiled (see Fig. 2–20) circular DNA molecule carrying an insert (see Fig. 5–8 for details). The right lane has the same plasmid digested with a restriction enzyme that cleaves the DNA twice, releasing the insert. Although smaller than the circular plasmid, the empty vector runs slower on the gel because the linear DNA offers more resistance to movement than the supercoiled circular plasmid. *C,* Polyacrylamide gel electrophoresis of the Arp2/3 complex, an assembly of seven protein subunits involved with actin polymerization (see Chapter 36 for details). All three samples are identical. In the left lane, the proteins are stained with the dye Coomassie blue. The proteins in the other two lanes were transferred to nitrocellulose paper; each reacted with an antibody to one of the subunit proteins (ARPC2 and ARPC1). The position of the bound antibody is determined with a second antibody coupled to an enzyme that produces light and exposes a piece of film black. This method is called chemiluminescence. (*B,* Courtesy of V. Sirotkin, Yale University. *C,* Courtesy of H. Higgs, Dartmouth Medical School.)

These **epitope** tags can be used to purify the protein or to localize the protein on gel blots or in cells. Other popular additions include fusion with a fluorescent protein, such as GFP (described earlier), for localization in cells. Fusions with the enzyme **glutathione S-transferase (GST)** are widely used for affinity chromatography and binding assays. GST binds tightly to glutathione, which can be immobilized on beads.

If the molecule of interest is part of an organelle, centrifugation can be used to isolate the organelle. Typically, the crude cellular homogenate is centrifuged multiple times at a succession of higher speeds (and therefore forces). Particles move in a centrifugal field according to their mass and shape. Large particles such as nuclei pack into a pellet at the bottom of the centrifuge tube at low speeds, whereas high speeds are required to pellet small vesicles. These pellets may be enriched in particular organelles, but are never pure. Next, the impure pellet is centrifuged for many hours in a tube containing a concentration gradient of sucrose. In **sedimentation velocity** gradients, particles are centrifuged in a gradient of sucrose (e.g., 5% sucrose in buffer at the top of the tube, increasing to 20% sucrose at the bottom). Because the motion of particles in a centrifugal field depends on the square of the radius (think of a spinning ice skater), the further down the tube the particle travels, the faster it will go. However, the motion of particles in a centrifugal force field also depends on the difference between their density and that of the surrounding medium.

box 5–3

CHROMATOGRAPHY

- **Affinity chromatography** (Fig. 5–6) is the most selective method. A ligand that binds the target molecule is attached covalently to a solid matrix. When a complex mixture of molecules passes through the column, the target molecule binds, whereas most of the other molecules flow through. After washing the column, the target protein is eluted by competition with free ligand or changing conditions, such as changes in pH or salt concentration.

- **Gel filtration** separates molecules on the basis of size. Inert beads of agarose, polyacrylamide, or other polymers are manufactured with pores of a particular size. Large molecules are excluded from the pores and elute first from the column in a volume (void volume) equal to the volume of buffer outside the beads in the column. Small molecules, such as salt, penetrate throughout the beads and elute much later in a volume equal to the total volume of the column. Molecules of intermediate size penetrate the beads to an extent that depends on their molecular radius. This parameter, called the **Stokes radius,** can be measured quantitatively if the column is calibrated with standards of known size. Such molecules elute between the void volume and the total volume.

- **Ion exchange chromatography** utilizes charged groups attached covalently to inert beads. These charged groups may be positive (e.g., the tertiary amine, diethylaminoethyl [DEAE]) or negative (e.g., carboxylate or phosphate). Ionic interactions retain oppositely charged solutes on the surface of the column particles provided the ionic strength of the buffer is low. Typically, a gradient of salt is used to elute bound solutes.

- Other types of chromatography media are widely used. Crystals of calcium phosphate, called hydroxyapatite, bind both proteins and nucleic acids, which can be eluted selectively by a gradient of phosphate buffer. Beads with hydrophobic groups, such as aromatic rings, absorb many proteins in concentrated salt solutions. They can be eluted selectively by a declining gradient of salt.

- The resolution of all chromatography methods depends on the size of the particles (usually beads) that form the immobile phase in the column. Resolution improves with small particles, but so does the resistance to flow. Therefore, high pressures are used to maintain good flow rates in the most high-resolution systems.

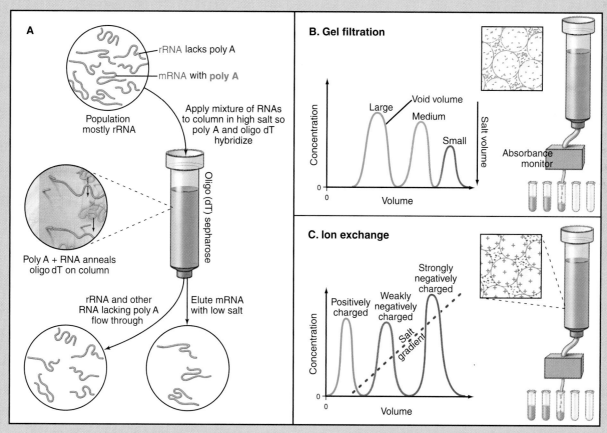

Figure 5–6 Chromatography. *A,* Affinity chromatography to purify poly A mRNAs with poly dT attached to beads. A mixture of RNAs is extracted from cells and applied to the column in a buffer containing a high concentration of salt. Only poly (A)$^+$ mRNA binds and is then eluted with buffer containing a low concentration of salt. rRNA, ribosomal RNA. *B,* Gel filtration chromatography separates molecules on the basis of size. Large molecules are excluded from the beads and travel through the column in the void volume outside the beads. Smaller molecules penetrate the beads depending on their size. Tiny molecules, such as salt, completely penetrate the beads and elute in a volume (the salt volume) equal to the size of the bed of beads. Material eluting from the column is monitored for absorbance to measure concentration and then collected in tubes in a fraction collector. *C,* Anion exchange chromatography. The beads in the column have a positively charged group that binds negatively charged molecules. A gradient of salt elutes bound molecules depending on their affinity for the beads. For cation exchange chromatography, the beads carry a negative charge.

Thus, the increasing density of sucrose gradient tends to slow the particle down. Ideally, the two factors counteract one another so that the particle moves at a constant rate, yielding the best separation. In **sedimentation equilibrium** gradients, particles move until their density equals that of the gradient, at which point they move no further, regardless of how long or hard they are spun. Membrane-containing organelles can be isolated in this way in sucrose gradients, but certain particles, such as DNA or RNA molecules, are denser than sucrose. They can be centrifuged to equilibrium in gradients of dense salts, such as cesium chloride. The small differences in size and buoyant density among many of the membrane-bound organelles limit the resolution of subcellular fractionation by sedimentation velocity and sedimentation equilibrium, so additional methods are useful in purifying preparations of organelles. For example, antibodies specific for a molecule on the surface of an organelle can be attached to a solid support and used to bind the organelle. Contaminating material can then be washed away.

Once a protein of interest has been purified, the path to its gene(s) is relatively direct. Traditionally, each constituent polypeptide was cut into fragments by proteolytic enzymes, after which these fragments were isolated by chromatography and their amino acid sequence determined by Edman degradation (see Chapter 2). Given some amino acid sequence, the corresponding gene can then be identified in a data base or isolated using oligonucleotide probes as the assay (see next section). However, increasingly, polypeptides are now being identified by **mass spectrometry.** Proteins are fragmented by cleavage at specific sites with a proteolytic enzyme, such as trypsin, and the molecular masses of the fragments produced are measured exactly in a mass spectrometer. Because the exact masses of all predicted tryptic fragments of all proteins whose gene sequences are known can be calculated from the sequence data bases, in many cases, the exact masses of all of the fragments obtained from a given polypeptide are sufficient to identify the encoding gene. The sensitivity of these methods has been improved to the point where a stained protein band on a gel typically suffices to identify the corresponding gene.

Isolation of Genes and cDNAs

A variety of facile methods make isolation of specific nucleic acids relatively routine. Genomic DNA is isolated from whole cells by selective extraction. mRNAs are purified by affinity chromatography, taking advantage of their polyadenylate (poly A) tails (see Chapter 15), which bind by base pairing to poly dT attached to an insoluble matrix (Fig. 5–6A). Because DNA is easier to work with than RNA (e.g., it can be cleaved by

restriction endonucleases and cloned), RNAs are usually converted to **complementary DNA (cDNA)** by reverse transcriptase, a DNA polymerase that uses RNA as a template.

Several options exist to purify a particular DNA from a complex mixture.

1. The **polymerase chain reaction (PCR)** uses DNA polymerase and two primers (oligonucleotides, each complementary to one of the ends of a DNA sequence) to synthesize a strand of DNA complementary to another DNA strand (Fig. 5–7A). This reaction is repeated to double the number of copies. Because the DNA duplex product must be dissociated at high temperature before each round of duplication, development of this method depended upon the cloning of DNA polymerases from bacteria that live at ultra-high temperatures (which do not denature these spe-

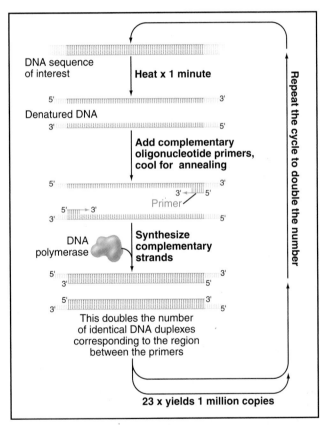

Figure 5-7 Polymerase chain reaction. From the top, double-stranded DNA with a sequence of interest is denatured by heating to separate the two strands. An excess of oligonucleotide primers complementary to the ends of the sequence of interest are added and allowed to bind by base pairing. DNA polymerase synthesizes complementary strands starting from the primers. This cycle is repeated many times to amplify the sequence of interest. Use of a DNA polymerase from a thermophilic bacterium allows many cycles at high temperature without losing activity.

cial DNA polymerases). Repeated steps of synthesis and denaturation allow a huge amplification in the amount of DNA present. Design of the primers requires knowledge of the sequence of the gene of interest, which may be available from data bases or which may be guessed from the sequence of the same gene in a related species or a similar gene in the same species. If the reaction is successful, a single sequence is amplified in quantities sufficient for cloning, sequencing, or large-scale biological production by expression in a bacterium (see later discussion). At its best, PCR is so sensitive that DNA sequences from a single cell can be cloned and characterized.

2. The DNA segment of interest can be isolated by **cloning** in a bacterial virus or plasmid (Fig. 5–8A). Such cloning strategies use **"libraries"** of DNA sequences, highly complex mixtures typi-

cally having more than 10^6 different cDNAs or genomic DNA fragments. These DNA molecules are transferred into the genome of a virus (usually a bacteriophage) or into a plasmid, a circular DNA molecule that is capable of replication in a host bacterium. The viruses or plasmids are diluted and introduced into susceptible bacteria, which grow on agar in petri dishes. In the case of viral vectors, cycles of virus infection and cell lysis in a continuous layer of bacteria produce small clear spots devoid of bacteria, called plaques. For plasmids, conditions are chosen in which only those bacteria carrying a plasmid will grow to form a colony. To clone the DNA sequence of interest, the DNA in the plaques or colonies is transferred to a membrane and tested for hybridization to a DNA probe complementary to the sequence of interest. This probe may be either a chemically

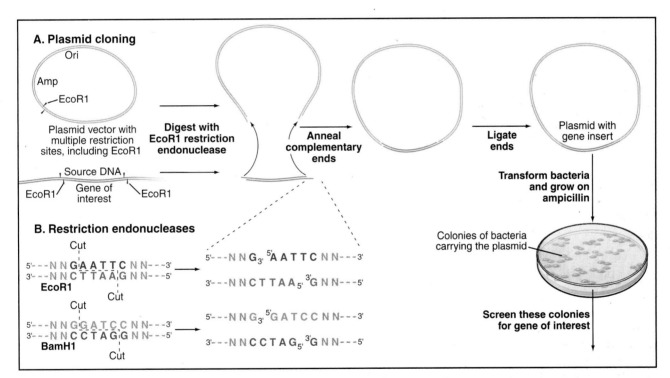

Figure 5-8 DNA cloning. *A,* Cloning of a segment of DNA into a plasmid vector. The vector is a circular DNA molecule with an origin of replication (Ori) that allows it to replicate in a host bacterium. Most vectors also include one or more genes conferring antibiotic resistance, in this example, resistance to ampicillin (Amp). This enables one to select only those bacteria carrying a plasmid by the ability to grow in the presence of ampicillin. Vectors also contain a sequence of DNA with multiple restriction enzyme digestion sites (see part *B*) for the insertion of foreign DNA molecules. In this example, a single restriction enzyme, EcoR1, is used to cut both the source DNA and the plasmid vector, leaving both with identical overhangs. The ends of the insert and the cut vector anneal together by base pairing and are then ligated together by a ligase enzyme, forming a complete circle of DNA. Plasmids are introduced into bacteria, which are then grown on ampicillin to select those with plasmids. Colonies of bacteria are screened for those containing the desired insert using, for example, DNA probes for sequences specific to the gene of interest. Figure 5–5*B* shows gel electrophoresis of a plasmid carrying an insert before and after digestion with a restriction enzyme to liberate the insert from the vector. *B,* Sequence-specific cutting of DNA with restriction enzymes. EcoR1 and BamH1 are two of the hundreds of different restriction enzymes that recognize and cleave specific DNA sequences. These two restriction enzymes recognize a palindrome of six symmetrical bases. Note that these enzymes leave overhangs with identical sequences on both cut ends that are useful for base pairing with DNA having the same cut. Other restriction enzymes recognize and cut from 4 to 10 bases.

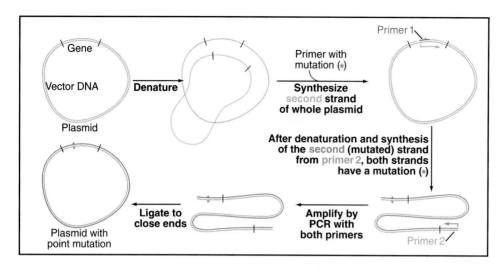

Figure 5-9 In vitro mutagenesis of cloned DNA. This is one of several types of PCR methods used to change one or more nucleotides (* in this example) in a cloned gene using a primer with altered bases. In this particular method, primer 1 has the altered base and is used to duplicate the entire plasmid. Primer 2 is used to synthesize the whole plasmid from the other end. After amplification with both primers, the two ends are ligated together and the plasmid is produced in quantity by growth in bacteria.

synthesized oligonucleotide based on sequences in a data base, or be derived from the coding sequence of the protein of interest. Most commonly, the probe is a small piece of cloned DNA generated by PCR or obtained from a repository. Plaques or colonies reactive with the probe are physically removed from the petri dish, and then the viruses (or cells bearing plasmid) are diluted. The process is repeated a few times until all of the plaques or colonies carry the sequence of interest.

3. An alternative approach, called **"expression cloning,"** typically uses a cDNA library that has been inserted into a viral vector next to a bacterial promoter and translational start codon (see Chapter 18), so that the host bacterium will copy the DNA, starting at the 5' end of the clone, into mRNA and synthesize the protein. In this case, viral plaques are transferred to a membrane and probed with a specific antibody recognizing the protein of interest. If it works (as it does for vertebrate genes) this is the quickest and easiest form of cloning. However, there are pitfalls, particularly when cloning genes from organisms whose preference for the use of particular codons differs from that of *Escherichia coli*. In yeasts, a modification of this method involves introducing plasmid libraries into a mutant strain, and then looking for sequences that will rescue the mutant cells. More sophisticated versions of expression cloning have been used, for example, to introduce cDNA libraries into vertebrate cells and then to look for expression of a particular trait, such as a membrane channel.

Once a gene or cDNA has been cloned, it is sequenced and used to predict the sequence of the encoded protein. Of course, analysis of a DNA sequence cannot reveal post-translational modifications of a protein, such as phosphorylation, glycosylation, or proteolytic processing. Such modifications, which are often critical for protein function, can only be identified by biochemical analysis of proteins from cells.

Cloned cDNAs are also used to express native or modified proteins in bacteria or other cells for biochemical analysis or antibody production. This approach has two advantages. First, the quantity of protein produced is often greater than that from a natural source. Second, cloned DNA can readily be modified to make amino acid substitutions and other alterations that are useful for studying protein function (Fig. 5–9). The behavior of mutant proteins in cells can provide evidence for the role of a given protein in particular cellular functions. Thus, biochemical, genetic, and molecular cloning approaches may be applied collectively to reveal the function of proteins.

■ Molecular Structure

Primary Structure

DNA sequences are now determined by automated dye-termination methods (Fig. 2–18). The same method, when applied to cDNAs, is used to deduce the sequence of proteins and structural RNAs. Protein sequencing by Edman degradation is still useful to detect modified amino acids (Fig. 2–5), but mass spectrometry is faster and more sensitive.

Subunit Composition

Gel electrophoresis of many isolated proteins has revealed that they consist of more than one polypeptide chain. Their stoichiometry can be determined from the size and intensity of the stained bands on the gel, but the only way to determine the total number of subunits is to measure the molecular weight of the native protein or protein assembly. The definitive method is a sedimentation equilibrium experiment carried out in an analytical ultracentrifuge. A sample of purified material is centrifuged at relatively low speed in a rotor that allows the measurement of the mass concentration from the top to bottom of the sample cell. At equilibrium, the sedimentation of the material toward the bottom of the tube is balanced by diffusion from the region of high concentration at the bottom of the tube. This balance between sedimentation and diffusion uniquely defines the molecular weight of the particle. A less direct approach is to measure the **sedimentation coefficient** (the parameter relating the rate of sedimentation to the centrifugal force) directly during centrifugation at high speed, and to measure the diffusion coefficient separately, most often by analytical gel filtration (see Fig. 5–6B). These two parameters are used to calculate the molecular weight. (Note that neither measurement separately is sufficient to measure molecular weights, despite numerous assertions that they are sufficient!) An advantage of the latter approach is that it can be used with impure material, provided an assay is available that is applicable to the two types of measurements. Light scattering can also be used to estimate molecular weights.

Atomic Structure

X-ray crystallography and **nuclear magnetic resonance (NMR)** spectroscopy (see Chapter 2; Fig. 2–8) are used to determine the atomic structure of proteins and nucleic acids at atomic resolution. Although structures as large as the ribosome (see Fig. 18–7) and viruses (see Figs. 4–11 and 4–13) have been determined by x-ray crystallography, some large structures are outside the size range of these high-resolution methods. They can be studied by electron microscopy of single particles or regular assemblies. In favorable cases, atomic structures of the parts of a large assembly can be fit precisely into lower resolution reconstructions from electron micrographs (see Figs. 39–5 and 39–9).

▌ Partners and Pathways

It is hard to think of a cellular molecule that functions in isolation, as virtually all cellular components are parts of assemblies, networks, or pathways. Thus, a major challenge in defining biological function is to place each molecule in its physiological context with all of its molecular partners. The classic example of such an endeavor is the biochemical mapping of the

major metabolic pathways (see Fig. 10–15 and any biochemistry textbook). Genetics played a prominent role in the discovery of the network of proteins that control the cell cycle (see Chapter 43). Currently, signaling, regulation of gene expression, and the control of development are pathways of particular interest.

Biochemical Methods

Once a molecule of interest is purified, finding partners is often the next step. One needs a method to separate the probe molecule bound to partners from free molecules. One approach is to use **affinity chromatography** with the probe molecule attached to an insoluble support, such as agarose gel filtration beads with a chemical cross-linking reagent. A popular variation is to express a probe protein fused to another protein that binds with high affinity to a small molecule attached to beads. GST is popular for this use. A crude cellular extract can be run through a column with immobilized probe molecule and washed, and bound molecules can be eluted with high salt, extremes of pH, specific ligands, or, if necessary, with denaturing agents, such as urea. Eluted proteins can be analyzed by gel electrophoresis and can be identified with antibodies, sequencing, or mass spectrometry. Bound nucleic acids can be cloned and sequenced. Alternatively, beads with attached probe molecules can be mixed with the crude extract and then centrifuged in a pellet along with bound molecules. Varying the concentration of such beads is a simple way to measure the affinity of the probe for its various partners.

Antibodies are frequently used to separate a protein and its partners from crude extracts. An antibody specific for the probe molecule is attached directly or indirectly to a bead and used to bind the protein of interest. This is called **immunoprecipitation.**

Genetics

Given a mutation in a gene of interest, two genetic tests are used to search for partners: (1) identification of a second mutation that suppresses the effects of the primary mutation (a **suppressor mutation,** Fig. 5–10A); and (2) identification of a second mutation that makes the phenotype more severe, often lethal (an **enhancer mutation,** Fig. 5–10B). A specialized class of enhancer mutations, called **synthetic lethal mutations,** are particularly useful in the analysis of genetic pathways in yeast. In this case, mutations in two genes in the same pathway, if present in the same cell, even as heterozygotes (i.e., each cell having one good and one mutant copy of each gene), cannot be

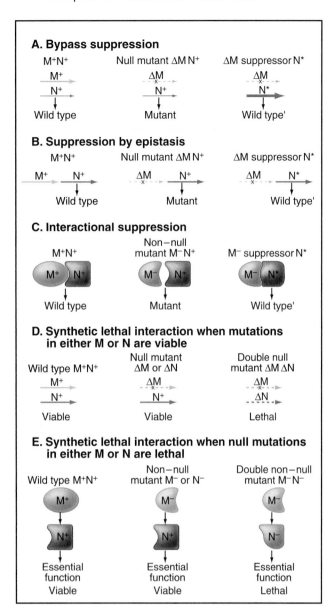

Figure 5–10 Analysis of genetic interactions between two genes, M and N. The sizes of the arrows indicate the level of function of the gene product, usually a protein. The phenotype is indicated for each example. Mutant phenotype means an altered function dependent on gene products M and N. In the diagram, + indicates a wild-type allele, * indicates a suppressor allele, and Δ indicates a null mutation. A, Bypass suppression. Gene products M and N operate in parallel, with M making the larger contribution. Loss of M yields a mutant phenotype because N alone does not provide sufficient function. Mutation N* enhances the function of N, allowing it to provide function on its own. B, Suppression by epistasis. Products M and N act in series on the same pathway. Loss of M function blocks the pathway. Mutation N* allows N to function without stimulation by product M. C, Interactional suppression. Function requires interaction of gene products M and N. Mutation M⁻ interferes with the interaction. Suppressor mutation N* allows product N* to interact with A⁻. D, Synthetic lethal interaction when null mutations in either M or N are viable. The products of genes M and N operate in parallel to provide function. N provides sufficient function in the absence of M (ΔM) and vice versa. Loss of both M and N is lethal. E, Synthetic lethal interaction when null mutations in either M or N are lethal. Products M and N function in series. N can provide residual function even when M is compromised by mutation M⁻, and vice versa. When both M and N are compromised (M⁻, N⁻), the pathway provides insufficient function for viability. (Redrawn from Guarente L: Synthetic enhancement in gene interaction: A genetic tool come of age. Trends Genet 9:362–366, 1993. Copyright 1993, with permission from Elsevier Science.)

tolerated, and so the cell dies. It is thought that each mutation lowers the level of production of some critical factor just a bit, and that the combination of the two effectively means that the output of the pathway is insufficient for survival. These tests can be made with existing collections of mutations by crossing mutant organisms. Alternatively, one can seek new mutations created by a second round of mutagenesis. The results depend on the architecture of the particular pathway (see Fig. 5–10). If the products of the genes in question operate in a sequence, analysis of single and double mutants will often reveal their order in the pathway. For essential genes in haploid organisms, a conditional allele of the primary mutation simplifies the experiment. Synthetic interactions (suppressor or lethal mutations) may also be driven by overproduc-

tion of wild-type genes on a plasmid. Caution is required in interpreting suppressor and enhancer mutations, given the complexity of cellular systems and the possibility of unanticipated consequences of the mutations.

Another approach is called a **two-hybrid assay** (Fig. 5–11). This assay depends on the observation that some transcriptional activators have two discrete functions: binding to target sites on DNA and recruitment of the transcriptional apparatus (see Chapter 14). Provided that both activities are associated with the 5' end of a gene, that gene will be expressed, even if the activities are on two different proteins. For this assay, the protein whose interactors are to be identified is cloned into a "bait" vector, fusing it to a protein containing a region of a yeast protein that recognizes

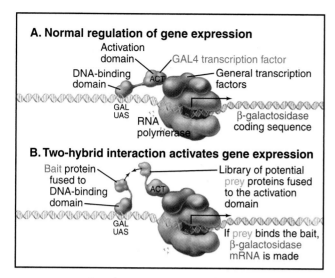

A. Normal regulation of gene expression

Activation domain

DNA-binding domain

GAL4 transcription factor

ACT

General transcription factors

GAL UAS

RNA polymerase

β-galactosidase coding sequence

B. Two-hybrid interaction activates gene expression

Bait protein fused to DNA-binding domain

ACT

Library of potential prey proteins fused to the activation domain

GAL UAS

If prey binds the bait, β-galactosidase mRNA is made

Figure 5–11 *A* and *B,* One version of the yeast two-hybrid assay for interacting proteins. Interaction between bait protein A and prey protein B brings together the two halves of a transcription factor required to turn on the expression of β-galactosidase. The DNA-binding domain of the GAL4 transcription factor binds a specific DNA sequence: GAL UAS. Generally, a library of random cDNAs or gene fragments is used to express test prey proteins as fusions with the activation domain.

particular "target" DNA sequences. A DNA construct for this so-called bait protein is introduced into yeast cells, which now have the "bait" protein localized to specific sites on the chromosomes. Into this population of cells is now introduced a plasmid library in which cDNA sequences have been cloned into a "prey" vector so that they are fused to a nuclear localization sequence and to an "activator domain" that will recruit the transcriptional apparatus. If the "bait" and "prey" proteins bind to one another, the activator sequences are carried to the target genes, which are then expressed. There are many forms of this assay. One produces an enzyme that produces a colored product, so positive colonies can be identified visually. In another version, the target gene encodes a gene essential for production of a particular amino acid, so that only cells in which a bait-prey interaction has occurred will grow on agar plates lacking that amino acid. Putative interactions must be tested carefully to define specificity, as false-positive results are common. Moreover, some valid interactions are missed owing to false-negatives.

Genomics

The advent of **microarrays** (Fig. 5–12), on which the expression of thousands of genes can be monitored in parallel, revealed that the expression of genes contributing proteins to a particular pathway is often modulated in parallel as conditions change. For example,

nearly 300 genes for constituents of the endoplasmic reticulum are turned on together in response to unfolded proteins in the lumen of the endoplasmic reticulum (see Fig. 20–10).

Rates and Affinities

Information about reaction rates is important for two reasons. First, reaction rates are required to account for the dynamic aspects of any biological system. Second, although the methods in the previous section usually provide initial clues about pathways, knowledge of reactant concentrations and **rate constants** is actually the only way to verify biochemical pathways. Fortunately, just two types of reactions occur in biology: first-order reactions, such as conformational changes and dissociation of molecular complexes, and second-order reactions between two molecules. Chapter 3 explains the rate constants for such reactions, the relationship of rate constants to the equilibrium constant for a reaction, and the relationship of the equilibrium constant to thermodynamics. Despite their importance, rate constants and the physiological concentrations of the molecules in a pathway are usually the least understood aspects of most biological systems. A common impediment is the lack of an assay with sufficient sensitivity and time resolution to measure reaction rates. Optical methods, such as those using fluorescence, are usually the best and can be devised for many processes.

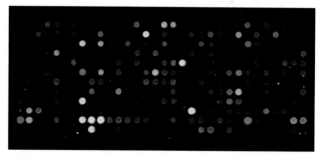

Figure 5–12 cDNA microarray for large-scale analysis of gene expression. PCR was used to make cDNA copies of mRNAs from two parts of the human brain. The cDNAs from cerebral cortex mRNAs were labeled with a red fluorescent dye, whereas those from the cerebellum were labeled with a green fluorescent dye. A mixture of equal proportions of the two fluorescent cDNA preparations was reacted with 384 different known cDNAs arrayed in tiny spots on a glass slide. The fluorescence bound cDNAs were imaged with a microscopic fluorescent scanner similar to a confocal microscope. Yellow spots bound equal quantities of cDNAs from the two sources. Red spots bound more cDNA from the cortex, indicating a higher concentration of those mRNAs. Green spots bound more cDNA from the cerebellum, indicating a higher concentration of those mRNAs. (Courtesy of C. Barlow and M. Zapala, Salk Institute, La Jolla, CA.)

Tests of Physiological Function

Reconstitution of Function from Isolated Components

The classic biochemical test of function is **reconstitution** of a biological process from purified components. This involves creating conditions in the test tube where isolated molecules can perform a complex process normally carried out within a cell. The difficulty of the task reflects the complexity of the function; successful efforts reveal the cellular requirements and mechanisms involved in the process. Examples of successful tests include reconstitution of ion channel function in pure lipid membranes (see Chapter 9), protein synthesis and translocation of proteins into the endoplasmic reticulum (see Chapter 20), and motility of bacteria powered by assembly of actin filaments (see Chapter 40).

Anatomical Tests

No biological process can be understood without knowing where the components are located in the cell. Often, cellular **localization** of a newly discovered molecule provides the first clue about its function. This accounts for why cell biologists put so much effort into localizing molecules in cells. Cell fractionation, fluorescent antibody staining, and expression of GFP fusion proteins are all valuable approaches, illustrated by numerous examples in this book. GFP fusion proteins are particularly valuable, since observing their behavior in live cells reveals their dynamics. A powerful ancillary maneuver is to photobleach the GFP fusion proteins in one part of a cell and observe how the fluorescent proteins in other parts of the cell redistribute with time (FRAP-fluorescence recovery after photobleaching). Of course, it is highly desirable to demonstrate that the GFP fusion protein is fully functional, that is, that it can replace the native protein through a gene replacement. It is important to bear in mind that this is not usually done for most vertebrate proteins where the genetics necessary to perform such tests is difficult or impossible. For more detailed localization, antibodies can be adsorbed to small gold beads and used to label specimens for electron microscopy (see Fig. 31–7).

Diverse cellular components, including RNA, proteins, and lipids, can be labeled with fluorescent dyes to study their intracellular localization and dynamics. Fluorescent RNAs and proteins can be microinjected into cells. Fluorescent lipids can be inserted into the outer leaflet of the plasma membrane in living cells; from there, they move to appropriate membranes and then mimic rather faithfully the behavior of their natural lipid counterpart.

Physiological Tests

Although often obscured by technical jargon, just three methods are available to test for physiological function: (1) reducing the concentration of active protein; (2) increasing the concentration of active protein; and (3) replacing the native protein with a protein with altered biochemical properties. Biochemical, pharmacological, and genetic methods are available for each test, with the genetic methods often yielding the cleanest results. These experiments are most revealing when robust assays are available to measure quantitatively how the cellular process under investigation functions when the concentration of native protein is varied or an altered protein replaces the native protein. When done well, these experiments provide extremely valuable constraints for quantitative models of biological systems, as described in the next section.

The most definitive way to reduce the concentration of active protein is to prevent its expression. This option is available if the protein is not required for viability. If a protein is essential, one can replace it with an altered version that is fully active under a certain set of conditions and completely inactive under other conditions. Proteins that are active at one temperature and inactive at another are widely used. Even then, it is difficult to control for the effects of temperature on all of the other processes in the cell. A second option is to put the expression of the protein under the control of regulatory proteins that are sensitive to the presence of a small molecule, such as a vitamin or hormone. Then, expression of the protein can be turned on and off at will. This is commonly done for vertebrate cells using promoters of gene expression that are engineered so that they can be turned on or off by the antibiotic tetracycline, which alters the ability of a bacterial protein (the tetracycline repressor) to bind to particular target sequences on DNA.

A new method to reduce the concentration of a particular protein is to target its mRNA for degradation by introducing a double-stranded RNA copy of part of its mRNA into the cytoplasm. This method is called RNAi, for RNA interference, since the biochemical processes that degrade the target RNA are used normally by animals, fungi, and plants for silencing the expression of foreign RNA, such as those introduced by viruses. Fragments from the double-stranded RNA guide an endonuclease to the targeted RNA, which is cleaved into short fragments, precluding translation.

Another strategy is to inhibit a particular protein with a drug, inhibitory peptide, antibody, or inactive partner protein. Drugs as probes for function have a long and distinguished history in biology, but their use is hampered by the difficulty of ruling out side effects, including action on other unknown targets. One wag has even asserted that "drugs are only specific for about a year," the time it takes for someone to find an effect on another cellular constituent. However, many drugs have the advantages that the onset of their action is rapid and their effects are reversible, so that one can follow the process of recovery when they are removed. Antibodies can be very specific, but the effects on their target must be fully characterized, and sufficient antibody must be introduced into the target cell (usually by the labor-intensive method of microinjection) to inactivate the target molecule. Alternatively, large molecules can be introduced by shearing cells suspended in the buffer containing the molecule. Proteins as large as antibodies enter through defects in the plasma membrane, which then reseal. This is called scrape loading or syringe loading. Some arginine-rich peptides, such as one from the HIV Tat protein, can also be used to carry inhibitory peptides across the plasma membrane into the cytoplasm. Other peptides can guide experimental peptides into various cellular compartments. It is also possible to inactivate pathways by the introduction of dominant negative mutants that can do part, but not all, of the job of a given protein. Particularly effective have been dominant negative mutants of protein kinases in which the active site is modified so that the protein can no longer act as a protein kinase. In cells these mutants bind to regulatory proteins and substrates, but do not phosphorylate them. This can block signal transduction pathways very effectively as the functional endogenous kinases are out-competed for their regulatory factors and substrates. Dominant negative mutants offer the advantage that they can be expressed in cells where they bind to and inhibit their target proteins. However, all too often, little is known about the concentrations of these dominant negative agents or the full range of their targets.

The concentration of active protein can be increased by **overexpression,** for example, driving the expression of the cDNA from a very active viral promoter. Some expression systems are conditional, being turned on, for example, by an insect hormone that does not activate any endogenous genes. Interpreting the consequences of overexpression tends to be more problematic than other approaches, as specificity of interactions with other cellular components can be lost at high concentrations.

Genetics is the best way to replace a native protein with a protein with altered biochemical properties. Such **gene replacement** requires homologous recombination in the genome, which is not readily available in all experimental systems (see Table 5–2). Examples of altered proteins include an enzyme with an altered catalytic function or a protein with altered affinity for a particular cellular partner. In the best cases, the altered protein is fully characterized before its coding sequence is used to replace that of the

wild-type protein, and the cellular concentration of the altered protein is confirmed to be the same as the wild-type protein. On the relatively long time scale of such experiments, interpreting the outcome may be compromised by the ability of cells to adapt to the change imposed by the gene substitution in unknown ways.

Mathematical Models of Systems

Even with an inventory of molecular components, their structures, concentrations, molecular partners, and reaction rates, and genetic tests for their contributions to a physiological process, one really does not know if a system operates according to one's expectations unless a mathematical model can match the performance of the cellular system over a range of conditions and, when challenged, with mutations in one or more component. In the best cases (bacterial metabolic pathways, bacterial chemotaxis, yeast cell cycle, muscle calcium transients, muscle cross-bridges), the mathematical models usually have fallen short of duplicating the physiological process. This means that some aspect of the process is incompletely understood or the assumptions in the mathematical model are incorrect. In either case, these failures offer important clues regarding the shortcomings of current knowledge and point the way toward improvements in underlying assumptions, experimental parameters, or mathematical models.

Selected Readings

Brent R, Finley RLJ: Understanding gene and allele function with two-hybrid methods. Ann Rev Genet 31:663–704, 1997.

Carthew RW: Gene silencing by double-stranded RNA. Curr Opin Cell Biol 13:244–248, 2001.

Celis J (Ed): Cell Biology: A laboratory handbook, vols I–III. New York: Academic Press, 1994.

Gariepy J, Kawamura K: Vectorial delivery of macromolecules into cells using peptide-based vehicles. Trends Biotechnol 19:21–28, 2001.

Guarente L: Strategies for the identification of interacting proteins. Proc Natl Acad Sci USA 90:1639–1641, 1993.

Guarente L: Synthetic enhancement in gene interaction: A genetic tool come of age. Trends Genet 9:362–366, 1993.

Inoué S: Video Microscopy. New York: Plenum Press, 1986.

Inoué S, Oldenbourg R: Microscopes. In Bass M, Van Stryland EW, Williams DR, Wolf WL: Handbook of Optics, vol II. New York: McGraw-Hill, Inc., 1995, pp 17.1–17.52.

International Human Genome Sequencing Consortium. Initial sequencing and analysis of the human genome. Nature

409:860–921, 2001. (Also see related articles in the same issue.)

Murphy DB: Fundamentals of Light Microscopy and Electronic Imaging. New York: Wiley-Liss, 2001, pp. 357.

Oliver SG: From gene to screen with yeast. Curr Opin Genet Dev 7:405–409, 1997.

Sambrook J, et al.: Molecular Cloning, 3rd ed. Plainview, NY: Cold Spring Harbor Laboratory, 2001.

Slayter EM: Optical Methods in Biology. New York: Wiley-Interscience, 1970.

Web site for biophysical methods, available at ⟨http://www.biophysics.org/society/btol⟩.

MEMBRANE STRUCTURE AND FUNCTION

chapter 6

MEMBRANE STRUCTURE AND DYNAMICS

Membranes make life possible by allowing cells to create an internal environment different from that outside. Membranes also divide the cytoplasm of eukaryotic cells into compartments called organelles, each with an internal composition optimized for certain biochemical activities. Biological membranes can separate these different environments because they are generally impermeable to macromolecules and selectively permeable to ions.

This chapter introduces features shared by all biological membranes: a **bilayer** of lipids; **integral proteins** that cross the bilayer; and **peripheral proteins** associated with the surfaces (Fig. 6–1D). The bilayer is a planar sandwich of lipids with hydrocarbon tails in the middle and polar head groups exposed to water on the surface. The hydrophobic interior of the bilayer is poorly permeable to ions and provides the barrier between compartments.

Integral proteins include a great variety of enzymes, adhesion proteins, receptors, ion channels, pumps, and solute carriers. Ion pumps (see Chapter 7) use a variety of energy sources to transport ions and other small solutes across membranes, creating solute concentration gradients across membranes. One class of pumps uses ATP hydrolysis to generate a transmembrane proton gradient or, alternatively, a proton gradient across the membrane to synthesize ATP. Carrier proteins (see Chapter 8) utilize energy from ion concentration gradients to drive the movement of solutes across membranes, up their concentration gradients. Ion-selective membrane channels (see Chapter 9) use ion gradients to produce electrical potentials across membranes. Because many hormones and other extracellular signaling molecules cannot penetrate a lipid bilayer, membranes contain protein receptors, which bind extracellular molecules and transmit signals across the membrane (see Chapter 26).

Peripheral proteins are found on the surfaces of the bilayer. Some peripheral proteins participate in enzyme reactions and signaling reactions. Others form a membrane skeleton on the cytoplasmic surface that reinforces the fragile lipid bilayer and attaches it to cytoskeletal filaments.

This chapter begins with a discussion of the lipid bilayer. It then considers examples of integral and peripheral membrane proteins before ending with a discussion of the dynamics of both lipids and proteins. The next three chapters introduce membrane pumps, carriers, and channels. Chapter 10 explains how pumps, carriers, and channels cooperate in a variety of physiological processes.

Development of Ideas about Membrane Structure

Our current understanding of membrane structure began in the 1920s, when it was first appreciated that cellular membranes consist of lipid bilayers (see Fig. 6–1A). Biochemists extracted lipids from red blood cells and found that these lipids spread out in a monolayer on the surface of a tray of water to cover an area sufficient to surround the cell twice. (Actually, offsetting errors—incomplete lipid extraction and an underestimation of the membrane area—led to the correct answer!) During the 1930s, cell physiologists realized that a bare lipid bilayer could not explain the mechanical properties of the plasma membrane, so they postulated a surface coating of proteins to reinforce the bilayer (see Fig. 6–1B). Early electron micrographs strengthened this view, since when viewed in cross sections, all membranes appeared as a pair of dark lines (interpreted as surface proteins and carbohydrates) separated by a lucent area (interpreted as

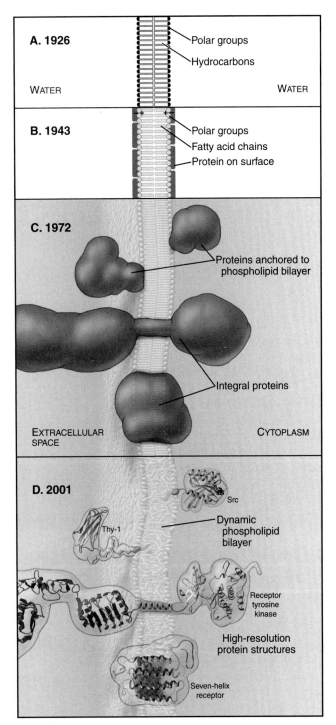

A. 1926

Polar groups
Hydrocarbons

WATER   WATER

B. 1943

Polar groups
Fatty acid chains
Protein on surface

C. 1972

Proteins anchored to
phospholipid bilayer

Integral proteins

EXTRACELLULAR
SPACE   CYTOPLASM

D. 2001

Src

Thy-1

Dynamic
phospholipid
bilayer

Receptor
tyrosine
kinase

High-resolution
protein structures

Seven-helix
receptor

Figure 6-1 Development of concepts in membrane structure. *A,* Gorder and Grendel model from 1926. *B,* Davson and Danielli model from 1943. *C,* Singer and Nicholson fluid mosaic model from 1972. *D,* Contemporary model with peripheral and integral membrane proteins. The lipid bilayer shown here and used throughout the book is based on an atomic model (see Fig. 6–5).

the lipid bilayer). By the early 1970s, two complementary approaches showed that proteins cross the lipid bilayer. First, electron micrographs of membranes split in two while frozen (a technique called freeze-fracturing) revealed protein particles embedded in the lipid bilayer. Later, chemical labeling of membrane proteins showed that many traverse the bilayer, exposing different parts of the polypeptide to the aqueous phase on the two sides. Light microscopy with fluorescent tags demonstrated that membrane lipids and some membrane proteins diffuse in the plane of the membrane. Quantitative spectroscopic studies showed that lateral diffusion of lipids is a rapid process, but that flipping from one side of a bilayer to the other is a slow one. The fluid mosaic model of membranes (see Fig. 6–1C) incorporated this information, showing transmembrane proteins floating in a fluid lipid bilayer. Subsequent work revealed the atomic structures of several proteins that span the lipid bilayer, the lipid anchors on some membrane proteins, and a network of cytoplasmic proteins that restricts the motion of many integral membrane proteins (see Fig. 6–1D).

Lipids

Cells produce a bewildering variety of lipids, which serve many essential roles. Lipids form the framework of biological membranes, act as tags to target proteins to membranes, store energy, and carry information as extracellular hormones and as intracellular second messengers in signal transduction. Lipids are relatively easy to recognize. They are roughly 100 to 1000 D in size and consist predominantly of aliphatic or aromatic hydrocarbons. However, the definition of a lipid is hazy at the boundaries. This chapter concentrates on major lipids found in biological membranes. Hundreds to thousands of minor lipids are also present. Any one of these obscure lipids may have an important biologic function that is not yet appreciated. For example, during the 1980s, a minor class of lipids with phosphorylated inositol head groups first attracted attention when investigators found that they had a role in signaling (see Chapter 28).

Phosphoglycerides

Phosphoglycerides are the main constituents of membrane bilayers (Fig. 6–2). (Phosphoglycerides are commonly called phospholipids, but this term is imprecise as other lipids also contain phosphate.) Phosphoglycerides have three essential parts: a three-carbon backbone of glycerol, two long-chain fatty acids esterified to carbons 1 and 2 (C_1 and C_2) of the glycerol, and phosphoric acid esterified to C_3 of the glycerol. By using several different fatty acids (Table 6–1), and by esterifying one of five different alcohols to the phosphate, cells make more than 100 major phosphoglycerides. In general, the fatty acids on C_1 have no or one double bond, whereas the fatty acids on C_2 have two or more double bonds. Each double bond creates a permanent bend in the hydrocarbon chain. The alcohol head groups, rather than the fatty acids, give phosphoglycerides their names:

- **phosphatidic acid** [PA] (no head group)
- **phosphatidylglycerol** [PG] (a glycerol head group)

Figure 6-2 Phosphoglycerides. *A,* Diagram of the parts of a phosphoglyceride and a space-filling model of phosphatidylcholine. *B,* Stick figures and space-filling models of the alcohol head groups. *C,* A saturated and an unsaturated fatty acid.

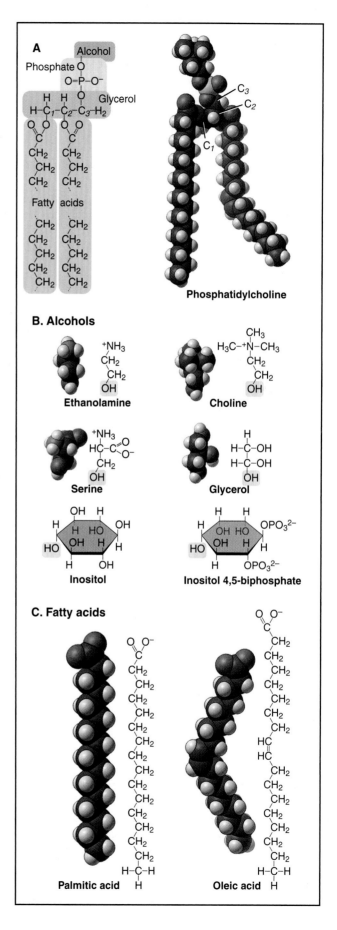

table 6-1

COMMON FATTY ACIDS OF MEMBRANE LIPIDS

Name	Carbons	Double Bonds (Positions)
Myristate	14	0
Palmitate	16	0
Palmitoleate	16	1 (Δ9)
Stearate	18	0
Oleate	18	1 (Δ9)
Linoleate	18	2 (Δ9, Δ12)
Linolenate	18	3 (Δ9, Δ12, Δ15)
Arachidonate	20	4 (Δ5, Δ8, Δ11, Δ14)

- **phosphatidylethanolamine** [PE] (an ethanolamine head group)
- **phosphatidylcholine** [PC] (a choline head group)
- **phosphatidylserine** [PS] (a serine head group)
- **phosphatidylinositol** [PI] (an inositol head group)

Head groups of phosphoglycerides have different charges and reactive groups that confer distinctive properties. All have a negative charge on the phosphate esterified to glycerol. Neutral phosphoglycerides—PE and PC—have a positive charge on their nitrogens, giving them a net charge of zero. PS has extra positive and negative charges, giving it a net negative charge like the other acidic phosphoglycer-ides (PA, PG, and PI). PI can be modified by esterifying one to five phosphates to the hexane ring hydroxyls. These **polyphosphoinositides** are highly negatively charged.

All phosphoglycerides have nonpolar tails and polar heads. In an aqueous environment, the tails associate to form a variety of structures that segregate them from water. From a biological perspective, by far the most important structure is the lamellar bilayer, with fatty acid chains lined up more or less normal to the surface and polar head groups exposed to water (see Fig. 6–1D).

The complicated metabolism of phosphoglycerides can be simplified as follows: enzymes can interconvert all phosphoglyceride head groups and remodel fatty acid chains. For example, three successive enzymatic methylation reactions convert PE to PC, whereas another enzyme exchanges serine for ethanolamine, converting PS to PE. Other enzymes exchange fatty acid chains after the initial synthesis of a phosphoglyceride. These enzymes are located on the cytoplasmic surface of the smooth endoplasmic reticulum. Biochemistry texts provide more details of these pathways.

Several minor membrane phospholipids are variations on this general theme. Plasmalogens have a fatty acid linked to carbon 1 of glycerol by an ether bond rather than an ester bond. They serve as sources of arachidonic acid for signaling reactions (see Chapter 28). Cardiolipin has two glycerols esterified to the phosphate of PA.

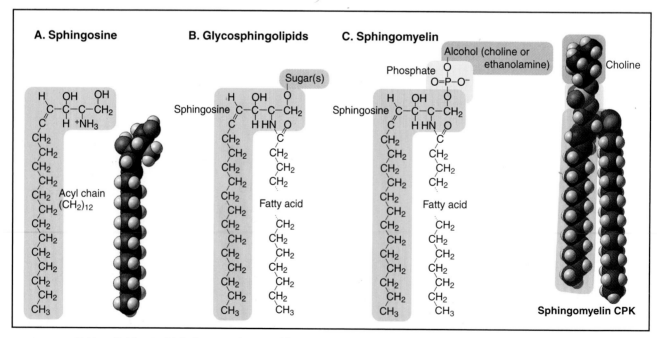

Figure 6-3 Sphingolipids. *A,* Stick figure and space-filling model of sphingosine. *B,* Diagram of the parts of a glycosphingolipid. *C,* Stick figure and space-filling model of sphingomyelin.

Sphingolipids

Most sugar-containing lipids of biological membranes are **sphingolipids.** Sphingolipids get their name from **sphingosine,** a nitrogen-containing base (Fig. 6–3) that is the structural counterpart of glycerol and one fatty acid of phosphoglycerides. Sphingosine carbons 1 to 3 have polar substituents. A double bond between C_4 and C_5 begins the hydrocarbon tail. Two variable features distinguish the various sphingolipids: the fatty acid attached by an amide bond to C_2 and the nature of the polar head groups esterified to the hydroxyl on C_1.

- The head groups of **glycosphingolipids** consist of one or more sugars. Some are neutral; others are negatively charged. Note the absence of phosphate. Sugar head groups of some glycosphingolipids serve as receptors for viruses.
- Alternatively, a phosphate ester can link a base to C_1. These so-called **sphingomyelins** have phosphorylcholine or phosphoethanolamine head groups just like PC and PE. Receptor-activated enzymes remove phosphorylcholine from sphingomyelin to produce the second messenger ceramide (see Chapter 28).

The physical properties of sphingolipids are similar to those of phosphoglycerides, with which they are found in many biologic membranes. The hydrocarbon tail of sphingosine and the fatty acid contribute to the hydrophobic bilayer, and polar head groups are exposed on the surface.

Cholesterol

Sterols are the third major class of membrane lipids. In animals, cholesterol (Fig. 6–4) is the major sterol. Plants, lower eukaryotes, and bacteria have other sterols in their membranes. Cholesterol is largely apolar, but in a bilayer, the hydroxyl on C_3 is oriented toward the surface. Cholesterol contributes to the fluidity of membranes by perturbing the packing of hydrocarbon chains in the bilayer.

Cholesterol is vital to metabolism, being situated at the crossroads of several metabolic pathways, including those that synthesize steroid hormones (such as estrogen, testosterone, and cortisol), vitamin D, and bile salts secreted by the liver. Cholesterol itself is synthesized (see Fig. 20–14) from **isopentyl** (5-carbon) building blocks that form 10-carbon **(geranyl),** 15-carbon **(farnesyl),** and 20-carbon **(geranylgeranyl) isoprenoids.** As described later, these isoprenoids are used as hydrocarbon anchors for many important membrane-associated proteins. Isoprenoids are also precursors of natural rubber and of cofactors present in visual pigments.

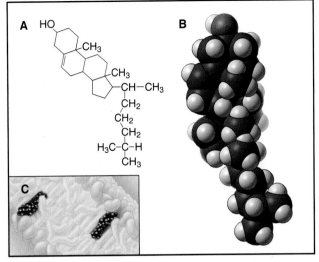

Figure 6–4 Cholesterol. *A,* Stick figure. *B,* Space-filling model. *C,* Disposition of cholesterol in a lipid bilayer with the hydroxyl oriented toward the surface. The rigid sterol nucleus tends to order fluid bilayers in the region between C_1 and C_{10} of the fatty acids, but promotes motion of the fatty acyl chains deeper in the bilayer owing to its wedge shape.

Glycolipids

Cells have three types of glycolipids: (1) sphingolipids (the predominant form); (2) glycerol glycolipids with sugar chains attached to the hydroxyl on C_3 of diglycerides; and (3) **glycosylphosphatidylinositols (GPI).** Some glycosylphosphatidylinositols simply have a short carbohydrate chain on the hydroxyl of inositol C_2. Others use a short sugar chain to link C_6 of phosphatidylinositol to the C terminus of a protein (see Fig. 6–9).

Triglycerides

Triglycerides are simply glycerol with fatty acids esterified to all three carbons. Lacking a polar head group, they are not incorporated into membrane bilayers. Instead, triglycerides form large, oily droplets in the cytoplasm that are a convenient way to store fatty acids as reserves of metabolic energy. In white adipose cells, specialized for lipid storage, the triglyceride droplet occupies most of the cytoplasm (see Chapter 30). Mitochondria oxidize fatty acids and convert the energy in their covalent bonds into ATP (see Chapter 10).

▌ Physical Structure of the Fluid Membrane Bilayer

A variety of biophysical methods have shown that lipids in a bilayer are highly dynamic. Fatty acid chains undergo internal motions on a picosecond time scale, and each phosphoglyceride diffuses laterally in the plane of the bilayer on a millisecond time scale. Rarely (about 10^{-5} s^{-1}), a neutral phosphoglyceride, such as PC, flips unassisted from one side of a bilayer to the other. Charged phosphoglycerides are slower. Proteins can facilitate this flipping in cellular membranes. Despite all the lateral movement of the molecules, phospholipid bilayers are stable and impermeable to polar or charged compounds, even those as small as Na^+ or Cl^-. This poor electrical conductivity is essential for many biological processes (see Chapters 7 to 10). Small, uncharged molecules, such as water and glycerol, pass slowly across lipid bilayers.

An atomic model of a phosphoglyceride bilayer (Fig. 6–5) accounts for the physical properties of biological membranes. The organization of the bilayer with the hydrocarbon chains on the inside and polar head groups facing the surrounding water arises naturally from the amphipathic nature of phosphoglycerides. The atomic model emphasizes the tremendous

disorder of the lipid molecules, as expected for a liquid. Polar head groups vary widely in their orientation, and some protrude far into water. At the atomic level, this makes the bilayer surface very rough. The average orientation of phosphorylcholine head groups nearly parallels the bilayer instead of sticking out into water. Hydrocarbon tails are highly irregular and far from straight, since about 25% of the bonds are in the bent (gauche) configuration. The molecular density is lowest in the middle of the bilayer.

Lipid molecules diffuse relatively rapidly in the plane of a bilayer. A typical diffusion coefficient for a membrane lipid is approximately 10^{-8} cm^2 s^{-1}, so given that the rate of diffusion is $2(D\ t)^{1/2}$ (t = time), a lipid molecule moves laterally about 1 $\mu m/s$ in the plane of the membrane. Thus, a diffusing lipid circumnavigates the membrane of a bacterium in a few seconds.

In the model, water penetrates the bilayer only to the level of the deepest carbonyl oxygens, leaving a

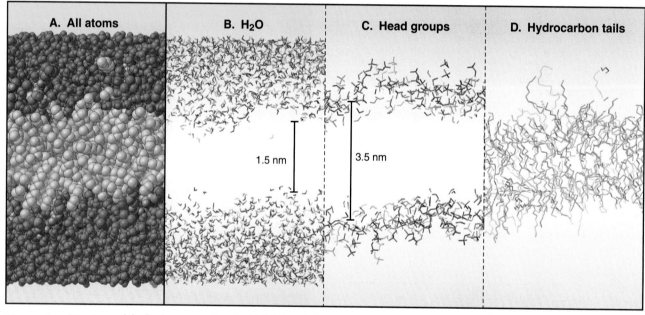

Figure 6–5 Atomic model of a hydrated phosphatidylcholine bilayer determined by simulation on a supercomputer. *A,* Space-filling model with all the atoms in the simulation. The water molecules are red. The polar regions of phosphatidylcholine (PC) from the carbonyl oxygen to the choline nitrogen are blue. Hydrocarbon tails are yellow. *B* to *D,* Stick figures. *B,* Water molecules only. *C,* Polar regions of PC from the carbonyl oxygen to the choline nitrogen only. *D,* Hydrocarbon tails only.

This model was calculated from first principles rather than experimental data, such as x-ray diffraction or NMR. This computational approach is both necessary and appropriate, as a lipid bilayer is a fluid without a regular structure. Such models account for virtually all molecular parameters (electron density, surface roughness, distance between phosphates of the two halves, area per lipid [0.6 nm^2], and depth of water penetration) of similar bilayers obtained by averaging techniques, including NMR, x-ray diffraction, and neutron diffraction. The simulation started with 100 PC molecules (based on an x-ray diffraction structure of PC crystals) in a regular bilayer with 1050 molecules of bulk phase water on each side. Taking into account surface tension and distribution of charge on lipid and water, the computer simulated the molecular motion of all atoms on a picosecond time scale using simple newtonian mechanics. After less than 100 picoseconds of simulated time (taking weeks of computation), the liquid phase of the lipids appeared. The model shown here is after 300 picoseconds of simulated time. (Courtesy of E. Jakobsson, University of Illinois, Urbana. Redrawn from Chiu S-W, et al.: Incorporation of surface tension into molecular dynamics simulation of an interface: A fluid phase lipid bilayer membrane. Biophys J 69:1230–1245, 1995.)

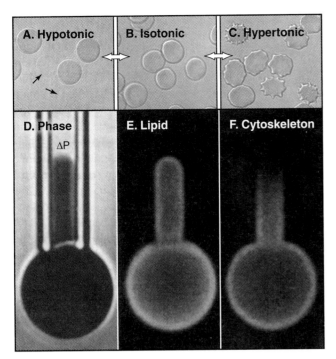

Figure 6-6 Membrane deformability illustrated by the plasma membrane of human red blood cells. *A* to *C,* Differential interference contrast light micrographs. In isotonic medium, the cell is a biconcave disk. In hypotonic medium, water enters the cytoplasm and the cell rounds up. The cell will burst *(arrows)* when the area of the membrane cannot accommodate the volume. In hypertonic medium, water leaves the cell and the membrane is thrown into spikes and folds. *D,* Phase contrast micrograph showing that the plasma membrane is flexible enough to be drawn by suction into a capillary tube. *E,* Fluorescence micrograph showing membrane lipids, marked with a fluorescent dye, evenly surround the membrane extension. *F,* The elastic membrane skeleton, marked with another fluorescent dye, stretches into the capillary, but not to the tip of the extension. (*D* to *F,* Courtesy of N. Mohandas, Lawrence Berkeley Laboratory, Berkeley, CA. Reference: Discher D, Mohandas N, Evans, E: Molecular maps of red cell deformation. Science 266:1032–1035, 1994.)

dehydrated plane about 1.5 nm thick in the center of the bilayer. Nevertheless, enough water moves across the bilayer to give it a modest permeability to water. Although not visible in the figure, water molecules near the bilayer tend to orient with their negative dipole toward the hydrocarbon interior. This generates an electrical potential (positive inside) between the hydrocarbon and the aqueous phase despite an oppositely oriented potential arising from the P–N dipole of the head groups. This inside positive potential may contribute to the barrier to the transfer of positively charged polypeptides across membranes (see Chapter 20).

The atomic model also accounts for the mechanical properties of membranes. Although bilayers neither stretch nor compress readily, they are very flexible owing to rapid fluctuations in the arrangement of the lipids. Thus, little force is required to deform bilayers into the complex shapes observed for cell membranes. Both these features are illustrated by the response of a red blood cell plasma membrane to changes in volume (Fig. 6–6). Because the membrane area is constant, a reduction in volume throws the membrane into folds, whereas swelling distends it to a spherical shape, until it eventually bursts. One can also draw out a narrow tube of membrane by sucking gently on the surface of a cell.

Biological membranes, consisting of a mixture of phosphoglycerides, sphingolipids, and cholesterol (Fig. 6–7), have physical properties similar to a bilayer of pure phosphatidylcholine—that is, limited permeability to ions, high electrical resistance, and the ability to self-seal. The length of fatty acids and the presence of unsaturated bonds strongly influence the physical properties of membranes. Fatty acids with 18 or more carbons are solid at physiological temperatures unless they contain double bonds. Hence, lipids in biological

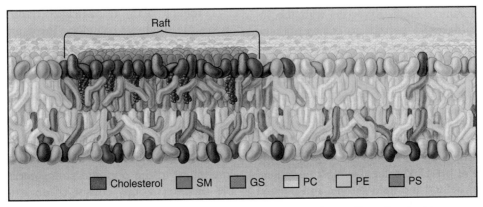

Figure 6-7 Drawing of the lipid composition of a plasma membrane illustrating the heterogeneity of the lipids and the asymmetrical distribution of the lipids between the two halves of the bilayer. Sphingomyelin (SM) and cholesterol form a small raft in the external leaflet. GS, glycosphingolipid; PC, phosphatidylcholine; PE, phosphatidylethanolamine; PS, phosphatidylserine.

anchored protein. If challenged by an antibody response from the host, the parasite sheds the protein by hydrolysis of the lipid anchor and expresses a variant protein to evade the immune system.

Electrostatic Interaction with Phospholipids

As postulated in the 1930s (see Fig. 6–1), a number of soluble cytoplasmic proteins bind the head groups of membrane lipids. The full range of these electrostatic interactions has yet to be explored, as the concept was largely neglected for two decades after the recognition of transmembrane proteins and the emergence of the fluid mosaic model of membranes. Annexins, a family of calcium-binding proteins implicated in membrane fusion reactions, bind tightly to phosphatidylserine. Myosin-I motor proteins (see Chapter 39) also bind strongly to phosphatidylserine, a possible step in targeting to cellular membranes.

Partial Penetration of the Lipid Bilayer

For years it was believed that no proteins partially penetrate the lipid bilayer. Either they traversed the membrane fully one or more times, or they bound to the surface. However, some peptide venoms (such as bee venom mellitin) intercalate into half of a lipid bilayer. Hydrophobic α-helices of prostaglandin H_2 synthase (see Chapter 28) are also postulated to anchor the enzyme to membranes by partially penetrating the lipid bilayer.

Association with Integral Proteins

Many peripheral proteins bind cytoplasmic domains of integral membrane proteins, such as catenins binding transmembrane cell adhesion proteins called cadherins. These protein–protein interactions may provide more specificity and higher affinity than do the interactions of peripheral proteins with membrane lipids. Such protein–protein interactions anchor the cytoskeleton to transmembrane adhesion proteins (see Chapter 32) and guide the assembly of coated vesicles during endocytosis (see Chapter 23). Protein–protein interactions also provide a way to transmit information across a membrane. Ligand binding to the extracellular domain of a transmembrane receptor can change the conformation of its cytoplasmic domain, promoting interactions with cytoplasmic, signal-transducing proteins (see Chapters 26 and 29).

The **membrane skeleton** on the cytoplasmic surface of the plasma membrane of human red blood cells (Fig. 6–10) provided the first insights regarding interaction of peripheral and integral membrane proteins. Two types of integral membrane proteins—an anion carrier called Band 3 and glycophorin—anchor a two-dimensional network of fibrous proteins to the membrane. The main component of this network is a long, flexible, tetrameric, actin-binding protein called

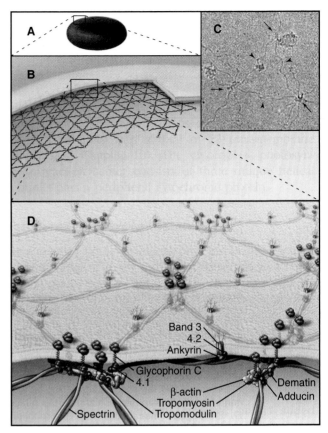

Figure 6–10 The membrane skeleton on the cytoplasmic surface of the red blood cell plasma membrane: whole cell (*A*), cut-away drawing (*B*), detailed drawing (*D*). Nodes consisting of a short actin filament and associated proteins interact with multiple spectrin molecules, which, in turn, bind to two transmembrane proteins: glycophorin and (via ankyrin) Band 3. *C*, An electron micrograph of the actin–spectrin network. (Courtesy of R. Josephs, University of Chicago.)

spectrin (after its discovery in lysed red blood cells, or "ghosts"; see Fig. 36–15). A linker protein called ankyrin binds tightly to both Band 3 and spectrin. About 35,000 nodes consisting of a short actin filament and associated proteins interconnect the elastic spectrin network. This membrane skeleton reinforces the bilayer, allowing a cell to recover its shape elastically after it is distorted by passage through the narrow lumen of blood capillaries.

Heterogeneous, Dynamic Behavior of Membrane Proteins

Several complementary methods can monitor the dynamic behavior of plasma membrane proteins (Fig. 6–11*A*). One approach—the one used originally—is to label proteins with a fluorescent dye, either by covalent modification or by attachment of an antibody with a bound fluorescent dye. After irreversibly bleaching fluorescent dyes in a small area of the mem-

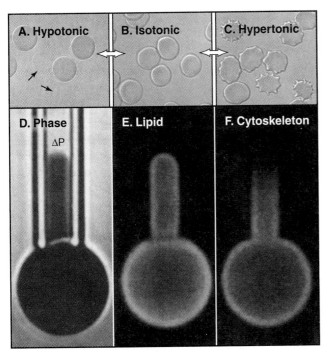

Figure 6-6 Membrane deformability illustrated by the plasma membrane of human red blood cells. *A to C,* Differential interference contrast light micrographs. In isotonic medium, the cell is a biconcave disk. In hypotonic medium, water enters the cytoplasm and the cell rounds up. The cell will burst *(arrows)* when the area of the membrane cannot accommodate the volume. In hypertonic medium, water leaves the cell and the membrane is thrown into spikes and folds. *D,* Phase contrast micrograph showing that the plasma membrane is flexible enough to be drawn by suction into a capillary tube. *E,* Fluorescence micrograph showing membrane lipids, marked with a fluorescent dye, evenly surround the membrane extension. *F,* The elastic membrane skeleton, marked with another fluorescent dye, stretches into the capillary, but not to the tip of the extension. (*D to F,* Courtesy of N. Mohandas, Lawrence Berkeley Laboratory, Berkeley, CA. Reference: Discher D, Mohandas N, Evans, E: Molecular maps of red cell deformation. Science 266:1032–1035, 1994.)

dehydrated plane about 1.5 nm thick in the center of the bilayer. Nevertheless, enough water moves across the bilayer to give it a modest permeability to water. Although not visible in the figure, water molecules near the bilayer tend to orient with their negative dipole toward the hydrocarbon interior. This generates an electrical potential (positive inside) between the hydrocarbon and the aqueous phase despite an oppositely oriented potential arising from the P−N dipole of the head groups. This inside positive potential may contribute to the barrier to the transfer of positively charged polypeptides across membranes (see Chapter 20).

The atomic model also accounts for the mechanical properties of membranes. Although bilayers neither stretch nor compress readily, they are very flexible owing to rapid fluctuations in the arrangement of the lipids. Thus, little force is required to deform bilayers into the complex shapes observed for cell membranes. Both these features are illustrated by the response of a red blood cell plasma membrane to changes in volume (Fig. 6–6). Because the membrane area is constant, a reduction in volume throws the membrane into folds, whereas swelling distends it to a spherical shape, until it eventually bursts. One can also draw out a narrow tube of membrane by sucking gently on the surface of a cell.

Biological membranes, consisting of a mixture of phosphoglycerides, sphingolipids, and cholesterol (Fig. 6–7), have physical properties similar to a bilayer of pure phosphatidylcholine—that is, limited permeability to ions, high electrical resistance, and the ability to self-seal. The length of fatty acids and the presence of unsaturated bonds strongly influence the physical properties of membranes. Fatty acids with 18 or more carbons are solid at physiological temperatures unless they contain double bonds. Hence, lipids in biological

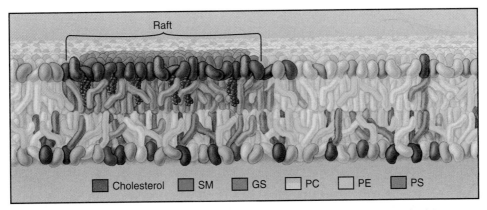

Figure 6-7 Drawing of the lipid composition of a plasma membrane illustrating the heterogeneity of the lipids and the asymmetrical distribution of the lipids between the two halves of the bilayer. Sphingomyelin (SM) and cholesterol form a small raft in the external leaflet. GS, glycosphingolipid; PC, phosphatidylcholine; PE, phosphatidylethanolamine; PS, phosphatidylserine.

membranes usually contain C16 saturated fatty acids and longer chain fatty acids with double bonds (C18 with one to three double bonds and C20 with four double bonds; see Table 6–1). Permanent bends created by double bonds and the presence of cholesterol contribute to bilayer fluidity by preventing tight packing of fatty acid tails in the middle of the bilayer.

Lipid composition varies considerably among various biological membranes. Moreover, lipids are usually distributed asymmetrically between the two halves of each bilayer. In plasma membranes, glycosphingolipids are outside and most phosphatidylserine is inside. PS asymmetry gives the cytoplasmic surface of the plasma membrane a net negative charge above and beyond that arising from the oriented water dipoles on the surface. This **lipid asymmetry** is established during biosynthesis of membranes (see Chapter 20) and is maintained as a result of the low rate of flipping of charged lipids from one side of a bilayer to the other.

Small islands of sphingolipids and cholesterol can form a separate phase in plasma membranes. These so-called **rafts,** which are about 50 nm in diameter, are held together in a more ordered phase by tight packing of saturated fatty acid tails and polar interactions of their head groups. Sphingolipids are predominantly in the outer leaflet of the bilayer; the lipids comprising the inner leaflet of rafts are not yet characterized. Rafts include transmembrane proteins, GPI-anchored proteins outside, and fatty acid–anchored proteins (such as Src tyrosine kinase) inside. Raft lipids and associated proteins diffuse together laterally on the membrane surface. Partitioning of plasma membrane proteins into raft and nonraft phases segregates some signaling molecules from each other.

Membrane Proteins

Integral membrane proteins cross the lipid bilayer, and peripheral membrane proteins associate with the inside or outside surfaces of the bilayer. Transmembrane segments of integral membrane proteins interact with hydrocarbon chains of the lipid bilayer and have few hydrophilic residues exposed on their transmembrane surfaces. Like other soluble proteins, peripheral membrane proteins have hydrophilic residues exposed on their surfaces and a core of hydrophobic residues. Chemical extraction experiments distinguish these two classes of membrane proteins. Alkaline solvents (e.g., 0.1 M carbonate at pH 11.3) solubilize most peripheral proteins, leaving behind the lipid bilayer and integral membrane proteins. Detergents, which interact with hydrophobic transmembrane segments, solubilize integral membrane proteins.

Integral Membrane Proteins

Atomic structures of about a dozen integral membrane proteins and primary structures of thousands of others show how proteins associate with lipid bilayers (Fig. 6–8). Many integral membrane proteins have a single peptide segment that fulfills the energetic criteria (Box 6–1) for a membrane-spanning α-helix. Glycophorin from the red blood cell membrane was the first characterized (see Fig. 6–8A). Nuclear magnetic resonance experiments established that the single **transmembrane segment** of glycophorin is an α-helix. This helix interacts more favorably with lipid acyl chains than with water. By analogy with glycophorin, it is generally accepted that single, 25-residue hydrophobic segments of other transmembrane proteins fold into α-helices. In many cases, independent evidence has confirmed that the single segment crosses the bilayer. For example, proteolytic enzymes might cleave the peptide at the predicted membrane interface. Potential glycosylation sites might be located outside the cell. Chemical or antibody labeling might identify parts of the protein inside or outside the cells.

The transmembrane helix of glycophorin has a strong tendency to form homodimers in the plane of the membrane. Dimers are favored because complementary surfaces on a pair of helices interact more precisely with each other than they interact with lipids. The increase in entropy associated with dissociation of lipids from interacting protein surfaces (comparable to the hydrophobic effect in water) drives the reaction.

Transmembrane segments of integral membrane proteins that cross the bilayer more than once are folded into α-helices or β-strands. Thus, all backbone amides and carbonyls are fully hydrogen-bonded to minimize the energy required to bury the backbone in the hydrophobic lipid bilayer. For the same reason, most amino acid side chains in contact with fatty acyl chains in the bilayer are hydrophobic.

Proteins with all α-helical transmembrane segments are the most common. These are found in bacteriorhodopsin (see Fig. 6–8B and the section on related seven-helix receptors in Chapter 26), pumps (see Chapter 7), carriers (see Chapter 8), many ion channels (see Chapter 9), cytochrome oxidase (see Chapter 10) and the photosynthetic reaction center (see Chapter 10). All these proteins have polar and charged residues in the plane of the bilayer, generally facing away from the lipid toward the interior of the protein, in contrast to the opposite arrangement in water-soluble proteins. Porins consist of an extended β-strand barrel with a hydrophobic exterior and a channel inside (see Fig. 6–8C). The acetylcholine receptor has one clear transmembrane helix that lines an aqueous

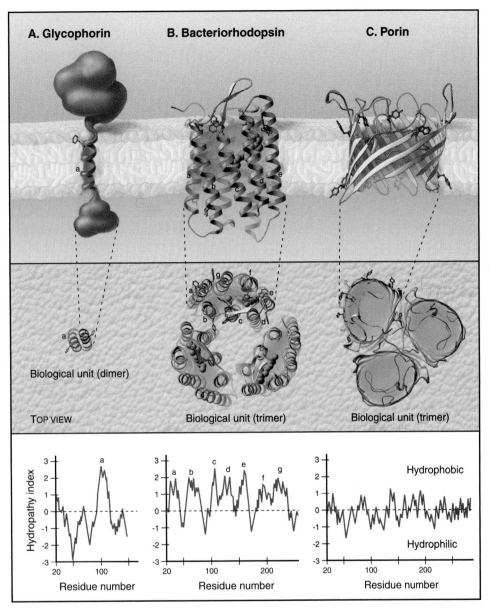

Figure 6–8 Structures of representative integral membrane proteins. *Top row,* Views across the lipid bilayer. *Middle row,* Views in the plane of the lipid bilayer. *Bottom row,* Hydrophobicity analysis. *A,* Glycophorin, a human red blood cell protein, has a single transmembrane α-helix. The extracellular and cytoplasmic domains are artistic conceptions. The transmembrane helices have a strong tendency to form homodimers in the plane of the membrane. (PDB file: 1MSR.) *B,* Bacteriorhodopsin, a light-driven proton pump from the plasma membrane of a halophilic bacterium, has seven transmembrane helices. This structure was first determined by electron microscopy of two-dimensional crystals and extended to higher resolution by x-ray diffraction. (PDB file: 1AT9.) *C,* Porin, a nonselective channel protein from the outer membrane of a bacterium, is composed entirely of transmembrane β-strands. This structure was determined by x-ray crystallography of three-dimensional crystals. (PDB file: 1PRN.) Hydropathy plots are calculated from the energy required to transfer an amino acid from an organic solvent to water. One sums the transfer free energy for segments of 20 residues. Segments with large, positive (unfavorable) transfer free energies (around 1.5 on this scale) are more soluble in the hydrophobic interior of a membrane bilayer than in water, and thus are candidates for membrane-spanning segments.

AMINO ACID SEQUENCES IDENTIFY CANDIDATE TRANSMEMBRANE SEGMENTS

Amino acid sequences of integral membrane proteins frequently provide important clues about segments of the polypeptide that cross the lipid bilayer. Each crossing segment must be long enough to span the bilayer with a minimum of charged or polar groups in contact with the lipid (see Fig. 6–8). Polar backbone amide and carbonyl atoms are buried in α-helices or β-sheets to avoid contact with lipid. In many transmembrane segments, aromatic residues project into the lipid near the level where acyl chains are bonded to the lipid head groups. A helix of 20 to 25 residues or a β-strand of 10 residues are long enough (3.0 to 3.8 nm) to span a lipid bilayer. Quantitative analysis of the side chain **hydropathy** (aversion to water) of the sequence of an integral membrane protein usually identifies one or more hydrophobic sequences long enough to cross a bilayer (see Fig. 6–8).

The approach works best for a protein like glycophorin, in which the single transmembrane helix has mostly apolar side chains surrounded by hydrocarbon chains. If a protein has multiple transmembrane helices, some may escape detection by hydrophobicity analysis because the helices may group together to surround a hydrophilic channel lined with charged and polar side chains. For example, two of seven transmembrane helices of bacteriorhodopsin contain charged residues facing the interior of the protein, and they barely qualify as transmembrane segments on the basis of their hydrophobicity. Transmembrane β-strands are even more challenging. None of the transmembrane strands of porin qualify in terms of hydrophobicity criteria because they are short and many contain polar residues. Only one of the four presumed transmembrane helices of the acetylcholine receptor has been confirmed in the low-resolution structure. The others may be β-strands. Soluble proteins generally lack hydrophobic sequences as long as 25 residues, but exceptions exist that may be misidentified as a transmembrane helix. Independent biochemical or structural data are required to confirm the identity of transmembrane polypeptides.

channel surrounded by other transmembrane segments that may be β-strands or α-helices (see Fig. 9–11).

Many transmembrane proteins consist of multiple subunits that associate in the plane of the bilayer. Bacteriorhodopsin self-associates to form extended two-dimensional crystals in the plane of the membrane. Bacterial and mitochondrial porins have three identical subunits, each with an aqueous pore. Many ion channels are formed by association of four similar or identical subunits with a pore at their interface. Acetylcholine receptors are a pentamer of identical or related subunits. Together, they form a cation channel that opens transiently when the neurotransmitter acetylcholine binds to the two α-subunits (see Chapter 9). Bacterial cytochrome oxidase is an assembly of four different subunits with a total of 22 transmembrane helices (see Chapter 10). The chloroplast photosynthetic reaction center consists of three unique helical subunits plus a peripheral cytochrome protein.

Peripheral Membrane Proteins

Six strategies bind peripheral proteins to the surfaces of membranes (Fig. 6–9). One of three different types of acyl chains can anchor a protein to a membrane by inserting into the lipid bilayer. Other proteins bind electrostatically to membrane lipids, and some insert partially into the lipid bilayer. Many peripheral proteins bind directly or indirectly to integral membrane proteins.

Isoprenoid Tails

A 15-carbon isoprenoid (farnesyl) tail is added posttranslationally to the side chain of a cysteine residue near the C terminus of the guanosine triphosphatase (GTPase) Ras (see Chapter 27) and many other proteins. The enzyme making this modification recognizes the target cysteine followed by two aliphatic amino acids plus any other amino acid (a CAAX recognition site). Membrane attachment by this farnesyl chain is required for Ras to participate in growth factor signaling (see Chapter 29).

Myristoyl Tails

Myristate, a 14-carbon saturated fatty acid, anchors the tyrosine kinase Src (see Chapter 27) and other proteins involved in cellular signaling to the cytoplasmic face of the plasma membrane. Myristate is added to the amino group of an N-terminal glycine during the biosynthesis of these proteins. Insertion of this single fatty acyl chain into a lipid bilayer is so weak ($K_d \sim 10^{-4}$ M) that additional electrostatic interactions between basic side chains of the protein and head groups of acidic phosphoglycerides are required to maintain attachment to the membrane. As a consequence, phosphorylation can dissociate some myristoylated proteins from membranes by competing with these secondary electrostatic interactions.

Glycosylphosphatidylinositol Tails

A short oligosaccharide–phosphoglyceride tail links a variety of proteins to the outer surface of the

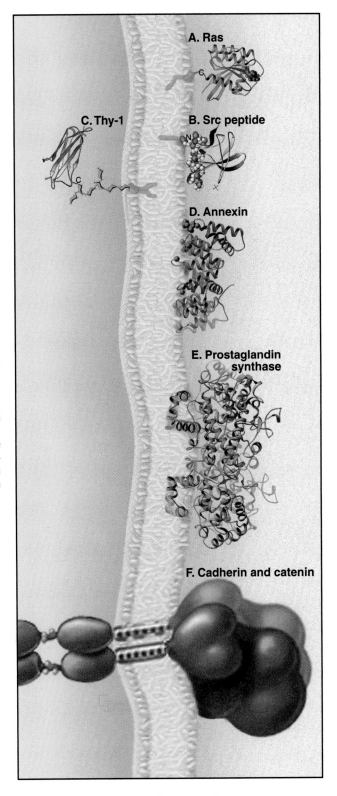

Figure 6-9 Six different ways for peripheral membrane proteins to associate with the lipid bilayer. *A,* A C-terminal isoprenoid tail attaches Ras to the bilayer. (PDB file: 121P.) *B,* An N-terminal myristoyl tail binds Src weakly to the bilayer. Electrostatic interactions between acidic lipids and basic amino acids stabilize the interaction. *C,* A C-terminal GPI tail anchors Thy-1 (similar to an immunoglobulin variable domain) to the bilayer. *D,* Electrostatic interactions with phospholipids bind annexin to the bilayer. (PDB file: 1A8A.) *E,* Hydrophobic helices of prostaglandin H$_2$ synthase are postulated to penetrate the lipid bilayer partially. (PDB file: 1CQE.) *F,* The peripheral protein α-catenin associates with the cytoplasmic portion of the transmembrane adhesion protein cadherin.

plasma membrane. The C terminus of these proteins is attached covalently to the oligosaccharide, and the two fatty acyl chains of phosphatidylinositol anchor the link to the lipid bilayer. In animal cells, this glycosylphosphatidylinositol (GPI) anchors important

plasma membrane proteins, including enzymes (acetylcholine esterase; see Chapter 10), adhesion proteins (T-cadherin; see Chapter 32), and cell surface antigens (Thy-1). The protozoan parasite *Trypanosoma brucei* covers itself with a high concentration of a GPI-anchored protein. If challenged by an antibody response from the host, the parasite sheds the protein by hydrolysis of the lipid anchor and expresses a variant protein to evade the immune system.

Electrostatic Interaction with Phospholipids

As postulated in the 1930s (see Fig. 6–1), a number of soluble cytoplasmic proteins bind the head groups of membrane lipids. The full range of these electrostatic interactions has yet to be explored, as the concept was largely neglected for two decades after the recognition of transmembrane proteins and the emergence of the fluid mosaic model of membranes. Annexins, a family of calcium-binding proteins implicated in membrane fusion reactions, bind tightly to phosphatidylserine. Myosin-I motor proteins (see Chapter 39) also bind strongly to phosphatidylserine, a possible step in targeting to cellular membranes.

Partial Penetration of the Lipid Bilayer

For years it was believed that no proteins partially penetrate the lipid bilayer. Either they traversed the membrane fully one or more times, or they bound to the surface. However, some peptide venoms (such as bee venom mellitin) intercalate into half of a lipid bilayer. Hydrophobic α-helices of prostaglandin H_2 synthase (see Chapter 28) are also postulated to anchor the enzyme to membranes by partially penetrating the lipid bilayer.

Association with Integral Proteins

Many peripheral proteins bind cytoplasmic domains of integral membrane proteins, such as catenins binding transmembrane cell adhesion proteins called cadherins. These protein–protein interactions may provide more specificity and higher affinity than do the interactions of peripheral proteins with membrane lipids. Such protein–protein interactions anchor the cytoskeleton to transmembrane adhesion proteins (see Chapter 32) and guide the assembly of coated vesicles during endocytosis (see Chapter 23). Protein–protein interactions also provide a way to transmit information across a membrane. Ligand binding to the extracellular domain of a transmembrane receptor can change the conformation of its cytoplasmic domain, promoting interactions with cytoplasmic, signal-transducing proteins (see Chapters 26 and 29).

The **membrane skeleton** on the cytoplasmic surface of the plasma membrane of human red blood cells (Fig. 6–10) provided the first insights regarding interaction of peripheral and integral membrane proteins. Two types of integral membrane proteins—an anion carrier called Band 3 and glycophorin—anchor a two-dimensional network of fibrous proteins to the membrane. The main component of this network is a long, flexible, tetrameric, actin-binding protein called

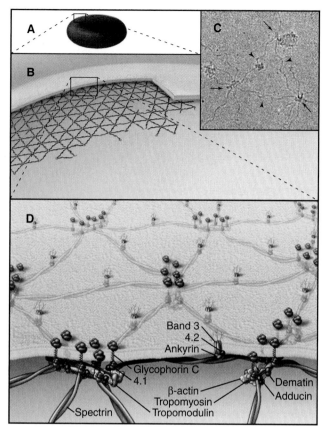

Figure 6–10 The membrane skeleton on the cytoplasmic surface of the red blood cell plasma membrane: whole cell (*A*), cut-away drawing (*B*), detailed drawing (*D*). Nodes consisting of a short actin filament and associated proteins interact with multiple spectrin molecules, which, in turn, bind to two transmembrane proteins: glycophorin and (via ankyrin) Band 3. *C*, An electron micrograph of the actin–spectrin network. (Courtesy of R. Josephs, University of Chicago.)

spectrin (after its discovery in lysed red blood cells, or "ghosts"; see Fig. 36–15). A linker protein called ankyrin binds tightly to both Band 3 and spectrin. About 35,000 nodes consisting of a short actin filament and associated proteins interconnect the elastic spectrin network. This membrane skeleton reinforces the bilayer, allowing a cell to recover its shape elastically after it is distorted by passage through the narrow lumen of blood capillaries.

Heterogeneous, Dynamic Behavior of Membrane Proteins

Several complementary methods can monitor the dynamic behavior of plasma membrane proteins (Fig. 6–11*A*). One approach—the one used originally—is to label proteins with a fluorescent dye, either by covalent modification or by attachment of an antibody with a bound fluorescent dye. After irreversibly bleaching fluorescent dyes in a small area of the mem-

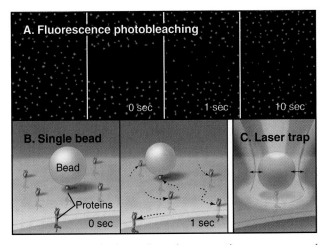

Figure 6-11 Methods used to document the movements of membrane proteins. *A,* Fluorescence recovery after photobleaching. *B,* Single-particle tracking. *C,* Optical trapping.

brane with a spot of intense light, one observes the fluorescence over time with a microscope. If the test protein is mobile, unbleached proteins from surrounding areas will move into the bleached area. This fluorescence recovery after **photobleaching** (FRAP) assay reveals that a fraction of the population of most membrane proteins diffuses freely in two dimensions in the plane of the membrane, but that a substantial fraction is immobilized, since the recovery from photobleaching is incomplete. The second approach is to label individual membrane proteins with antibodies or lectins (carbohydrate-binding proteins) attached to small particles of gold or plastic beads. High-contrast light microscopy can follow the motion of a particle attached to a membrane protein. Despite their size, the particles have minimal effects on diffusion of membrane proteins. The third method is an extension of this single-particle tracking. Instead of merely watching spontaneous movements, the investigator can grab a particle in an **optical trap** created by focusing an infrared laser beam through the microscope objective. Manipulation of particles with an optical trap reveals

what happens when force is applied to a membrane protein.

Membrane proteins exhibit a wide range of dynamic behaviors (Fig. 6–12). Some molecules diffuse freely. Others diffuse intermittently, alternating with periods of restricted movement. A substantial number of membrane proteins are immobilized, presumably by direct or indirect associations with the membrane skeleton or cytoskeleton. Others exhibit long-distance directed movements.

The whole population of a given type of membrane protein (e.g., a cell adhesion protein) may exhibit more than one class of dynamic behavior. For example, most proteins with GPI anchors diffuse freely, as expected from their association with the lipid bilayer, but a fraction of any GPI-anchored protein has restricted mobility. Some transmembrane proteins also diffuse freely, but a fraction may become trapped or immobilized at any time. Diffusing proteins must be free of interactions with the membrane skeleton and with anchored membrane proteins. Cell adhesion proteins (cadherins; see Chapter 32) and nutrient receptors (transferrin receptors; see Chapter 23) are examples of transmembrane proteins that diffuse intermittently. They alternate between free diffusion and temporary trapping for 3 to 30 seconds in local domains measuring less than 0.5 μm in diameter. In some cases, trapping depends on the cytoplasmic tails of transmembrane proteins, which are thought to interact reversibly with the cytoskeleton or with immobilized membrane proteins. Tugs with an optical trap show that the cages that confine these particles are elastic, as expected for cytoskeletal networks. Extracellular domains of these proteins may also interact with adjacent immobilized proteins. Immobilized proteins do not diffuse freely, and particles attached to them resist displacement by optical traps. Remarkably, the lipid bilayer can flow past immobilized transmembrane elements without disrupting the membrane. If the plasma membrane of a red blood cell is sucked into a narrow pipette (see Fig. 6–6), lipids of the fluid

Figure 6-12 Movements of proteins in the plane of membranes. *A,* Transient confinement by obstacle clusters. *B,* Directed movements. *C,* Transient confinement by the membrane skeleton. *D,* Free diffusion. (See Jacobson K, Sheets ED, Simson R: Revisiting the fluid mosaic model of membranes. Science 268:1441–1442, 1995, for more information.)

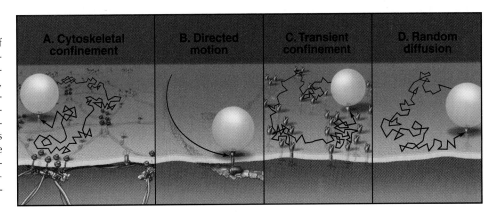

membrane bilayer extend uniformly over the protrusion, leaving behind the immobilized membrane proteins and the membrane skeleton.

Some membrane proteins undergo long-distance translational movements in relatively straight lines. Diffusion cannot account for these linear movements, so they must be powered by motor proteins attached to cytoplasmic domains. Because disruption of cytoplasmic actin filaments by drugs impedes these movements, myosins (see Chapter 39) are the most likely, but still unproved, motors for these movements. In some instances, members of the integrin family of adhesion proteins (see Chapter 32) use this transport system.

Movement of membrane proteins in the plane of the membrane is essential for many cellular functions. During receptor-mediated endocytosis, receptors are concentrated in coated pits before internalization (see Chapter 23). Similarly, transduction of many signals from outside the cell depends on formation of receptor dimers or trimers (see Chapter 26). Some freely diffusing receptor subunits may be brought together by binding extracellular ligands. In other cases, ligand binding changes the conformation of preexisting dimers in the membrane. In both cases, juxtaposition of the cytoplasmic domains of receptor subunits activates downstream signaling mechanisms, such as protein kinases. Similarly, clustering of adhesion receptors, allowed by movements in the plane of the plasma membrane, enhances binding of cells to their neighbors or to the extracellular matrix (see Chapter 32).

Selected Readings

Brown DA, London E: Functions of lipid rafts in biological membranes. Annu Rev Cell Dev Biol 14:111–136, 1998.

Casey PJ, Seabra MC: Protein prenyltransferases. J Biol Chem 271:5289–5292, 1996.

Dowhan W: Molecular basis for membrane phospholipid diversity: Why are there so many lipids? Annu Rev Biochem 66:199–232, 1997.

Edwards PA, Ericsson J: Sterols and isoprenoids: Signaling molecules derived from the cholesterol biosynthesis pathway. Annu Rev Biochem 68:157–186, 1999.

Gahmberg GG, Tolvanen M: Why mammalian surface proteins are glycoproteins. Trends Biochem Sci 21:308–311, 1996.

Jakobsson E: Computer simulation studies of biological membranes: Progress, promise and pitfalls. Trends Biochem Sci 22:339–344, 1997.

White SH, Wimley WC: Membrane protein folding and stability: Physical principles. Annu Rev Biophys Biomol Struct 28:319–365, 1999.

Zhang FL, Casey PJ: Protein prenylation: Molecular mechanisms and functional consequences. Annu Rev Biochem 65:241–270, 1996.

chapter 7

MEMBRANE PUMPS

Membrane Permeability: An Introduction

Although lipid bilayers provide a barrier to diffusion of ions and polar molecules larger than about 150 D, protein pores provide selective passages for these larger molecules across membranes. These proteins allow cells to control solute traffic across membranes, an essential feature of many physiological processes. Integral proteins that control membrane permeability fall into three broad classes—pumps, carriers, and channels—each with distinct properties (Fig. 7–1).

- **Pumps** are enzymes that utilize energy from adenosine triphosphate (ATP), light, or (rarely) other sources to move ions (generally, cations) and other solutes across membranes at relatively modest rates. They establish concentration gradients between membrane-bound compartments.
- **Carriers** are enzyme-like proteins that provide passive pathways for solutes to move across membranes down their concentration gradients from a region of higher concentration to lower concentration. Each conformational change in a carrier protein translocates a limited number of solutes across the membrane. Carriers use ion gradients as a source of energy to perform a remarkable variety of work. Some carriers use translocation of an ion down its concentration gradient to drive another ion or solute up a concentration gradient.
- **Channels** are ion-specific pores that typically open and close transiently in a regulated manner. When a channel is open, a flood of ions passes quickly across the membrane through the channel, driven by electrical and concentration gradients. The movement of ions through open channels controls the electrical potential across membranes,

so that changes in channel activity produce rapid electrical signals in excitable membranes of nerves, muscles, and other cells.

This chapter and the three that follow it consider, in turn, the three classes of proteins that control membrane permeability. Pumps are discussed first because they create the solute gradients required for the function of carriers and channels. The concluding chapter in this section, entitled Membrane Physiology, illustrates how pumps, carriers, and channels work together to perform a remarkable variety of functions. An important point is that differential expression of a subset of isoforms of these proteins in specific membranes allows differentiated cells to perform a wide range of complex functions.

Membrane Pumps

Protein pumps transport ions and other solutes across membranes up concentration gradients as great as 100,000-fold. Energy for this task can come from a variety of sources: light, oxidation-reduction reactions, or, most commonly, hydrolysis of ATP (Table 7–1). Energy is conserved in the form of transmembrane electrical or chemical gradients of the transported ion or solute. The potential energy in these ion gradients drives a variety of energy-requiring processes (Fig. 7–2). Most known biologic pumps translocate cations. Although they could just as well move anions, cations were selected during the evolution of early life forms 3 billion years ago.

Pumps are called **primary active transporters** because they transduce electromagnetic or chemical energy directly into transmembrane concentration gradients. Some carriers use ion gradients created by pumps to drive the uphill movement of other ions or

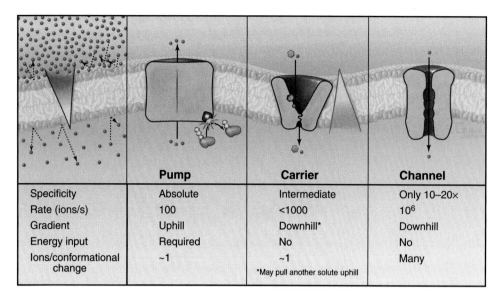

	Pump	**Carrier**	**Channel**
Specificity	Absolute	Intermediate	Only 10–20×
Rate (ions/s)	100	<1000	10^6
Gradient	Uphill	Downhill*	Downhill
Energy input	Required	No	No
Ions/conformational change	~1	~1	Many
		*May pull another solute uphill	

Figure 7-1 Properties of the three types of proteins that transport ions and other solutes across membranes. The triangle represents the concentration gradients of Na^+ (*blue*) and glucose (*green*) across the membrane.

solutes, so these are called **secondary transporters** (see Chapter 8). Channels are **passive transporters**, allowing net diffusion of ions and water only down their concentration gradients (see Chapter 9).

▌ Diversity of Membrane Pumps

A vast array of integral membrane proteins can capture energy from an external source to pump ions and other solutes across biologic membranes (see Table 7–1). The protein families differ in their energy sources and transported materials. Fortunately, these pumps had a limited number of common ancestors, providing a relatively simple classification and generalizations about their structures and mechanisms. Given the importance of pumps in establishing transmembrane electrochemical gradients, the simplicity of this list is remarkable. Its brevity may be attributable to the

fact that a single pump can drive a whole host of secondary reactions mediated by different carriers.

This chapter considers four representative pumps, with an emphasis on examples for which high-resolution structures are available. Chapter 10 provides additional details on H^+ translocation by redox-driven cytochrome *c* oxidase and the role of transport adenosinetriphosphatases (ATPases) in ATP synthesis by mitochondria and chloroplasts. Microbiology texts provide more information on pumps driven by decarboxylases and pyrophosphatases.

▌ Light-driven Proton Pumping by Bacteriorhodopsin

Owing to its simplicity, small size, and the availability of a high-resolution structure (Fig. 7–3), more is known about light-driven transport of protons by **bac-**

table 7–1

DIVERSITY OF MEMBRANE PUMPS*

Energy Source	Pump	Driven Substance	Distribution
Light	Bacteriorhodopsin	H^+	Halobacteria
	Halorhodopsin	Cl^-	Halobacteria
Light	Photoredox	H^+	Photosynthetic organisms
Redox potential	Electron transport chain NADH oxidase	H^+	Mitochondria, bacteria
		Na^+	Alkalophilic bacteria
Decarboxylation	Ion-transporting decarboxylases	Na^+	Bacteria
Pyrophosphate	H^+-pyrophosphatase	H^+	Plant vacuoles, fungi, bacteria
ATP	Transport ATPases	Various ions and solutes	Universal

*Each class of pumps has a different evolutionary origin and structure.

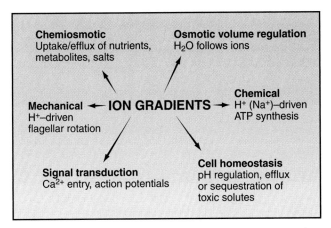

Figure 7-2 Cellular processes driven by the energy stored in ion gradients.

teriorhodopsin than about any other pump. This pump allows the halophilic (salt-loving) Archaea *Halobacterium halobium* to convert light energy into a proton gradient across its plasma membrane. The 26-kD pump packs into two-dimensional crystalline arrays in the plasma membrane. The polypeptide is folded into seven α-helices that cross the lipid bilayer. The light-absorbing chromophore retinal (vitamin A aldehyde), is bound covalently to the side chain of lysine 216 (Lys216) via a Schiff base. This chromophore makes the protein and the membrane purple.

Bacteriorhodopsin absorbs light and uses the energy to pump protons out of the cell. A proton-driven ATP synthase uses this proton gradient to make ATP (see later section). The proton pathway includes the side chains of aspartate 96 (Asp96), aspartate 85 (Asp85), glutamate 204 (Glu204), and the Schiff base. Local environments give the two aspartates remarkably different ionization constant (pK_a) values. Asp96 has a very high pK_a of about 10, so it can serve as a proton donor. Asp85 has a low pK_a of about 2, so it serves as a proton acceptor. Absorption of a photon changes the conformation of the retinal and the pK_a of the Schiff base. These four groups work together to transfer a single proton from the cytoplasm to the extracellular space.

1. The mechanism starts with retinal in the all-*trans* configuration and protons bound to the Schiff base and Asp96 at the hydrophobic, cytoplasmic end of the proton pathway.
2. Absorption of a photon isomerizes retinal to the 13-*cis* configuration and changes the conformation of the protein, favoring transfer of the Schiff base proton to Asp85.
3. Asp85 transfers the proton to Glu204, which releases the proton outside the cell.
4. A further conformational change reorients the Schiff base toward Asp96. The pK_a of Asp96 is

lower in this conformation, so a proton transfers from Asp96 to the Schiff base.
5. Asp96 is re-protonated from the cytoplasm.
6. The retinal re-isomerizes to the all-*trans* configuration in preparation for another cycle.

The net result of this cycle is rapid vectorial transport of a proton from the cytoplasm out of the cell. Steps 4 to 6 are rate limiting, occurring at a rate of about 100 s^{-1}. The other reactions are fast, provided an adequate flux of light. Retinal not only captures energy by absorbing a photon, but also acts as a switch that changes both the accessibility and affinities of the proton-binding groups in a sequential fashion.

In addition to bacteriorhodopsin, halobacterial plasma membranes contain two related proteins: halorhodopsin and sensory rhodopsin. Halorhodopsin absorbs light and pumps chloride into the cell. Interestingly, a single amino acid substitution can reverse the direction of pumping. Sensory rhodopsin couples light absorption by its bound retinal to phototaxis (swimming toward light) with a tightly coupled transducer protein. In the absence of this transducer protein—HtrI—sensory rhodopsin transports protons out of the cell much like bacterial rhodopsin. The design of these seven-helix transporters is remarkably similar to the large family of seven-helix receptors (see Chapter 26), especially the photoreceptor proteins that vertebrates use for vision (see Chapter 29).

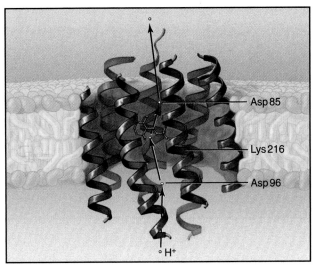

Figure 7-3 Proton pathway across the membrane through bacteriorhodopsin. The atomic structure, together with analysis of a wide array of mutations, reveals the pathway for protons through the middle of the bundle of helices. Further insights come from analysis of reaction intermediates, which differ in light absorption. A cytoplasmic proton binds successively to Asp96, the Schiff base linking retinal to lysine 216 (Lys216) and Asp85 before release outside the cell. Absorption of light by retinal drives conformational changes in the protein that favor the transfer of the proton across the membrane, up its concentration gradient.

table 7–2

ATP-DRIVEN TRANSPORT ATPASE PUMPS

Pump	Subunits	Distribution	Substrate	Function
F_0F_1 Family				
F_0F_1	8 or more	Mitochondria, chloroplasts, eubacteria, plasma membranes	H^+ (rarely Na^+)	ATP synthesis or ATP-driven H^+ pumping
V_0V_1	8 or more	Eukaryotic endomembranes	H^+ (rarely, N^+)	ATP-driven H^+ (or rarely, Na^+) pumping
P-type ATPase Family				
Na^+K^+-ATPase	2	Plasma membrane	3 Na^+ for 2 K^+	Generation of Na^+, K^+ gradient
H^+K^+-ATPase	2	Stomach and kidney plasma membranes	1 H^+ for 1 K^+	Gastric and renal H^+ secretion
SERCA Ca-ATPase	1	Sarcoplasmic reticulum, endoplasmic reticulum	2 Ca^{2+} for 2 H^+	Lowering of cytoplasmic Ca^{2+}
PMCA Ca-ATPase	1	Plasma membrane	1 Ca^{2+} for 1 H^+	Lowering of cytoplasmic Ca^{2+}
H^+-ATPase	1	Plasma membrane in yeast, plants, protozoa	1 H^+	Generation of proton gradient
ABC Transporters				
MDR1 P-glycoprotein	1	Plasma membrane	Drugs	Drug secretion
CFTR	1	Respiratory tract and pancreatic epithelial plasma membranes	ATP, Cl^-	Cl^- secretion
TAP1, 2	2	Endoplasmic reticulum	Antigenic peptides	Transport of antigenic peptides from cytoplasm into ER
MDR2	1	Liver cell apical plasma membrane	Phosphatidylcholine	Phosphoglyceride flippase, bile secretion?
STE6	1	Yeast plasma membrane	Mating pheromone peptide	Signaling for mating
HisQMP	4 + pp	Eubacteria plasma membrane	Histidine	Histidine uptake
PstSCAB	4 + pp	Eubacteria plasma membrane	Phosphate	Phosphate uptake
OppDFBCA	4 + pp	Eubacteria plasma membrane	Oligopeptides	Peptide uptake
HlyB	2	*Escherichia coli* plasma membrane	Hemolysin A (107-kD protein)	Hemolysin A uptake

pp, periplasmic protein.

ATP-Driven Pumps

Three families of transport ATPases (Table 7–2) are essential for the physiology of all forms of life. F_0F_1-ATPases and P-type ATPases differ in structure, but both generate electrical and/or chemical gradients across membranes. ABC transporters differ from the other pumps in both structure and function. They do not produce ion gradients but transport a much wider range of solutes across membranes. Inhibitory drugs have been useful in characterizing these pumps, and some are also used therapeutically (Table 7–3).

Free energy released by ATP hydrolysis puts a limit on the concentration gradient that these pumps can produce. If transport is electrically neutral (i.e., if it does not produce a membrane potential; see Chapter 9) the maximum gradient is about 100,000-fold. Such an extraordinary gradient is actually created by the electrically neutral H⁺K⁺-ATPase of gastric epithelial cells, which acidifies the stomach down to a pH of 2.

F₀F₁-ATPase Family

The two major subdivisions of this family are called F₀F₁-ATPases (or F-type ATPases) and V₀V₁-ATPases (or V-type ATPases) (Figs. 7–4 and 7–5). V₀V₁-ATPases, named for their location in the vacuolar system of eukaryotes, pump protons into organelles and out of Archaea. F₀F₁-ATPases of eubacteria, mitochondria, and chloroplasts generally run in the other direction, using proton gradients generated by other membrane proteins to drive ATP synthesis. However, purified F₀F₁-ATPases are freely reversible, using ATP hydrolysis to pump protons or proton gradients to synthesize ATP.

Phylogenetic analysis of the subunit polypeptides traces the origin of V-type ATPases to the precursor of

table 7–3	
TOOLS FOR STUDYING PUMPS	
Agent	**Target**
Cardiac glycosides* (e.g., ouabain, digitalis)	Na⁺K⁺-ATPase
Omeprazole*	H⁺K⁺-ATPase (parietal cell)
Oligomycin	F₀F₁-ATP synthase
*Used clinically as drugs.	

all contemporary life forms (see Fig. 1–1). F-type ATPase arose in eubacteria after their divergence from the Archaea-eukaryote lineage. Eukaryotes came to have both F-type ATPases and V-type ATPases when symbiotic eubacteria gave rise to mitochondria and chloroplasts. Two subtle points are of interest here.

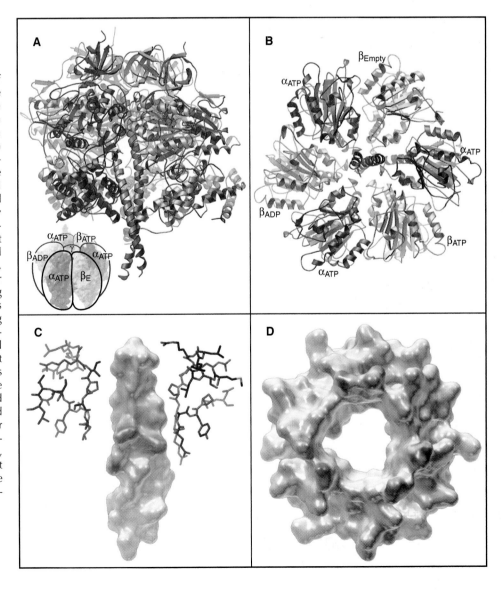

Figure 7–4 Atomic structure of mitochondrial F₁. *A,* Oblique view of a ribbon diagram with α-subunits in red, β-subunits in yellow, and the γ-subunit in blue. The γ-subunit forms an antiparallel coiled-coil. *B,* A ribbon diagram viewed from the membrane (*bottom*) side. All three α-subunits have a bound ATP. The β-subunits are empty or bind ATP or ADP. *C,* Space-filling model of the γ-subunit with the electrostatic potential indicated as blue for positive, red for negative, and grey for neutral. Part of the surrounding α- and β-subunits are shown as stick diagrams. *D,* Space-filling bottom view of the α- and β-subunits with the asymmetrical channel for the γ-subunit (not shown). Note that the surfaces of both the γ-subunit and the channel formed by the α- and β-subunits are hydrophobic and suitable to act as a molecular bearing. (PDB file: 1bmf. Reference: Abrams JP, Leslie AGW, Lutter R, Walker JE: Structure at 2.8 Å resolution of F₁-ATPase from bovine heart mitochondria. Nature 370:621, 1994.)

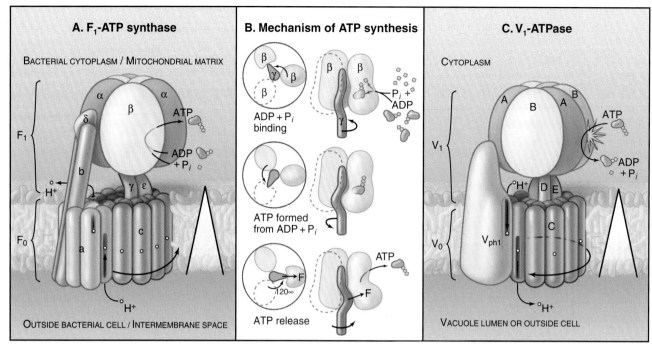

Figure 7–5 *A* to *C*, Models of the mitochondrial F_0F_1–ATP synthase and the V_0V_1 pump based on the atomic structure of F_1-ATPase and electron micrographs of the whole enzyme. Colors code the homologous subunits. F_0 is the oligomycin-sensitive factor. F_1 is the ATPase. Proton transfer across the membrane can drive ATP synthesis, or ATP hydrolysis can pump protons across the membrane. The text explains the reversible ATPase reaction. (Reprinted with permission from Nature. Reference: Elston T, Wang H, Oster G: Energy transduction in ATP synthesis. Nature 391:510–513, 1998. Copyright 1998, Macmillan Magazines Limited.)

First, a few eubacteria still have a V-type ATPase. Second, archaebacterial V-type ATPases function as ATP synthases similar to mitochondrial and eubacterial F-type ATP synthases.

F-type ATPases (ATP Synthases)

F-type ATPases of mitochondria, chloroplasts, and bacterial plasma membranes produce most of the world's ATP during aerobic metabolism (see Chapter 10). Redox-driven and light-driven pumps create proton gradients to drive ATP synthesis. Many bacteria can reverse this process, using the F-type ATPase to produce a proton gradient at the expense of ATP hydrolysis. Eukaryotes have elaborate mechanisms to inactivate the ATPase and prevent futile cycles of ATP synthesis and hydrolysis. For example, in mitochondria, an inhibitory protein binds the F_1-ATPase if the oxygen supply required to generate the proton gradient is compromised.

F_0F_1-ATPase has two parts (see Fig. 7–5). Water-soluble, globular F_1 catalyzes ATP hydrolysis or synthesis. F_0 is embedded in the membrane and passively conducts protons across the lipid bilayer. A stalk connects F_1 to F_0, providing a way to couple proton translocation to ATP synthesis. Given a higher concentration of protons outside the bacterium or mitochondrion

than inside, protons pass through F_0 and drive the synthesis of ATP by F_1. Conversely, in bacteria, ATP hydrolysis by F_1 can drive protons out of the cell.

The atomic structure of F_1 (see Fig. 7–4) suggested that rotation of a protein shaft couples proton fluxes in F_0 to ATP synthesis or, alternatively, couples ATP hydrolysis in F_1 to proton pumping by F_0. In the simplest case, bacterial F_1 consists of five different types of polypeptides in the ratio $\alpha_3\beta_3\gamma\delta\epsilon$. Mitochondrial F_1 has additional subunits. The α- and β-subunits are folded similarly and arranged alternately like segments of an orange around a hydrophobic shaft that is formed by the γ-subunit, which is folded back on itself to form a long, antiparallel, α-helical coiled-coil. The sleeve formed by α- and β-subunits is lined with hydrophobic residues. To accommodate the asymmetrical shaft, the surrounding α- and β-subunits have slightly different conformations. Each α- and β-subunit has an adenine nucleotide binding site. ATP bound stably to α-subunits does not participate in catalysis. Nucleotide binding sites on β-subunits catalyze ATP synthesis and hydrolysis.

Proton flux through the F_0 complex drives rotation of the γ-subunit inside F_1, providing energy to drive conformational changes in β-subunits that synthesize ATP (see Figs. 7–5 and 7–6). In the reverse reaction,

ATP hydrolysis drives rotation of the shaft, a process that can be observed directly by light microscopy. F_1 is attached to a glass coverslip, and an actin filament is attached to the free end of the γ-subunit. When ATP is added, the actin filament rotates around, driven by ATP hydrolysis by the β-subunits. Consistent with rotation of γ-subunits relative to F_1, a disulfide bond between β- and γ-subunits stops the F_1-ATPase; reduction of the disulfide bond restores activity. Assuming that this mechanism is correct, the γ-subunit rotates like the camshaft in a motor at a maximum rate of about 130 times per second (8000 rpm) in mitochondria and twice as fast in chloroplasts.

During ATP synthesis, the catalytic sites on the β-subunits participate cooperatively, in a sequence of steps. β-Subunits can be in one of three conformations—open, loose, and tight—which designations refer to their increasing affinities for adenine nucleotides. At any time in an F_1 molecule, one β-subunit is open, one is loose, and one is tight. All three subunits pass in lock step through the sequence of three states. ADP and inorganic phosphate (P_i) bind to the β-subunit in the loose conformation. Input of energy by the rotating γ-subunit converts this site to the tight conformation, which favors ATP synthesis from ADP and P_i. The next input of energy drives the tight state to the open state, which allows ATP to dissociate. All these transitions are reversible. With continued input of energy from proton translocations, F_1 moves through this cycle of states and produces ATP. On the other hand, in vitro or in bacteria, these reactions can pump protons at the expense of ATP hydrolysis.

The membrane-embedded F_0 complex consists of 12 to 15 protein subunits in the ratio ab_2c_{9-12}. The single a-subunit is thought to provide a channel for protons to move across the lipid bilayer to the 12 c-subunits surrounding the shaft. The c-subunits are simple hairpins of two α-helices with one residue, aspartate 61 (Asp61), which is particularly important for proton translocation. Reaction of Asp61 of a single copy of the c-subunit with the protein modification reagent DCCD completely inhibits H^+ conduction and ATP hydrolysis of the bacterial F_0F_1. This inhibition emphasizes the tight coupling of all the subunits of F_0F_1.

Each ATP synthesized or hydrolyzed is coupled to the transport of three or four protons. Given three ATP synthesized/hydrolyzed per complete F_1 cycle, 9 to 12 copies of c-subunits in F_0 provide the correct stoichiometry if each transports a single proton. Binding and release of protons at Asp61 is thought to drive rotation of the γ-subunits, which induces the conformational changes in F_1 that produce ATP. The mechanism driving the rotation of the "camshaft" is not known, but a molecular brace anchors F_1 to the a-subunit, allowing the c-subunits and the attached shaft to rotate inside F_1.

V-Type ATPases

Vacuolar ATPases (see Fig. 7-5) are found in the membranes bounding acidic compartments in eukaryotic cells, including clathrin-coated vesicles, endosomes, lysosomes (see Chapter 24), Golgi apparatus (see Chapter 21), secretory vesicles (including synaptic vesicles), and plant vacuoles. V-type pumps are also present in the plasma membranes of cells specialized to secrete protons, such as osteoclasts (see Chapter 34), macrophages, and kidney tubule intercalated cells.

V-type pumps have two functions. First, they acidify all the compartments just mentioned. The acidic pH promotes ligand dissociation from receptors in endosomes and activates lysosomal hydrolases, as well as many other reactions (see Chapter 24). Second, proton gradients across these membranes provide the energy source to drive H^+-coupled transport of other solutes, such as the uptake of neurotransmitters by synaptic vesicles (see Chapter 10).

Although similar in architecture to F_0F_1-ATPase, V-type pumps differ in three ways. First, eukaryotic

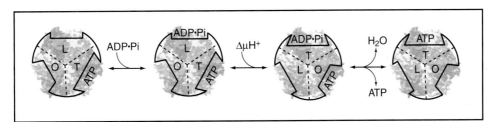

Figure 7-6 The binding change model for ATP synthesis by F_1. Each of the three β-subunits differs in conformation and affinity for nucleotides. The three subunits cycle in succession from the loose (L) state (that binds ADP and P_i), to the tight (T) state (that favors ATP synthesis) to the open (O) state (that releases ATP). Energy provided by the electrochemical gradient of protons ($\Delta\mu H^+$) is required for the γ-subunit to drive each successive transition from loose to tight. (Reference: Boyer PD. The ATP synthase—A splendid molecular machine. Annu Rev Biochem 66: 717–749, 1997.)

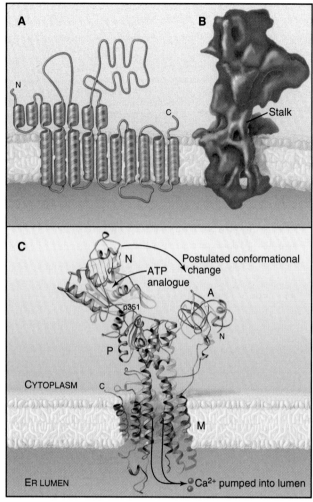

Figure 7-7 Models of P-type ATPase, the smooth endoplasmic reticulum calcium (SERCA)–ATPase from skeletal muscle. *A*, Topology of the polypeptide chain based on sequence analysis. The 100-kD protein spans the lipid bilayer 10 times, with most of the mass projecting into the cytoplasm. All P-type ATPases have a similar topology. Residues in transmembrane segments confer ion specificity. *B*, Three dimensional model at 8 Å resolution from electron micrographs of two-dimensional crystals formed in the absence of Ca^{2+}. *C*, Atomic structure from x-ray diffraction of crystals formed in the presence of Ca^{2+}. A, M, N, and P are domain names. The N domain must rotate to fit into the low-resolution structure without Ca^{2+} and for ATP in the active site to phosphorylate aspartic acid 351. The structure of the N domain is similar to another enzyme, haloacid dehalogenase. (*B*, Reprinted with permission from Nature. From Toyoshima CH, Stokes DL: Three-dimensional cryoelectron microscopy of the calcium ion pump in the sarcoplasmic reticulum membrane. Nature 362:469,1993. Copyright 1993, Macmillan Magazines Limited. *C*, PDB file: 1EUL. Reprinted with permission from Nature. Reference: Toyoshima C, Nakasako M, Nomura H, Ogawa H: Crystal structure of the calcium pump of sarcoplasmic reticulum at 2.6 Å resolution. Nature 405:647–655, 2000. Copyright 2000, Macmillan Magazines Limited.)

V-type pumps are exclusively proton pumps that cannot make ATP. Second, isolated V_1 complex has no ATPase activity. Finally, the V_o complex alone has no H^+-transporting activity. Most protein subunits of

V-type pumps are homologues of their counterparts from F-type pumps, but an ancient duplication of the original gene for c-subunits made the c-subunits of eukaryotic V-type pumps twice as large as those in F-type pumps. The six copies of V-type c-subunits provide the same total number of membrane-spanning helices as the 12 F-type c-subunits, but each has only one glutamate equivalent to Asp61. Accordingly, V-type pumps transport only 1 to 2 H^+ per ATP hydrolyzed.

P-Type Cation Pumps: E_1E_2-ATPases

All living organisms depend upon P-type ATPases (see Table 7–2) to pump cations across membranes. Their name comes from the fact that they utilize a high-energy covalent **β-aspartyl phosphate intermediate.** They are also called E_1E_2-ATPases from a description of their mechanism.

Eukaryotic P-type ATPases use ATP hydrolysis to generate the primary ion gradients across the plasma membrane that are required for the function of channels and most cation-coupled transport. In animal cells, **Na^+K^+-ATPase** produces the primary gradients of Na^+ and K^+. In plants and fungi, the functional homologue H^+-ATPase generates a proton gradient. Production of these primary ion gradients is expensive, consuming up to 25% of total cellular ATP. Other eukaryotic P-type ATPases acidify the stomach and clear cytoplasm of the second messenger, Ca^{2+}. Other bacterial P-type ATPases scavenge K^+ and Mg^{2+} from the medium and export Ca^{2+}, Cu^{2+}, and toxic heavy metals.

The sarco(endo)plasmic reticulum **Ca^{2+}-ATPase** (SERCA1) is particularly abundant in the sarcoplasmic reticulum of skeletal muscle (see Chapter 42). It can be purified in large quantities, allowing determination of both its atomic structure (Fig. 7–7) and its enzyme mechanism (Fig. 7–8). Other P-type ATPases consist of homologous α-subunits with large cytoplasmic domains and a minimum of six transmembrane helices. Eukaryotic P-type ATPases, such as the Na^+K^+- and Ca^{2+}-ATPases have 10 transmembrane helices. The cytoplasmic N domain binds ATP and transfers its γ-phosphate to aspartic acid 351 in the P domain. Transmembrane helices bind two Ca^{2+} ions and transfer them across the lipid bilayer. Many P-type ATPase are about 110 kD, like the Ca-ATPase, but some are larger or smaller owing to variable features. Na^+K^+-ATPase and H^+K^+-ATPase require 50-kD β-subunits for transport. The glycosylated β-subunit has a single transmembrane segment with most of its mass outside the cell.

To pump Ca^{2+} at the expense of ATP hydrolysis, the Ca^{2+}-ATPase cycles between two conformations: E_1, which allows access to the Ca^{2+} binding sites from the cytoplasm and E_2, which allows access from the lumen of the endoplasmic reticulum. The crystal struc-

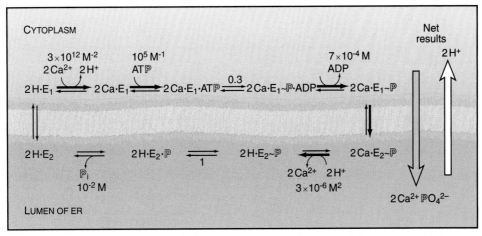

Figure 7–8 Reaction mechanism of the SERCA-ATPase. The E stands for enzyme, having two conformations: E_1 and E_2. E_1 has the Ca^{2+}-binding site oriented toward the cytoplasm. E_2 has the Ca^{2+}-binding site oriented toward the lumen of the endoplasmic reticulum. Ca^{2+} binds E_1 on the cytoplasmic side. Subsequent binding of ATP and phosphorylation of the enzyme drive the enzyme toward the E_2 state and transport Ca^{2+} up a steep concentration gradient into the lumen of the endoplasmic reticulum. Dephosphorylation of the enzyme favors a return to the E_1 state.

ture has two Ca^{2+} bound side by side midway across the transmembrane domain within a cluster of four helices and may correspond to the species $2Ca\text{-}E_1$. Possible pathways to both sides of the membrane exist within these transmembrane helices. The structures of the other intermediates are not known, but the enzyme mechanism is understood in great detail (see Fig. 7–8). Starting in the lower left corner of Figure 7–8 without bound Ca^{2+} or ATP, the E_2 and E_1 conformations of the protein are in equilibrium. If cytoplasmic Ca^{2+} ions are available, they bind cooperatively to the E_1 conformation with micromolar affinity. Ca^{2+} binding activates the enzyme, favoring utilization of bound ATP to form a phosphoenzyme intermediate. This must involve a substantial reorientation of the N domain from that in the crystal structure to bring bound ATP into contact with aspartate 351 (Asp351) in the P domain, since Asp351 is 2.5 nm away from the ATP analogue bound to the N domain in the crystal. The equilibrium constant for phosphorylation is near unity. The free energy of ATP hydrolysis is conserved in the β-aspartyl phosphate phosphoenzyme intermediate, which favors the E_2 conformation. The E_2 conformation exposes the Ca^{2+} binding sites to the lumen of the endoplasmic reticulum and reduces the affinity for Ca^{2+} by several orders of magnitude. Ca^{2+} dissociates into the lumen, completing its uphill transfer from the cytoplasm. The phosphorylated intermediate is hydrolyzed and phosphate dissociates, completing the cycle. Because the cycle transfers 2 Ca^{2+} into the lumen and 2 H^+ out, it generates an electrical potential (see Chapter 9). In the steady state, the Ca^{2+} gradient is maintained, but the H^+ gradient dissipates

owing to H^+ permeability across the membrane and to the buffering capacity of the lumen. All reactions in the pathway are reversible, so a large gradient of Ca^{2+} across the membrane can drive the synthesis of ATP.

All P-type ATPases work the same way as the Ca^{2+}-ATPase, but with adaptations to pump other ions. For example, the E_1 conformation of the Na^+K^+-ATPase of eukaryotic plasma membranes picks up 3 Na^+ from the cytoplasm. The $P\text{-}E_2$ conformation releases these Na^+ one after another outside the cell and then binds 2 K^+. Dephosphorylation of the phosphoenzyme favors the E_1 conformation, which releases K^+ in the cytoplasm.

P-type ATPases are involved in some human diseases. Mutations in Ca^{2+}-ATPase cause muscle stiffness and cramps. Mutations in Cu^{2+}-ATPases cause two inherited diseases: **Menkes' syndrome,** in which patients are copper-deficient owing to impaired intestinal absorption, and **Wilson's disease,** in which the inability to remove copper from the liver is toxic. Omeprazole and related drugs are used to treat ulcers by inhibiting gastric H^+K^+-ATPase. Drugs called **cardiac glycosides** strengthen the heartbeat by inhibiting the cardiac isoform of Na^+K^+-ATPase (see Chapter 10). These drugs are commonly used to treat congestive heart failure.

ABC Transporters

ABC transporters form the largest and most diverse family of ATP-powered pumps (see Table 7–2). For example, the genome of baker's yeast encodes no fewer than 30 putative ABC transporters, compared

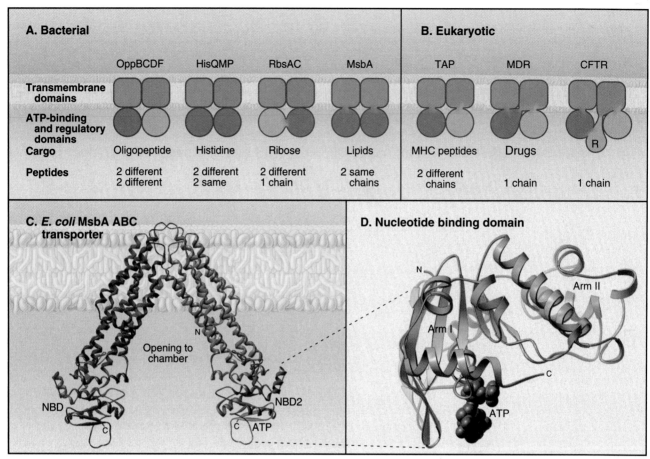

Figure 7–9 Models of the family of ABC transporters. *A* and *B*, Domain organization. Each transporter has two ATP-binding domains in the cytoplasm (*purple circles*) and two transmembrane domains, each consisting of 6 α-helices (*blue* or *pink squares*). CFTR has an additional regulatory (R) domain in the cytoplasm. The four domains required for activity may be four separate polypeptides or may be incorporated in several ways into polypeptides with two or four domains. *C*, Ribbon diagram of the atomic structure of *E. coli* MsbA, which transfers phospholipids across the bilayer. About 100 residues of the nucleotide-binding domain (NBD) are disordered and not shown. *D*, Atomic model of the nucleotide-binding domain, HisP, of the histidine transporter of *Salmonella typhimurium*. Arm I of the L-shaped protein binds ATP. Arm II associates with membrane-spanning domains. (*C*, PDB file: 1JSQ. Reference: Chang G, Roth CB: Structure of MsbA from *E. coli*: Homolog of the multidrug resistance ATP binding cassette (ABC) transporters. Science 293:1793–1800, 2001. *D*, PDB file: 1bOu. Reprinted with permission from Nature. Reference: Hung L-W, et al, Crystal structure of the ATP-binding subunit of an ABC transporter. Nature 396:703–707, 1998. Copyright 1998, Macmillan Magazines Limited.)

with 16 P-type ATPases, one F-type ATPase, and one V-type ATPase. In *Escherichia coli,* ABC transporters are the largest gene family. ABC transporters are found in all known organisms. Various family members are located in the plasma membrane, endoplasmic reticulum, and, most likely, other organelles. Each ABC transporter is specific for one or a few related substrates, but the whole family has an enormous range of substrates, including inorganic ions, sugars, amino acids, complex polysaccharides, peptides, and even proteins. Specialized members of the family act as ion channels (e.g., the **cystic fibrosis transmembrane regulator, CFTR**) or regulate other membrane proteins, such as the sulfonylurea receptor.

ABC transporters have a modular design (Fig. 7–9). Each half consists of a bundle of α-helices that spans the six times bilayer and continues into the cytoplasm, with the nucleotide-binding domain capping the cytoplasmic end of the bundle. Two sequences in the nucleotide-binding domain give the family its name **(ATP-binding cassette).** The Walker A motif (GXXGXGKS/T, where X is any residue) is also called a P loop, since it binds the γ-phosphate of ATP in ABC transporters and other ATP-binding proteins. The Walker B motif ($RX_{6-8}F_4D$, where F is any hydrophobic residue) interacts with Mg^{2+} bound to ATP. Motif B is typically separated from motif A by 100 to 150 residues.

Various "experiments" of evolution show that the parts of the gene corresponding to the four independently folded domains can be arranged in nearly every way imaginable. Regardless, the protein products assemble into pumps presumed to have similar structures, either by association of up to four subunits or by folding of a single polypeptide. Some bacterial transporters utilize additional extracellular subunits that bind and concentrate transported substances in the vicinity of the pump. Some vertebrate ABC transporters have an additional cytoplasmic domain involved in regulation by phosphorylation.

The structure of the MsbA phospholipid transporter (see Fig. 7–9B) suggests how ABC transporters might work. The transmembrane domains form a chamber lined by charged and hydrophobic side chains known to interact with transported substrates. In the structure without bound ATP, the chamber is open to the cytoplasm and laterally to the inner leaflet of the bilayer. It is postulated that ATP binding and hydrolysis drive a cycle of conformational changes that brings the nucleotide-binding domains together and exposes substrates in the chamber to the extracellular leaflet of the bilayer or the extracellular space, allowing them to escape. In the simplest cases, flippases like MsbA move phospholipids from one leaflet of the bilayer to the other, while yeast STE6 transports a small, prenylated pheromone peptide out of the cell. Bacterial permeases pump nutrients to the cell, and **TAP1** and **TAP2** pump peptide fragments of antigenic proteins into the lumen of the endoplasmic reticulum.

Other family members are more problematic. The vertebrate cystic fibrosis transmembrane conductance regulator (CFTR; see Fig. 7–9B) looks like a pump and acts like a channel. It allows Cl⁻ to move down its concentration gradient out of the cell. ATP binding and hydrolysis by the nucleotide-binding domains may open and shut this channel. Mutations in CFTR are responsible for cystic fibrosis (see Chapter 10).

The **multiple drug resistance** proteins (**MDR1** and **MDR2**) are ABC transporters that provide a challenge for cancer chemotherapy (Fig. 7–10). In about half of the cases in which chemotherapy fails to cure cancer in humans, the cause is the emergence of clones of tumor cells that overexpress an MDR. Normal cells use a low level of MDR1 to export an unknown substance, perhaps a steroid, phospholipid, or some other hydrophobic molecule. However, MDR can transport many hydrophobic compounds, including some chemotherapeutic drugs. These drugs enter cells by dissolving in the membrane, and they subsequently poison vital cellular processes. Cells that overexpress MDR survive by pumping the drug out as fast as it diffuses into the cell.

The multiple drug resistance protein 2 (MDR2) is another unconventional pump located in the apical plasma membrane of liver cells. It is a flippase that moves phosphatidylcholine from the inner to the outer half of the lipid bilayer, perhaps in preparation for secretion in bile.

Some even less conventional ABC transporters appear to regulate ion channels. The sulfonylurea receptor (SUR) ABC transporter is required for the function of an ATP-sensitive potassium channel (K_{ATP}) that regulates insulin secretion. SUR binds drugs called

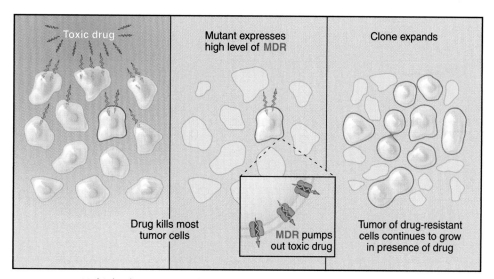

Figure 7-10 Multiple drug resistance in cancer chemotherapy. In a population of tumor cells, most are sensitive to killing by a chemotherapeutic drug. However, variants that express high levels of the ABC transporter, MDR, can clear the cytoplasm of the drug. A clone of these variant cells may expand, allowing the tumor to grow in the presence of the drug.

sulfonylureas that are used to treat forms of diabetes involving inadequate insulin secretion. These drugs activate secretion by inhibiting the K_{ATP} channel (see Chapter 9).

▌ Selected Readings

Abrams JP, Leslie AGW, Lutter R, Walker JE: Structure at 2.8 Å resolution of F_1-ATPase from bovine heart mitochondria. Nature 370:621, 1994.

Aravind L, Galperin MY, Koonin EV: The catalytic domain of the P-type ATPase has the haloacid dehalogenase fold. Trends Biochem Sci 23:127–128, 1998.

Boyer PD: The ATP synthase—A splendid molecular machine. Annu Rev Biochem 66:717–750, 1997.

Chang G, Roth CB: Structure of MsbA from E. coli: A homolog of the multidrug resistance ATP binding cassette (ABC) transporters. Science. 293:1793–1800, 2001.

Haupts U, Tittor J, Oesterhelt D: Closing in on bacteriorhodopsin: Progress in understanding the molecule. Annu Rev Biophys Biomol Struct 28:367–399, 1999.

Higgins CF, Linton KJ: The xyz of ABC transporters. Science. 293:1782–1784, 2001.

Inesi G. Teaching active transport at the turn of the twenty-first century: Recent discoveries and conceptual changes. Biophys J 66:554, 1994.

Junge W, Lill H, Engelbrecht S: ATP synthase: An electrochemical transducer with rotary mechanics. Trends Biochem Sci 22:420–423, 1997.

Lanyi J: Bacteriorhodopsin as a model for proton pumps. Nature 375:461, 1995.

MacLennan DH, Rice WJ, Green NM: The mechanism of Ca^{2+} transport by the sarco(endo)plasmic reticulum Ca^{2+}-ATPases. J Biol Chem 272:28815–28818, 1997.

Nakamoto RK, Ketchum CJ, Al-Shawi MK: Rotational coupling in the F_0F_1 ATP synthase. Annu Rev Biophys Biomol Struct 28:205–234, 1999.

Spudich JL, Lanyi JK: Shuttling between two protein conformations: The common mechanism for sensory transduction and ion transport. Curr Opin Cell Biol 8:452, 1996.

Stevens T, Forgac M: Structure, function and regulation of the vacuolar (H^+)-ATPase. Annu Rev Cell Dev Biol 13:779–808, 1998.

Stock D, Leslie AGW, Walker JE: Molecular architecture of the rotary motor in ATP synthesis. Science 286:1700–1705, 1999.

Toyoshima G, Nakasako M, Nomura H, Ogawa H: Crystal structure of the calcium pump of sarcoplasmic reticulum. Nature 405:647–655, 2000.

chapter 8

MEMBRANE CARRIERS

Carriers are integral membrane proteins that allow substrates to move across lipid bilayers along electrochemical gradients without making or breaking chemical bonds (Fig. 8–1). Carriers, also known as facilitators, are said to catalyze secondary reactions, which distinguishes them from pumps that catalyze primary transport reactions requiring energy from ATP hydrolysis, electron transport, or absorption of light. The phrase "catalyze secondary reactions" is used advisedly, since carriers work step-by-step more like enzymes than like channels, which simply provide a pore. Carriers frequently use ion gradients created by pumps to perform work in so-called chemiosmotic cycles (see Chapter 10).

Carriers provide pathways for solutes to move down their own concentration gradients from higher concentration to regions of lower concentration. More remarkably, carriers can also provide a pathway for substrates to move up concentration gradients, provided that their passage through the carrier is coupled to the transport of another substrate down its electrochemical gradient. Glucose provides good examples of both downhill and uphill movement through different carriers. The GLUT1 carrier allows glucose to move down its concentration gradient from plasma into red blood cells. On the other hand, the SGLT1 carrier uses a gradient of Na^+ established by ATPase pumps to move glucose up its concentration gradient into intestinal cells. All carrier-mediated reactions are reversible, so that substrates can move in either direction across the membrane, depending on the polarity of the driving forces.

Like pumps, carriers are found in all membranes, wherever cells need to exchange molecules for metabolism, storage, or extrude wastes.

Structure of Carrier Proteins

Many of the thousands of carrier proteins known from gene sequences consist of a single polypeptide with 12 (rarely, 10 or 14) hydrophobic segments (Table 8–1 and Fig. 8–2). Regardless of the substances transported, about one third of these carrier proteins are classified as members of the **major facilitator superfamily** and are likely to have arisen from a common ancestor. These carriers are active as monomers. Carriers in mitochondria and chloroplasts are half as long, with six hydrophobic segments. Homodimers of these shorter polypeptides are thought to form a structure equivalent to the longer polypeptides.

Direct experimental evidence strongly supports a carrier model with 12 transmembrane α-helices. Spectroscopic experiments show that 60% to 70% of the polypeptide is α-helical, enough to form 12 transmembrane helices. Experiments with parts of carrier proteins fused to a reporter protein confirm that the hydrophobic segments span the membrane and that both the N-terminus and the C-terminus are in the cytoplasm.

The sequences of the two halves of 12-helix carrier polypeptides are homologous to each other. This likely represents duplication of an ancestral gene, which coded for a six-helix protein that formed functional dimers similar to those in mitochondria and chloroplasts. This gene duplication and fusion had two advantages. First, it allowed the two halves of the gene to diversify separately to increase substrate specificity. Divergence has been extensive, leaving less than 30% identical residues in the two halves of all sequenced carriers. Second, a single polypeptide simplifies assembly of a functional carrier, as two half-

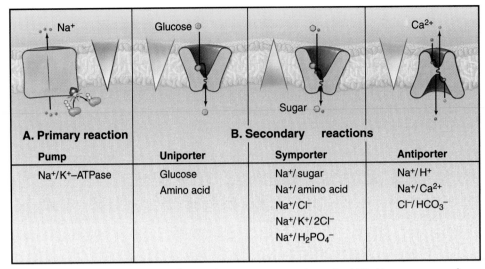

A. Primary reaction	B. Secondary reactions		
Pump	**Uniporter**	**Symporter**	**Antiporter**
Na⁺/K⁺–ATPase	Glucose Amino acid	Na⁺/sugar Na⁺/amino acid Na⁺/Cl⁻ Na⁺/K⁺/2Cl⁻ Na⁺/H₂PO₄⁻	Na⁺/H⁺ Na⁺/Ca²⁺ Cl⁻/HCO₃⁻

Figure 8–1. *A* and *B*, Primary and secondary transport reactions. An ATP-driven pump produces a gradient of an ion, such as Na⁺, across a membrane. The triangles represent gradients of Na⁺ (*purple*), glucose (*green*), sugar (*blue*) and Ca²⁺ (*light blue*) across the membrane. This ion gradient drives secondary transport reactions mediated by carriers. Uniporters allow an ion or other solute to move across the membrane down its concentration gradient. Symporters and antiporters couple transport of an ion (Na⁺ in this example) down its concentration gradient with the transport of a solute (glucose or Ca²⁺ in these examples) up its concentration gradient. Antiporters carry out these reactions in succession, picking up Na⁺ outside, reorienting, dissociating Na⁺ inside, picking up Ca²⁺ inside, reorienting, and releasing Ca²⁺ outside.

sized subunits do not have to find each other. If the two halves of a 12-helix carrier are expressed in the same cell, they can assemble functional carriers, but less efficiently than the intact protein.

Genetic experiments on **LacY,** the lactose carrier of *Escherichia coli*, provide important clues about the three-dimensional arrangement of the 12 helices in the lipid bilayer. Investigators selected mutants of LacY that allow the bacteria to grow on α-glycosides rather than on lactose, the normal β-glycoside substrate for LacY. The mutations map to 6 of the 12 transmembrane helices, suggesting that these helices line a channel where the mutated residues bind substrate. In fact, the mutations in each segment are spaced so that they align on one side of a helix. A complementary approach is to introduce single-cysteine residues by mutagenesis throughout a carrier and to test which ones can react with hydrophilic probes that pass through the pore. Again, residues along a subset of helices are found in the pore. The field awaits atomic structures to provide further insights regarding mechanisms.

No one knows exactly how a substrate uses a carrier to cross a membrane, but models (see Fig. 8–2*C*) generally suggest that substrates first bind to a part of the pore exposed to the aqueous phase on one side of the membrane. All models assume that a significant conformational change closes the pathway at one end and opens it at the other end, allowing the substrate to escape on the other side of the membrane.

Carrier Physiology and Mechanisms

Investigators have identified about 500 different reactions attributable to secondary transporters and characterized about a dozen carriers well enough to understand their mechanisms. These model systems (see Table 8–1) provide a framework to divide carriers into three broad classes (Fig. 8–3) based on mechanism:

- **Uniporters** transport a single substrate that moves alone down its concentration gradient. This reaction is also called **facilitated diffusion**, facilitated in the sense that the carrier provides a low-resistance pathway across a poorly permeable lipid bilayer. GLUT carriers for glucose are an example of a uniporter found in mammalian tissues.
- **Antiporters** exchange substrates in opposite directions across a membrane. The driving ion moves in one direction, the driven substance in the other. The mitochondrial ANC exchanger for ADP and ATP is an antiporter.
- **Symporters** allow two or more substrates to move together in the same direction across a membrane. The driving ion and the driven sub-

table 8–1

EXAMPLES OF CARRIER PROTEINS

Carrier	Subunits	Distribution	Substrate	Function
Uniporters				
GLUT1	1×12 helix	Red blood cells	Glucose	Glucose uptake
GLUT4	1×12 helix	Fat, muscle	Glucose	Insulin-responsive glucose uptake
UCP	2×6 helix	Mitochondria	H^+	Uncoupling protein, thermal regulation
Antiporters				
NHE-1	1 or 2×12 helix	Kidney, gut	Na^+/H^+	Acid-base balance
Band 3	1×14 helix	Red blood cells	HCO_3^-/Cl^-	Acid-base balance
UhpT	1×12 helix	*E. coli*	P_i/glucose 6-phosphate	Glucose 6-phosphate uptake
NCE	1×12 helix	Muscle	$3\ Na^+/Ca^{2+}$	Ca^{2+} homeostasis; regulation of heart contractility
ANC	2×6 helix	Mitochondria	ADP/ATP	ATP, ADP exchange
TPE	2×7 helix	Chloroplast	P_i/2 PGA	ATP generation
Symporters				
LacY	1×12 helix	*E. coli*	H^+/lactose	Lactose uptake
NKC1	1×12 helix	Kidney, gut, lung	$Na^+/K^+/2\ Cl^-$	NaCl regulation, fluid secretion
SGLT1	1×12 helix	Gut	Na^+/glucose	Glucose uptake
Various	1×12 helix	Central nervous system neurons	$Na^+/Cl^-/\gamma$-gamma-aminobutyric acid (GABA)	Neurotransmitter reuptake

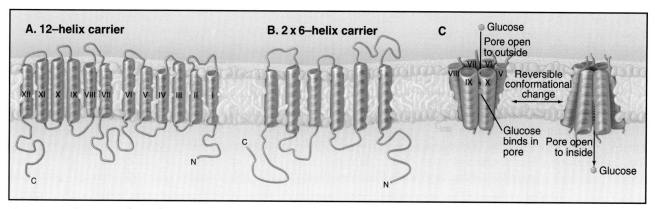

Figure 8–2. Structure of membrane carrier proteins. *A,* Transmembrane topology of a 12-helix carrier protein. *B,* Transmembrane topology of a six-helix carrier peptide that dimerizes to form a functional protein. *C,* A hypothetical model of transport carried out by reorientation of transmembrane helices. The model shows just 6 of the 12 transmembrane helices of carrier.

Figure 8–3. *A to C,* Carrier hypothesis with kinetic intermediates of three classes of carrier. C_o has the substrate binding site oriented toward the outside of the cell. C_i has the substrate binding site oriented inside. S, S_1, S_2, and Na are substrates. The arrows indicate transitions among the intermediates. Transport occurs when a substrate binds on one side of the membrane and is released on the opposite side after the carrier changes conformation.

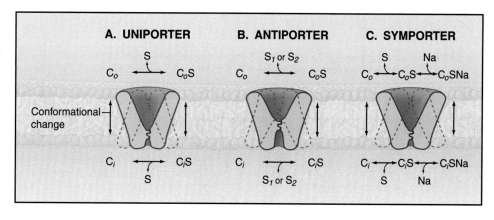

table 8-2

TOOLS FOR STUDYING CARRIERS

Agent	Target
Furosemide*	$Na^+/K^+/2\ Cl^-$ symporter
Amiloride*	Na^+/H^+ antiporter
SITZ, DITZ	HCO_3^-/Cl^- antiporter
Cytochalasin B	GLUT isoforms
Phloretin	GLUT isoforms
Phlorizin	SGLT isoforms

*Used clinically as a drug.

stance move together across the membrane. This is also known as **cotransport**. Examples are the *E. coli* LacY protein and the mammalian Na⁺-coupled glucose transporters.

Dividing carriers into these three classes should not obscure the important point that these proteins are remarkably similar. In fact, relatively simple mutations can convert a carrier from one class to another.

A few carriers are more complicated than is indicated by this classification. For example, neurotransmitter carriers catalyze both antiporter and symporter reactions, with Na⁺ and Cl⁻ going in one direction and a neurotransmitter in the opposite direction. This example also makes the important general point that the stoichiometry of antiporter and symporter reactions need not be one-to-one. Table 8–1 provides other examples.

All three classes of carriers use similar mechanisms to transfer bound substrates across membranes. This follows naturally from having a common evolutionary ancestor and similar architectures. They work like enzymes, binding substrates on one side of mem-

branes, undergoing a conformational change that reorients this binding site, and releasing substrate on the opposite side of the membrane. Substrate concentrations on the two sides determine the direction of net transfer across the membrane. Whether a carrier is a uniporter, antiporter, or symporter depends simply on the number of substrate binding sites and the rate and equilibrium constants for the various species to reorient across the membrane. The actual rate of transfer depends on the concentrations of substrates. A limited number of specific inhibitors (Table 8–2) have been useful in establishing physiological functions of carriers.

Uniporters

The prefix "uni-" indicates that a single substrate moves across the membrane along its own electrochemical gradient. Nonelectrolytes, such as glucose, use uniporters simply to move across membranes down a chemical gradient. Movement of charged substrates is influenced by the membrane potential and by pH gradients in the case of weak acids or bases.

Classic experiments with **GLUT1** in the plasma membrane of red blood cells led to the carrier concept in the 1950s. Human red blood cells are convenient to use because they express high concentrations of GLUT carriers and because blood banks can provide large quantities of cells. The time course of radioactive glucose accumulation (Fig. 8–4A) shows that transport is stereospecific for D-glucose and that net transport stops when the concentrations of D-glucose are equal inside and out. Slow equilibration of L-glucose across the membrane probably represents passive diffusion across the lipid bilayer, as this rate is predicted from

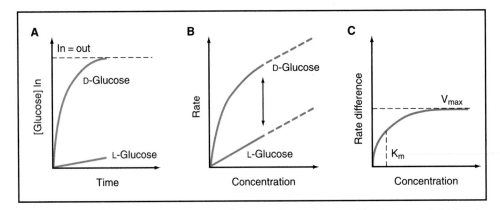

Figure 8-4. Experiments on transport of radioactive glucose into red blood cells establishing the existence of membrane carriers. *A,* Time course of the uptake of D- and L-glucose. *B,* Rate of uptake of D- and L-glucose as a function of extracellular concentration. Uptake of L-glucose is by diffusion across the lipid bilayer. *C,* Rate of uptake of D-glucose corrected for diffusion as a function of extracellular concentration. The curve is similar to the dependence of an enzyme on substrate concentration, yielding the maximum rate (V_{max}) at high substrate concentration and the apparent affinity of the carrier (K_m) for the substrate at half the maximal rate; see Chapter 3.

the solubility of glucose in membrane lipids. This experiment showed that something in the membrane causes an acceleration in the rate of glucose entry, giving rise to the concept of facilitated diffusion.

The dependence of the initial rate of D-glucose entry on its concentration (see Fig. 8–4B) provided evidence for a specific, saturable, carrier molecule in the membrane. Because the rate of D-glucose entry includes both diffusion across the bilayer and movement through a carrier, the L-glucose rate must be used to correct for the rate of diffusion. Once this is done, the rate of facilitated D-glucose entry has a hyperbolic dependence on the concentration of D-glucose (see Fig. 8–4C). This concentration dependence is just like a bimolecular binding reaction (see Chapter 3) or the rate of a simple enzyme mechanism that depends on the rate of substrate binding to the enzyme (see Chapter 3). Thus, the substrate concentration at the half-maximal velocity provides an estimate of the affinity of the carrier for the substrate. At high substrate concentrations, the substrate binding sites on the carrier are saturated and the rate plateaus at a maximal velocity owing to rate-limiting conformational changes. These enzyme-like properties, along with the ability to stop facilitated transport with protein inhibitors, suggest that carriers are proteins with specific binding sites for their substrates.

The carrier hypothesis is now understood in terms of carrier proteins embedded in the lipid bilayer; these proteins bind substrate and undergo readily reversible first-order transitions between at least two different conformations (see Fig. 8–2C). One conformation exposes a substrate binding site on one side of the membrane. Another conformation exposes a binding site on the other side. Thus, a single substrate molecule can bind on one side of the membrane and release on the other, thus moving across the membrane. (The carrier does not physically diffuse across the membrane as formerly believed.)

Net transport requires a concentration gradient, as the conformational change that reorients substrate binding sites is reversible, and substrate can move either way. The rates of substrate movement depend on the rates of formation of substrate-carrier complex on the two sides of the membrane. The rates of these second-order reactions depend directly on the substrate concentrations, so the binding sites of the carrier are more fully occupied on the uphill side, and the net movement of substrate is therefore in the downhill direction. When substrate concentrations are the same on the two sides, exchange continues without net movement because the carrier is equally saturated on both sides of the membrane.

This simple carrier model clarified a large body of confusing information and clearly distinguished carriers from channels for the first time. The original carrier model for the GLUT1 uniporter also led directly to kinetic schemes for antiporters and symporters (see Fig. 8–3B and C).

Carrier mechanisms involve a series of reversible reactions, including rate-limiting conformational changes in the carrier that move substrates across the membrane. Carriers generally translocate substrates at rates of 10^{-1} to 10^3 s^{-1}, similar to enzyme reactions, whereas channels transfer ions at rates of 10^6 to 10^9 s^{-1} during the brief times that they open (see Chapter 9).

Chapter 10 describes how fat and muscle cells use glucose uniporters to take up glucose from the blood after a meal. Chapter 30 explains how uncoupling protein, a proton uniporter in mitochondria, generates heat in brown fat cells when animals arise from hibernation and mammalian infants are born.

Antiporters

Antiporters translocate two different substrates and use a concentration gradient of one substrate to drive another substrate up its concentration gradient. Like uniporters, these carriers undergo reversible, conformational changes that expose substrate binding sites on one or the other side of a membrane. Two modifications of the uniporter mechanism provide a model for antiporters (Fig. 8–3B). First, two substrates, S_1 and S_2, compete for binding antiporters. Second, a substrate-free carrier cannot undergo the conformational changes required to change the orientation of its binding sites. These differences make transport of two substrates dependent upon each other in an obligate fashion.

For example, the heart $3Na^+/Ca^{2+}$ exchanger binds either Na$^+$ or Ca^{2+} and uses the large Na$^+$ gradient across the plasma membrane to drive the transport of Ca^{2+} out of the cytoplasm up a concentration gradient. On the outer surface of the cell, the carrier binds three Na$^+$. After the conformational change that reorients the binding site, the three Na$^+$ dissociate inside and one Ca^{2+} binds. Reorientation of the binding site carries this Ca^{2+} to the outer surface of the cell, where it dissociates. (In addition to the substrate concentrations, the membrane potential must also be taken into account, as this exchange is not electrically neutral, and the potential may affect the binding of one or both substrates to the carrier.)

Antiporters generally exchange like substrates: cations for cations, anions for anions, sugars for sugars, and so on. The Na$^+$/H$^+$ antiporter of kidney, gut, and most other cells allows cells to manipulate their internal pH. Band 3 antiporter of red blood cells exchanges Cl$^-$ for HCO$_3^-$. Carbon dioxide produced in tissues by oxidative reactions diffuses into red blood cells, where a cytoplasmic enzyme—carbonic anhydrase—transforms carbon dioxide into HCO_3^-. The antiporter provides a way for the HCO_3^- to return to the plasma, where it is carried to the lungs as the bicarbonate anion. UhpT antiporter (uptake of hexose phosphate transporter) allows *E. coli* to scavenge glucose 6-phosphate from the medium in exchange for inorganic phosphate. Antiporters in mitochondria, consisting of dimers (each with six helices like the presumed ancestor of all carriers), exchange cytoplasmic ADP for ATP synthesized by these organelles.

Symporters

The prefix "sym-" indicates that two substrates are transported in the same direction. A simple extension of the uniporter mechanism provides a model for symporters (see Fig. 8–3C). Like uniporters, the carrier has two conformations with substrate binding sites open to either side of the membrane. The binding site may be free or occupied by a single substrate, like a uniporter, but in addition, two substrates can bind together. A second difference is that transmembrane reorientation of substrate binding sites is much more favorable for free carrier and carrier with two bound substrates than carrier with only one bound substrate. This feature of symporters minimizes leaks of one substrate across the membrane.

E. coli LacY symporter (also called lac permease) is a well-characterized 12-helix carrier that uses a proton gradient across the plasma membrane to drive accumulation of lactose. The proton gradient is created by the respiratory chain under aerobic conditions, or by the F-type ATPase pump under anaerobic conditions (see Chapter 10). Protons move down their concentration gradient as lactose moves up its concentration gradient into the cell. Mutations in LacY can cause internal leaks that uncouple sugar transport from proton movements. Vertebrate SGLT1 symporter carries out a comparable reaction for intestinal epithelial cells using the Na^+ gradient to take up glucose from the lumen of the gut (Chapter 10).

Two key experiments (Fig. 8–5) established the symporter concept. The first demonstrated that extracellular Na^+ was required for intestinal cells with the SGLT1 transporter to accumulate D-glucose against a concentration gradient. This experiment left open the possibility that Na^+ simply activates the carrier in some way without being used directly to drive glucose accumulation. Second, an experiment with LacY demonstrated that sugar and cation move across the membrane together. Not only was a proton gradient required for sugar transport, but a high concentration of another sugar (a nonmetabolizable lactose analogue) in the medium could drive H^+ into the cell along with the sugar. Additional experiments confirmed that the

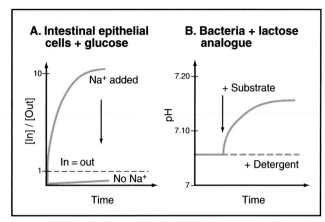

Figure 8–5. Experimental evidence for the existence of symporters. *A*, Effect of Na^+ on uptake of radioactive glucose by apical plasma membrane vesicles isolated from intestinal epithelial cells containing the Na^+/glucose symporter SGLT1. The addition of Na^+ to the external buffer strongly favors glucose uptake against its concentration gradient. *B*, Cotransport of protons and lactose by bacteria expressing LacY H/lactose symporter. Bacteria are suspended in weakly buffered medium. Lactose added to the medium moves into the cells and down its concentration gradient. Protons accompany the lactose through the symporter, raising the pH of the medium. If detergent makes the membrane permeable, the pH does not change.

stoichiometry of the reaction was one lactose transported in for every H^+ transported in. (Because this transport reaction is not electrically neutral, the membrane potential is a factor, and another pathway must be available to balance the charge [e.g., by carrying K^+ in the opposite direction].) These experiments established that both substrates move together across the membrane with a fixed stoichiometry and that a concentration gradient of either can drive the other. Parallel experiments on plasma membrane vesicles isolated from vertebrate kidney cells showed that Na^+ moving inward down its electrochemical gradient can drag glucose in with it. When the Na^+ concentration is equal on the two sides, the carrier facilitates the movement of glucose across the membrane, but not its net accumulation.

Selected Readings

Kaback HR: In and out with lac permease. Int Rev Cytol 137A:97–125, 1992.

Kaback HR, Wu J: From membrane to molecule to the third amino acid from the left with a membrane transport protein. Q Rev Biophys 30:333–364, 1997.

Kaplan JH: Molecular biology of carrier proteins. Cell 72:13–18, 1993.

Kramer R: Functional properties of solute transport systems: Concepts and perspectives. Biochim Biophys Acta 1185:1–34, 1994.

Malandro MS, Kilberg MS: Molecular biology of mammalian amino acid transporters. Annu Rev Biochem 65:305–336, 1996.

Maloney PC: Bacterial transporters. Curr Opin Cell Biol 6: 571–582, 1994.

Orlowski J, Grinstein S: Na^+/H^+ exchangers of mammalian cells. J Biol Chem 272:22373–22376, 1997.

Turk E, Wright EM: Membrane topology motifs in the SGLT cotransporter family. J Membr Biol 159:1–20, 1997.

Walmsley AR, Barrett MP, Bringaud F, Gould GW: Sugar transporters from bacteria, parasites and mammals: Structure-activity relationships. Trends Biochem Sci 23: 476–480, 1998.

Wright EM, Loo DDF, Turk E, Hirayama BA: Sodium cotransporters. Curr Opin Cell Biol 8:468–473, 1996.

chapter 9

MEMBRANE CHANNELS

Channels are integral membrane proteins with transmembrane pores that allow particular ions or small molecules to cross a lipid bilayer. Some channels are open constitutively, but most open just part time. Each time a channel opens, thousands to millions of ions diffuse down their electrochemical gradient across the membrane. Carriers and pumps are orders of magnitude slower, since they use rate-limiting conformational changes to transport each ion (see Chapters 7 and 8).

The ability to control diffusion across membranes allows channels to perform three essential functions (Fig. 9–1). First, certain channels cooperate with pumps and carriers to transport water and ions across cell membranes. This is required to regulate cellular volume and for secretion and absorption of fluid, as in salivary glands, kidney, inner ear, and plant guard cells. Second, ion channels regulate the **electrical potential** across membranes. The sign and magnitude of the membrane potential depend on ion gradients created by pumps and carriers (see Chapters 7 and 8) and the relative permeabilities of various channels (Appendix 9–1). Open channels allow unpaired ions to diffuse down concentration gradients across a membrane, separating electrical charges and producing a **membrane potential.** Coordinated opening and closing of channels change the membrane potential and produce an electrical signal that spreads rapidly over the surface of a cell. Nerve and muscle cells use these **action potentials** for high-speed communication. Third, other channels admit Ca^{2+} from outside the cell or from the endoplasmic reticulum into the cytoplasm where it triggers a variety of processes (see Chapter 28), including secretion (see Chapter 22) and muscle contraction (see Chapter 42).

Cells control channel activity in two ways. Long term, each cell type expresses a unique repertoire of channels from among hundreds of channel genes. **Excitable cells,** such as nerve and muscle, express plasma membrane voltage-gated channels to produce action potentials. Epithelial cells express Na^+ channels, Cl^- channels, K^+ channels, and water channels to produce the salt and water fluxes required for secretion and reabsorption of fluids in glands and the kidney. In the short term, cells open and shut specific types of channels in response to physiological or environmental stimuli. Some channels respond to changes in membrane potential. Others respond to intracellular or extracellular ligands or to mechanical forces.

Channels are important in medicine. Ion channels are targets of powerful drugs and toxins, including curare, tetrodotoxin ("voodoo toxin"), paralytic shellfish toxins, cobra toxin, local anesthetics, antiarrhythmic agents, and, probably, general anesthetics (see Table 9–1). Defects in ion channel genes cause many inherited disorders, including some cardiac arrhythmias and kidney stones. The human autoimmune disorder myasthenia gravis targets ion channels.

This chapter covers 10 large families of plasma membrane channels. Other chapters discuss cystic fibrosis transmembrane regulator Cl^- channels (see Chapters 7 and 10), gap junction channels used for communication between adjacent cells (see Chapter 33), and intracellular Ca^{2+} release channels that participate in signal transduction (see Chapters 28 and 42). Understanding channels requires not only information about their structure and activity, but also some knowledge of electrical phenomena. Appendices 9–1 to 9–3 contain essential technical information about electrophysiology.

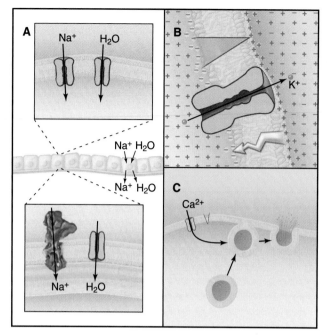

Figure 9-1 Functions of membrane channels. *A,* Transport of salt and water across an epithelium by water channels in both the apical and basolateral membranes, a Na+ channel in the apical membrane, and a Na+ pump in the basolateral membrane. *B,* Regulation of membrane potential. The triangle represents the concentration difference of K+ across the membrane. The zigzag arrow represents the membrane potential, negative inside. *C,* Ca2+ signaling in secretion.

Channel Proteins and Genes

Physiologists introduced the concept of channels in the 1950s to explain ion currents during action potentials. Proof that channels are integral membrane proteins followed in the 1970s with isolation of the acetylcholine receptor and the voltage-gated Na+ channel. The great diversity of channels was revealed initially by cloning complementary DNAs (cDNAs) using functional assays and homology with known channels. Ul-

timately, the full repertoire of channels emerged from sequenced genomes.

A new channel can be characterized by expressing its cDNA in a test cell and then making electrical recordings of ion currents from the cell or patches of its membrane (see Appendix 9–1). If expression of a single channel protein fails to reproduce the channel activity observed in the cell of origin, auxiliary subunits are probably required. Historically, investigation of channel functions has relied on toxins and drugs that inhibit particular channels more or less specifically (Table 9–1). Some of these agents are also used therapeutically. This approach is often limited by a lack of specificity or lack of an inhibitor. Mutations, including those in human disease, provide definitive tests for physiological functions, with some surprising results.

The inventory of channels is currently in the thousands and growing rapidly owing to genome sequencing. Known channels vary widely in the signals that they mediate, their modes of activity, their physiological roles, and their regulation. The historical nomenclature for channels, which varies according to the ion transported, mode of regulation, physiological role, or drug sensitivity, is often ambiguous. Fortunately, knowledge of channel protein primary structures (and a few atomic structures) has clarified evolutionary relationships and provided a framework to classify most plasma membrane channels into a few large families (Fig. 9–2).

A limited number of genes in early forms of life appear to have given rise to most channel genes. For example, the gene for a simple prokaryotic channel with just two transmembrane segments (called S5 and S6) is the progenitor of a huge family of channels with 2 to 24 transmembrane segments. Some channels with two transmembrane segments acquired features to provide for rectified ion fluxes (see later section), extracellular ligand binding (neuropeptides and ATP), and intracellular ligand binding (cyclic adenosine

Figure 9-2 Classification of channel proteins. This scheme is based on primary structure, atomic structures (where known), and postulated evolutionary origins. The predicted transmembrane topology has the extracellular side at the top and uses rectangles to indicate helices labeled "S" or "M." P loops are shown as a short helix and loop between two transmembrane helices. S4 voltage-sensing helices are pink. Drawings on the right indicate the known (or likely) subunit composition. Pores are located in the center of each ensemble of subunits except for chloride channels and aquaporins, where the pore is contained within each subunit. In many cases, it is possible to trace the origins of a channel family back to prokaryotes. In other cases, family members are known only in vertebrate organisms. In most families, relatively recent gene duplications and divergence have given rise to multiple isoforms of each type of channel. Channel nomenclature is not uniform. Some names indicate the transported ion (Na+, K+, Ca2+, Cl−), whereas others signify the regulatory modality (i.e., voltage-gated [VG] or neurotransmitter-gated), a physiological role (intracellular calcium release), drug binding (ryanodine receptor), or some other feature. ClC, chloride channel; ENaC, epithelial sodium channel; GABA, γ-amino butyric acid; 5-HT, 5-hydroxytryptamine; IC, intracellular ligand; IP3, inositol triphosphate; Kir, potassium inward rectifier; nAch, nicotinic acetylcholine; R, receptor; Ryanodine, a chemical that binds calcium-release channels; VG, voltage-gated; XC-ATP, extracellular ATP-gated channel.

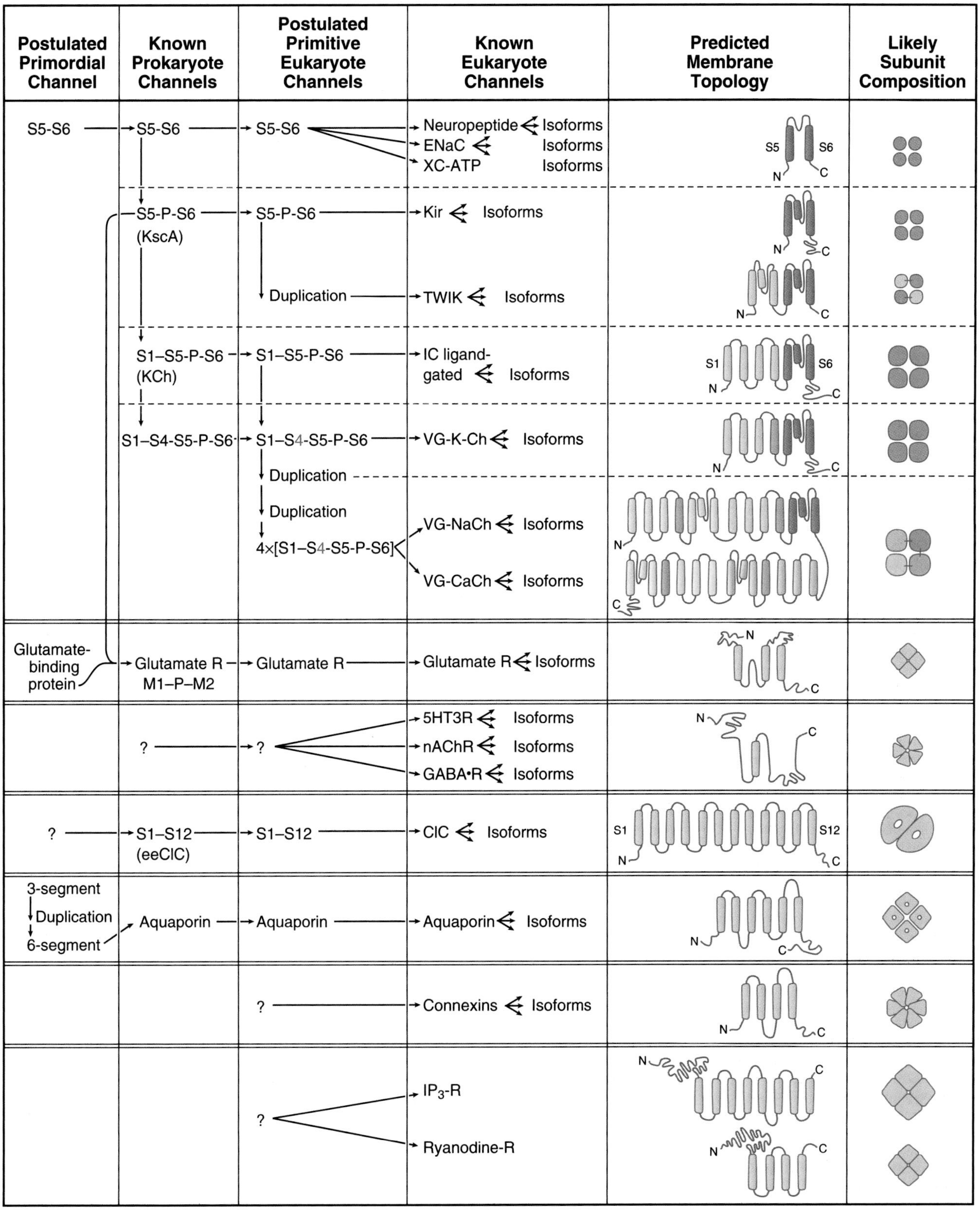

Postulated Primordial Channel	Known Prokaryote Channels	Postulated Primitive Eukaryote Channels	Known Eukaryote Channels	Predicted Membrane Topology	Likely Subunit Composition
S5-S6	S5-S6	S5-S6	Neuropeptide ⇐ Isoforms ENaC ⇐ Isoforms XC-ATP Isoforms		
	S5-P-S6 (KscA)	S5-P-S6	Kir ⇐ Isoforms		
		Duplication	TWIK ⇐ Isoforms		
	S1–S5-P-S6 (KCh)	S1–S5-P-S6	IC ligand-gated ⇐ Isoforms		
	S1–S4-S5-P-S6	S1–S4-S5-P-S6	VG-K-Ch ⇐ Isoforms		
		Duplication			
		Duplication 4×[S1–S4-S5-P-S6]	VG-NaCh ⇐ Isoforms VG-CaCh ⇐ Isoforms		
Glutamate-binding protein	Glutamate R M1–P–M2	Glutamate R	Glutamate R ⇐ Isoforms		
	?	?	5HT3R ⇐ Isoforms nAChR ⇐ Isoforms GABA·R ⇐ Isoforms		
?	S1–S12 (eeClC)	S1–S12	ClC ⇐ Isoforms		
3-segment ↓ Duplication 6-segment	Aquaporin	Aquaporin	Aquaporin ⇐ Isoforms		
		?	Connexins ⇐ Isoforms		
		?	IP$_3$-R Ryanodine-R		

Figure 9-2 *See legend on opposite page*

table 9–1

EXAMPLES OF CHANNEL-BLOCKING AGENTS

Compound (Chemical Class)	Source	Physiological Effect
Sodium Channel Blockers		
Tetrodotoxin (alkaloid)	Japanese puffer fish Pacific salaman-ders	Paralyzes skeletal muscle
Saxitoxin (alkaloid)	Dinoflagellates	Paralyzes skeletal muscle
μ-Conotoxins (peptide)	Maine snails	Paralyzes skeletal muscle
Batrachotoxin (alkaloid)	Arrow poison frogs	Paralyzes skeletal muscle
Lidocaine	Chemical synthesis	Reduces cardiac and nerve excitability
Potassium Channel Blockers		
Quaternary amino alkanes	Chemical synthesis	Blocks K-currents, nerve excitability
Calcium Channel Blockers		
Dihydropyridines	Chemical synthesis	Reduces excitability of L-type channels of striated muscles
Omega-conotoxin (peptide)	Pacific cone snail	Inhibits N-type channels in the nervous system; blocks synaptic transmission
Nicotinic Acetylcholine Receptor		
α-Bungarotoxin (peptide)	Snake	Blocks neuromuscular transmission; paralyzes skeletal muscle
α-Cobra toxin	Cobra	Blocks neuromuscular transmission; paralyzes skeletal muscle
Curare	The vine strychnos toxifera	Blocks neuromuscular transmission; paralyzes skeletal muscle

monophosphate [cAMP], G proteins). A simple duplication of one of these genes yielded channels with four segments. Even before the emergence of eukaryotes, addition of four segments (S1 to S4) yielded channels with six transmembrane segments. Acquisition of positive charges by S4 provided for voltage sensitivity. Two rounds of gene duplication and divergence produced voltage-gated channels consisting of four domains, each with six transmembrane segments, such as voltage-gated Na^+ channels. Water channels originated in prokaryotes by duplication of a gene that encoded three hydrophobic transmembrane segments. The extracellular domain of glutamate-gated channels originated as a bacterial glutamate-binding protein. The transmembrane domain of other ligand-gated channels may be related to bacterial mechanosensitive channels, a second family of channels with two transmembrane segments but a different fold than the S5/S6 channels. Double-barreled Cl^- channels also had a bacterial ancestor. The origins of gap junction connexins, calcium release channels, and single transmembrane segment channels are still obscure.

Channels in higher eukaryotes are products of multigene families that arose from multiple rounds of gene duplication and divergence. Alternative splicing also enriches the variety of channels. Combining different subunit isoforms in one channel creates increased specialization. All of this diversity suggests a sophistication of function that is difficult to demonstrate with current assays. For example, channels that produce action potentials in neurons cannot substitute for their counterparts in skeletal muscle. The reason for this is not known.

Channel Structure

The simplest channel subunits have a single transmembrane segment. For example, small bacterial peptides (gramicidin, alamethicin, and colicins, which are made to kill other species) can assemble to form highly selective and conductive channels. Gramicidin A (a 13-residue peptide) forms K^+-selective channels that may even be rendered voltage dependent by substitution of one or two amino acids.

Most channel proteins span the lipid bilayer two or more times. Some are single, large polypeptides, but many consist of multiple subunits. Most of the transmembrane segments of large channels probably contribute to regulation rather than pore formation.

Although the structures of most channels have yet to be determined, atomic structures of the transmembrane domains of a few channels suggest some general principles of pore formation and selectivity. Atomic structures of cytoplasmic and extracellular domains of other channels (see later section) provide important clues about how they are regulated.

KcsA, a K^+ channel with two transmembrane segments, is a model for the whole family of **S5/S6 channels** (Fig. 9–3). This channel, from the eubacterium *Streptomyces lividans,* consists of four identical subunits, each with two transmembrane helices connected by a **P loop** (for permeability) consisting of a short third helix and a crucial strand that makes the **selectivity filter.** The transmembrane helices are packed close together on the cytoplasmic side of the bilayer, but they splay apart on the extracellular side to make room for the **pore** helices and selectivity filter. A continuous pore extends across the membrane. The narrowest part is formed by a sequence of three residues (GYG) conserved in essentially all K^+ channels. Arranged in a straight strand highly reinforced by surrounding residues, the backbone carbonyls of these three residues line a pore 1.2 nm long and about 0.2 nm in diameter, just wide enough to accommodate a dehydrated K^+ ion. This passage distinguishes between K^+ and Na^+ with a fidelity of 10,000 to 1 even though Na^+ (with a diameter of 0.095 nm) is smaller than K^+ (0.133 nm in diameter). K^+ fits so perfectly into the pore that the pore oxygens replace the water shell of K^+ without an energy penalty, whereas the smaller Na^+ binds more strongly to its hydration shell than to the pore. The selectivity filter accommodates two K^+ ions, a local concentration exceeding that inside or outside the cell by more than 10-fold, so it actually concentrates K^+. However, it does not impede diffusion through the pore, since electrostatic repulsion between these closely spaced ions forces them apart. The remainder of the pore is lined with hydrophobic groups, but a cavity in the middle of this passage accommodates a hydrated K^+, in an environment with a negative electrostatic potential that is thought to reduce the electrostatic barrier to the ion as it crosses the membrane, as predicted by earlier physiological studies.

The atomic structure of the mechanosensitive channel, **MscL** (Fig. 9–4), from *Mycobacterium tuberculosis*, has revealed another topology for a channel polypeptide that might be relevant to ligand-gated ion channels, which also consist of five subunits surrounding a central pore. Like KcsA, each subunit of MscL has two transmembrane helices, one of which forms the walls of the pore. However, the polypeptide is threaded in the opposite direction from KcsA. Like KcsA, aromatic side chains extend into the lipid near the surfaces of the bilayer. A third C-terminal helix extends the pore 4 nm into the cytoplasm. The central pore is lined with polar residues except at its narrowest constriction where I14 and V21 reduce the diameter to about 0.2 nm. This is postulated to be the gate that opens and closes in response to physical tension in the surrounding lipid bilayer. Tension might pull the helices apart from each other and allow ions to move across the membrane. These channels lack a selectivity filter like that of KcsA, passing cations indiscriminately at high rates.

Water and glycerol channels consist of a tetramer of identical subunits. Each subunit has a narrow cen-

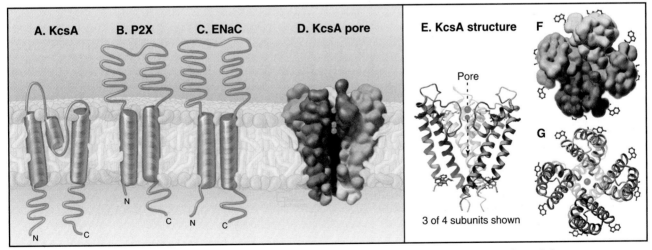

Figure 9–3 Channels with two transmembrane segments and the atomic structure of KcsA, a K^+ channel from *Streptomyces lividans. A–C,* Drawings of transmembrane topology. The short helix and loop between the two transmembrane helices of KcsA are collectively known as a P loop owing to their participation in the permeability of the pore. *D,* Space-filling model of KcsA with each subunit shaded a different color and with a cut-away view to expose the central pore. *E to G,* Ribbon and space-filling models of KcsA. The central pore is 4.5 nm long. Starting on the extracellular side, the pore consists of a negatively charged vestibule; a selectivity filter, 1.2 nm in length, that accommodates two dehydrated K^+ ions in a single-file fashion *(blue),* a central cavity with space for a single hydrated K^+ (not shown); a hydrophobic section; and a negatively charged cytoplasmic vestibule. Aromatic side chains (shown as stick figures) at both ends of the two transmembrane helices project radially into the lipid. (PDB file: 1BL8; reference: Doyle DD et al: The structure of the potassium channel: Molecular basis of K^+ conduction and selectivity. Science 280:69–77, 1998.)

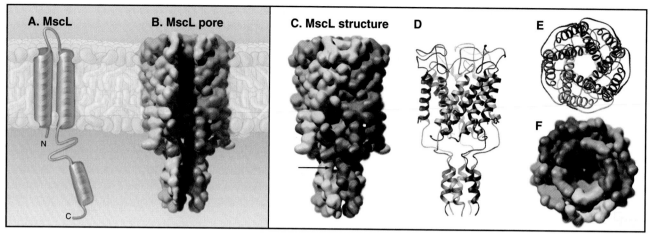

Figure 9-4 Atomic structure of MscL, a mechanosensitive channel from *Mycobacterium tuberculosis. A,* Subunit topology. Ribbon model with each subunit shaded a different color. *B,* Space-filling model with each subunit shaded a different color and a cut-away view to expose the central pore, which is 8 nm long. *C* to *F,* Space-filling and ribbon models. The arrow indicates the probable ion entry site on the cytoplasmic side of the pore. (PDB file: 1MSL; reference: Chang G, et al: Structure of the MscL homolog from *Mycobacterium tuberculosis*: A gated mechanosensitive ion channel. Science 282:2220–2226, 1998.)

tral pore surrounded by transmembrane α-helices (see Fig. 9–12). The pore accommodates the transported molecule to the exclusion of other molecules.

Channel Activity

Channel pores can be either open or closed (Fig. 9–5). Open channels, also called the **active state**, pass selected ions across the membrane at rates approaching their diffusion in water. Closed channels have a different conformation that does not pass ions or water. Most (if not all) channels also have an **inactivated state** in which part of the channel protein or an impermeant ion blocks the pore of an otherwise open channel, preventing ion diffusion. Inactivation makes a channel unresponsive to conditions that favor the active state. Voltage-gated Na^+ channels provide a good example; they cycle from closed to open and then inactivate before returning to the closed state.

Selectivity in the Open State

Open channels vary widely in their ability to discriminate among ions. Highly selective channels, such as voltage-gated K^+, Na^+, and Ca^{2+} channels, pass ions without bound water. Less selective channels, like the nicotinic acetylcholine receptor, are equally permeable to Na^+ and K^+, which probably pass through as hydrated ions. Gap junction channels pass most molecules smaller than 800 D without discrimination (see Chapter 33).

Extensive physiological data and the structure of KcsA suggest that channels achieve their selectivity by virtue of the fact that particular dehydrated ions bind

the channel filter equally well as their water shell. Ions that fit poorly in the pore are rejected, as it is energetically unfavorable to shed their hydration shell. The **ion flux** through an open channel (at a fixed membrane potential) is approximately proportionate to the ion concentration on the side from which the ions

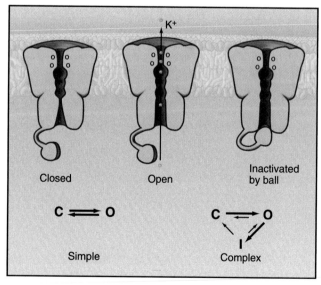

Figure 9-5 Functional states of a typical ion channel embedded in a lipid bilayer. Closed channels are inactive. Open channels are active, forming a selective pore for particular ions across the bilayer. The pore rejects other ions because of inappropriate size or charge. Either the channel protein itself or a large ion can inactivate channels by blocking the pore. In this example, an inactivation ball blocks the pore to inactivate the channel. Simple channels switch between two conformations: open and closed. Complex channels switch from closed to open to inactivated and then back to closed without returning to the open state.

migrate. The maximum rate of ion flux—10^6 to 10^8 ions/second—is limited by the time required for binding and dissociation at specific sites as an ion traverses the pore. At this high rate, channels discriminate between selected ions that bind and rejected ions that do not during an interaction lasting only 10 to 100 nanoseconds! Ions may move in single file through the pore, driven in part by electrostatic repulsion between the ions.

Transition Between the Closed, Open, and Inactivated States

Conformational changes physically open and close the pore in channel proteins. It is speculated that the pore opens and closes at a discrete spot where it is narrowest, but no example is available of atomic structures in the open and closed states.

Switching between conducting and nonconducting states is called **gating**. Gating determines channel activity because channels generally do not open partway or change their ion selectivity. Transitions between closed and open states are so fast that channels are effectively either fully open or fully closed (Fig. 9–6). The steady-state **probability of being open** (P_o) is simply the fraction of the total time that the channel is open. For a given channel, the fraction of time in the open state determines the ion flux. Because channels act independently, the total flux across a membrane depends on the number of channels open at a given time.

Some channels fluctuate spontaneously between open and closed, but in most cases, local physiological conditions, considered in detail in the following sections, control gating from moment to moment. External or internal ligands open some channels. The membrane potential opens and closes other channels without affecting the conductance of the open channels. Mechanical force gates some channels. Cells also use the full range of signaling mechanisms (see Chap-

ters 25 to 28) from phosphorylation to second messengers to guanosine-triphosphate (GTP)-binding proteins to influence the probability that particular channels open or close. By modulating the sensitivity of various channels, cells modify the behavior of their membranes and their responses to external conditions. This modulation makes channels in general, and membrane excitability in particular, highly adaptable. Chapter 10 illustrates how channel modulation regulates the heart rate, changes the efficiency of communication between nerve cells, and adapts cells to some stresses.

In some cases, a process called **inactivation** stops the flux of ions through active channels. The pore of an inactivated channel remains in the open conformation so it admits ions, but a part of the channel itself or an ion blocks the pore and prevents ions from crossing the membrane (see Fig. 9–5). Flexible cytoplasmic domains inactivate voltage-gated channels (see later discussion) by plugging the open pore. Large organic or inorganic ions, such as polyamines and Mg^{2+}, block other open channels simply by binding within and occluding the pore. The membrane potential influences ion blocking because it drives ions into or out of channels. A blocking ion that binds an open channel and dissociates slowly turns off the channel for a long time. Blockers that dissociate on a millisecond time scale cause the current through the channel to flicker on and off multiple times every time the channel opens. Even faster blocking events cannot be resolved but reduce the rate at which ions move through active channels. Local anesthetics are pharmacological channel blockers. Binding sites for blocking ions can be found on the outside, the inside, or both sides of the membrane, depending on the channel.

Transient channel openings lasting a few milliseconds change the membrane potential, but not the cytoplasmic ion composition, because so few ions cross the membrane (see Appendices 9–2 and 9–3). This is energy efficient because ion gradients created by energy-requiring pumps are not dissipated. Longer openings of tens of milliseconds can alter the ion composition of the cell. For example, voltage-gated Ca^{2+} channels remain open long enough to change the intracellular Ca^{2+} concentration and trigger cellular events (see Chapter 28). They are among the few channels that convert electrical signals to chemical signals.

Channels with One Transmembrane Segment

The simplest known channel is found in the membrane envelope of influenza virus. This **M_2 channel** consists of four small subunits, each with but one transmembrane helix. After an infected cell takes the virus into an endosome (see Chapter 23), the acidic

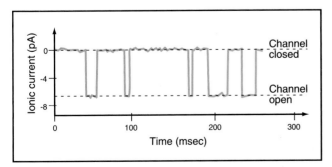

Figure 9–6 Patch recording of a single cation channel molecule. This time course shows the current that results when a single channel opens and closes at random. When open, it conducts Na^+ ions at a rate of about 36×10^6 per second, yielding a current of -6 pA. The transitions between open and closed are so fast that they appear instantaneous on this time scale.

environment opens the channel, allowing protons to enter the virus and to begin to disassemble the protein shell around the genome. The antiviral drug amantadine blocks these channels.

Vertebrates also have simple channel proteins of about 130 residues with a single transmembrane segment and no sequence homology with other known channels. These **minK** channels participate in the formation of voltage-gated, K^+-specific channels with low conductance that open slowly when the membrane depolarizes and close very slowly. minK subunits assemble with a second type of subunit with a conventional P loop called KvLQT1 and HERG, both implicated in disorders of cardiac rhythm. Both subunits contribute to the pore of the channel. Mice lacking the minK gene have defects in hearing and balance. Epithelial cells in the inner ear fail to secrete the K^+-rich fluid required for the function and viability of hair cells that transduce sound waves.

Mechanosensitive Channels

MscL (see Fig. 9–4) is an example of the simplest known channels that open in response to stretching the plasma membrane. They pass large fluxes of cations nonspecifically, allowing the cell to accommodate to swelling. These channels are widespread in prokaryotes and are also found in eukaryotes. It is speculated, but not yet proven by structural studies, that the transmembrane helices of these proteins may be the evolutionary precursors of ligand-gated ion channels (see later section).

S5/S6 Cation Channels with Two Hydrophobic Transmembrane Segments

This widespread family of S5/S6 channels, including KcsA (see Fig. 9–3), share two transmembrane helices and have a common evolutionary origin (see Fig. 9–2). The two transmembrane helices are equivalent to S5 and S6 of larger-channel proteins. Viewed functionally, they are quite heterogeneous and would not have been recognized as being related. All are cation channels and none are gated by voltage, but they vary in most other ways. For example, epithelial Na^+ channels are not gated at all, whereas peptides, ATP, and mechanical force gate other family members.

Inward Rectifier Potassium Channels

Four subunits form a channel, with the M2 (equivalent to S6) helix and P loop lining a K^+-selective pore. Several channels in this family (Kir2.1, Kir2.3, Kir3

family, and Kir4.1) are **inward rectifiers.** A rectifier is an electronic component that passes current preferentially in one direction. Inward rectifier K^+ channels pass K^+ into the cell when the membrane potential is below E_K (see Appendix 9–2), a membrane potential that is not achieved physiologically. Above the resting potential, these K^+ channels pass only a small K^+ current out of the cell when they open. The reason is that impermeant cytoplasmic cations, Mg^{2+}, and polyamines (ornithine metabolites having net positive charges of 2+ to 4+) bind to negatively charged residues on the cytoplasmic end of the S6 segment of open channels and block the passage of K^+. Despite their low permeability, these channels help to maintain the resting membrane potential in many cells and to repolarize excitable cells during an action potential.

Divergence from a common ancestor created a number of families of related channels with differing physiological properties.

- Kidney Kir1.1 channels provide a pathway for K^+ to leave renal conducting duct cells for the urine. Accordingly, they are constitutively open and not blocked by cytoplasmic ions.
- Kir2 channels in the heart and brain contribute to maintaining the resting membrane potential by keeping it from being hyperpolarized. They are constitutively active with inward rectification sensitive to membrane potential.
- Kir3 or Kir3.1 and Kir3.4 channels in the pacemaker cells of the heart regulate heart rate under the control of trimeric GTP–binding proteins (see Chapter 10).
- *Cytoplasmic* ATP regulates Kir6.2 channels in the pancreas. These channels, also called K_{ATP} channels, have a novel function requiring interaction with a member of the ABC transporter family, the **sulfonylurea receptor (SUR).** High blood glucose levels raise cytoplasmic ATP concentrations, which closes Kir6.2 channels. This pushes the membrane potential toward threshold for opening a Ca^{2+} channel, which triggers insulin secretion. Sulfonylurea drugs used to treat diabetes mellitus promote insulin secretion by inhibiting these ATP-sensitive channels.

Epithelial Sodium Channels

Epithelial Na^+ channels accelerate the rate-limiting step in Na^+ transport, an essential process that moves salt and water across epithelia in a number of organs (see Fig. 9–1A). Typically, epithelial Na^+ channels in the apical plasma membrane provide pores for Na^+ to diffuse down its concentration gradient into the cytoplasm, and Na^+/K^+-ATPases in the basolateral plasma membrane pump Na^+ out of the cell into the underlying extracellular space. Water follows Na⁺ through water channels. Renal collecting tubules use this strategy to resorb salt and water. Lung epithelial cells do the same to clear fluid from air spaces. Mice with knockout mutations in the lung epithelial Na⁺ channel gene die at birth with fluid in their lungs.

Epithelial Na⁺ channels consist of multiple α-, β-, and γ-subunits, but their stoichiometry is not known. All have two hydrophobic segments thought to be transmembrane helices, but no verified P loops. The second putative helix probably lines a pore that is 10 times more permeable to Na⁺ than to K⁺. The channel opens and closes randomly for relatively long periods, between 0.5 and 5 seconds, unaffected by the membrane potential or any known natural ligand. The drug **amiloride** blocks epithelial Na⁺ channels, so they are called amiloride-sensitive Na⁺ channels to distinguish them from voltage-gated Na⁺ channels. The steroid hormone **aldosterone,** produced in response to salt loss, increases the plasma membrane content of Na⁺ channels and the rate of Na⁺ resorption by the kidney.

Liddle's syndrome illustrates the importance of epithelial Na⁺ channels. Mutations in the C-terminal tails of the β- or γ-subunits of epithelial Na⁺ channels increase the open time of the channels, leading to excess salt and water resorption by the kidney. Humans with these mutations develop severe high blood pressure at a young age. Hypersecretion of aldosterone by adrenal tumors has similar effects.

ATP-Gated Channels

Vertebrates express at least seven protein subunits for cation channels that open in response to *extracellular* ATP. This may be surprising, as ATP is usually considered to be an intracellular energy carrier. However, ATP is stored along with neurotransmitters in many types of synaptic vesicles, so it is released at such synapses, including sympathetic nerves that innervate blood vessels and nerves involved with pain perception. These ATP-gated "purinergic" channels are called P2X receptors to distinguish them from P2Y receptors, members of the seven-helix family that are coupled to GTP-binding proteins. The subunit composition and stoichiometry are unknown. No ATP-binding site is obvious in the primary structure. The lack of specific inhibitors has impeded research on the function of these channels.

Peptide-Gated Channels

The discovery of channels gated by small peptides in the nervous systems of invertebrates was unanticipated, as all previously known channels gated by extracellular ligands bound small amines or amino acids. These channels are also unusual because they are se-

lective for Na⁺ and sensitive to amiloride. They are related to epithelial Na⁺ channels. The human brain expresses related proteins, but little is known about their functions.

Channels with Four Transmembrane Helices

Although discovered only recently, K⁺ channels with four transmembrane segments and two P loops (see Fig. 9–2, TWIK) are abundant in the genome, with 40 to 50 genes in *C. elegans*. Two of these subunits presumably form a channel with four domains similar to KcsA. They help establish the resting potential of the plasma membrane by allowing K⁺ to leak out of the cell, independent of the membrane potential. These leak channels are activated by volatile anesthetics, leading to hyperpolarization of the membrane and reduced excitability.

Voltage-Gated Cation Channels

Voltage-gated channels have two main functions. First, voltage-gated K⁺ and Na⁺ channels produce action potentials in excitable cells (see Chapter 10). Depolarization of the membrane opens these channels transiently, driving the membrane potential first toward the Na⁺ equilibrium potential (see Appendix 9–2) and then back toward the K⁺ equilibrium potential. Second, voltage-gated Ca²⁺ channels convert electrical signals into chemical signals when they admit Ca²⁺ to the cytoplasm, where it acts as a second messenger (see Chapter 28) to stimulate secretion, activate protein kinases, trigger muscle contraction, or influence gene expression.

Voltage-gated channels share a common domain structure (see Figs. 9–2 and 9–7). Each domain consists of six transmembrane helices, including S5, a P loop, and S6, surely folded like KcsA. In K⁺ channels and a bacterial Na⁺ channel, these domains are four separate polypeptides that associate noncovalently as homo-oligomers or hetero-oligomers. Na⁺ and Ca²⁺ channels consist of four similar but nonidentical domains connected in a single polypeptide. Voltage-gated channels have additional specialized domains and/or subunits, but the four main domains carry out the basic functions.

In each domain, the P loop and S5/S6 form the pore and selectivity filter. Transplantation of a P loop (S6 is required in some cases) from one channel to another yields a chimeric channel with the ion conductance of the foreign P loop. The arrangement of the surrounding helices S1 to S4 is not yet known, but they are probably tilted like S5 and S6. Extensive evi-

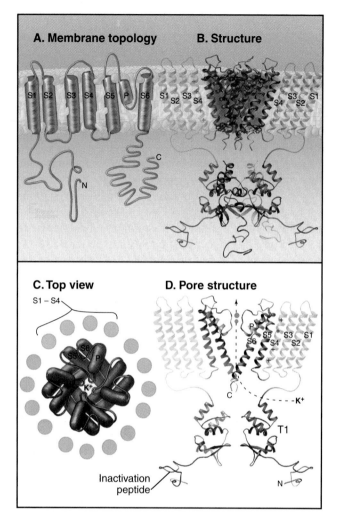

A. Membrane topology **B. Structure**

C. Top view **D. Pore structure**

S1 – S4

Inactivation peptide

Figure 9–7 Voltage-gated potassium channels. *A,* Subunit transmembrane topology. Each of four subunits has six transmembrane α-helices with a P loop between S5 and S6, similar to KcsA. *B,* Ribbon diagram based on atomic structures of KcsA (for S5, P, S6), T1, and the N-terminal inactivation peptide. S1 to S4 are shown as hypothetical helices lateral to the central pore-forming S5, P, S6. *C,* Top view of the hypothetical arrangement of the six helices in each of the four subunits. *D,* Side view of two subunits showing the central pore. Positively charged segment S4 senses the membrane potential. The T1 domain of K⁺ channels controls the assembly of four separate subunits into a functional channel. (PDB files: KcsA 1BL8, T1 domain 1td1, inactivation peptide 1ztr. Courtesy of S. Choe, Salk Institute for Biological Studies, La Jolla, CA.)

dence implicates S4 as part of the **voltage sensor** that couples membrane depolarization to channel opening.

The probability that a voltage-sensitive channel is open depends on the membrane potential (Fig. 9–8). The transition is sharp, likely because all four domains respond in a cooperative fashion. A negative internal membrane potential stabilizes the closed state. Segment S4 has a positively charged lysine or arginine every third or fourth residue, so these residues line up on one face of the helix. This S4 sequence is the "signature" of voltage-gated channels. Clever spectro-

scopic measurements show that, as the membrane potential depolarizes to −50 mV, the S4 helix rotates about 180 degrees, bringing the positive charges closer to the external side of the membrane. This physical movement, which can be detected as a **"gating current,"** initiates the conformational change that opens the channel.

Inactivation is accomplished by flexible parts of these channels, either a ball and chain at the N-terminus of some K⁺ channels (see Fig. 9–7) or a loop between the domains of Na⁺ channels. Inactivation depends upon membrane depolarization in the sense that the channel must first open to expose a binding site for the **inactivation peptide,** which then occludes the pore and blocks conduction. As a result, the channel opens only transiently. Less is known about the transition from the inactivated state to the closed state, but a conformational change must occlude the pore before the ball dissociates from the cytoplasmic side of the pore.

Potassium Channels

All known voltage-gated K⁺ channels assemble from four α-subunits. Each subunit forms a voltage-gated channel domain with helices S1 to S6 and a P loop (see Fig. 9–7). These tetramers have a square profile surrounding a central pore. Sequencing of the *Drosophila shaker* gene first revealed the architecture of these α-subunits.

Vertebrates and invertebrates use three strategies to produce voltage-gated K⁺ channels with diverse physiological properties, such as the rate of inactivation. First, they express many different K⁺ channel proteins from about 20 genes (in *C. elegans*), aug-

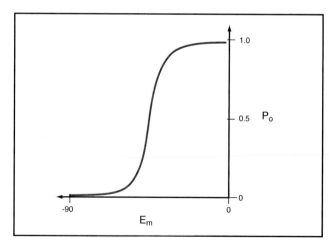

Figure 9–8 Graph of the open probability (P_o) of a voltage-gated Na⁺ channel as a function of membrane potential (E_m). Essentially, all channels are closed at the resting potential of −70 mV and all are open above a threshold potential of about −40 mV.

mented by alternate splicing of messenger RNAs (mRNAs). All metazoons appear to have four subfamilies of voltage-sensitive K+ channels. T1 domains near the N-termini of these subunits restrict formation of tetramers to subunits from the same subfamily. Second, some K+ channels are heterotetramers, providing a combinatorial strategy with the potential to produce thousands of different tetramers. Third, soluble β-subunits associate with the cytoplasmic side of some α-subunits and modify the behavior of the K+ channel tetramer. One type of voltage-gated K+ channel has a Ca²⁺ binding site at the C-terminus. Signaling events that raise cytoplasmic Ca²⁺ make these channels more sensitive to membrane depolarization, reducing the excitability of the membrane.

Shaker K+ channels are voltage-gated and rapidly inactivated by a ball on a chain carried on the N-termini of either α- or β-subunits. These residues form a globular domain tethered to the rest of the protein by a flexible linker. After a channel opens, a ball from any α- or β-subunit may inactivate the channel by binding to a site near the S4/S5 loop. Amputation of these N-terminal residues eliminates inactivation, but a soluble peptide consisting of residues 6 to 46 can rescue inactivation by binding open channels.

Mutations in the gene for the cardiac K+ channel, called HERG, cause an autosomal dominant human disease called **long QT syndrome.** The QT interval is the time between depolarization and repolarization of the heart muscle on electrocardiograms. HERG codes for a heart K+ channel of the delayed-rectifier type, which is responsible for repolarizing the membrane during action potentials (see Chapter 10). Affected patients have a mixture of normal and defective K+ channels. Mutant channels open more slowly in response to depolarization of the membrane, prolonging the action potential and predisposing the patient to abnormal cardiac rhythms and sudden death. Some HERG mutations also cause deafness.

Na⁺ Channels

Voltage-gated Na+ channels consist of one large α-subunit of four domains linked in series, each with S1 to S6 helices and a P loop (see Fig. 9–2, VG-NaCh). The 260-kD protein is 25% to 30% carbohydrate. These α-subunits alone form voltage-gated Na+ channels in vertebrate hearts and other organs. In some tissues, one or more small (39-kD) β-subunits help target α-subunits to their proper places in the cell or modify channel behavior.

Vertebrates express more than 10 Na+ channel isoforms that share many common features: transient activation by membrane depolarization, selectivity for Na+ over K+ and other monovalent ions, and the ca-

pacity to propagate action potentials. They differ slightly in their sensitivity to local anesthetics and neurotoxins. Neurons, cardiac muscle, and neonatal skeletal muscle express isoforms with a polypeptide insert between domains I and II containing five to seven phosphorylation sites that modulate channel activity.

Voltage-gated Na+ channels depolarize the plasma membrane during action potentials (see Chapter 10), so their distribution effectively defines the excitable regions of nerve cell membranes. When activated by membrane depolarization, Na+ channels cycle from closed to open to inactivated in 1 to 2 msec. At the threshold voltage, most Na+ channels open synchronously over a narrow range of membrane potential (see Fig. 9–8). Open channels are selectively permeable to Na+ (P_{Na}/P_K = 20 to 45). In 1 to 2 msec after opening, the channel inactivates when a short cytoplasmic segment between domains III and IV binds to and blocks the open pore. The channel remains inactivated until the membrane repolarizes. Then the channel rearranges to the closed state, without reopening. Inactivation does not depend on membrane potential, but because it rarely occurs unless the channel is open, inactivation appears to be voltage dependent.

Local anesthetics and a variety of neurotoxins block Na+ channels, inhibiting generation of action potentials. Several of these agents are specific for Na+ channels in particular tissues. For example, Na+ channels of sensory nerves and cardiac muscle cells are sensitive to local anesthetics, such as lidocaine and procaine. They bind to Na+ channels in the open state and block passage of Na+. Because they reduce the excitability of cardiac muscle, local anesthetics are used to treat potentially fatal disorders of cardiac rhythm. Anyone who has had dental work knows that local anesthetics also block the perception of painful stimuli. Snails use paralytic toxins to paralyze their prey, and puffer fish toxins are a health hazard for those who eat this fish.

Mutations in the gene for a heart Na+ channel are another cause of long QT syndrome in humans. Patients have a mixture of normal and defective Na+ channels. Most of the time, the mutant channels open and close normally, but occasionally, they fail to inactivate, sustaining the inward Na+ current that depolarizes the membrane. These rare abnormal events in a large population of Na+ channels delay the repolarization of the membrane, prolong the action potential, and predispose the patient to abnormal cardiac rhythms and sudden death.

Calcium Channels

Ca²⁺ channels are structurally the most complex voltage-gated ion channels (see Fig. 9–2, VG-CaCh).

Heart Ca^{2+} channels were first purified using their affinity for dihydropyridine drugs, so they are also called **dihydropyridine receptors.** The α_1-subunit has four internally homologous domains with sequence features similar to a Na^+ channel. It forms voltage-gated, Ca^{2+}-selective channels. The α_2-subunit is a glycoprotein with no homology to other known channel subunits. Its role is uncertain, but coexpression of α_2 appears to be essential for assembly and normal gating kinetics of α_1. The roles of the other, smaller peptide subunits designated β, γ, and δ are less well characterized.

Like voltage-gated Na^+ channels, Ca^{2+} channels are activated by membrane depolarization, inactivated by a first-order process, and returned to the resting state when the membrane repolarizes. Inactivation is generally slower than for Na^+ channels.

Ca^{2+} channels have numerous functions. First, in some cells, Ca^{2+} channels contribute to membrane depolarization during action potentials. Given the very low Ca^{2+} concentration inside cells (see Chapter 28), open Ca^{2+} channels have a powerful effect on membrane potential. During an action potential, Ca^{2+} currents supplement Na^+ currents in vertebrate heart cells and replace Na^+ currents in heart pacemaker cells (see Chapter 10) and some invertebrate neurons.

Second, given their long activity cycles, Ca^{2+} channels can convert electrical signals (membrane depolarization) into chemical signals by raising the cytoplasmic Ca^{2+} concentration. In cardiac muscle, Ca^{2+} triggers the release of Ca^{2+} from internal stores to stimulate contraction (see Chapters 10 and 42). In nerve terminals, an influx of Ca^{2+} triggers the secretion of neurotransmitters (see Chapter 10). In some neurons, changes in postsynaptic Ca^{2+} levels are associated with changes in the strength of synaptic signals. These changes constitute one level of synaptic learning (see Chapter 10).

Third, plasma membrane Ca^{2+} channels act as voltage sensors in skeletal muscle. Action potentials stimulate Ca^{2+} channels, which use direct physical contact to activate **Ca^{2+} release channels** located in the endoplasmic reticulum (see Chapter 42). The released Ca^{2+} stimulates contraction.

To carry out these diverse physiological functions, vertebrate cells express a variety of Ca^{2+} channel proteins with different physiological properties. Traditionally, Ca^{2+} channels have been divided into three classes, termed N, T, and L, based on the voltage required for activation, open channel currents, inactivation kinetics, and sensitivity to drugs (Table 9–2). For example, only L-type calcium channels are sensitive to dihydropyridines, which are used therapeutically to dilate blood vessels by relaxing smooth muscle. N-type Ca^{2+} channels resist dihydropyridines but are blocked selectively and nearly irreversibly by ω-conotoxin, which prevents neurotransmitter release at some synapses. Although this classification is still useful, the continued discovery of channels with novel properties has blurred these distinctions. Now cDNA cloning, expression, and characterization of single molecules provide more discrimination.

Chloride Channels

Investigators have found a large family of chloride channels (ClCs) in organisms ranging from bacteria to yeast and animals. These ClCs are implicated in membrane excitability, volume control, and epithelial transport. The transmembrane topology is not well defined, but the subunits have about 12 transmembrane segments.

The best known member of the family is ClC0 from skeletal muscle. Like voltage-gated cation channels, ClC0 channels open when the membrane depolarizes and then inactivate. In contrast to cation channels, which have a single conductance state, active Cl^- channels conduct at two levels: 10 or 20 pS. Their proposed structure explains this unusual behavior (see Fig. 9–2). Two subunits each have a pore with a conductance of 10 pS. When active, either one or both subunits conduct Cl^-. This differs from other ion channels, which form a single pore in the middle of a ring of four or five subunits. Porins (see Fig. 4–10) of the

table 9–2			
CALCIUM CHANNEL CLASSIFICATION			
Type	**Distribution**	**Functions**	**Blockers**
L-type	Cardiac muscle; skeletal muscle	Excitation-contraction coupling	Dihydropyridines
N-type	Some heart cells; sympathetic neurons; central nervous system presynaptic terminals	Neurotransmitter secretion	Omega-conotoxin
T-type	Neurons	Neuron excitation	Ni^{2+}

outer mitochondrial membrane and bacterial cell walls and the aquaporins (see later section) are the only other channels thought to have multiple pores within one channel protein.

Mutations in Cl⁻ channel genes cause several human diseases. Defective skeletal muscle ClC1 channels cause recessive and dominant myotonias. Mutations in kidney ClC5 channels predispose individuals to the formation of kidney stones.

Channels Gated by Intracellular Ligands

Families of channels gated by cytoplasmic Ca^{2+}, cyclic nucleotides, or β/γ-subunits of trimeric GTPases (see Chapter 27) diverged from K^+ channels relatively recently in evolution, about the time of divergence of animals from fungi. Their sequences are similar to each other (see Fig. 9–2, LC ligand-gated), and none are known in lower eukaryotes.

Ca^{2+}-activated K^+ channels are first cousins of voltage-gated K^+ channels. They have six transmembrane segments and a P loop. The Ca^{2+}-binding protein, **calmodulin** (see Chapter 28), binds constitutively to the cytoplasmic tail following S6. Ca^{2+}, entering the cytoplasm through the plasma membrane or released from intracellular stores (see Chapter 28), binds this associated calmodulin and activates the channel by making it more sensitive to membrane depolarization. Expression from different genes and alternative splicing produce a variety of these channels with different physiological properties.

Cyclic nucleotide–gated ion channels have six membrane-spanning segments with a P loop and a C-terminal cyclic nucleotide–binding domain homologous with bacterial cyclic nucleotide–binding proteins (Fig. 9–9). Four of these subunits, some of which may be different isoforms, form a functional channel. Cyclic nucleotide that binds to its cytoplasmic receptor domain opens a pore for Na^+ and Ca^{2+} and depolarizes the membrane. Changes in cyclic nucleotide concentration provide a sharp on/off switch, as ligand must occupy at least three of the four subunits to open the channel. Ca^{2+} entering the cytoplasm binds to calmodulin associated with the N-terminal cytoplasmic segment of the protein (see Chapter 28). This provides negative feedback to the channel.

Ion channels gated by intracellular cyclic nucleotides are particularly important in sensory systems, including olfaction and vision (see Chapter 29). Odorant molecules stimulate olfactory sensory neurons by binding plasma membrane seven-helix receptors. These receptors work through trimeric GTPases to increase the cytoplasmic concentration of cyclic adenosine monophosphate (cAMP). cAMP opens cAMP-

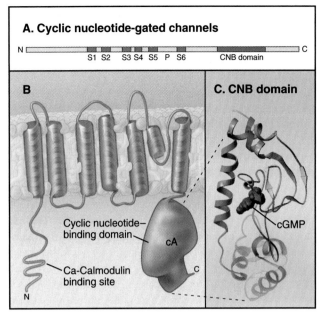

Figure 9-9 Cyclic nucleotide–gated cation channels. *A*, Domain architecture with six predicted transmembrane helices (S1 to S6), a P loop, and a C-terminal cyclic nucleotide–binding domain. *B*, Predicted transmembrane topology of each of the four identical subunits. The N-terminal cytoplasmic domain has a binding site for calcium-calmodulin. *C*, Atomic structure of the bacterial cyclic nucleotide–binding protein, CAP, which is homologous to the ligand-binding domains of these channels. cGMP, cyclic guanosine monophosphate. (PDB file: 3gap.)

gated cation channels, depolarizes the membrane, and fires an action potential. Visual transduction also uses a cyclic nucleotide–gated channel. Light activates a seven-helix receptor, leading to a decline in cytoplasmic cyclic guanosine monophosphate (cGMP). This closes cGMP-gated channels, hyperpolarizing the photoreceptor plasma membrane and reducing the secretion of neurotransmitter.

Ion Channels Gated by Extracellular Ligands

Channels gated by chemicals mediate communication between nerve terminals and other nerves or muscles. This communication takes place at specializations called synapses, which facilitate chemical transmission (see Chapter 10). On the sending side, presynaptic terminals are specialized for exocytosis of chemicals called neurotransmitters, which they package in small synaptic vesicles. Neurotransmitters include acetylcholine, serotonin, glutamic acid, glycine, and γ-aminobutyric acid (GABA) (see Fig. 10–7). When an action potential arrives at a nerve terminal, voltage-gated Ca^{2+} channels admit Ca^{2+} to the cytoplasm, causing synaptic vesicles to fuse with the plasma membrane, releasing transmitter outside the cell. Transmitters diffuse to the postsynaptic membrane in microseconds.

On the receiving side, the transmitter activates ligand-gated ion channels in the postsynaptic membrane. Many of these receptor-channels appear to have diverged from a common ancestor, but glutamate receptors had a separate bacterial origin. Some ligand-gated channels stimulate action potentials in the postsynaptic membrane by admitting cations, which drive the membrane potential toward threshold. Others inhibit action potentials by admitting Cl⁻, which hyperpolarizes the postsynaptic membrane.

Stimulation of ligand-gated channels is transient because of an inactivating conformational change called desensitization and because neurotransmitters are rapidly removed from the synaptic cleft between the cells (see Chapter 10). An extracellular enzyme degrades acetylcholine. Carriers (see Chapter 8) remove all other neurotransmitters by pumping them back into the presynaptic cell.

Glutamate Receptors

Glutamate receptors depolarize the postsynaptic membrane when glutamate binding opens a cation channel permeable to both Na⁺ and K⁺ (see Chapter 10). This depolarization of the plasma membrane excites the cell by activating voltage-sensitive sodium channels to trigger an action potential. Eukaryotic glutamate receptor channels (Fig. 9–10) have an extracellular ligand-binding domain and four hydrophobic segments: M2 is a P loop between transmembrane helices M1 and M3. Four subunits form a channel with their P loops on the cytoplasmic side of the plasma membrane, rather than outside like KcsA and its many relatives. A change in the conformation of the extracellular domain induced by glutamate binding opens a pore through the middle of the channel. Successive binding of glutamate to each of the four subunits opens the pore in steps (although binding is usually too fast to resolve these partially open states).

Multiple genes, alternative splicing, and RNA editing (see Chapter 15) all provide a diversity of glutamate receptor subunits, which assemble into homomeric and heteromeric channels distributed to different parts of the nervous system. Three families of isoforms are sensitive to different pharmacological agonists in addition to glutamate: *N*-methyl-D-aspartate **(NMDA)**, α-amino-3-hydroxy-5-methyl-4-isoxazole propionate **(AMPA)**, or **kainate**. NMDA receptors are more permeable to Ca²⁺ than Na⁺ and K⁺. Because excess intracellular Ca²⁺ can be damaging, overstimulation of NMDA receptors by glutamate released from cells during strokes, or constitutive activation of NMDA receptors by point mutations, can lead to neuronal death.

Eukaryotic glutamate receptor channels apparently originated in eubacteria by fusion of genes for a peri-

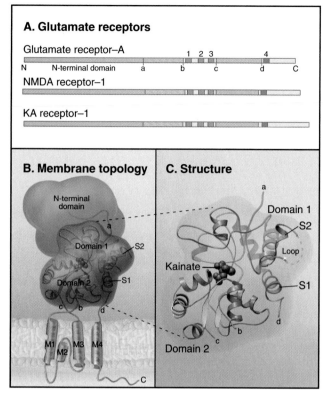

Figure 9–10 Glutamate-gated ion channels. *A*, Domain organization with the glutamate-binding domain between a and b and four predicted transmembrane segments M1 to M4. M2 is probably a cytoplasmically oriented P loop. *B*, Transmembrane topology and orientation of the atomic structure of the glutamate-binding domain. The N-terminal domain is shown approximately to scale. Four of these subunits are thought to constitute a channel similar to an inverted K⁺ channel. *C*, Atomic structure of the ligand-binding extracellular domain from the vertebrate kainate (KA) receptor. (PDB file: 1gr2. Reprinted with permission from Nature. Reference: Armstrong N, Sun Y, Chen G-Q, Gouaux E: Structure of a glutamate-receptor ligand-binding core in complex with kainate. Nature 395:913–917, 1998. Copyright 1998, Macmillan Magazines Limited.)

plasmic amino acid–binding protein (similar to *Escherichia coli* glutamine-binding protein) and an S5/P/S6 potassium channel similar to KcsA. Cyanobacteria have such a glutamate-gated, potassium-selective channel with only two transmembrane segments and a P loop similar to an inverted KcsA channel. The domain organization of plant glutamate receptors is similar to animal brain glutamate receptors. Glutamate receptors participate in the response of developing plants to light.

Nicotinic Acetylcholine Receptor

From a physiological standpoint, the best characterized ligand-gated channel is an excitatory cation channel—the nicotinic acetylcholine receptor from the plasma membrane of skeletal muscle cells. This receptor triggers action potentials that stimulate muscle con-

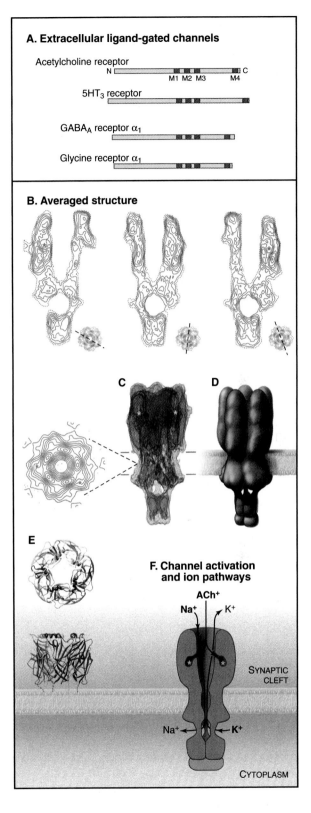

Figure 9-11 Nicotinic acetylcholine receptor. *A,* Domain organization of the acetylcholine receptor and related receptors gated by neurotransmitters. The second hydrophobic segment M2 forms a transmembrane helix. The conformations of the other transmembrane segments are not known. *B,* Structure of the pentameric nicotinic acetylcholine receptor from the electric organ of the electric ray determined by electron microscopy at a resolution of 0.46 nm. The four different kinds of subunits $(\alpha_2\beta\gamma\epsilon)$ in these pentameric channels have homologous sequences but distinct structures even at this resolution. The density maps are sections perpendicular to the membrane through the subunits indicated in the cross-sections to the lower right of each map. The two red α-subunits each have a deep cavity marked with an asterisk where acetylcholine binds. All five subunits come close together within the membrane bilayer to form a pore opened by acetylcholine binding. A cross-section of the pore at the lower left shows an M2 α-helix contributed by each of the five subunits lining the pore. *C,* Three-dimensional density map. *D,* Space-filling surface representation. *E,* Ribbon diagrams showing top and side views of the atomic structure of a pentameric acetylcholine binding protein from a snail. This cylindrical structure is homologous with the N-terminal, extracellular domain of the nicotinic acetylcholine receptor. *F,* Central section through the pore showing the passage for Na^+ into the cell and K^+ out of the cell. A 43-kD protein called rapsyn (*blue*) binds on the cytoplasmic side. (*A to D, F,* Structural maps courtesy of N. Unwin, MRC Laboratory of Molecular Biology, Cambridge, England; reference: Miyazawa A, Fujioshi Y, Stowell M, Unwin N. Nicotinic acetylcholine receptor at 4.6 Å resolution: Transverse tunnels in the channel wall. J Mol Biol 288: 765–786, 1999. *E,* PDB file: 1I9B. Reference: Brejc K, van Dijk WJ, Klaassen RV, et al: Crystal structure of an ACh-binding protein reveals the ligand-binding domain of nicotinic receptors. Nature 411:269–276, 2001.)

traction (see Chapters 10 and 42). It is called the nicotinic acetylcholine receptor because it also binds **nicotine.** Related nicotinic acetylcholine receptors in the central and peripheral nervous system are thought to be targets in tobacco addiction.

The muscle nicotinic acetylcholine receptor is a pentamer of four different, but homologous, subunits with the composition $\alpha_2\beta\gamma\epsilon$ (Fig. 9–11). Each subunit has a large N-terminal extracellular segment, four hydrophobic sequences (M1 to M4), and a large cytoplasmic segment between M3 and M4. The M2 segment of each of the five subunits forms an α-helix that lines the ion pore like staves of a barrel. Negative side chains on M2 may contribute to the cation selectivity of the pore. The other three hydrophobic segments of each subunit may be membrane-spanning α-helices or a β-sheet. A crystal structure of a pentameric molluscan acetylcholine-binding protein provides a model for the N-terminal extracellular domains. The 210 residues are folded into a highly twisted β-sandwich of 10 strands with the conserved residues forming a hydrophobic core. Muscle cells and some central nervous system neurons express more than two dozen different isoforms of nicotinic acetylcholine receptors, most with a mixture of subunits but some with five identical subunits.

Acetylcholine binding in deep cavities in the two α-subunits opens a transmembrane pore that is more permeable to K^+ and Na^+ than to Ca^{2+}. Active channels cause the membrane potential to collapse toward a reversal potential around 0 mV. This triggers a self-propagating action potential in the muscle plasma membrane with nearly 100% efficiency (see Fig. 10–8).

Many toxins bind nicotinic acetylcholine receptors, blocking transmission of impulses between motor nerves and skeletal muscle (see Table 9–1). **α-Bungarotoxin** has been used to characterize the receptor. **Curare** is a powerful muscle relaxant used during surgery because it blocks acetylcholine-binding sites without opening the channel. Local anesthetics, such as procaine, bind within the channel and block ion conductance.

Some people produce autoimmune antibodies to nicotinic acetylcholine receptors, resulting in a disease called **myasthenia gravis.** When antibody binds to the receptor, the skeletal muscle internalizes the receptor, reducing its response to acetylcholine and causing weakness.

Other Neurotransmitter Receptors

Receptors activated by the neurotransmitters GABA or glycine consist of five subunits with sequences similar to nicotinic acetylcholine receptors. They are Cl^- channels that hyperpolarize the postsynaptic membrane. Several isoforms of GABA receptors bind **benzodiazepines,** drugs used to treat depression. They increase the probability that the channel will open. **Strychnine** inhibits glycine receptors, making neural circuits oversensitive to stimulation. Channels opened by 5-hydroxytryptamine (serotonin) consist of five similar subunits.

Capsaicin Receptors

The receptor that responds to the hot substance in chili peppers (a chemical called capsaicin) is a novel calcium channel with six transmembrane segments and a putative P loop. High temperatures also activate these channels, explaining why the chemical and thermal stimuli yield the same sensation.

Water Channels

Water channels, called **aquaporins,** are the most recently discovered family of channel proteins. Although postulated years ago by physiologists to explain the water permeability of certain cell membranes, they eluded isolation until investigators tested a small hydrophobic protein from red blood cells for water channel activity. When expressed in frog eggs, this protein made the eggs permeable to water so that they swelled and burst when placed in hypotonic media. Knowledge of this protein rapidly led to the characterization of a family of related proteins from many species.

Aquaporins are an ancient family of proteins found in bacteria, fungi, plants, and animals. A related channel transports glycerol across bacterial membranes. All known family members have six hydrophobic segments, thought to be α-helices, that cross the lipid bilayer (Fig. 9–12). The two halves of the protein arose by a gene duplication, since their sequences are remarkably similar. These features have been conserved from bacteria to humans. Four identical subunits form a stable tetramer in the plane of the membrane. Each tetramer has four separate water pores. Hydrogen bonding of waters with a pair of asparagine residues at a narrow point in the pore allows the channel to be selective for water.

Water diffuses relatively slowly across lipid bilayers, so membranes are barriers to water movement unless they contain water channels. Aquaporins provide highly permeable pores across membranes. About 10 water molecules line up in a pore about 0.3 nm in diameter. Osmotic pressure created by pumps, carriers, and the macromolecular composition drives water through the pore at rates exceeding 10^9 water molecules per second. This explains why red blood cells rapidly swell and shrink passively, depending on the osmolarity of the surrounding fluid (see Fig. 6–8). As far as it is known, most water channels have no gates, so they are open constitutively.

Various human tissues express six different aquaporin isoforms. Aquaporin-1 is found in red blood cells, renal proximal tubules, blood vessel endothelial cells, and the choroid plexus (which makes spinal fluid in the brain). A few humans carry mutations that inactivate aquaporin-1; remarkably, homozygotes have no symptoms despite the low water permeability of their red blood cells (and presumably other tissues that depend on this isoform). Aquaporin-2 is required for renal collecting ducts to reabsorb water. One patient with inactivating mutations in both aquaporin-2 genes suffered from severe water loss, called nephro-

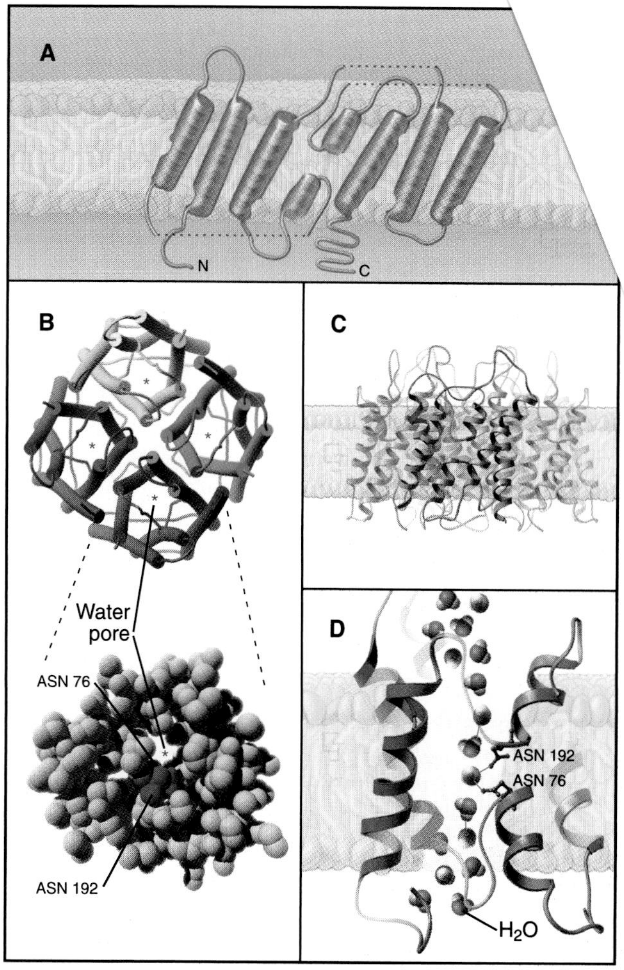

Figure 9–12 Water channels. *A*, Membrane topology of aquaporin-1 deduced from the primary structure. The two halves of the polypeptide have similar sequences but are inverted relative to each other. *B*, Atomic structure determined by electron crystallography, showing for identical units, each with a pore *(red asterisk)*. *C*, Ribbon diagram. *D*, Detail of the water pore, with a chain of water molecules crossing the membrane. Two asparagines in the middle of the pore hydrogen bond one water. (Courtesy of P. Agre, Johns Hopkins Medical School. PDB file: 1FQY; reference: Murata K, Mitsuoka K, Hirai T, et al: Structural determinants of water permeation through aquaporin-1. Nature 407:599–605, 2000.)

genic diabetes insipidus. **Antidiuretic hormone** (vasopressin) controls the placement of aquaporin-2 in the collecting duct membrane. It activates a seven-helix receptor, causing cytoplasmic vesicles storing aquaporin-2 to fuse with the plasma membrane. This increases the permeability of apical plasma membranes to water, allowing it to move from the urine into the hypertonic extracellular space of the renal medulla. Reaction of sensitive cysteine residues with mercuric chloride closes the water pores of aquaporins. This explains how mercurials, used therapeutically as diuretics in the past, inhibit the reabsorption of water filtered by the kidney. The reversible inhibition of aquaporins with mercurials provides a test for their participation in physiological processes.

Water channels are also important in plants, which depend on water to maintain turgor and to expand cells in growing tissues. When the stomata in the leaves are open, water moves continuously from roots through xylem vessels and cells in tissues to exit from leaves as vapor. The movement across cell and tonoplast membranes depends on water channels. Water deprivation induces expression of tonoplast aquaporins in some plants and may provide a mechanism for plants to compete for water when it is scarce.

Porins

Porins are channels with wide, water-filled pores found in the outer membranes of gram-negative bacteria and mitochondria. The subunits are composed of an antiparallel barrel of 16 or 18 β-strands that cross the membrane (see Fig. 6–8C). One to three of the loops connecting the strands extend into the center of the barrel and line the pore. The functional molecule consists of three identical subunits.

Most porins are relatively nonselective pores for small, water-soluble molecules, although some are specific for certain solutes, such as sugars. *E. coli* uses a related protein with 22 transmembrane β-strands to transport iron complexes across the outer membrane. A central "cork" domain occludes the lumen of this β-barrel. Interactions across the periplasmic space with plasma membrane proteins open and close the pore. A variety of viruses use bacterial porins as receptors.

ELECTRICAL RECORDINGS IN BIOLOGY

Analysis of electrical activity across biological membranes requires sensitive methods to detect electrical potential differences and the flow of current on a rapid time scale. Physiologists and clinicians use four general methods, with different sensitivities, to detect electrical activity of single channels (patch electrodes), cell membranes (microelectrodes and fluorescent dyes), and whole tissues (extracellular electrodes).

Single Channel Recordings with Patch Electrodes. "Patch-clamp microelectrodes" (Fig. 9–13*A*) provide the best way to characterize the behavior of individual channels. A small-diameter, fire-polished glass capillary is pressed, with suction, onto the surface of a cell, forming a high-resistance seal (10–50 gigaohm). The membrane patch is small enough to contain just a few ion channels. The electrode becomes part of an electric circuit that can measure current or voltage across the membrane. The high-resistance seal between micropipette and membrane ensures that more electrical current (composed of ions) flows through a single open channel than leaks in around the side of the electrode. When a channel opens, a sensitive ammeter connected to the micropipette records the direction and magnitude of ion flow through the channel as an electrical current. Patch electrodes give direct information about both current and the time that individual channels spend open or closed.

Variations of the patch-clamp technique provide access to channel properties. Leaving the membrane patch on the cell (cell-attached configuration) reveals properties of the channels in their cellular context. Lifting the membrane patch off the cell (excised-patch configuration) exposes the cytoplasmic surface of the membrane to ions, enzymes, or second messengers that the investigator adds to the bath. Similarly, the investigator can test the effects of potential ligands, drugs, and ions in the micropipette.

Measurement of Membrane Potentials with Intracellular Microelectrodes and Fluorescent Dyes. A glass capillary is drawn to a fine tip ($\sim$0.5 μm), filled with a conducting solution (3 M KCl), and inserted through the plasma membrane. The tip penetrates the cell with minimal damage, and the membrane seals tightly around it. The microelectrode is connected to a meter to record current and voltage (see Fig. 9–13*B*). Alternatively, the investigator can apply a patch electrode to the cell surface and suck forcefully to breach the membrane, putting the micropipette in continuity with the cytoplasm for recordings from the rest of the membrane.

Two microelectrodes inserted into a beaker of saline register no potential difference. If one electrode is inserted into a cell, the meter registers a potential difference of -60 to -90 mV inside the cell relative to the bath. This **membrane potential** arises from the combined action of many membrane pumps, carriers, and

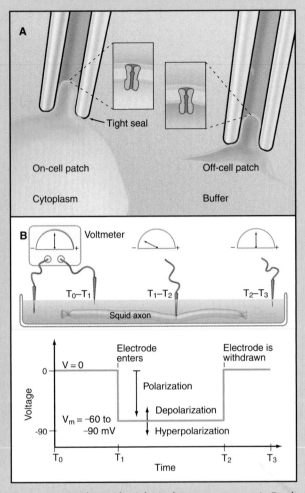

Figure 9–13 Electrophysiological measurements. *A,* Patch electrode. Fine-tipped glass micropipettes form a tight seal with a small patch of plasma membrane. The salt solution inside the pipette conducts current flowing through an open channel in the patch for recording. Lifting the patch of membrane off the cell exposes the cytoplasmic surface of the membrane to experimental manipulation from the bath. Solutes in the micropipette can stimulate the extracellular face of the membrane. *B,* Measurement of membrane potentials and currents with microelectrodes. A fine-tipped micropipette penetrates the plasma membrane of a cell and is part of a circuit that can record either membrane potential or current flowing across the membrane. To measure membrane potential, a voltmeter in the circuit records the voltage inside the cell relative to the bath and follows any changes that occur when ion channels open and close. To measure current, an electronic feedback device is placed in the circuit to hold the membrane potential at a constant value. Under these "voltage-clamped" conditions, the feedback device provides current to balance any current that results from opening of membrane channels. The current from the feedback device is a record of current across the membrane.

appendix 9–1

ELECTRICAL RECORDINGS IN BIOLOGY *Continued*

channels. Thus, the membrane potential is an ensemble property of a large number of individual molecules. Microelectrodes can measure the membrane potential on a submillisecond time scale.

New fluorescent dyes provide an optical signal that is sensitive to membrane potential. This is the only convenient approach for acquiring information about the spatial distribution of potential charges.

Extracellular Electrical Measurements. Synchronous electrical activity of thousands of cells produces small elec-

trical currents outside the cells, which can be recorded with extracellular electrodes or even with electrodes on the surface of the body. Physicians take advantage of this phenomenon to record the ensemble electrical activity of the heart (**electrocardiogram** [ECG]), brain (**electroencephalogram** [EEG]), and muscle (**electromyogram** [EMG]). These recordings reflect the behavior of thousands of cells, so they provide little information about events at molecular or cellular levels.

appendix 9–2

THE BIOPHYSICAL BASIS OF MEMBRANE POTENTIALS

The membrane potential arises from separation of charges across an insulating surface (Fig. 9–14). The lipid bilayer provides the insulation required to separate charges. Either pumps or channels can produce unpaired charges. Pumps that transport unpaired ions generate membrane potentials directly. Channels that pass unpaired ions can use ion concentration gradients across membranes to generate membrane potentials. The concentration gradient provides a diffusional force to drive ions through channels. Because channels are ion specific, an excess of charge builds up after very few ions cross a membrane. This excess charge creates a membrane potential and stops the net movement of additional ions across the membrane.

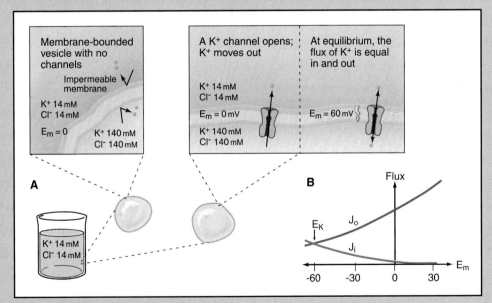

Figure 9–14 Membrane potential. *A,* Production of a membrane potential, Em, by a K+-selective ion channel and a 10-fold potassium chloride concentration gradient across a membrane. The three panels illustrate the situations without a channel, when a channel first opens, and at equilibrium. *B,* Dependence of K+ fluxes out of the vesicle (J_o) and into the vesicle (J_i) as a function of membrane potential (E_m). K+ passes into the vesicle (driven by the concentration gradient) and out of the vesicle (driven by the voltage across the membrane). At a potential of −60 mV, these fluxes are balanced. This is called the resting potential, or E_K. If the membrane potential is greater than −60 mV, the flux of K+ into the vesicle (driven by the concentration gradient) exceeds the flux out of the vesicle (driven by the voltage across the membrane). This pushes the potential toward E_K.

Appendix continued on following page

appendix 9–2

THE BIOPHYSICAL BASIS OF MEMBRANE POTENTIALS *Continued*

This discussion starts with a qualitative description of forces behind membrane potentials and then develops a quantitative account of membrane potentials with single or multiple types of ion channels.

Diffusion Potentials. An impermeable membrane enclosing concentrated potassium chloride is suspended in a bath of more dilute potassium chloride (see Fig. 9–14). If the membrane contains a pore that is *selectively permeable* for bidirectional diffusion of K$^+$, the concentration gradient drives K$^+$ out of the membrane compartment. Because Cl$^-$ cannot pass through this selective pore or the membrane bilayer, the inside compartment loses positive charge. Charge imbalance creates an electrical field, negative inside, called the **membrane potential.** By convention, extracellular voltage is defined as zero.

Force provided by the membrane potential influences the diffusion of ions through the pore in both directions. The positive potential outside opposes the diffusion of K$^+$ out of the vesicle and drives K$^+$ into the vesicle, up its concentration gradient. Net K$^+$ efflux continues until a charge imbalance builds up a membrane potential large enough to drive K$^+$ influx at the same rate that the concentration gradient drives K$^+$ efflux. The electrical potential required to stop net ion movement is called the **equilibrium potential** for K$^+$, or **Nernst potential,** E_K.

Quantitative Relationships. The quantitative description of membrane potentials by the Nernst equation is *the* central concept of electrophysiology. This relationship between an ion concentration gradient and a balancing membrane potential is derived as follows, using K$^+$ as an example.

The concentration gradient provides the first force. J_o is the rate (expressed in ions per second) of efflux through the K$^+$-selective pore. J_i is the rate of influx. The fluxes are proportionate to the concentrations on the side from which the ions come. The ratio of these rates is equal to the ratio of the inside and outside K$^+$ concentrations, K_i and K_o:

$$\frac{J_o}{J_i} = \frac{K_i}{K_o}$$

A typical cell has a $K_i : K_o$ ratio of about 35.

The membrane potential provides a second force. A positive potential gives a positive ion a higher energy, driving it down the electrical gradient. A negative potential has the opposite effect. The difference in electrical energy per mole of ions is equal to *zFE,* where *z* is the valence (+1 for K$^+$), *F* is the faraday constant (10^5 coulombs/mol), and *E* is the potential in volts. This difference in energy enters the equation for the flux ratio as an exponential term (the "Boltzmann factor"), with the electrical energy difference divided by the thermal energy:

$$\frac{J_o}{J_i} = \frac{K_i e^{zFE/RT}}{K_o}$$

where *R* is the gas constant and *T* is the absolute temperature.

The K$^+$ fluxes in and out are equal when

$$\frac{K_i e^{zFE/RT}}{K_o} = 1$$

This famous Nernst equation can be rearranged to give the equilibrium (Nernst) potential in terms of the ion concentrations.

$$E_K = \frac{RT}{zFK_i} \ln K_o$$

RT is the thermal energy of a mole of particles. The ratio *RT/zF* has the dimensions of voltage and provides the electrical potential that gives a mole of charged particles with valence *z* an electrical energy *(zFE)* equal to the thermal energy *(RT).* At physiological temperatures, its value is about 25 mV for univalent ions where *z* = 1. The ratio of *RT/zF* establishes the range of potentials (tens of millivolts) that occur in cells.

Another form of the Nernst equation is more convenient. Since ln (x) = 2.3 log (x), and 2.3 *RT/F* = 60 mV at 30°C, the Nernst equation can be rewritten as

$$E_K = \frac{60\ \text{mV}}{z} \log K_o/K_i$$

Thus, the membrane potential is −60 mV when the K$^+$ concentration inside is 10 times the concentration outside.

Nernst Potential for Various Ions. The Nernst potential can be calculated for each ion known to have a selective channel in cell membranes: Na$^+$, K$^+$, Ca^{2+}, and Cl$^-$ (see Fig. 9–15). Given physiological gradients of these ions across the plasma membrane, the membrane potential could range from −98 to +128 mV, depending on which channels are open. In resting cells, only K$^+$ channels are open, so the resting membrane potential is close to E_K. Thus, variation of extracellular K$^+$ concentration changes the membrane potential. In vertebrates, the normal extracellular K$^+$ concentration is about 4 mM, but it varies from 2 mM to >8 mM in disease states. This four-fold variation in K_o changes the membrane potential by 30–37 mV, enough to affect cellular processes that are sensitive to the membrane potential. Other channels open and close selectively in response to extracellular or intracellular ligands, membrane potential, physical forces, or other factors (see text). Selective activation of channels is responsible for action potentials and other behavior of excitable membranes (see Chapter 10).

appendix 9–3

CHARGING AND DISCHARGING THE MEMBRANE

Opening or closing ion channels influences the membrane potential and the flux of ions across the membrane. This discussion explains how movement of just a few ions allows cells to change their membrane potential without dissipating ion gradients across the membrane. Consequently, flux through a few ion channels rapidly changes the membrane potential during action potentials. The result of opening multiple channels with different ion selectivities and concentration gradients is also explained.

Membrane Capacitance. The membrane potential (E) produced by a given net charge inside the cell (Q) depends on the physical properties of the membrane, summarized in a constant called **capacitance** (C).

$$E = \frac{Q}{C}$$

Capacitance depends on membrane area, thickness (physical separation between internal and external charges), and dielectric constant. If the capacitance is large, many ions must move to change the membrane potential. For cell membranes, the capacitance is approximately 1 μF/cm^2. One farad is 6 × 10^{18} charges per volt.

Charge Movement for a Small Cell. The following calculation shows why *ion concentration gradients change little during most electrical events in cells.* This is important to obviate the requirement for excessive energy to restore ion gradients. A cell that is 18 μm in diameter might have a capacitance of 10^{-11} F, or 6 × 10^7 charges per volt of membrane potential. Thus, movement of 6 million positive charges out of the cell produces a membrane potential of −0.1 volt, or −100 mV. A cell of this size with an internal concentration of 150 mM K$^+$ contains about 2.7 × 10^{11} K$^+$, so movement of less than one out of 40,000 K ions from inside to outside creates a large membrane potential. This fraction of ions is far less for large cells owing to their smaller ratio of surface area to volume. Thus, little energy is required for a large change in membrane potential, such as an action potential. When ion channels open, few ions cross the membrane before an opposing electrical field develops and retards further flux.

In Chapters 7 and 8, pumps and carriers were also noted to produce opposing membrane potentials when moving ions across membranes. This can be avoided by opening ion channels that short-circuit the change in membrane potential by providing pathways for counterions to move in the same direction or similar ions to move in the opposite direction across the membrane.

Rate of Charge Movement Through Channels. A current is the rate of movement of charge. The ionic current (I) across a membrane is taken as *positive* when charges move *outward.* According to this definition, the equation for conservation of charge in a cell is

$$\frac{dQ}{dt} = -I$$

A positive current reduces the net charge inside the cell, and vice versa. Including the relationship for capacitance ($E = Q/C$), the equation relates the current to the rate of change of membrane potential:

$$\frac{dE}{dt} = \frac{-I}{C}$$

Because channels conduct about 6 × 10^6 charges per second, a single open channel changes E at a rate of −100 mV/sec on this 18-μm cell.

Because most channels occur at densities of 50–200/μm^2, an 18-μm cell will have 50,000–200,000 channels. If a few channels open together, the membrane potential rapidly approaches the Nernst potential for the selected ion. This explains why most electrical events in cells transpire in a millisecond time frame. Because the rate of current flow through ion channels is not limiting, the time course of electrical events depends on the kinetics of channel opening and closing. This focuses attention on factors that control whether channels are open or closed, also known as **gating.**

Net Current Through Ion-Selective Channels. Another way to describe ionic current across a membrane is

$$I = ze_o(J_o - J_i)$$

where e_o is the elementary charge. The dependence of current on membrane potential for real channels is complicated (see Fig. 9–14B), so electrophysiologists approximate this current-voltage relationship of channels by a linear relationship, such as Ohm's law ($E = IR$):

$$I = g(E - E_{ion})$$

where g is **conductance** (inverse of resistance) and E_{ion} is the **reversal potential** of a particular ion channel (the potential at which current reverses from out to in). For perfectly selective pores, the reversal potential for each ion equals its Nernst potential, even in the face of other ionic gradients. The unit used for current is siemens (equivalent to 1 ampere per volt). Most channels have currents in the picosiemens range (10^{-9} S).

For a simple pore, a plot of current versus membrane potential is linear, with no current at E_{ion}; real channels are more complicated. Typical plots of current versus voltage deviate from a straight line. This is called **rectification.** Deviation may be attributable to voltage-dependent conformational changes in the channel protein or to nonpermeant ions blocking the pore.

Appendix continued on following page

appendix 9–3

CHARGING AND DISCHARGING THE MEMBRANE *Continued*

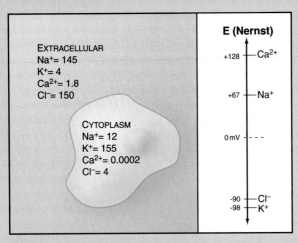

EXTRACELLULAR
$Na^+ = 145$
$K^+ = 4$
$Ca^{2+} = 1.8$
$Cl^- = 150$

CYTOPLASM
$Na^+ = 12$
$K^+ = 155$
$Ca^{2+} = 0.0002$
$Cl^- = 4$

E (Nernst)

+128 — Ca^{2+}

+67 — Na^+

0 mV - - - -

-90 — Cl^-
-98 — K^+

Figure 9-15 Physiological ion concentrations and membrane potentials. Ion concentrations in the cytoplasm and outside a typical vertebrate cell. The scale on the right shows the corresponding equilibrium membrane potentials (Nernst potentials) that would result if channels for each one of these ions opened.

Each channel contributes independently to the total current, so given *n* channels on a cell membrane, the total current is

$$I = ng(E - E_{ion}).$$

Opening Na^+ and K^+ channels has opposite effects because the ion concentration gradients are reversed. The Nernst potential for Na^+ is about +65 mV in a typical cell, given a 10-fold excess of Na^+ outside the cell. Current through an Na^+ channel is negative (i.e., inward) at membrane potentials below E_{Na}. Thus, if a Na^+ channel opens on a cell in which *E* equals 0, the membrane potential rises toward E_{Na}.

Consequence of Multiple Channel Types Opening Simultaneously. More than one type of open channel creates a situation more complicated than the *equilibrium* described by the Nernst potential for a single ion species (Figs. 9–15 and 9–16). Consider a cell with physiological ion gradients and two channels—one open K^+ channel and one open Na^+ channel—having conductances of g_K and g_{Na}. The total current through these two channels is the sum of the individual currents:

$$I_{total} = g_K(E - E_K) + g_{Na}(E - E_{Na})$$

Note from this relationship that current is zero at the midpoint between E_K and E_{Na}, and the line has twice the slope of a single channel (i.e., twice the conductance).

Which channel predominates? The equation for I_{total} can also be written as

$$I_{total} = g_{eff}(E - E_{eff})$$

where the effective conductance g_{eff} and reversal potential E_{eff} are given by

$$g_{eff} = g_K + g_{Na}$$

and

$$E_{eff} = \frac{g_K E_K}{g_K + g_{Na}} + \frac{g_{Na} E_{Na}}{g_K + g_{Na}}$$

The two channels together act like a single channel with an effective conductance equal to the sum of their conductances and a reversal potential that is the

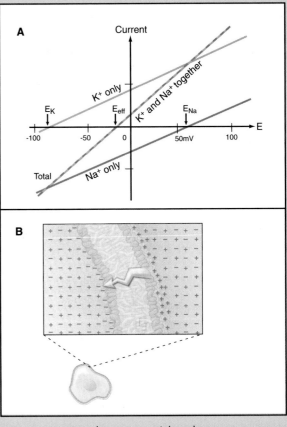

Figure 9-16 Membrane potential and currents across a membrane with two types of channels. *A,* Dependence of currents on membrane potential resulting from opening either K^+ channels or Na^+ channels individually or together. In contrast to Figure 9–14*B,* which shows ion fluxes in each direction, this is a plot of net current. E_K and E_{Na} are the equilibrium potentials (zero current) when only potassium or sodium channels are open. When both types of channels are open, the equilibrium potential (E_{eff}) is midway between the equilibrium potentials of the two types of channels. *B,* Distribution of positive (*red*) and negative (*blue*) ions across the plasma membrane and around a cell having a negative membrane potential. Excess negative charge builds up near the inside of the membrane, with the excess positive charge near the outside.

appendix 9–3

CHARGING AND DISCHARGING THE MEMBRANE *Continued*

weighted average of their reversal potentials, that is, weighted by their relative conductances (see Fig. 9–16A).

Goldman, Hodgkin, and Katz formulated another equation for *E*. It uses permeability (P, in units of cm/sec) to describe the membrane potential:

$$E = \frac{RT}{F} \ln \frac{P_{Na}[Na]_o + P_K[K]_o + P_{Cl}[Cl]_o + \ldots}{P_{Na}[Na]_i + P_K[K]_i + P_{Cl}[Cl]_i + \ldots}$$

This equation summarizes the concepts presented here about membrane potentials. Just *two factors* determine the membrane potential: (1) the **concentration gradients** of different ions (e.g., the Nernst potentials for each ion) and (2) the relative permeabilities of the membrane to these ions. When all Na^+ and Cl^- channels are closed (P_{Na}, $P_{Cl} = 0$), the equation reduces to the Nernst relationship for K. When all K^+ and Cl^- channels are closed (P_K, $P_{Cl} = 0$), the equation collapses to the Nernst relationship for Na^+.

In nerve cells, the resting membrane is most permeable to K^+ but also slightly permeable to Na^+, so the resting potential is near E_K. Opening more K^+ channels or lowering extracellular K^+ makes the resting potential more negative. Opening more Na^+ channels or raising extracellular Na^+ makes the resting potential more positive.

Charge Redistribution by Electrical Conduction. Most cellular ions have balancing counterions, whereas unpaired ions contributing to membrane potentials are confined to boundary layers near the membrane (see Fig. 9–16B). Like-charged ions repel one another, so unpaired ions tend to accumulate at boundaries where they can move no farther.

During electrical events, unpaired ions redistribute over membrane surfaces by electrical conduction at rates much faster than diffusion. It works as follows. Ions are always in motion, exchanging places. Introduction of extra ions sets off a chain of movements as neighbors repel each other, resulting in rapid spread of unbalanced charge near the membrane. Diffusion of the entering ions over to the membrane would take much longer than this electrical wave. Thus, electrical signaling is the fastest signaling process in cells.

▌ Selected Readings

Agre P, Bonhiver M, Borgnia MJ: The aquaporins, blueprints for cellular plumbing systems. J Biol Chem 273:14659–14662, 1998.

Armstrong CM, Hille B: Voltage-gated ion channels and electrical excitability. Neuron 20:371–380, 1998.

Biggin PC, Roosild T, Choe S: Potassium channel structure: Domain by domain. Curr Opin Struct Biol 2000.

Brejc K, van Dijk WJ, Klaassen RV, et al: Crystal structure of an Ach-binding protein reveals the ligand-binding domain of nicotinic receptors. Nature 411:269–276, 2001.

Bretweiser G: Mechanisms of K^+ channel regulation. Membrane Biol 152:1–11, 1996.

Brown DA: The acid test for resting potassium channels. Curr Biol 10:R456–459, 2000.

Catterall WA: Molecular properties of a superfamily of plasma membrane cation channels. Curr Opin Cell Biol 6:607–615, 1994.

Cooper EC, Jan LY: Ion channel genes and human neurological disease: Recent progress, prospects and challenges. Proc Natl Acad Sci USA 96:4759–4766, 1999.

Dutzler R, Campbell EB, Cadene M, et al: X-ray structure of a ClC chloride channel at 3.0 Å reveals the molecular basis of anion selectivity. Nature 415:287–294, 2002.

Gadsby DC: Two-bit anion channel really shapes up. Nature 383:295, 1996.

Hille B: Ion Channels of Excitable Membranes. Sunderland, MA: Sinauer Associates, 1992.

Hockerman GH, Peterson BZ, Johnson BD, Catterall WA: Molecular determinants of drug binding and action on L-type calcium channels. Annu Rev Pharmacol Toxicol 37:361–396, 1997.

Nichols CG, Lpatin AN: Inward rectifier potassium channels. Annu Rev Physiol 59:171–191, 1997.

North RA: Families of ion channels with two hydrophobic segments. Curr Opin Cell Biol 8:474–483, 1996.

Sukharev SI, Blount P, Martinac B, Kung C: Mechanosensitive channels of *Escherichia coli*: The MscL gene, protein, and activities. Annu Rev Physiol 59:633–657, 1997.

Unwin N: Neurotransmitter action: Opening of ligand-gated ion channels. Cell 72:31–41, 1993.

Zagotta WN, Siegelbaum SA: Structure and function of cyclic nucleotide-gated channels. Annu Rev Neurosci 19:235–263, 1996.

chapter 10

MEMBRANE PHYSIOLOGY

This chapter describes how pumps, carriers, and channels cooperate in living systems. These three components often work together in circuits or cycles. Pumps establish chemical and electrical gradients of ions across membranes. Channels regulate membrane permeability to these ions to maintain the electrical potential (see Chapter 9) required for membrane excitability. Carriers use ion gradients as a source of energy to drive transport as well as to do other work (Fig. 7–1). Coupling ion fluxes through pumps and carriers to do work is called a **chemiosmotic cycle.** In **oxidative phosphorylation** and **photosynthesis,** energy from the breakdown of nutrients or from absorption of photons is used to energize electrons. During tunneling of these electrons through transmembrane proteins, energy is partitioned off to create a proton gradient that drives a chemiosmotic cycle to synthesize adenosine triphosphate (ATP).

Selective expression of a repertoire of pumps, carriers, and channels in specific membrane compartments enables cells to build sophisticated machines from a stockpile of standard components. If the pumps, carriers, and channels produced by a cell are known, it is relatively easy to explain complicated physiological processes by applying general principles for the operation of these membrane proteins. The examples in this chapter will also show how defects in pumps and channels cause disease and how pharmacologic manipulation of channels can alleviate symptoms of disease.

▎Chemiosmotic Cycles

A simple chemiosmotic cycle couples a cation transporting pump to solute transport by a carrier (Fig. 10–1). The membrane could be a plasma membrane or an organelle membrane. The driving reaction is called the primary transport step, indicating an input of energy and, in most cases, some chemical reaction. Other reactions are called secondary transport reactions, indicating that no chemistry is involved. The transported substrate is the same chemically on both sides of the membrane. Although simple in concept, the importance and power of chemiosmotic cycles should not be underestimated. They operate in every membrane of every cell.

Pumps use energy derived from ATP hydrolysis, light absorption, or another chemical reaction (see Table 7–1) to move ions in one direction across a membrane. This raises the concentration of a cation (C^+) on one side and depletes it on the other side of a membrane-bounded compartment. An ion gradient is characterized by both a chemical term, the concentration gradient, and an electrical gradient (the membrane potential discussed in Chapter 9). The electrochemical potential across a membrane represents a reservoir of power and a capacity to do work, also known as ion-motive forces. A mechanical analogue is using a pump to fill an elevated reservoir with fluid.

Carriers and other membrane proteins use the potential energy of ion gradients to drive other processes. This is analogous to using fluid flow out of a reservoir to drive a turbine, which puts the energy to use for other types of work. Many carriers use energy derived from the downhill passage of one substrate to transport one or more other substances up their concentration gradients across the same membrane barrier. In Figure 10–1, the carrier links the transport of substrate S to the movement of cation C down its gradient. Recirculation of cations allows the cell to accumulate substrate against its concentration gradient. In addition to the osmotic work illustrated in the figure, chemiosmotic cycles can also do chemical work.

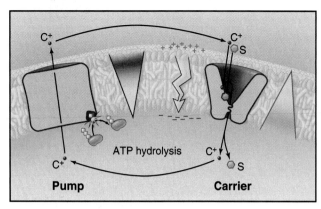

Figure 10-1 A model chemiosmotic cycle in a membrane surrounding a closed space. An ATP-driven pump transports a cation C^+ out of the compartment. The energy derived from ATP is stored as a concentration gradient of C^+ *(red triangle)* and a membrane potential *(yellow arrow)* across the membrane. The carrier uses the electrochemical gradient of C^+ to drive the transport of both C^+ and a solute up a concentration gradient *(green triangle)* across the membrane.

During both oxidative and photosynthetic phosphorylation, proton cycles drive ATP synthesis by F_0F_1-ATP synthases. Chemiosmotic cycles can also perform mechanical work. The electrochemical gradient of protons across the plasma membrane drives rotation of bacterial flagella (see Chapter 41).

Chemiosmotic cycles using protons dominate the biological world. Most bacterial cycles involve proton pumps, proton-linked carriers, or other proton-linked events. The same is true of lower eukaryotes, fungi, and plants. Plasma membranes of plant cells have a powerful proton pump and a collection of proton carriers. Proton chemiosmotic cycles are also characteristic of most eukaryotic organelles, including the Golgi apparatus, endosomes, lysosomes, mitochondria, and chloroplasts. Animal cell plasma membranes are a major exception because they use predominately sodium ions for their chemiosmotic cycle.

▌ Epithelial Transport

Net transport across an epithelium depends on tight junctions (see Chapter 33) that seal the extracellular space between the cells (Fig. 10-2). These junctions separate two extracellular compartments. The **apical compartment** is the free surface (e.g., the skin) or the lumen of the organ (e.g., the intestine, respiratory tract, or kidney tubules). The **basolateral compartment** lies between epithelial cells and is continuous with the underlying connective tissue and its blood vessels. Tight junctions seal the extracellular space, inhibiting diffusion of solutes, including glucose, between the apical and basolateral compartments of the extracellular space. The extent of this seal varies from

very tight to leaky. Tight junctions also separate the plasma membrane into apical and basolateral domains, restricting the movement of integral membrane proteins between these domains.

Glucose Transport in the Intestine, Kidney, Fat, and Muscle

A chemiosmotic cycle transports glucose uphill from the lumen of the intestine to the blood (see Fig. 10-2). Tight junctions restrict movement of glucose between the epithelial cells, so all of the glucose must move through the cytoplasm. Glucose transport across the epithelial cells requires the following components:

- Na^+K^+-ATPase, located in the basolateral plasma membrane

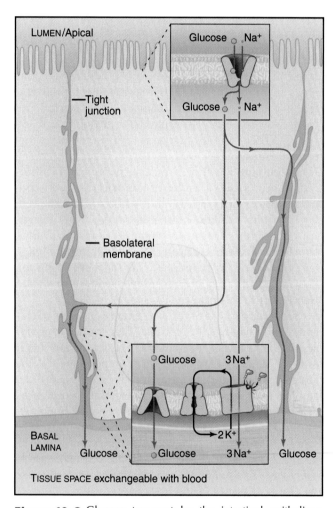

Figure 10-2 Glucose transport by the intestinal epithelium. Tight junctions seal the epithelium of polarized epithelial cells. Na^+K^+-ATPase pumps *(square icon)* in the basolateral plasma membrane drive Na^+/glucose symporters in the apical plasma membrane *(upper inset)* and glucose uniporters in the basolateral plasma membrane *(left icon in lower inset)* to move glucose from the lumen of the intestine to the blood. Basolateral K^+ channels *(middle icon)* recycle K^+ pumped into the cell.

- SGLT1 Na$^+$/glucose symporter, restricted to the apical plasma membrane
- GLUT5 uniporter, restricted to the basolateral plasma membrane

The molecular composition of the membrane domains explains the mechanism of glucose transport. Na$^+$K$^+$-ATPases produce Na$^+$ and K$^+$ gradients across the plasma membrane by continuously pumping Na$^+$ out of and K$^+$ into the cell at the expense of ATP hydrolysis. SGLT Na$^+$/glucose symporters use Na$^+$ moving inward down its electrochemical gradient to accumulate high internal concentrations of glucose from the lumen. In this step, energy is expended (dissipation of the Na$^+$ gradient) to move glucose uphill. GLUT uniporters on the basolateral membrane simply facilitate movement of cytoplasmic glucose down its concentration gradient into the blood. In the gut, this process provides for the uptake of glucose from food. Renal proximal tubule cells use a similar strategy to recapture glucose filtered from blood, transporting it across the tubule cell and back into the blood.

Glucose uptake by fat and muscle cells offers a different perspective. These tissues are designed to take up glucose from the blood when it is plentiful following a meal. Mammals have genes for six isoforms of the classical D-glucose uniporter. The GLUT4 isoform is important because it is regulated by insulin. Muscle and fat express GLUT4 but store it internally in membrane vesicles. After a meal, elevation of blood glucose stimulates secretion of insulin into blood. Signal transduction mechanisms (see Fig. 29–7) lead to fusion of these GLUT4 vesicles with the plasma membrane. That increases the rate of glucose transport into fat and muscle by 5- to 20-fold, lowering the blood glucose concentration and providing these cells with glucose, which they then convert to glycogen and triglycerides for storage.

Salt and Water Transport in the Kidney

In a section of the kidney tubule called the loop of Henle, the epithelium uses Na$^+$K$^+$-ATPase pumps and Na$^+$/K$^+$/2Cl$^-$ symporters to reabsorb NaCl that is filtered from blood into the excretory pathway (Fig. 10–3). Without this provision, salt would be lost in urine. Tight junctions seal this epithelium, so that salt must pass through the cells to reach the blood. Na$^+$/K$^+$/2Cl$^-$ symporters in the apical plasma membrane provide a way for NaCl to enter the cell down its concentration gradient. Abundant Na$^+$K$^+$-ATPases in the basolateral plasma membrane (5000/μm^2) create a Na$^+$ gradient to drive the symporter and to clear the cytoplasm of Na$^+$ accumulated from the tubule lumen. KCl that enters with Na$^+$ through the Na$^+$/K$^+$/2Cl$^-$ symporter leaves the cell through channels: K$^+$ channels

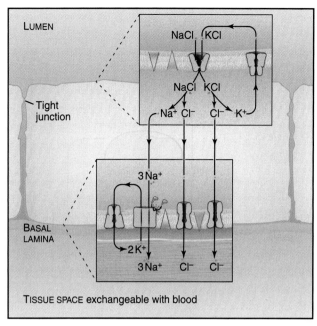

Figure 10–3 Sodium chloride transport by the epithelium of the kidney tubule. Tight junctions seal the space between these polarized epithelial cells of the thick ascending limb of the loop of Henle. Na$^+$K$^+$-ATPase pumps *(square icon)* in the basolateral plasma membrane drive Na$^+$/K$^+$/2Cl$^-$ symporters in the apical plasma membrane. K$^+$ channels in the apical plasma membrane and K$^+$ channels and Cl$^-$ channels in the basolateral plasma membrane provide paths for K$^+$ to circulate and for Cl$^-$ to follow Na$^+$ across the cell from the lumen of the tubule to the blood compartment.

in apical and basolateral membranes and Cl$^-$ channels in basolateral membranes.

A drug used to treat congestive heart failure—furosemide—inhibits the Na$^+$/K$^+$/2Cl$^-$ symporter in the loop of Henle. A weak heart leads to accumulation of fluid in the lungs (causing shortness of breath) and other tissues (causing swelling of ankles). Inhibition of the Na$^+$/K$^+$/2Cl$^-$ symporter reduces NaCl reabsorption, so the kidney produces large quantities of urine, clearing excess fluid from the body and relieving symptoms.

Cystic Fibrosis as a Transporter Disease

Normally, cells in the lung and gastrointestinal tract use a complicated selection of familiar pumps and carriers to secrete salt and water at their apical surfaces (Fig. 10–4). Na$^+$K$^+$-ATPases in the basolateral membrane set up an electrochemical gradient of Na$^+$, which is exploited by basolateral membrane Na$^+$/K$^+$/2Cl$^-$ symporters to take in Na$^+$, along with K$^+$ and Cl$^-$ anions. The inward movement of Na$^+$ down its electrochemical gradient drives the entry of K$^+$ and Cl$^-$ up their gradients. This brings excess potassium chloride into the cell. (The K$^+$ brought in by both the Na$^+$K$^+$-

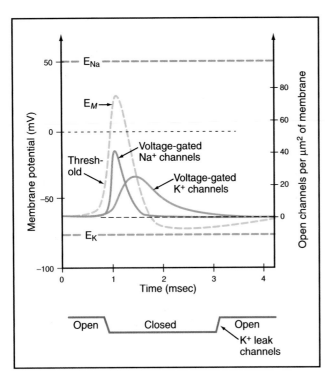

Figure 10-6 The time course of an action potential passing a measuring electrode inserted through the plasma membrane of a squid giant axon. Spread of an action potential from an adjacent area of the membrane brings the membrane potential E_m, to threshold, triggering the action potential at this point on the membrane. The other curves show the conductance of the membrane at this point for Na^+ and K^+ expressed as the concentration of open channels. The lower trace shows the times during which K^+ leak channels open and close at this point. E_{Na} is the Na^+ equilibrium potential, and E_K is the K^+ equilibrium potential.

relationship between conductance and voltage. From these relationships, measured under controlled conditions, they could calculate the membrane response to virtually any experimental condition. To explain these changes in permeability, they postulated the existence of ionic channels. The voltage clamp provided a direct measure of this channel activity. This approach also revealed the behavior of channels held at a potential more positive than their resting potential.

Three Channels Generating Action Potentials

Voltage-gated Na^+ and K^+ channels open and close in sequence to produce action potentials. Depending on the type of open channel, the membrane potential varies in time between the K^+ equilibrium potential (E_K) and the Na^+ equilibrium potential (E_{Na}) (see Chapter 9). Because membrane depolarization activates these ion channels, and because the response spreads this depolarization, triggering an action potential initiates a cascade of reactions that moves over the membrane, first to depolarize and then to repolarize the membrane. In nerves, just three types of voltage-

gated channels are required to generate action potentials.

- K^+-selective leak channels of the Kir family and the TWIK family are open at resting potentials. Kir channels are blocked by cytoplasmic Mg^{2+} when the membrane depolarizes.
- Voltage-gated Na^+ channels are closed at the resting potential but open if the membrane depolarizes to about -40 mV. They open only transiently because a first-order inactivation reaction closes the pore, even if the membrane potential is at or above zero. These channels return to the closed state without passing again through the open state.
- Delayed-rectifier voltage-gated K^+ channels have a low probability of being open at the resting potential. They respond to membrane depolarization by opening, but they do so more slowly than do Na^+ channels. They stay open long enough to allow the membrane potential to approach E_K.

The properties of these channels explain the time course of an action potential as follows:

Stage 1. At rest, the membrane is slightly permeable to K^+ but not to other ions, so the resting potential is near E_K, about -70 mV. K^+-selective leak channels and a few open voltage-gated K^+ channels contribute to this basal K^+ permeability.

Stage 2. If the membrane is depolarized and reaches the threshold potential, K^+-selective leak channels *close* and voltage-gated Na^+ channels *open*. Because the membrane is permeable only to Na^+, and because many Na^+ channels open, Na^+ moves into the cell and the membrane potential rapidly approaches E_{Na}, about $+45$ mV.

Stage 3. After 1 to 2 msec, Na^+ channels spontaneously *inactivate* and slowly responding delayed-rectifier K^+ channels *open*. Now the membrane is strongly and selectively permeable to K^+, so K^+ moves out of the cell and the membrane potential reverses all the way to E_K, about -80 mV. K^+ channels are less synchronized than Na^+ channels, so the membrane potential falls more slowly than it rises.

Stage 4. Delayed-rectifier K^+ channels close progressively as the membrane repolarizes, and K^+-selective leak channels open, returning the membrane potential to the resting voltage, just above E_K.

During an action potential, the membrane voltage changes by 100 to 150 mV in 1 to 2 msec. The membrane bilayer is approximately 7 nm thick, so this voltage corresponds to a field variation on the order of 150,000 volts/cm in 1 to 2 msec. Such strong forces elicit conformational changes in membrane proteins, such as voltage-gated ion channels.

- SGLT1 Na$^+$/glucose symporter, restricted to the apical plasma membrane
- GLUT5 uniporter, restricted to the basolateral plasma membrane

The molecular composition of the membrane domains explains the mechanism of glucose transport. Na$^+$K$^+$-ATPases produce Na$^+$ and K$^+$ gradients across the plasma membrane by continuously pumping Na$^+$ out of and K$^+$ into the cell at the expense of ATP hydrolysis. SGLT Na$^+$/glucose symporters use Na$^+$ moving inward down its electrochemical gradient to accumulate high internal concentrations of glucose from the lumen. In this step, energy is expended (dissipation of the Na$^+$ gradient) to move glucose uphill. GLUT uniporters on the basolateral membrane simply facilitate movement of cytoplasmic glucose down its concentration gradient into the blood. In the gut, this process provides for the uptake of glucose from food. Renal proximal tubule cells use a similar strategy to recapture glucose filtered from blood, transporting it across the tubule cell and back into the blood.

Glucose uptake by fat and muscle cells offers a different perspective. These tissues are designed to take up glucose from the blood when it is plentiful following a meal. Mammals have genes for six isoforms of the classical D-glucose uniporter. The GLUT4 isoform is important because it is regulated by insulin. Muscle and fat express GLUT4 but store it internally in membrane vesicles. After a meal, elevation of blood glucose stimulates secretion of insulin into blood. Signal transduction mechanisms (see Fig. 29–7) lead to fusion of these GLUT4 vesicles with the plasma membrane. That increases the rate of glucose transport into fat and muscle by 5- to 20-fold, lowering the blood glucose concentration and providing these cells with glucose, which they then convert to glycogen and triglycerides for storage.

Salt and Water Transport in the Kidney

In a section of the kidney tubule called the loop of Henle, the epithelium uses Na$^+$K$^+$-ATPase pumps and Na$^+$/K$^+$/2Cl$^-$ symporters to reabsorb NaCl that is filtered from blood into the excretory pathway (Fig. 10–3). Without this provision, salt would be lost in urine. Tight junctions seal this epithelium, so that salt must pass through the cells to reach the blood. Na$^+$/K$^+$/2Cl$^-$ symporters in the apical plasma membrane provide a way for NaCl to enter the cell down its concentration gradient. Abundant Na$^+$K$^+$-ATPases in the basolateral plasma membrane (5000/μm^2) create a Na$^+$ gradient to drive the symporter and to clear the cytoplasm of Na$^+$ accumulated from the tubule lumen. KCl that enters with Na$^+$ through the Na$^+$/K$^+$/2Cl$^-$ symporter leaves the cell through channels: K$^+$ channels

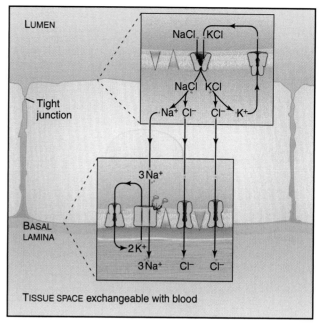

Figure 10–3 Sodium chloride transport by the epithelium of the kidney tubule. Tight junctions seal the space between these polarized epithelial cells of the thick ascending limb of the loop of Henle. Na$^+$K$^+$-ATPase pumps (square icon) in the basolateral plasma membrane drive Na$^+$/K$^+$/2Cl$^-$ symporters in the apical plasma membrane. K$^+$ channels in the apical plasma membrane and K$^+$ channels and Cl$^-$ channels in the basolateral plasma membrane provide paths for K$^+$ to circulate and for Cl$^-$ to follow Na$^+$ across the cell from the lumen of the tubule to the blood compartment.

in apical and basolateral membranes and Cl$^-$ channels in basolateral membranes.

A drug used to treat congestive heart failure—furosemide—inhibits the Na$^+$/K$^+$/2Cl$^-$ symporter in the loop of Henle. A weak heart leads to accumulation of fluid in the lungs (causing shortness of breath) and other tissues (causing swelling of ankles). Inhibition of the Na$^+$/K$^+$/2Cl$^-$ symporter reduces NaCl reabsorption, so the kidney produces large quantities of urine, clearing excess fluid from the body and relieving symptoms.

Cystic Fibrosis as a Transporter Disease

Normally, cells in the lung and gastrointestinal tract use a complicated selection of familiar pumps and carriers to secrete salt and water at their apical surfaces (Fig. 10–4). Na$^+$K$^+$-ATPases in the basolateral membrane set up an electrochemical gradient of Na$^+$, which is exploited by basolateral membrane Na$^+$/K$^+$/2Cl$^-$ symporters to take in Na$^+$, along with K$^+$ and Cl$^-$ anions. The inward movement of Na$^+$ down its electrochemical gradient drives the entry of K$^+$ and Cl$^-$ up their gradients. This brings excess potassium chloride into the cell. (The K$^+$ brought in by both the Na$^+$K$^+$-

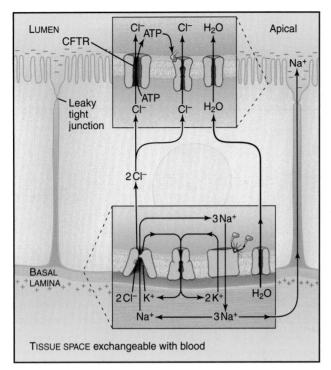

Figure 10-4 Salt and water transport across the epithelium lining the respiratory tract. Leaky tight junctions partially seal the space between these polarized epithelial cells. Na+K+-ATPase pumps in the basolateral plasma membrane drive Na+/K+/2Cl− symporters in the basolateral plasma membrane. CFTR Cl− channels in the apical plasma membrane allow Cl− to move into the lumen, creating a negative electrical potential that pulls Na+ between the cells into the lumen. CFTR also releases ATP, which activates additional Cl− channels. Water follows sodium chloride into the lumen through water channels and between the cells. Basolateral K+ channels allow K+ to circulate.

ATPase and the Na+/K+/2 Cl− symporter recycles after exiting from the cell by way of channels in the basolateral plasma membrane. Thus, K+ is merely catalytic.) Excess Cl− is left inside the cell. The cystic fibrosis transmembrane regulator (CFTR) protein, an ABC pump, in the apical plasma membrane acts as a Cl− channel. In response to the appropriate signals, the channel opens and Cl− moves down its electrochemical gradient out of the cell, carrying charge to the outside. The whole epithelium becomes polarized, with the lumen electrically negative relative to the connective tissue. This electrical driving force allows Na+ to move between cells, from the blood compartment through leaky tight junctions to the surface of the epithelium. Sodium chloride on the apical surface creates an osmotic force that draws water down its concentration gradient from inside to outside through water channels (see Chapter 9). A balance between this fluid secretion and fluid reabsorption normally keeps the surface of the epithelium properly hydrated, allowing the cilia to clear the lung of bacteria and

secretions and the ducts of the pancreas to secrete digestive enzymes.

Patients with cystic fibrosis have mutations in CFTR that cause defects in apical Cl− transport and secretion. Their lungs are too dry as a result of this imbalance in fluid secretion and reabsorption on the surface of epithelia. This situation is life-threatening because cilia in the respiratory tract cannot move sticky, dry, mucus containing bacteria and viruses out of the lungs, thereby predisposing to respiratory infections. Sticky secretions in the pancreatic ducts also interfere with the secretion of digestive enzymes by the pancreas. Many different mutations in the CFTR gene cause the disease. By far the most common mutation (67% of cases) deletes the codon for phenylalanine 508 (F508). The resulting protein is temperature-sensitive, not folding properly at 37°C and failing to negotiate the secretory pathway to the plasma membrane. Patients with two copies of this mutation on chromosome 7 have classic cystic fibrosis. Heterozygotes with one normal gene (about 5% of the population) have no symptoms. Combination of this ΔF508 mutation with a number of other mutations in the other copy of the gene vary in the severity of their pancreatic problems, but still have typical lung disease.

Cellular Volume Regulation

Cells employ both short- and long-term strategies involving pumps, carriers, and channels to maintain a constant volume (Fig. 10–5). These compensatory mechanisms are required because water channels and the intrinsic (low) permeability of lipid bilayers to water allow water to move across the plasma membrane if the osmotic strength of its environment changes even a small amount. Water moves to maintain an osmotic equilibrium, as illustrated for red blood cells in Figure 6–6. In a hypotonic medium, water moves into a cell to dilute the cytoplasm. In a hypertonic medium, water moves out to concentrate the cytoplasm. Mechanisms employed to compensate for these volume changes are well defined, but how cells sense volume changes or trigger these responses is less clear.

Animal cells respond acutely to loss of water by activating Na+/H+ antiporters, Cl−/HCO3− antiporters, and/or Na+/K+/2Cl− symporters that bring potassium chloride and sodium chloride into the cell. Water follows, returning the cell to its original volume in minutes. The acute response to swelling activates K+ channels, Cl− channels (ClC-3), and/or a K+/Cl− symporter, taking potassium chloride and water out of the cell. Compensation by moving inorganic ions works in the short run but is not an acceptable long-term solution because changes in the internal concentrations of

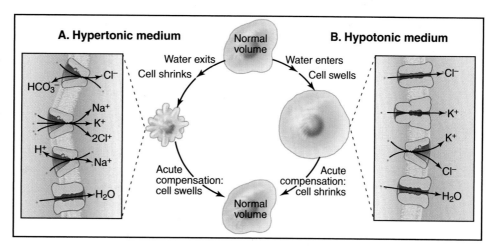

Figure 10-5 Acute cellular volume control. *A,* Cell is placed in hypertonic medium. *B,* Cell is placed in hypotonic medium. Cells compensate for volume changes by activating channels and carriers to move inorganic ions into or out of the cell. Water follows passively through channels and across the lipid bilayer.

K^+, Na^+, and Cl^- affect the membrane potential and other physiological processes.

In the long term, cells use small organic molecules called osmolytes to adjust the osmotic strength of cytoplasm and to maintain their volume. Osmolytes include amino acids, polyalcohols (sorbitol and inositol), and methylamines that do not interfere with cellular biochemistry or membrane excitability. Adjustment of osmolyte concentrations takes longer than for ions as it requires synthesis or degradation of transport proteins. In response to swelling, cells immediately activate channels that allow osmolytes and Cl^- to escape from cytoplasm; this is followed later by a reduction in the number of plasma membrane Na^+/osmolyte symporters. In response to shrinking, cells close the osmolyte channels and synthesize additional Na^+/osmolyte symporters.

▌ Excitable Membranes

Regulation of membrane potential is particularly important in higher organisms, which use electrical signals generated by membrane channels for communication in their nervous and muscular systems. For example, reading and understanding this page depends upon rapid creation and processing of electrical and chemical signals by cells in the visual system and brain. Ion channels produce the key event, a transient change in electrical potential of the plasma membrane, called an action potential. These energy-efficient electrical signals are the fastest means of communication in the body, spreading over the plasma membrane at tens of meters per second. Similarly, action potentials trigger skeletal muscle contraction, control the timing of the heartbeat, and coordinate the peristaltic motions of the gut and contractions of the uterus.

Electrical excitability is not limited to nerves and muscles. Eggs use a form of action potential as an early step in blocking fertilization by more than one sperm. Chemotaxis by macrophages and secretion of insulin and other hormones both depend on electrical excitability. The reader should be familiar with the appendices in Chapter 9 to appreciate the following material.

Description of an Action Potential

If a microelectrode drives a small positive or negative current into a cell, a second microelectrode a short distance away detects a small voltage response. These electrotonic potentials decline rapidly with distance.

In striking contrast to these small local currents, if the plasma membrane of an excitable cell, such as nerve or muscle, is depolarized beyond a certain level, called a **threshold,** the membrane responds over a few milliseconds with a large, stereotyped change in membrane potential, called an **action potential** (Fig. 10–6). Voltage-gated ion channels generate this powerful electrical signal that spreads rapidly (10 m/sec) over the entire plasma membrane. During an action potential, the membrane potential can reach a peak of +40 to 50 mV before repolarizing to the resting potential. Because action potentials are self-triggering, they travel without dissipation over long distances. This high-speed transmission is very efficient, requiring only a few ions.

The molecular events during an action potential were first characterized around 1950 in squid giant axons using microelectrodes coupled to an electronic feedback circuit. This clever "voltage clamp" holds the membrane potential constant by providing the cell with electrical current to compensate for changes in ion currents. Investigators discovered that changes in permeability to Na^+ and K^+ ions produced action potentials. Changing one variable at a time, they determined the time and voltage dependence of ion-specific conductance. They also determined the

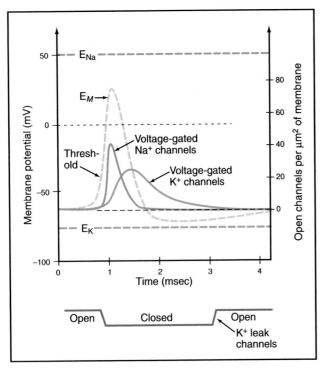

Figure 10–6 The time course of an action potential passing a measuring electrode inserted through the plasma membrane of a squid giant axon. Spread of an action potential from an adjacent area of the membrane brings the membrane potential E_m, to threshold, triggering the action potential at this point on the membrane. The other curves show the conductance of the membrane at this point for Na^+ and K^+ expressed as the concentration of open channels. The lower trace shows the times during which K^+ leak channels open and close at this point. E_{Na} is the Na^+ equilibrium potential, and E_K is the K^+ equilibrium potential.

relationship between conductance and voltage. From these relationships, measured under controlled conditions, they could calculate the membrane response to virtually any experimental condition. To explain these changes in permeability, they postulated the existence of ionic channels. The voltage clamp provided a direct measure of this channel activity. This approach also revealed the behavior of channels held at a potential more positive than their resting potential.

Three Channels Generating Action Potentials

Voltage-gated Na^+ and K^+ channels open and close in sequence to produce action potentials. Depending on the type of open channel, the membrane potential varies in time between the K^+ equilibrium potential (E_K) and the Na^+ equilibrium potential (E_{Na}) (see Chapter 9). Because membrane depolarization activates these ion channels, and because the response spreads this depolarization, triggering an action potential initiates a cascade of reactions that moves over the membrane, first to depolarize and then to repolarize the membrane. In nerves, just three types of voltage-

gated channels are required to generate action potentials.

- K^+-selective leak channels of the Kir family and the TWIK family are open at resting potentials. Kir channels are blocked by cytoplasmic Mg^{2+} when the membrane depolarizes.
- Voltage-gated Na^+ channels are closed at the resting potential but open if the membrane depolarizes to about -40 mV. They open only transiently because a first-order inactivation reaction closes the pore, even if the membrane potential is at or above zero. These channels return to the closed state without passing again through the open state.
- Delayed-rectifier voltage-gated K^+ channels have a low probability of being open at the resting potential. They respond to membrane depolarization by opening, but they do so more slowly than do Na^+ channels. They stay open long enough to allow the membrane potential to approach E_K.

The properties of these channels explain the time course of an action potential as follows:

Stage 1. At rest, the membrane is slightly permeable to K^+ but not to other ions, so the resting potential is near E_K, about -70 mV. K^+-selective leak channels and a few open voltage-gated K^+ channels contribute to this basal K^+ permeability.

Stage 2. If the membrane is depolarized and reaches the threshold potential, K^+-selective leak channels *close* and voltage-gated Na^+ channels *open*. Because the membrane is permeable only to Na^+, and because many Na^+ channels open, Na^+ moves into the cell and the membrane potential rapidly approaches E_{Na}, about $+45$ mV.

Stage 3. After 1 to 2 msec, Na^+ channels spontaneously *inactivate* and slowly responding delayed-rectifier K^+ channels *open*. Now the membrane is strongly and selectively permeable to K^+, so K^+ moves out of the cell and the membrane potential reverses all the way to E_K, about -80 mV. K^+ channels are less synchronized than Na^+ channels, so the membrane potential falls more slowly than it rises.

Stage 4. Delayed-rectifier K^+ channels close progressively as the membrane repolarizes, and K^+-selective leak channels open, returning the membrane potential to the resting voltage, just above E_K.

During an action potential, the membrane voltage changes by 100 to 150 mV in 1 to 2 msec. The membrane bilayer is approximately 7 nm thick, so this voltage corresponds to a field variation on the order of 150,000 volts/cm in 1 to 2 msec. Such strong forces elicit conformational changes in membrane proteins, such as voltage-gated ion channels.

Membrane Depolarization: The Stimulus for Action Potentials

The initial depolarization of the plasma membrane that triggers an action potential can arise from activation by a neurotransmitter (see the section that follows) or spread of an action potential from an adjacent membrane or from an adjacent cell through a gap junction. Membrane depolarization must exceed a certain threshold to trigger an action potential. Threshold arises directly from the properties of the ion channels. Depolarization less than threshold activates a few Na^+ channels, producing a small inward Na^+ current, but it also activates some delayed-rectifier K^+ channels, resulting in K^+ efflux. If the Na^+ conductance is small relative to the K^+ conductance, outward currents predominate and the membrane repolarizes. Depolarization greater than threshold activates additional Na^+ channels, yielding inward Na^+ currents greater than outward K^+ currents, at least briefly. This further depolarizes the membrane, amplifying activation of Na^+ channels and producing the cascade of channel activation that makes action potentials an all-or-nothing event.

■ Synaptic Transmission

Nerves use chemical messengers called **neurotransmitters** (Fig. 10–7) to communicate rapidly with other neurons and effector cells, such as skeletal muscle and glands. This chemical communication occurs at sites called synapses (Figs. 10–8 and 10–9), where the sending cell is specialized to secrete a particular neurotransmitter and the receiving cell is specialized to respond to that neurotransmitter. The sending side is referred to as **presynaptic,** whereas the receiving side is designated **postsynaptic.** Small vesicles containing neurotransmitter pack the presynaptic nerve terminal. **Neurotransmitter receptors** concentrate in the postsynaptic plasma membrane. Analysis of synaptic transmission reveals much about the mechanisms of secretion (see Chapter 22), signal transduction, and psychoactive drugs that affect behavior.

Neurotransmitters are generally small organic molecules with an amino group, including acetylcholine, norepinephrine, 5-hydroxytryptamine (serotonin), and the amino acids glycine and glutamic acid (see Fig. 10–7). Secretory mechanisms are similar at all synapses, but each neurotransmitter requires different biochemical machinery for synthesis, packaging in synaptic vesicles, and reception by the postsynaptic cell. These differences among the various types of synapses make it possible to modify synaptic transmission selectively at a subset of synapses using a particular transmitter, such as in treatment with psychoactive drugs.

This section compares two types of synapses that use ligand-gated ion channels: the neuromuscular junction and central nervous system (CNS) synapses. These examples show how pumps, carriers, and channels work together to ensure synaptic transmission.

In addition to activating ligand-gated ion channels, most neurotransmitters also stimulate particular seven-helix receptors (see Fig. 10–7). For example, acetylcholine stimulates the seven-helix **muscarinic acetylcholine receptor,** which uses a trimeric G-protein intermediary to activate Kir3.1 K^+ channels. Glutamate stimulates seven-helix **"metabotropic" receptors,** which also act through trimeric G proteins. Disruption

Transmitter	Structure	Receptors	
		Channels	Seven-helix
Acetylcholine	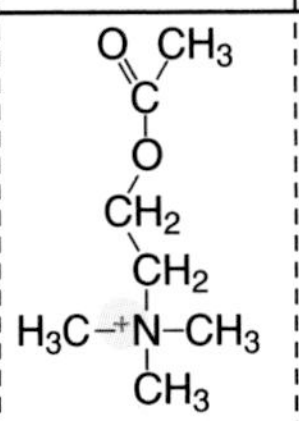	Excitatory (nicotinic) Na^+/K^+ channel	Muscarinic receptor
Dopamine	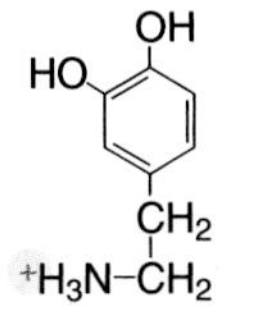	—	Dopamine receptor
γ-Aminobutyric acid (GABA)	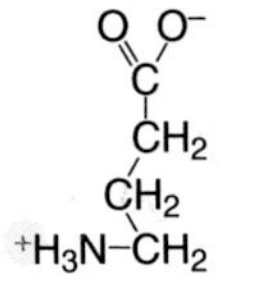	Inhibitory Cl^- channel	β-type GABA receptor
Glutamate	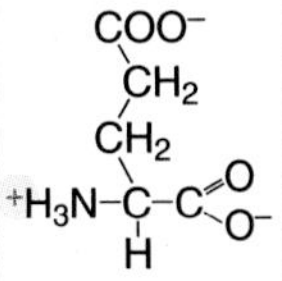	Excitatory Na^+/K^+ channel or $Na^+/K^+/Ca^{2+}$ channel	Metabotropic glutamate receptor
Glycine	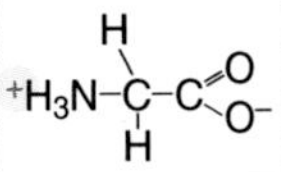	Inhibitory Cl^- channel	—
Norepinephrine	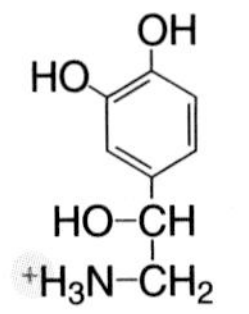	—	Adrenergic receptor
Serotonin	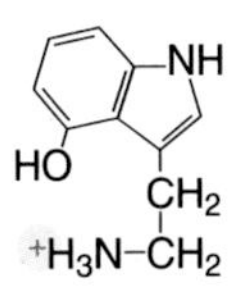	Excitatory Na^+/K^+ channel	Serotonin receptor

Figure 10–7 Neurotransmitters and their ligand-gated ion channels and seven-helix receptors.

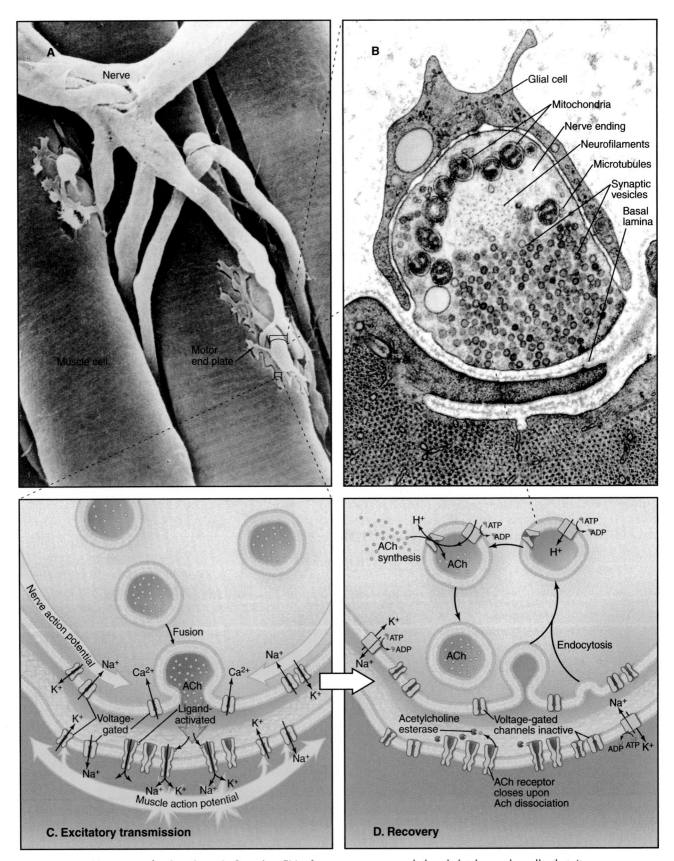

Figure 10-8 Neuromuscular junction. *A,* Scanning EM of a motor nerve and the skeletal muscle cells that it innervates. *B,* EM of a thin section of a frog neuromuscular junction. *C,* Excitatory synaptic transmission. The nerve action potential opens voltage-gated calcium channels. Entry of Ca²⁺ triggers fusion of a synaptic vesicle containing acetylcholine (ACh) with the plasma membrane. Acetylcholine binds and opens postsynaptic channels on the muscle cell which trigger an action potential. *D,* Recovery includes acetylcholine hydrolysis, recycling of synaptic vesicle membranes, and loading of synaptic vesicles with new acetylcholine. (*A,* Courtesy of Don Fawcett, Harvard Medical School. *B,* Courtesy of J.E. Heuser, Washington University.)

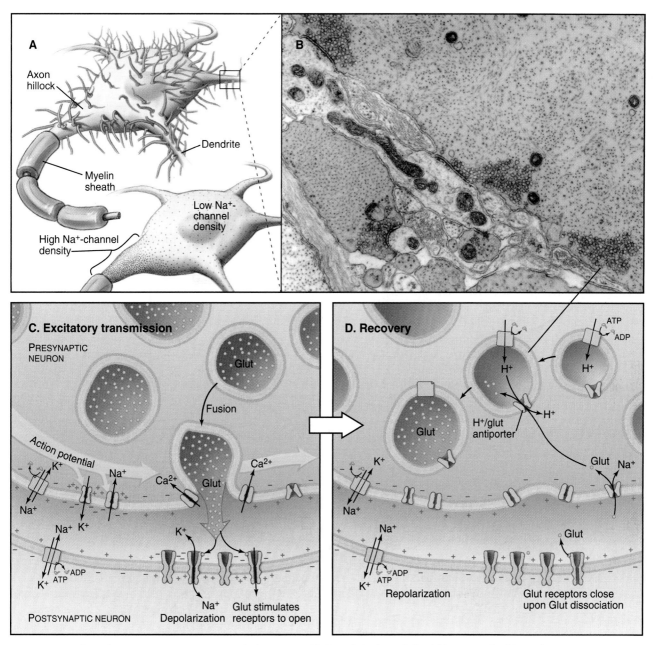

Figure 10-9 Central nervous system synapses. *A,* A neuron with its cell body and dendrites covered with a mixture of excitatory and inhibitory synapses. A high density of voltage-gated Na+ channels in the proximal part of the axon, called the axon hillock, favors the generation of an action potential when the sum of postsynaptic potentials brings the axon hillock to threshold. *B,* An electron micrograph of a thin section of brain showing synapses with vesicles *(green)* clustered in the presynaptic axon. *C,* Synaptic transmission at a CNS excitatory synapse. A presynaptic action potential opens voltage-gated Ca2+ channels. Entry of Ca2+ stimulates fusion of synaptic vesicles filled with glutamate (Glut) with the plasma membrane. Glutamate binds and opens postsynaptic AMPA receptors that generate a local postsynaptic potential change. *D,* Recovery from excitatory stimulation includes retrieval of glutamate by a presynaptic Na+/glutamate symporter and concentration of glutamate in synaptic vesicles by a H+/glutamate antiporter. (*B,* Courtesy of Don Fawcett, Harvard Medical School.)

of the gene for metabotropic glutamate receptors leaves mice with defects in coordination and learning.

Neuromuscular Junction

Motor neurons in the spinal cord and brainstem control contraction of skeletal muscle cells (see Chapter 42). Long axons from these neurons terminate in synapses on skeletal muscle cells, called neuromuscular junctions (see Fig. 10–8*A* and *B*). Every neuronal action potential that reaches a neuromuscular junction produces an action potential that spreads over the surface of the muscle cell and initiates contraction. This highly reliable, one-to-one communication depends on chemical transmission by **acetylcholine** between the nerve and muscle.

Figure 10–8*C* illustrates the membrane proteins required for neuromuscular transmission. Both the nerve terminal and muscle depend on Na^+K^+-ATPase and Ca^{2+}-ATPase pumps to maintain gradients of Na^+, K^+, and Ca^{2+} across their plasma membranes. Both presynaptic and postsynaptic cells need voltage-gated Na^+ channels and K^+ channels for action potentials. Additionally, the presynaptic membrane requires voltage-gated Ca^{2+} channels. Highly concentrated nicotinic acetylcholine receptors in the postsynaptic membrane ($\sim 20,000/\mu m^2$) transduce the arrival of extracellular acetylcholine into membrane depolarization.

A neuronal action potential initiates synaptic transmission by admitting Ca^{2+} into the presynaptic terminal through voltage-gated Ca^{2+} channels. Within less than 1 msec, Ca^{2+} triggers fusion of **synaptic vesicles** containing acetylcholine with the plasma membrane. Within microseconds, acetylcholine in the synaptic cleft between the cells reaches millimolar concentrations and binds the acetylcholine receptors.

Weak but cooperative binding of acetylcholine to two subunits of the **acetylcholine receptor** (see Fig. 9–11) opens a nonselective cation channel. The open pore is about equally permeable to K^+ and Na^+ and less permeable to Ca^{2+}, so the membrane potential collapses toward a reversal potential of about 0 mV. This is above threshold for triggering a self-propagating action potential in the muscle plasma membrane with nearly 100% efficiency. The muscle action potential activates voltage-sensitive Ca^{2+} channels that trigger Ca^{2+} release from the smooth endoplasmic reticulum and set off contraction (see Chapter 42).

Two different mechanisms terminate activation of acetylcholine receptors. An extracellular enzyme, **acetylcholinesterase,** rapidly degrades free acetylcholine, usually depleting acetylcholine from the synaptic cleft in a few milliseconds. Acetylcholine then dissociates from the receptor, closing the channel. During prolonged exposure to acetylcholine, a conformational change in the acetylcholine receptor increases its affinity for bound acetylcholine and closes the channel. In this **desensitized state,** acetylcholine dissociates only when its extracellular concentration is very low. Once acetylcholine dissociates, the receptor slowly returns to rest.

Nerve terminals retrieve synaptic vesicle membrane by endocytosis (see Chapter 23). Cytoplasmic enzymes synthesize new acetylcholine. A V-type ATPase proton pump acidifies the lumen of synaptic vesicles, providing an electrochemical potential to drive an acetylcholine/H^+ antiporter, which concentrates acetylcholine in vesicles.

Central Nervous System Synapses

Synaptic transmission between neurons in the CNS differs fundamentally (see Fig. 10–9) from the efficient, one-to-one coupling at neuromuscular junctions, where every presynaptic action potential triggers a postsynaptic action potential. CNS neurons receive synaptic inputs from many neurons. Synapses cover the surface of dendrites and the cell body (see Fig. 10–9*A*). Some synapses excite the postsynaptic cell by opening ligand-gated cation channels that depolarize the membrane locally. Such small, local changes tend to push the membrane toward threshold for an action potential. Other synapses are inhibitory, hyperpolarizing the postsynaptic membrane locally by opening ligand-gated Cl^- channels. These changes are inhibitory, since they drive the membrane potential away from threshold. From moment to moment, neurons spatially average excitatory and inhibitory stimuli and fire action potentials when the combined effects of these opposing stimuli exceed threshold potential in the proximal part of the axon, called the **axon hillock.** Both the pattern and frequency of action potentials carry information in the brain.

Transmission at chemical synapses in the CNS depends on cooperation of pumps, carriers, and channels (see Fig. 10–9*C* and *D*). ATPase pumps maintain concentration gradients of Na^+, K^+, and Ca^{2+} across both presynaptic and postsynaptic plasma membranes. Voltage-gated K^+ and Na^+ channels establish the resting membrane potential and fire action potentials. Neurotransmitters activate ligand-gated channels that control the postsynaptic membrane potential. Carriers in the presynaptic membrane and adjacent supporting cells terminate transmission by removing neurotransmitter from the synaptic cleft.

Incoming information takes the form of action potentials that arrive at synapses. As in the neuromuscular junction, action potentials open voltage-gated Ca^{2+} channels in the presynaptic membrane. This transient rise in cytoplasmic Ca^{2+} can trigger the fusion of synaptic vesicles with the presynaptic plasma membrane, releasing transmitter, but the probability of successful fusion is lower than at neuromuscular junctions. After vesicle fusion transmitter diffuses to its receptors in the postsynaptic membrane.

Transmitters activate ligand-gated channels that cause a local, short-lived change in membrane potential, called a **postsynaptic potential** (PSP). At **excitatory synapses,** the neurotransmitter **glutamate** activates receptors that open **cation channels** that depolarize the membrane. However, in contrast to the neuromuscular junction, individual PSPs do not fire action potentials. First, individual PSPs only raise the membrane potential a few millivolts, so they do not bring the postsynaptic membrane to threshold. Second, dendritic and cell body plasma membranes contain few voltage-gated Na^+ channels. Furthermore, **inhibitory synapses** on the same cell counteract excitatory synapses by secreting **glycine** or γ-**aminobutyric acid** (GABA) to activate **Cl^- channels** that hyperpolarize the membrane, taking it farther from threshold.

Excitatory and inhibitory PSPs spread passively over the postsynaptic membrane and generate an action potential only when their sum at a particular time brings the membrane potential at the axon hillock to threshold (see Fig. 10–9A). The axon hillock is located at the base of each axon. This part of the plasma membrane is particularly sensitive to voltage owing to a high concentration of voltage-gated Na^+ channels. At threshold, they open, depolarizing the membrane (see Fig. 10–6). Delayed-rectifier K^+ channels then repolarize the membrane in preparation for following action potentials. Each action potential is identical and spreads out along the axon.

Because bringing the axon hillock to threshold requires multiple excitatory postsynaptic potentials, the frequency of the postsynaptic output depends on the intensity of the presynaptic input. In fact, the frequency of postsynaptic action potentials is proportional to the intensity of the presynaptic input above a threshold. This proportionality depends on additional voltage-gated K^+ channels that suppress the firing rate at low levels of stimulation.

Removal of neurotransmitters from the synaptic cleft terminates activation of postsynaptic receptors (see Fig. 10–8D). Na^+K^+-ATPase pumps provide a Na^+ gradient to drive symporters that return neurotransmitters to their presynaptic cells. Within the presynaptic cell, a second proton-driven chemiosmotic cycle concentrates transmitter in synaptic vesicles. A V-type, proton-translocating ATPase acidifies the lumen of the synaptic vesicle and establishes the proton electrochemical gradient across the vesicle membrane to drive the antiporter.

Modification of CNS Synapses by Drugs and Disease

Because transport systems that retrieve glutamate from the synaptic cleft and repackage it in vesicles determine the duration of synaptic stimulation, inhibiting these transport processes with drugs prolongs stimulation at particular classes of CNS synapses with profound effects on brain function and behavior. A plasma membrane dopamine transporter is the main target of **cocaine.** Cocaine also inhibits transporters for serotonin and norepinephrine. Tricyclic **antidepressants** inhibit norepinephrine uptake, and other drugs inhibit serotonin uptake. These drugs have dramatic effects on the symptoms of depression as well as a range of milder psychiatric disorders. Millions of people benefit from these drugs, even though the physiological consequences of transporter inhibition are incompletely understood.

Excess stimulation of *N*-methyl-D-aspartate (NMDA) receptors rapidly kills postsynaptic neurons, likely owing to the deleterious effects of excess cytoplasmic Ca^{2+}. This occurs when glutamate is released from ischemic brain tissue during a stroke. Such damage may contribute to neuron death in degenerative diseases of the nervous system, such as amyotrophic lateral sclerosis and Alzheimer's disease.

Acetylcholine secreted by neurons and **nicotine** from tobacco modulate synaptic transmission in the CNS. In the CNS, acetylcholine acts on *presynaptic* terminals, rather than participating directly in fast synaptic transmission like it does at the neuromuscular junction. Nicotinic acetylcholine receptors in the *presynaptic* plasma membrane are highly permeable to Ca^{2+}, so their stimulation admits Ca^{2+} into the presynaptic terminal. This enhances both the spontaneous release of neurotransmitter and release in response to action potentials. The isoform composition of CNS acetylcholine receptors differs from that of muscles. Some are homopentamers of α-subunits. Others are heteropentamers of α- and β-subunits. These ligand-gated channels may account for the enhancing effects of nicotine on learning and memory, but also for tobacco addiction. Loss of CNS neurons secreting acetylcholine may contribute to dementia in Alzheimer's disease.

Modification of CNS Synapses by Use

The pattern of stimulation at glutamate-mediated synapses in the CNS can produce long-term changes that enhance or reduce the efficiency of synaptic transmission (Fig. 10–10). The **hippocampus,** a region of the vertebrate cerebral cortex known to participate in **memory** processes, is particularly favorable for observing this simple form of cellular learning. Intense stimulation by excitatory glutamate synapses (20 pulses over a period of 200 msec) strengthens subsequent responses to stimulation of these synapses for days or weeks. This is called **long-term potentiation (LTP).** Conversely, slow, prolonged stimulation at glutamate synapses reduces the response for hours. This is called **long-term depression (LTD).**

These adaptations to use attract considerable attention because high-order brain functions, such as learning and memory, are believed to depend on changes in the flow of impulses through neural circuits, and the changes in transmission during LTP and LTD occur on an appropriate time scale. Their mechanisms and their actual relation to learning and memory have generated intense investigation.

LTP involves two types of glutamate receptors, **AMPA receptors** and **NMDA receptors** (see Chapter 9) found in postsynaptic specializations called dendritic spines (see Fig. 10–10). AMPA receptors open and close rapidly in response to glutamate. When open, they admit Na^+ to depolarize the postsynaptic plasma membrane. The slow response of NMDA receptors to

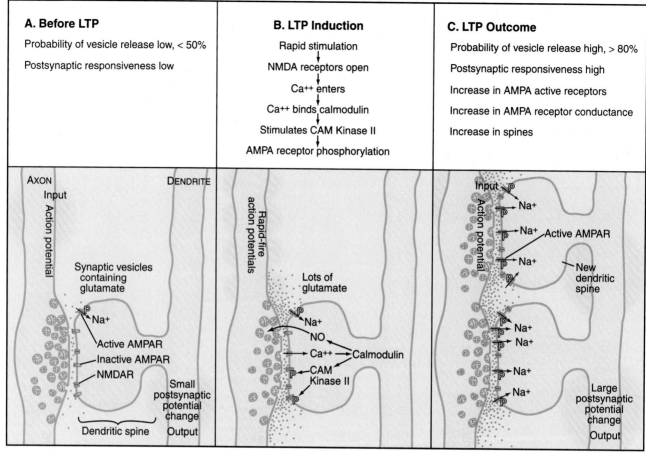

Figure 10–10 Mechanism of long-term potentiation (LTP) of synaptic transmission at excitatory synapses in the hippocampus. *A*, Prior to LTP, postsynaptic responses to presynaptic action potentials are unreliable and small. *B*, Some acute responses to vigorous stimulation. *C*, After induction of LTP, postsynaptic responses are more reliable and larger. AMPAR and NMDAK are two classes of glutamate receptors; NO is nitric oxide; CAM Kinase II is calcium-calmodulin Kinase II.

glutamate depends on the membrane potential as partial depolarization is required to displace an extracellular Mg^{2+} ion blocking the channel. This dual dependence on glutamate and membrane potential makes NMDA receptors coincidence detectors, responsive to rapid stimulation or stimulation at nearby excitatory synapses. When open, NMDA receptors admit Ca^{2+} into the postsynaptic cell.

In principle, LTP and LTD might alter the efficiency of synaptic transmission by changing glutamate release from the presynaptic cell or responsiveness of the postsynaptic cell to glutamate. In fact, a wide range of experiments suggests that both presynaptic and postsynaptic changes contribute. The best documented presynaptic change is an increase in the probability that an action potential will stimulate the fusion of a glutamate-containing synaptic vesicle with the plasma membrane. In the resting state, exocytosis of these vesicles is unreliable. LTP increases the probability of exocytosis from less than 0.5 to greater than 0.8. In addition, the postsynaptic side responds more robustly to glutamate owing to a higher concentration of AMPA receptors with enhanced conductance when

open and to additional synapses with the stimulating axon.

The mechanisms bringing about these changes are incompletely understood, but the following is well established. LTP depends on stimulation of NMDA receptors and Ca^{2+} entry. Within the postsynaptic dendritic spine, Ca^{2+} activates processes that initiate and maintain LTP. Within seconds, Ca^{2+} binds calmodulin (see Chapter 28) and triggers events dependent on calcium-calmodulin, including activation of protein kinases, such as CAM-kinase II (see Chapter 27) and production of the gas nitric oxide (NO) (see Chapter 28). Phosphorylation of AMPA receptors by CAM-kinase II increases their responsiveness to glutamate, perhaps accounting for "waking up silent synapses." LTP also recruits AMPA receptors to the synapse. NO and perhaps other extracellular messengers, such as eicosanoids (see Chapter 28), may provide feedback to the presynaptic terminal to modify its exocytosis efficiency. Within minutes, LTP induces target dendrites to grow filopodia and spines; these are presumed to account for the increased number of synapses observed after an hour or so. Extension of these processes and remodeling of the shape of dendritic spines depend on actin filament assembly (see Chapters 36 and 41). Over the longer term, the postsynaptic cell activates gene transcription and protein synthesis, bringing about further changes that stabilize the changes that enhance synaptic transmission.

LTD appears, in many ways, to be the reverse of LTP, with less reliable presynaptic exocytosis and less responsive postsynaptic AMPA receptors. It, too, depends on NMDA receptors, but the biochemical basis for the synaptic changes is even less well understood.

▌ Cardiac Membrane Physiology

Spontaneous Action Potentials of Pacemaker Cells

Intrinsically excitable **pacemaker cells** in the **sino-atrial node** drive rhythmic contractions of the heart (see Fig. 42–19). The membrane potential of these cells drifts spontaneously toward threshold, setting off action potentials about once each second (Fig. 10–11). Cardiac action potentials spread via **gap junctions** (see Chapter 33) from cell to cell throughout the heart, activating contraction in a reproducible pattern.

Spontaneous action potentials of cardiac pacemaker cells are more complicated than those of nerves. Seven different plasma membrane channels determine their frequency:

1. *Voltage-gated Na^+ channels.* As in nerves, these channels rapidly activate at membrane potentials above threshold and then rapidly inactivate.
2. *T-type, voltage-gated Ca^{2+} channels.* These low-conductance channels activate transiently at membrane potentials more negative than Na^+ channels, about −70 mV.
3. *L-type, voltage-gated Ca^{2+} channels.* These high-conductance channels slowly activate and inactivate when the membrane depolarizes to about −40 mV. Sympathetic nerve stimulation sensitizes these channels to membrane depolarization. Dihydropyrines block these channels.
4. *Delayed-rectifier, voltage-gated K^+ channels.* As in nerves, these channels activate and inactivate slowly in response to membrane depolarization. Sympathetic nerves stimulate these channels.
5. *Kir3.1 inward-rectifier K^+ channels.* These channels conduct K^+ over a limited range of membrane potential, between about −30 and −80 mV. Parasympathetic nerve stimulation activates these channels.
6. *Kir6.2 inward-rectifier K^+ channels.* Normal levels of cytoplasmic ATP inhibit these channels. Depletion of cytoplasmic ATP activates these channels.
7. *Nonselective K^+/Na^+ channels.* Repolarization of the membrane activates these channels.

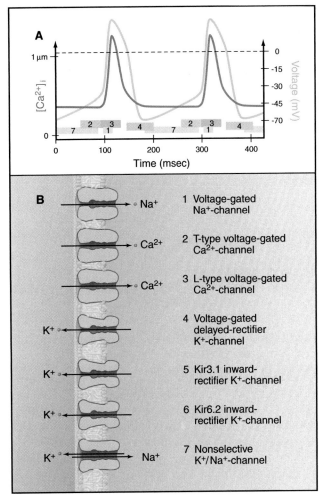

Figure 10–11 Mechanism of spontaneous cardiac pacemaker action potentials. Sequential activation and inactivation of seven different plasma membrane channels account for the time course of action potentials and cytoplasmic Ca^{2+} transients in pacemaker cells of the sinoatrial node. *A*, Time courses of the fluctuations in membrane potential *(orange)* and cytoplasmic Ca^{2+} concentration *(blue)*. Colored boxes indicate when the various channels enumerated in *B* are open. Kir3.1 and Kir6.2 are inactive under these conditions. *B*, Channels contributing to pacemaker activity.

These channels produce a spontaneous cycle of pacemaker action potentials. At the threshold potential (about −40 mV), voltage-gated Na^+ channels open synchronously and rapidly depolarize the membrane. As they inactivate, L-type Ca^{2+} channels open, prolonging the depolarization and admitting Ca^{2+}; this, in turn, triggers contraction by releasing more Ca^{2+} from internal stores (see Chapter 42). As these Ca^{2+} channels slowly inactivate, delayed-rectifier K^+ channels open and drive the membrane potential toward E_K, the K^+ equilibrium potential. As the membrane potential reaches a minimum, delayed-rectifier K^+ channels inactivate, but the two Kir channels open. In the absence of other channel activity, the membrane potential would remain near E_K, but the nonselective Na^+/K^+ channels open and the membrane slowly de-

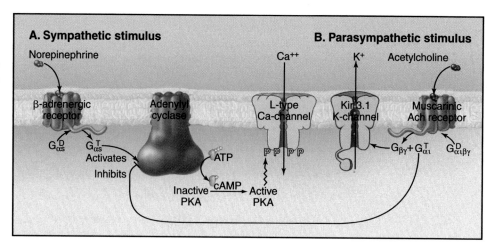

Figure 10–12 Regulation of the rate of cardiac pacemaker cells by sympathetic (A) and parasympathetic (B) nerves. D stands for GDP associated with G protein α-subunits; T stands for GTP; PKA is protein kinase A; cAMP is cyclic adenosine monophosphate. GTP-Gα$_s$ stimulates adenylyl cycle. GTP-Gα$_i$ inhibits adenylyl cyclase.

polarizes, drifting toward threshold. T-type Ca²⁺ channels contribute to the slow, spontaneous depolarization. At threshold, the cycle repeats.

Regulation of Heart Rate by G Proteins and Phosphorylation

Regulation of pacemaker cells by autonomic nerves is an example of the widespread regulation of channels by G proteins and phosphorylation (Fig. 10–12). Neurotransmitters from the two parts of the autonomic nervous system have opposite effects on the frequency of cardiac contraction. The resting rate reflects a compromise in the competition between these two inputs. Acetylcholine from **parasympathetic nerves** slows the heartbeat, whereas norepinephrine from **sympathetic nerves** speeds the rate and increases the strength of contraction. These neurotransmitters modify their target channels indirectly by activating two different seven-helix receptors (see Chapter 26).

Norepinephrine increases the heart rate by modulating L-type Ca²⁺ channels. Norepinephrine that binds to plasma membrane β-adrenergic receptors activates G proteins (see Chapter 29), which stimulate **adenylyl cyclase,** the enzyme that makes cyclic adenosine monophosphate (cAMP) (see Chapter 28). This second messenger stimulates cyclic **AMP–dependent protein kinase** (PKA) (see Chapter 27) to phosphorylate cytoplasmic residues of L-type, voltage-gated Ca²⁺ channels in the plasma membrane. Phosphorylated Ca²⁺ channels are more likely to open than nonphosphorylated channels. Phosphorylation increases the rate at which the membrane potential drifts toward threshold. This increases the frequency of action potentials of pacemaker cells, and the heart rate.

Acetylcholine released by parasympathetic nerves activates Kir3.1 inward-rectifier K⁺ channels that slow the heartbeat. It binds to different seven-helix receptors, called muscarinic acetylcholine receptors (because they bind muscarine), to distinguish them from

the nicotinic acetylcholine receptors. Acetylcholine binding to muscarinic receptors activates a trimeric G protein, different from that activated by norepinephrine. Two G-protein subunits, comprising the Gβγ complex, dissociate from the Gα$_i$ subunit and activate Kir3.1/3.4 channels. When open, these channels reduce the rate at which the membrane potential drifts toward threshold. In addition the Gα$_i$ subunit inhibits cyclic AMP production and reduces Ca²⁺ channel phosphorylation. This decreases the probability that Ca²⁺ channels are open, contributing to a lowering of the heart rate. If the energy supply of the heart is compromised, ATP levels fall. This activates Kir6.2 channels, which reduce the rate of spontaneous depolarization and the heart rate until ATP levels are restored.

Regulation of Cardiac Contractility

A set of channels similar to those in the sinoatrial node generate action potentials in cardiac muscle cells and stimulate contraction. Cardiac muscle cells can generate spontaneous action potentials, but they have fewer T-type Ca²⁺ channels and more Kir K⁺ channels, so the rate of spontaneous action potentials is lower than that of pacemaker cells. Except in disease, pacemaker cells drive action potentials throughout the rest of the heart. Sympathetic nervous stimulation, acting through cyclic AMP–dependent protein kinase, strengthens cardiac contraction. Phosphorylated L-type Ca²⁺ channels admit more Ca²⁺ to activate the contractile machinery more fully. The same kinase activates delayed-rectifier K⁺ channels, which prevent activated Ca²⁺ channels from prolonging the action potential. This allows heart muscle cells to keep up with stimuli generated at a higher rate from pacemaker cells. Cyclic AMP–dependent protein kinase also enhances contractility by phosphorylating proteins of the contractile apparatus and smooth endoplasmic reticulum (see Chapter 42).

Therapeutic Effect of Digitalis in Congestive Heart Failure

In congestive heart failure, cardiac contraction fails to produce enough force to maintain adequate circulation of blood. **Cardiac glycosides,** such as digitalis (from the foxglove plant), ameliorate this common human condition by inhibiting an isoform of Na^+K^+-ATPase in the plasma membrane of heart cells (Fig. 10–13). Plasma membrane L-type Ca^{2+} channels and endoplasmic reticulum Ca^{2+} release channels activate contraction by transiently increasing cytoplasmic Ca^{2+}. Calcium ATPase pumps (see Fig. 7–7) in smooth endoplasmic reticulum clear most of this Ca^{2+} from cytoplasm, but plasma membrane Na^+/Ca^{2+} antiporters, driven by the plasma membrane Na^+ gradient, contribute as well.

Digitalis and related compounds, such as ouabain, strengthen cardiac contraction indirectly by inhibiting an isoform of Na^+K^+-ATPase found in the cardiac plasma membrane. Reduced sodium pump activity lowers the electrochemical gradient of Na^+ across the plasma membrane and provides less driving force for Na^+ to exchange for Ca^{2+}. The result is a slightly higher steady-state concentration of Ca^{2+} in cytoplasm, which strengthens contraction. A drug that targets Ca^{2+} export directly would be desirable, but thus far, researchers have failed to find a satisfactory inhibitor.

The success of cardiac glycosides depends upon their selectivity for the α_2 isoform of the α-subunit of the Na^+K^+-ATPase, which is expressed in heart, skeletal muscle, and fat. This α_2 isoform is much more sensitive to cardiac glycosides than the α_1 isoform. Although the α_2 isoform represents a minority of cardiac sodium pumps, its inhibition lowers the Na^+ gradient across the heart cell plasma membrane without deleterious effects on other tissues. One reason may be that the Na^+/Ca^{2+} symporter that works with the sodium pump in the heart is not expressed in skeletal muscle or fat.

Oxidative Phosphorylation by Mitochondria

Structure and Evolution of Mitochondria

Mitochondria arose when a *Eubacterium* set up residence in a primitive nucleated eukaryotic cell (see Fig. 1–1). The closest extant relatives of this bacterium are *Rickettsia*, intracellular parasites with a genome of 1.1 megabase pairs that cause typhus and Rocky Mountain spotted fever. Over more than a billion years, most of the bacterial genes moved to the nucleus of host eukaryotes. The pace of gene transfer to the nucleus varied considerably, but all known mitochondria retain some bacterial genes in a chromosome that varies from 366,924 bp in the plant *Arabidopsis* to 16,569 bp in humans to only 5966 bp in *Plasmodium*. Most mitochondrial chromosomes are circular. These small genomes encode RNAs and proteins essential for mitochondrial function, including subunits of proteins responsible for production of ATP. The highly paired-down human mitochondrial genome encodes only 13 proteins and just enough tRNAs to translate these genes. In other mitochondrial genomes, protein genes range from just 3 in *Plasmodium* to 97 in a protozoan. Vertebrate cells contain about 1000 copies of mtDNA. Nuclear genes encode the remaining components of mitochondria, including the machinery to synthesize proteins in the mitochondrial matrix. All the products of nuclear genes are transported into mitochondria after synthesis in cytoplasm (see Figs. 19–2 and 19–3).

Mitochondria consist of membrane compartments, one inside the other, separated by a space (Fig. 10–14). The **inner membrane** surrounds the **matrix.** Each membrane and compartment has a distinct protein composition. The inner membrane is thrown up into folds called **cristae** that vary in number and shape depending upon the species, tissue, and metabolic state. Cristae may be tubular or flattened sacs that appear to be connected to the peripheral part of the inner membrane by specialized junctions.

Mitochondria use a combination of pumps, carriers, electron transport proteins, and enzymes to convert energy extracted from the chemical bonds of nutrients into ATP. This section of the chapter focuses on the inner membrane and matrix, which produce ATP. Porins in the **outer membrane** provide channels for passage for molecules of less than 5000 D, including most metabolites required for ATP synthesis. The inner membrane is only selectively permeable; in fact, its

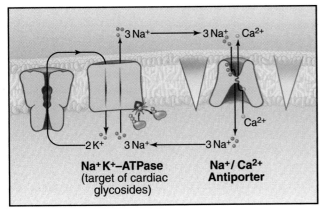

Figure 10–13 The chemiosmotic cycle that helps clear Ca^{2+} from the cytoplasm of cardiac muscle cells. Na^+K^+-ATPase pumps create a Na^+ gradient (*purple triangle*) to drive the Na^+/Ca^{2+} antiporter to transport Ca^{2+} up its concentration gradient (*blue triangle*) out of the cell. Cardiac glycosides inhibit the cardiac isoform of Na^+K^+-ATPase, raising the concentration of cytoplasmic Ca^{2+} and strengthening cardiac contraction. K^+ channels (*left*) allow K^+ to circulate.

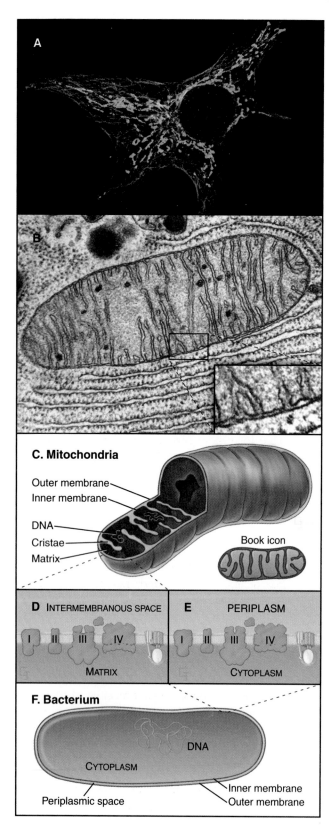

C. Mitochondria

Outer membrane
Inner membrane
DNA
Cristae
Matrix

Book icon

D INTERMEMBRANOUS SPACE

I II III IV

MATRIX

E PERIPLASM

I II III IV

CYTOPLASM

F. Bacterium

DNA

CYTOPLASM

Periplasmic space

Inner membrane
Outer membrane

Figure 10–14 Cellular distribution and structure of mitochondria. *A,* Fluorescence light micrograph of a Cos-7 tissue culture cell with mitochondria labeled with green fluorescent antibody to the β-subunit of the F1-ATPase and microtubules labeled red with an antibody. *B,* Electron micrograph of a thin section of a mitochondrion. *C* to *F,* Drawings of the compartments of a mitochondrion compared with a *Eubacterium.* (*A,* Courtesy of Michael Yaffee, University of California, San Diego; *B,* Courtesy of Don Fawcett, Harvard Medical School.)

impermeability to H$^+$ and other intermediates in the energy-converting reactions is key to the operation of the system.

Synthesis of ATP by Oxidative Phosphorylation

As the main site of energy conversion into ATP, mitochondria receive energy-yielding chemical intermediates from two main metabolic pathways: **glycolysis** and **fatty acid oxidation** (Fig. 10–15). Both pathways feed into the **citric acid cycle** of energy-yielding reactions in the mitochondrial matrix:

- The glycolytic pathway in cytoplasm converts the six-carbon sugar, glucose, into pyruvate, a three-carbon substrate for pyruvate dehydrogenase, a large, soluble, enzyme complex in the mitochondrial matrix. The products of pyruvate dehydrogenase (carbon dioxide, the reduced form of nicotinamide adenine dinucleotide [**NADH**] and acetyl coenzyme A [-CoA]) are released into the matrix. NADH is a high-energy electron carrier (see Fig. 10–15). **Acetyl-CoA** is a two-carbon metabolic intermediate that supplies the citric acid cycle with energy-rich bonds.
- Breakdown of lipids yields fatty acids linked to acetyl-CoA by a thioester bond and transported across the inner membrane of mitochondria, using carnitine in a shuttle system. In the matrix, acyl-carnitine is reconverted to acyl-CoA. Enzymes in the matrix degrade fatty acids two carbons at a time in a series of oxidative reactions that yield NADH, the reduced form of flavin adenine dinucleotide (**FADH$_2$**) (another energy-rich electron carrier associated with an integral membrane enzyme complex), and acetyl-CoA for the citric acid cycle.

Breakdown of acetyl-CoA during one turn of the citric acid cycle produces three molecules of NADH, one molecule of FADH$_2$, and two molecules of carbon dioxide. Energetic electrons donated by NADH and FADH$_2$ drive an **electron transport pathway** in the inner mitochondrial membrane that powers a chemiosmotic cycle to produce ATP (Fig. 10–16). Electrons use two routes to pass through three protein complexes in the inner mitochondrial membrane. Starting with NADH, electrons pass through complex I to complex III to complex IV. Electrons from FADH$_2$ pass through complex II to III to IV. Along both routes, energy is partitioned off to transfer multiple protons (at least 10 electrons per NADH oxidized) across the inner mitochondrial membrane from the matrix to the inner membrane space. The resulting electrochemical gradient of protons drives ATP synthesis (see Fig. 7–3).

This process is called **oxidative phosphorylation,** since molecular oxygen is the sink for energy-bearing electrons at the end of the pathway and since the reactions add phosphate to ADP. Oxidative phosphorylation is understood in remarkable detail thanks to atomic structures of ATP synthase and two of four electron transfer complexes. Nuclear genes encode most of the protein subunits of these complexes, but mitochondrial genes are responsible for a few key subunits.

Bacteria have homologues of all of the key proteins in mitochondrial oxidative phosphorylation (see Fig. 10–14). Although many changes have accumulated during the divergent evolution of bacteria and eukaryotes, both bacteria and mitochondria have retained the essential features of oxidative phosphorylation. Thus bacteria are useful model systems with which to study these common mechanisms. Plasma membranes of bacteria and inner membranes of mitochondria have equivalent components, whereas the bacterial cytoplasm corresponds to the mitochondrial matrix.

Energy enters this pathway in the form of electrons produced when NADH is oxidized to NAD$^+$, releasing one H$^+$ and two electrons (see Fig. 10–16). If the proton and electrons were to combine immediately with oxygen, their energy would be lost as heat. Instead, these high-energy electrons are separated from the protons and then passed along the electron transport pathway, before finally recombining to reduce molecular oxygen to form water. Along the pathway, electrons associate transiently with a series of oxidation/reduction acceptors, generally, metal ions associated with organic cofactors, such as hemes in cytochromes and iron-sulfur centers (2Fe2S) and copper centers in complex IV. Electrons move along the transport pathway at rates of up to 1000 s^{-1}. To travel at this rate through a transmembrane protein complex spanning a 35-nm lipid bilayer, at least three redox cofactors are required owing to the fact that the efficiency of quantum mechanical tunneling of electrons between redox cofactors falls off rapidly with distance. Two cofactors, even with optimal orientation, are too slow.

Step by step, electrons lose energy as they move along the transport pathway. In three complexes along the pathway, energy given up by the electrons is used to pump protons from the matrix to the inner membrane space. This establishes an electrochemical proton gradient across the inner mitochondrial membrane that is used by **ATP synthase** to drive ATP production. Direction is provided to the movements of electrons by the progressive increase in electron affinity of the acceptors. The final acceptor, oxygen (at the end of the pathway), has the highest affinity.

The first component of the electron transport pathway is **complex I** (also called NADH:ubiquinone oxidoreductase). This is the largest element in the

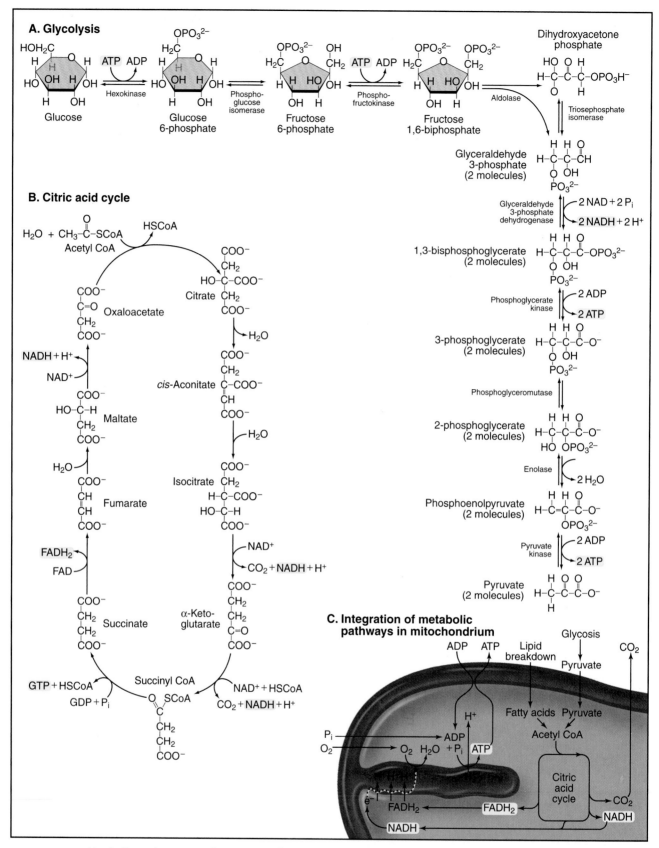

Figure 10–15 Metabolic pathways supplying energy for oxidative phosphorylation. *A,* Glycolysis. *B,* Citric acid cycle. Production of acetyl-CoA by the glycolytic pathway in cytoplasm and fatty acid oxidation in the mitochondrial matrix drive the citric acid cycle in the mitochondrial matrix. This energy-yielding cycle is also called the Krebs cycle after the biochemist H. Krebs. NADH and FADH$_2$ produced by these pathways supply high-energy electrons to the electron transport chain. *C,* Overview of metabolic pathways. Energy-rich metabolites are highlighted in yellow.

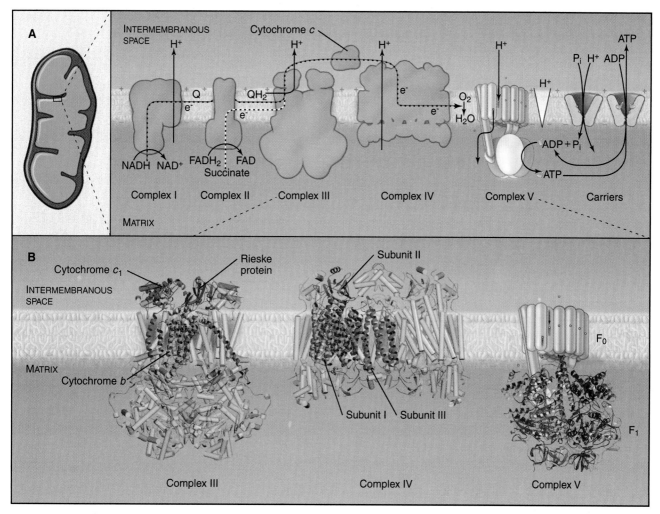

Figure 10-16 Chemiosmotic cycle of the respiratory electron transport chain and ATP synthase. *A,* The left panel shows a mitochondrion for orientation. The right panel shows the electron transport system of the inner mitochondrial membrane. Red and yellow arrows trace the pathway of electrons through the four complexes. Black arrows show the sites of proton translocation between the matrix to the intermembranous space. The stoichiometry is not specified, but at the last step, four electrons are required to reduce oxygen to water. ATP synthase uses the electrochemical proton gradient produced by the electron transport reactions to drive ATP synthesis. *B,* The available atomic structures of the electron transport chain are shown. In the cytochrome bc₁ complex III, the 3 of 11 mitochondrial subunits used by bacteria are shown as ribbon models. The supporting subunits found in mitochondria are shown as cylinders. The four subunits of complex IV encoded by the mitochondrial genome are shown as ribbon models. They form the functional core of the complex, which is supported by additional subunits shown as cylinders. See Figure 7–4 for further details of ATP synthase (Complex V). (*B,* Images of Complex III and Complex IV courtesy of M. Saraste, European Molecular Biology Laboratory, Heidelberg, Germany. Reference: Zhang Z, et al: Electron transfer by domain movement in cytochrome bc₁. Nature 392:677–684, 1998. PDB file: 1BCC. Reference: Yoshikawa S, et al: Redox-coupled crystal structural changes in bovine heart cytochrome c oxidase. Science 280:1723–1729, 1998. PDB file: 2OCC.)

pathway (mol wt >900 kD) consisting of more than 40 different protein subunits in vertebrates with a number of bound organic (quinols) and inorganic (iron-sulfur centers) acceptors for electrons. Bacterial complex I has 14 subunits. Most fungi have a complicated complex I, but budding yeasts have lost the genes for most of complex I. They get along with some simple NADH dehydrogenases that do not pump protons. For each molecule of NADH oxidized, com-

plex I transfers four protons from the matrix into the inner membrane space. Only a low-resolution structure is available based on electron microscopy.

The second component of the electron transport pathway is **complex II** or succinate:ubiquinone reductase, a transmembrane enzyme that makes up part of the citric acid cycle. Complex II couples oxidation of succinate (a four-carbon intermediate in the citric acid cycle) to fumarate with reduction of flavin adenine dinucleotide (FAD) to FADH$_2$. Complex II does not pump protons, but transfers electrons from FADH$_2$ to ubiquinone. Reduced ubiquinone carries these electrons to complex III.

The third component of the electron transport pathway is **complex III,** also called **cytochrome bc$_1$.** This well-characterized, transmembrane protein complex consists of 11 different subunits. The homologous bacterial complex has only three of these subunits, the ones that participate in energy transduction in mitochondria. Eight other subunits surround this core. Complex III couples the oxidation and reduction of ubiquinone to the transfer of protons from the matrix across the inner mitochondrial membrane. Energy is supplied by electrons that move through the cytochrome-b subunit to a subunit with a 2Fe2S redox center. This subunit then rotates into position to transfer the electron to cytochrome c$_1$, another subunit of the complex. Cytochrome c$_1$ then transfers the electron to the water-soluble protein, cytochrome c, in the intermembranous space (or periplasm of bacteria).

Cytochrome oxidase, complex IV, takes electrons from four cytochrome c molecules to reduce molecular oxygen to two waters, as well as to pump four protons out of the matrix. Mitochondrial genes encode the three subunits that form the core of the enzyme, carry out electron transfer, and translocate protons. Nuclear genes encode the surrounding 10 subunits.

The electrochemical proton gradient produced by the electron transport chain provides energy to synthesize ATP. Chapter 7 explained how the rotary ATP synthase (Complex V) can either use ATP hydrolysis to pump protons or use the transit of protons down an electrochemical gradient to synthesize ATP. The proton gradient across the inner mitochondrial membrane drives rotation of the γ-subunit. The rotating γ-subunit physically changes the conformations of the α- and β-subunits, bringing together ADP and inorganic phosphate to make ATP. An antiporter in the inner membrane exchanges cytoplasmic ADP for ATP synthesized in the matrix.

Mitochondria and Disease

Dozens of mutations in mitochondrial DNA (mtDNA) have been linked to rare human diseases (also see Fig. 19–4). The situation is complicated by the existence of about 1000 copies of mtDNA per vertebrate cell. A mutation in one copy would be of no consequence, but segregation of mtDNAs may lead to cells in which mutant mtDNAs predominate, yielding large, defective proteins. A recurring point mutation in a subunit of complex I causes some patients to develop sudden onset of blindness in middle age owing to death of neurons in the optic nerve. Other patients with the

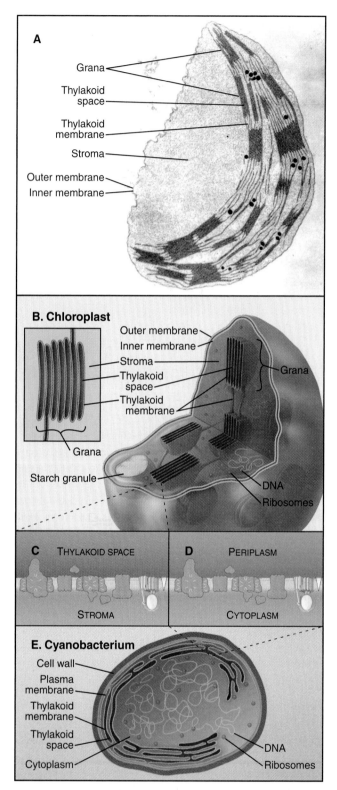

Figure 10-17 Morphology of chloroplasts and cyanobacteria. *A,* Electron micrograph of a thin section of a spinach chloroplast. *B,* Drawing of a chloroplast. *C* and *D,* Block diagrams comparing the machinery in the photosynthetic membranes of chloroplasts and cyanobacteria. *E,* Drawing of a cyanobacterium illustrating the internal folds of the plasma membrane to form photosynthetic thylakoids. (*A,* Courtesy of K. Miller, Brown University.)

same mutation in a larger fraction of mtDNA molecules suffer from muscle weakness and mental retardation as children. Mutations in the genes for subunits of ATP synthase cause muscle weakness and degeneration of the retina. Mutations in nuclear genes for mitochondrial proteins cause similar symptoms.

Photosynthesis by Bacteria and Chloroplasts

Structure and Evolution of Photosynthesis Systems

Photosynthetic *Eubacteria* and chloroplasts of algae and plants (Fig. 10–17) use **chlorophyll** to capture the remarkable amount of energy carried by single photons to boost electrons to an excited state. These high-energy electrons drive a chemiosmotic cycle to make NADPH and ATP, energy currency used by all cells. Photosynthetic organisms use ATP and the reducing power of NADPH to synthesize three-carbon sugar phosphates from carbon dioxide. Glycolytic reactions (see Fig. 10–15) running backward use this three-carbon sugar phosphate to make six-carbon sugars and more complex carbohydrates for use as metabolic energy sources and structural components. Some Archaea, such as *Halobacteria halobium,* and some recently discovered *Eubacteria* use a completely different light-driven pump lacking chlorophyll to generate a proton gradient to synthesize ATP. Retinol associated with bacteriorhodopsin absorbs light to drive proton transport (see Fig. 7–3).

Photosynthesis originated approximately 3.5 billion years ago in a *Eubacterium,* most likely a gram-negative purple bacterium. These bacteria evolved the components to assemble a transmembrane complex of proteins, pigments, and oxidation/reduction cofactors called a **reaction center** (Fig. 10–18). Reaction centers absorb light and initiate an electron transport pathway that pumps protons out of the cell. Such photosystems turn sunlight into electrical and chemical energy with 40% efficiency, better than any man-made photovoltaic cell. Given their alarming complexity and physical perfection, it is remarkable that photosystems emerged only a few hundred million years after the origin of life itself.

Broadly speaking, photosynthetic reaction centers of contemporary organisms can be divided into two different groups (Fig. 10–19). The reaction centers of purple bacteria and green filamentous bacteria utilize the pigment pheophytin and a quinone as the electron acceptor, like **photosystem II** of cyanobacteria and chloroplasts. The reaction centers of green sulfur bacteria and heliobacteria have iron-sulfur centers as electron acceptors, similar to **photosystem I** of cyanobacteria and chloroplasts.

Cyanobacteria are unique among bacteria in that they have both types of photosystems as well as a manganese enzyme that splits water, releasing from two water molecules four electrons, four protons, and oxygen. Coupling this enzyme to photosynthesis was a pivotal event in the history of the earth, as this reaction is the source of most of the oxygen in the earth's atmosphere.

Chloroplasts of eukaryotic cells arose from a symbiotic cyanobacterium. Much evidence indicates that this event occurred just once, giving all chloroplasts a common origin. However, to account for chloroplasts in organisms that diverged prior to the acquisition of chloroplasts, one must also postulate lateral transfer of chloroplasts from, for example, a green alga to *Euglena.* Alternatively, cyanobacteria may have colonized eukaryotic cells on up to three different occasions, giving rise to organelles that evolved into chloroplasts (see Fig. 1–1).

Chloroplasts have retained up to 250 original bacterial genes on circular genomes, whereas many bacterial genes were lost or moved to the nucleus of host eukaryotes. Chloroplast genomes encode subunits of many proteins responsible for photosynthesis and chloroplast division, ribosomal RNAs and proteins, and a complete set of tRNAs. Chloroplast proteins encoded by nuclear genes are transported post-translationally into chloroplasts (see Fig. 19–5) after their synthesis in cytoplasm.

The organization of cyanobacterial membranes explains the architecture of chloroplasts (see Fig. 10–17). In cyanobacteria, light-absorbing pigments, as well as protein complexes involved with electron transport and ATP synthesis, are concentrated in invaginations of the plasma membrane. The F1 domain of ATP synthase faces the cytoplasm, and the lumen of this membrane system is periplasmic. This internal membrane system remains in chloroplasts but is separated from the inner membrane (the former plasma membrane). These **thylakoid membranes** contain photosynthetic hardware and enclose the thylakoid membrane space. Like the bacterial plasma membrane, the chloroplast **"inner membrane"** is a permeability barrier, containing carriers for metabolites. The inner membrane surrounds the **stroma,** the cytoplasm of the original symbiotic bacterium, a protein-rich compartment devoted to synthesis of three-carbon sugar phosphates, chloroplast proteins, and all plant fatty acids. The stroma also houses the genomes and stores starch. The **outer membrane,** like the comparable bacterial and mitochondrial membranes, has large pore channels that allow free passage of metabolites.

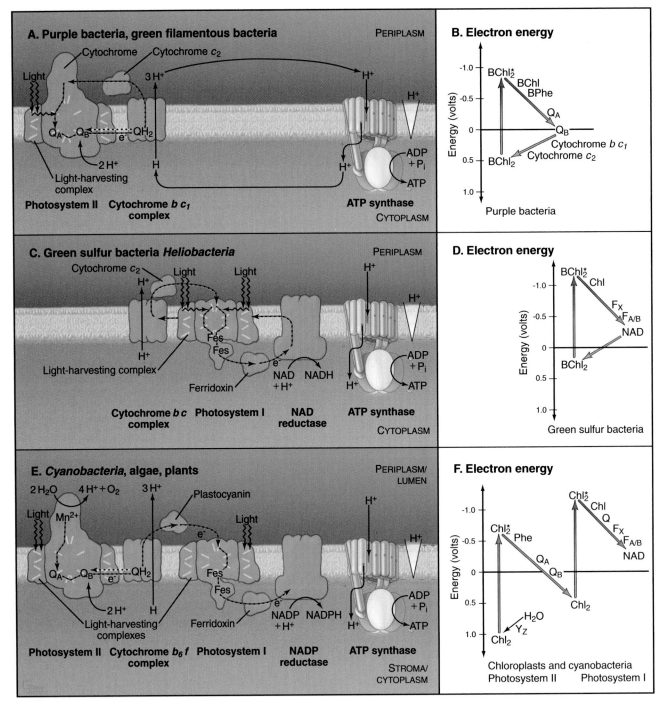

Figure 10-18 Comparison of photosynthetic components, electron transport pathways, and chemiosmotic cycles to make ATP. *A* and *B*, Photosystem II only. *C* and *D*, Photosystem I only. *E* and *F*, Both photosystem II and photosystem I. The diagrams in figure parts *B*, *D*, and *F* show the energy levels of electrons in the three types of photosynthetic organisms. Vertical arrows show excitation of an electron by an absorbed photon. Arrows sloping to the right show electron transfer pathways through each reaction center. Arrows sloping to the left show electron transfer steps outside the reaction centers. (*A*, *C*, and *E*, Reference: Kramer DM, Schoepp B, Liebl U, Nitschke W: Cyclic electron transfer in *Heliobacillus mobilis*. Biochemistry 36:4203–4211, 1997. *B*, *D*, and *F*, Reference: Allen JP, Williams JC: Photosynthetic reaction centers. FEBS Lett 438:5–9, 1998.)

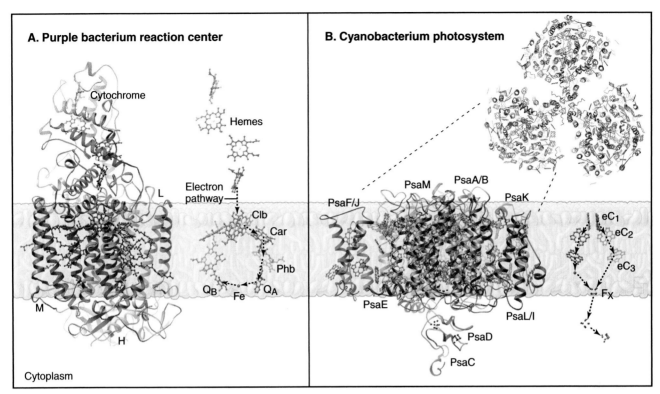

Figure 10-19 Structures of photosystem hardware. *A,* Ribbon diagram of photosystem II from the purple bacterium, *Rhodopseudomonas viridis,* with ball and stick models of chlorophyll and other cofactors to the right in their natural orientations. Similar core subunits L and M each consist of five transmembrane helices. This pair of subunits binds four molecules of chlorophyll-b (Clb); two molecules of bacteriopheophytin-b (Phb); one nonheme iron (Fe); two quinones (Q_A, Q_B); and one carotenoid (Car) in a rigid framework. A cytochrome with four heme groups binds to the periplasmic side of the core subunits. Subunit H associates with the core subunits via one transmembrane helix and with their cytoplasmic surfaces. The atomic structure of this photosynthetic reaction center was the Nobel prize work of J. Diesenhoffer, R. Huber and H. Michel. *B,* Ribbon diagram of photosystem I of *Synechococcus elongatus,* with ball and stick models of chlorophyll and other cofactors to the right in their natural orientations. This trimeric complex consists of three identical units, each composed of 11 polypeptide chains. Within each of these units, this 4Å structure includes 43 α-helices, 89 chlorophylls, a quinone, and three iron-sulfur centers, but lacks amino acid side chains, carotenoids, and some parts of the polypeptide chains. The photosynthetic reaction center consists of the C-terminal halves of the two central subunits *(PsaA/PsaB; red-brown)* associated with six chlorophylls, one or two quinones, and a shared iron-sulfur cluster. Plastocyanin or cytochrome c_6 on the lumen side donates electrons to reduce the P700 special pair chlorophylls (eC_1) of the reaction center. Light energizes an electron, which passes successively through two other chlorophylls, a quinone and the shared iron-sulfur cluster *(red)*, F_x. The electron then transfers to the iron-sulfur clusters of the accessory subunit PsaC on the stromal side of the membrane. The surrounding eight subunits *(red, grey)*, associated with about 80 chlorophylls, comprise the core antenna system, forming a nearly continuous ring of α-helices around the reaction center. Absorption of light by additional light-harvesting complexes and these antenna subunits puts chloroplast electrons into an excited state. This energy passes from one pigment to the next until it eventually reaches the reaction center. (*A,* Reference: Diesenhoffer J, Michel H: The photosynthetic reaction center from the purple bacterium *Rhodopseudomonas viridis.* Science 245:1463–1473, 1989. Copyright of Deisenhoffer & Michel, 1988, Nobel Foundation. PDB file: 1PRC. *B,* Reference: Schubert W-D, Klukas O, Krauss N, et al: Photosystem I of *Synechococcus elongatus* at 4Å resolution: Comprehensive structure analysis. J Molec Biol 272:741–769, 1997. PDB file: 2PPS.)

Light and Dark Reactions

Photosynthetic mechanisms capture energy from photons to drive two types of reactions:

- **"Light reactions"** depend on continuous absorption of photons. These reactions occur in or on the surface of thylakoid membranes. They include generation of high-energy electrons, electron transport to make NADPH, creation of a proton gradient across the thylakoid membrane for the chemiosmotic synthesis of ATP, and generation of oxygen.

- **"Dark reactions"** convert carbon dioxide into three-carbon sugar phosphates. These reactions continue for some time in the dark. However, they depend on ATP and NADPH produced by light reactions, so they eventually stop when ATP and NADPH are exhausted in the dark. These reactions account for most of the carbon dioxide converted to carbohydrates on earth. (Specialized prokaryotes drive carbon fixation by oxidation of hydrogen sulfide and other inorganic compounds.)

All photosynthetic systems use similar mechanisms to capture energy from photons (see Fig. 10–18). Pigments associated with transmembrane proteins in photosynthetic reaction centers absorb photons and use the energy to boost electrons to a high-energy, **excited state.** Subsequent electron transfer reactions partition this energy in several steps to generate a proton gradient across the membrane. Generation of this proton electrochemical gradient and chemiosmotic production of ATP are similar to oxidative phosphorylation (see Fig. 10–16).

Specific photosynthetic systems differ in the complexity of the hardware, the source of electrons, and the products (see Fig. 10–18). Most photosynthetic bacteria use either photosystem I or II to create a proton gradient to synthesize ATP. Cyanobacteria and green plants use both types of reaction centers in series to raise electrons to an energy sufficient to make NADPH in addition to ATP. These advanced systems also use water as the electron donor and produce molecular oxygen as a byproduct.

Energy Capture and Transduction by Photosystem II

The reaction center from the purple bacterium *Rhodopseudomonas viridis* (see Fig. 10–19) is a model for the more complex photosystem II of chloroplasts. This bacterial reaction center consists of just four subunits. A cytochrome subunit on the periplasmic side of the membrane donates electrons. Two core subunits form a rigid transmembrane framework to bind 10 redox cofactors in orientations that favor transfer of high-energy electrons from two "special" chlorophylls through a secondary **chlorophyll *b*** and **pheophytin *b*** to a **quinone.**

Photosynthesis begins with absorption of a photon by the special pair chlorophylls. Photons in the visible part of the spectrum are quite energetic, 40 to 80 kcal mol^{-1}, enough to make several ATPs. The purple bacterium reaction center absorbs relatively low-energy, 870-nm red light. The energy elevates an electron in the special pair chlorophylls to an excited state. In an organic solvent, the excited state would decay rapidly (10^9 s^{-1}), and the energy would dissipate as heat or emission of a less energetic photon by fluorescence or phosphorescence. However, reaction centers are optimized to transfer excited-state electrons rapidly and efficiently from the special pair chlorophylls to a secondary chlorophyll *b* (3×10^{-12} sec), then to pheophytin (200×10^{-12} sec) and then to tightly bound quinone A (200×10^{-12} sec). Transfer is by **quantum mechanical tunneling** right through the protein molecule. Because the tunneling rate falls off quickly with distance, four redox centers must be spaced close together to allow an energetic electron to transfer across the lipid bilayer faster than spontaneous decay of the excited state.

On the cytoplasmic side of the membrane, two electrons transfer from quinone A to loosely bound quinone B (100×10^{-9} sec), where they combine with two protons to make a high-energy **reduced quinone,** QH$_2$. In purple bacteria, these cytoplasmic protons are taken up through water-filled channels in the reaction center, contributing to the proton gradient.

QH$_2$ has a low affinity for the reaction center and diffuses in the hydrophobic core of the bilayer to the next component in the pathway, the chloroplast equivalent of the mitochondrial cytochrome bc$_1$ complex III. As in mitochondria, passage of energetic electrons through this complex releases protons from QH$_2$ on the periplasmic side of the membrane, adding to the electrochemical gradient. The electron circuit is completed by transfer of low-energy electrons from complex bc$_1$ to a soluble periplasmic protein, cytochrome c_2. Electrons then move to the cytochrome subunit of the reaction center, which supplies special pair chlorophylls with electrons for the photosynthetic reaction cycle.

The net result of this cycle is the conversion of the energy of two photons into transport of three protons out of the cell. A diagram of the energy levels of the various intermediates in the cycle (see Fig. 10–18B) shows how energy is partitioned after an electron is excited by a photon and then moves, step by step, through protein-associated redox centers back to the ground state.

The proton electrochemical gradient established by photosynthetic electron transfer reactions is used to drive an ATP synthase similar to those of nonphotosynthetic prokaryotes and mitochondria.

Light Harvesting

Reaction center chlorophylls absorb light themselves, but both chloroplasts and bacteria increase the efficiency of light collection with proteins that absorb light and transfer the energy to a reaction center. Most of these **light-harvesting complexes** are small, transmembrane proteins that cluster around a reaction center, although some bacteria and algae also have soluble light-harvesting proteins. Transmembrane, light-harvesting proteins consist of a few α-helices associated with multiple chlorophyll and carotenoid pigments (see Fig. 10–18C and Fig. 10–19B). The use of different pigments broadens the range of wavelengths absorbed. Multiple pigments increase the efficiency of photon capture. Leaves are green because chlorophylls and carotenoids absorb purple and blue wavelengths (<530 nm) as well as red wavelengths (>620 nm), reflecting only yellow-green wavelengths in between.

Light absorbed by light-harvesting proteins boosts pigment electrons to an excited state. This energy (but not the electrons) moves without dissipation by **fluorescence resonance energy transfer** from one closely spaced pigment molecule to another, and eventually to the special pair chlorophylls of a reaction center. This rapid (10^{-12} sec), efficient process transfers energy captured over a wide area to a reaction center to initiate a cycle of electron transfer and energy transduction.

Energy Capture and Transduction by Photosystem I

Green sulfur bacteria and heliobacteria have reaction centers similar to photosystem I of cyanobacteria and chloroplasts. Generation of a proton gradient by photosystem I has many parallels with photosystem II. Direct absorption of light or resonance energy transfer from surrounding light-harvesting complexes excites special pair chlorophylls in photosystem I (see Fig. 10–18C and D). Excited-state electrons move rapidly within the reaction center from these chlorophylls through two accessory chlorophylls and to an iron-sulfur center. The pathway includes a quinone in cyanobacteria and chloroplasts. Electrons then move to the iron-sulfur center of a subunit on the cytoplasmic side of the membrane. The subsequent events in green sulfur bacteria and heliobacteria are still under investigation but are thought to include electron transfer by the soluble protein ferridoxin to an NAD reductase, followed by transfer by a lipid intermediate to cytochrome bc complex, and then back to the reaction center via a cytochrome c.

Oxygen-Producing Synthesis of NADPH and ATP by Dual Photosystems

Chloroplasts and cyanobacteria combine photosystem II and photosystem I in the same membrane to form a system capable of accepting low-energy electrons from the oxidation of water and producing both a proton gradient to drive ATP synthesis and reducing equivalents in the form of NADPH (see Fig. 10–18E and F). Both photosystems are more elaborate in dual systems than in single systems. Although plant photosystem II, with more than 25 protein subunits, is much more complicated than the homologous reaction center of purple bacteria, the arrangement of transmembrane helices and chlorophyll cofactors in the core of the plant reaction center is similar to the simple reaction center of purple bacteria.

Photosynthesis begins when the special pair chlorophylls of photosystem II are excited by direct absorption of light or by resonance energy transfer from surrounding light-harvesting complexes (see Fig. 10–18E and F). Electrons come from splitting two waters into molecular oxygen and four protons. Excited-state electrons tunnel through the redox cofactors and combine with protons from the stroma (or cytoplasm in bacteria) to reduce quinone QB to QH_2, a high-energy electron donor. QH_2 diffuses to complex b_{6-f}, the chloroplast equivalent of the mitochondrial bc_1 complex. Passage of electrons through complex b_{6-f} releases protons from QH_2 into the thylakoid lumen (or bacterial periplasm), contributing to the proton gradient across the membrane.

Complex b_{6-f} donates electrons from QH_2 to photosystem I. Direct absorption of 680-nm light or resonance energy transfer from surrounding light-harvesting complexes boosts special pair chlorophyll electrons to a very high-energy, excited state (Fig. 10–18F). Excited-state electrons pass through chlorophyll and iron-sulfur centers of photosystem I to the iron-sulfur center of the redox protein, ferridoxin, on the cytoplasmic/stromal surface of the membrane. The enzyme NADP reductase combines electrons from ferridoxin with a proton to form NADPH, the final product of this tortuous electron transfer pathway powered at two way stations by absorption of photons. Uptake of stromal protons during NADPH formation contributes to the transmembrane proton gradient for the synthesis of ATP. Antiporters in the inner membrane exchange ATP for ADP, as in mitochondria.

Synthesis of Carbohydrates

ATP and NADPH produced by light reactions drive the unfavorable conversion of carbon dioxide into sugars. This is the first step in the earth's annual production of about 10^{10} tons of carbohydrates by photosynthetic organisms. This process is very expensive, consuming three ATPs and two NADPHs for each carbon dioxide added to the five-carbon sugar ribulose 1,5-bisphosphate. The responsible enzyme, **ribulose phosphate carboxylase** (called RUBISCO), is the most abundant protein in the stroma and may be the most abundant protein on earth. The products of combining the five-carbon sugar with carbon dioxide are two molecules of the three-carbon sugar, 3-phosphoglycerate.

An antiporter in the inner chloroplast membrane exchanges 3-phosphoglycerate for inorganic phosphate, so 3-phosphoglycerate can join the glycolytic pathway in the cytoplasm (see Fig. 10–15). Driven by this supply of 3-phosphoglycerate, the glycolytic pathway runs backward to make six-carbon sugars, which are used to make disaccharides such as sucrose to nourish nonphotosynthetic parts of the plant, the glucose polymer **starch** to store carbohydrate, and **cellulose** for the extracellular matrix.

Selected Readings

Allen JP, Williams JC: Photosynthetic reaction centers. FEBS Lett 438:5–9, 1998.

Bergles DE, Diamond JS, Jahr CE: Clearance of glutamate inside the synapse and beyond. Curr Opin Neurobiol 9:293–298, 1999.

Blankenship RE, Hartman H: The origin and evolution of oxygenic photosynthesis. Trends Biochem Sci 23:94–97, 1998.

Bliss TVP, Collingridge GL: A synaptic model of memory: Long-term potentiation in the hippocampus. Nature 361:31–39, 1993.

Bortolotto ZA, Fitzjohn SM, Collingridge GL: Roles of metabotropic glutamate receptors in LTP and LTD in the hippocampus. Curr Opin Neurobiol 9:299–304, 1999.

Deisenhofer J, Michel H: The photosynthetic reaction center from the purple bacterium *Rhodopseudomonas viridis*. Science 245:1463–1473, 1989.

Frey TG, Mannella CA: The internal structure of mitochondria. Trends Biochem Sci 25:319–324, 2000.

Gray MW, Burger G, Lang BF: Mitochondrial evolution. Science 283:1476–1481, 1999.

Katz AM: Physiology of the Heart, 2nd ed. New York: Raven Press, 1992.

Kim JH, Huganir RL: Organization and regulation of proteins at synapses. Curr Opin Cell Biol 11:248–254, 1999.

Lisman JE, Fallon JR: What maintains memories? Science 283:339–340, 1999.

Mannella CA, Marko M, Butte K: Reconsidering mitochondrial structure: New views of an old organelle. Trends Biochem Sci 22:37–38, 1997.

McGehee DS, Role LW: Memories of nicotine. Nature 383:670–671, 1996.

McManus ML, Churchwell KB, Strange K: Regulation of cell volume in health and disease. N Engl J Med 333:1260–1266, 1995.

Michel H, Behr J, Harrenga A, Kannt A: Cytochrome C oxidase: Structure and spectroscopy. Ann Rev Biophys Biomolec Struct 27:329–356, 1998.

Moser CC, Keske JM, Warncke K, et al: Nature of biological electron transfer. Nature 355:796–802, 1992.

Record MT, Courtenay ES, Cayley DS, Guttman HJ: Responses of *E. coli* to osmotic stress: Large changes in amounts of cytoplasmic solutes and water. Trends Biochem Sci 23:143–150, 1998.

Rhee K-H, Morris EP, Barber J, Kuhlbrandt W: Three-dimensional structure of the plant photosystem II reaction centre at 8Å resolution. Nature 396:283–286, 1998.

Saraste M: Oxidative phosphorylation at the *fin de siècle*. Science 283:1488–1493, 1999.

Scheffler IE: Mitochondria. New York: J. Wiley & Sons, 1999.

Schubert W-D, Klukas O, Krauss N, et al: Photosystem I of *Synechococcus elongatus* at 4Å resolution: Comprehensive structure analysis. J Molec Biol 272:741–769, 1997.

Severs NJ: The cardiac muscle cell. Bioessays 22:188–199, 2000.

Stevens CF: Strengths and weaknesses in memory. Nature 381:471–472, 1996.

Thompson SM: Synaptic plasticity: Building memories to last. Current Biol 10:R218–221, 2000.

Wallace DC: Mitochondrial diseases in man and mouse. Science 283:1482–1488, 1999.

STORAGE AND EXPRESSION OF GENETIC INFORMATION

chapter 11

INTRODUCTION TO NUCLEAR AND CHROMOSOMAL STRUCTURE AND FUNCTION

The nucleus is the intracellular compartment within which DNA replication and RNA transcription and processing occur. The presence of a discrete nuclear compartment constitutes a fundamental difference between eukaryotes and the prokaryotes, which have their DNA in a distinct region of cytoplasm that is not bounded by a membrane. This difference has a profound influence on cellular physiology. In the absence of a physical boundary between the DNA and the cytoplasm in prokaryotes, the processes of transcription and translation can be coupled directly, with ribosomes attaching to a nascent messenger RNA (mRNA) even before it is fully copied from the DNA template.

Eukaryotes evolved mechanisms to transport substances across the nuclear membrane to allow RNA transcription in the nucleus and its translation in cytoplasm. This intervening transport step provided an additional level of control in the regulation of gene expression and allowed the evolution of structurally complex genes.

Chapter 12 begins the discussion of the nucleus by considering the organization of the DNA into discrete **chromosomes,** each consisting of a single, long, DNA molecule (Fig. 11-1). Every species has a characteristic number of chromosomes that are visualized as separate entities only during cell division. For example, humans have 46 chromosomes that contain, in total, about 6.6×10^9 base pairs of DNA. Between 1996 and 2000, the sequences of the DNA molecules that comprise the genomes of several fungi, the nematode worm *Caenorhabditis elegans*, the fruit fly *Drosophila melanogaster*, the plant *Arabidopsis thaliana*, and humans were essentially completely determined. These sequences have revealed the distribution of the regions of DNA that encode proteins and RNAs, as well as extensive noncoding regions. Two specific DNA structures are essential for the maintenance of

chromosome integrity: **centromeres** and **telomeres.** Centromeres consist of DNA sequences which, together with their attendant proteins, regulate the segregation of chromosomes during cell division. Telomeres are specialized structures that protect the ends of chromosomes and permit complete replication of the chromosomal DNA.

Given the spacing of 3.4 Å per base pair in B-form DNA, each human cell contains more than 2 m of DNA packaged in a nucleus only 5 to 20×10^{-6} m in diameter! Thus, DNA must be extensively folded to fit it into a nucleus. Together, the DNA plus its packaging proteins are called **chromatin.** Chapter 13 considers the various levels of chromatin packaging. The most basic levels of this packaging (up to a 40-fold reduction in the length of the DNA fiber) are accomplished by interactions between the DNA and histone proteins to make nucleosomes and the 30-nm fiber. Higher levels of packaging of the chromatin fiber are not well understood. Current models propose that this higher-order packing occurs by folding the chromatin fiber into loop domains containing 60,000 to 100,000 base pairs of DNA. These models postulate that the base of each loop domain is defined by discrete DNA segments that interact with a protein skeleton of the nucleus (called the nuclear matrix, nucleoskeleton, or chromosome scaffold). Nuclei contain two broad classes of chromatin: **heterochromatin,** which is highly condensed throughout the cell cycle and is generally inactive in transcription, and **euchromatin,** which is less condensed and contains actively transcribed genes.

Chapter 14 discusses RNA transcription, the initial step in recovering the information encoded in the chromosomal DNA. Three cellular RNA polymerases have characteristic tasks: **polymerase I** transcribes ribosomal RNAs; **polymerase II** transcribes all mRNAs

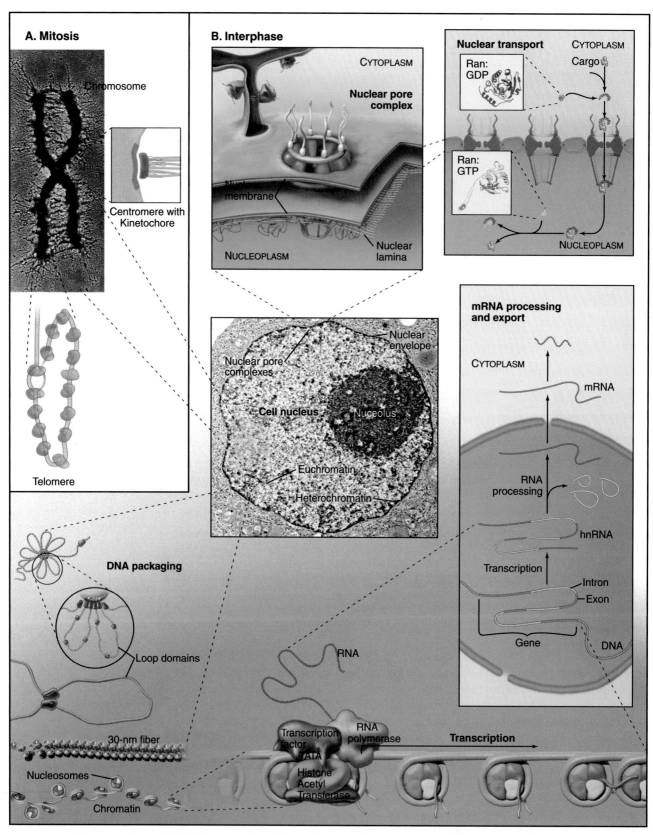

A. Mitosis

Chromosome

Centromere with Kinetochore

Telomere

B. Interphase

CYTOPLASM

Nuclear pore complex

Nuclear membrane

NUCLEOPLASM

Nuclear lamina

Nuclear transport

CYTOPLASM

Cargo

Ran: GDP

Ran: GTP

NUCLEOPLASM

Nuclear envelope

Nuclear pore complexes

Cell nucleus

Nuceolus

Euchromatin

Heterochromatin

DNA packaging

Loop domains

30-nm fiber

Nucleosomes

Chromatin

Transcription factor

RNA polymerase

Transcription

TATA

Histone Acetyl Transferase

RNA

mRNA processing and export

CYTOPLASM

mRNA

RNA processing

hnRNA

Transcription

Intron

Exon

Gene

DNA

Figure 11-1 Summary diagram highlighting a number of the topics covered in Chapters 12 to 16. *A*, Condensed mitotic chromosome, showing the two major structural specializations: the centromere, which regulates chromosome behavior in mitosis, and the telomere, which protects the ends of the chromosomal DNA molecules (Chapter 12). *B*, Major features of the structure and physiology of the interphase cell nucleus (shown in the thin section at the center). *Top center,* Structure of the nuclear envelope (Chapter 16). *Top right,* Movement of macromolecules between the nucleus and cytoplasm (Chapter 16). *Bottom,* Levels of packaging of the DNA fiber into chromatin and its transcription into RNA (Chapters 13 and 14). *Right middle,* Processing of RNA transcripts to yield mature RNAs (Chapter 15). GTP, guanine triphosphate; GDP, guanine diphosphate; hnRNA, heterogeneous nuclear RNA; TATA, DNA sequence in gene control region.

plus a number of small RNA molecules involved in RNA processing; and **polymerase III** transcribes transfer RNAs (tRNAs) and the smallest ribosomal RNAs. The discussion focuses on the ways in which these transcriptional processes are regulated in eukaryotic cells. Eukaryotic genes contain both upstream (5') and downstream (3') regulatory regions that are not transcribed into RNA. The region of the chromosome located just upstream from the start site of transcription is termed the **promoter.** Control regions that function from a distance to stimulate transcription are known as **enhancers.** These regulatory sequences form the binding sites for specific proteins that either stimulate or repress transcription. In addition, the chromatin organization of the DNA template and the location of specific sequences within the nucleus also influence the efficiency of transcription.

The initial products of transcription of most eukaryotic genes are extensively modified before they are suitable for export into the cytoplasm. Chapter 15 explains that this **RNA processing** is required, in part, because some regions of the initial RNA copy of a eukaryotic gene do not appear in the final mRNA; that is, genes are divided into coding (exon) and noncoding (intron) regions. Introns are removed before export of the mRNA from the nucleus. Other essential RNA-processing events include cleavage and polyadenylation of the 3' end of mRNA, the addition of 5' cap structures, and a host of sometimes bizarre editing events. Both the RNA substrates for these events and many enzymes that carry out the reactions are packaged into ribonucleoprotein (RNP) particles by specific proteins, but RNAs themselves may carry out a number of the enzymatic reactions.

The structure and physiology of the nucleus are discussed in Chapter 16. The boundary of the nucleus, known as the **nuclear envelope,** is composed of inner and outer nuclear membranes, separated by a perinuclear space that is continuous with the lumen of the endoplasmic reticulum. The inner nuclear membrane is closely associated with a protein layer called the **nuclear lamina.** This entire nuclear envelope is traversed by symmetrical annulate structures termed **nuclear pore complexes**. These pores are the site of transport between the nucleus and cytoplasm, with newly processed RNAs heading out to the cytoplasm and newly translated proteins wending their way into the nucleus. Macromolecules destined to traffic across the nuclear envelope typically contain within their sequences short regions, called **nuclear localization sequences** and **nuclear export sequences,** that bind to specific adapter and receptor proteins that transport them through the nuclear pore. The mechanism of this transport is now understood in detail, including the role of a small guanosine triphosphatase (GTPase) called **Ran** that regulates the direction of movement.

The nucleus contains a number of prominent substructures, the most prominent of which is the **nucleolus**. This is the site not only of ribosomal RNA (rRNA) transcription from a tandem array of ribosomal RNA genes, but also of processing and ribosome assembly. In addition to nucleoli, nuclei contain several other specialized regions. These are less well understood and have, in some cases, been identified solely on a morphologic basis. Factors associated with RNA processing are found in 300 to 500 discrete sites distributed throughout the nucleus, known as speckles. Nuclei also contain several other regions with distinctive substructures, including cajal bodies (formerly known as coiled bodies) and promyelocytic leukemia morphonuclear leukocyte (PML) nuclear bodies. Although their functions are not known, the presence of these and other specialized nuclear subdomains suggests that functional compartmentalization of the nucleus may contribute to regulation of nuclear functions.

Selected Readings

Adams MD, Celniker SE, Holt RA, et al: The genome sequence of *Drosophila melanogaster*. Science 287:2185–2195, 2000.

Chervitz SA, Aravind L, Sherlock G, et al: Comparison of the complete protein sets of worm and yeast: Orthology and divergence. Science 282:2022–2028, 1998.

Craig JM, Earnshaw WC, Vagnarelli P: Mammalian centromeres: DNA sequence, protein composition, and role in cell cycle progression. Exp Cell Res 246:249–262, 1999.

Kuo MH, Allis CD: Roles of histone acetyltransferases and deacetylases in gene regulation. Bioessays 20:615–626, 1998.

Lamond AI, Earnshaw WC: Structure and function in the nucleus. Science 280:547–553, 1998.

Lee TI, Young RA: Transcription of eukaryotic protein-coding genes. Annu Rev Genet 34:77–137, 2000.

Lewis JD, Tollervey D: Like attracts like: Getting RNA processing together in the nucleus. Science 288:1385–1389, 2000.

Mattaj IW, Englmeier L: Nucleocytoplasmic transport: The soluble phase. Annu Rev Biochem 67:265–306, 1998.

McEachern MJ, Krauskopf A, Blackburn EH: Telomeres and their control. Annu Rev Genet 34:331–358, 2000.

Ryan KJ, Wente SR: The nuclear pore complex: A protein machine bridging the nucleus and cytoplasm. Curr Opin Cell Biol 12:361–371, 2000.

Smit AF: The origin of interspersed repeats in the human genome. Curr Opin Genet Dev 6:743–748, 1996.

Vignali M, Hassan, AH, Neely KE, Workman JL: ATP-dependent chromatin-remodeling complexes. Mol Cell Biol 20:1899–1910, 2000.

chapter 12

CHROMOSOME ORGANIZATION

Chromosomes are enormous DNA molecules that can be propagated stably through countless generations of dividing cells (Fig. 12–1). Genes are the reason for the existence of the chromosomes, but in higher eukaryotes, they actually make up only a small fraction of the chromosomal DNA. Much of the DNA apparently serves no informational role and so is referred to as noncoding.

In addition to the genes, only three classes of specialized DNA sequences are needed to make a fully functional chromosome: (1) a centromere; (2) two telomeres; and (3) an origin of replication for approximately every 100,000 bp of DNA. Centromeres regulate the partitioning of chromosomes during mitosis and meiosis. Telomeres protect the ends of the chromosomal DNA molecules and ensure their complete replication. Origins of replication are discussed in Chapter 45. The structure of genes is considered in Chapter 14. Box 12–1 lists a number of key terms presented in this chapter.

Chromosome Morphology and Nomenclature

Chromosomes from somatic cells of higher eukaryotes are only visualized directly during mitosis. Each mitotic chromosome consists of two **sister chromatids** that are held together at a waist-like constriction called the **centromere**. The portions of the chromosomes that are not in the centromere itself are called "chromosomal arms" (Fig. 12–2).

One DNA Molecule per Chromosome

Each eukaryotic chromosome contains one DNA molecule that stretches from one end (**telomere**) to the other. In organisms with small chromosomes, including budding yeast, the intact chromosomal DNA may be resolved by pulsed-field gel electrophoresis into a characteristic series of bands (Fig. 12–3). This method permits the visualization of intact chromosomal DNA up to the size of the largest chromosome of the fission yeast (5.5 million base pairs). However, even the smallest human chromosome, which is about 40 million base pairs long, is too large to resolve by this technique.

The Organization of Genes on Chromosomes

Since the mid 1970s, much effort world-wide has been devoted to determining the complete sequences of the chromosomes of a wide variety of organisms (see Fig. 1–1), ranging from simple viruses to humans. One major goal of this effort—the complete sequence of the gene-rich portions of the human genome—has been completed in draft form and is expected to be finished by 2003. Together, sequencing efforts completed to date have already generated an enormous bank of data on the genetic composition of simple and complex organisms.

The complex genomes sequenced range in size from 1,042,519 base pairs for the intracellular parasite *Chlamydia trachomatis* to 120 million base pairs for the fruit fly *Drosophila melanogaster*. These genomes contain anywhere from 834 predicted genes (for the intracellular parasite *Rickettsia prowazekii*) to 18,266 predicted genes (for the nematode worm *Caenorhabditis elegans*) to 30,000 to 40,000 genes for humans. However, because gene prediction algorithms are still being developed, only rough estimates of gene number are available, even for completely sequenced genomes. As a rule of thumb, the bacterial genomes tend to make very efficient use of space, with about 90% of the genome being devoted to coding sequences. The re-

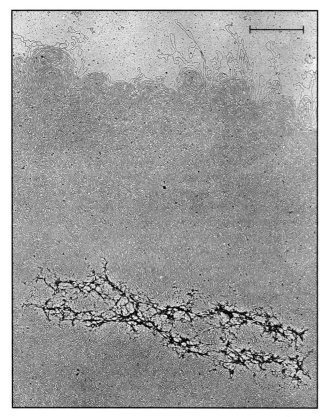

Figure 12-1 Electron micrograph of a chromosome from which most proteins were extracted, allowing DNA *(thin lines)* to spread out from the residual scaffold. Enormous amounts of DNA are packaged in each chromosome; this image shows less than 30% of the DNA of this chromosome. (From Paulson JR, Laemmli UK: The structure of histone-depleted chromosomes. Cell 12:817, 1977. Copyright 1977, with permission from Elsevier Science.)

maining 10% is mostly taken up by sequences involved in gene regulation. One notable exception to this is *R. prowazekii*, for which only 76% of the genome is thought to be devoted to coding sequences. The likely explanation for this is that this intracellular parasite is still in the process of shedding unneeded genes (it derives many of its metabolic functions from the host cell). Thus, much of the noncoding DNA may be remnants of unneeded genes undergoing various stages of gradual degradation and loss.

The first eukaryotic genome to be sequenced was the budding yeast *Saccharomyces cerevisiae*. The 12 million base pair genome of this organism is subdivided into 16 chromosomes ranging in size from 230,000 to more than 1 million base pairs (see Fig. 12–3). The genome contains about 6200 predicted genes, of which at least 4665 have been shown to be transcribed into RNA. About 75% of the budding yeast genome is found in coding sequences, with the remainder in regulatory regions, repeated DNAs, and intervening sequences (introns) (Fig. 12–4). Introns, which are removed by a sophisticated splicing mechanism (see Chapter 15), are present in about 5% of the

genes. Large-scale analysis of the budding yeast DNA sequence reveals the existence of periodic fluctuations in relative content of G + C base pairs, and also in gene density. A similar fluctuation has been postulated to explain the banding structure of chromosomes from higher eukaryotes (see Chapter 13).

The first sequence of the genome of a multicellular eukaryote (*C. elegans*) revealed a number of important organizational differences from the budding yeast. First, although the genome is eight times larger (97 million base pairs distributed in six chromosomes), the nematode has only about three times more genes than the budding yeast. This means that only about 27% of the genome is occupied by coding regions. An almost identical percentage is occupied by introns, which occur at an average of about five per gene. The function of the remainder of the genome is not known, although some of the sequences are likely to be involved in gene regulation. As might be expected for a multicellular organism, worms contain many genes that are not seen in the single-celled yeast. These include molecules involved in cell-cell signaling, such as nuclear hormone receptors, cell-cell adhesion molecules, and components involved in the programmed cell death pathway.

The second genome sequence of a multicellular

---

box 12–1

KEY TERMS

Chromatin: DNA plus the proteins that package it within the cell nucleus

Chromosome: A DNA molecule with its attendant proteins that moves as an independent unit during mitosis and meiosis. Before DNA replication, each chromosome consists of a single DNA molecule plus proteins and is called a *chromatid*. After replication, each chromosome consists of two identical DNA molecules plus proteins. These are called *sister chromatids*. Chromosomal DNA molecules are usually linear but can be circular in organelles, bacteria, and viruses.

Centromere: The chromosomal locus that regulates the movements of the chromosomes during mitosis and meiosis. The centromere is defined by specific DNA sequences plus proteins that bind to them. In higher eukaryotes, the centromere of mitotic chromosomes can be visualized as a constricted region where sister chromatids are held together most closely.

Kinetochore: The centromeric substructure that binds microtubules and directs the movements of chromosomes in mitosis

Telomere: The specialized structure at either end of the chromosomal DNA molecule that ensures the complete replication of the chromosomal ends and protects the ends within the cell

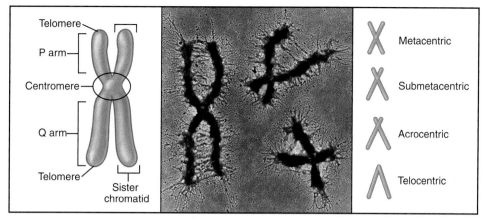

Figure 12-2 Anatomy of mitotic chromosomes from higher eukaryotes. *Left,* The principal structural features of chromosomes. *Center,* An electron micrograph of human mitotic chromosomes. *Right,* A diagram of the various classes of chromosomes. At mitosis, chromosomes of higher eukaryotes consist of sister chromatids held together at the centromeric region. Chromosomes are classified based upon the position of the centromere relative to the arms. In *metacentric* chromosomes, the centromere is located midway along the chromatid. In *submetacentric* chromosomes, the centromere is located asymmetrically so that each chromatid can be divided into short (**P**) and long (**Q**) arms. In *acrocentric* chromosomes, the centromere is located near the end of the arms. In *telocentric* chromosomes, the centromere appears to be located very near the end of the chromatid.

eukaryote (*D. melanogaster*) showed important differences from the worm sequence. Most surprisingly, the fly, despite its more complex body plan and life cycle, has about one-third fewer genes than the worm, and only about twice as many as the budding yeast. As a result, only about 13% of the *Drosophila* genome is occupied by DNA that codes for proteins. About half of the fly genes identified to date appear to be related to proteins found in the human genome, and of 289 genes presently associated with human diseases, 177 have clearly recognized homologues in the fly. This underscores the usefulness of the fly, with its powerful genetics, as a model organism for the study of human disease.

Figure 12-3 Pulsed-field gel electrophoresis of budding yeast chromosomes. Intact cells embedded in a block of agarose are treated under very gentle conditions with proteases and detergents to free the chromosomal DNA from other cellular constituents. The DNA is then moved under the influence of an electrical field out of the agarose block and directly into an agarose gel. The technique uses a specialized gel apparatus in which the direction and strength of the electrophoretic field is varied periodically. This technique permits the separation of very long DNA molecules (of up to several million base pairs). (Courtesy of P. Hieter, University of Vancouver.)

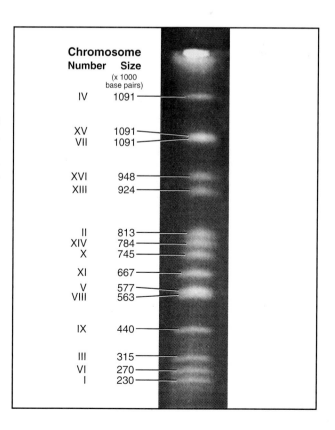

Chromosome Number	Size (x 1000 base pairs)
IV	1091
XV	1091
VII	1091
XVI	948
XIII	924
II	813
XIV	784
X	745
XI	667
V	577
VIII	563
IX	440
III	315
VI	270
I	230

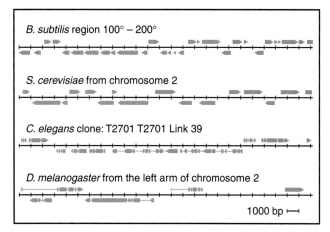

B. subtilis region 100° – 200°

S. cerevisiae from chromosome 2

C. elegans clone: T2701 T2701 Link 39

D. melanogaster from the left arm of chromosome 2

1000 bp ⊢—⊣

Figure 12-4 Comparison of the sequence organization of a typical bacterium *(B. subtilis)*, the budding yeast *S. cerevisiae*, the nematode worm *C. elegans*, and the fruit fly *D. melanogaster*. Each line shows a comparison of the gene densities over a 25,000-bp region of the chromosome, chosen at random. Regions of genes encoding a product are shown as thick orange arrows.

The draft sequence of the human genome, published early in 2001, showed a further tendency for genes to occupy an ever-decreasing percentage of the DNA. Humans apparently have far fewer genes than predicted: about 35,000 as opposed to recent predictions of up to 100,000 (Table 12–1). These genes occupy only about 5% of the chromosomes. In contrast, ancient repeated-sequence elements appear to occupy about 50% of the genome, as discussed in a later section. To put this all in perspective, every million base pairs of DNA sequenced yielded 483 genes in *S. cerevisiae*, 197 genes in *C. elegans*, 117 genes in *D. melanogaster*, and only 12 to 15 genes in humans. As is the case for all complex eukaryotes, human genes are broken up into regions that appear in mature RNA molecules (exons) and regions that are removed by splicing (introns) (see Chapter 15). The average human protein-coding gene is 28,000 base pairs long and has 8 exons that average only 145 base pairs separated by introns averaging a bit over 3,000 base pairs in length. It is therefore not surprising that the identification of genes in genomic DNA sequence is a complex art that is still in its infancy and that current estimates of human gene numbers are very error prone.

The first two human chromosomes to be sequenced "completely" (excluding regions containing large amounts of repetitive DNA, such as centromeres) were numbers 21 and 22. On chromosome 22, prediction programs revealed the presence of 545 genes in the 33.4×10^6 base pairs sequenced, whereas on chromosome 21, the predictions revealed the presence of only 225 genes spread over the 33.8×10^6 base pairs. This relatively small number of genes may explain, in part, why humans with three copies of chromosome 21 are viable (Down syndrome), whereas those with three copies of chromosome 22 are not. How can there be so few genes on such large chromosomes? On chromosome 21, one region of 7 Mb (which is almost twice the size of the entire *E. coli* chromosome) has no identified genes.

Noncoding DNA in Eukaryotic Genomes

Eukaryotic genomes range in size from 1.2×10^7 base pairs in a budding yeast to 5×10^{10} base pairs in some amphibians (see Table 12–1). Organisms with large genomes contain more genes than organisms with smaller genomes, but they also contain large amounts of noncoding DNA. The function, if any, of this noncoding DNA remains an important unsolved question.

table 12–1
AMOUNTS OF DNA IN VARIOUS GENOMES

Organism	Haploid Genome Size (bp)	Predicted Number of Protein-Coding Genes
Rickettsia prowazekii (endoparasitic bacterium)	1,111,523	834
Escherichia coli (free-living bacterium)	4,639,221	4288
Bacillus subtilis (free-living bacterium)	4,214,810	4100
Saccharomyces cerevisiae (budding yeast)	12,052,000	6144
Caenorhabditis elegans (nematode worm)	9.7×10^7	18,266
Drosophila melanogaster (fruit fly)	1.4×10^8	13,338
Mus musculus (house mouse)	2.7×10^9	?
Xenopus laevis (South African clawed frog)	3.1×10^9	?
Homo sapiens (human)	3.3×10^9	~35,000
Triturus cristatus (salamander)	2.2×10^{10}	?

Interspersed Families of Repetitive DNA

Eukaryotic genomes contain large amounts of **repetitive DNA** sequences that are present in many copies (thousands, in some cases). By contrast, coding regions of genes (which are typically present in a single copy per haploid nucleus) are referred to as **unique-sequence DNA**.

Repetitive DNA shows two patterns of distribution in the chromosomes. **Satellite DNAs** are clustered in discrete areas, such as the centromeres. Other types of repetitive DNA are dispersed throughout the genome. In humans, the bulk of this dispersed repetitive DNA is composed of **SINES** (*s*hort *in*terspersed repeated *s*equences) and **LINES** (*l*ong *in*terspersed repeated *s*equences).

SINES and LINES, plus other similar DNA families, account for up to 45% of the human genome. The Alu class of SINES, with a consensus sequence of about 300 bp, constitutes about 13% of the total DNA. (A consensus sequence is the average arrived at by comparing a number of different sequenced DNA clones.) LINES, with a consensus sequence of 6 to 8 kb, make up about 20% of the genome. Interestingly, SINES and LINES have quite different distributions along the chromosomes. LINES are concentrated in gene-poor regions of the chromosomes with a relatively higher content of A:T base pairs. In contrast, the Alu SINES are concentrated in gene-rich regions with a relatively higher content of G:C base pairs.

Both LINES and SINES show similarities to mobile genetic elements termed **retroposons** that move (transpose) from one place in the DNA to another through production of an RNA intermediate. Upon completion of a transposition event, the original retroposon remains in its original chromosomal location, whereas the newly generated element (which may be either full-length or partial) is inserted at a new site in the genome.

Most LINE and SINE elements in the genome appear to be nonfunctional. Either they represent only partial copies of the progenitor element, or they have accumulated mutations that prevent them from encoding functional proteins. It is thought that, over time, mutations accumulate to such an extent that the LINE or SINE is no longer recognizable by its sequence, and it sinks into the background of anonymous noncoding DNA. The physiological role, if any, of these elements is as yet unknown. One possibility is that they do not do anything advantageous and are analogous to an infection of the DNA that is tolerated as long as it does not move into genes that are essential for life. This is called the "**selfish DNA**" hypothesis. Although unlikely, these elements could conceivably have im-portant functions that simply have not yet been identified.

The Centromere: Overview

The **centromere** is at the heart of all chromosomal movements in mitosis and meiosis, as it is the region where the chromosome becomes attached to the spindle (the microtubule-based apparatus upon which chromosomes move; see Chapter 47). The centromere also has an important role in monitoring the attachment of the chromosomes to the mitotic spindle and controlling the progress of cells through mitosis. The centromere is a nucleoprotein structure, and both DNA and proteins are essential to its function.

In chromosomes of higher eukaryotes, the centromere may be visualized directly as a waist-like stricture or **primary constriction** where the two sister chromatids are most intimately paired. Several abundant families of repetitive DNAs are concentrated in the centromeres of human chromosomes. The chromatin of centromeres is entirely composed of **constitutive heterochromatin**, a special type of chromatin that is not transcribed and that remains condensed throughout the cell cycle. (For a discussion of heterochromatin, see Chapter 13.)

Embedded in the surface of the centromeric heterochromatin is a button-like structure called the **kinetochore**, the function of which is to direct chromosomal movements in mitosis (Fig. 12–5). When a thin section of the centromere is examined by electron microscopy, the kinetochore appears to have up to

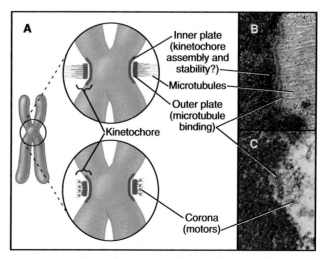

Figure 12–5 Kinetochore structure. *A*, A diagram of the major layers of the kinetochore. *B*, Thin-section electron micrograph of a kinetochore with attached microtubules. *C*, Thin-section micrograph of an unattached kinetochore (*B*, Courtesy of J. B. Rattner, University of Calgary.)

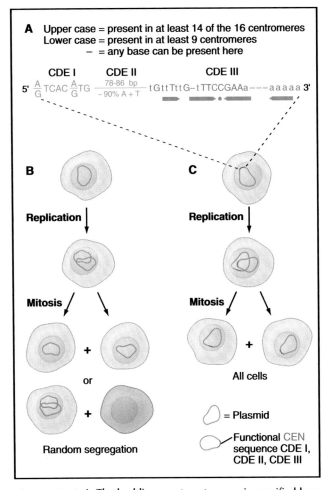

A Upper case = present in at least 14 of the 16 centromeres
     Lower case = present in at least 9 centromeres
          – = any base can be present here

Figure 12-6 *A,* The budding yeast centromere is specified by a 125-bp sequence, with three conserved DNA elements (CDE I to CDE III). CDE I and CDE III bind proteins in a sequence-specific manner. CDE III has mirror symmetry: a central C (*dot*) is flanked by two regions of complementary DNA sequence (*arrows*). All that seems to be important about CDE II is its abundance of A and T nucleotides and its overall length. *B* and *C,* The assay for mitotic stability of a plasmid used to clone CEN DNA from most budding yeast chromosomes. The plasmid carries a gene encoding an enzyme involved in adenine metabolism. When the plasmid is present, colonies are white. If the plasmid is lost, the colonies become red as a result of the accumulation of a byproduct of adenine metabolism. If the plasmid is capable of replication but lacks a centromere, the colonies will be mostly red, reflecting the inefficient segregation of the plasmid at mitosis *(B)*. If the plasmid carries a functional centromere, the colonies will be white, as the plasmid will be successfully transmitted at nearly every division *(C)*.

four layers. An innermost dense **inner plate** is continuous with the surface of the centromeric heterochromatin. This structure contains appreciable amounts of DNA. A protein-rich **outer plate** is separated from the inner plate by a narrow **unstained area**, which comprises the third layer of the kinetochore. These three layers are all that is seen of the kinetochore when chromosomes have attached microtubules. However, in kinetochores that are free of microtubules, a fourth

layer, the **fibrous corona**, is seen to radiate outward from the outer plate. The fibrous corona is the location of microtubule motor proteins (see Chapter 37) that move chromosomes during mitosis.

The multilayered kinetochore structure is only visible during mitosis. During interphase, the centromere persists as a condensed ball of heterochromatin, indistinguishable from other areas of condensed chromatin within the nucleus. The distinct kinetochore structure forms on the surface of the centromere during the stage of mitosis called prophase (see Chapter 47), reaching its mature state following nuclear envelope breakdown when the chromosome comes in contact with microtubules at the onset of mitotic prometaphase.

Variations in Centromere Organization Among Species

Each chromosome has particular DNA sequences, called **CEN** sequences, that specify protein-binding sites required for assembly of the kinetochore. CEN sequences are autonomous; if inserted into circular DNA molecules (plasmids), they can render them capable of interacting with the mitotic spindle and segregating during mitosis (Fig. 12–6). The best understood CEN sequences come from the budding yeast *S. cerevisiae* and the fission yeast *Schizosaccharomyces pombe.* Surprisingly, these two distantly related yeasts have evolved extremely different solutions to the organization of CEN sequences.

CEN sequences from all 16 chromosomes of budding yeast have a common organization based around three conserved sequence elements. These are designated (in the 5′ to 3′ direction) **CDE I** (*c*entromere *D*NA *e*lement I, 8 bp), **CDE II** (78 to 86 bp), and **CDE III** (25 bp). This organization is diagrammed in Figure 12–6. A 125-bp region spanning CDE I to CDE III is sufficient to direct the efficient segregation of the yeast chromosomes, which can reach a size of more than 1 million base pairs.

Even though the three chromosomes of *S. pombe* chromosomes are only 1.8- to 13-fold larger (3.5 to 5 million base pairs) than their counterparts in *S. cerevisiae,* the centromeres of fission yeast are 300- to 600-fold larger (Fig. 12–7). The smallest *S. pombe* centromere is 35,000 base pairs across, whereas the largest spans 110,000 base pairs. Fission yeast centromeres are also much more complex than their counterparts from budding yeast. The former each contain a central core of unique-sequence DNA that is 4 to 7 kb long, flanked by complex arrays of repeated sequences. In general, genes that are inserted into the *S. pombe* centromere undergo transcriptional repression, a feature also commonly observed with centromeres of higher eukaryotes, including mammals. This repression of gene expression seems to correlate with centromere function: a number of mutants that reduce the repression of inserted genes also impair centromere function. This suggests that fission yeast centromeres must occur in a particular chromatin environment to function as kinetochores.

Studies of *S. pombe* centromeres have revealed an additional level in the regulation of centromere function. *S. pombe* centromeric DNA apparently must undergo an **epigenetic** activation event to function as a centromere. Epigenetic events are inheritable properties of chromosomes that cannot be explained by changes in the nucleotide sequence. They are thought to be explained either by enzymatic modification of the DNA (e.g., methylation of cytosine), or by stable association of proteins with the DNA. There is increasing evidence that epigenetic mechanisms play an essential role in the assembly of centromeres in higher eukaryotes, including humans.

The best characterized, naturally occurring centromeric DNA for any metazoan comes from the fruit fly *D. melanogaster*. Studies in which the fly's X chromosome has been fragmented into ever-smaller pieces have revealed that this centromere is contained within a stretch of roughly 420,000 base pairs. This is mostly composed of simple-sequence satellite DNAs, but several "islands" of more complex DNA are interspersed throughout the region. These islands are rich in repeats and transposable DNA elements. No sequences have been found that look like the yeast centromeres, and, in fact, no sequences have been found in this region that are unique to the fly centromeres: all sequences found so far at centromeres can also be found on the chromosome arms. Thus, it appears that something other than the simple DNA sequence may be responsible for conferring centromere activity on this region of the chromosome. This conclusion is supported by the observation that an adjacent region of the X chromosome that is not normally part of the centromere can, under certain circumstances, acquire centromere function. This has been interpreted as supporting epigenetic models for centromere function.

Mammalian Centromere DNA

CEN DNA, as defined by the functional criteria outlined in Figure 12–6, has not yet been identified from any vertebrate. This may be primarily attributable to the large size and complex organization of the vertebrate centromere. For example, the centromere of chromosome 21 (the smallest human chromosome at ≈ 40 million base pairs) has been estimated to encompass >5 million base pairs. This entire region appears to be composed of highly repeated satellite DNA sequences.

Satellite DNA is composed of many thousands of copies of short DNA sequences that are clustered together in "head-to-tail" arrays in various regions of the chromosome (Fig. 12–8). The principal satellite DNAs of mouse and man are concentrated primarily (but not exclusively) in the centromeric regions of the chromosomes.

The major human centromeric satellite DNA, **α-satellite**, is a complex family of repeated sequences that constitute approximately 5% of the genome. Monomers 171 base pairs long are organized into higher-order repeats (Fig. 12–9). Some of the monomers have a conserved 17-bp sequence (the "CENP-B box"), which forms the binding site for a centromeric protein called CENP-B (see later section). The organization of higher-order repeats varies greatly from chromosome to chromosome, and more than 30 distinct repeats, comprising 2 to 32 monomers, have been described. Each chromosome has one or a few types of higher-order repeats of α-satellite DNA.

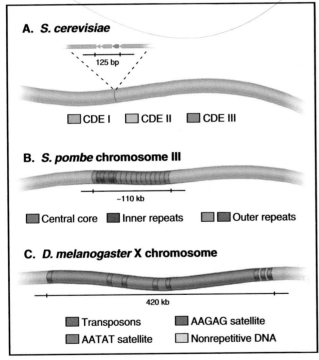

Figure 12–7 Organization of the centromeric DNAs of budding yeast, fission yeast, and fruit fly. *A,* The budding yeast **point centromere** is specified by a 125-bp sequence. *B,* The fission yeast **regional centromeres** all contain central core DNA flanked by complex arrays of repeated sequences. Embedded within these repeated sequences are a number of genes encoding transfer RNAs, not shown here. The minimum region required to construct a functional centromere in fission yeast artificial chromosomes is about 10 kb in length and includes the central core DNA plus a portion of the flanking repeated DNA. *C,* The fruit fly also has a regional centromere encompassing 420 kb. This is rich in satellite DNA and contains a number of transposable elements. Interestingly, both the satellite DNAs and transposons are also found at other, noncentromeric, regions of the chromosomes.

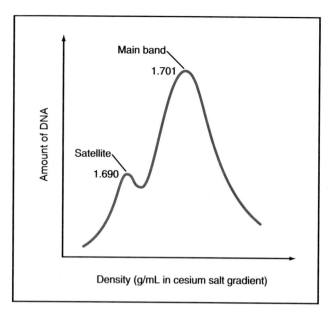

Figure 12–8 Identification of mouse satellite DNA by buoyant density centrifugation. Cellular DNA was sheared into small fragments and centrifuged at high speed in a density gradient formed from concentrated cesium salts. In this density equilibrium protocol, each piece of DNA stops moving in the density gradient when its density matches that of the cesium solution. The density at which the DNA forms a band is determined by its content of G:C and A:T base pairs. When fragments of mouse DNA are centrifuged to equilibrium on such gradients, it is found to be distributed in two peaks: a major broad peak and a distinct "satellite" peak. The "satellite" peak contains a homogeneous population of a highly repeated DNA sequence referred to as the major satellite. This is located at the centromeres of mouse chromosomes.

The entire centromeric region of certain chromosomes may be composed of α-satellite monomers, with little or no interspersed DNA of other types. The amount of α-satellite DNA at different centromeres varies widely: from as little as 300,000 base pairs on the Y chromosome to up to 5 million base pairs on chromosome 7. In addition, the α-satellite DNA content of a given chromosome can vary by more than a million base pairs in different individuals. Thus, whatever the function of α-satellite DNA may be, clearly, a wide variation in local organization is tolerated.

Human chromosomes also contain several other families of satellite DNA. Classical satellites I to IV, which together constitute 2% to 5% of the genome, are composed of divergent repeats of the sequence GGAAT. These satellites occur in blocks more than 20,000 base pairs long that are immediately adjacent to the centromeres of chromosomes 1, 9, and 16 and that may be found at much lower levels near most centromeres. The region adjacent to the centromere of chromosome 9 apparently contains 7 to 10 million base pairs of satellite III sequence. The long arm of the Y chromosome also contains huge amounts of satellite III DNA (up to 40% of its total DNA).

What is the human equivalent of yeast CEN DNA? The best candidate thus far is α-satellite, which occurs at all natural centromeres. In support of this idea, it has been observed that α-satellite DNA arrays introduced into cells can occasionally form tiny minichromosomes with functional centromeres. However, these mammalian artificial chromosomes, even though much smaller than natural chromosomes, are very much larger than the input DNA molecules and have proven difficult to characterize in molecular detail. Thus, the exact composition of their centromeric DNA is not yet determined.

Contrary to the idea that humans have a defined CEN DNA like budding yeast, noncentromeric DNA can acquire the ability to act as a centromere in some individuals. Very rarely in such individuals, a partial chromosome functions normally in mitosis, despite the fact that the normal centromere has been lost. Such chromosomes have acquired a new centromere or **neocentromere** in a new location on one of the chromosome arms. One neocentromere has apparently been cloned and sequenced in its entirety and has been shown to be composed of the normal DNA that exists at that location on the arm of chromosome 10.

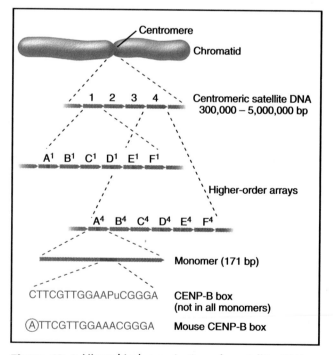

Figure 12–9 Hierarchical organization of α-satellite DNA at human centromeres. The numbers (1 to 4) indicate higher-order repeats of α-satellite DNA. These may contain from 2 to 32 monomers (indicated by A[1], B[1], etc.). DNA sequences of adjacent monomers within a repeat (A[1], B[1], C[1], for example) may differ by as much as 40% from one another. DNA sequences of monomers occupying identical positions within the higher-order repeats (A[1], A[4], etc.) are nearly 99% identical to one another. The red box (sequence shown at the bottom) represents the binding site for centromeric protein CENP-B.

This strongly supports models in which the centromere is specified by epigenetic markers, rather than the exact DNA sequence per se. It could be that the linkage observed between α-satellite DNA and centromeres actually reflects a propensity of α-satellite DNA to acquire the epigenetic mark, rather than a sequence-specific mechanism as occurs in *S. cerevisiae*.

Centromere Proteins of the Budding Yeast

Many functions of centromeres are accomplished as a result of the binding of specialized proteins to the CEN DNA sequences. In all, over 30 kinetochore-associated proteins are now known in the budding yeast. The best characterized factors that bind to CEN DNA in the budding yeast include CBF 1 and 3 (*c*entromere-*b*inding *f*actor binding to CDE I or CDE III), Mif2P, and Cse4p (Fig. 12–10).

CBF 1 is a protein with a molecular weight of 39,000 that is homologous to the helix-loop-helix family of DNA-binding proteins (see Chapter 14). When the gene for CBF 1 is disrupted, cells are viable, but the rate of chromosome loss during mitosis increases by about 10-fold. Thus, the interaction of CBF 1 with CDE I is not essential for chromosome partitioning in mitosis but does increase the fidelity of the process.

Two proteins, termed Mif2P and Cse4p, bind to CDE II. The function of Mif2p is not known; however, Cse4p is a specialized histone H3. Current evidence suggests that the core of the yeast kinetochore is a specialized nucleosome involving Cse4p. (Nucleosomes are described in further detail in Chapter 13).

CBF 3 binding to CDE III is essential for centromere function, as single base-pair changes in CDE III that block CBF 3 binding can lower chromosome transmission fidelity by a factor of 10^5. **CBF 3** consists of four subunits of 110, 64, 58, and 23 kD (see Fig. 12–10). All of the genes encoding these polypeptides are essential for the life of the cell.

CBF 3 is required for the binding of microtubules to the yeast centromere. The three largest subunits of CBF 3 apparently make up the core of the yeast kinetochore, possibly with p64 making the primary contact with CDE III DNA. In vivo, p58 appears to be essential for regulation of kinetochore assembly. The kinetochore can only assemble if p58 is phosphorylated, and recruitment of the p58 kinase appears to be the essential role of p23. In addition, a complex containing p23 appears to mediate the destruction of p58 via the ubiquitin/proteasome pathway. Thus, regulation of p58 levels may be an important aspect of kinetochore assembly. Neither the centromere components that interact with microtubules nor the motor proteins that move the chromosomes during mitosis have yet been identified conclusively.

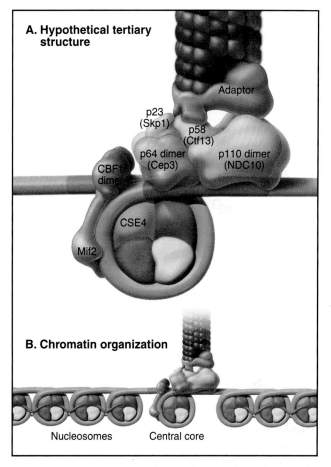

Figure 12–10 *A,* Artist's rendering of a hypothetical model for the organization of the budding yeast kinetochore. CDE II *(orange)* corresponds to roughly one turn of DNA around a nucleosome (see Chapter 13). This means that CDE I *(blue)* and CDE III *(red)* may be located next to one another, so that CBF 1 and CBF 3 may interact with one another. The proteins that bind to these DNA sequences are discussed in the text. *B,* The region of DNA containing CDE I to III is packaged in a specialized chromatin structure flanked by an ordered array of nucleosomes (see Chapter 13).

Mammalian Centromere Proteins

Several proteins located at the human centromere have now been characterized. These proteins, designated CENPs (*cen*tromere *p*roteins), are recognized by autoantibodies present in the sera of certain individuals with rheumatic diseases (Figs. 12–11 and 12–12).

CENP-A (MW = 17,000), like yeast Cse4p, is a special variant subtype of histone H3 (see Chapter 13). CENP-A appears to be involved in establishment of a specialized nucleosomal structure in the inner kinetochore plate. CENP-A is essential for life and is required for CENP-C to target to the kinetochore.

CENP-B (MW = 65,000) is distributed throughout the centromeric heterochromatin beneath the kinetochore plate. CENP-B binds specifically to a 17-bp sequence (the CENP-B box) in α-satellite DNA (see Fig.

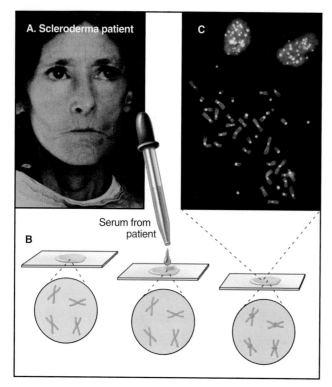

Figure 12–11 Some patients with scleroderma have autoantibodies recognizing centromeric proteins. Scleroderma ("hard skin") is a serious connective tissue disease associated with excessive deposition of collagen in the skin and walls of blood vessels. Note the "purse string" appearance of the skin surrounding the mouth of this patient (A). When serum from a patient with anticentromere antibodies is added to chromosomes on a slide (B) and bound antibodies are detected with a fluorescent probe, the centromeric regions of the chromosomes "light up" (C). Anticentromere antibodies are useful to identify patients at risk for serious autoimmune disease. Up to 20% of the population has a mild condition, Raynaud's phenomenon (hypersensitivity of the skin to cold), that is occasionally a precursor to scleroderma. Sensitive assays for anticentromere antibodies revealed that patients with Raynaud's phenomenon plus these autoantibodies have increased risk of progression to scleroderma. (A, Reprinted from the Clinical Slide Collection on the Rheumatic Diseases, copyright 1991, 1995, 1997. Used by permission of the American College of Rheumatology.)

12–9). The consequences of this binding are not known, but the protein may play a role in establishing the overall structure of the centromeric heterochromatin. Disruption of the mouse gene for CENP-B has revealed that the protein is not essential for centromere function or chromosome segregation.

CENP-C (MW = 107,000) is a DNA-binding protein concentrated in the inner kinetochore plate that is essential for kinetochore assembly. CENP-C shares several limited regions of protein similarity to budding yeast Mif2p. CENP-C is involved in the assembly and function of the kinetochore. CENP-C is only present at centromeres that actually function in spindle attachment in mitosis (Fig. 12–13). Genetic knockout exper-

iments have revealed that the CENP-C gene is essential for life, and that microinjection of antibodies recognizing CENP-C into cells causes the cells to become arrested in mitosis. These injected cells have chromosomes with aberrant kinetochore structures that are either abnormally small or lack the characteristic multilayered structure altogether.

The Ends of the Chromosomes: Why Specialized Telomeres Are Needed

The ends of chromosomal DNA molecules pose at least two problems that cells solve by packaging the chromosome ends into specialized structures called **telomeres.** First, it is essential that cells distinguish the ends of a chromosome from breaks in DNA. When cells detect DNA breaks, they stop their progression through the cell cycle and repair the breaks by joining the ends together (see Chapter 46). Telomeres keep normal chromosome ends from inducing cell cycle arrest and from being joined to other DNA ends by the repair machinery. Second, telomeres permit the chromosomal DNA to be replicated out to the very end (see later discussion).

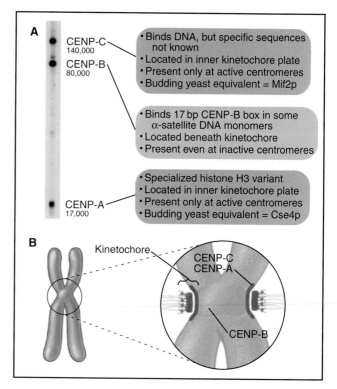

Figure 12–12 Human CENP autoantigens. *A*, Centromere proteins detected with anticentromere antibodies from a scleroderma patient on an immunoblot following SDS gel electrophoresis of chromosomal proteins. *B*, Drawing of the localization of centromere proteins at the kinetochore.

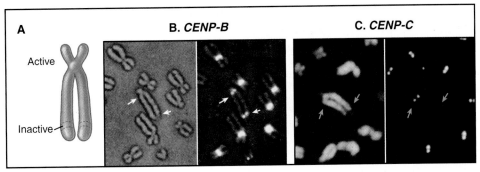

Figure 12-13 Demonstration that the CENP-C protein is only found at functional centromeres. An unusual chromosome was discovered during prenatal screening of a fetus that sonography had indicated to be abnormal. This chromosome consisted of two copies of the maternal chromosome 13 linked end to end. It thus contained two centromeres, and so was termed dicentric. Such dicentric chromosomes are normally very unstable during mitosis, as the two centromeres on one chromatid often become attached to opposite spindle poles. This causes the chromosome to be stretched and ultimately break. In the case of this particular dicentric chromosome, one of the centromeres has somehow become inactivated (it may have lost its epigenetic mark). This chromosome thus behaves perfectly normally in mitosis. When the distribution of centromere proteins at the active and inactive centromeres was compared, it was found that CENP-B was present at both, but that CENP-C was only present at the active centromere. *A*, Organization of the dicentric chromosome. *B*, Phase-contrast view of chromosomes from the amniocytes *(left)*. Phase-contrast view taken with superimposed antibody staining for CENP-B *(right)*. *C*, DNA stain of a different chromosome spread *(left)*. Staining with antibody specific for CENP-C *(right)*.

The Structure of Telomeric DNA

Telomeres in all organisms tested to date (with the exception of certain flies) are composed of many repeats of short DNA sequences. The sequence 5′ TTAGGG 3′ is found at the ends of chromosomes of a wide range of organisms, from human to rattlesnake to the fungus *Neurospora crassa*. In the human, roughly 650 to 2500 copies of this sequence are found at the end of each chromosome, yielding a total length of about 4000 to 15,000 bp (this varies in different tissues). Different telomere sequences have been noted in protozoans, yeasts, and higher plants.

The telomeric repeat is organized in a unique orientation with respect to the chromosome end. Thus, the end of every chromosome has one G-rich strand and one complementary C-rich strand. The G-rich strand always makes up the 3′ end of the chromosomal DNA molecule. Thus, the very 3′ end of the chromosome always has the following structure: ....(TTAGGG)-OH. Furthermore, the end of the chromosome is not a blunt structure; the G-rich strand ends in a single-stranded overhang that is approximately 200 bp long. Under certain conditions in vitro, this single-stranded telomeric DNA can adopt a four-stranded structure; however, this unusual structure does not seem to occur in vivo. Instead, recent evidence suggests that the single-stranded DNA may "invade" the double helix of telomeric repeats, causing the ends of chromosomes to form large loops, called t loops (see later discussion).

How Telomeres Replicate the Ends of the Chromosomal DNA

One role of telomeres is to prevent the erosion of the end of the chromosomal DNA molecule during each round of replication (see Chapter 45). All DNA replication proceeds with a polarity of 3′ to 5′ on the template DNA (5′ to 3′ in the newly synthesized DNA). Furthermore, all DNA polymerases (but not RNA polymerases) work by elongating a preexisting stretch of double-stranded nucleic acid. During cellular DNA replication, this is achieved by making a short RNA primer and then elongating the RNA: DNA duplex with DNA polymerase. The primer is subsequently removed and the newly opened gap is filled by a DNA polymerase elongating from the next upstream DNA end (Fig. 12–14).

If the very end of the chromosomal DNA is replicated from an RNA primer that sits on the very end of the DNA molecule, it follows that when this primer is removed, there is no upstream DNA on which to put a primer. How, then, is the DNA underneath the last RNA primer replicated? Years of searching for a DNA polymerase that could operate in the opposite direction proved fruitless. The answer that ultimately emerged turned out to be both elegant and unexpected.

Many cells have an enzymatic activity whose specific function is to lengthen the 3′ end of the chromosomal DNA. This activity is referred to as **telomerase.** Telomerases are enzymes that contain both protein and RNA subunits. The sequences of these

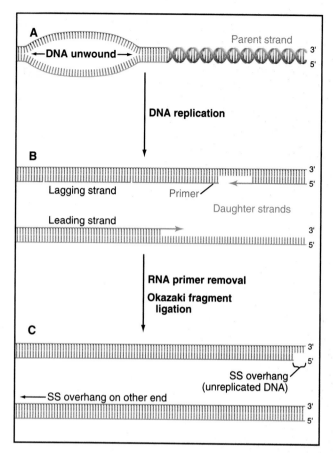

Figure 12-14 *A* to *C,* The DNA replication problem at chromosome ends. DNA polymerases cannot initiate the formation of DNA on a template de novo: they can only extend preexisting nucleotide strands (see Chapter 45). In contrast, RNA polymerases can initiate synthesis without a primer. As a result, all replicating DNA chains start from a short region of RNA, which is used to "prime" the DNA polymerase. The enzyme starts by creating an RNA: DNA junction and then laying down DNA. The RNA "primer" is later degraded and the gap is filled in by DNA polymerase, which uses the next upstream DNA end as a primer. How is the DNA underneath the very last primer to be replicated?

components provide an essential clue as to how this enzyme works.

The sequence of the human telomere is TTAGGG. When the sequence of human telomerase RNA was examined, it was found to contain the region AUCCCAAUC, which could base-pair with the TTAGGG repeat at the end of the chromosome. This observation led to a proposal for the mechanism of telomerase action (Fig. 12–15). In brief, the enzyme uses its own RNA as a template for the synthesis of DNA, which it attaches to the end of the chromosome. This hypothesis has been confirmed by studies that show that alterations in the sequence of the telomerase RNA lead to alterations in the telomere sequence at the end of the chromosome.

According to this model, the telomerase actually synthesizes DNA from an RNA template. Thus, telo-

merase is a member of a class of DNA polymerases called **reverse transcriptases**. These enzymes were first described in certain RNA tumor viruses known as retroviruses, and also appear to be involved in the movement of the LINE retroposons.

Telomerases have been characterized from budding yeast, mice, humans, and two ciliated protozoans. The enzymes consist of at least two protein subunits complexed to the RNA. The telomerase RNA varies in size and sequence between species, with the human RNA, hTR, being 450 nucleotides long. hTR is complexed with two polypeptides: TP1 (a 240-kD protein of unknown function that specifically binds telomerase RNA) and hTERT (a 127-kD protein that is *te*lomerase *r*everse *t*ranscriptase). Active human telomerase can be reconstituted in vitro from purified hTR and hTERT in the presence of a cell-free lysate from reticulocytes (which appears to provide essential protein-folding factors).

Telomerase is subject to tight biological regulation, with active enzyme being detected in only a few normal tissues in adult humans. These include the intestine and testis. In addition, about 85% of cancer cells express active telomerase. In cells that lack telomerase, an alternative pathway, thought to involve DNA recombination, can help to maintain the telomeric repeats at chromosome ends. Paradoxically, hTR and TP1 are not tightly regulated. They are detected in many tissues, most of which lack telomerase activity. By contrast, the expression of hTERT correlates tightly with telomerase activity. Furthermore, introduction of a DNA-encoding hTERT into telomerase-negative cells is sufficient to convert those cells to telomerase-positive. This has extremely important consequences for the growth of the cells (see Fig. 12–17).

Structural Proteins of the Telomere

Telomeres provide special protected ends for the chromosomal DNA molecule, in part by coating the end of the DNA molecules with protective proteins and, possibly, by adopting a specialized DNA loop structure. In organisms in which telomeric DNA sequences are relatively short, these sequences are packaged into a specialized chromatin structure. In mammals, in which the telomeric sequences are much longer, the bulk of the telomeric DNA is packaged into chromatin with a specialized shortened internucleosomal spacing (see Chapter 13).

Three types of proteins associate with telomeres (Fig. 12–16). The first binds in a sequence-specific manner to the double-stranded telomeric repeats. In budding yeast, the best known such protein is Rap1p. Mammals have two proteins of this type: TRF1 and

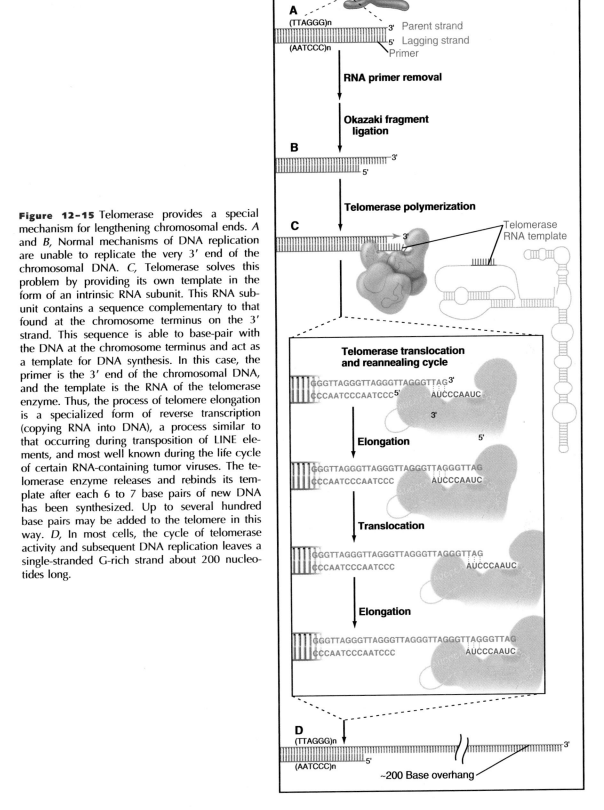

Figure 12-15 Telomerase provides a special mechanism for lengthening chromosomal ends. *A* and *B,* Normal mechanisms of DNA replication are unable to replicate the very 3' end of the chromosomal DNA. *C,* Telomerase solves this problem by providing its own template in the form of an intrinsic RNA subunit. This RNA subunit contains a sequence complementary to that found at the chromosome terminus on the 3' strand. This sequence is able to base-pair with the DNA at the chromosome terminus and act as a template for DNA synthesis. In this case, the primer is the 3' end of the chromosomal DNA, and the template is the RNA of the telomerase enzyme. Thus, the process of telomere elongation is a specialized form of reverse transcription (copying RNA into DNA), a process similar to that occurring during transposition of LINE elements, and most well known during the life cycle of certain RNA-containing tumor viruses. The telomerase enzyme releases and rebinds its template after each 6 to 7 base pairs of new DNA has been synthesized. Up to several hundred base pairs may be added to the telomere in this way. *D,* In most cells, the cycle of telomerase activity and subsequent DNA replication leaves a single-stranded G-rich strand about 200 nucleotides long.

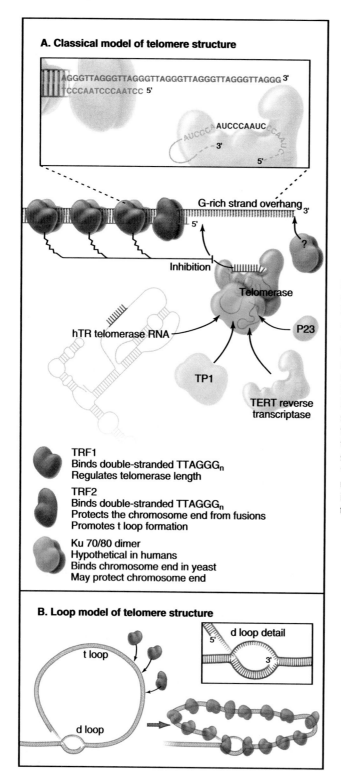

A. Classical model of telomere structure

AGGGTTAGGGTTAGGGTTAGGGTTAGGGTTAGGGTTAGGG 3'
TCCCAATCCCAATCC 5'

AUCCCA AUCCCAAUC

G-rich strand overhang 3'

5'

?

Inhibition

Telomerase

hTR telomerase RNA

P23

TP1

TERT reverse transcriptase

TRF1
Binds double-stranded $TTAGGG_n$
Regulates telomerase length

TRF2
Binds double-stranded $TTAGGG_n$
Protects the chromosome end from fusions
Promotes t loop formation

Ku 70/80 dimer
Hypothetical in humans
Binds chromosome end in yeast
May protect chromosome end

B. Loop model of telomere structure

t loop

d loop detail
5'
3'

d loop

Figure 12-16 *A*, The proposed structure of the end of a human chromosome. TRF1 and TRF2 bind to the double-stranded $(TTAGGG)_n$ repeats at telomeres. TRF1 somehow regulates the action of telomerase. TRF2 is responsible for protecting the integrity of chromosomal ends. If it is lost, chromosomes fuse with one another, and many abnormalities are seen. In yeast, a protein called Ku binds to the ends of the DNA. This may not be the case in vertebrates, since recent evidence suggests that the chromosome end may be protected by formation of a specialized t loop structure. *(B)*. This loop forms when the single-stranded G-rich 3' end of the chromosome "invades" the double-stranded portion of the telomere, base pairing with one strand and *d*isplacing the other (D loop). TRF2 can promote formation of t loops in vitro.

TRF2 (*t*elomere *r*epeat *f*actor). These proteins have essential roles in telomeric structure and function. TRF1 can regulate telomerase activity, thus helping to maintain the proper length of telomeres. A similar function has been proposed for Rap1p in budding yeast, where the telomeres appear to elongate only until they create a threshold number of binding sites for this protein. Mammalian TRF2 appears to protect the chromosome ends; interference with the binding of this protein to telomeres results in a loss of the G-strand overhangs and a dramatic increase in the tendency of chromosomes to fuse end to end. This may be because TRF2 can promote the formation of a special looped configuration of DNA in which the single-stranded G-strand overhang is base-paired with "upstream" DNA (see Fig. 12–16*B*).

Telomeric proteins of the second class bind to the single-stranded DNA of the G-strand overhang. The telomere-binding protein of the ciliated protozoan *Oxytricha* has two subunits (α and β) whose function is not known. In budding yeast, Cdc13p and Est1p bind to the G-strand overhang. Cdc13p protects the end of the recessed C-rich strand at telomeres. In *cdc13* mutants, the C-rich strand is rapidly degraded, with lethal consequences for the cell. Est1p appears to regulate telomerase activity. Equivalent proteins have yet to be described in humans.

Proteins of the third class bind to the very end of the DNA. Thus far, these proteins have been shown to function only in yeast and ciliates, where the telomere DNA may not form t loops. The identification of these proteins was very surprising, given that one essential role of telomeres is to make the ends of the DNA *not* resemble DNA breaks. In budding yeast, it is clear that a heterodimer of two proteins termed Ku70/Ku80 (70,000 and 80,000 D, respectively; Ku refers to the initials of an autoimmune patient whose serum was first used to identify these proteins) is an essential component of chromosome ends. However, this protein is also an essential component of DNA double-strand break repair and specialized DNA recombination pathways, both of which involve ligating DNA molecules together—just what is *not* desired at telomeres! At yeast telomeres, the Ku dimer actually performs a protective function (in mutants lacking Ku, telomeres shorten dramatically), and it also seems to have a role in assembly of the specialized chromatin structure that is found at telomeres. It now appears that chromosome ends are, in fact, recognized by the breakage repair machinery, but that some aspect of the telomeric structure changes the function of this machinery so that it assumes an end-blocking role, rather than an end-joining role.

One further aspect of telomeric function appears to be the proper location of the chromosome ends within the cell. In budding yeast, telomeres show a preferential tendency to cluster together at the nuclear periphery. Mutants in the telomere-binding SIR proteins, or in regions of the histones with which they intersect, disrupt this clustering. This results in activation of genes that are normally silenced when located in close proximity to telomeres. Thus, positioning of the telomere within the nucleus may be used to sequester genes into compartments where their transcriptional activity is repressed.

Telomeres, Aging, and Cancer

Although the average length of telomeric repeats in humans is about 4000 bp, this length varies. Chromosomes of older individuals have shorter telomeres and gametes have longer telomeres. This suggests the interesting possibility that chromosomes might lose telomeric sequences during the life of an individual.

The relationship between telomere length and aging is most readily studied in cultured cells. Normal cells in culture grow for only a limited number of generations (often called the Hayflick limit) before undergoing **senescence** (this involves cessation of growth, enlargement in size, and expression of marker enzymes, like β-galactosidase). Because normal somatic cells lack telomerase activity, their telomeres shorten by about 50% before the cells senesce. Senescent cells stop dividing before their telomeres become critically short. In some cases, it is possible to force the senescent cells to resume proliferation (e.g., by expressing certain viral oncogenes). These "driven" cells continue to divide and their telomeres continue to shorten until a **crisis** point is reached. In crisis, cells suffer chromosomal instability (chromosomal fusions and breaks can occur) and cell death. In populations of human cells in crisis, very rarely (in about 1 in a million cases), cells appear that once again grow normally. These cells express telomerase. These observations with cultured cells led to the suggestion that senescence might occur in cells when the telomeric repeats of one or more chromosomes are reduced to some critical level.

If this model is right, it suggests very interesting (and controversial) implications for the regulation of cell life. Suppose that telomerase is only active in the germ line, so that all gametes have long telomeres. Now, if the enzyme were inactivated in somatic cells, this would effectively provide every cell lineage with a limitation to how many times it could divide before loss of telomeric sequences causes it to become senescent. Provided that the starting telomeres were sufficiently long and that telomerase were expressed in unusual tissues, like testis and intestine, in which rapid division occurs throughout the life of the individual, this would have no deleterious effect on the life span of the organism. In fact, such a mechanism might provide an important advantage by minimizing the chances that a clone of cells would escape from the normal regulation of growth control and become cancerous.

This model has recently been tested in two ways. First, mice were prepared in which the gene coding for the RNA component of telomerase was disrupted. Surprisingly, these mice were healthy and fertile for six generations in the complete absence of telomerase.

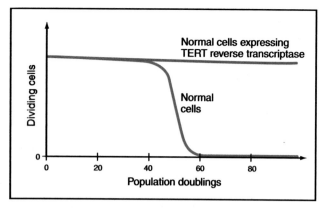

Figure 12-17 Introduction of hTERT, the human reverse transcriptase subunit of telomerase, into normal cells is sufficient to overcome the senescence limit and immortalize the cells. These cells are not transformed into invasive cancer cells; instead, they act like normal cells that can now grow indefinitely.

Their cells could also be transformed into cancer cells. However, at the sixth generation, the mice abruptly became sterile as a result of cell death in the male germ line. This experiment thus showed that telomerase is not needed for the day-to-day life of a mammal, but clearly, it is needed for the survival of the species. In a second experiment, the hTERT reverse transcriptase subunit of telomerase was introduced into normal cells growing in culture. This caused an increase in the level of active telomerase with dramatic results. Instead of undergoing senescence, these cells kept dividing in culture, apparently indefinitely (Fig. 12–17). However, unlike cancer cells, which are also immortal, these cells did not acquire the ability to cause tumors.

Thus, this experiment showed convincingly that telomeres are part of a mechanism that regulates the proliferative capacity of somatic cells.

∎ Selected Readings

Craig JM, Earnshaw WC, Vagnarelli P: Mammalian centromeres: DNA sequence, protein composition, and role in cell cycle progression. Exp Cell Res 246:249–262, 1999.

Doolittle RF: Microbial genomes opened up. Nature 392:339–342, 1998.

Dujon B: The yeast genome project: What did we learn? Trends Genet 12:263–270, 1996.

Evans SK, Bertuch AA, Lundblad V: Telomeres and telomerase: At the end, it all comes together. Trends Cell Biol 9:329–331, 1999.

Gottschling DE, Stoddard B: Telomeres: Structure of a chromosome's aglet. Curr Biol 9:R164–167, 1999.

International Human Genome Sequencing Consortium: Initial sequencing and analysis of the human genome. Nature 409:860–921, 2001.

McEachern MJ, Krauskopf A, Blackburn EH: Telomeres and their control. Annu Rev Genet 34:331–358, 2000.

Pidoux AL, Allshire RC: Centromeres: Getting a grip of chromosomes. Curr Opin Cell Biol 12:308–319, 2000.

Rubin GM, et al.: Comparative genomics of the eukaryotes. Science 287:2204–2215, 2000.

Shay JW, Zou Y, Hiyama E, Wright WE: Telomerase and cancer. Hum Mol Genet 10:677–685, 2001.

Smit AF: The origin of interspersed repeats in the human genome. Curr Opin Genet Dev 6:743–748, 1996.

Sullivan BA, Blower MD, Karpen GH: Determining centromere identity: Cyclical stories and forking paths. Natl Rev Genet 2:584–596, 2001.

chapter 13

DNA PACKAGING IN CHROMATIN AND CHROMOSOMES

Chromosomal DNA molecules are thousands of times longer than the nuclear diameter and must, therefore, be highly folded throughout the cell cycle. This folding is accomplished by combining the DNA with structural proteins to make **chromatin**. A hierarchy of levels of chromatin folding compacts the DNA but permits transcriptional machinery access to those regions of the chromosome required for gene expression.

The first level of folding involves coiling DNA around a protein core to yield a **nucleosome**. This shortens DNA about seven-fold relative to naked DNA. The string of nucleosomes is next folded into a shorter, thicker filament, called a **30-nm fiber**, which is about 40-fold shorter than naked DNA. This is further folded into fibers, 100 to 300 nm in diameter, that are thought to be organized into **loop domains** of 15,000 to 100,000 base pairs. Specific regions of DNA may anchor these loop domains to proteins of the **nuclear matrix** or **chromosome scaffold**.

▋ The First Level of Chromosomal DNA Packaging: The Nucleosome

The continuous DNA fiber of each chromosome links hundreds of thousands of nucleosomes in series. Individual nucleosomes can be isolated following cleavage of DNA between neighboring particles. Random digestion of chromatin by enzymes called nucleases initially yields a mixture of particles consisting of one or more nucleosomes containing multiples of about 200 base pairs of DNA (Fig. 13–1). Continued nuclease cleavage gives an unstable particle containing 166 base pairs of DNA (two full turns of DNA around a protein core). Further cleavage yields a stable particle with 146 base pairs of DNA (1.75 turns of the DNA around

the protein core). The latter is called a **nucleosome core particle** (see Fig. 13–1).

The isolated nucleosome core particle is disk-shaped, with DNA coiled in a left-handed superhelix around an octamer of **core histones**. This octamer consists of a central tetramer composed of two closely linked **H3**: **H4** heterodimers, flanked on either side by an **H2A**: **H2B** heterodimer (Table 13–1). Each core histone has a compact domain of 70 to 100 amino acid residues and a flexible N-terminal "tail" of approximately 30 residues. High-resolution x-ray structural analysis of the nucleosome core particle and isolated histone octamer has revealed that the compact histone domains are composed of a characteristic Z-shaped "histone fold" consisting of a long α-helix flanked by two shorter α-helices (Fig. 13–2). Interactions between adjacent central helices stabilize the various dimer pairs. Nucleosomal DNA winds around the protein core, following a helical path along the surface of the octamer. At two places, DNA kinks slightly away from the core. These distortions alter the structure of the nucleosomal DNA, giving it a repeat periodicity of 10.2 base pairs per turn, rather than the 10.5 base pairs per turn that are characteristic of DNA free in solution.

The amino-terminal portions of the histones (**N-terminal tails**) are important for interactions both inside and outside the nucleosome. They project outward from the cylindrical faces of the nucleosomal core, as well as through minor groove "tunnels" where the two turns of the DNA superhelix line up so that adjacent regions of minor groove are paired.

Although these N-terminal tails are not ordered either in crystals or in solution, they are among the most highly conserved regions of these very highly conserved proteins, as they serve two essential functions. First, by promoting interactions between nucleo-

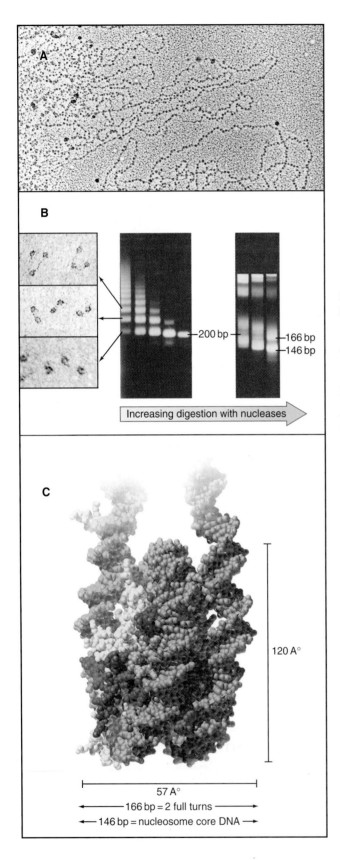

A

B

200 bp

166 bp
146 bp

Increasing digestion with nucleases

C

120 A°

57 A°

166 bp = 2 full turns

146 bp = nucleosome core DNA

Figure 13-1 Nucleosomes. *A,* Electron micrograph showing chromosomal loops covered in nucleosomes, which under these conditions look like beads on a string. *B,* Nuclease digestion of chromosomes releases fragments containing varying numbers of nucleosomes *(left),* in which the DNA fragments vary by multiples of 200 base pairs *(center).* More extensive nuclease digestion results in production of the nucleosome core particle, with 146 bp of DNA *(right). C,* The crystal structure of the nucleosome core particle. The DNA wraps around a compact core of histones. (*B, left panel,* Composite of excerpts from Woodcock CL, Sweetman HE, Frado LL: Structural repeating units in chromatin. II. Their isolation and partial characterization. Exp Cell Res 97:111–119, 1976; *center and right panels,* exerpts from Allan J, Cowling GJ, Harborne N et al: Regulation of the higher-order structure of chromatin by histones H1 and H5. J Cell Biol 90:279–288, 1981. *C,* PDB file: 1 aoi.)

table 13–1

PROPERTIES OF HISTONES

Histone	Molecular Weight	Number of Amino Acids	Net Positive Charge
H2A	13,960	129	+15
H2B	13,774	125	+19
H3	15,342	135	+20
H4	11,282	102	+16
H1	23,000	224	+58

Note: The core histones, H3 and H4 in particular, are highly conserved in evolution among eukaryotes. For example, pea and mammalian H4 differ in only 2 of 102 amino acids. H1 histones are much more variable. The histone octamer contains 162 positive charges that, together with small cations such as Mg^{2+} and polyamines, neutralize the negative charges on the DNA phosphates.

somes, the N-terminal tails permit the nucleosomes to pack into the compact 30-nm fiber. Histones from which tails have been removed by protease treatment can assemble into nucleosomes but cannot pack into 30-nm fibers. Second, specific modifications of these N-terminal tails are used initially during chromatin assembly and then later on to regulate the accessibility of the DNA within the chromatin fiber to the transcription, replication, and repair machinery (see later section).

Regulation of Chromatin Structure by the Histone N-terminal Tails

Human nuclei contain roughly 3.3×10^7 nucleosomes packed more or less tightly along the DNA. Despite the fact that more than 70% of the molecular surface of nucleosomal DNA is accessible to solvent, most protein regulatory factors bind nucleosomal DNA 10- to 10^4-fold less well than naked DNA. Thus, nucleosomes establish a general environment in which DNA replication and gene transcription are repressed. As a result, eukaryotes must elaborate strategies to manipulate DNA accessibility. (Chapter 14 deals with this regulation in more detail than the general aspects covered here.)

The N-terminal histone tails provide a molecular "handle" to manipulate DNA accessibility in chromatin (Fig. 13–3). Proteins called transcription factors regulate gene expression by binding specific DNA sequences in promoter regions adjacent to the coding sequences of genes and recruiting transcriptional machinery (RNA polymerases and associated proteins) to the gene. Many transcription factors recruit a type of protein complex, called a **coactivator,** that facilitates loading of transcriptional apparatus onto the gene. Several coactivators are enzymes that modify the N-terminal histone tails. One coactivator, the 1800-kD yeast SAGA complex, contains at least seven proteins, including a histone acetyltransferase called Gcn5, which transfers acetate groups from acetyl coenzyme A (CoA) to the ϵ-amino groups of lysine-14 and lysines-8 and -16 in the N-terminal tails of histones H3 and H4, respectively (Fig. 13–4). Acetylation reduces the net positive charge of the N-terminal domain, causing the chromatin to "loosen" and adopt a conformation more favorable to transcription. Histone acetylation is crucial for life; indeed, yeast cells die if these three lysines are mutated to arginines, thus preserving their positive charge but preventing them from being acetylated.

Histone acetylation provides the transcriptional apparatus a toe-hold in chromatin. For most yeast genes,

Figure 13-2 Secondary structure of the histones within the core particle. *A,* A ribbon diagram shows that each histone protein in the octameric core of the nucleosome has a characteristic α-helical structure (the histone fold). Portions of the flexible N-terminal portions of the histones, which have a critical role in regulating chromatin structure, did not occupy a unique location in the crystal and do not appear in this structure. *B,* The histone octamer surrounded by one of the two turns of DNA. (Adapted from Luger K, Mäder AW, Richmond RK, et al: Crystal structure of the nucleosome core particle at 2.8 Å resolution. Nature 389: 251–260, 1997.)

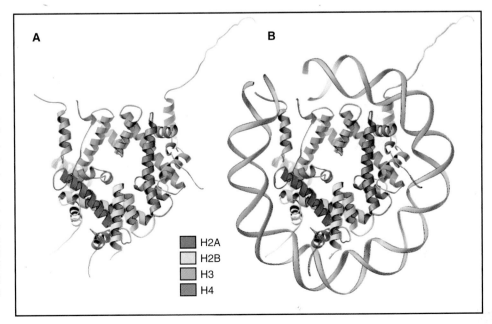

A   B

H2A
H2B
H3
H4

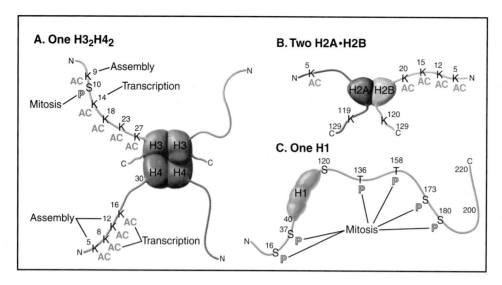

Figure 13-3 The amino- and carboxy-terminal domains of the histones are sites for numerous protein modifications involved in regulating nucleosome assembly, transcription, and mitotic chromosome condensation. The sites on one H3 and one H4 are shown. AC, acetylation of lysine (K); P, phosphorylation; S, serine; T, threonine.

this appears to be sufficient to permit transcription to occur. However, genetic studies indicate that, for certain genes, acetylation of N-terminal histone tails must be followed by further remodeling of chromatin to permit efficient transcription.

Complex protein "machines" remodel chromatin, using energy from ATP hydrolysis to alter nucleosome structure or to move nucleosomes around, or both. Two large "machines" in yeast—RSC (remodels the structure of chromatin) with 15 subunits, and SWI/SNF (switch/sniff) with 11—share a key subunit, a protein called SWI2/SNF2. This enzyme is related to proteins that utilize ATP to unwind the DNA helix. *Drosophila* has at least three smaller complexes that share a common subunit—ISWI (imitation of switch)—which re-

sembles SWI2/SNF2. How these "machines" work is not known, but presumably, they use ATP hydrolysis to loosen the association of the histone octamer with DNA. Several of these complexes contain actin and/or actin-related proteins (see Chapter 36). How these contribute to chromatin remodeling is not known. Interestingly, one *Drosophila* complex, NURF (nucleosome remodeling factor), uses the N-terminal histone tails as handles to act on nucleosomes.

Histone Acetylation and Nucleosome Assembly

During DNA replication, existing nucleosomes are partitioned randomly between daughter DNA strands. Newly assembled nucleosomes then fill the gaps. His-

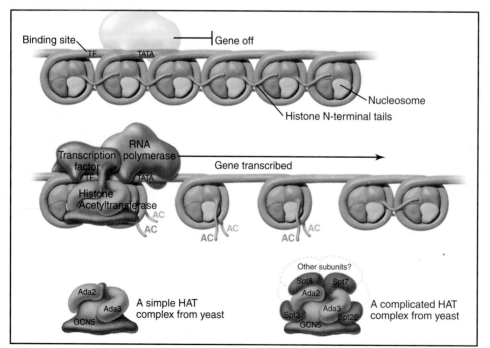

Figure 13-4 Acidic transcription factors *(purple)* bind specific DNA sequences and recruit coactivators to the 5' ends of genes. Many of these coactivators have histone acetyltransferase (HAT) activity and work by acetylating the N-terminal tails of the core histones, thereby loosening the chromatin structure and promoting the binding and activation of the RNA polymerase holoenzyme (see Chapter 14). The coactivators vary in composition and complexity from the relatively simple HAT complex *(bottom left)* to the huge and elaborate SAGA complex *(bottom right)*. AC, acetylation. TATA, DNA sequence in the gene promoter (see Chapter 14). GCN5, Ada2, Ada3, Spt3, Spt7, Spt8, and Spt20 are the names of budding yeast genes whose products are found in these complexes.

tone acetylation has an important role during de novo nucleosome assembly, which occurs in parallel with DNA replication and repair. The N-terminal tails of newly translated H3 and H4 are modified in the cytoplasm by a histone acetyltransferase called HAT1, resulting in acetylation of lysine-9 of H3 and lysine-5 and lysine-12 of H4, sites distinct from those involved in transcriptional activation. Acetylated histones associate with chromatin assembly factor, CAF1, then move into the nucleus and associate with DNA to organize about 120 base pairs into a nascent nucleosome. This nucleosome is completed through the binding of two H2A: H2B heterodimers and maturation of H3 and H4 by removal of acetyl groups by a specific histone deacetylase, HDAC1. Histones are accompanied throughout this journey from HAT1 to CAF1 to HDAC1 by escort molecules p46 and p48, which bind to H4 and may serve as adapters between histones and various factors necessary for chromatin assembly.

Linker DNA and the Linker Histone H1

When examined by electron microscopy at low ionic strength, nucleosomal chromatin resembles a string of beads measuring about 10 nm in diameter, with **linker DNA** extended between adjacent nucleosomes (see Fig. 13–1). Each nucleosome in chromosomes is typically associated with about 200 base pairs of DNA. Subtracting 166 base pairs for two turns around the histone octamer, this leaves 34 base pairs of linker DNA between adjacent nucleosomes. Linker DNA can vary widely. In mammals, nucleosomes in neurons are closely packed, with no extra linker DNA, whereas those in the adjacent glial cells are separated by 34 base pair linkers. The reason for this variation is unknown.

A fifth histone, **H1** or **linker histone**, binds to linker DNA between nucleosomes. H1 histones differ from core histones in that they have a globular central domain flanked by unstructured basic domains at both the N- and C-termini (see Fig. 13–3). One H1 molecule typically sits at the side of each nucleosomal core where the DNA molecule enters and exits the structure (Fig. 13–5).

Levels of H1 phosphorylation at serines and threonines throughout the N- and C-terminal histone tails rise two- to three-fold during mitosis owing to the action of cdk1:cyclin B, the master cell cycle regulatory kinase (see Chapter 43). H1 phosphorylation was long thought to be essential for mitotic chromosome condensation, but mitotic chromosomes actually can condense normally without H1. Core histone H3 is also phosphorylated at serine-10 during mitosis, but the role of this modification is also unknown.

Mammals have at least seven variant forms (called subtypes) of H1 histones (H1$_{a-e}$, H1^o, and H1$_t$, the

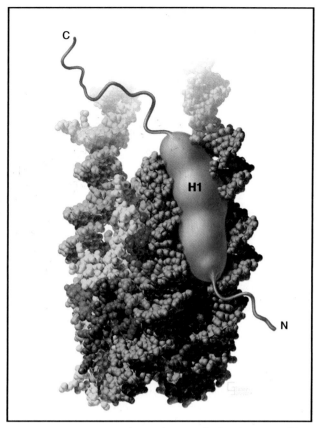

Figure 13-5 Artist's rendition showing the binding site of histone H1 on the nucleosome, near the site where DNA strands enter and exit the core particle.

latter found exclusively in the testis in developing sperm). All encode proteins of similar molecular weight whose amino acid sequences vary by about 15% to 20%. Different H1 subtypes may be expressed simultaneously in individual cells, and there is some evidence that they may partition to different regions of the chromatin. It was long thought that these subtypes might be important in regulating gene expression. For example, cells entering the nondividing G$_o$ state (see Chapter 43) make an H1 subtype called H1^o, which was thought to repress DNA replication and transcription. However, gene knockout experiments yielded the surprising finding that mice lacking H1^o survive without any obvious ill effects, as do *Tetrahymena* (a ciliated protozoan) lacking linker histone altogether. Thus, the role of H1 linker histone remains enigmatic.

▌ The Second Level of Chromosomal DNA Packaging: The 30-nm Fiber

Levels of chromatin structure beyond the nucleosome are poorly understood. For example, the **30-nm fiber** is a condensed filament of nucleosomes that can be

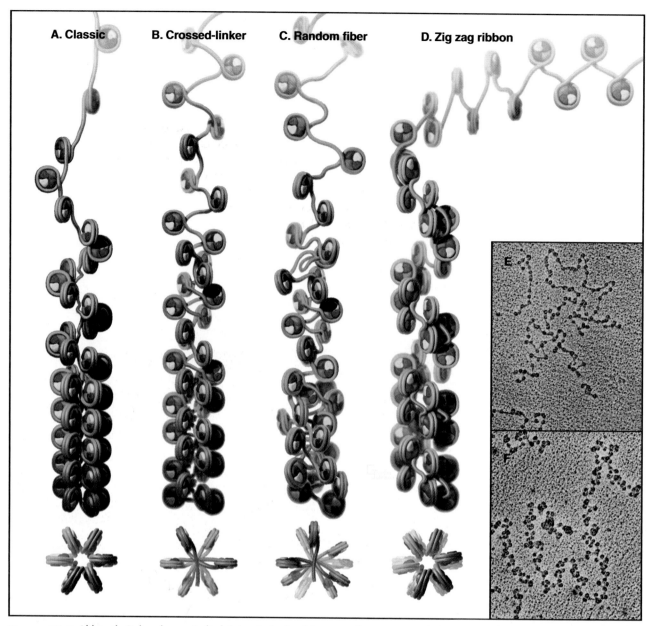

Figure 13-6 Although it has been studied intensively for 30 years, the structure of the 30-nm chromatin fiber remains controversial. *A* to *D,* Various models of the 30-nm fiber: classic solenoid (a type of helix), crossed-linker solenoid, random fiber, and zig-zag ribbon. The classic solenoid model has been widely favored but continues to be challenged. *E* and *F,* Histone H1 causes a compaction of the chromatin filament. *E,* Chromatin spread for electron microscopy following removal of histone H1: the 100-nm fiber or so-called "beads on a string." *F,* A similar preparation with H1 present: the 30-nm fiber. (*E* and *F,* From Thoma F, Koller T: Influence of histone H1 on chromatin structure. Cell 12:101–107, 1977.)

observed by electron microscopy. Investigators agree that disk-shaped nucleosomes are arranged with their flat faces roughly parallel to the long axis of the filament, but they disagree about how nucleosomes pack into this filament. Models range from a relatively ordered helical solenoid, to a twisted helical ribbon, to a random zig-zag aggregation of nucleosomes (Fig. 13–6). This controversy arises in part because chromatin fibers are very fragile and easily damaged during preparation for structural studies.

Higher Levels of Chromosomal DNA Packaging in Interphase Nuclei

Dense packing of macromolecules in the nucleus makes it very difficult to observe the details of higher-level folding of chromatin fibers directly. For this reason, studies of higher-order chromatin organization traditionally depended largely on studies of mitotic chromosomes. This is now changing, as new methods allow one to observe conformations of particular regions of chromosomes in the nuclei of living cells.

Experiments in which specific DNA loci are visualized within fixed nuclei by in situ hybridization can be used to estimate the degree of chromatin compaction within interphase nuclei. The physical distance between two DNA sequences separated by a known number of base pairs can be used to calculate the extent of compaction of the DNA between them. For regions of DNA up to about 250,000 base pairs apart, the chromatin fiber is shortened about two- to three-fold relative to the 30-nm fiber. When sequences are separated by tens of millions of base pairs, the shortening increases by another 20- to 30-fold. This suggests that there are at least two levels of chromatin folding beyond the 30-nm fiber.

The organization of particular chromatin fibers can be observed by fluorescence microscopy of living cells after labeling with a fluorescent marker, such as the jellyfish green fluorescent protein (GFP) (Fig. 13–7). This approach reveals that chromosome arms are dynamic, changing both their structure and location as cells traverse the cell cycle. At times in the cycle when the chromosome arm becomes relatively more decondensed, it is possible to observe the presence of a fiber, 100 to 300 nm in diameter, that has been referred to as a **chromonema fiber,** and may be the next level of chromatin packing above the 30-nm fiber. Similar fibers are seen in electron micrographs of interphase cells, but it is not yet known if the chromonema fiber or some other structure is the highest level of chromatin folding in interphase nuclei.

Higher-Order Chromosomal Structure in Mitotic Chromosomes

Studies of mitotic chromosomes and specialized chromosomes from fruit flies and other organisms suggest that chromosomes have large-scale structural domains composed of chromatin loops containing thousands to millions of base pairs. For example, some tissues of *Drosophila* larvae are composed of huge polyploid cells. These cells have nuclei with giant **polytene chromosomes,** each consisting of more than 1000 identical DNA molecules packed side by side in precise linear register. Examination by light microscopy reveals that polytene chromosomes have a complex pattern of thousands of bands (Fig. 13–8) representing domains of differentially compacted chromatin. Each band contains one or several genes and potentially constitutes a domain for gene expression. Stress or hormones that stimulate gene expression cause certain bands to lose their compact shape and puff out laterally. Such **puffs** are composed of hundreds of identical chromatin loop domains, all of which are being actively transcribed (see Fig. 13–8).

Although polytene chromosomes provide the clearest demonstration of structural domains along a chromosome, the arms of normal diploid mitotic chromosomes also appear to have a domain substructure. This is seen when chromosomes are subjected to G-banding (Fig. 13–9). G-banded human chromosomes from the early (prometaphase) stage of mitosis have up to 2000 discrete bands seen by this technique. Although the structural basis for the bands is not known, G-banding is important because this structural organization, seen on mitotic chromosomes, correlates with a functional domain organization of the chromosome arms during interphase. DNA within dark G-bands replicates later in S phase than does DNA in light G-bands. In addition, actively transcribed genes are more highly concentrated in light G-bands.

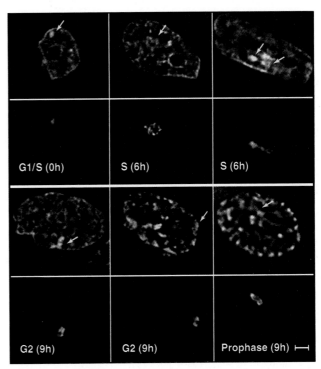

G1/S (0h) S (6h) S (6h)

G2 (9h) G2 (9h) Prophase (9h) ⊢━┥

Figure 13–7 Direct visualization of changes in the compaction and location of a chromosome arm in a living cell. DNA molecules carrying the binding sites for a specific DNA-binding protein were integrated into the chromosomes of a cell at random and caused to amplify into large arrays, which, in some cases, corresponded to whole chromosome arms. These cells were then induced to express the DNA-binding protein as a fusion to jellyfish green fluorescent protein (GFP). In the lower panel at each time point, the fluorescently labeled chromosome arm can be seen to change both its degree of condensation and its position within the nucleus as a function of the cell cycle. The upper panels show total DNA stained with DAPI. DNA replication occurs in the S phase, which is separated from mitosis (cell division) by the G_1 and G_2 gap phases (see Chapter 43). (Reproduced from Li G, Sudlow G, Belmont AS: Interphase cell cycle dynamics of a late-replicating, heterochromatic homogeneously staining region: Precise choreography of condensation/decondensation and nuclear positioning. J Cell Biol 140:975–989, 1998, by copyright permission of the Rockefeller University Press.)

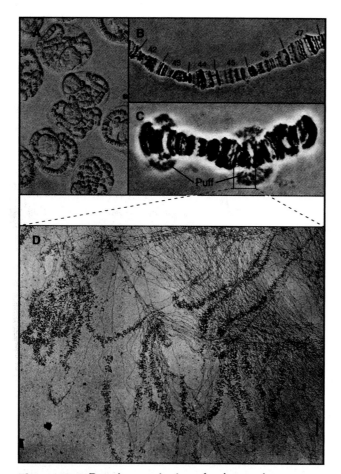

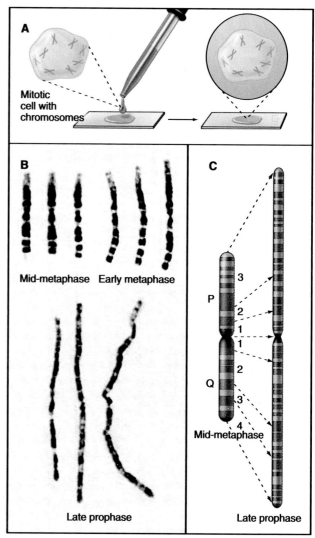

Figure 13-8 Domain organization of polytene chromosomes. Once fly larvae achieve a certain size, most cells stop dividing and larval growth proceeds via an increase in the size of individual cells. To keep the protein synthesis machinery of these huge cells supplied with messenger RNA, DNA replication is uncoupled from cell division so that, ultimately, the cells contain many times the normal complement of cellular DNA (i.e., they are *polyploid*). In certain tissues, the numerous copies of the chromosomes are maintained in strict alignment with respect to one another, making giant *polytene* chromosomes, the best known of which occur in the salivary gland. *A*, Giant polytene chromosomes are visible within isolated salivary gland nuclei. *B*, A portion of a high-resolution map of the *Drosophila* polytene chromosomes. *C*, Polytene chromosome showing puffs. The inset box shows an area analogous to that used in panel *D*. *D*, Electron micrograph of puff showing transcribing DNA loops. These loops are covered with a "fuzz" corresponding to growing RNA chains coated with proteins. (*A*, From Robert M: Isolation and manipulation of salivary gland nuclei and chromosomes. Methods Cell Biol 9:377–390, 1975. *B*, Courtesy of Margarete Heck, University of Edinburgh. *C*, From Andersson K, Mahr R, Bjorkroth B, et al: Rapid reformation of the thick chromosome fiber upon completion of RNA synthesis at the Balbiani ring genes in Chironomus tentans. Chromosoma 87:33–48, 1982. *D*, Reprinted from Lamb MM, Daneholt B: Characterization of active transcription units in Balbiani rings of Chironomus tentans. Cell 17:835–848, 1979. Copyright 1979, with permission from Elsevier Science.)

Figure 13-9 Chromosome banding reveals the complex and reproducible multidomain substructure of mitotic chromosome arms. *A*, Mitotic cells are dropped on a slide to spread the chromosomes. In G-banding, chromosomes are given harsh treatments, such as exposure to concentrated sodium hydroxide, proteases, or high temperatures, and then are stained with Giemsa dye. The chromosome arms then exhibit a characteristic pattern of light and dark bands. *B*, Photographs of G-banded human chromosome 2 from cells in late prophase, early metaphase, and mid-metaphase. Several examples are shown for each stage, illustrating the reproducibility of the banding patterns. *C*, Diagram summarizing the metaphase and prophase patterns. Because G-banding patterns are reproducible, this technique provides a way to identify individual chromosomes unambiguously. This was a major factor in the development of the field of *cytogenetics*, which is the study of the correlation between the structure of the chromosomes and genetics. (*B* and *C*, Adapted from Yunis JJ, Sawyer JR, Ball DW: The characterization of high-resolution G-banded chromosomes of man. Chromosoma. 67:293–307, 1978.)

The regularity of chromatin higher-order structure in mitotic chromosomes is easily seen when specific cloned regions of the genome are localized by in situ hybridization. When regions of up to about 1 million base pairs are highlighted by this method, they are distributed across the width of the chromosome in a sharp band similar to the bands of polytene chromosomes (Fig. 13–10). Smaller regions appear as spots

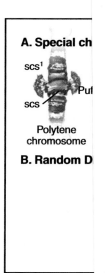

A. Special ch

scs¹

scs   Pu

Polytene
chromosome

B. Random D

Figure 13-16 Scs
somes. Biochemic;
binding sites for DI
red eye pigment p
injected into eggs
locations. White e
the chromosome a
thereby turning it
showed that scs e
inactive chromatin

matin and activ
than by setting
expression is ins
some.

The first bc
elements (for sp
a chromosomal
puffs following
13–16). Scs elen
elements by ins
either side of a
randomly into tl
bryos. In this e;
though it were
mosomal domai1
have an unusual
appear to be fre
to one side of tl
and named BE,
factor, 32 kD).
along Drosophila
between the ban
eral function in
pression. Furthe
whether boundai
ing gene expres
important role in
S/MARs were
ent assay—asso(

on the chromatids. Both bands and spots are distributed symmetrically on the two sister chromatids. This
indicates that the chromatin fiber is folded similarly in
both sister chromatids.

The Loop Domain Model for Chromosome Domain Organization

From the observations discussed earlier, chromatin appears to have a reproducible, higher-order packing
arrangement in nuclei and mitotic chromosomes.
Other studies suggest that chromatin loops, containing
an average of 15,000 to 100,000 base pairs, provide
the structural basis for these large-scale chromatin domains. This is called the **loop domain model** (Fig.
13–11).

Chromosome loop domains are best seen in
lampbrush chromosomes, found in oocytes of
many species (Fig. 13–12). Lampbrush chromosome
loops are sites of intense transcriptional activity as oocytes stockpile huge stores of the components needed
for rapid cell division during early development of the
fertilized egg. The loops are particularly visible because each DNA loop is coated with many RNA transcripts, together with proteins that package them.

But do such loops exist in normal somatic chromosomes? If chromosomes are swelled in hypotonic
solutions, it is readily apparent that loops of chromatin
radiate outward from the central chromatid axis (see
Fig. 13–11C). Alternatively, if stripped of histones, isolated chromosomes consist of an enormous pool of
DNA surrounding a residual structure that retains the
general shape of chromosome arms. In certain cases,
it is possible to trace individual loops of DNA radiating outward from the central structure (see Fig.
13–11B). Similar looped structures can be seen if interphase nuclei are depleted of histones.

Further refinements of direct fluorescence labeling
methods are needed to observe the chromatin higher-
order structure within living cells at higher resolution.
Meanwhile, a great deal of effort has been put into
studying the proteins and DNA sequences that may be
responsible for higher-order chromatin packaging.

Mitotic Versus Interphase Chromosomes

At first glance, mitotic chromosomes and interphase nuclei appear to be dramatically different. However, much
of this apparent difference is attributable to the absence
from mitotic chromosomes of many components associated with RNA transcription and processing that actually
make up the bulk of the nuclear constituents.

Present data are consistent with models in which
both interphase and mitotic chromosomes are organized into similar, higher-order loop domains, with the
main difference between the two states being in the
degree of aggregation of the loops (see Fig. 13–11A).

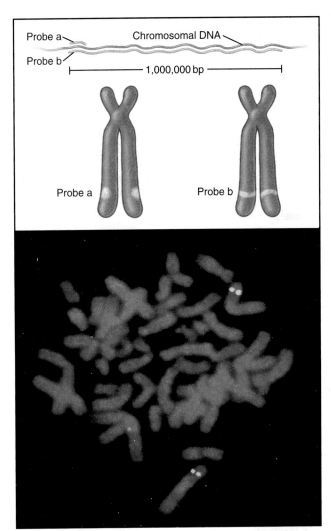

Figure 13-10 *Upper panel,* Fluorescence in situ hybridization
(FISH) performed on mitotic chromosomes. Chromosomes are
spread on a slide as in Figure 13–9. Following chemical fixation steps to preserve the chromosomal structure, the chromosomal proteins are removed by digestion with proteases and the
genomic DNA strands are melted (separated) by heating. Next,
a "probe DNA" *(yellow)* is added. This probe DNA is single-
stranded, so that it can base-pair (hybridize) to its complementary sequences in the chromosome. The probe DNA is chemically labeled with biotin. Next, the sites of hybridization on the
chromosomes are detected with fluorescently labeled avidin, a
protein from egg white that binds to biotin with extremely high
affinity. The sites of avidin-binding appear yellow, whereas the
remainder of the chromosomal DNA is counterstained with a red
dye. *Lower panel,* The micrograph shows FISH analysis using a
probe from near the von Hippel Lindau locus. (*Lower panel,* Courtesy of Jeanne Lawrence, University of Massachusetts, Amherst.)

Such changes would presumably be driven by specialized proteins, such as the condensins (see later section) that have an essential role in mitotic chromosome condensation.

Currently, it is widely assumed that conclusions
about chromatin organization, derived from studies of
mitotic chromosomes, will be broadly relevant to interphase chromosome structure and vice versa.

chromos
many o
function
separate
Whateve
somes, t
and off
Thus it i
    Mem
fold prot
mosome
protein:
be ident
of minic
of these
fined as
tain SMC
mosome
    One
tial for
Other SI
regulatio
proteins
sion, and
proteins
rial chror
    The
condensi
peptides,
SMC poly
α-helical
in Fig. 1.

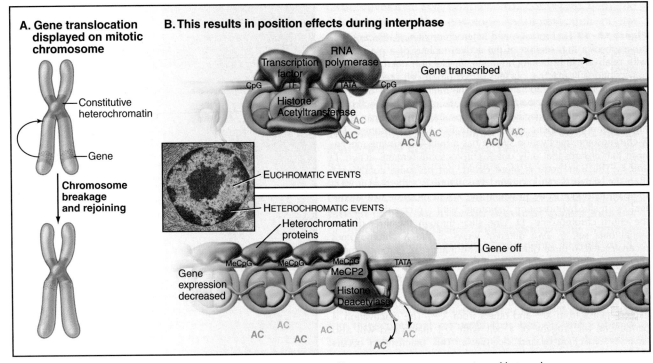

Figure 13–19 Position effect—the effect of moving a transcriptionally active gene next to a region of heterochromatin. The active gene is now repressed through a mechanism involving (among other things) DNA methylation and deacetylation of histone H4. *A,* The relative position of the gene is shown on mitotic chromosomes as it would be determined by in situ hybridization (see Fig. 13–10). *B,* Diagrammatic representation of the effects of this gene translocation on transcription of the gene during interphase. In the translocated example *(lower),* heterochromatin proteins spread over the active sequences and recruit activities that methylate CpG (MeCpG) residues and deacetylate the histones. Histone deacetylation induces a change in chromatin compaction that represses binding of proteins required for transcription. AC, acetylation. (*Inset,* Reference: Fawcett DW: The Cell, Philadelphia: WB Saunders, 1981.)

A. Con

N
C   NTP

Cdk1:cyclin

**B. Chro
    con**

Proph
chron

Figure 13
including
which is r
kinase, use
final levels
unknown n
adenosine (

5-methyl-cytosine is recognized by several specific binding proteins. One of these, MeCP2 (<u>m</u>ethyl <u>cyto-sine–binding protein</u>), represses expression of nearby genes when it binds to methylated DNA by recruiting a deacetylase complex that removes acetyl groups from the core histone N-terminal tails, thereby making the chromatin less accessible to the transcriptional apparatus (Fig. 13–19). Genes inactivated in facultative heterochromatin have a greater degree of methylation of their CpG islands and lower degree of acetylation of histone H4 than their counterparts in active chromatin.

DNA methylation is involved in a second, very specific type of gene silencing known as **imprinting.** Imprinted genes are expressed from a single chromosome contributed by either the mother or father (paternal or maternal imprinting, respectively; the imprinted gene is "off"). The detailed mechanism is not known, but imprinted alleles have been shown to have elevated levels of DNA methylation in their associated CpG islands.

Heterochromatin also contains specific proteins that suppress transcription. If an actively transcribed gene is moved into close proximity to constitutive heterochromatin by a chromosomal rearrangement, transcription from the gene is repressed (see Fig. 13–19). This "**position effect**" demonstrates that transcriptional inactivity of heterochromatin is not solely the result of a lack of genes, but also reflects an *active* suppression of transcription.

Heterochromatin protein 1 (HP1), first identified in *Drosophila,* is one component involved in the down-regulation of transcription by heterochromatin. HP1 appears to be a widely used, structural adapter protein involved in the regulation of chromatin structure. The amino-terminal region of HP1 contains a motif of 50 amino acids called a **chromo domain** (<u>chrom</u>atin <u>mo</u>dification <u>o</u>rganizer) that targets HPI to nucleosomes containing histone H3 methylated on lysine 9, a form of H3 associated with inactive chromatin. Chromo domains are found on many nuclear proteins, including the important *Polycomb* family proteins. *Polycomb* proteins are important in development because they help to confirm the identity of particular body segments. In each segment, certain pattern-determining genes are turned on while others are turned off. *Polycomb* family proteins do not turn genes on and off; however, they apparently lock the genes that are off in a silent state. *Polycomb* proteins can establish a stable chromatin conformation in which gene expression is repressed, even through many generations of cell division. The fact that HP1 and *polycomb* proteins share the chromo domain motif suggests that heterochromatin may participate in the long-term regulation of gene expression that is essential for development of complex organisms.

Large-Scale Structural Compartmentation of the Nucleus

In addition to the existence of higher-order structural domains within each chromosome, it now appears that the nucleus possesses further levels of organization. For example, individual chromosomes occupy discrete territories within cell nuclei and do not intermingle with one another to any appreciable extent. This was originally seen for the giant polytene chromosomes in *Drosophila* but is equally true for chromosomes in human somatic cells (Fig. 13–20). Genes being actively transcribed are usually located at the periphery of the domains, as are factors involved in RNA processing (see Chapter 15).

To date, the question of whether chromosomes occupy preferred positions within the cell nucleus remains little explored even though it could potentially have important implications for the regulation of gene expression in tissues. In neurons, the X chromosome is usually positioned near the nuclear envelope, but generally, chromosomes do not appear to have favored nuclear locations. Figure 13–20 shows one particularly clear example of a correlation between gene location in the nucleus and its transcriptional activity. These experiments with living cells also have revealed that chromosome territories can change their conformation (i.e., become more compact or more stretched out), and even change their location within nuclei (see Fig. 13–7). At the large-scale domain level, movements are slow and appear to be correlated with replication of DNA. This fits with earlier observations that the distribution of centromeres changes across the cell cycle. During G_1 phase, centromeres tend to cluster together and to be located toward the periphery of the nucleus. During S phase, they tend to be much more dispersed and to move into the nuclear interior. Currently, there is no explanation for the mechanisms underlying this movement of chromosomes within the nucleus. The phenomenon is of particular interest in view of the observations that, upon activation, certain genes can relocate from regions ("compartments") of the nucleus where transcription is relatively infrequent

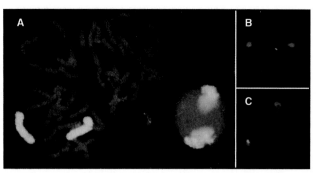

Figure 13-20 Organization of chromosomes within mammalian cell nuclei probed by in situ hybridization. *A,* Chromosome 4 occupies a discrete domain within the cell nucleus. Chromosome painting involves in situ hybridization with complex mixtures of DNA probes that come from all along a particular chromosome, performed under conditions in which the repeated sequences that are common to numerous chromosomes do not contribute to the image. *Left,* Spread chromosomes from a mitotic cell with the two chromosomes 4 appearing "painted." *Right,* An interphase nucleus showing two discrete territories occupied by chromosome 4. *B* and *C,* The CD4 gene *(green)* is located in the nucleoplasm in cells where it is expressed *(B)* but is associated with centromeric heterochromatin in cells where it is silent *(C).* (From Lamond AI, Earnshaw WC: Structure and function in the nucleus. Science 280:547–553, 1998, F1ACD.)

into areas where transcription is favored (see Fig. 13–20*B* and *C*). This provides a further level at which gene expression can be controlled.

Conclusions

The packaging of the DNA into nuclei and chromosomes remains one of the least understood areas of cell biology. Researchers have determined the structure of the nucleosome in molecular detail and are beginning to understand a good deal about how manipulation of nucleosomes promotes transcription of the DNA. However, levels of chromatin and nuclear organization beyond the nucleosome remain largely unmapped and unknown. Clearly, this is an important area to watch for future developments.

Selected Readings

Bell AC, Felsenfeld G: Stopped at the border: Boundaries and insulators. Curr Opin Genet Dev 9:191–198, 1999.

Belmont AS: Visualizing chromosome dynamics with GFP. Trends Cell Biol 11:250–257, 2001.

Belmont AS, Dietzel S, Nye AC, et al: Large-scale chromatin structure and function. Curr Opin Cell Biol 11:307–311, 1999.

Bird AP, Wolffe AP: Methylation-induced repression—belts, braces, and chromatin. Cell 99:451–454, 1999.

Brown CE, Lechner T, Howe L, et al: The many HATs of transcription coactivators. Trends Biochem Sci 25:15–19, 2000.

Earnshaw WC: Mitotic chromosome structure. BioEssays 9: 147–150, 1988.

Hennig W: Heterochromatin. Chromosoma. 108:1–9, 1999.

Hirano T: Chromosome cohesion, condensation, and separation. Annu Rev Biochem 69:115–144, 2000.

Jenuwein T, Allis CD: Translating the histone code. Science 293:1074–1080, 2001.

Koshland D, Strunnikov A: Mitotic chromosome condensation. Annu Rev Cell Dev Biol 12:305–333, 1996.

McGhee JD, Felsenfeld G: Nucleosome structure. Ann Rev Biochem 49:1115–1156, 1980.

Naar AM, Lemon BD, Tjian R: Transcriptional coactivator complexes. Annu Rev Biochem 70:475–501, 2001.

Ramakrishnan V: Histone structure and the organization of the nucleosome. Ann Rev Biophys Biomol Struct 26:83–112, 1997.

Varga-Weisz PD, Becker PB: Chromatin-remodeling factors: machines that regulate? Curr Opin Cell Biol 10:346–353, 1998.

Workman JL, Kingston RE: Alteration of nucleosome structure as a mechanism of transcriptional regulation. Annu Rev Biochem 67:545–579, 1998.

chapter 14

GENE EXPRESSION

Each organism, whether it has 600 genes *(Myco-plasma)*, 6000 genes (budding yeast), or 30,000 genes (humans), depends on reliable mechanisms to turn these genes on and off. This is called regulation of gene expression. In simple organisms, like bacteria and yeast, environmental signals, such as temperature or nutrient levels, control much of gene expression. In multicellular organisms, genetically programmed gene expression controls development from a fertilized egg. Within these organisms, cells send each other signals that control gene expression either through direct contact or via secreted molecules, such as growth factors and hormones.

Given the vast number of genes, even in simple organisms, regulation of gene expression is complicated. Fortunately, work over the past 20 years has revealed many important general principles that have simplified our thinking about gene expression. Proteins called **transcription factors** turn genes on or off by binding to particular DNA sequences adjacent to the sequences encoding the protein or RNA product of the gene. Transcription factors are numerous, representing approximately 6% of human genes. They are also quite diverse, binding to a wide range of DNA regulatory sites. Fortunately, they fall into a limited number of families with similar structures and binding mechanisms. Three types of DNA-dependent RNA polymerases respond to these regulatory proteins and copy DNA sequence into RNA. Regulation of transcription factors is achieved by variations in a limited number of mechanisms that control their synthesis, transport from the cytoplasm into the nucleus, and activity through post-translational modifications or binding to small molecular ligands.

The most important level of regulation is transcrip-

tion initiation, the first step in production of RNA transcripts. The past decade has seen the discovery of hundreds of key components in this process. This chapter examines the basic features of eukaryotic transcription units and the basal transcription machinery. Regulatory transcription factors that control the expression of several selected genes are discussed in the context of how external signals can reprogram patterns of gene expression. Finally, the chapter addresses the mechanisms by which mutation of transcription factor genes leads to human disease.

The Transcription Cycle

Synthesis of RNA by **RNA polymerases** is a cyclic process that can be broken down into three sets of events: initiation, elongation, and termination (Fig. 14–1). Each of these events consists of multiple individual steps. In the first step of the **initiation** process, RNA polymerase locates and binds to the chromosome near the beginning of the gene, forming a **preinitiation complex** at a sequence termed a **promoter.** This binding must be highly specific to distinguish promoter from nonpromoter DNA. Next, a conformational change in the polymerase-promoter complex results in formation of an **open complex** in which the DNA duplex is unpaired, allowing RNA polymerase access to nucleotide bases that are complementary to the start of the message. After formation of a phosphodiester bond between the first two complementary ribonucleotides, the polymerase translocates one base and repeats the process of phosphodiester bond formation, resulting in **elongation** of the nascent RNA. The elongation reaction cycle continues at an average rate of about 20 to 30 nucleotides per second until the complete gene has been transcribed. Elongation is not

Chapter by Jeffrey L. Corden.

215

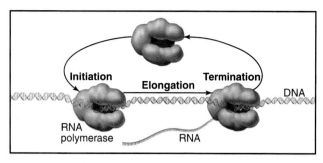

Figure 14-1 The transcription cycle. The transcription reaction consists of three basic steps in which the RNA polymerase initiates transcription at the promoter, elongates the nascent RNA copy of one of the DNA strands, and terminates transcription upon completion of the message.

a uniform reaction, however, as RNA polymerase pauses at certain sequences, which is an important regulatory step in transcription.

The final step in the transcription cycle is **termination.** In this reaction, the polymerase reaches a signal on DNA that causes an extended pause in elongation. Given enough time and the appropriate sequence context, the nascent transcript dissociates from the elongating RNA polymerase and the DNA template returns to a base-paired conformation. Ultimately, RNA polymerase dissociates from the template and is free to begin a new search for a promoter.

The Transcription Unit

The gene-coding and regulatory (*cis*-acting) DNA sequences that direct transcription initiation, elongation, and termination are collectively called a **transcription unit.** Figure 14–2 shows a simple RNA polymerase II transcription unit encoding the human hemoglobin β-chain. Although only a small fraction of this region encodes the β-globin polypeptide, the adjacent regulatory sequences are crucial for proper expression of β-globin. Genetic defects resulting in decreased β-globin production are called β-thalassemias. Such mutations can occur either in the coding region, resulting in an unstable or truncated polypeptide, or in the adjacent control regions, leading to low levels of transcription or aberrant processing of the newly synthesized RNA (see Chapter 15). Thus, the transcription unit can be thought of as a linked series of modules, all of which must be functional for the gene to be transcribed at the correct level.

Each of the steps in the transcription cycle can potentially serve as the target of regulatory molecules. The frequency of initiation varies among different promoters as dictated by the need for the gene product. The initiation reaction is most often regulated presumably because this prevents synthesis of messages that encode unneeded products. Elongation and termination can also be regulated, as can the splicing and

further processing of messenger RNAs (mRNAs) discussed in Chapter 15. The sum of these nuclear regulatory steps, together with cytoplasmic regulation of mRNA stability and translation efficiency, contributes to the wide variation seen in the abundance of different mRNAs and proteins in particular types of cells.

Biogenesis of RNA

A typical eukaryotic cell contains about two to three times more RNA than genomic DNA. This RNA is composed of molecules, usually several hundred to several thousand nucleotides long, that are distributed between the nucleus, where RNA synthesis occurs, and the cytoplasm, where RNA is used to synthesize proteins. Cells have three different types of RNA: (1) **ribosomal RNA (rRNA;** see Chapter 18), the most abundant type, making up about 75% of the total; (2) small, stable RNAs, such as **transfer RNA (tRNA;** see Chapter 2), **small nuclear RNAs (snRNA;** see Chapter 15), involved in splicing and **5S rRNA,** which comprise about 15%; and (3) **mRNA** and its precursor **hnRNA** (heterogeneous nuclear RNA), which account for only 10%.

Transcription of cellular RNA takes place in the nucleus and is linked to subsequent steps that process the nascent transcript in preparation for its eventual function (see Chapter 15 for a complete discussion of these steps). For mRNA precursors, this includes methylation and capping of the 5′ end of the nascent tran-

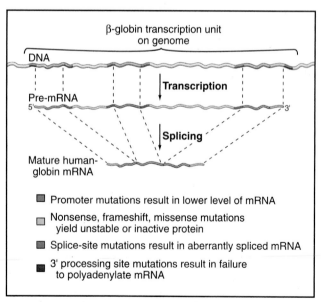

Figure 14-2 The transcription unit of a protein coding gene. The nucleotide sequence of one of the two DNA strands is transcribed into a complementary pre-mRNA copy. The pre-mRNA is processed by removing introns and splicing together the protein-coding exons *(orange).* The DNA sequences required for expression of a functional β-globin protein are indicated in different colors. Mutations in any of these sequences can lead to decreased β-globin expression.

script. Most messages are also spliced to remove introns; the 3' end of the message is then cleaved, and a stretch of adenosine residues is added. The mRNA is then transported to the cytoplasm where it serves as the template for protein synthesis.

Ribosomal RNA is synthesized from a set of tandemly repeated genes as a single molecule, which is cleaved to give the final 28S, 5.8S, and 18S RNAs (Fig. 14–3). These are assembled, together with 5S RNA and about 80 proteins, into ribosomes in the nucleolus. Transfer RNA is synthesized in the nucleus and transported to the cytoplasm, where it is charged with amino acids prior to participating in protein synthesis (see Chapter 18). snRNAs are synthesized and processed in the nucleus. From there, they migrate to the cytoplasm, where they acquire essential proteins, and then return to the nucleus, where they function in the enzymatic reactions of RNA processing (splicing; see Chapter 15). The postsynthetic processing pathway that a particular transcript follows is dictated, in part, by the transcription machinery that is used to initiate and elongate the transcript and by certain features of the nascent RNA.

Three Eukaryotic RNA Polymerases

Three different RNA polymerases transcribe the three classes of eukaryotic RNA (Fig. 14–4A). These polymerases can be distinguished experimentally on the basis of their sensitivity to the fungal toxin α-**amanitin,** with RNA polymerase II being the most sensitive and RNA polymerase I being the most resistant. RNA polymerase I localizes to the nucleolus, where it synthesizes rRNA. RNA polymerase II synthesizes mRNA in the nucleoplasm and several snRNAs involved in RNA splicing. RNA polymerase III synthesizes tRNA, 5S rRNA, and the 7S RNA of the signal recognition particle (see Chapter 18). RNA polymerase I synthesizes one species, whereas RNA polymerase III synthesizes several hundred species of highly abundant transcripts. The pool of mRNAs is more complex, however. Most cells have approximately 20,000 different species of mRNA. The relative abundance of individual mRNAs can vary widely from just a few copies to more than 10,000 copies per cell. Thus, RNA polymerase II must recognize thousands of different promoters and transcribe them with widely varying efficiency. In contrast, RNA polymerases I and III are specialized for the high-volume transcription necessary to produce rRNAs (>100,000 copies per cell) and other abundant, small, stable RNAs.

The RNA polymerases are multi-subunit enzymes with combined molecular weights of nearly 500,000 D. The three eukaryotic RNA polymerases are composed of up to 10 different subunits, most of which are unique to each enzyme (see Fig. 14–4A). The sub-

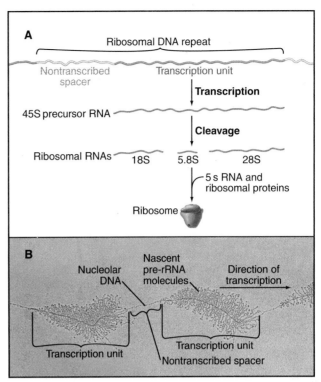

Figure 14–3 Ribosomal RNA transcription unit. Ribosomal RNA is transcribed from a set of transcription units arrayed as tandem copies of the same transcription unit. *A,* Map showing the arrangement of sequences in a typical ribosomal DNA repeat. *B,* Electron micrograph showing two active rRNA transcription units. Note that each transcription unit is transcribed by multiple RNA polymerases. As the polymerases traverse the gene, the attached nascent RNA is extended, giving a tree-like appearance. (*B,* Courtesy of Yvonne Osheim, University of Virginia, Charlottesville.)

units assemble into a structure that is roughly spherical, with a diameter of approximately 150Å. The most prominent feature is a cleft that is 25Å wide, large enough to accommodate the DNA template (see Fig. 14–4B). The active site is located on the back wall of the cleft. The framework of this structure is provided by the two largest subunits that comprise the two lobes that clamp down on the template DNA.

The multiple eukaryotic RNA polymerases apparently originated through duplication of primordial subunit genes, followed by evolution of specialized functions. Specialization was balanced, however, by the need to retain the structural elements required for RNA synthesis. In each eukaryotic RNA polymerase, the largest subunits are homologous to the bacterial β'- and β-subunits that make up the catalytic core of prokaryotic RNA polymerases (Fig. 14–4C). The structure of a bacterial RNA polymerase reveals that the most conserved residues are located on the inner surfaces of the enzyme where they are likely to be involved in the synthesis of RNA (Fig. 14–4D).

Transcription does not necessarily require such large enzymes. Bacteriophages have evolved structur-

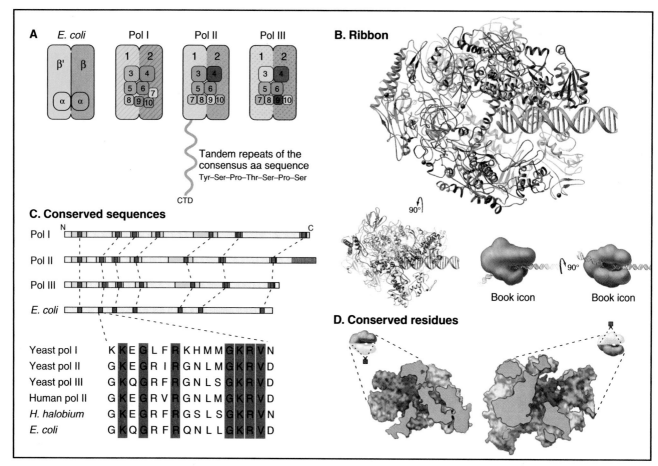

Figure 14–4 Multiple RNA polymerases. *A,* Eukaryotic cells have three different polymerases that share three common subunits (numbers 5, 6, and 8) and have a number of other related, but distinct, subunits (indicated by related colors and distinct shading). *B,* A ribbon diagram of the structure of RNA polymerase II showing the arrangement of different subunits (colored as in part *A*). Metal ions are indicated as red balls. A prominent cleft, large enough to accommodate a DNA template, is formed between the two largest subunits. The model DNA fragment is shown for size comparison only. *C,* Conserved amino acid sequences are dispersed throughout the largest subunits. Red rectangles indicate sequences conserved among both prokaryotes and eukaryotes. Yellow rectangles represent sequences conserved among the three different eukaryotic RNA polymerases. *H. halobium* is *Halobacterium halobium. D,* Conserved residues are located on the inner surface of the RNA polymerase. (*B,* PDB file: 1I50; Reference: Cramer P, Bushnell DA, Kornberg RD: Structural basis of transcription: RNA polymerase II at 2.8 angstrom resolution. Science 292:1863–1876, 2001. *D,* From Zhang G, Campbell EA, Minakhin L, et al: Crystal structure of *Thermus aquaticus* core RNA polymerase at 3.3 Å resolution. Cell 98:811–824, 1999.)

ally distinct, DNA-dependent RNA polymerases that are one-fifth the size of the eukaryotic enzymes, yet are able to carry out complete transcription cycles. The complexity of the eukaryotic enzymes is likely attributable to the need for regulation, with additional subunits acting as sites for interaction with regulatory proteins. Domains that differ among the three types of eukaryotic RNA polymerase are likely to be involved in certain functions, such as interaction with cofactors that are unique to a particular class of polymerase. One example of a class-specific domain is found in the largest subunit of RNA polymerase II, which has an unusual repetitive **carboxyl-terminal domain (CTD)** made up of tandem repeats of the consensus heptapeptide TyrSerProThrSerProSer. This domain has been implicated in the formation of an RNA polymerase II complex that contains many of the cofactors

needed for initiation. The CTD is highly phosphorylated in vivo, and the timing of CTD phosphorylation suggests that this modification may be involved in the transition between the initiation and elongation steps of transcription. The CTD also binds to pre-mRNA processing factors, suggesting that it plays a role in coupling transcription and the subsequent processing of the nascent mRNA.

Basal RNA Polymerase Promoters

A promoter can loosely be defined as the sum of DNA sequences necessary for transcription initiation. This definition is not sufficient, however, as most genes are regulated (positively or negatively) at the transcription initiation level. Thus, a distinction must be made between **basal levels of transcription** (in the absence of any regulatory factors) and **regulated** (activated or repressed) **transcription** directed by the function of gene regulatory proteins. Both basal and regulated levels can vary from promoter to promoter depending on the precise sequence of the promoter DNA and the abundance of its associated factors. Strong promoters drive the expression of genes whose products are required in abundance, whereas weaker promoters are tailored for expression of rare proteins or RNAs. In multicellular organisms, a promoter may direct expression at an intermediate level in some cells, at an activated level in others, and at a repressed level in yet others.

Eukaryotic RNA polymerase I and II promoter elements are situated similarly to those in *Escherichia coli,* just upstream of the transcription start site. In contrast, RNA polymerase III promoters contain key promoter elements within the transcribed sequences.

RNA polymerase I recognizes a single type of promoter located upstream of each copy of the long tandem array of pre-rRNA coding sequences (Fig. 14–5*A*). The core element of this promoter overlaps the transcription start site. An upstream control element located approximately 100 bp from the start site stimulates transcription. RNA polymerase I is not required in yeast cells that contain a pre-rRNA gene under control of an RNA polymerase II promoter. Therefore, if RNA polymerase I does recognize other promoters, these transcripts are not required for viability.

Comparison of the first eukaryotic protein-coding gene sequences revealed a conserved consensus sequence located approximately 30 bp upstream of the transcription start site of most RNA polymerase II–transcribed genes (Fig. 14–5*B*). This consensus sequence—TATAAAA—is called a **TATA box** and shows some similarity to the bacterial "Pribnow box" which is located about 10 bp upstream from all bacterial genes. In addition to the TATA box, a less conserved promoter element, the **initiator,** is found in the vicinity of the transcription start site of many genes. RNA polymerase II–transcribed genes that do not contain TATA boxes often contain strong initiator elements. Together, these two elements account for the basal promoter activity of most protein-coding genes. Additional sequences upstream and downstream of the TATA box have been identified in some promoters.

Two types of RNA polymerase III promoters have been identified; in both, key elements lie within the transcribed sequences (see Fig. 14–5). tRNA genes contain two 11-bp elements, the A box and B box, centered about 15 bp from the 5′ and 3′ ends of the coding sequence, respectively. The 5S-rRNA gene contains a single internal element, the C box, located in the center of the coding region.

General Transcription Factors

Purified eukaryotic RNA polymerase on its own cannot initiate transcription from promoters known to be active in vivo. Specific in vitro transcription can be obtained in extracts from nuclei, and fractionation of such extracts has led to the identification of additional factors necessary for specific transcription by purified RNA polymerase in vitro. Most of these factors are unique to each RNA polymerase and, because they are required for transcription of most promoters (within each class), they are termed **general transcription factors (GTFs)**. GTFs are remarkably conserved among different eukaryotes, and several are present in *Archaea.* Although most of the factors required for transcription by each class of polymerase are distinct, there is at least one factor, first identified as the *TATA box–binding protein* (TBP), that is common to all three polymerase systems. The following discussion focuses on both the similarities and differences in transcription initiation involving the three forms of eukaryotic RNA polymerase.

RNA Polymerase II Factors

The RNA polymerase II GTFs comprise more than 20 polypeptides with an aggregate molecular weight of more than 10^6 D. Table 14–1 lists the known human GTFs. The genes encoding these basal transcription factors have been cloned, and the role of the different factors in transcription initiation has been established.

Before RNA polymerase II can initiate transcription in vitro, an ordered assembly of factors at the pro-

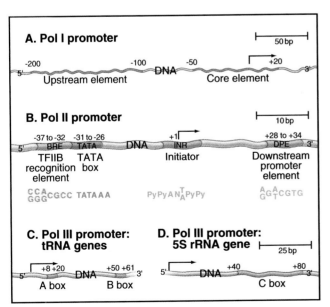

Figure 14–5 *A* to *D,* Eukaryotic promoters. The three RNA polymerases recognize different promoter sequences. Positions of promoter elements are indicated with respect to the start of transcription (+1). For the RNA polymerase II promoter elements, the consensus sequences are shown. Not all polymerase II promoters contain all of these elements.

table 14–1

SUMMARY OF EUKARYOTIC RNA POLYMERASE II GENERAL TRANSCRIPTION FACTORS

Factor	No. of Subunits	Subunit M_r (KDa)	Functions
TFIIA	3	12,19,35	Stabilizes binding of TBP and TFIIB
TFIIB	1	25	Binds TBP, selects start site, and recruits polymerase II
TFIID	12	15–250	Interacts with regulatory factors
(TBP)	1	38	Subunit of TFIID. Specifically recognizes the TATA box
TFIIE	2	34,57	Recruits TFIIH
TFIIF	2	30,74	Binds polymerase II and TFIIB
TFIIH	9	35–98	Unwinds promoter DNA; phosphorylates CTD (C-terminal domain of RNA polymerase II)
Polymerase II	12	10–220	Catalyzes RNA synthesis
Total	42	~1,000	

TBP, TATA box–binding protein

moter must occur. Assembly of the RNA polymerase II **preinitiation complex** (Fig. 14–6*A*) begins with the binding of TFIID, a large factor (~700 kD) consisting of a TBP and a set of **TBP-associated factors** called **TAFs**. TBP alone is sufficient for basal transcription, whereas TAFs apparently serve as targets for further activation of transcription (see subsequent sections). TBP is the first polypeptide in the basal transcription machinery to recognize a specific DNA sequence during the initiation process. DNA binding is provided by a highly conserved C-terminal 180–amino acid domain whose structure, complexed with TATA box promoter DNA, has been determined by x-ray crystallography. TBP is a saddle-shaped monomer with an axis of 2-fold symmetry (see Fig. 14–6*B*). The interacting surface of TBP (corresponding to the underside of the "saddle") binds to the minor groove of the TATA sequence, which is splayed open in the process. A pronounced DNA bend at each end of the TATAAA element is produced by the binding of TBP (see Fig. 14–6*C*).

The TFIID–TATA box complex serves as a binding site for additional positive and negative regulators. **TFIIA** associates with the TBP-DNA complex and serves two functions. First, it stabilizes the TBP-DNA interaction. Second, TFIIA prevents the binding of repressors that arrest further initiation complex formation. TFIIA contacts DNA upstream from the TATA box and makes limited contacts with TBP. Much of the surface of TBP and TFIIA remains accessible for interaction with other GTFs and regulatory proteins.

The next step in assembly of the initiation complex is binding of **TFIIB,** which binds to one side of TBP and makes contacts with DNA upstream and downstream of the TATA box (see Fig. 14–6*D*). Mutations in the yeast gene encoding TFIIB show altered mRNA start-site selection, indicating that TFIIB establishes the spacing between the TATA box and the transcription start site. TFIIB interacts directly with TBP and RNA polymerase II and is thus essential for the next steps in initiation complex assembly.

RNA polymerase II enters into the preinitiation complex (see Fig. 14–6*A*) in association with **TFIIF.** This factor is related to bacterial σ-factor and acts to stabilize the interaction of RNA polymerase II with TFIIB and TBP. In addition, TFIIF binds to free polymerase and prevents interactions with nonpromoter DNA sites.

TFIIE and **TFIIH** are the final general factors to enter the preinitiation complex. Binding of these factors results in more stable protein DNA contacts in the vicinity of the transcription start site. In addition, TFIIH contains a number of subunits with enzymatic activities, including both 5′–3′ and 3′–5′ helicase, DNA-dependent adenosine triphosphatase (ATPase), and CTD kinase activities. RNA polymerase II initiation requires hydrolysis of the β-γ phosphate bond in adenosine triphosphate (ATP), a reaction catalyzed by each of the TFIIH activities and not seen during initiation by RNA polymerases I or III. Both the helicase and CTD kinase activities of TFIIH are stimulated by TFIIE.

The TFIIH **helicase** activity uses the energy from ATP hydrolysis to unwind a short stretch of promoter DNA at the transcription start site. This unpairing of DNA allows RNA polymerase II to recognize the template strand, bind the complementary nucleotides, and synthesize the first few phosphodiester bonds. For some promoters, the requirement for TFIIH unwinding activity is obviated if the template is negatively supercoiled. In such cases, unwinding energy is stored in

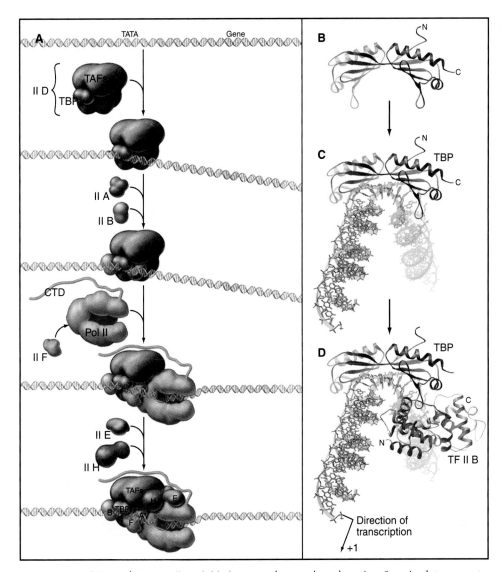

Figure 14-6 RNA polymerase II preinitiation complex on the adenovirus-2 major late promoter DNA. The sequential assembly of general transcription factors leads to a preinitiation complex with the promoter region in the closed complex *(A)*. Helicase activities present in TFIIH use the energy of ATP to unwind the promoter, leading to formation of an open complex. Binding of TBP *(B)* leads to a pronounced bend in the DNA *(C)*. TFIIB interacts both upstream and downstream of the TATA box and directs RNA polymerase to the transcription start site *(D)*. (TBP + DNA coordinates [parts *B, C,* and *D*], Courtesy of Stephen Burley, Rockefeller University. PDB file: 1VOL.)

the DNA conformation, and RNA polymerase II requires only TBP and TFIIB for initiation.

TFIIH contains eight polypeptides, several of which have functions outside of transcription initiation. The protein kinase activity that phosphorylates the CTD is Cdk-activating kinase (Cak), itself a Cdk-cyclin complex that phosphorylates and activates other cyclin-dependent kinases (see Chapter 43). In the initiation complex, phosphorylation of the CTD is thought to release the CTD from interactions with GTFs, allowing the transition to the transcription elongation phase. Other TFIIH subunits have been identified as components of the DNA repair machinery. Several genes encoding TFIIH subunits are mutated in diseases affect-

ing human DNA excision repair, suggesting that TFIIH may serve to link transcription to DNA repair (see later section).

Holoenzyme

The ordered assembly of GTFs in vitro requires a substantial number of specific protein-protein interactions. In vivo, many of these steps are consolidated through the assembly of large macromolecular complexes containing RNA polymerase II, several of the GTFs, other factors that alter chromatin structure, and various additional transcription factors. One of these complexes, the **mediator,** contains more than 20 polypeptides

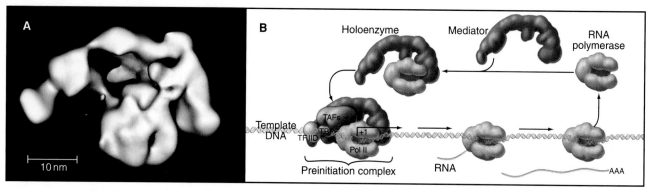

Figure 14-7 RNA polymerase II holoenzyme. *A,* The three-dimensional structure of the yeast holoenzyme, reconstructed from electron micrographs of particles preserved in negative stain. *B,* The mediator complex assists RNA polymerase II in locating promoters through interactions with factors bound to promoter proximal and/or enhancer sequences. Interaction with TFIID, bound at the TATA box, is important in assembling a productive complex. TFIID is thought to remain bound to the TATA box and to facilitate subsequent rounds of initiation. (*A,* Courtesy of Joshua Davis and Francisco Asturias, Scripps Research Institute, La Jolla, CA.)

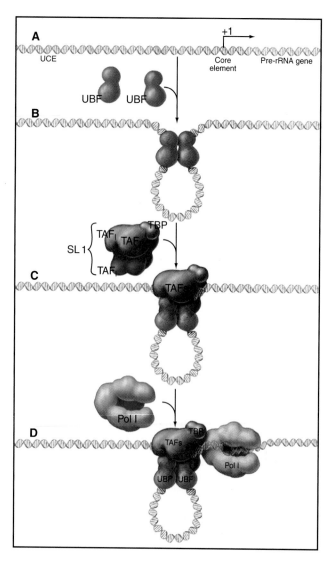

Figure 14-8 RNA polymerase I preinitiation complex. Ribosomal RNA promoters *(A)* assemble a preinitiation complex consisting of an upstream binding factor (UBF) *(B)* and a multi-subunit factor called SL1 *(C)* that contains TBP. Together, these factors recruit RNA polymerase I *(D).* UCE, upstream control element.

(many with unknown functions) but lacks RNA polymerase II. Mediator reversibly interacts with RNA polymerase II to form a **holoenzyme** (Fig. 14–7) that, unlike the bacterial RNA polymerase holoenzyme, does not contain all of the factors necessary for initiation, as it requires TBP for promoter recognition. RNA polymerase II holoenzyme responds to transcription activators (described in a subsequent section) in vitro, suggesting that one role for the multitude of proteins in this complex is to offer multiple interaction sites for recruitment of holoenzyme to the promoter. The presence of chromatin-remodeling factors (see subsequent section) suggests that changes in template structure could be another holoenzyme function.

RNA Polymerase I Factors

Initiation at RNA polymerase I promoters can also proceed through an ordered assembly of transcription factors (Fig. 14–8). The **upstream binding factor** binds to the **upstream control element** and to part of the core element, which are brought together by DNA looping. This initial complex is stabilized by **selectivity factor 1** (SL1), which is a complex of TBP with three RNA polymerase I–specific TAFs.

RNA Polymerase III Factors

The assembly of RNA polymerase III initiation complexes varies on different promoters (Fig. 14–9). Initiation at tRNA genes begins with the binding of **TFIIIC**

to the A and B boxes. **TFIIIB** then binds upstream of the A box at a sequence determined both by the interaction with TFIIIC and by the DNA-binding capacity of TBP. Once the TFIIIC-TFIIIB complex is assembled, RNA polymerase III can initiate transcription. Multiple rounds of initiation can occur on the stable DNA-TFIIIC-TFIIIB complex.

Transcription of 5S rRNA genes requires an additional factor called **TFIIIA**. This protein was the first transcription factor and the first zinc finger protein to be identified. TFIIIA recognizes the C box located near the center of the 5S rRNA–coding region. TFIIIC then binds by making contacts on each side of TFIIA, in much the same way that the A and B boxes are contacted on tRNA genes. Finally, TFIIIB binds through interactions with TFIIIC and DNA, and the resulting preinitiation complex is recognized by RNA polymerase III.

Other Initiations

In addition to the three classical transcription systems, there are several other forms of transcription initiation that warrant mention. First, not all RNA polymerase II promoters contain the TATA box element. In these cases, the initiator element provides the primary sequence target, and its recognition requires the function of one of several auxiliary factors that are thought to bind to the initiator. Despite the lack of a TATA box, these promoters still require TBP, presumably because it serves to stabilize the binding of required TAFs.

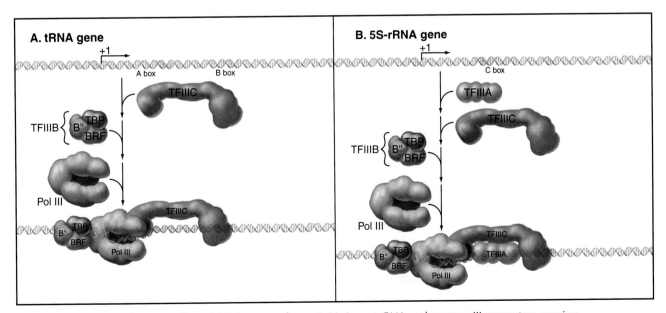

Figure 14–9 RNA polymerase III preinitiation complexes. Initiation at RNA polymerase III promoters requires recognition of sequences within the transcribed sequences. These sequences differ for tRNA and 5S ribosomal genes. *A,* In the case of tRNA genes, only TFIIIC is required for specific binding. *B,* For 5S genes, the internal element is recognized by the specific DNA-binding factor TFIIIA. BRF, TFIIB-related factor.

Another unusual set of promoters drives expression of the snRNA genes. These promoters contain binding sites for both RNA polymerase II and RNA polymerase III factors, and they can be transcribed by either polymerase. Like other eukaryotic promoters, TBP is required for transcription. Unlike the other systems, the snRNA promoters recruit a novel TBP complex, SNAP-C, which contains a unique set of TAFs.

Summary of the Eukaryotic Basal Transcription Machinery

Despite the evolutionary divergence of the multiple eukaryotic RNA polymerases and the specialization of each polymerase for a unique set of promoters, the fundamental mechanisms of transcription have been conserved. This conservation is reflected not only in similar sequences of the subunits of the polymerases themselves, but in the presence of TBP and TFIIB homologues among the GTFs used by each class of polymerase. Indeed, *Archaea,* which have only a single RNA polymerase, contain both TBP and TFIIB. This observation suggests that initiation mechanisms employing GTFs evolved before the duplication of the RNA polymerases.

Why are so many factors required to make a transcript? It seems likely that part of the complexity is necessary to generate multiple sites for interaction of regulatory factors that could either activate or repress the assembly or function of the preinitiation complex. A second role for the complex set of factors could be in targeting the polymerases to specific sites in the nucleus. Finally, some of the factors could act subsequent to initiation by loading elongation, splicing, or termination factors onto the RNA polymerases.

■ Transcription Elongation and Termination

Until now, the discussion of transcription has focused on the recognition of potential promoter sites on DNA and the formation of the first few phosphodiester bonds creating the nascent transcript. The final stage of initiation leads to successful elongation and movement of the polymerase away from the promoter. This process of **promoter clearance** is associated with structural changes in the polymerase that prepare the enzyme for efficient RNA synthesis and render it susceptible to the action of factors that can regulate the elongation process. Such regulatory factors, together with structural features of the nascent transcript, influence the elongation process and can trigger the termination of transcription and the dissociation of the ternary elongation complex containing the DNA template, nascent RNA, and RNA polymerase.

The Catalytic Cycle

The DNA-dependent RNA polymerases catalyze synthesis of an RNA polymer from ribonucleoside 5'-triphosphates (ATP, guanosine triphosphate [GTP], cytidine triphosphate [CTP], and uridine triphosphate [UTP]) according to the following reaction:

$$(NMP)_n + NTP \longrightarrow (NMP)_{n+1} + PP_i$$

where $(NMP)_n$ is the RNP polymer, NTP is one of the three ribonucleoside 5'-triphosphates, and PP_i is pyrophosphate. Polymerase extends the RNA chain in the 5' to 3' direction by adding ribonucleotide units to the chain's 3' end. Selection of the incoming NTP is directed by the DNA template and takes place at the transcription bubble, an unpaired segment of the DNA template (see Fig. 14–10B). The 3' hydroxyl group acts as a nucleophile, attacking the α-phosphate of the incoming NTP in a reaction similar to that seen in DNA replication (see Chapter 45, Fig. 45–2). This reaction proceeds in vivo at a rate of 20 to 30 nucleotides per second. At this rate, polymerase takes more than 17 hours to synthesize a single transcript from the mammalian dystrophin gene, which is more than 2.4 million base pairs long. Clearly, the elongation complex must be very stable!

The Transcription Elongation Complex

Efficient synthesis of RNA requires balancing two competing demands. First, the elongation complex (Fig. 14–10) must be very stable because if the complex prematurely dissociates, polymerase must restart transcription from the promoter. The complex must also be loosely bound so that the polymerase can easily translocate along the DNA template. The structure of RNA polymerase is well designed to meet these needs. The cleft formed at the interface between the two largest subunits is open when the polymerase is in the initiation complex. Once the first few RNA phosphodiester bonds are formed, the polymerase undergoes a conformational change. Subunits at the outer edge of the cleft close like jaws to encircle the DNA template. In this structure, the front end of the transcription bubble is positioned at the back wall of the cleft, close to a magnesium ion that forms part of the catalytic center. A nearby channel is thought to allow access to nucleoside triphosphate substrates.

Pausing, Arrest, and Termination

RNA polymerase does not elongate at a constant rate, but rather synthesizes RNA in short spurts between long pauses. Such reversible pausing constitutes the rate-limiting step in elongation, is dependent on the sequence of the RNA being transcribed, and is regulated by factors that interact with RNA polymerase.

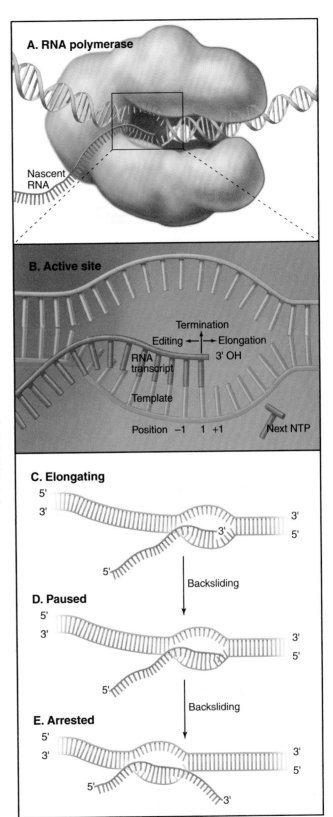

Figure 14-10 Transcription elongation. *A,* Model of the transcription elongation complex consisting of RNA polymerase, template DNA, and nascent RNA transcript. RNA polymerases interact with the template upstream and downstream of the transcription bubble. *B,* The active site of RNA polymerase positions the growing end of the nascent transcript in the appropriate location for the addition of the next nucleoside triphosphate (NTP). After each single nucleotide addition, the polymerase may translocate forward and repeat the nucleotide addition *(C),* slide backward and pause for a variable time *(D),* slide further backward allowing removal of the transcript and termination of transcription *(E).*

With each nucleotide addition reaction, polymerase has three choices. Moving forward, the polymerase can incorporate another nucleotide. Alternatively, the polymerase can move in the reverse direction. In this process, the 3' end of the growing chain is displaced from the DNA template. This pause may be short, and the polymerase may move forward again and continue synthesis. If conditions are not appropriate for elongation, the polymerase may move back several more bases. Such backtracking extrudes a segment of the nascent transcript from the transcription bubble. This segment can be removed from the transcript by ribonuclease activity present at the active site of the polymerase. This activity is stimulated by specific elongation factors and is thought to provide the polymerase with the capacity to edit out incorrectly incorporated nucleotides.

Long pauses can lead to complete removal of the nascent transcript, collapse of the transcription bubble, and dissociation of the RNA polymerase from the DNA template. This form of termination is important for ensuring that only the intended gene is transcribed. In an alternative pathway, endonucleolytic cleavage of the end of the nascent transcript results in a new 3' end located in the active site. In this case, transcription can continue until the eventual termination signal is reached.

Gene-Specific Transcription

Promoter Proximal and Enhancer Elements

The development of in vivo techniques for analyzing eukaryotic promoter function has led to the discovery of a number of regulatory elements in addition to the TATA box. In these experiments, plasmids containing a promoter or its mutated derivative are reintroduced into eukaryotic cells by transfection or microinjection. Transcription directed by the cloned promoter is detected by one of several approaches that allow the transgene product to be identified from among the background of cellular transcripts. In one approach (Fig. 14–11A), the promoter drives expression of a bacterial reporter gene like chloramphenicol acetyltransferase (CAT) or β-galactosidase, which can conveniently be assayed in extracts from transfected cells that contain little or no background activity. This approach applies only to RNA polymerase II, which produces translatable mRNAs. A more direct analysis, applicable to transcription by all three RNA polymerases, makes use of specific RNA or DNA probes to quantify precisely RNAs transcribed from the transgene. Such experiments have demonstrated that basal promoter elements are insufficient for full expression of these reporter genes. Analysis of regions of DNA upstream of the transcription start site has suggested the exis-

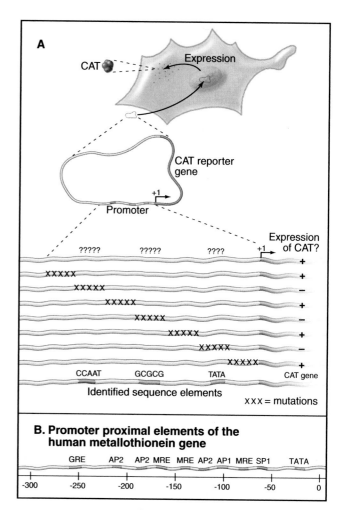

Figure 14–11 RNA polymerase II promoter regulatory elements. *A*, In vivo assays are used to identify key regulatory sequences. In the example shown, a promoter is placed in front of a gene encoding chloramphenicol acetyltransferase (CAT) and the resulting plasmid is transfected into cultured cells. This bacterial enzyme is easily assayed in eukaryotic cells because there is no endogenous activity. Targeted clusters of mutations, strategically placed throughout the promoter region, are tested for their effect on expression of the reporter gene. Mutations that reduce expression define important regulatory elements. *B*, The region immediately upstream of the metallothionein gene contains binding sites for several transcription factors. The elements are named for the factor that binds there: GRE (glucocorticoid response element), MRE (metal response element), and AP1, AP2, and SP1 (which bind factors of the same name).

tence of additional promoter elements. For RNA polymerase II, these elements fall into two classes. The first class of elements, located 50 to 100 bp upstream of the start of transcription, is termed promoter proximal elements. The second class, termed enhancers, is located at variable distances up to about 10 kb from the start of transcription.

Promoter proximal elements are short (~10 bp) sequences that serve as specific binding sites for transcription regulatory proteins. One example of a promoter proximal element is the CCAAT box in the promoter of the herpes simplex virus thymidine kinase gene. This site was identified by a technique called linker-scanning (see Fig. 14–11*A*) in which clustered mutations are introduced at regular intervals in the promoter. Mutations that result in a decrease in transcription define important sequences. In the case of the thymidine kinase promoter, the CCAAT and the TATAAA sequences are required for full transcription. Thymidine kinase expression also requires the sequence GGCGCC, which serves as the binding site for SP1, a transcription factor involved in expression of a number of so-called housekeeping genes whose products are involved in normal cellular functions. These promoter proximal elements are present in many different genes where they are necessary for constitutive expression.

Other promoter proximal elements are involved in regulated expression. Elements that confer response to cellular stress or exposure to heavy metals are also located in promoter proximal positions. Most promoters contain several different promoter proximal elements. This allows for complex regulation of transcription levels by varying the relative abundance or activity of the various factors. Figure 14–11*B* shows the location of regulatory elements directly upstream of the human metallothionein gene, whose product protects cells from the toxic effects of metals. The large number of regulatory sites suggests that this gene can be regulated by a variety of different mechanisms.

The first **enhancer** sequence was discovered in the promoter of the simian virus 40 early genes. This regulatory element has several features that distinguish it from other promoter elements. First, an enhancer increases the rate of initiation from a basal promoter even if it is located up to 10 kb away from the promoter. Second, enhancers work even if located internal to or downstream of the promoter. Finally, the enhancer element will work in either orientation relative to the promoter (Fig. 14–12). Enhancer elements are found in the vicinity of many but not all genes, but in most cases, the enhancer works in a cell type–specific fashion. An example is a sequence in an intron of the immunoglobulin heavy chain gene that enhances transcription in lymphocytes but not in other cells. This regulation of enhancer function is likely to be accomplished by changes in the levels of various enhancer-binding factors in different tissues.

Enhancers are considerably more complicated than promoter proximal elements and are, in fact, clusters of regulatory elements similar to the proximal elements. Apparently, there is a synergistic effect of clustering these sites that yields a more potent activating element and distinguishes enhancers from promoter proximal elements. Both enhancers and pro-

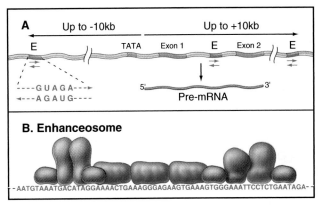

Figure 14–12 Enhancer elements. *A,* These condensed clusters of factor-binding sites can influence expression when located far from the promoter in either the upstream or downstream position. In addition, they work in either orientation with respect to transcription. *B,* Model enhancer showing the tight packing of several different DNA-binding proteins. These complexes fold into structures that have been called enhanceosomes.

moter proximal elements can be grafted onto different basal promoters and maintain their function. The enhancer can stimulate transcription from any basal promoter through protein-protein interactions that create a loop in the intervening DNA. Thus, even though an enhancer may be more than 1000 bp away from the start site of transcription, it is thought that proteins bound to the enhancer make direct physical contact with proteins bound near the transcription start site.

Gene-Specific Transcription Factors

To recognize specific DNA sequences like those present in promoter proximal and enhancer elements, a protein must be capable of "reading" DNA sequences. The 1990s witnessed the identification and characterization of hundreds of gene-specific transcription factors. Current estimates indicate that approximately 6% of the coding capacity of the human genome is devoted to transcription factors that recognize specific DNA sequences. However, even this large number of factors is not sufficient to allow each gene to be regulated by a unique factor. The apparent solution to this problem is to regulate individual genes through combinations of regulatory elements. Thus, the particular combination of factors that binds to a promoter can represent a unique regulatory set that allows a cell to respond very specifically to external signals. Most of the factors identified to date are activators. This is likely attributable to the need to overcome the generally repressive effect of chromatin (see later discussion). Specific repressors have also been identified and will be discussed here. How these factors bind DNA and regulate the function of the basal transcription machinery is the subject of the following sections.

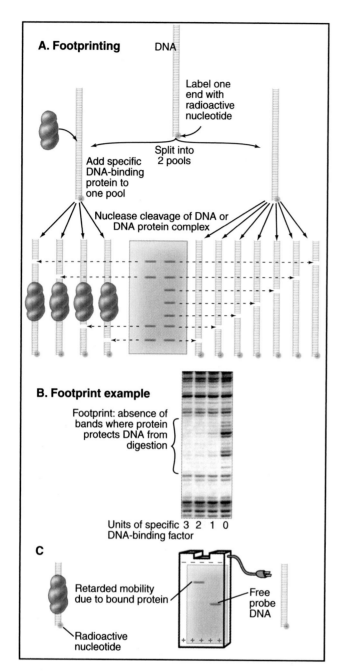

A. Footprinting   DNA

Label one end with radioactive nucleotide

Split into 2 pools

Add specific DNA-binding protein to one pool

Nuclease cleavage of DNA or DNA protein complex

B. Footprint example

Footprint: absence of bands where protein protects DNA from digestion

Units of specific   3 2   1   0
DNA-binding factor

C

Retarded mobility due to bound protein

Free probe DNA

Radioactive nucleotide

Figure 14-13 Two techniques for identifying proteins that bind to specific DNA sequences. *A,* and *B,* Footprinting assay. A fragment of DNA thought to contain a binding site is radiolabeled at one end of one strand. The labeled probe is then split into two fractions and the DNA-binding protein is added to one fraction. The two samples are then randomly cleaved with nuclease or chemical reagents in such a way as to cleave only one bond per DNA fragment. High-resolution electrophoresis is used to separate the cleaved fragments, and autoradiography reveals a ladder of fragments differing in length by a single base. *B,* Protein bound to DNA protects a limited region of DNA from cleavage, as revealed by the absence of bands in the radioactive ladder. *C,* Electrophoretic mobility shift assay. A short (20- to 50-bp), double-stranded DNA fragment is radiolabeled and bound to a protein sample. The complex is electrophoresed in a non-denaturing gel. The large protein bound to the DNA retards its mobility in the gel compared with the free DNA.

Methods for Identifying and Isolating Transcription Factors

Rapid progress in identifying and characterizing transcription factors has been made possible by the development of techniques that allow the detection and characterization of specific DNA-protein complexes. The first of these techniques is termed DNA footprinting. In this assay, protein is mixed with DNA that is radioactively labeled at one end (Fig. 14–13*A*). The resulting DNA-protein complex is then lightly digested with deoxyribonuclease to give, on average, one random cut per DNA molecule. The resulting population of cleaved DNA molecules is then stripped of protein and separated by gel electrophoresis. The area protected by a specific DNA-binding protein appears as a blank area or "footprint" that results from the protein blocking access of the nuclease in the binding region, thus leaving a gap in the family of digestion products of differing lengths.

A less precise but more versatile method of visualizing protein-DNA complexes is the DNA mobility shift assay (Fig. 14–13*C*). The principle of this technique is that fragments of DNA with a bound protein move more slowly during gel electrophoresis than the same DNA fragments without bound protein.

Both techniques allow detection of specific DNA-binding proteins in crude cellular extracts and thus can be used as assays for protein purification. Amino acid sequences of a purified DNA-binding protein can then be used to generate probes for cloning the gene that encodes the factor. Transcription factors can also be cloned directly by screening expression libraries with labeled DNA oligonucleotides corresponding to the sequence of the regulatory element and detecting proteins that bind to them. These approaches have been used to isolate hundreds of specific DNA-binding proteins that play specific roles in transcription regulation.

Transcription Factors as Modular Proteins

In addition to interaction with specific DNA sequences, transcription factors must interact both with regulatory molecules and the basal transcription machinery. Functional domains in transcription factors have been mapped by dissecting the factor genes and testing the different domains in vivo (Fig. 14–14). The surprising result of this type of analysis is that many transcription factors are modular proteins with discrete functional domains that can be exchanged without impairing activity. For example, exchanging the DNA-binding domains of the glucocorticoid and estrogen receptors creates a hybrid factor that recognizes estrogen-responsive promoters but activates transcription in response to glucocorticoid hormone. DNA-binding do-

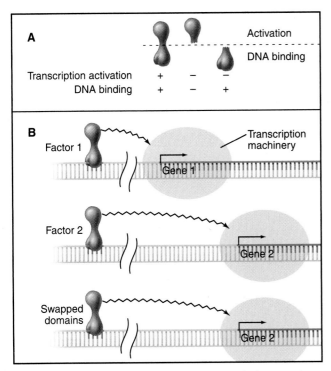

Figure 14-14 Transcription factors consist of discrete, functional modules. *A,* Domain characterization. Although the entire factor is required for activation, the bottom domain is sufficient for DNA binding. *B,* Domain swapping. The activation domain of one factor (activating gene 1) can be fused to the DNA-binding domain of a heterologous factor (activating gene 2). The resulting chimeric factor will only activate genes containing the recognition site for the DNA-binding domain (gene 2).

mains from bacterial regulatory proteins can also be engineered to perform as eukaryotic factors by grafting them to the activating domain from a eukaryotic factor. Such chimeric factors will stimulate transcription as long as two functions are maintained: specific DNA binding and transcription activation.

DNA-Binding Domains

Gene-specific transcription factors must bind to and release from their target DNA sequences with an appropriate specificity and affinity. This recognition problem involves structural, kinetic, and thermodynamic considerations. Structural studies have yielded important information about such protein-DNA interactions, in particular, the description of the complementary surfaces involved (shape recognition) and the chemistry of these surfaces (chemical recognition). Although at a coarse level, DNA structure appears monotonous, protein structure is more variable. Thus, it is not surprising that a variety of protein structures have evolved surfaces that are complementary to DNA and that display amino acid residues suitable for binding specific DNA sequences through unique three-dimen-

sional networks of hydrogen bonds, as well as van der Waals, hydrophobic, and electrostatic interactions.

The richest source of DNA sequence variation comes from the chemical groups present within the major groove. Specific DNA-binding proteins probe the major groove of double-stranded DNA with a small structural domain (usually, an α-helix) whose shape is complementary to the surface topography of a particular DNA sequence. The correct DNA sequence is recognized through multiple interactions between amino acid side chains in the recognition helix and the chemical groups on the edges of DNA bases in the major groove. Single amino acid changes in the recognition helix can change the sequence that is recognized. Protein-DNA complexes are stabilized by additional contacts between amino acid side chains and deoxyribose rings and phosphate groups.

The recognition domains of specific transcription factors typically interact with only 3 to 6 bp of DNA. Given the size and complexity of the typical mammalian genome, a sequence must be approximately 16 bp long to occur by chance only once. How then can genes be specifically recognized among the very large number of close but nonidentical sequences? There are several answers to this question. First, the recognition protein can either use several recognition domains or it can dimerize with itself or other DNA-binding proteins. Both of these strategies increase the length of the specific sequence to be recognized. The specific recognition sequences need not be contiguous, and, in fact, multiple recognition domains may sterically block each other unless they are spaced slightly apart. Binding of protein dimers can lead to recognition of sequences with two-fold rotational symmetry.

DNA-binding proteins can be grouped into families based on the structure of the domains used for DNA sequence recognition (Fig. 14-15). These include the **helix-turn-helix (HTH)** proteins, the **homeodomains, zinc finger** proteins, **steroid receptors, leucine zipper** proteins, and the **helix-loop-helix (HLH)** proteins. Although these families include most of the known transcription factors, there remain other, uncharacterized recognition domains. It is clear that nature has evolved a number of alternative strategies for specific sequence recognition. Within a given family, the recognition domain of each transcription factor has an amino acid sequence that targets the protein to a particular DNA sequence. Conversely, the same promoter element can be recognized by members of different families. The following sections discuss some of the more common eukaryotic DNA-binding domains.

Homeodomain

This motif was discovered in *Drosophila* proteins that regulate development and has been found in a wide

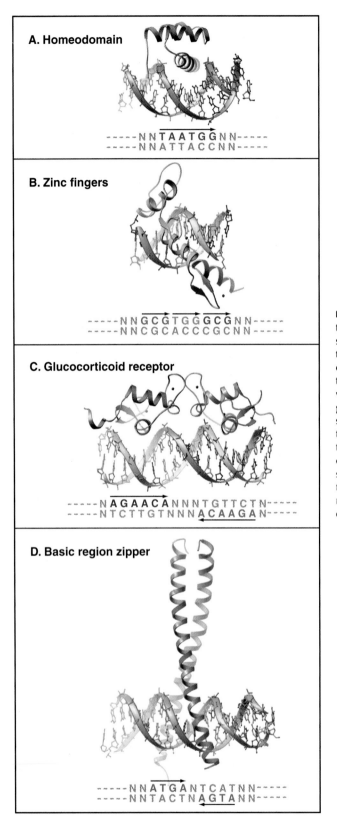

A. Homeodomain

```
-----NNTAATGGNN-----
-----NNATTACCNN-----
```

B. Zinc fingers

```
-----NNGCGTGGGCGNN-----
-----NNCGCACCCGCNN-----
```

C. Glucocorticoid receptor

```
-----NAGAACANNNTGTTCTN-----
-----NTCTTGTNNNACAAGAN-----
```

D. Basic region zipper

```
-----NNATGANTCATNN-----
-----NNTACTNAGTANN-----
```

Figure 14–15 Molecular structures of transcription factor DNA-binding domains. Recognition of specific DNA sequences requires interactions between amino acid side chains in the protein and chemical groups on the DNA bases. In each of the examples shown here, an α-helix interacts with specific bases through contacts in the major grove. *A*, The homeodomain α-helix recognizes a specific six-base sequence. *B*, A protein with three-zinc fingers recognizes three consecutive three-base sequences. *C*, The glucocorticoid receptor forms a dimer that recognizes the same six-base sequence in opposite orientations spaced three bases apart. *D*, A leucine zipper factor dimerizes to recognize a pair of four-base sites with opposite orientation spaced one base apart.

range of different eukaryotic transcription factors, including more than 150 in the human genome. The 60–amino acid domain forms a stable structure that can bind DNA specifically. Recognition is provided by a helix-turn-helix (HTH) motif composed of two helices, one of which sits in the major groove of the DNA-binding site contacting a recognition sequence of 6 bp (see Fig. 14–15A). The HTH structure is not a stable domain on its own but exists as part of a larger DNA-binding domain, such as the homeodomain. Additional binding affinity is provided in the homeodomain by a flexible arm that interacts with the minor groove.

Zinc Finger Proteins

The zinc finger protein sequence (see Fig. 14–15B), first identified in the RNA polymerase III basal factor TFIIIA, has since been found in a variety of different RNA polymerase II factors, including more than 600 human transcription factors. Each "finger" consists of a 30-residue sequence with conserved pairs of cysteines and histidines that bind a single zinc ion. The tip of the finger sticks into the major groove where it contacts three bases. Most zinc finger proteins contain multiple fingers, allowing longer sequences to be recognized in order to increase specificity. A similar structure is present in the steroid hormone receptor family, although in this case, the zinc ion is coordinated by four cysteine residues and the finger structure is composed of two helices rather than one. Steroid hormone receptors also contain a dimerization domain, allowing recognition of sequences with dyad symmetry (Fig. 14–15C).

Leucine Zipper Proteins

Leucine zipper domains are made up of two subdomains: a basic region that recognizes a specific DNA sequence and a series of repeated leucine residues (leucine zipper) that mediate dimerization. These domains form a continuous α-helix that can dimerize through formation of a coiled-coil structure involving specific contacts between hydrophobic leucine zipper domains (see Figs. 14–15D, 2–12B, and 2–12C). CAAT/enhancer binding protein (CEBP), the factor that recognizes the CCAAT sequence, was the first member of this family to be discovered. Dimers of leucine zipper proteins recognize short, inverted, repeat sequences. The zipper family comprises many members, some of which can cross-dimerize and recognize asymmetrical sequences. Another family of factors comprises the helix-loop-helix (HLH) proteins, which have the same type of basic region but differ in that they have two helical dimerization domains separated by a loop region.

Dimerization

An important aspect of transcription factor function is the ability to associate with other factors. Such associations can both expand the repertoire of DNA sequences that can be specifically recognized and inhibit the recognition of other sites. In the case of the leucine zipper proteins shown in Figure 14–16, one can

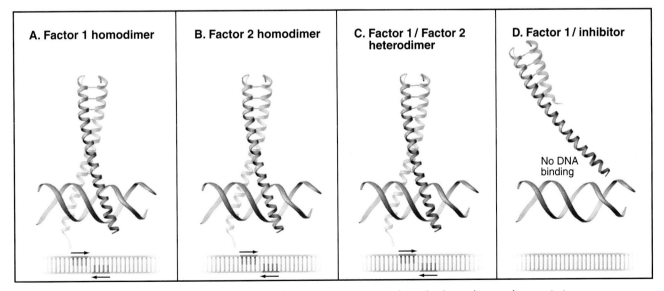

A. Factor 1 homodimer **B. Factor 2 homodimer** **C. Factor 1 / Factor 2 heterodimer** **D. Factor 1 / inhibitor**

No DNA binding

Figure 14–16 Transcription factor dimers that recognize novel targets. A and B, The homodimers of transcription factors 1 and 2 recognize different sites containing inverted four-base recognition elements. C, Heterodimers formed by factors 1 and 2 recognize a novel class of asymmetrical sites consisting of two different half-sites. D, Subunits that dimerize through formation of leucine zippers but lack the DNA-binding helix can act as inhibitors of the activating subunit.

see that formation of a heterodimer leads to recognition of a site that is different from either of the sites recognized by the two homodimers. Increasing the number of factors that can form heterodimers allows a small number of factors to recognize a large number of binding sites.

Leucine zipper factors can also be inhibited by dimerizing. In the case shown in Figure 14–16D, one of the activating factors interacts with an inhibitory factor consisting of a leucine zipper dimerization domain lacking a DNA-binding domain. In the absence of a second DNA-binding domain, this dimer cannot recognize the DNA-binding site. Expression of such a truncated protein would, therefore, inhibit the function of the full-length factor.

Transcriptional Activation

DNA binding of a transcription factor per se does not activate transcription. This function is provided by a separate domain that somehow interacts with the basal transcription machinery to elevate the rate of transcription. The most well-characterized activation domain is an acidic domain derived from the herpesvirus VP16 protein. This domain activates transcription when added to a wide variety of different DNA-binding domains in a number of different cell types. Other types of activator domains have been characterized as being proline-rich or glutamine-rich.

One of the major unsolved problems in transcription is the mechanism by which transcription factors activate transcription. It seems likely that some contact between the activation domain and the basal machinery is involved, but whether this interaction is direct or occurs through intermediary factors is currently under study. Given the diversity in activation domains, there are likely to be several activation mechanisms. The discovery that TAFs (see Fig. 14–6) are not required for basal transcription suggests that they could serve as a target for activators. Components of the mediator (see Fig. 14–7) and of coactivators have also been implicated.

How interactions between widely separated regulatory complexes can lead to an increased frequency of initiation is not known. One popular model is that the enhancer and basal machinery come into contact through the looping of DNA (Fig. 14–17A). This could account for the action of enhancer proteins bound at sites thousands of base pairs from the start of transcription. Interaction between the two DNA-protein complexes may lead to a more stable preinitiation complex and, thus, to higher rates of RNA polymerase II initiation.

Another feature of the activation process that is not understood is the nature of the interaction between multiple bound factors. Most promoters contain

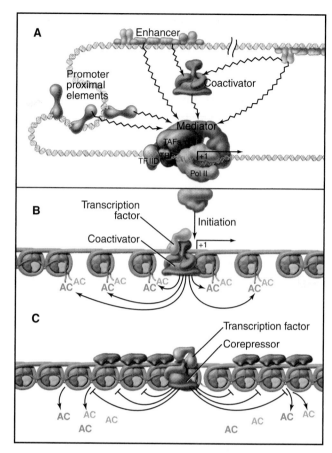

Figure 14–17 Transcription activation mechanisms. *A,* Contact between transcription activators and mediator or TAF subunits, or both, leads to stable preinitiation complexes and elevated transcription. In some cases, a coactivator acts as an intermediary in this process. *B,* Histone acetylases in a coactivator loosen chromatin in the vicinity of the promoter, allowing assembly of preinitiation complexes. *C,* Recruitment of histone deacetylases in a corepressor represses transcription by compacting the chromatin in the vicinity of the promoter.

several binding sites for regulatory factors. When more than one factor is bound at an upstream site, the activation level can be higher than the sum of activation by individual transcription factors. The molecular basis of this synergistic effect is unknown, but the implication is that there are multiple targets for activators in the basal machinery.

Chromatin and Transcription

The DNA in eukaryotic cells associates with an equal mass of protein to form chromatin (see Chapter 13). For years, the sole function of chromatin was thought to be compaction of DNA. More recent studies have indicated an additional functional role of chromatin proteins in regulation of gene expression.

The most obvious influence of chromatin on transcription is the ability of nucleosomes to restrict access of transcription proteins to the DNA template. This property is observed in the relative resistance of transcriptionally inactive regions of the genome to digestion by nucleases and in the localization of unexpressed genes in highly condensed heterochromatin. Furthermore, artificially shutting off histone synthesis results in an increase in the basal expression of many genes.

Gene activation often involves disruption or displacement of nucleosomes. Several types of activation have been proposed. The free energy of binding of transcription factors (approximately −12 to −15 kcal/mol) is thought to be sufficient to displace the histone complex. This direct binding requires that the recognition site be accessible on the surface of the nucleosome, a situation that could be regulated by the precise positioning of the nucleosome with respect to the DNA sequence in a process called **phasing.** Because the typical factor-binding site is only about 10 bp, binding of a single transcription factor does not readily displace an entire nucleosome. The presence of multiple factor-binding sites may exert a cooperative disruptive effect by simultaneously releasing several regions at once.

For some promoters, the mere presence of the correct factors may not be sufficient to open the chromatin at the promoter. Several mechanisms for destabilizing nucleosomes have been described. Some transcription factor complexes contain **histone acetylases** that modify the positively charged amino terminal histone tails, thereby weakening the interaction of the nucleosome with DNA (see Fig. 14–17B). Other regulatory complexes contain **histone deacetylases** that are recruited to promoters for the purpose of repressing transcription (see Fig. 14–17C).

Several ATP-dependent nucleosome destabilization mechanisms have been described (see Chapter 13). The yeast SWI/SNF complex that is required for the expression of many genes contains an ATP-dependent nucleosome-destabilizing activity. SWI/SNF binds to the RNA polymerase II holoenzyme complex, suggesting a mechanism for bringing the nucleosome-destabilizing complex to promoters.

Gene activation by nucleosome disruption can be counteracted by factors that stabilize chromatin. Reporter genes placed near yeast telomeres are silenced in a fashion that is dependent on the distance from the telomere. **Silencing** also occurs at yeast mating-type loci. These negative effects in broad regions of chromatin are brought about by recruitment of histone deacetylases that maintain these heterochromatin domains (see Chapter 13).

Modulation of Transcription Factor Activity

Regulation of transcription initiation is of fundamental importance in controlling gene expression. In many cases, the availability of factors that bind to specific sites in promoters is the switch that turns a gene on. Various strategies to control the binding of specific factors have been discovered. One of the most straightforward means of regulation is synthesis of the specific factor (Fig. 14–18A). In this situation, the genes targeted by the factor are not activated until the factor is itself expressed. This method requires a preceding level of transcription regulation and translation of the mRNA encoding the specific factor. All of these steps take some time; thus, this regulatory scheme is not used in situations in which rapid responses are required. Rather, this approach seems to be employed more commonly in regulating developmental pathways. The following section discusses transcription factor cascades.

Several mechanisms are used to regulate the activity of existing transcription factors. The advantage of these mechanisms is that specific genes can be activated rapidly without the need to synthesize the factor. One mechanism involves the formation of an active factor from two inactive subunits (see Fig. 14–18D).

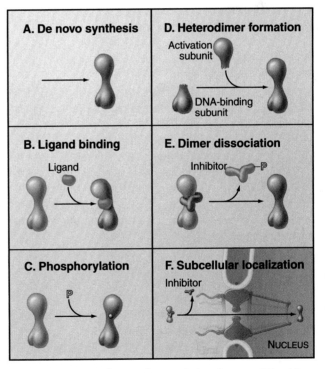

Figure 14–18 Regulation of transcription factor activity. Many strategies have evolved to regulate transcription factors in response to specific signals. A, The availability of a factor may be controlled by expressing it, de novo, only when it is needed. B, Factors may be synthesized in an inactive state and depend on a small molecule (ligand) for activity. C, Transcription factors synthesized in an inactive state can be activated by postsynthetic modification, such as phosphorylation. D, Some factors require an appropriate partner for activity. E, Constitutively active factors can be held in check by associating with inhibitory subunits. F, Active factors can be sequestered in the cytoplasm by blocking their transport to the nucleus.

In this mechanism, the association can be regulated either through synthesis or by modification of preexisting subunits leading to their association. Binding of small-molecule ligands is another means of controlling transcription factor activity (see Fig. 14–18*B*). In this mechanism, the binding of the ligand induces a conformational change that leads to DNA binding and transcription activation. Interaction of transcription factors with inhibitory subunits is also used to regulate factor activity (see Fig. 14–18*E*). The DNA binding or activation potential is held in check until the appropriate signal leads to dissociation of the inhibitory factor. Covalent modification—for example, by phosphorylation—is also used to convert inactive transcription factors to a functional form (see Fig. 14–18*C*). Finally, the ability of transcription factors to bind DNA may be regulated by restricting their localization to the cytoplasm (Fig. 14–18*F*). These regulatory schemes are not mutually exclusive, and many regulatory pathways (see the examples that follow) employ several different levels of regulation.

Transcription Factors and Signal Transduction

One of the hallmarks of eukaryotic gene regulation is the ability of cells to respond to a wide range of external signals. Cells detect the presence of hormones, growth factors, cytokines, cell surface contacts, and many other signals. This information is then transmitted to the nucleus, where appropriate changes in expression of specific genes are executed. Transcription factors represent the final step in these signal transduction pathways; the following sections discuss several specific examples. Chapter 29 covers several other signaling pathways that regulate gene expression.

Steroid Hormone Receptors

Regulation of gene expression by steroid hormone receptors involves both ligand-binding and inhibitory subunits. This family of receptors includes transcription factors with a common sequence organization consisting of a specific DNA-binding domain, a ligand-binding domain that regulates DNA binding, and one or more transcription activation domains. The ligands that regulate these factors are small, lipid-soluble hormone molecules that act by diffusing through cell membranes and binding directly to the transcription factor (Fig. 14–19*A*). The steroid hormones, retinoids, thyroid hormone, and vitamin D bind to distinct members of the receptor family, enabling these factors to recognize sequences in the promoters of genes that are destined for activation. The specific sites of action

in promoter DNA, termed **hormone response elements** (HREs), are related to either AGAACA or AGGTCA (see Fig. 14–15*C*). Specificity of the response is generated by the spacing and relative orientation of the binding sites. Steroid receptors usually bind to inverted repeats separated by three nucleotides, whereas some other receptors prefer direct repeats of similar sites. The nuclear receptors can bind as homodimers, although recent evidence suggests that heterodimers actually prevail in vivo. In addition to heterodimerizing with other members of the nuclear receptor family, interactions with other types of transcription factors could serve to link the steroid response to other pathways that signal through cell surface receptors.

Steroid hormone receptors are blocked from interacting with DNA by heat shock protein 90 (Hsp90) (see Fig. 18–14). This protein is a molecular chaperone that keeps the receptor ligand-binding domain in a conformation ready to bind the ligand but unable to enter the nucleus. Hormone binding to the receptor dissociates Hsp90 and frees the receptor's DNA-binding domain. The free ligand–bound receptor moves from the cytoplasm to the nucleus, where it binds its cognate HRE and activates transcription.

Cyclic Adenosine Monophosphate (cAMP) Signaling

Changes in gene expression often develop in response to the binding of signal molecules to cell surface receptors. Binding of ligand induces a structural change in the receptor that sets off a chain of events that leads to changes in transcription. Protein phosphorylation plays an important role in this process.

One of the best understood examples of transcriptional regulation through cell surface receptor signaling is the adenyl cyclase system. The binding of ligand to some seven-helix receptors results in an increase in synthesis of **cAMP**, which, in turn, activates **protein kinase A** (see Fig. 29–3). The promoters of cAMP-regulated genes contain a conserved DNA sequence element, called a **cAMP response element (CRE),** that mediates the transcriptional response to cAMP. A transcription factor, termed cAMP response element–binding **(CREB)** protein, binds the CRE specifically. CREB protein is a member of the leucine zipper family and binds the CRE as a dimer. The DNA-binding domain of CREB protein can be exchanged with other DNA-binding domains without loss of cAMP responsiveness. This indicates that cAMP does not work by altering the DNA binding of CREB protein; rather, it suggests that cAMP alters the transcription activation function. Recent experiments have identified a site in the activation domain of CREB protein that is phosphorylated by the protein kinase A. Mutation of serine

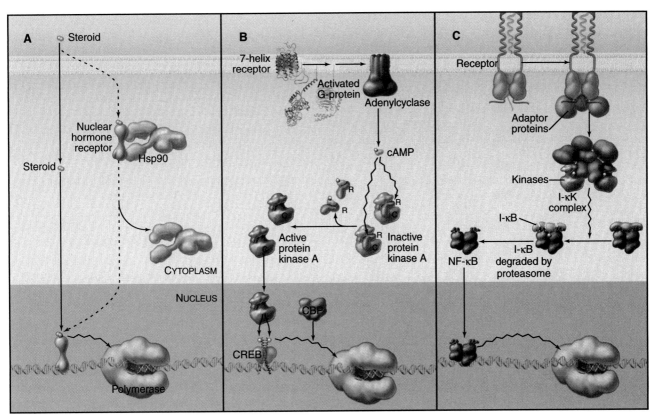

Figure 14-19 Transcription factors as targets of signal transduction pathways. External signals are transmitted by a variety of pathways that eventually impinge on transcription factors. *A*, Steroid hormones diffuse through the cell membrane and bind to the hormone receptor in the cytoplasm (estrogen) or, more commonly, the nucleus. Hormone binding induces a conformational change that renders the receptor competent to activate transcription. *B*, Ligands bound to the extracellular surface of seven-helix receptors initiate a pathway that leads to the activation of protein kinase A that moves to the nucleus where it phosphorylates transcription factor CREB. (C, catalytic subunit of PKA. R, regulatory subunit of PKA that is dissociated from C by binding cAMP. R is shown smaller than actual size.) *C*, In a third strategy, constitutively active transcription factors are kept sequestered in the cytoplasm until a signaling pathway is activated. In this example, the transcription factor NF-κB is bound to an inhibitor called I-κB. Activation of the pathway leads to phosphorylation of I-κB, which targets the inhibitory subunit for destruction by the proteasome. The free NF-κB is transported to the nucleus, where it activates the transcription of target genes.

133 to alanine results in a CREB protein that cannot be phosphorylated and cannot activate transcription of CRE-containing genes. Phosphorylation of serine 133 leads to a conformational change in CREB protein that allows it to interact with a protein named CBP (CREB-binding protein). CBP is an adaptor that recruits the transcription machinery leading to transcription of target genes. Thus, the signal generated by binding of a ligand to a cell surface receptor is transduced to a DNA-binding factor that activates transcription of genes containing the appropriate regulatory elements.

Cytokine Signaling

NF-κB, a transcription factor present in many cell types, is held in an inactive form in the cytoplasm through interaction with an inhibitor called **I-κB.** When B lymphocytes (see Chapter 30) are stimulated to produce antibody, NF-κB binds to an enhancer in the immunoglobulin κ-chain gene and activates tran-

scription. The stimulatory signal leading to NF-κB activity is transmitted through a protein kinase cascade that eventually phosphorylates I-κB, signaling its destruction by proteolysis. This event unmasks the NF-κB nuclear localization signal, leading to its transport to the nucleus, where it activates transcription of immunoglobulin genes. NF-κB is present in many cell types, where it is the target of signal transductory cascades involving inflammation.

Transcription Factor Cascades

The signal transduction cascades are designed to relay information from the external environment to the nucleus, where changes in gene expression can be affected. In simple eukaryotes, these changes often result in changes in expression of genes important for survival (e.g., heat shock responses or changes in metabolic pathways). In more complicated eukaryotes, signaling pathways often lead to expression of new

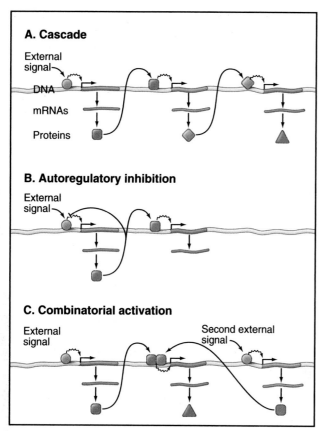

A. Cascade

External
signal
DNA

mRNAs

Proteins

B. Autoregulatory inhibition

External
signal

C. Combinatorial activation

External
signal

Second external
signal

Figure 14-20 Regulatory circuits. The complex patterns of gene expression observed in multicellular organisms arise from interactions among thousands of transcription activators and repressors. Several examples of these interactions are illustrated in this figure. *A*, Transcription factors activate other factors, leading to a cascade of changes in gene expression. In this example, expression of a new transcription factor leads to activation of a number of genes, often including additional transcription factors. The end result is a series of changes in the pattern of gene expression. *B*, Some transcription factors can act either as activators or repressors. In this example, the external signal leads to expression of a new factor. This factor goes on to activate expression of other genes while at the same time repressing its own expression. In this way, the initial signal is quenched. *C*, Activation may require more than one signal. In this example, activation of the middle gene depends on the presence of two activators. Each of these transcription factors is activated by different external signals. Thus, the middle gene is only activated when both signaling pathways are active.

transcription factors, which lead to yet more changes in gene expression. Figure 14–20*A* shows an example of such a cascade of gene expression. In this example, the external signal leads to expression of a factor that, among other targets, activates another transcription activator. This factor itself is able to activate a new set of genes containing yet another transcription factor. In Figure 14–20*B*, the transcription factor feeds back and inhibits its own expression, thus limiting the response to a single round. Other modifications of the transcription cascade involve the integration of signals (see Fig. 14–20*C*).

The response of tissue culture cells to growth-promoting stimuli is an example of this type of transcription factor cascade. Cell growth is a tightly regulated process that is dependent on a number of external cues, including growth factors, hormones, and contact with adjacent cells. Growth-promoting signals are relayed through signal transduction pathways to the nucleus, where they result in changes in gene expression that lead to cell division. The regulatory network involved in this process has been delineated through studying genes that are expressed in response to growth factors. Several sets of genes form a cascade of gene expression that eventually leads to mitosis. The first genes activated in response to growth factors are the **immediate early genes** (see Chapter 44). Transcription of these genes is not dependent on translation, but seems to be the direct result of changes in protein function induced by the signal transduction pathway. Two of the best characterized transcription factors are products of the immediate early genes *jun* and *fos*. These two genes, first discovered as retroviral oncogenes, encode leucine zipper proteins that form a heterodimer and bind to the consensus sequence TGA(GC)TCA. These sites are also known as AP1 sites because they bind *a*ctivator *p*rotein 1, which is the Fos-Jun heterodimer. AP1 sites are located upstream of many delayed early genes and regulate their expression. **Delayed early genes** encode a wide range of proteins, including additional transcription factors and proteins needed for nucleotide and DNA synthesis. These genes are not needed in resting cells and are, therefore, not expressed. Transcription factors expressed as delayed early genes act later in the cascade to activate yet another set of target genes. These genes encode proteins needed to prepare cells for division.

In summary, signals from growth factors stimulate transient expression of Fos and Jun, which then sets off a cascade of transcription factor expression leading to a round of cell division. Whether subsequent rounds of division occur can depend on the duration of the original stimulus and response. In this scenario, the initial cascade is dependent on the presence of an extreme second signal. The involvement of Fos and Jun in regulation of growth explains the hijacking of these genes by a number of viruses that transform cells and cause cancer. In these viruses, the cellular gene has been captured and is either expressed to higher levels or is mutated so that it is no longer dependent on external regulatory signals.

Transcription Factors in Development

In the preceding sections, the discussion centered on how external signals can lead to changes in gene expression in the nucleus, which, in turn, lead to changes in cell function. A critical step in this genetic program is the regulation of one transcription factor by another. Such cascades of transcription factor activity are fundamental to gene regulation in development.

Early cell divisions in multicellular organisms create different types of daughter cells through expression of different sets of genes in each daughter cell. In this case, the level of expression of a gene is governed by two types of information. First, the environment of the cell sends signals that are transduced to the nucleus; these signals impinge on the transcription machinery to change the pattern of gene expression. The way in which the nucleus interprets the transduced signals depends on the set of transcription factors that preexist within it. Thus, in addition to external signals, the history of the cell dictates which genes will respond to which signals.

The exact program of transcription factor interaction during development is extremely complicated and is certainly beyond the scope of this chapter. The underlying principles of these pathways are worth considering, however. One important observation is that developmentally regulated transcription factors are often autoregulatory (see Fig. 14–20*B*). For factors that activate their own expression, this form of regulation acts as a switch that leads to continued expression after the initial stimulus is gone. Another important property of developmentally regulated transcription factors is that they are, in turn, regulated by several different factors. This allows complicated combinatorial signals to dictate expression (see Fig. 14–20*C*). For example, some transcription factors activate certain promoters while repressing others. The basis of this contradictory property is thought to be the ability of transcription factors to cooperate with each other when bound at the same promoter. This cooperation can be either positive or negative. This allows the expression of a target gene to be regulated both by external signals (e.g., proximity of an adjacent cell that expresses a signaling molecule) and by the preexistence of a given factor in the cell. In this way, only cells of a certain lineage that are located in a certain area of an embryonic segment are able to express the gene. As more of the transcription factors involved in development are discovered, the challenge will be to decipher the complicated combinatorial interactions among them.

▌ Transcription Factors and Human Disease

Advances in genomics and human genetics have demonstrated that mutations within specific genes are responsible for the pathogenesis or clinical features of particular human diseases. Multicellular organisms devote a significant fraction of their genome to encoding the transcription apparatus and attendant regulatory factors. Therefore, it is not surprising that mutations in some of the thousands of genes involved in transcription result in clinical phenotypes. The following examples indicate that mutations in either gene-specific or general transcription factors can contribute to disease.

Androgen Receptor

A nuclear hormone receptor, androgen receptor, binds the androgen testosterone and regulates expression of genes involved in the development of male secondary sexual characteristics. As with other transcription factors, the androgen receptor has DNA-binding and transcription activation domains. In addition, the androgen receptor has a ligand-binding domain that binds testosterone and regulates the DNA-binding properties of the factor. Because the androgen receptor gene is located on the X chromosome, it has been possible to identify many otherwise recessive mutations in the gene in males (which have only one copy of the X).

Mutations that alter different parts of the androgen receptor cause different clinical phenotypes. The most severe mutations cause **androgen insensitivity syndrome** (AIS), a condition in which individuals with a 46,XY chromosome constitution develop secondary female sexual characteristics. In this syndrome, androgens are synthesized but the receptor fails to respond. Single missense mutations in the ligand-binding domain can weaken or eliminate ligand binding. Alternatively, ligand binding may be normal, but the mutation may weaken or eliminate DNA binding. Some AIS mutations are associated with male breast cancer.

Another type of mutation in the androgen receptor causes a neuromuscular disease called spinal and bulbar muscular atrophy (Kennedy's syndrome). This X-linked disease involves wasting of the proximal limb muscles, as well as changes in facial muscles. The molecular basis of the disease is an expansion of a series of repeated CAG (glutamine) codons in the amino-terminal transcription activation domain. Normally, this region encodes 11 to 31 consecutive glutamine residues in different individuals. The number of repeats in patients with Kennedy's syndrome ranges from 40 to 52. The mechanism by which the expanded polyglutamine domain results in motor neuron damage has not been determined.

TFIIH and Human Disease

As discussed in a previous section, the general RNA polymerase II transcription factor TFIIH is a multisubunit factor containing both RNA polymerase II C-terminal domain (CTD) kinase and DNA helicase activities. In addition to its role as a transcription factor,

TFIIH plays a role in DNA repair and may serve to direct DNA repair to transcriptionally active regions in the genome.

Mutations in TFIIH subunits are associated with a set of rare human disorders (**xeroderma pigmentosum,** Cockayne's syndrome, and trichothiodystrophy), each linked to defects in nucleotide excision repair of DNA damaged by ultraviolet light or chemical mutagens. Mutations in these diseases map to the genes encoding two different TFIIH helicase activities. Presumably, the alterations in these activities cause changes in DNA unwinding, either in the transcription initiation reaction or in the process of nucleotide excision repair. Some mutations are more selective for the DNA repair function, whereas other TFIIH mutations cause little or no DNA repair phenotype, but rather seem to affect the TFIIH transcription function. The latter mutations cause wide-ranging defects, as might be expected for a defect in a general transcription factor.

▌ Selected Readings

Cramer P, Bushnell DA, Kornberg RD: Structural basis of transcription: RNA polymerase II at 2.8 angstrom resolution. Science 292(5523):1863–1876, 2001.

Dilworth FJ, Chambon P: Nuclear receptors coordinate the activities of chromatin remodeling complexes and coactivators to facilitate initiation of transcription. Oncogene 20(24):3047–3054, 2001.

Garvie CW, Wolberger C: Recognition of specific DNA sequences. Molec Cell 8:937–946, 2001.

Gnatt AL, Cramer P, Fu J, et al: Structural basis of transcription: An RNA polymerase II elongation complex at 3.3 Å resolution. Science 292(5523):1876–1882, 2001.

Lee TI, Young RA: Transcription of eukaryotic protein-coding genes. Annu Rev Genet 34:77–137, 2000.

Lemon B, Tjian R: Orchestrated response: A symphony of transcription factors for gene control. Genes Dev 14(20):2551–2569, 2000.

Myers LC, Kornberg RD: Mediator of transcriptional regulation. Annu Rev Biochem 69:729–749, 2000.

Ptashne M, Gann A: Transcriptional activation by recruitment. Nature 386(6625):569–577, 1997.

Reinberg D, Orphanides G, Ebright R, et al: The RNA polymerase II general transcription factors: Past, present, and future. Cold Spring Harbor Symp Quant Biol 63:83–103, 1998.

Roeder RG: Role of general and gene-specific cofactors in the regulation of eukaryotic transcription. Cold Spring Harbor Symp Quant Biol 63:201–218, 1998.

chapter 15

PROCESSING
OF EUKARYOTIC RNAS

RNAs serve many functions. **Messenger RNAs (mRNAs)** direct protein synthesis, **transfer RNAs (tRNAs)** bring the correct amino acid to the growing protein chain, and **ribosomal RNAs (rRNAs)** provide the catalytic center for protein synthesis. In addition, RNAs also remove introns (some U RNAs, and group I and II RNAs), process the 5′ ends of tRNAs (RNase P), serve in rRNA modification and cleavage (most U RNAs, small nucleolar RNAs), and cleave other RNAs (e.g., hammerhead RNA). RNAs can even direct changes in the primary sequence of mRNAs (e.g., guide RNAs in trypanosomes) and regulate developmental pathways (as in *Drosophila* sex determination).

Genes that encode various RNAs are transcribed in the nucleus (a few are transcribed in mitochondria) by RNA polymerase I, II, or III, but the primary transcripts are virtually never the mature, active species. Instead, these larger precursor RNAs (pre-RNAs) are processed by various reactions, including cleavage, joining, and chemical modification, to acquire their final forms. In fact, the size discrepancy of precursor and mature RNAs was the first evidence for RNA processing in eukaryotes. Interestingly, these post-transcriptional processing reactions are frequently directed or even catalyzed by other RNAs.

Maturation events vary according to the identity of the RNA. Pre-mRNA processing involves 5′ capping, 3′ polyadenylation, and internal splicing. The 18S, 5.8S, and 28S rRNAs of the ribosome are excised from a common precursor and then undergo methylation and pseudouridylation. tRNAs, which are also processed from larger precursors, undergo cleavage at both ends, addition of nucleotides at their 3′ ends, numerous base modifications, and often, splicing. At the other

extreme, eukaryotic 5S RNAs require no processing or only limited trimming of their 3′ end. In contrast, in prokaryotes, the primary mRNA transcript is used directly to specify translation, whereas 5S RNA is cleaved from a larger pre-rRNA precursor. In both eukaryotes and prokaryotes, steady-state concentrations of mature RNAs are dictated by a combination of their rates of synthesis, processing, and turnover (Table 15–1).

Processing of Transcripts Synthesized by RNA Polymerase II

RNA polymerase II (pol II) is responsible for producing all mRNAs, some small nuclear RNAs (snRNAs), and numerous small nucleolar RNAs (snoRNAs) (see Chapter 14). Most pol II transcripts undergo similar events during pre-mRNA processing (Fig. 15–1). However, mRNAs for the major histones (see Chapter 13) and the snRNAs and snoRNAs undergo different kinds of maturational reactions. Although genes and their transcripts vary greatly in size, an average mammalian mRNA is approximately 2 kb. By contrast, its nuclear precursor, called **heterogeneous nuclear RNA (hnRNA),** is 2 to 20 times that length (Fig. 15–2). Ultimately, only about 10% of a typical hnRNA molecule enters the cytoplasm; the rest is degraded in the nucleus. hnRNAs are turned into mRNAs by a process that involves changing both the 5′ and 3′ ends of the molecule and removing segments from the middle. These various events are specified on the nascent hnRNA as it emerges from the polymerase.

5′ Capping

Because all RNA is synthesized in the 5′ to the 3′ direction, researchers were startled to find that no 5′ ends could be detected on eukaryotic mRNAs. Instead,

---

Chapter by Barbara Sollner-Webb, with help in figure design from Christine Smith and WCE.

table 15–1

RNA AMOUNTS AND RATES OF SYNTHESIS IN AN AVERAGE VERTEBRATE CELL LINE*

Type of RNA	RNA Polymerase	Percent of Steady-state Cellular RNA	Percent of RNA Synthesis	Percent of Genome Used	Mean Size (kb)	Half-life
Nuclear rRNA precursors	Pol I	5	39	0.1	14	Hours
Cytoplasmic rRNA		70	–	0.05	6 (in total)	Days
Nuclear hnRNA	Pol II	7	58	20	1–100	Minutes
Cytoplasmic mRNA		3	–	1–2	0.5–10	Hours
Small, stable RNAs (mostly tRNAs)	Pol III	15	3	0.2	0.1	Days

*Numbers are approximate.

the initial 5' triphosphate moiety of the primary transcript becomes joined to a guanosine (G) residue in an unusual 5'-5' triphosphate linkage, leaving a free 3' hydroxyl terminus on the 5' end of the mRNA (Fig. 15–3*A*). The reverse G is then methylated on the N^7 position of the base, and the first and sometimes the second nucleotides of the original RNA are methylated on the 2'-O position of the ribose. The resultant structure is called a **5' cap.**

The 5' cap forms early in transcription while the nascent transcript is about 20 to 30 nucleotides long, and the enzymes that specify the capping (see Fig. 15–3*B*) are part of the RNA pol II complex. The mRNA cap acts as a landing pad for specific proteins and serves several functions:

1. It helps define the 5' boundary of the first intron (see later discussion) to ensure proper splicing.
2. It assists in the transport of mRNAs from the nucleus to the cytoplasm.
3. It aids in translational initiation by binding the eIF-4E translation factor and directing protein synthesis to begin at the first AUG of the mRNA.
4. It stabilizes the mRNA and makes it resistant to degradation by 5' exonucleases (see later section).

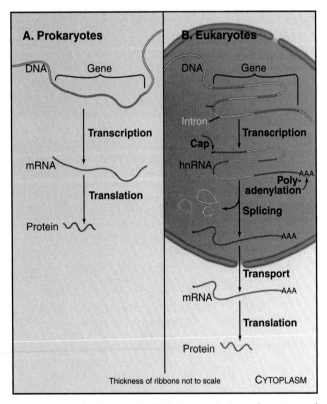

Figure 15–1 From gene to RNA to protein in prokaryotes and eukaryotes. *A,* In prokaryotes, the newly synthesized mRNA can be used immediately for translation into protein. *B,* In eukaryotes, the mRNA is processed in the nucleus prior to export to the cytoplasm for translation. The processing events include 5' capping, 3' cleavage and polyadenylation, and splicing to remove introns.

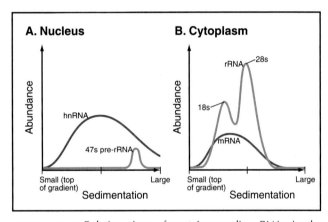

Figure 15–2 Relative sizes of protein-encoding RNAs in the nucleus and cytoplasm—early evidence for RNA processing. Panels *A* and *B* illustrate the distribution of RNAs that have been resolved by sucrose gradient centrifugation (which separates molecules based on their size and shape; see Chapter 5). *A,* In the nucleus, hnRNA (mostly pre-mRNA) is relatively abundant, a widely diverse population of thousands of species that vary tremendously in size. Nucleolar 47S pre-rRNA (14,000 nucleotides) is shown in blue; 28S mature rRNA (about 4,000 nucleotides) would migrate to the position of the vertical line at the midpoint of the x axis. *B,* In the cytoplasm, mRNA is considerably smaller and rRNA transcripts are much more abundant (about 40-fold more so than mRNA). This is because much of the mass of each hnRNA is removed by processing prior to its export to the cytoplasm and because rRNAs are much more stable than most mRNAs.

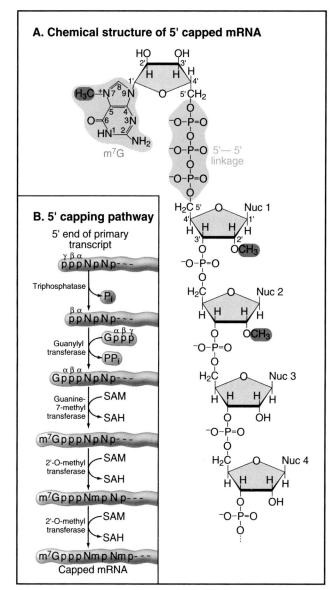

A. Chemical structure of 5' capped mRNA

B. 5' capping pathway

Figure 15-3 A 7-methyl guanosine cap blocks the 5' ends of mRNAs and leaves a 3' OH. *A*, Newly synthesized mRNAs acquire a protective cap shortly after they emerge from the polymerase. The cap is formed by attachment of an inverted G via an unusual 5'-5'-triphosphate linkage. In addition methyl groups are added *(red shading)*: one at the N^7 position of the inverted G, one on the 2' OH of the first nucleotide (Nuc1) of the initial transcript, and generally another on the 2' OH of the second nucleotide (Nuc2). *B*, Messenger RNA capping is a multistep process. First the 5' phosphate is removed by a triphosphatase, and guanylyl transferase adds the inverted monophosphate G. Next, methyl transferases to the S-adenosyl methionine (SAM) transfer the methyl group from N^7 position of the inverted G (m^7G) and the 2' OHs of the first and second nucleotides (Nm), releasing S-adenosyl homocysteine (SAH).

3' Polyadenylation

At the other end of a mature mRNA from the 5' cap is a stretch of 50 to 200 A residues. This region of **"poly A"** is not encoded in the genome but is added through processing events in the nucleus. RNA pol II produces a primary transcript that often extends thousands of nucleotides beyond the end of the mature mRNA. Once the 3' portion of the mRNA is transcribed, the poly A signal sequence (which includes an AAUAAA motif in metazoans, and a somewhat more degenerate A/U-rich region in yeast) directs a large multiprotein complex to cleave the pre-mRNA about 25 nucleotides downstream of the AAUAAA. A string of A residues (~200 in humans and ~100 in yeast) is then added to the 3' end of the nascent RNA (Fig. 15–4*A*). The poly A tail becomes complexed with poly A binding protein at a stoichiometry of 1 molecule per 10 to 20 A residues. The downstream portion of the cleaved pre-mRNA, which lacks a 5' cap and a 3' poly A, is rapidly degraded by exonucleases.

Polyadenylation serves a number of functions, including the following:

1. It stimulates transcription termination, often far downstream of the poly A signal
2. It facilitates removal of the 3'-most intron (see later discussion)
3. It assists in transport of mRNA to the cytoplasm
4. It occasionally generates two mRNAs from the same primary transcript through selection of alternative poly A sites. This can allow the regulated synthesis of related proteins with different C-terminal sequences, the best known example of which is the switch from the membrane-bound to

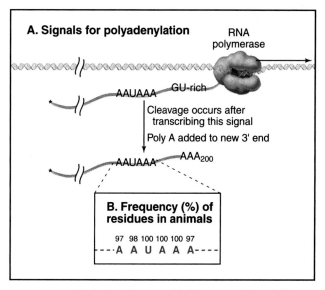

A. Signals for polyadenylation

B. Frequency (%) of residues in animals

97 98 100 100 100 97
- - - A A U A A A - - - -

Figure 15-4 Poly A tails are added to pre-mRNAs following transcription. *A*, After pol II transcribes the protein-coding region of the gene, it encounters and transcribes two sequence elements—AAUAAA and a GU-rich region—which serve as signals to a 3' end processing complex that cleaves the nascent RNA, releasing it from the transcription complex. The newly created 3' end is then modified by the subsequent addition of up to 200 adenosine (A) residues. *B*, The poly A signal is highly conserved in vertebrates.

the secreted form of immunoglobulins during B cell maturation.

5. It protects the mRNA from degradation (see later discussion)

6. It contributes to translation initiation of eukaryotic mRNAs. This was an unexpected finding as translation begins near the 5′ end, far from the poly A tail. Participation of the 3′ end in translation initiation implies that the two ends of the mRNA interact or communicate with each other.

Furthermore, in the laboratory, poly A tails allow isolation of mRNA (which constitutes only about 2% of total RNA) by affinity chromatography on columns with immobilized poly dT (see Fig. 5–6*A*).

Pre-mRNA Splicing

By the early 1970s, a puzzling set of observations emerged. Cytoplasmic mRNAs were found to be much shorter than their nuclear hnRNA counterparts, despite the fact that both possessed 5′ caps and 3′ poly A

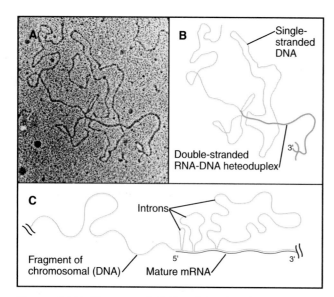

Figure 15–5 Discovery of RNA splicing by electron microscopy. *A,* In this electron micrograph, isolated mature mRNA encoding an adenovirus structural protein was hybridized to a portion of the viral chromosome. The RNA:DNA hybrid (called a heteroduplex) is characterized by a thick region from which single-stranded loops extend. Because the introns are no longer present in the mature mRNA, the regions of the chromosome where they are encoded cannot hybridize to the mRNA and form single-stranded loops. *B,* Artist's interpretation. The cross-shaped structure at the 3′ end of this molecule is a technical artifact. *C,* Simplified drawing showing the pattern of base-pairing between the genomic DNA and the mature mRNA. (*A* and *B,* From Berget SM, Berk AJ, Harrison T, et al: Spliced segments at the 5′ termini of adenovirus-2 late mRNA: A role for heterogeneous nuclear RNA in mammalian cells. Cold Spring Harbor Symp Quant Biol 42:523–529, 1978. See also Chow L, Gelinas R, Broker T, et al: An amazing sequence arrangement at the 5′ ends of Ad2 mRNA. Cell 12:1–8, 1977.)

tails. How could hnRNAs be shortened to mRNAs while retaining both ends? The answer came in 1977 with the discovery of RNA splicing (Fig. 15–5). Most higher eukaryotic mRNAs (and many lower eukaryotic mRNAs as well) are encoded in the genome in a hyphenated form. Blocks of protein-coding sequences, called **exons,** are separated by intervening sequences, called **introns,** that range in length from about 75 to more than 10,000 nucleotides. The **primary transcript** is a copy of the entire gene, containing introns as well as exons; the introns are then removed in a process called **pre-mRNA splicing.**

In unicellular eukaryotes, introns are generally short; rarely are more than four found in a gene, and many genes have none. By contrast, mammalian genes have an average of 8 introns, but can contain more than 50, and these can be very large, particularly in comparison to the small size of mammalian internal exons. An extreme example is the human dystrophin gene, mutations in which causes the disease muscular dystrophy (see Fig. 42–9). This gene is more than 2 million bp long and contains more than 65 introns that separate the exons constituting a mature mRNA that is 14,000 nucleotides long.

Splicing Mechanism

The sequence elements that direct intron removal are short motifs near either end of the intron (Fig. 15–6*A*). Almost invariably, the first two residues of the intron (at the **5′ splice site,** also called the **splice donor**) are GU and the last two residues of the intron (at the **3′ splice site,** also called the **splice acceptor**) are AG. Flanking residues in the exons also show conservation. In addition, a key A residue (at the **branch point** of the intron) is located within a conserved sequence element, about 30 nucleotides upstream of the 3′ splice site. The following section describes the sequence of reactions that occurs during splicing, as well as how the process is facilitated by other RNAs and proteins.

Analysis of splicing reactions in cell-free extracts has revealed that the process involves two transesterification reactions. **Transesterification** refers to an ester bond [in this case, a phosphodiester bond] that is attacked by the oxygen of an activated hydroxyl group. Because one phosphodiester bond is broken while another is formed, the bond energy of the reaction is conserved. The reader is also referred to the section on group I and II splicing that follows. In the first transesterification reaction, the 2′ OH of the branch site A residue (which has been physically strained to activate it) makes a nucleophilic attack on the 5′ splice site. This liberates the upstream exon (see Fig. 15–6*B*) and links the A in an unusual 2′-5′ bond to the 5′ end of the intron while retaining the usual 3′-5′ and 5′-3′ bonds that link it to its neigh-

Figure 15-6 Nonprotein coding regions (introns) are spliced out of pre-mRNAs following polymerase II transcription. *A,* Three conserved sequence elements—the 5' splice site, the branch site, and the 3' splice site—help direct intron removal. The most conserved sequences of the 5' and 3' splice sites are the GU and AG at the two ends of the intron; numbers above indicate the extent of sequence conservation. The branchpoint contains a key adenosine (A) residue that plays a central role in the splicing process. In mammals, the sequences surrounding this A residue are much less conserved than in yeast, and there is a tract of more than 10 pyrimidine residues (Py) between the branchpoint and the 3' splice site. *B,* The sequence of events in pre-mRNA splicing (see text for description). Note the unusual structure of the branchpoint A, with all of its OHs (5', 3', and 2') involved in phosphodiester linkages to form the branched structure of the lariat *(inset).*

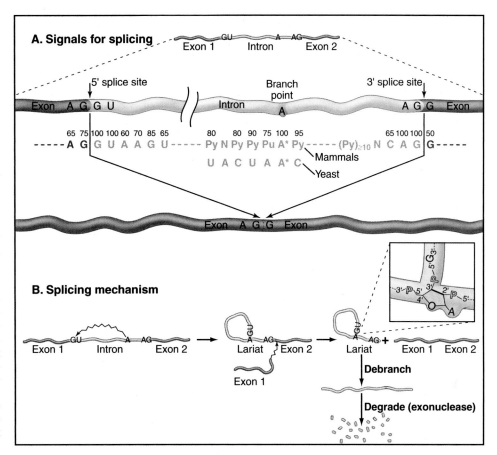

bors. Consequently, the intron forms an intramolecular loop called a **lariat.** In the second transesterification reaction, the 3' end of the liberated upstream exon attacks the 3' splice site and covalently joins the upstream and downstream exons, thereby completing the splicing-out of the intron. The liberated lariat intron is then converted to a linear molecule by a debranching enzyme and is rapidly degraded.

snRNAs and the Spliceosome

The splicing reaction is carried out by a large RNA-protein complex, called the spliceosome, which is similar in size to the ribosome. The key components of the spliceosome are five *small nuclear ribonucleoprotein* particles (**snRNPs,** pronounced "snurps"). Each snRNP consists of an **snRNA** (U1, U2, U4, U5, and U6 are used in pre-mRNA splicing) associated with about 10 to 20 polypeptides. Some proteins are shared by the various snRNPs, such as the seven Sm proteins, which are recognized by antibodies found in certain patients with the autoimmune disease systemic lupus erythematosus. Other snRNP proteins associate with only one particular snRNA. Spliceosomes also contain many accessory proteins, including hnRNP proteins that rapidly package nascent hnRNAs and SR proteins. The latter are rich in serine (S) and arginine

(R) residues and bring together other splicing factors and snRNPs via protein-protein interactions. Analysis of pre-RNA processing (*prp*) mutants in yeast has implicated at least 100 proteins in splicing. This constitutes about 2% of the yeast genome, underscoring the complexity of RNA splicing and its importance to the cell.

A combination of pre-mRNA:snRNA and snRNA:snRNA base-pairing interactions, along with additional stabilization provided by proteins, aligns the 5' and 3' splice sites and the branch region in the proper configuration for splicing (Fig. 15–7). Each snRNP has a distinct and timely role. The U1 snRNP initially recognizes the 5' splice site by base-pairing to the surrounding consensus sequence. The U2 snRNP then associates with the branch region, causing the branchpoint A to bulge out. In yeast, this involves U2 base-pairing to a very conserved branch consensus sequence (UACUAAC), whereas in mammals (where the sequence surrounding the branch A is less conserved [see Fig. 15–6]), recognition by U2 is facilitated by U2-associated factor (U2AF), a protein that binds a cluster of U and C residues (called the polypyrimidine tract) in the 3' portion of the intron. The pre-mRNA/U1/U2 complex is then joined by a U4/U5/U6 tri-snRNP complex. U5 brings the ends of the exons together, and the U4, whose role is to act as a chaperone, releases

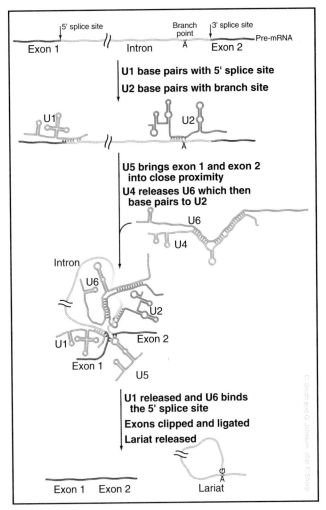

Figure 15-7 Small nuclear RNAs interact with the pre-mRNA to orchestrate the splicing of introns. As the newly transcribed mRNA is emerging from the polymerase, U1 and U2 snRNPs bind through RNA:RNA base pairing to the 5' splice and branch sites, respectively. Although shown here as individual snRNAs, they are part of a large RNP complex. In mammals, U2 binding is assisted by the U2AF protein, which interacts with the polypyrimidine tract and 3' splice site. U5 snRNA enters as part of a tri-snRNP complex with U4 and U6 snRNAs and uses its prominent stem loop structure to base-pair with the last two nucleotides of exon 1 and the first two nucleotides of exon 2. This brings together the two phosphodiester bonds that must be broken and reformed during the splicing reaction. Acting like a chaperone, U4 initially base-pairs extensively with U6. This interaction is then disrupted so that U6 can interact with U2 near the activated branchpoint A. As U5 and U6 form these interactions with the pre-mRNA, U1 leaves, allowing U6 access to the 5' splice site (not shown). Through a transesterification reaction, the phosphodiester bond at the 5' splice site is broken, and eventually exon 1 is joined to exon 2, resulting in the mature mRNA product and the lariat intron.

U6, which then displaces U1, base-pairing at the 5' end of the intron. U6 also binds U2, thereby bringing the branchpoint A and the 5' end of the intron together. U6 is considered to play the most central role in the splicing reaction. Together these interactions

strain and activate the branchpoint A of the pre-mRNA and trigger the first transesterification reaction. Note the dynamic nature of the various RNA:RNA interactions in the spliceosome as the reaction proceeds.

Recently, a parallel set of minor snRNPs was identified. These catalyze the splicing of a class of unusual introns that do not follow the "GU/AG rule" but instead contain "AU/AC" at their 5' and 3' splice sites. In this case, U11 and U12 take the place of U1 and U2, U4$_{atac}$ and U6$_{atac}$ take the place of U4 and U6, and the U5 snRNP is shared by both splicesomes. Splicing of AU/AC introns appears to be mechanistically analogous to normal splicing.

Exon Definition

Given the facts that the 5' and 3' splice sites and branch site are defined by rather short and degenerate consensus sequences and introns are often longer than 10 kb, accurate identification of exon-intron boundaries would appear to be a nearly impossible task. Comparison of complementary DNA (cDNA) and genomic sequences of many genes has demonstrated that the linear order of exons in genes is always maintained in the mRNA. That is, if the order of exons in the chromosome is a-b-c-d-e-f-g, the order in the mRNA can be b-d-f but never b-f-d. Despite this restriction, introns are often spliced out from the hnRNA in a temporal sequence that is quite different from that in which they were transcribed. Further confounding matters is the fact that pre-mRNAs generally contain not only the "correct" 5' and 3' splice sites but other "cryptic" 5' or 3' splice sites that can be used in certain circumstances. For example, if a 5' or 3' splice site is deleted experimentally, the new transcript often is still spliced, but at a site that would otherwise not be used.

How does the splicing machinery keep all this straight and avoid splicing together the wrong regions of the mRNA, particularly in an hnRNA with many large introns? One clue to proper splice site identification was derived from the observation that internal exons are commonly less than 300 nucleotides long. This raised the possibility that the two ends of each *exon* are identified, rather than the ends of the introns. For example, a pair of 3' and 5' splice sites across a single small exon might be recognized more easily than a pair of splice sites flanking the often-enormous intron (see Fig. 15-1). This process, called **exon definition,** would allow the splicing machinery to assemble in a rapid, well-orchestrated manner during transcription of the gene. If pairing happened during transcription, a 5' splice site would be paired with the next 3' splice site on a nascent transcript before additional downstream, potentially confusing, 3' splice sites are even synthesized. Subsequent to this pairing, the splicing reactions could occur in any order, before or after the entire pre-mRNA has been transcribed.

Although most pre-mRNAs are transcribed in a few minutes, the actual removal of introns and joining of the exons may take more than 30 minutes to complete. Communication between the splicing machinery and the 5′ cap and poly A tail complexes also appears to help define the first and last exons.

Although splicing, as well as capping and polyadenylation, can be reconstituted as individual reactions in vitro, the three processes are closely associated with pol II transcription in vivo. This occurs because processing factors bind the **C-terminal domain (CTD)** of RNA pol II and then associate with the nascent RNA chain as it emerges from the enzyme (Fig. 15–8). RNAs transcribed in vivo by a pol II lacking the CTD—which consists of multiple repeats of a 7 amino acid sequence (see Chapter 14)—undergo only limited capping, splicing, or polyadenylation. An attractive theory for explaining recognition of exons in the correct order is that splicing factors that recognize one exon, and hence a 5′ splice site, remain attached to the CTD as the intron is transcribed. When the next exon is transcribed, it is recognized by splicing factors also on the CTD, placing the 5′ splice site and 3′ splice site in close proximity for rearrangement across the introns. Thus, the CTD of RNA pol II may act as a scaffold upon which the splicing complexes are assembled in a coordinated fashion. In this scenario, exons are naturally brought together in the same linear order in which they are transcribed, independent of the temporal order in which the subsequent splicing reactions take place.

Evolutionary Advantages of Splicing

Pre-mRNA splicing is clearly an ancient process: it occurs in eukaryotes, *Archaea,* and a bacteriophage of *Escherichia coli,* although it has not been found in *Eubacteria.* Identically placed introns in the human and corn triose phosphate isomerase gene imply that this split gene existed before plants and animals diverged, about 800 million years ago (see Fig. 1–1). Some researchers of evolution believe that the progenitor organism from which current prokaryotes and eukaryotes were derived utilized introns that were lost in the evolution of current *Eubacteria,* but others believe that splicing only evolved later. It is likely that the extensive splicing machinery just described evolved from specialized **RNA enzymes (ribozymes)** that are capable of splicing themselves (see the later section on group II introns). The greater complexity of the trans-acting spliceosome may have evolved as a mechanism to make this process applicable to a much wider selection of RNA transcripts, without the need to encode the complete ribozyme within each intron.

What do cells gain by investing all of this genetic information and energy in splicing? Splicing certainly

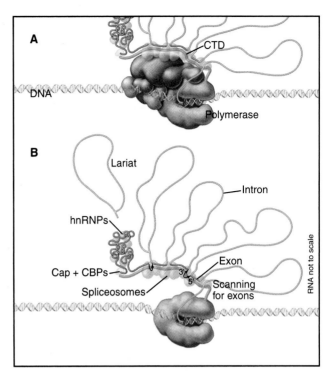

Figure 15–8 The carboxy-terminal domain (CTD) of RNA pol II acts as a scaffold that coordinates the events of pre-mRNA processing. *A,* Transcribing RNA polymerase holoenzyme with associated general transcription factors. *B,* In this view, the transcription factors have been stripped away, revealing that scanning for splice sites and binding of the factors needed for the actual events of splicing are occurring in complexes associated with the CTD. The 5′ cap forms early and with cap binding protein (CBP) remains associated with the CTD throughout transcription. Note that the spliceosomes and hnRNPs are not shown to scale. Along the RNA molecule, exons are shown in red and introns in gray.

complicates the synthesis of mRNA. However, it may serve evolution by favoring the creation of new genes with new functions through "exon shuffling." Because genomes frequently undergo recombination, genes with new functions could conveniently be created from segments of existing functional units (exons) by recombination almost anywhere within their large flanking introns. In some instances, such as the immunoglobulin genes and the pyruvate kinase gene, exons encode amino acid sequences that fold into independent structural domains of proteins. Thus, on an evolutionary time scale, the presence of large introns could facilitate recombination to create new genes encoding proteins with new specificities.

Alternative Splicing and Trans-splicing

Splicing also offers cells an opportunity to "customize" gene products to meet different specialized needs. This can readily be accomplished by **alternative splicing** (Fig. 15–9A), in which the use of different splice donor and/or acceptor sites allows for the

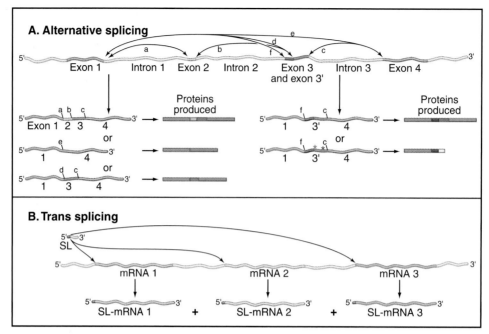

Figure 15–9 Alternative and trans-splicing are variations on the theme of splicing. *A,* This panel shows a number of the possible mRNA and protein products of a gene whose mRNA is subject to alternative splicing. In the examples shown at the left, by skipping one or more internal exons, alternative splicing provides a mechanism for producing related proteins with different combinations of amino acid "modules" encoded by different exons. Alternate 3′ splice sites can also be used. In the examples shown at the right, a different splice acceptor site is used, redefining the 5′ end of one exon. This often causes the exon to be read in a different reading frame *(blue asterisk),* thereby changing the amino acid sequence of the protein. If the alternative reading frame has a stop codon *(red asterisk)* this results in a truncated protein. For simplicity, the poly A at the 3′ end of each mRNA is not shown. *B,* Trans-splicing occurs between two separate RNA molecules. Many of the genes in *Trypanosomes* and *Nematodes* are encoded in a polycistronic manner (i.e., there is more than one coding region per pre-mRNA). To release each individual mRNA from its precursor transcript, a branchpoint A residing upstream of each mRNA attacks a 5′ splice site that is provided by the spliced leader (SL) RNA. Instead of a lariat intermediate, this forms a Y intermediate. The 3′ OH of the liberated upstream portion of the SL-RNA then acts like an upstream exon and attacks the phosphodiester at the 3′ splice site, thus splicing the short SL-RNA *(red)* to each mRNA. Messenger RNA 3′ ends are generated by polyadenylation (not shown).

production, from a single gene, of multiple mRNAs with partly overlapping genetic information, each encoding a distinct polypeptide. Multiple alternative 5′ splice sites can be joined to a common 3′ splice site, and multiple alternative 3′ splice sites can be joined to a common 5′ splice site. In this way, partial or whole exons can be added or deleted. Thus, an exon of one mRNA can be in an intron of an alternatively spliced mRNA. Although first discovered in viruses, alternative splicing also occurs in cellular transcripts, especially in higher eukaryotes. In humans, about one in four pre-mRNAs is alternatively spliced.

Although some transcripts are alternatively spliced in all cell types, others are differently spliced in particular cells, allowing different tissues to produce specialized forms of particular proteins. Alternative splicing of common primary transcripts produces tissue-specific mRNAs for troponin T, tropomyosin, calcitonin, and many brain neuropeptides. Furthermore, alternative splicing can yield tissue-specific mRNAs encoding

transcription factors that influence the differential expression of other genes. In fact, it is through alternative splicing that the sex of the fruit fly *Drosophila* is determined.

How are alternative splice sites selected? It has been observed that the flanking regions of most alternatively spliced exons match poorly with canonical splicing consensus sequences. This means that variations in the abundance of a limiting splicing factor can determine whether such a poorly defined exon is included or excluded in the mature mRNA. For example, when the alternative splicing factor (ASF) was initially purified, it turned out to be a known splicing factor (SF2), which had previously been shown to play a general role in splicing. In another example, in *Drosophila*, a cascade of genes (called *sex lethal, transformer, transformer 2,* and *double sex*) are transcribed equally but spliced differently in males and females. A high X chromosome:autosome ratio initiates this splicing cascade. When present, each encoded protein enhances or represses splicing of the subsequent gene's transcript in a female-specific manner. With this appropriate splicing, the fly is female; otherwise, the default pathway is for a male fly.

Although all known splicing of nuclear transcripts in higher eukaryotes takes place intramolecularly (i.e., within a single transcript), in certain lower eukaryotes, notably the trypanosomatids, intermolecular splicing between exons of two different transcripts occurs instead. This so-called **trans-splicing** joins a common spliced *leader RNA* (SL-RNA, which corresponds to the 5′ exon) from one primary transcript to various coding exons from other pre-mRNAs (see Fig. 15–9*B*). The mechanism is similar to pre-mRNA splicing except that SL-RNA appears to function both as the donor exon and in place of U1 RNA. The nematode worm *Caenorhabditis elegans* uses both trans-splicing and cis-splicing, and it even utilizes more than one kind of SL-RNA.

mRNA Transport and Degradation

The rate of synthesis of any given protein depends greatly on the cytoplasmic concentration of its mRNA, which is determined by the balance between the rates of its production and degradation. After processing is completed, mRNA is transported through nuclear pores to the cytoplasm (see Fig. 16–16) where it can direct protein synthesis (see Fig. 18–18) until it is degraded (Fig. 15–10). Spliceosome components, bound to introns, may prevent transport until processing has been completed. Upon exiting the nucleus, many but not all hnRNP proteins dissociate from mRNA.

Studies of yeast mRNAs, which are typically shorter-lived than those of mammals, have provided general insights into mechanisms of mRNA degradation. Initially, mRNA molecules are resistant to degradation, but their 3′ poly A tracts shorten steadily with time. Once the poly A is reduced to approximately 10 nucleotides (probably too short to bind the protective poly A binding protein), the 5′ end of the mRNA is rapidly decapped, yet another example of communication between the 3′ and 5′ regions of an mRNA. Following decapping, the RNA molecule is rapidly degraded from both ends by exonucleases, including ones that cleave from the 5′ end, and the exosome (see later section) which cleaves from the 3′ end. The poly A shortening rate varies for different mRNAs, determining their relative half-lives and thus their steady-state concentration.

Although a major route for mRNA turnover in yeasts, and probably in higher organisms, this is not the only one. Some RNAs get decapped without prior deadenylation, others get degraded without prior decapping, and still others get degraded starting from an internal cleavage event. In fact, the most long-lived

cellular RNAs (rRNAs, 5S RNA, and tRNAs) are neither capped nor polyadenylated. They evidently are protected from degradation by tight secondary structures and associations with specific proteins. (See the section that follows on snoRNA processing.)

Although mRNA turnover has, to date, received much less experimental attention than mRNA production, it is likely to be as important in determining the amount of protein made from a gene. Vertebrate mRNA half-lives range from a few minutes (e.g., the c-fos immediate early gene mRNA; see Fig. 44–11) to a few hours (most mRNAs) to a few days (e.g., globin mRNA in reticulocytes and ovalbumin mRNA in chicken oviduct cells). Several mechanisms specify this wide range of degradation rates. Many mRNAs with very short half-lives, such as those encoding certain growth factors, cytokines, and lymphokines (see Chapters 26 and 29), have a series of AU-rich elements located within their 3′ untranslated regions. These elements bind specific proteins that target these RNAs for degradation by the exosome complex (see Fig. 15–10).

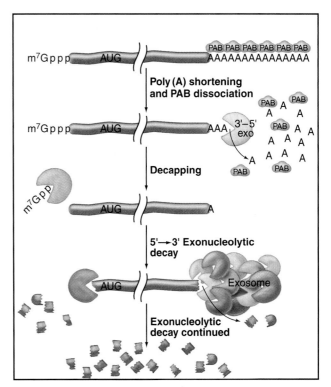

Figure 15–10 Messenger RNA degradation is a multi-step regulated process. As mRNAs age in the cytoplasm, the length of their 3′ poly A tails gradually decreases, releasing the poly A binding (PAB) proteins, which helped the 3′ end of the mRNA associate with the 5′ cap structure. Without the PAB proteins, the RNA begins to be degraded by 3′–5′ exonucleases. It also rapidly loses its 5′ cap and is degraded by 5′-3′ exonucleases. Without such physical interactions between the 5′ and 3′ ends or other mechanisms to protect them (such as bound factors or secondary structures), cytoplasmic RNAs are rapidly degraded.

The half-lives of some mRNAs are regulated in response to differing needs of the cell. For instance, binding of the hormone prolactin to receptors on mammary gland cells increases the half-life of the mRNA encoding the milk protein casein from 1 to 40 hours, which stimulates milk production. In another example, the cellular concentration of iron regulates the half-life of the mRNA encoding the mammalian transferrin receptor (required for iron import into cells; see Chapter 23). High concentrations of cytoplasmic iron cause release of a protective protein (the iron-responsive element binding protein) from the mRNA, making it susceptible to cleavage and degradation.

Messenger RNAs containing premature nonsense (stop) codons are specifically degraded through a more general mechanism known as **nonsense-mediated decay.** This is thought to protect cells against potentially damaging truncated proteins that would result from translation of mRNAs containing stop codons in the middle of their reading frames. This has long been an enigma because this selective decay is seen for spliced mRNA in nuclei as well as the cytoplasm, despite the fact that the ability to read codons in frame was thought to be solely a cytoplasmic property. Recent evidence for some translation occurring also in the nucleus may help provide the explanation.

Another form of RNA degradation still under active investigation is called **RNA interference (RNAi).** Through this process, perfect duplex RNA (such as natural viral RNA or a duplex RNA a researcher has intentionally generated in a cell) is cleaved into 21 nucleotide fragments which direct cleavage of cytoplasmic mRNA to which they are complementary. In some cases, the duplex RNA is also self propagating. Using RNAi researchers can specifically deplete cells of selected mRNAs. For experiments on mammalian cells, to avoid complications, 21 nucleotide fragments are introduced as preformed duplexes. RNAi is being used in a large scale genomic screen to inactivate all 18,000 genes of *Caenorhabditis elegans.*

Other Kinds of Processing of Pol II Transcripts

Histone 3′ End Formation

Although most eukaryotic mRNAs acquire 3′ poly A tails, mRNAs encoding the major histone proteins undergo a different kind of 3′ end processing. Located within the 3′ untranslated region of the histone pre-mRNA is a conserved sequence element that base-pairs with the U7 snRNP (Fig. 15–11A). This recruits factors that cleave, to generate the mature 3′ end of histone mRNA. Why do only histone mRNAs lack a 3′ poly A tail? Perhaps it is because these mRNAs are only needed during S phase of the cell cycle when they are transcribed, translated, and rapidly degraded. Their lack of a poly A tail may facilitate their rapid

turnover, preventing production of histone proteins after DNA replication has been completed. By contrast, minor histone variants that are synthesized throughout the cell cycle have normal poly A tails.

snRNAs and snoRNAs

RNA pol II also transcribes many snRNAs, including most U RNAs. Some, like the U RNAs of the spliceosome, are localized in the nucleoplasm and are called snRNAs, whereas others, like U3 and U8 (which are involved in rRNA processing; see the section that follows), are localized in the nucleolus and are termed **snoRNAs** (small *n*ucle*o*lar RNAs). The term **U RNA** originally referred to U residue-rich RNA but has evolved to describe any RNA that is relatively small and resides in the nucleus when mature.

The primary transcripts of the abundant pol II-transcribed U snRNAs (U1–U5 and U7) acquire a distinctive 5′ cap. Like that of pre-mRNAs, their cap starts with the addition of a reverse G residue, which becomes methylated on the N^7 position and then 2′-O methylated on the first residue of the original RNA (see Fig. 15–11B). These U snRNAs are then temporarily exported to the cytoplasm where the cap acquires two more methyl groups on the reverse G, forming a 2,2,7 trimethyl G cap, rather than the 7-methyl-G cap of pre-mRNA molecules. The U snRNAs that will become part of the spliceosome bind a group of proteins called Sm proteins and are then reimported to the nucleus. The autoantibody that recognized the Sm proteins (from a patient with systemic lupus erythematosus) provided an important tool aiding in the initial characterization of the splicing machinery. U snoRNAs also undergo cap trimethylation, although this evidently occurs within the nucleus.

It used to be thought that all functional RNAs transcribed by RNA pol II retained the 5′ cap that is added to the primary transcript. This theory was disproven with the discovery of a large new class of RNAs that are transcribed by RNA pol II but are located within introns of other genes and then processed out of them (see Fig. 15–11D). These small RNAs localize to the nucleolus and, together with associated proteins, form **snoRNPs** (*s*mall *n*ucle*o*lar *r*ibo*n*ucle*o*protein particles). In mammals, the more than 100 different intron-encoded snoRNPs are used in rRNA processing and modification (see later section). Yeast has an analogous set of snoRNAs, some of which are intron-encoded and some of which are transcribed from their own promoters.

These intron-encoded snoRNAs are of two basic types—called C/D and H/ACA snoRNAs according to their conserved elements, which also determine the proteins they bind. These proteins bind while the snoRNAs are still in their intronic precursor form and are retained after their host intron has been spliced

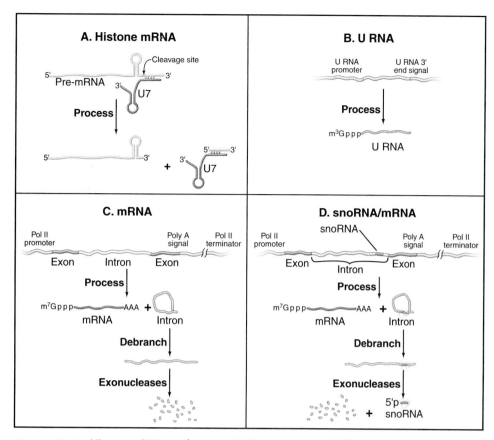

Figure 15–11 Histone mRNAs and some snRNAs are processed differently from other polymerase II transcripts. *A,* Messenger RNAs encoding histone proteins that bind the newly replicated DNA in S phase are not polyadenylated like other mRNAs. Instead, their 3′ ends are cleaved in a process guided by the U7 snRNP. U7 base-pairs with a specific sequence downstream of a highly conserved stem loop structure present in these histone mRNAs. Cleavage then occurs between the U7 base-pairing and the base of the stem loop. *B,* Some U RNAs undergo minimal processing, acquiring only a distinctive 5′ cap structure after transcription. Most, however, also require at least a 3′ processing cleavage. *C,* Messenger RNAs are processed by 5′ capping, 3′ cleavage and polyadenylation, and generally splicing (see Fig. 15–6). *D,* Small nucleolar RNAs involved in rRNA modification typically reside in the introns of other abundantly transcribed genes in mammals and are released during splicing. Here, an average snoRNA of about 200 bases is encoded in an average intron (for humans) of about 3000 bases. Following debranching, exonucleases trim the ends of the intron, releasing the snoRNAs, which are protected from complete degradation by their secondary structure and the presence of bound proteins.

and debranched. What defines the ends of each snoRNA during processing is not known, but it is likely that these bound proteins may help to block the progression of nucleases that otherwise rapidly degrade excised debranched introns. Interestingly, most genes whose introns contain snoRNAs encode proteins that are part of, or associate with, ribosomes. Although this could reflect a functional association—somehow coordinating levels of ribosomal components with the machinery that helps produce ribosomes—it appears more likely that, since cells require several thousands of copies of snoRNAs, they must derive from highly transcribed genes, such as those encoding the highly abundant proteins required for transcription. The existence of this new class of RNA, generated by a previously unknown processing mechanism and acting

in a previously unknown manner, was quite unanticipated.

Processing of Transcripts Synthesized by RNA Polymerase III

RNA polymerase III (pol III) is responsible for synthesizing a rather diverse set of transcripts—5S rRNA, tRNAs, U6 snRNA, signal recognition particle RNA 7SL, and a few small cytoplasmic RNAs (called Y RNAs, as opposed to the U RNAs located in the nucleus). In addition to serving a wide range of functions, the transcripts synthesized by pol III show a great diversity in the processing they undergo.

5S RNA Processing

5S rRNA joins with 28S and 5.8S rRNAs to form the large subunit of the ribosome (see Fig. 18–6). However, unlike the other rRNAs, 5S RNA is encoded by a separate gene, is transcribed by a different polymerase, and has a different processing fate (see the following section on 18S, 5.8S, and 28S rRNA processing). In fact, 5S RNA has the simplest life history of any eukaryotic transcript. It is not capped but retains the 5' triphosphate from transcription initiation, the only mature eukaryotic RNA known to do this. Neither is it spliced or polyadenylated. Its ends are presumably protected from degradation by a tightly base-paired secondary structure and associated proteins, as is the case with other stable rRNAs. In some species, the primary transcript of the 5S RNA gene is already the fully mature product, making it the only known example of a eukaryotic cytoplasmic RNA that undergoes no processing. In other species, the 3' end of the primary transcript is trimmed by nuclease action to generate the mature form. This minimal processing of

5S rRNA in eukaryotes contrasts with the situation in prokaryotes, where 5S RNA is transcribed as part of the large pre-rRNA and requires processing of both ends, while mRNAs are used without any processing.

tRNA Processing

Pre-tRNAs require considerable processing before reaching their mature form: their 5' and 3' ends are cleaved, nucleotides are added to their 3' ends, numerous modifications are made to specific internal residues and, in many cases, internal introns are spliced out (Fig. 15–12).

The 5' ends of tRNAs from organisms spanning all three domains of life result from an endonucleolytic cleavage catalyzed by a ribonucleoprotein complex, **RNase P.** Eukaryotic RNase P consists of a highly conserved RNA and nine proteins that recognize the hairpin structure of a pre-tRNA. The RNA component of some bacterial RNase P species can catalyze this reaction in vitro without protein cofactors, but this activity has not been demonstrated for the eukaryotic enzyme. (Additional information on RNA enzymes is presented in the section on Group I and Group II introns.) Intriguingly, it appears that much of the tRNA processing occurs in the nucleolus, not in the nucleoplasm, as had been thought for decades.

At their 3' end, all tRNAs acquire a terminal CCA trinucleotide that is needed for the aminoacylation reaction, which charges the tRNA with an amino acid (see Fig. 18–4). In eukaryotes, RNA pol III terminates transcription downstream of the 3' end of the mature tRNA; the extra 3' sequences are then removed by nuclease action and a terminal CCA is added by RNA nucleotidyl transferase (also known as CCA-adding enzyme) (see Fig. 15–12B). The La protein, which binds the poly U tract at the 3' end of pre-tRNAs and other pol III transcripts, is important for proper 3' end processing.

Collectively, tRNAs make up the most highly modified class of RNAs, with nearly 100 different kinds of **nucleoside modifications** possible at various internal positions. These modifications—which range from simple methyl additions (e.g., 1-methylguanosine) to elaborate moieties (e.g., 2-methylthio-N6-threonylcarbamoyladenosine)—are introduced by chemical alteration of the originally transcribed nucleotide without breakage of the phosphodiester backbone. The enzymology of these modifications is often complex, and different proteins may catalyze the same nucleoside modification at two different positions in the tRNA. Modified nucleosides are believed to add versatility and specificity to tRNA action.

Common among pre-tRNAs in eukaryotes (and *Archaea*) is the presence of a small intron one nucleotide 3' of the anticodon (see Fig. 15–12C). Transfer

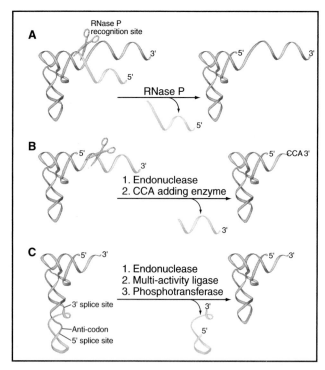

Figure 15-12 Transfer RNAs require extensive processing before they function in translation. *A,* Transcription of tRNA genes produces precursor tRNAs that have extensions at both their 5' and 3' ends. RNaseP cleaves the precursor tRNAs, yielding their mature 5' ends. *B,* The 3' ends of tRNAs are also processed by endonucleolytic cleavage. Subsequently, the sequence CCA is added. A 3' CCA is a universal feature of all tRNAs. *C,* Some tRNA genes contain introns that are removed by a series of reactions carried out by protein enzymes (RNA molecules are not involved) (see text for description of the mechanism). The green bar shows the anticodon, which is typically located one base away from the 5' splice site.

RNA splicing was actually the first kind of intron removal discovered. It is mechanistically distinct from pre-mRNA splicing, utilizing no RNA cofactors, transesterification reactions, or lariat intermediates. Instead, tRNA introns are removed by the action of protein enzymes. First, an endonuclease clips both ends of the intron, generating 2′-3′ cyclic phosphate and 5′ OH termini. These ends are not direct substrates for a ligase but become joined in a rather complex set of reactions: the 5′ terminus of the downstream exon becomes phosphorylated; the 2′-3′ cyclic phosphate of the upstream exon is converted into a 2′ phosphate, liberating its 3′ OH; and then these newly created 3′ OH and 5′ phosphate ends are joined by ligation. In yeast, all three of these reactions are catalyzed by the same protein. A separate enzyme then removes the 2′ phosphate remaining at the end of the upstream exon. Interestingly, the multifunctional tRNA ligase also participates in removing at least one intron in a pre-mRNA, at a site that lacks a GU/AG or AT/AC consensus. Thus, nature uses two completely different mechanisms to remove intervening sequences from transcripts.

Small RNA Processing

Unlike most major U RNAs, which are pol II transcripts, U6 snRNA, MRP RNA (see later section), and a number of other small RNAs are transcribed by pol III. U6 is the most evolutionarily conserved snRNA and also the most intimately involved in identifying the 5′ splicing site. The 5′ end of the U6 transcript retains its α phosphate, which is protected by an O-methylation, unlike the 2,2,7 trimethylguanosine cap that forms on the major snRNAs transcribed by pol II. Internal residues become modified much as rRNAs do in the nucleolus (see the section that follows). At the 3′ end, the oligo U where transcription terminates is first extended with non-templated U residues in a reaction that depends on the La auto-antigen and is then shortened to five U residues with a terminal 2′-3′ cyclic phosphate. This allows binding of a complex of seven proteins (Lsm, *like* the *Sm* proteins on the other U-snRNPs) needed for the U4/U5/U6 tri-snRNP to assemble and function in splicing. Although less is known about the processing of the other pol III-transcribed small RNAs, they, too, acquire a γ methyl cap and undergo some 3′ end trimming.

▌ Processing of Polymerase I Transcripts

Observed for more than 100 years and located within the nucleus of all eukaryotic cells is a large, electron-dense region, called the nucleolus, where ribosome synthesis largely occurs. Early electron microscopy of nucleoli that had been dispersed in solutions of low ionic strength revealed a series of structures resembling **Christmas trees** (Fig. 15–13*A*). What is now known is that each "Christmas tree" represents a single rDNA repeat unit (i.e., ribosomal RNA gene, of which there are ~100 to 200 in tandem array) being transcribed by RNA pol I. The rDNA forms the trunk, nascent pre-rRNA makes up the branches, and processing complexes containing the U3 snoRNA that rapidly bind the newly synthesized rRNA at a far 5′ processing site form 5′ terminal "balls," which appear as ornaments.

From these long precursor molecules (~47S or about 14 kb in mammals; ~35S or about 7 kb in yeast) are then cleaved the 18S, 5.8S, and 28S rRNAs that will form the small and large subunits of the ribosome. In these endonucleolytic and exonucleolytic processing events, variably sized **external** and **internal transcribed spacers** (**ETS** and **ITS,** respectively) are removed and then degraded, similar to the fate of pre-mRNA introns (see Fig. 15–11*B*). Cleavages occur within the transcribed spacers as well as at their ends. Surprisingly, the cleavage events at many of the processing sites seem fundamentally different. Pre-rRNAs are also processed by modification of nearly 200 specific rRNA residues. Also, about 80 ribosomal proteins rapidly bind pre-rRNA in the nucleolus, and a few additional proteins bind to the 18S region in the cytoplasm. Because it is so abundant in the cell, pre-rRNA was the first transcript recognized to generate mature species by RNA processing, and many of its major hallmarks were already identified prior to the recombinant DNA revolution.

It has been known for some time that snoRNPs are involved in cleaving the large pre-rRNA transcript (see Fig. 15–13*B*), although there appear to be some differences in their utilization in yeast and mammals. U3 snoRNP is important for a very early cleavage—the first pre-rRNA processing event in mammals—at a site within the 5′ ETS where the balls of the Christmas trees form (in mammals, this processing also involves the U14, U17, and E3 snoRNAs). U3 also helps with cleavage in ITS1, and U22 and U14 (in yeast) assist in releasing 18S rRNA. U14 may also serve as a chaperone to help fold an internal portion of the 18S region in mammals. U8 functions by helping cleavage within ITS1 and the 3′ ETS, while in yeast, MRP and RNase III are involved in processing in these regions. Interestingly, MRP is another RNP that has a related RNA and shares eight common proteins with RNase P (see the earlier discussion of tRNA processing). Furthermore, MRP cleaves eukaryotic pre-rRNA at a site similar to the one where RNase P cleaves prokaryotic pre-rRNA in liberating a tRNA. Following these specific endonucleolytic cleavages, the ends are trimmed by 5′ to 3′ and 3′ to 5′ exonucleases (see the section on the exosome that follows).

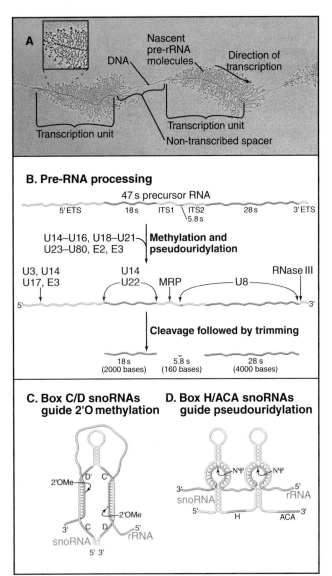

Figure 15-13 Following transcription by polymerase I in the nucleolus, rRNAs undergo extensive cleavage and modification before they function in protein synthesis. *A,* This electron micrograph shows rDNA genes in the process of being transcribed by numerous polymerase I complexes. The genes are organized in tandem arrays with spacers in between them. As the polymerases move along the gene, the transcripts get longer and branch out from the DNA "trunk," giving the Christmas tree appearance. The "ornaments" at the ends of the branches *(see inset)* correspond to RNA processing complexes. *B,* As the rRNA transcripts emerge from pol I, they interact with well over a hundred snoRNAs as well as over a hundred ribosomal and preribosomal proteins. Some snoRNAs (specifically, U3, U14, U17, E3, U22, MRP, U8, and RNase III) are involved in cleavage of the transcripts into 18S, 5.8S, and 28S rRNAs. However, the vast majority are required to target specific sites within the rRNA for methylation and pseudouridylation. Note that the sizes of transcripts shown here are as found in humans, but so far, RNase MRP and RNase III action has been characterized only in budding yeast. *C* and *D,* Small nucleolar RNAs, characterized by conserved sequence elements called boxes C and D, are involved in rRNA methylation, which occurs at the 2′ position of selected ribose moieties, while snoRNAs containing elements called H and ACA are required for pseudouridylation (NΨ, which rotates uridine residues to form a carbon-carbon linkage to the ribose, rather than the traditional N-C linkage). These conserved sequence elements are shown in green. Both kinds of snoRNAs form extensive base-pairing interactions with rRNA and use this sequence specificity to select the residues within the rRNA to be modified. Box C/D snoRNAs position the rRNA residue to be methylated 5 bp *(red dot)* upstream of their box D (and D′) sequences. Some C/D snoRNAs direct methylation of two different rRNA sites (shown here): others direct only one. Box H/ACA snoRNAs use their stem loop structures to place the uridine residue to be rotated precisely opposite the base of their top stem. (*A,* Courtesy of Yvonne Osheim, University of Virginia, Charlottesville.)

Recently, well over 100 additional snoRNPs have been found to play a role in rRNA processing. They serve as guide RNAs that target about 110 specific sites for **2′-O methylation** and about 95 sites for **pseudouridylation** in mammals (somewhat fewer in yeast) (see Fig. 15–13*B*). These snoRNAs each contain one or more regions of 10 to 20 nucleotides complementary to a site of rRNA that is targeted for modification (see Fig. 15–13*C* and 15–11*C*). These base-pairing regions are located at precise positions relative to the modifications they direct. The snoRNAs that direct 2′-O methylation are characterized by sequence elements, called boxes C and D, which bind the 2′-O-methylase fibrillarin, whereas those that direct pseudouridylation contain boxes H and ACA and bind the pseudouridine synthase dyskerin. These methylations and pseudouridylations occur rapidly following transcription and are confined to the most highly con-

served portions of the rRNA, where they may fine-tune its folding. Curiously, some snRNAs also undergo such snoRNA-guided methylation, possibly while in the nucleolus. Thus in pre-rRNA processing, the newly synthesized transcript associates with numerous small RNAs that help to fold, cleave, and modify the 18S, 5.8S and 28S RNAs, which with their assembled proteins are exported to the cytoplasm for use in translation as the small and large ribosomal subunits.

The Exosome

A theme common throughout RNA processing, regardless of whether a transcript is synthesized by pol I, II, or III, is that exonucleases remove unwanted regions of RNA. There are exonucleases that degrade in the 5′ to 3′ direction and others that degrade in the 3′ to 5′

direction. Recently, a large complex was discovered to contain numerous 3'-5' exonucleases (e.g., 11 in yeast) that are important for processing a wide variety of RNAs; the function of the complex depends on all those proteins. This **exosome** (see Fig. 15–10) trims 3' precursors of rRNAs, snRNAs, and snoRNAs, and degrades unspliced pre-mRNAs and rRNA spacer regions.

Group I and Group II Introns

The earlier sections describe how introns are removed from eukaryotic pre-mRNAs by transesterification reactions using large RNA/protein complexes, or from pre-tRNAs by protein-based endonuclease and ligase enzymes. In another fascinating kind of splicing, also present in eukaryotes (and prokaryotes, too), the introns themselves catalyze their own release. These self-cleaving RNAs, known as group I and group II introns, fold into specialized structures that carry out two transesterification reactions similar to those of pre-mRNA splicing (Fig. 15–14A and B).

Group I Introns

In 1981, researchers studying the ciliate *Tetrahymena* were shocked to discover that a 413-nucleotide intron was capable of catalyzing its own removal from an rRNA precursor molecule. Until that time, all known enzymes were proteins, but here was a catalytic RNA. This rRNA intron can direct multiple RNA breakage/joining reactions and can even act on other RNA molecules. Hence, it is a true RNA enzyme, a **ribozyme.** This *Tetrahymena* intron has since become the prototype for a family of self-splicing RNAs, known as **group I introns,** which are found in pre-rRNAs from other unicellular eukaryotes, in pre-mRNAs from the mitochondria and chloroplasts of many lower organisms, and in the mitochondria of higher plants. They are even present in bacteriophage T4.

Despite significant differences in their primary sequences, the various group I family members fold into a conserved tertiary structure capable of carrying out two phosphodiester cleavage reactions quite similar to pre-mRNA splicing. However, instead of an attack at the 5' splice site by an internal A residue, the nucleophile is a noncovalently bound guanosine, from guanosine triphosphate (GTP), guanosine diphosphate (GDP), or guanosine monophosphate (GMP) (compare Fig. 15–14A with Fig. 15–6B). The 3' OH of this guanosine cofactor attacks and releases the upstream exon, which then attacks at the 3' splice site, joining the two exons. Numerous Mg^{2+} ions are important for folding the intron into a tertiary structure that holds the 5' and 3' exon junctions in close proximity via

base-pairing to its "internal guide sequence." In addition, a binding pocket for the guanosine cofactor is created near a coordinated Mg^{2+} ion that helps activate the attacking hydroxyl. The only requirements for the in vitro group I splicing reaction are externally added guanosine and Mg^{2+}. However, in vivo it appears that group I introns are also aided by specific proteins.

Because the bond energy is conserved in transesterification reactions, no external energy is needed, and the group I splicing reaction is completely reversible. Under appropriate conditions, group I introns can not only splice and cleave RNA, but can also catalyze a number of reactions, including endonucleolytic cleavage, DNA and RNA ligation, and even RNA chain polymerization. Thus, there is a precedent for envisioning that, at the dawn of evolution, before DNA and proteins, a self-replicating RNA "life form" could have evolved. This is the basis of the **"RNA world"** hypothesis.

Group II Introns

Group II introns comprise a second class of self-splicing introns. Thus far, they have only been found in the mitochondria and chloroplasts of plants and fungi, and although most are located in protein-coding genes, group II introns are also present in a few tRNA and rRNA genes. Group II splicing has been of particular interest to evolutionary biologists because of the intriguing parallels between it and pre-mRNA splicing (see the legend for Fig. 15–14).

Similar to group I introns, RNAs belonging to the group II class of introns fold into a distinct tertiary structure. Under nonphysiological conditions (moderately high temperature and high Mg^{2+} concentration), a number of group II introns are capable of splicing themselves out of their host RNAs in the absence of any protein. However, they require additional trans-acting factors to do this in vivo. Indeed, unspliced fungal group II introns encode maturation proteins that assist in their excision. The transesterification reactions undertaken by group II introns exactly parallel those of nuclear pre-mRNA splicing. First, the 5' splice site is attacked by an internal "branchpoint" adenosine which creates a lariat intermediate (compare Figs. 15–14B and 15–6B). The liberated upstream exon then attacks the 3' splice site, ligating the two exons together. The striking difference between the two kinds of splicing is that even in vitro, pre-mRNA splicing requires U1, U2, U4, U5, and U6, about 100 protein factors, and energy input.

Interestingly, the intramolecular secondary structure of the group II intron forms a catalytic center that closely resembles the intermolecular base-pairing of snRNAs in the spliceosome (see Fig. 15–14C). This

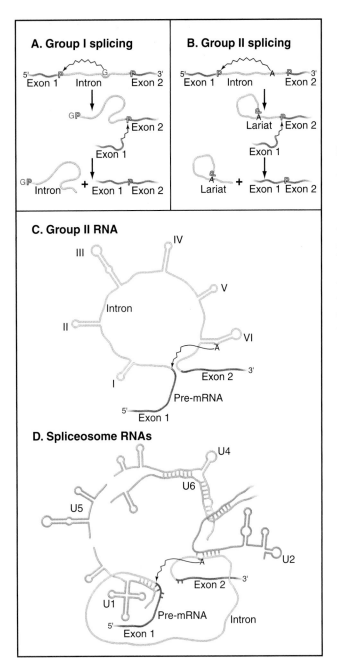

Figure 15-14 Group I and II introns are catalytic RNAs. *A,* Group I introns remove themselves from their precursor RNAs via a two-step mechanism. First, a G (*red,* in the form of GTP, GDP, GMP, or even just G) binds a pocket within the intron that aligns it so that its 2' OH can attack the phosphodiester at the 5' splice site. Then, similar to the mechanism for pre-mRNA splicing, the 2' OH of the released exon 1 attacks the phosphodiester at the 3' splice site, thus joining the two exons together. *B,* Group II splicing is even more similar to pre-mRNA splicing than group I. An adenosine (A) near the 3' end of the group II intron attacks at the 5' splice site, a lariat intermediate is formed, and then the two exons are joined. (Compare this figure with Fig. 15–6.) *C and D,* Group II introns fold into specialized structures that are capable of carrying out splicing in the absence of protein. Many RNA researchers have speculated that the combination of splicing snRNAs interacting with a pre-mRNA intron may be related evolutionarily to group II introns (compare Fig. 15–14*C* and *D*). Specifically, Domain VI of Group II, like the U2:branch region duplex, activates the branch A residue by placing it in a bulged configuration; Domain V, like the U6:U2 duplex, assists in bringing the branch A to the 5' splice site by base pairing; and Domain III, like U5, base-pairs with both the 5' and 3' exon regions at the splice sites.

has led to the hypothesis that group II elements located in introns were the ancestors of the machinery used in pre-mRNA splicing. During evolution, the catalytically active group II elements may have become removed from the intron and dispersed onto several distinct small snRNAs. Through base-pairings and protein-mediated interactions, these RNAs come together in the spliceosome to create a group II–like catalytic center that can act on many different pre-mRNAs. In fact, splicing of an intron in *Chlamydomonas* appears to be an intermediate case, where the catalytic center is made up by three distinct RNAs.

Other Ribozymes

In nature, there are many other catalytically active RNA forms, including the hammerhead (see Fig. 2–24) and hairpin structures of certain viral RNAs. These ribozymes catalyze cleavage of RNA by nucleophilic attack, targeted by base-pairing and tertiary interactions. Their small size (50 to 100 nucleotides) has helped crystallographers to determine their three-dimensional structures, which has allowed a detailed view of the events during catalysis.

In addition, the hammerhead ribozyme is proving

useful to scientists because it need not be formed by intramolecular base-pairing, but can arise by intermolecular base-pairing between catalytic and substrate domains. This has allowed researchers to design catalytic domains that base-pair with substrate RNAs of interest and direct their specific cleavage, thus forming a sequence-specific designer restriction endonuclease for RNA.

RNA Editing

The term **RNA editing** describes a diverse series of recently discovered but mechanistically unrelated post-transcriptional processing events through which the primary sequence of an RNA is changed in ways other than those described earlier. These include both nucleotide modifications and insertions/deletions.

Nucleotide Alterations

There are a few cases in which a mammalian nuclear-encoded mRNA acquires a base substitution. The hu-

man apolipoprotein B mRNA initially encodes a long protein, but in an event that serves to regulate this gene's expression into protein, a single C to U change converts a CAA glutamine codon into a UAA termination codon, causing translation to stop halfway through the mRNA. This editing results from a specific deamination (Fig. 15–15A), catalyzed by a deaminase enzyme that is targeted by a motif in the adjoining RNA. There are at least two other examples of this kind of C to U deamination in mammalian mRNA.

Mitochondrial and chloroplast genes of some lower eukaryotes and plants exhibit much more frequent, yet still highly specific, C to U changes in their mRNAs. The enzymatic basis of these changes and their mode of recognition remain to be determined, but clearly, a single conserved sequence motif, like that in apolipoprotein B, is not involved. Transfer RNAs in certain organisms as diverse as marsupials, the protozoa *Acanthamoeba,* and the parasite Leishmania also exhibit a specific C to U conversion.

Another kind of RNA editing involving nucleotide modification in eukaryotic cells results from a double-

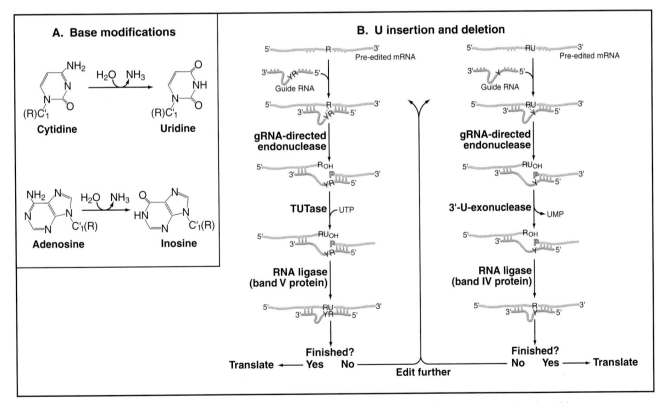

Figure 15–15 RNA editing alters mRNA coding sequences. *A,* The coding potential of an mRNA can be altered by deamination: the amino group at position 4 of C is replaced with a carbonyl, thus turning it into U. A similar reaction occurs at position 2 of A residues, which produces the base inosine. *B,* Uridine (U) residues are inserted into, and less frequently deleted from, mRNA coding regions in *Trypanosome* mitochondria via a mechanism that involves binding of a guide RNA (gRNA), cleavage of the mRNA, addition of a few to several Us by terminal uridylyl transferase (TUTase) or removal of terminal Us by a 3'-U-exonuclease, and then ligation. Curiously, even though these reactions apparently follow very similar pathways and are catalyzed by a common seven-protein complex, completely distinct endonucleases, U addition or U removal, and ligase activities are used by the two pathways.

strand RNA adenosine deaminase activity that selectively converts A to I residues in double-strand regions of certain RNAs (see Fig. 15–15A). In the glutamate receptor mRNA, a codon is altered in this manner as part of a regulatory strategy. The inability of the resultant inosine to hydrogen-bond with the previously complementary uridine residue also serves to unwind the modified RNA region.

Nucleotide Insertions and Deletions

Trypanosomes and related organisms are parasitic protozoans that exhibit probably the most bizarre form of RNA processing. There, U residues become inserted into, and occasionally deleted from, mitochondrial transcripts at precise sites (see Fig. 15–15). This creates AUG initiation codons, creates termination codons, corrects encoded frame shift mutations, and can even create much of the protein coding sequence. Although some mitochondrial transcripts undergo no editing, and some undergo editing in only a small region, about one-third exhibit massive editing. In cytochrome oxidase subunit III, for example, more than half of the protein-encoding nucleotides of the mature mRNA are U residues added by editing. These U residues are inserted in blocks of 1 to a few residues at about 150 specific sites throughout the protein coding region. Note that if only one too many or one too few U residues were to be inserted at any site, a frame shift would result, yielding a nonfunctional mRNA. This is certainly an unexpected way to create an mRNA coding region.

The specificity of this U insertion remained a mystery until small RNA molecules, called **guide RNAs,** were identified. These guide RNAs contain a 5′ region that is complementary to the editing substrate RNA and that can anchor to the pre-mRNA. Adjoining this, their central region is complementary to the edited version of the adjoining sequence, and it evidently guides the U insertions and deletions, which are demarcated by mismatches with the pre-edited mRNA sequence. Many overlapping guide RNAs are needed to direct editing in almost all mRNAs.

It was originally thought that the requisite breakage and rejoining of the pre-mRNA phosphodiester backbone was attributable to transesterification reactions (like mRNA and rRNA splicing), but it has since become clear that this editing occurs by nuclease and ligase action (see Fig. 15–15). First, the guide RNA directs endonuclease cleavage at the editing site (the 5′ end of the mRNA region base-paired with the guide RNA's anchor region). Then, for U deletion, the extra U residues are removed by a 3′ U-specific exonuclease. For U insertion, U residues are added to the 3′ cleaved end by a terminal U transferase. Next, RNA

ligases reseal the partially edited mRNA. Finally, base-pairing between the mRNA and the guide RNA zips up to the next editing site, and the next editing cycle is initiated. However, if the editing was not correct, the base-pairing does not extend beyond, and that position is re-edited. A functional editing complex that catalyzes both U insertion and U deletion has been isolated. It contains only seven different polypeptides, a surprisingly small number, relative to the spliceosome. The editing complex also exhibits all the enzymatic activities described earlier. Unexpectedly, the activities that catalyze the corresponding steps of U deletion and U insertion all appear to be different, suggesting that U deletion and U insertion may have evolved separately, only later becoming joined in the same complex. Trypanosome RNA editing also has evolutionary implications because any change to an A, C, or G in an edited mRNA region would require at least two concerted mutations in the DNA, one in the sequence encoding the pre-mRNA and another in the relevant guide RNA.

A less understood but equally intriguing second case of insertional RNA editing occurs in mitochondrial mRNAs, tRNAs, and rRNAs of the acellular slime mold, *Physarum polycephalum*. These transcripts undergo nucleotide insertion, roughly one every 30 nucleotides. Rather than being strictly one kind of residue, *Physarum* editing is primarily C insertion, but can occasionally be A, G, and U insertion. Neither putative conserved recognition signals nor guide RNAs have been found, and recent data indicate that this processing may be closely coupled with transcription, rather than being post-transcriptional, as in trypanosome editing.

▌ Conclusion

Both the wide variety of RNA molecules present in a eukaryotic cell and also the various processing events that are required before these transcripts can function have been described. An interesting theme throughout has been the way that RNA molecules are intimately involved in carrying out various cleavages and modifications that occur during maturation; in some instances, the RNAs catalyze reactions in the absence of any protein. Although many of the processing events appear to be mere trimming, it is likely that they also play a role in assessing whether a functional RNA has been synthesized. In addition, it is interesting that many of the fascinating, noncanonical forms of RNA processing are found in mitochondria, evolutionary vestiges of early prokaryotic endosymbiants, that are not under the same selective pressure as free living organisms. Perhaps these varied kinds of RNA processing are very ancient, reflecting hold-overs from an earlier evolutionary period. Since many of these events appear to occur only in small groups of organisms, there likely are other unexpected forms of RNA processing waiting to be discovered.

▌ **Selected Readings**

Abelson J, Trotta CR, Li H: tRNA splicing. J Biol Chem 273: 12685–12688, 1998.

Gott JM, Emeson RB: Functions and mechanisms of RNA editing. Annu Rev Genet 34:499–531, 2000.

Hastings ML, Kainer AR: Pre-mRNA splicing in the new millennium. Curr Opin Cell Biol 13:302–309, 2001.

Lafontaine DL, Tollervey D: The function and synthesis of ribosomes. Nat Rev Mol Cell Biol 2:514–520, 2001.

Minvielle-Sebastia L, Keller W: mRNA polyadenylation and its coupling to other RNA processing reactions and to transcription. Curr Opin Cell Biol 11:352–357, 1999.

Mitchell P, Tollervey D: mRNA turnover. Curr Opin Cell Biol 13:320–325, 2001.

Proudfoot N: Connecting transcription to messenger RNA processing. Trends Biochem Sci 25:290–293, 2000.

Sharp PA: Split genes and RNA splicing. Cell 77:805–815, 1994.

Shatkin AJ, Manley JL: The ends of the affair: Capping and polyadenylation. Nat Struct Biol 7:838–842, 2000.

Sollner-Webb B: Trypanosome RNA editing: Resolved. Science 273:1182–1183, 1996.

Weinstein LB, Steitz JA: Guided tours: From precursor snoRNA to functional snoRNP. Curr Opin Cell Biol 11: 378–384, 1999.

Will CL, Lührmann R: Spliceosomal UsnRNP biogenesis, structure and function. Curr Opin Cell Biol 13:290–301, 2001.

chapter 16

NUCLEAR STRUCTURE AND DYNAMICS

The nucleus, first described in 1831, houses the chromosomes together with the machinery for DNA replication and RNA transcription and processing (Fig. 16–1). Because eukaryotic genes are transcribed into RNAs containing intervening sequences that must be removed by splicing in order to assemble mature RNA molecules, it is necessary to ensure that immature RNAs are kept apart from the translational apparatus. This sequestration of immature RNAs is one function of the nuclear envelope, two concentric membranes that separate the nucleus and cytoplasm. In addition to regulating the movement of RNAs, this nuclear envelope regulates the movement of proteins, such as transcription factors, in and out of the nucleus. Thus, this double membrane has an important role in the control of gene expression and the cell cycle.

This chapter describes what is known about the structure of the nucleus, the nuclear envelope, and the transport of macromolecules in and out of the nucleus. Much is known about the mechanisms of DNA replication (see Chapter 45), RNA transcription and processing (see Chapters 14 and 15), and nuclear trafficking of macromolecules. Paradoxically, less is known about the structural organization of the nucleus and the role of its specialized subcompartments in these nuclear functions.

Overall Organization of the Nucleus

Studies in which entire individual chromosomes are labeled by in situ hybridization (chromosome painting; see Fig. 13–20) reveal that chromosomes occupy discrete, compact regions within the nucleus. These **chromosome territories** are separated by a network of channels with a much lower chromatin concentration, the **interchromosomal domain**. Most RNA transcription, processing, and transport are thought to occur in interchromosomal domain channels. Because these channels occupy only a small fraction of the nuclear volume, the effective concentration of factors in the interchromosomal domain is increased, thereby promoting assembly of large macromolecular complexes for transcription and splicing.

General Organization of Components Involved in RNA Processing

RNA transcription and processing occur at approximately 10,000 discrete sites spread throughout the average mammalian nucleus. These sites likely correspond to structures, originally observed by electron microscopy on the surface of regions of condensed chromatin, called **perichromatin fibrils**. Perichromatin fibrils contain RNA polymerase II plus associated splicing factors and RNA packaging proteins.

Factors involved in RNA processing are distributed in nuclei in a characteristic pattern in which bright **speckles** are seen against a more diffuse background of nucleoplasmic staining (Fig. 16–2). The diffuse staining probably corresponds to splicing factors associated with perichromatin fibrils at the thousands of sites where RNA transcription and processing take place. In contrast, the speckles correspond to clusters of **interchromatin granules**, particles 200 to 250 Å in diameter that are distributed throughout the interchromosomal domain. Interchromatin granules contain aggregates of small nuclear ribonucleoproteins (snRNPs) (see Chapter 15) and other protein factors involved in RNA processing.

Considerable evidence suggests that speckles are

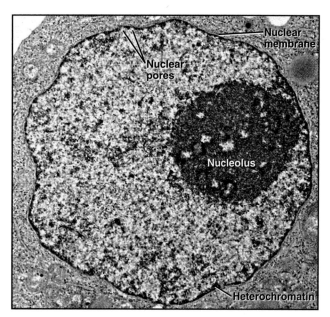

Figure 16-1 Electron micrograph of a thin section of a nucleus from a cancer cell with the major features labeled. (Courtesy of Scott Kaufmann, Mayo Clinic, Rochester, MN.)

storage depots for inactive splicing components, although this is contested (see later discussion). Speckles are less prominent in cells that transcribe RNA at high levels, and they become strikingly prominent when RNA processing is inhibited (see Fig. 16–2). Furthermore, studies in which components involved in RNA processing were labeled with green fluorescent protein and observed in vivo reveal that factors involved in RNA processing can cycle between speckles and sites of transcription.

Although metabolic labeling experiments indicate that speckles are not sites of active transcription, messenger RNAs (mRNAs) for certain genes accumulate either within or immediately adjacent to speckles. Other mRNAs are seldom or never seen associated with speckles. This is interpreted to show that certain speckles (or regions intimately associated with them) are involved in one or more steps in mRNA maturation and transport. It remains to be established whether the speckles simply store inactive factors or participate more actively in mRNA metabolism.

When cells enter mitosis, RNA processing factors redistribute diffusely throughout the cytoplasm, and speckles disperse. During telophase, processing factors reaggregate in the cytoplasm into punctate structures termed mitotic interchromatin granule clusters. These are subsequently imported into the nucleus at the completion of mitosis.

Present along with speckles in the interchromosomal domain are 1 to 10 **Cajal bodies** (formerly known as coiled bodies), compact structures about

1 μm in diameter (see Fig. 16–2) that resemble balls of tangled threads in the electron microscope. Cajal bodies contain high concentrations of many factors involved in mRNA processing, as well as a number of nucleolar components, but lack non-snRNP protein-splicing factors that are present in speckles. They also contain an 80-kD human autoantigen of unknown function, called p80-coilin. In contrast to speckles, Cajal bodies disperse when transcription and splicing are blocked, and they are particularly prominent in rapidly growing cells with high levels of gene expression. However, like speckles, some Cajal bodies disassemble during mitosis and reform during the G_1 phase after transcription is reinitiated.

The role of Cajal bodies remains enigmatic. In some cell types, a subset of the Cajal bodies co-localize with genes encoding certain of the U snRNAs involved in RNA processing (see Chapter 15). This discovery has led to a proposal that Cajal bodies might regulate snRNA gene expression.

Mammalian nuclei also contain about 10 to 20 bodies, varying in size from 0.3 to 1 mm, that are variously known as promyelocytic leukemia (**PML bodies**), PODs (PML oncogenic domains), or nd10 (nuclear domain 10). These structures have attracted attention because of their link with human acute promyelocytic leukemia (APL). Many patients with APL carry a translocation between chromosomes 15 and 17 that produces a fusion between a protein called PML and the retinoic acid receptor alpha (RARα). This fusion protein is termed PML-RARα. Antibodies to PML protein stained subnuclear structures that were given the name PML bodies. PML bodies are often, although not always, juxtaposed with Cajal bodies (see Fig. 16–2). In APL cells, PML bodies are "shattered" into many tiny punctate foci scattered throughout the nucleus. However, when APL cells are treated with drugs that are clinically effective in the treatment of APL, such as retinoic acid and arsenic trioxide, the PML bodies reform and the PML-RARα fusion protein is degraded. This reveals a very interesting link between these structures and the cancerous phenotype. At present, the function of PML bodies remains unknown.

Cell nuclei also contain other discrete subregions with distinctive structural organizations or biochemical composition, or both (see Fig. 16–2 and Table 16–1). Although little is known about the functions of several of these nuclear domains, they are noteworthy because they reveal that the nucleoplasm is not a homogeneous "soup" in which the chromatin and nucleolus are immersed. Rather, the nucleus appears to be organized into discrete structural subdomains. Future experimentation will determine whether these domains, like the nucleolus (see later discussion), reflect the functional compartmentalization of the nucleoplasm.

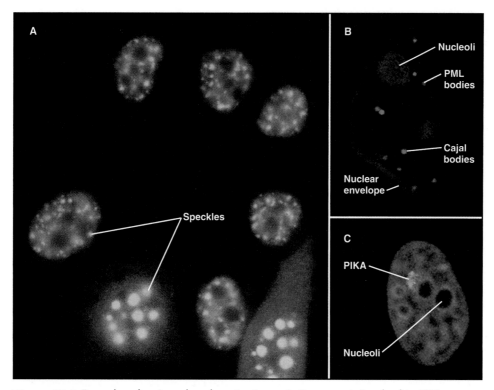

Figure 16-2 Examples of major subnuclear structures. *A,* Components involved in RNA processing are scattered throughout the nucleus, but concentrated in domains called speckles that are rich in interchromatin granules. Inhibition of RNA processing causes splicing components to accumulate in enormous concentrations of interchromatin granule clusters. Several cells were injected with a short oligonucleotide that disrupts the function of the U1 snRNP in RNA processing (see Chapter 15), and were then stained with an antibody recognizing the Sm splicing components *(green).* The injected cells were marked by introducing an inert fluorescent dextran marker into the cytoplasm *(red). B,* Nucleus with simultaneous staining of nucleoli *(blue),* PML nuclear bodies *(red),* Cajal bodies *(green),* and the nuclear envelope *(purple). C,* Nucleus with simultaneous staining of DNA *(blue)* and the polymorphic interphase karyosomal association (PIKA) *(red).* Nucleoli appear as unstained areas. A number of proteins involved in the sensing and repair of DNA damage concentrate in the PIKA. *(A,* Courtesy of David Spector, Cold Spring Harbor Lab, NY. *B,* Courtesy of Angus Lamond, University of Dundee, Scotland.)

The Nucleolus—The Most Prominent Nuclear Subdomain

The nucleolus, first identified more than 150 years ago, is the most conspicuous and best characterized substructure within the nucleus. The nucleolus is a specialized region surrounding transcriptionally active ribosomal RNA (rRNA) genes. Within this region occur the bulk of the steps for ribosome biogenesis, from the transcription and processing of rRNA to the initial assembly of ribosomal subunits. The ribosome is a complex macromolecular machine with four different structural RNA molecules and about 85 proteins that are assembled into two subunits (see Chapter 18 and Figs. 18–6 and 18–7). rRNA transcription by RNA polymerase I comprises nearly one-half of total cellular RNA synthesis in some cell types. This high level of synthesis is necessary to produce several million ribosomes in each cell cycle. rRNA (most of it in ma-

ture ribosomes) typically constitutes approximately 80% of total stable cellular RNA in vertebrates. Interestingly, other stable RNAs are also processed in the nucleolus.

Ribosomal Biogenesis in Functionally Distinct Regions of the Nucleolus

The nucleolus contains three morphologically distinct regions (Fig. 16–3). The rRNA genes, together with significant amounts of RNA polymerase I and its associated transcription factors, are largely concentrated in **fibrillar centers**. It is generally thought that ribosomal genes that are actively undergoing transcription lie near the border between the fibrillar centers and the **dense fibrillar component** that surrounds them. The **granular component** is the site of pre-ribosome assembly and is made up of densely packed clusters

table 16–1

MAJOR NUCLEAR SUBDOMAINS

Structure	Description
Cajal bodies	Formerly known as coiled bodies. About 1 μm in diameter, Cajal bodies have a coiled fibrous substructure. First identified by electron microscopy, up to 8 of these structures are seen per cell. They contain a characteristic protein called p80-coilin (M_r 80 kD). They may be involved in regulation of certain small nuclear RNA genes.
GEMs	GEMs are usually found paired with coiled bodies, which they may overlap. They contain the survival of motor neurons (SMN) protein, which is encoded by the gene mutated in spinal muscular atrophy, a severe, inherited, human, muscular wasting disease. SMN and its cofactors SIP1 appear to play an essential role in biogenesis of snRNPs (see Chapter 15).
Nuclear bodies	The function of nuclear bodies, which are seen as 5 to 20 spots within the nucleus, is unknown. They were originally observed in electron micrographs of cells following hormonal treatments. However, it is not clear that all nuclear bodies described in various cell types are structurally or functionally homologous. A marker antigen for some types of nuclear bodies (called PBC 95K - M_r 95 kD) is recognized by autoantibodies from patients with primary biliary cirrhosis. Some may correspond to PML bodies.
Nucleolus	The nucleolus is the site of rRNA transcription and processing, as well as of preribosomal assembly.
PIKA	The polymorphic interphase karyosomal association (PIKA) may be up to 5 μm in diameter during G_1 phase, but its morphology and number vary across the cell cycle. It appears to correspond to sites of sensing or repair of DNA damage.
PML bodies	Also known as PODs and ND10, 10 to 15 of these structures are scattered throughout the nucleus. They are identified with autoantibodies to an antigen called ND (MW 53,000) and also with antibodies to the PML protein. Their function is unknown, but morphologic studies show a strong link with the cancerous phenotype in cells from patients with acute promyelocytic leukemia (see text).
Speckles	Speckles are concentrations of components involved in RNA processing. They correspond to clusters of interchromatin granules seen by electron microscopy. They may serve as storage depots of splicing factors, or they may play a more active role in mRNA metabolism.

of pre-ribosomal particles that are 15 to 20 nm in diameter.

Ribosomal RNA loci on several chromosomes have a modular organization, with genes alternating with spacer regions (see Fig. 15–13). The repeat unit in this array (gene plus spacer) is approximately 40,000 base pairs in humans. Humans have approximately 300 to 400 copies of the ribosomal DNA (rDNA) repeat unit located in clusters on chromosomes 13, 14, 15, 21, and 22. In a typical somatic cell, only a fraction of these genes is actively transcribed. An additional rRNA, 5S, is encoded by distinct genes and transcribed by RNA polymerase III.

A very simple yet efficient mechanism guarantees that a proper balance is achieved between the RNA components of the two ribosomal subunits. The major RNA components of both the small and large ribosomal subunits are encoded by a single precursor RNA molecule. In humans, this 13,000-base precursor is commonly described by its sedimentation coefficient in sucrose gradients as 45S. Following its transcription, the RNA precursor is processed in a series of cleavages to yield the 18S, 5.8S, and 28S rRNA molecules. In addition to the cleavages, rRNA processing also involves extensive base modifications to introduce ap-

proximately 100 2'-O-methyl ribose and approximately 90 pseudouridine residues per molecule (see Chapter 15). The earliest stages of rRNA processing probably occur in the dense fibrillar component of the nucleolus. Later stages take place in the granular component. Ribosomal protein synthesis occurs in the cytoplasm on free ribosomes, and the newly synthesized proteins are transported into the nucleus for assembly into ribosomes, also in the granular component.

Disassembly of the Nucleolus During Mitosis

The nucleolus disassembles during each mitotic cycle, starting with the dispersal of the dense fibrillar and granular components during prophase. This disassembly is apparently driven by specific phosphorylation of nucleolar proteins. Ultimately, the fibrillar centers alone remain associated with the mitotic chromosomes, forming what are termed **nucleolus-organizing regions** (widely known by the abbreviation **NOR**s; Fig. 16–4). The nucleolar proteins nucleolin and RNA polymerase I remain bound at NORs during mitosis. NORs are often the sites of a prominent **secondary constriction** of the chromosome. (The primary constriction is the centromere.)

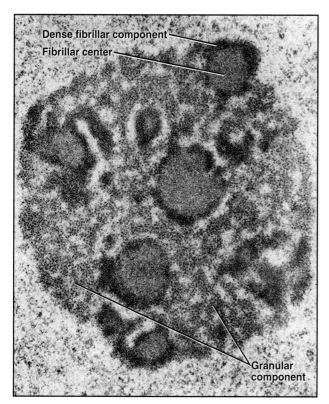

Figure 16–3 Electron micrograph of a thin section of a typical nucleolus. The fibrillar centers, dense fibrillar component, and granular component are indicated. (From Fawcett DW: The Cell. Philadelphia: WB Saunders, 1981, Figure 134.)

Nucleolar reformation after mitosis begins with the formation of aggregates termed **prenucleolar bodies**. These associate with the NORs to reform nucleoli in a process requiring transcription of the rRNA genes. Apparently, the nascent transcripts, rather than the ribosomal genes, form the nucleation point for assembly of the nucleolus in each cell cycle. This link between ribosomal gene transcription and formation of the nucleolus was clearly demonstrated by microinjecting antibodies to RNA polymerase I into mitotic cells. Injected cells were unable to transcribe rRNA and did not reform nucleoli in the next G_1 phase.

Structure of the Nuclear Envelope

The nuclear envelope provides a selectively permeable barrier between the nuclear compartment and the cytoplasm (Fig. 16–5). Nuclear pores that bridge both membranes control movements of macromolecules both ways across the barrier. One purpose of this barrier and transport system is to ensure that only fully processed mRNAs are delivered to ribosomes for translation into protein. In addition, various chromosomal events, including DNA replication and expression of certain genes, are regulated, at least in part, by

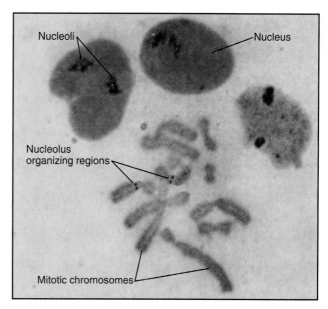

Figure 16–4 Use of silver staining to visualize the nucleolus in interphase nuclei and the nucleolus organizer regions on mitotic chromosomes of the rat kangaroo. (From Robert-Fortel I, Junera HR, Geraud G, et al: Three-dimensional organization of the ribosomal genes and Ag-NOR proteins during interphase and mitosis in PtK1 cells studied by confocal microscopy. Chromosoma 102:146–157, 1993, Figure 2c.)

changes in the ability of factors to move from the cytoplasm into the nucleus. In fact, cellular DNA replication requires an intact and functional nuclear envelope. Disassembly of the nuclear envelope is a critical aspect of mitosis in higher eukaryotes, as this releases the chromosomes so that they can be segregated to the

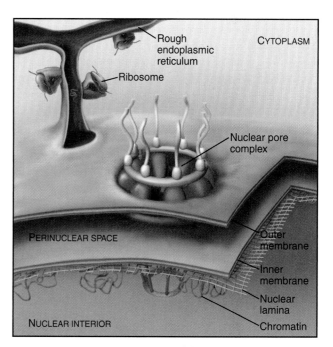

Figure 16–5 Summary overview of the organization of the nuclear envelope.

daughter cells by the cytoplasmic mitotic spindle. Mitotic segregation of chromosomes to daughter cells takes place with the nucleus in some lower eukaryotes including yeasts.

The nuclear envelope is composed of two concentric lipid bilayers termed the **inner and outer nuclear membranes**. The outer nuclear membrane is continuous with the rough endoplasmic reticulum and shares its functions. For example, it has ribosomes attached to its outer surface. A fibrous **nuclear lamina** of intermediate filaments supports the inner nuclear membrane and mediates its interactions with chromatin. The inner and outer nuclear membranes are separated by a **perinuclear space** about 30 nm that is continuous with the lumen of the endoplasmic reticulum. **Nuclear pore complexes** bridging both nuclear membranes provide the sole route for communication between the nucleus and cytoplasm.

Structure and Assembly of the Nuclear Lamina

The nuclear lamina is a protein meshwork, approximately 30 to 80 nm thick, that is composed of inter-

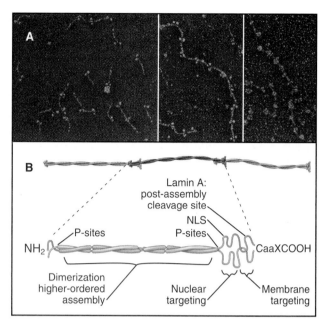

Figure 16–7 Lamin organization and assembly. *A*, Several stages in the assembly of isolated lamin B dimers into filaments in vitro. The dimers at left have two globular heads at the c-terminal end of a rod that is 52 nm long. *B*, Diagram of the structural organization of the nuclear lamins. The sequence CaaXCOOH (see text) is a signal for the attachment of a farnesyl group. NLS, nuclear localization sequence; P-sites, phosphorylation sites that regulate lamina disassembly in mitosis. (*A*, From Heitlinger E, Peter M, Haner M, et al: Expression of chicken lamin B2 in Escherichia coli: Characterization of its structure, assembly, and molecular interactions. J Cell Biol 113:485–495, 1991, by copyright permission of the Rockefeller University Press.)

mediate filament proteins called **nuclear lamins** (Fig. 16–6). Like other intermediate filament proteins (see Chapter 35), nuclear lamins have a central, rod-like domain that is largely composed of α-helical coiled-coil flanked by two globular domains (Fig. 16–7). Lamin molecules self-associate to form 10-nm intermediate filaments. Mammals express two classes of lamin subunits. **Lamin A** and **lamin C** are derived from a common pre-mRNA by alternative splicing (see Chapter 15). Members of the **lamin B** family are the products of distinct genes.

Lamin gene expression depends on the cell type and stage of development. All nuclei of higher eukaryotes, including early embryos, have a lamina containing lamin B-like subunits. The content of A and C lamins varies. They typically appear only later in development as cells begin to differentiate. This variation in lamina composition may affect chromosome organization, possibly contributing to different patterns of gene expression.

The C–terminal globular domain contains a nuclear localization sequence (see later section) that ensures the rapid import of newly synthesized lamin precursors into the nucleus. Within the nucleus, lamins acquire a post-translational modification that targets

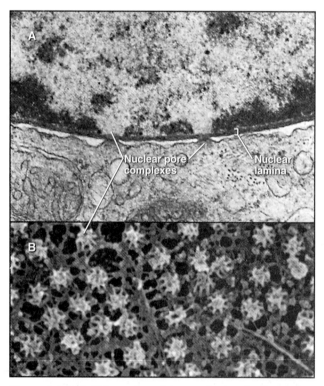

Figure 16-6 *A*, Thin-section electron micrograph of a nuclear envelope with a prominent nuclear lamina and nuclear pores. *B*, Field emission scanning electron micrograph of the inner surface of an amphibian oocyte nuclear envelope. The nuclear pores are prominent, protruding above the underlying nuclear lamina. (*A*, Reference: Fawcett DW. The Cell. Philadelphia: WB Saunders, 1981, Figure 156 (upper). *B*, From Zhang C, Jenkins H, Goldberg MW, et al: Nuclear lamina and nuclear matrix organization in sperm pronuclei assembled in Xenopus egg extract. J Cell Sci 109:2275–2286, 1996, Figure 5a.)

them to the nuclear envelope. The modification involves the enzymatic addition of a hydrophobic hydrocarbon tail (a C15-isoprenoid group called **farnesyl**) to each lamin polypeptide (see Chapter 6). The farnesyl group is added to a characteristic amino acid motif called the CaaX box (Ca$_1$a$_2$X, where C refers to cysteine located four amino acids from the carboxy terminus; a$_1$ refers to any aliphatic amino acid; a$_2$ refers to valine, isoleucine, or leucine; and X refers usually to methionine or serine) at the carboxy terminus of the protein (see Fig. 16–7). This motif was first recognized in the *ras* proteins involved in intracellular signaling (see Chapter 29). Lamin subunits lacking a CaaX box are unable to assemble on the inner nuclear membrane and instead form aggregates in the nuclear interior. Following the assembly of lamin A into the lamina, the C-terminal 18 amino acids are clipped off, removing the farnesyl group. For B-type lamins, the aaX residues are removed, leaving a protein with the farnesyl group remaining attached at its carboxy terminus. The presence or absence of the farnesyl tag may account, in part, for different solubility properties of lamins A and B during mitosis.

In addition to the farnesyl tails on lamin B, the lamina appears to be tethered to the inner nuclear membrane by interactions with integral membrane proteins (see later section). The surface of the lamina facing the nuclear interior also interacts with the chromosomes. Thus, the lamina and its associated proteins may not only serve as a structural support for the nuclear envelope but may also influence chromosome distribution and function within the nucleus. Interestingly, in mice, loss of lamin A causes disruption of the nuclear envelope and leads to a type of muscular dystrophy. Mutations in the lamin A gene may also cause certain types of muscular dystrophy.

Local concentrations of lamins also appear transiently inside the nucleus throughout the cell cycle. Intranuclear lamin A spots are most prominent in G$_1$, whereas those with lamin B are most prominent during S, when they co-localize with sites of replication. Lamin B spots do not co-localize with lamin A spots. The role of these intranuclear concentrations of lamins is unknown, but they may be localized regions of nuclear matrix (see Chapter 13) with roles in RNA transcription and DNA replication.

Proteins of the Inner Nuclear Membrane

Integral membrane proteins anchor the lamina to the inner nuclear membrane. These proteins are the 58-kD lamin B receptor and LAPs (Fig. 16–8). Two unrelated genes—LAP1 and LAP2—produce a number of polypeptides with distinct structural and functional properties as a result of extensive alternative splicing of the primary transcripts. Lamin B binds to the lamin B re-

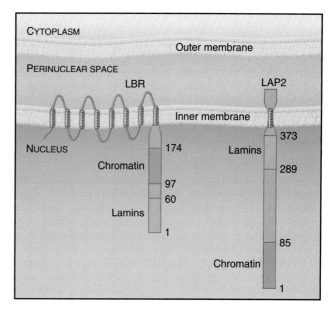

Figure 16–8 Diagram of the topology of two major proteins of the inner nuclear membrane, the lamin B receptor (LBR), and lamina-associated protein 2 (LAP2). The regions of these proteins that bind lamins are shown in yellow. Regions that associate with chromatin are shown in blue. Numbers refer to amino acid residue position, with 1 being the NH$_2$ terminus.

ceptor and lamina-associated proteins (LAPs) 1 and 2. Lamins A and C bind to LAP1. Although different in many respects, the lamin B receptor and LAP2b (the former with eight membrane-spanning domains, the latter with one) share some features. Both bind lamin B and chromatin. Both are suggested to play important roles in the reassembly of the nuclear envelope after mitosis. In addition, both exist in multiprotein complexes containing associated protein kinases. These factors suggest that phosphorylation regulates these proteins.

Several surprising observations suggest that these proteins may do much more than simply anchor lamins to the nuclear envelope. The hydrophobic region of the lamin B receptor resembles a yeast enzyme involved in cholesterol biosynthesis, and it can actually function enzymatically when expressed in yeast. LAP2 apparently can be processed to release a 49–amino acid polypeptide called thymopoetin that functions as a T-cell differentiation factor. In addition, a portion of LAP2 resembles emerin, the nuclear envelope protein that is defective in individuals with Emery-Dreifuss muscular dystrophy.

Integral proteins of the inner nuclear membrane, such as the lamin B receptor, enter the nucleus by diffusing in the plane of the membrane from their site of synthesis in the rough endoplasmic reticulum (ER). In the rough ER, the protein is highly mobile, rapidly diffusing to the nuclear envelope, along the membrane lining the nuclear pores, and thence to the inner nuclear membrane. There, the protein becomes fixed in place, presumably by binding to the lamina or

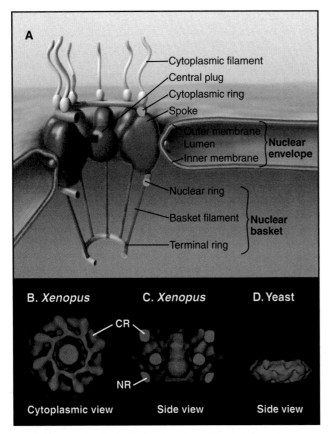

Figure 16-9 *A*, Three-dimensional model of the nuclear pore complex. The pore has eight-fold symmetry, with a central channel and eight peripheral channels. The cytoplasmic and nuclear filament networks contain components that function in docking of transport complexes to the pores. *B to D*, Three-dimensional reconstruction of the nuclear pore complexes from the frog *Xenopus laevis* and the budding yeast. The yeast pore complex is smaller than the amphibian complex. This structure is very difficult to observe by electron microscopy, partly because it is very fragile and partly because the structure contains both protein and lipid, which may limit access to stains. *CR*, cytoplasmic ring; *NR*, nuclear ring. (*B* and *C*, From Akey CW, Radermacher M: Architecture of the Xenopus nuclear pore complex revealed by three-dimensional cryo-electron microscopy. J Cell Biol 122:1–19, 1993, by copyright permission of the Rockefeller University Press. *D*, From Yang Q, Rout MP, Akey CW: Three dimensional architecture of the isolated yeast nuclear pore. Molec Cell 1:223–234, 1998.)

chromatin. Chromatin binding by lamin B receptor may involve interactions with the heterochromatin protein HP1 (see Chapter 13).

Nuclear Pore Complexes

All traffic between the nucleus and cytoplasm passes through elaborate channels, called **nuclear pore complexes**, that bridge both the inner and outer nuclear membranes (Fig. 16–9). These cylindrical channels have eight-fold rotational symmetry and an overall diameter of about 130 nm. The pore is composed of three concentric rings. A barrel-like **luminal ring** is

embedded in the nuclear envelope. The luminal ring is flanked by the **nuclear** and **cytoplasmic rings**, which are embedded in the inner and outer nuclear membranes, respectively. The nuclear ring appears to be anchored to the nuclear lamina. Eight filaments project outward from the nuclear and cytoplasmic rings. The cytoplasmic filaments are 30 to 50 nm long and are often highly twisted in appearance. By comparison, the nuclear filaments are longer (~100 nm) and are joined at their outer end by a fibrous ring, much like the wire that secures the cork on a champagne bottle. This structure is called the **nuclear basket**. Both sets of filaments appear to be involved in docking of macromolecules to be transported through the pore.

The three rings are linked by eight columns or **spokes**, so called because of their appearance when the pore is viewed end-on. The spokes are complex structures that have a protuberance projecting toward the center of the cylinder (see Fig. 16–9). The inner ends of these adjacent bulges fuse together, making a central ring with an opening about 55 nm in diameter. This is thought to be the opening through which all regulated traffic passes in and out of the nucleus. In addition, smaller vertical channels with a diameter of 10 nm separate the spokes at the perimeter of the pore complex.

A central plug or granule occupies the large hole through the central ring in many (although not all) pore complexes. This has been suggested, variously, to be material in transit through the pore, a transporter that actively moves nuclear components through the pore, or a structural artifact caused by the shriveling of the various pore-associated filaments during preparation of the samples for electron microscopy. The significance of this plug remains to be determined.

Vertebrate nuclear pore complexes are large structures with a mass of approximately 120 million Da that contain multiple copies of approximately 100 proteins. Yeast nuclear pores are similar in overall structure but lack a number of peripheral structures present in vertebrate pores. Biochemical analyses of isolated yeast nuclear pore complexes reveal that they are composed of approximately 30 proteins, most of which have now been identified. Six of these proteins account for more than 25% of the total mass and are likely to be largely responsible for the structural framework of the pore.

The most abundant class of nuclear pore proteins is known as **nucleoporins** (Fig. 16–10). The structurally diverse nucleoporins contain regions of repeated amino acid sequences that end in the dipeptide FG (phenylalanine-glycine). Two common examples include XFXFG and GLFG, but other repeats may also be found. It has been suggested that these repeats may be important for interactions with molecules as they transit the pores. Many nucleoporins are glyco-

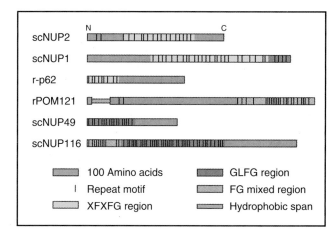

Figure 16-10 Sequence organization of the nucleoporins, the structural components of the nuclear pores. Nucleoporins contain combinations of repeated sequences as shown. Letters refer to the amino acids (see Fig. 2–4). They may be somehow involved in helping cargo to traffic through the pores.

proteins bearing *O*-linked *N*-acetylglucosamine attached to serine or threonine residues. These sugar residues are directly exposed to the cytosol and are added to the proteins by a cytosolic enzyme that is distinct from the glycosyl transferases that lie within membrane-bound compartments of the secretory pathway (Chapter 20).

Three experiments show that nucleoporins are required to transport proteins into the nucleus. First, antibodies to nucleoporins inhibit transport by isolated nuclei or when injected into live cells. Second, lectins (proteins that bind specifically to sugars like those on the nucleoporins) such as wheat germ agglutinin inhibit transport in similar experiments. Third, reconstitution experiments show that the well-characterized, highly conserved nucleoporin **p62** (62kD; its budding yeast counterpart is called Nsp1p) is essential for transport. p62 and two other nucleoporins, p54 and p58, form part of a rod-like complex 50 to 60 nm long. This complex binds in the central region of the cytoplasmic and nuclear faces of the pore complex. Nuclear pore complexes can be assembled in the absence of the p62 complex using the *Xenopus* egg extract system (Chapter 43). These pores appear structurally normal but are inactive in transport.

▌ Traffic Between Nucleus and Cytoplasm

More than 1 million molecules per minute pass through the 3000 to 5000 nuclear pores of a typical growing cell. Traffic heading out of the nucleus includes mRNAs, ribosomes, and transfer RNAs (tRNAs), all of which must be transported to the cytoplasm to function in protein synthesis. Traffic headed into the nucleus includes nuclear and ribosomal proteins.

Other molecules follow more complex routes. snRNPs are exported to the cytoplasm to acquire essential protein components; they must then be reimported into the nucleus. Individual pores can simultaneously transport components in both directions.

Nuclear pores are gated structures with a constitutive channel about 9 nm in diameter through which solutes and small proteins (up to ~60 kD) can diffuse passively. However, they can also open up dramatically, allowing macromolecular complexes of up to 20 to 25 MDa to pass. Surprisingly, despite the presence of the constitutive channels, almost all physiological traffic through the pores, even of small molecules, is a facilitated process involving specific carrier proteins.

The pore gate opens to a maximum of 25 nm, but larger particles can squeeze through, provided they are deformable. This is well documented for export of a well-studied enormous RNA of 35 to 40 kb that associates with roughly 500 packaging proteins to make an RNP particle about 50 nm in diameter. The RNP is deformed into a rod-like structure that measures 25 × 135 nm as it passes through the pore (Fig. 16–11). Rigid particles apparently cannot exceed the 25-nm limit.

Proteins that are imported into the nucleus bear a **nuclear localization sequence (NLS),** also called a nuclear localization *signal,* that is recognized by specific carrier proteins (Figs. 16–12 and 16–13). The

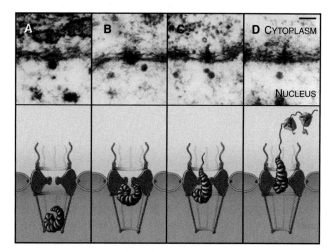

Figure 16-11 *A* to *D*, Electron micrographs *(upper panels)* and an artist's rendition *(lower panels)* show a large RNP particle become deformed as it traverses across the nuclear envelope *(top,* cytoplasm; *bottom,* nucleus). This RNA encodes a secreted protein, with a molecular weight of about 1,000,000 D, from the salivary gland of the fly *Chironomous tentans.* Once in the cytoplasm, the 5' end of the RNA docks with ribosomes and begins synthesis of its protein even before the passage of the remainder of the RNP through the pore has been completed. (From Mehlin H, Daneholt B, Skoglund U: Translocation of a specific premessenger ribonucleoprotein particle through the nuclear pore studied with electron microscope tomography. Cell 69:605–613, 1992, Figure 2. Copyright 1992, with permission from Elsevier Science.)

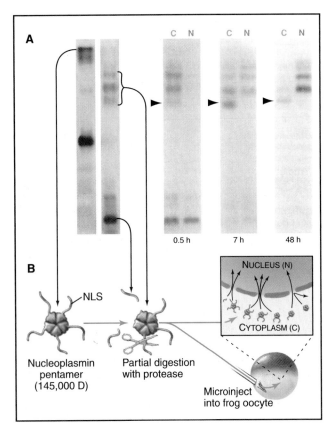

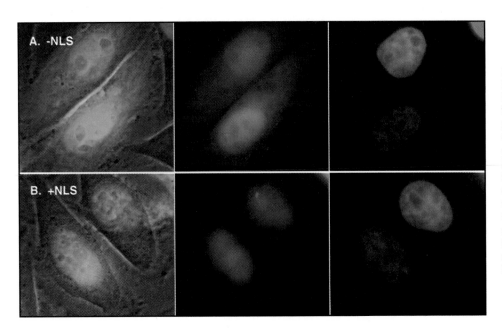

Figure 16–12 Identification of a nuclear localization sequence (NLS) on the protein nucleoplasmin. This 29,000-kD protein exists in vivo as a pentameric complex with a molecular weight of 145,000. The monomer is small enough to diffuse passively through the nuclear pores, but the pentamer is too large to do so. A, Gentle cleavage of the pentamer with a protease removes a relatively small peptide from one end of the protein *(left two gel lanes)*. When the cleaved pentamers were labeled with radioactivity and injected into the cytoplasm of a *Xenopus* oocyte, it was found that four species were produced that could still migrate into the nucleus, and one species was produced that could not *(right three pairs of gel lanes)*. B, The interpretation of this experiment is that each nucleoplasmin polypeptide contains a "tail" that can be removed by proteolysis, and that this tail contains a nuclear localization sequence. Each pentamer can migrate into the nucleus as long as it retains at least one polypeptide with a tail. Tail-less pentamers *(arrowheads in A)* remain stuck in the cytoplasm. C, cytoplasm; N, nucleus. (A, From Dingwall C, Sharnick SV, Laskey RA: A polypeptide domain that specifies migration of nucleoplasmin in the nucleus. Cell 30: 449–458, 1982. Copyright 1982, with permission from Elsevier Science.)

various known types of NLS vary in complexity. The most common is a patch of basic amino acids similar to the sequence PKKKRKV (single-letter amino acid code; see Fig. 2–4), first identified on the simian virus 40 (SV40) large T antigen. A point mutation, yielding PK*N*KRKV, inactivates this sequence as a signal for nuclear transport. A related type of NLS features two smaller patches of basic residues separated by a variable spacer (<u>KR</u>PAATKKAGQA<u>KKKK</u> [critical residues are underlined]). These two types of sequences are referred to as basic NLSs.

Basic nuclear localization sequences function autonomously and can direct the migration of a wide range of model molecules into the nucleus in vivo. In one extreme example, when coated with nucleoplasmin, a protein with a basic NLS, colloidal gold parti-

Figure 16–13 A protein (the inhibitor of CAD nuclease, or ICAD, see Chapter 49) was fused to the green fluorescent protein (GFP) and expressed in cultured cells. A, A mutant form of the ICAD:GFP fusion protein lacking the ICAD nuclear localization sequence (NLS) accumulates randomly throughout the cell. B, The intact ICAD: GFP fusion protein with NLS accumulates quantitatively in the nucleus. (Courtesy of K. Samejima, University of Edinburgh.)

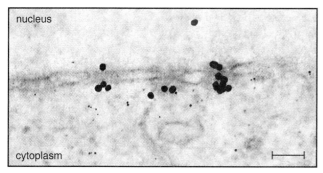

Figure 16-14 The nuclear localization sequence of nucleoplasmin can even cause large colloidal gold particles to be transported into the cell nucleus. A thin-section electron micrograph shows gold particles coated with nucleoplasmin crossing the nuclear envelope by passing through the nuclear pore complexes. Much smaller gold particles coated with bovine serum albumin (BSA) remain in the cytoplasm. Both sets of gold particles were microinjected into the cytoplasm of *Xenopus* oocytes, and the cells were processed 1 hour later for electron microscopy. *Upper,* nucleus; *lower,* cytoplasm. Bar is 0.1 μm. (From Dworetzky SI, Lanford RE, Feldherr, CM: The effects of variations in the number and sequence of targeting signals on nuclear uptake. J Cell Biol 107:1279–1287, 1988, by copyright permission of the Rockefeller University Press.)

cles up to 23 nm in diameter are transported through nuclear pores (Fig. 16–14).

Many proteins exported from the nucleus bear a **nuclear export sequence (NES)** that is recognized by carriers related to those used for nuclear import (Fig. 16–15). Like import signals, these signals vary in size and complexity. One example of a leucine-rich sequence that is recognized by the carrier CRM1 is provided by the human immunodeficiency virus I Rev protein (LQLPPLERLTL). Certain RNA sequences or structures may also serve as NESs.

A third type of signal—a nuclear retention signal (NRS)—is present on a number of proteins that bind to immature RNAs. These proteins hold immature RNAs in the nucleus and must be removed before mature RNAs can be exported to the cytoplasm. This mechanism allows the nuclear envelope to segregate immature, unprocessed RNAs from the protein-synthetic machinery in the cytoplasm.

The following is a brief description of protein import into the nucleus. A protein with an NLS (known as **cargo**) is recognized by an **adapter** molecule. This complex binds to an **import receptor,** forming a tripartite complex, which then passes through pores into the nucleus. There, the cargo and adapter are displaced from the import receptor. The adapter then releases its cargo and is transported back to the cytoplasm as the cargo of an export receptor. Import receptors also shuttle back through pores, where they can meet more cargo/adapter complexes. This general picture runs in reverse for the case of molecules that are exported from the nucleus. Note that not all im-

port and export events require adapters; some cargo can bind directly to import and export receptors.

The key to this system is that it is *vectorial;* nuclear components are transported into the nucleus while components that function in the cytoplasm are

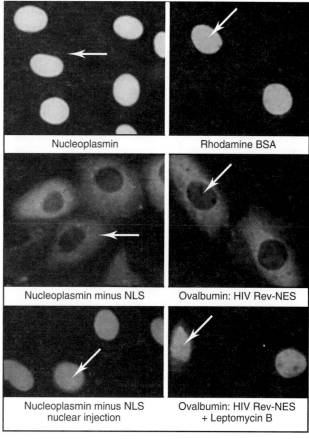

Figure 16-15 Demonstration of the existence of specific nuclear import and export signals on proteins. *Left,* Nuclear import. Nucleoplasmin microinjected into the cytoplasm rapidly migrates into the nucleus *(top).* Nucleoplasmin lacking its NLS, when microinjected into the cytoplasm, stays in the cytoplasm *(middle).* Nucleoplasmin lacking its NLS microinjected into the nucleus stays in the nucleus *(bottom).* *Right,* Nuclear export. Fluorescently labeled bovine serum albumin (BSA) microinjected into the nucleus stays in the nucleus *(top).* When ovalbumin, to which the NES of the HIV (the virus that causes AIDS) Rev protein has been conjugated, is microinjected into the nucleus, it rapidly migrates into the cytoplasm *(middle).* In the presence of leptomycin B, a drug that inhibits the activity of the nuclear export receptor CRM1, ovalbumin to which the NES of the HIV Rev protein has been conjugated, if microinjected into the nucleus, stays in the nucleus *(bottom).* (*Left,* From Dingwall C, Robbins J, Dilworth SM, et al: The nucleoplasmin nuclear location sequence is larger and more complex than that of SV-40 large T antigen. J Cell Biol 107:841–849, 1988, by copyright permission of the Rockefeller University Press. *Right,* Reprinted with permission from Nature. Fukuda M, Asano S, Nakamura T, et al: CRM1 is responsible for intracellular transport mediated by the nuclear export signal. Nature 390:308–311, 1997, Figure 1*b* [without lower right panel]. Copyright 1997, Macmillan Magazines Limited.)

table 16–2

PROTEINS INVOLVED IN NUCLEAR TRAFFICKING

Protein Type	Description
Adapters	
importin α*	An import adapter, importin α interacts with importin β during nuclear transport and binds basic NLSs. Humans have at least five distinct importin α genes, expressed in a tissue-specific manner.
snurportin 1	This adapter binds the trimethyl G cap structure on snRNPs during import. It also interacts with importin β during nuclear transport.
hnRNP A1	This protein has a major role in the export of mRNA from the nucleus. The molecule is extremely abundant (10^8 copies/cell) and active (10^5 copies/min shuttling between the nucleus and cytoplasm).
Importin β-Related Molecules Involved in Import	
importin β	A founder member of the large family of nuclear trafficking receptors, importin β binds various adapters and interacts with nucleoporins during import. RanGTP regulates binding to adapters.
transportin	Transportin imports mRNA-binding proteins into the nucleus.
Importin β-Related Molecules Involved in Export	
CAS	CAS recycles importin α and snurportin 1 to the cytoplasm.
CRM1	CRM1 exports proteins with leucine-rich NESs and also U snRNAs. It is a target of the fungal toxin leptomycin B.
Exportin-t	This protein is involved in tRNA export.
Directionality Factors	
Ran	A small Ras-family GTPase, Ran binds importin-related nuclear trafficking receptors, as well as a number of regulatory proteins.
RanGAP1	This protein stimulates GTP hydrolysis by Ran in cytoplasm (GAP = GTPase-activating protein).
RCC1	RCC1 is the nuclear GTP exchange factor (GEF) for Ran. It stimulates release of GDP from Ran.
RanBP1	RanBP1 is a cytoplasmic protein that binds RanGTP and acts with RanGAP1 to stimulate GTP hydrolysis by Ran.
RanBP2	A major component of the cytoplasmic filaments of the nuclear pore, RanBP2 has four Ran-binding domains. It also binds RanGAP1 and may locally convert cytoplasmic RanGTP to RanGDP so that it can return to the nucleus.
NTF2	A 10-kD protein, NTF2 binds RanGDP and promotes its recycling back to the nucleus.

*The importin molecules were discovered independently and termed karyopherins.

transported out. This means that each carrier picks up its cargo on one side of the nuclear envelope and deposits it on the other. This directionality is regulated by a simple yet elegant system involving a small guanine triphosphatase (GTPase) and its associated factors.

Components of Nuclear Import and Export

The nuclear import and export system is complex, but the general principles of its operation are simple. To understand how it works, this section first introduces several of the components (Table 16–2) and then describes one type of transport in detail.

Adapters

Adapters bind to the NLS or NES sequences on target molecules and also to particular regions on receptors. The best known adapter is **importin α** (also known as karyopherin α), which is responsible for recognition of small basic NLS sequences. An example of a different type of adapter is the heterogeneous nuclear ribonucleoprotein (hnRNP) A1 protein, which has a major role in the export of mRNA from the nucleus. It is likely that many more diverse types of adapters remain to be discovered.

Receptors

Currently, all known nuclear trafficking receptors are related to **importin β**, the import receptor for proteins bearing a basic NLS. At least eight members of the importin β family are known in vertebrates (14 in yeast). Some of these function in nuclear import, whereas others function in export. In addition to binding adapters (or occasionally, binding directly to cargo), receptors bind to components of the nuclear pore and to a small GTPase called **Ran**. Chapter 27 introduces GTPases in detail.

Directionality/Recycling Factors

Nuclear trafficking receptors know what side of the nuclear membrane they are on as a result of interactions with Ran and its bound nucleotide cofactor. RanGTP (Ran with bound GTP) *dissociates* import complexes but is required *to form* export complexes. The system imparts directionality because RanGTP is converted to RanGDP (Ran guanine diphosphate) in the cytoplasm and RanGDP is converted to RanGTP in the nucleus.

Protein cofactors required to stimulate the hydrolysis of GTP bound to Ran are confined to the cytoplasm. Like other small GTPases (see Chapter 27), Ran has low intrinsic GTPase activity, but interactions with binding proteins (RanBP1 or RanBP2) and a GTPase-activating protein called **RanGAP1** stimulate GTP hydrolysis. RanBP1 is anchored in the cytoplasm. RanBP2 is a component of the fibers projecting from the nuclear pore into the cytoplasm. This huge (>350 kD) protein can bind up to four Ran molecules as well as RanGAP1 and may provide a structural scaffolding for the conversion of RanGTP into RanGDP at the surface of the pore. Because RanBP1 and RanBP2 are both anchored in the cytoplasm, RanGTP is efficiently converted to RanGDP only in cytoplasm.

RanGDP must reenter the nucleus to be recharged with GTP. RanGDP transport into the nucleus requires the small protein nuclear transport factor 2 (NTF2). Back in the nucleus, Ran must release its bound GDP to acquire GTP. GDP dissociation is slow but is stimulated by a guanine nucleotide exchange factor (GEF). This protein, called **RCC1** (regulator of chromosome condensation 1), is tightly associated with chromatin throughout the cell cycle. This allows nuclear import to resume immediately after the nuclear envelope reforms at the end of mitosis.

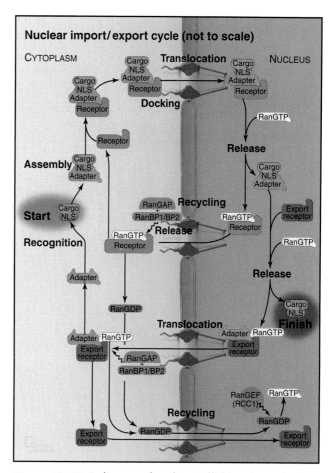

Figure 16-16 A diagram of nuclear trafficking shows the integration of the two half-cycles of import and export of proteins. See text for a more detailed explanation.

How the Import Cycle Works

Consider the import into the nucleus of a typical protein bearing a basic nuclear localization sequence (Figs. 16–16 and 16–17). In the cytoplasm, the adapter importin α recognizes and binds the NLS on this cargo. The cargo/adapter complex first binds to the import receptor importin β, and then, in a process known as docking, the ternary complex binds to the cytoplasmic filaments of the nuclear pore. The tripartite complex is transferred through the pore in a process that is not understood, but which may involve interactions of importin β with nucleoporins bearing the XFXFG repeats. Despite the fact that this transport involves a significant structural rearrangement of the pore during opening of the gate, it now appears that the transport event itself may not require ATP or GTP hydrolysis.

In the nucleus, the cargo/importin α/importin β complex encounters RanGTP. RanGTP binds to importin β, displacing the cargo/importin α complex from it. Importin β/RanGTP then shuttles back through the pore to the cytoplasm. In the nucleus, the cargo/importin α complex encounters a nuclear export receptor called **CAS.** CAS binds tightly to importin α, provided RanGTP is present. Binding of CAS and RanGTP releases the cargo, which is now free to do its job in the nucleus. Because CAS is an export receptor, the importin α/CAS/RanGTP complex now follows a reverse route through the nuclear pores back into the cytoplasm. (Molecules such as importin α function as adapters in one direction and cargo in the other.)

The cargo is now in the nucleus, but the system is stalled. The import receptor, importin β, is back in the cytoplasm, but in a complex with RanGTP that is unable to bind further cargo for import into the nucleus. The import adapter, importin α, is also in the cytoplasm, but it is locked in a complex with the CAS export receptor and RanGTP. The solution to this problem is simple. Through the action of RanBP1, RanBP2, and RanGAP1, the RanGTP is converted to RanGDP. This is released by importin β, which is now ready for further action in nuclear import. In addition, hydrolysis of RanGTP causes the importin α/CAS/RanGTP complex to fall apart. This allows CAS to shuttle back into the nucleus for further work as an

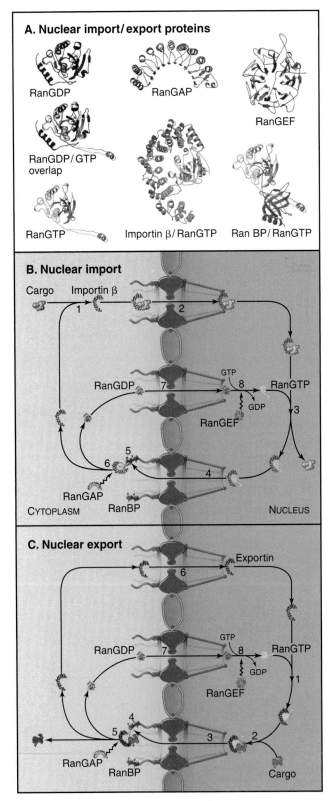

Figure 16–17 Nuclear trafficking molecules. *A,* Crystal structures of components involved in nuclear transport. *B* and *C,* The two half-cycles of import and export of cargo with scale drawings of the proteins, key structural transitions, and the order of events enumerated. (Ribbon models provided by F. Wittinghoffer, MPI Dortmund, Germany.)

export receptor, and it frees up importin α to bind more cargo and function as an import adapter.

Although there are a number of names to remember, the nuclear trafficking system is actually quite straightforward, being regulated by the state of the guanine nucleotide bound by Ran. Cargo that is meant to be imported into the nucleus is released from its carriers in the presence of high levels of RanGTP. Conversely, cargo that is meant to be exported to the cytoplasm is picked up by its carriers only in the presence of high levels of RanGTP and is released when the Ran is converted to RanGDP.

Regulation of Transport Across the Nuclear Envelope

Cells regulate nuclear trafficking in several ways. The first of these is to change the number of pores. In rat liver, there are 15 to 20 pores per μm^2 of nuclear envelope ($\sim$4000 per nucleus). This number can be shifted up or down depending on the transcriptional activity in the nucleus. In growing cells, the number of nuclear pores appears to increase concomitant with entry into S phase.

Traffic across the nuclear envelope may be regulated by masking or unmasking nuclear localization sequences. A nuclear protein with a masked NLS is trapped in the cytoplasm. A classical example is the regulation of transcription factor NF-κB by IκB. IκB binds to NF-κB and covers up its NLS. Because IκB also has a nuclear export signal, the NF-κB:IκB complex is entirely cytoplasmic. Following an appropriate signal (see Fig. 14–19*C*), IκB is degraded. This uncovers the NLS on NF-κB, allowing it to enter the nucleus where it activates genes involved in immune and inflammatory responses.

Phosphorylation can also affect NLS function. Phosphorylation adjacent to a basic NLS inhibits nuclear import. This provides a mechanism to regulate the ability of a particular cargo to enter the nucleus in response to cell cycle or other cues that can be coupled to specific protein kinase activation.

A third mechanism by which traffic across the nuclear envelope is regulated is by anchoring components on one side of the nuclear membrane. One example is nuclear retention signals on RNPs that hold immature RNAs in the nucleus until their processing is completed. A related mechanism regulates the activity of several developmental transcription factors, which are restrained in the cytoplasm unless specific stimuli release them for entry into the nucleus. One example is provided by *dorsal*, the transcription factor regulating the establishment of the dorsal-ventral axis in developing *Drosophila melanogaster* embryos (Fig. 16–18). If *dorsal* protein is transported into the nucleus,

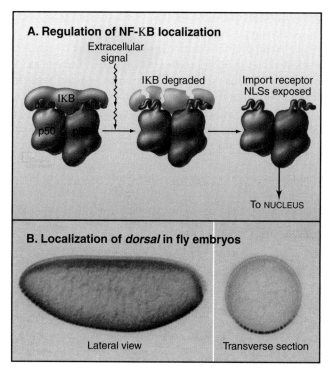

Figure 16-18 *A*, Regulation of NF-κB localization. The transcription factor NF-κB is kept in the cytoplasm as a result of interactions with its inhibitor IκB. IκB holds NF-κB in the cytoplasm in two ways. When it binds NF-κB, it covers up the NF-κB NLS. Second, IκB contains a nuclear export signal, so that any NF-κB associated with it that happens to enter the nucleus is rapidly exported to the cytoplasm. *B*, Localization of the *dorsal* transcription factor in *Drosophila* embryos. These images represent a longitudinal *(left)* and cross-sectional *(right)* view of wild-type embryos. The *dorsal* protein is stained with specific antibody, which appears as dark spots where it has become concentrated in the cell nuclei in the ventral portion of the embryo. (*B*, From Roth S, Stein D, Nusslein-Volhard, C: A gradient of nuclear localization of the dorsal protein determines dorsoventral pattern in the Drosophila embryo. Cell 59:1189–1202, 1989, Figure 2 *e* and *f*.) Copyright 1989, with permission from Elsevier Science.

cells develop into tissues normally found on the ventral surface of the embryo. If this factor remains in the cytoplasm, the cells develop into dorsal tissues. Entry of this protein into the nucleus is under the control of other regulatory factors, which appear to function by tethering the *dorsal* protein in the cytoplasm unless specific signals are given for its release.

▌Disassembly and Reassembly of the Nuclear Envelope During Mitosis

The sudden and dramatic disassembly of the nuclear envelope is one of the hallmarks of mitosis in higher eukaryotes (Fig. 16–19). The mechanism of this disassembly is not entirely understood, but disassembly of the nuclear lamina is thought to contribute to the process.

Two post-translational modifications of the lamins drive mitotic disassembly of the lamin filaments:

1. Cdk1:cyclin B kinase (and possibly other kinases as well) phosphorylate two serine residues that flank the central rod domain (see Fig. 16–7) of all three lamin subunits. Replacement of these serines with alanine residues blocks lamina disassembly at mitosis.

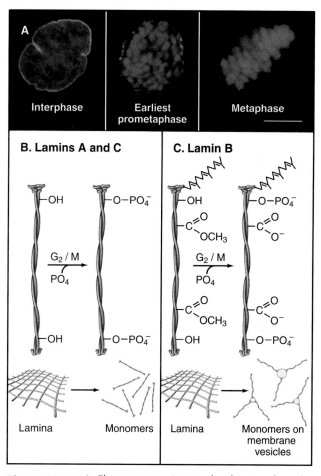

Figure 16-19 *A*, Fluorescence micrographs showing the solubilization of the nuclear lamina during mitosis. The lamins *(green)* are concentrated at the nuclear periphery in interphase cells and are distributed throughout the cytoplasm of a mitotic cell. *B* and *C*, Summary of the regulation of lamina disassembly during mitosis. Lamin disassembly in mitosis is regulated by post-translational modification of the proteins. *B*, Lamins A and C are phosphorylated on sites that flank the central α-helical rod domains in the lamin dimer. *C*, Lamin B is phosphorylated in a similar way, but also undergoes methylation of key carboxyl residues during interphase. Lamin B is also modified by the addition of a hydrophobic farnesyl group *(top)* that helps it to remain associated with membranes during mitosis. Not shown to scale. (*A*, Courtesy of Kumiko Samejima, University of Edinburgh.)

2. On lamin B, methyl groups are removed from one or more carboxyl groups that are normally present as esters during interphase. Lamins A and C are not methylated. Remethylation of these groups is required at the end of mitosis before lamin B will reassemble into the lamina.

In mitosis, lamin A disassembles to soluble complexes that are dispersed throughout the cytoplasm of the cell. B-type lamins also disperse, but the proteins remain associated with membrane vesicles that also contain the lamin B receptor.

Because lamina disassembly and reassembly is driven by a cycle of reversible modifications, the lamins can be used for multiple rounds of nuclear assembly. However, this raises an intriguing problem. If, as indicated earlier, the farnesylated CaaX motif is required to mediate the assembly of *newly synthesized* lamin A into a lamina structure, how can the mature lamin A from which this motif has been removed target to the lamina during nuclear reassembly? The answer to this question is not known.

Nuclear envelope reassembly occurs during late anaphase and telophase of mitosis (see Chapter 47), initiating with the binding of membrane vesicles to the surface of the highly condensed chromosomes. Electron microscopy reveals that several types of vesicles are involved, and binding of vesicles containing the lamin B receptor is an early event. Small amounts of the lamins also bind to the chromosomal surface at this time. Fusion of the vesicles results in production of an intact double-membrane structure around the mass of condensed chromosomes. Once nuclear pores reform, the bulk of the soluble lamin subunits are then transported into the reforming nucleus, and the chromosomes partially decondense. Transport of the lamins into the nucleus is essential for progression of the cell into the next S phase. If the process is blocked, the chromatin remains highly condensed, and the cells experience a cell cycle arrest. This suggests that the lamina has a role in organizing the higher-order structure of the nuclear periphery that is essential for cell cycle progression.

Nuclear pores disassemble along with the rest of the nuclear envelope each time higher eukaryotic cells pass through mitosis. During mitosis, the pore subunits are scattered throughout the cytoplasm. They come back together during the early stages of nuclear envelope reassembly during telophase. Pores start to form as soon as nuclear membrane vesicles start to fuse and flatten on the surface of the chromosomes, well before the chromosomes are surrounded by an intact nuclear envelope. By examining various stages of nuclear envelope assembly using a high-resolution field emission scanning electron microscope, it has been possible to describe a number of prospective intermediates in pore complex assembly. Pore assembly is necessarily an early event in nuclear reassembly after mitosis, as the pores provide the sole avenue for other essential nuclear components to gain access to the interior of the growing nucleus.

▌ Selected Readings

Azuma Y, Dasso M: The role of Ran in nuclear function. Curr Opin Cell Biol 12:302–307, 2000.

Hood JK, and Silver PA: In or out? Regulating nuclear transport. Curr Opin Cell Biol 11:241–247, 1999.

Hutchison CJ, Alvarez-Reyes M, Vaughan OA: Lamins in disease: Why do ubiquitously expressed nuclear envelope proteins give rise to tissue-specific disease phenotypes? J Cell Sci 114:9–19, 2001.

Lamond AI, Earnshaw WC: Structure and function in the nucleus. Science 280:547–553, 1998.

Lewis JD, Tollervey D: Like attracts like: Getting RNA processing together in the nucleus. Science 288:1385–1389, 2000.

Matera AG: Nuclear bodies: Multifaceted subdomains of the interchromatin space. Trends Cell Biol 9:302–309, 1999.

Mattaj IW, Englmeier L: Nucleocytoplasmic transport: The soluble phase. Annu Rev Biochem 67:265–306, 1998.

Nigg EA: Nucleocytoplasmic transport: Signals, mechanisms and regulation. Nature 386:779–787, 1997.

Pemberton LF, Blobel G, Rosenblum JS: Transport routes through the nuclear pore complex. Curr Op Cell Biol 10:392–399, 1998.

Rout MP, Wente SR: Pores for thought: Nuclear pore complex proteins. Trends Cell Biol 4:357–365, 1994.

Stuurman N, Heins S, Aebi U: Nuclear lamins: Their structure, assembly, and interactions. J Struct Biol 122:42–66, 1998.

BIOGENESIS, TRAFFIC, AND FUNCTIONS OF CELLULAR MEMBRANE SYSTEMS

chapter 17

INTRODUCTION TO MEMBRANE COMPARTMENTS

Cells are continuously engaged in their own biosynthesis. A proliferating cell must double its complement of DNA, RNA, protein, glycoconjugate, and lipid constituents before division. Quiescent cells must degrade and then replace RNA, enzymes, structural proteins, and lipids, which have variable, but shorter, lifetimes than the cell itself. Many cells also produce proteins or glycoconjugates for export.

Consider this example: a liver cell (called a hepatocyte) has an average life span of about 1 year. Over the decades-long life of a human, stem cells must divide to replenish the supply of hepatocytes. The individual proteins that make up the cell have shorter functional lifetimes than the cell itself and so must be degraded and replaced more frequently—some every hour, others every day, and some every few weeks or months—in a process collectively called **protein turnover.** Membrane lipids also undergo turnover; some lipid species have lifetimes measured in minutes. A primary function of hepatocytes is to produce and secrete serum proteins, such as transferrin, an iron-carrying protein, and low-density lipoprotein (LDL), a cholesterol-carrying particle, which are used by other cells. Each day, a liver cell secretes an amount of serum proteins equal to its total content of proteins. Finally, hepatocytes actively import macromolecules from the bloodstream for degradation or for transport to the bile. All these activities consume energy, which must be provided continuously.

The various activities of biosynthesis, degradation, and energy production that support these operations are each compartmentalized in eukaryotic cells. Subcellular compartments, called organelles, are specialized for unique functions and are recognizable by

their distinctive chemical compositions. The abundance or size of an intracellular compartment varies between different cell types within a multicellular organism, as each has developed to perform distinct, specialized functions (Fig. 17–1). An organelle often holds a monopoly on performing a given task; for example, endoplasmic reticulum (ER) synthesizes membrane protein and lipid, lysosomes degrade proteins, and mitochondria produce the cell's chemical energy. This division of labor has many advantages, but also presents many challenges in terms of coordination of cellular activities, organelle biosynthesis, and cell division.

Advantages of Compartments

An organelle is surrounded by a semipermeable membrane that establishes a microenvironment in which enzymes, cofactors, and substrates can be concentrated, increasing the rates of macromolecular interactions. Moreover, the chemical environments on either side of a semipermeable membrane can be controlled to establish the appropriate ionic milieu (pH, divalent cation concentration, redox potential) or ionic asymmetry (pH, ionic and/or electrical gradient) required for a specific task. This microenvironment is generated, in part, by organelle-specific pumps (see Chapter 7), carriers (see Chapter 8), and channels (see Chapter 9). Enzymes that are embedded in an organelle membrane can more efficiently mediate chemical reactions because diffusion of substrates and products is reduced from three dimensions to two dimensions. For hydrophobic substrates and products, the advantage of being embedded in a compartmental membrane is obvious: they can be kept away from water molecules. Compartmentalization also enables potentially dangerous activities to be sequestered, such as degradative

Chapter by Sandra L. Schmid, based on an original draft by Ann L. Hubbard, J. David Castle, and Pat Shipman.

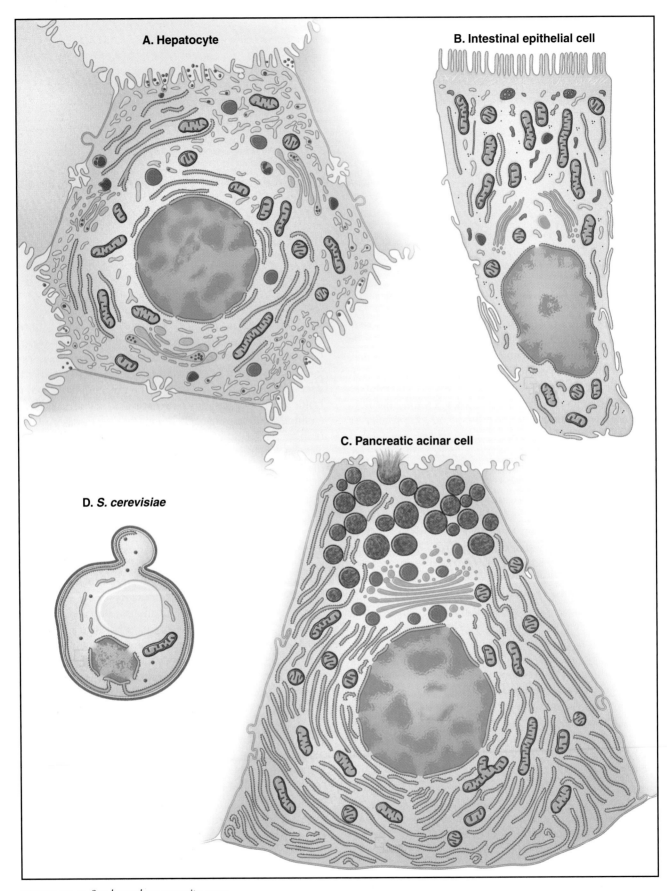

A. Hepatocyte

B. Intestinal epithelial cell

C. Pancreatic acinar cell

D. *S. cerevisiae*

Figure 17-1 *See legend on opposite page*

enzymes in lysosomes, oxidative enzymes in peroxisomes, and death-promoting activities in the intermembrane space of mitochondria.

▌ Origins of Compartments

Compartmentalization of ancestral prokaryotic cells enabled the first eukaryotes to increase in size, to capture energy more efficiently, and to regulate gene expression in more complex ways. Tracing the origins of compartments has been the subject of lively and insightful speculation; a brief discussion of some of the key issues is warranted to help the reader appreciate the significance of organelles and to identify the possible interrelationships (Fig. 17–2).

Heterotrophic organisms (those capable of obtaining nutrients from a variety of sources) acquired the ability to hydrolyze complex organic macromolecules (including their own components), thus providing themselves with the building blocks for new macromolecules. These ancestral prokaryotes were compartmentalized in the sense that biosynthesis occurred inside the cell, whereas digestion mostly occurred outside. Such an organization required the export of the digestive machinery (hydrolytic enzymes either attached to the cell surface or as free secretory products) and the import of the products of digestion (see Fig. 17–2A and inset). Thus, targeting and translocation of proteins across membranes was the first innovation leading to compartmentalization. Present-day bacteria transport proteins across membranes after they are completely synthesized, suggesting that this post-translational translocation (see Chapter 19) was the original primitive strategy.

Functionally distinct subdomains within the primitive prokaryotic plasma membrane could have been created by lateral segregation of protein complexes. In present-day bacteria, regions of the plasma membrane involved in energy production are indeed spatially segregated from those involved in protein translocation. One speculation is that invaginations of the subdomains of the plasma membrane involved in the synthesis of membrane lipids and in protein translocation

could have generated an intracellular biosynthetic organelle that survives today as the endoplasmic reticulum. Similarly, internalization of secreted hydrolytic enzymes, together with nutrients from the environment, might have created a primitive lysosome derived from the plasma membrane (see Fig. 17–2B). This would increase the efficiency of digestion and absorption of macromolecular nutrient sources would increase because the two processes could be coupled and concentrations maintained. The existence of two intracellular organelles would create the need for transport vesicles, the lipid and protein components of which could be synthesized in the progenitor ER. Transport vesicles could serve not only as carriers, exporting products to the cell surface or vacuole and importing raw materials, but also as protective devices that segregate digestive enzymes from the surrounding cytoplasm. Once multiple destinations existed, targeting instructions had to be provided to distinguish among alternate routes.

This "divide-and-specialize" strategy could have been employed a number of times, refining the internal membrane system. Eventually, the export and digestive pathways would have separated from each other and from the lipid synthetic and protein translocation machinery (see Fig. 17–2C). With each separation, it would become necessary to insert a new level of intercommunicating vesicles and a new set of targeting instructions. Regardless of the evolutionary pathway, the outcome of these events was the development of a vacuolar system consisting of the ER, the center for protein translocation and lipid synthesis; the Golgi complex and secretory pathway, for post-translational modification and distribution of biosynthetic products to different destinations; and the endosome/lysosome system, for uptake and digestion.

Several other important developments were essential in the ontogeny of compartments (see Fig. 17–2D). First, the ER was further refined to create the nuclear envelope housing the genome, the defining characteristic of the eukaryotic cell. This enabled the cell to develop a much more complex genome and to segregate transcription from translation. Second, translocation into the ER became coupled to protein syn-

Figure 17–1 Compartmentalization in functionally diverse eukaryotic cells. All eukaryotic cells have a full complement of the organelles required for energy production, metabolism, biosynthesis, and degradation; however, the numbers or overall size of each intracellular compartment varies depending on the function of the cell. *A*, The hepatocyte is a polarized cell specializing in constitutive secretion, transcytosis, and processing of serum proteins. It has amplified organelles along both the biosynthetic and endocytic pathways. Golgi stacks are oriented toward the "apical" surfaces, which correspond in this tissue to the bile canaliculi seen at the cell–cell contacts. *B*, The intestinal epithelial cell lines the boundary between the outside and the inside of the organism. Its two plasma membrane surfaces, which must interact with very different environments, are functionally and structurally distinct. *C*, The pancreatic acinar cell, which is specialized for regulated secretion, has a greatly enlarged ER, Golgi apparatus, and secretory granule compartments. *D*, The biosynthetic and endocytic compartments of *Saccharomyces cerevisiae*, baker's yeast, are maintained at minimum size to facilitate rapid cell division. Nuclear pores are larger than scale.

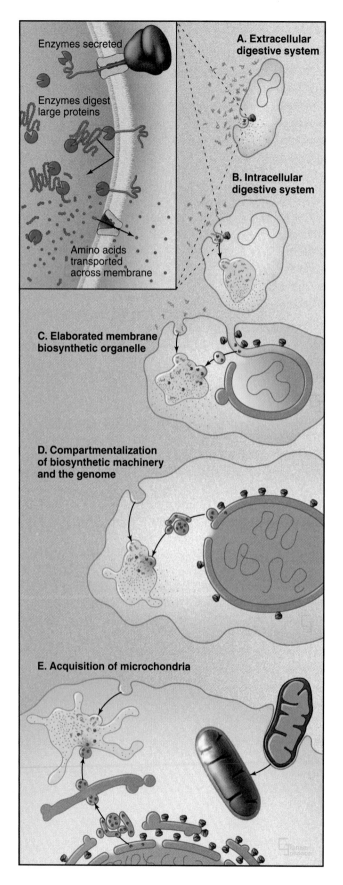

Enzymes secreted

Enzymes digest
large proteins

Amino acids
transported
across membrane

**A. Extracellular
digestive system**

**B. Intracellular
digestive system**

**C. Elaborated membrane
biosynthetic organelle**

**D. Compartmentalization
of biosynthetic machinery
and the genome**

E. Acquisition of microchondria

thesis (cotranslational), particularly in higher eukaryotes; the machinery used was modified from that in prokaryotes. Third, as oxygen appeared in the atmosphere, new and separate compartments were added to exploit this powerful oxidant. Peroxisomes arose as centers for oxidative degradation, particularly of products of lysosomal digestion that could not be reutilized for biosynthesis (e.g., D-amino acids, uric acid, xanthine). Mitochondria arose as centers where oxygen could be used to extract additional energy from metabolites and convert it into adenosine triphosphate (ATP) for biosynthesis and work. Mitochondria (and chloroplasts, found in plant cells) were initially bacteria that were ingested by a so-called "protoeukaryote" (see Fig. 17–2E and Fig. 1–1). A stable, endosymbiotic relationship evolved, enabling the bacterium to function as an energy producer within the cytoplasm of its host. The mitochondrial progenitor brought along its own genome, most of which moved to the nucleus during subsequent evolution. It is not clear whether peroxisomes arose in the same way as mitochondria (but earlier in evolution) or as a new specialization of the existing eukaryotic vacuolar compartment. No prokaryotic remnants have been detected in peroxisomes. The advent of oxygen also made possible the synthesis of cholesterol and its incorporation into membranes, particularly the plasma membrane and its communicating partners. It has been argued that incorporating cholesterol into membranes thickens them without compromising their fluidity; a strong yet flexible cell surface in the absence of a cell wall may have been an important factor that enabled early cells to increase in size.

Challenges Associated with Compartmentalization

Although advantageous, compartmentalization and the resulting division of labor also created some problems for the eukaryotic cell. As the compartments are not autonomous, their activities must be integrated to benefit the whole cell. Thus, mechanisms are required to transport material between compartments and across the membranes surrounding them. Some organelles are connected in functional series, termed pathways, which allow material to move from one to the next in a vectorial manner (Fig. 17–3). All nucleated cells

Figure 17–2 A to E, Speculative model for the evolution of intracellular compartments. The driving force is presumed to be the acquisition and degradation of essential nutrients from complex macromolecules present in increasingly dilute solution.

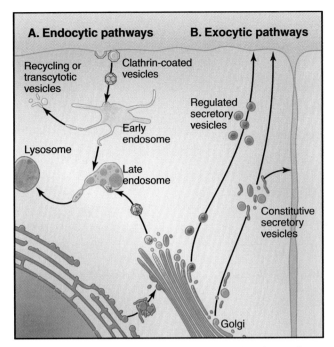

A. Endocytic pathways

B. Exocytic pathways

Recycling or transcytotic vesicles

Clathrin-coated vesicles

Regulated secretory vesicles

Early endosome

Lysosome

Late endosome

Constitutive secretory vesicles

Golgi

Figure 17-3 Cellular compartments involved in biosynthesis/exocytosis/endocytosis are functionally linked to the biosynthetic and endocytic pathways respectively. Membrane transport through these two pathways is balanced to establish and maintain compartment size and to ensure the doubling of cellular membrane content before division.

have these pathways. The exocytic or **secretory pathway** coordinates organelle biosynthesis and secretion, whereas the **endocytic pathway** regulates the cell's interactions with its environment. The two pathways operate coordinately in protein and lipid turnover. The static snapshots of cellular compartments seen in fixed (dead) cells belie the dynamic aspects of the organelles and their pathways.

The mechanisms to move molecules between organelles and across membranes are central topics in cell biology. The pumps (see Chapter 7), carriers (see Chapter 8), and channels (see Chapter 9) that transport small molecules across organelle membranes are topics of previous chapters. Transport of proteins and lipids between organelles, in a process collectively termed **vesicular trafficking,** is the major subject of the following chapters. The process begins in the cytoplasm with protein synthesis (discussed in Chapter 18). Proteins that do not reside in the cytoplasm must be exported to their final destination—the nucleus,

mitochondria, or the ER—if the protein is to be secreted or will reside in an organelle along either the exocytic or endocytic pathway (see Chapter 19). Newly synthesized proteins deposited in the ER must be transported and delivered through the Golgi apparatus and along the exocytic pathway to their target organelle, where they take up residence (see Chapters 20 and 21). Vesicular trafficking along the endocytic pathway (discussed in Chapter 22) to lysosomes allows the cell to interact with and sample its environment, to obtain nutrients, and to remodel its membranes. A consequence of compartmentalization is that membrane proteins and molecules within the lumen of intracellular organelles are topologically segregated from the cytoplasm and so must be transported in carrier vesicles. Moreover, several mechanisms are used to maintain organelle identity despite the extensive flux of membrane material along both endocytic and exocytic pathways. The mechanisms governing protein sorting—the formation of transport vesicles at one organelle and their targeting and fusion to the next organelle in the series—apply at each stage of transport. The basic steps, which will be introduced in Chapter 20 as they come into play during the first vesicular trafficking events that occur between the ER and Golgi compartments, involve the following: (1) sorting signals direct proteins into transport vesicles; (2) coat proteins (e.g., COPI, COPII, or clathrin/AP complexes), which assemble from the cytoplasm, recognize specific sorting signals, recruit cargo for transport, and help to deform the membrane; and (3) membrane proteins called v- and t-SNARES on the vesicle and target membrane, respectively, direct fusion and accurate delivery through mutual recognition. Importantly, each of these events—coat assembly, cargo recruitment, vesicle budding, vesicle docking, and fusion—is supervised by families of GTPases that coordinate and monitor the fidelity of membrane-trafficking events. These mechanisms must have evolved coordinately with the increasingly complex compartmentalization of the cell.

Selected Readings

DeDuve C: The birth of the complex cell. Sci Am 274:50–57, 1996.

DeDuve C: Blueprint for a cell. Burlington, NC: Neil Patterson/London: Portland Press, 1991.

chapter 18

PROTEIN SYNTHESIS AND FOLDING
IN THE CYTOPLASM

The nuclear genome contains information specifying thousands of proteins. Whatever their final destination—nucleus, cytoplasm, membrane-bound organelles, or extracellular space—these proteins are synthesized in the cytoplasm. (The few proteins encoded by genes in mitochondria and chloroplasts are synthesized in those organelles.) The biochemical synthesis of proteins is called **translation,** as the process translates sequences of nucleotides in a **messenger RNA (mRNA)** into the sequence of amino acids in a polypeptide chain. Translation of mRNA requires the concerted actions of small **transfer RNAs (tRNAs)** linked to amino acids, **ribosomes** (complexes of RNA and protein), and many soluble proteins. Several proteins regulated by GTP hydrolysis orchestrate the interactions of these components. Ultimately RNA bases in the ribosome catalyze the formation of the peptide bond. Folding newly synthesized polypeptides requires additional factors, referred to as **chaperones.** It has been proposed that the bulk of the evolution of the translation apparatus occurred after the basic mechanisms were established, to provide greater precision. This perspective seems to explain the extraordinary complexity of the process. This chapter describes the major components of the protein synthetic machinery and how they work together to produce functional proteins. It concludes by considering the process of protein folding in cells.

Protein Synthetic Machinery

Messenger RNA

mRNAs have three parts: nucleotides at the 5′ end that provide binding sites for the machinery that initiates

polypeptide synthesis; nucleotides in the middle that specify the sequence of amino acids in the polypeptide; and nucleotides at the 3′ end that regulate the stability of the mRNA (see Chapters 14 and 15). Within the protein-coding region, successive triplets of three nucleotides, called **codons,** specify the sequence of amino acids. The **genetic code** relating nucleotide triplets to amino acids is, with a few minor exceptions, universal. Particular amino acids are encoded by one to four different triplets (Fig. 18–1). An **initiation codon** (AUG) specifies methionine, which begins all polypeptide chains. In addition, any one of three **termination codons** (UAA, UGA, UAG) stop peptide synthesis.

Eukaryotic and bacterial mRNAs differ in three ways. First, eukaryotic mRNAs encode one protein and bacterial mRNAs generally encode more than one protein. Second, most eukaryotic (and eukaryotic viral) mRNAs are modified on their 5′ end with methyl groups, which form a "cap" (Fig. 18–2). This **5′ cap** is stable throughout the life of the mRNA and protects the 5′ end against attack by nucleases. Third, most eukaryotic mRNAs have a tail of 50 to 200 adenine residues added post-transcriptionally to the 3′ end. The **poly-A tail** may protect the mRNA from degradation in the cytoplasm and increase reinitiation of transcription. Bacterial mRNAs lack 5′ caps or 3′ poly-A tails.

Many single-stranded mRNAs have some secondary structure (see Chapter 2) stabilized by hydrogen-bonding of complementary bases. During protein synthesis, this secondary structure must be systematically disrupted to allow each codon to be read by pairing with the anticodon in the appropriate RNA.

Transfer RNA

tRNAs are adapters that deliver amino acids to the translation machinery by matching mRNA codons with

Chapter by William E. Balch and TDP, based on an original draft by Ann L. Hubbard, J. David Castle, and Pat Shipman.

	Second Position				
	U	**C**	**A**	**G**	
U	UUU ⎫ Phe UUC ⎭ UUA ⎫ Leu UUG ⎭	UCU ⎫ UCC ⎬ Ser UCA ⎪ UCG ⎭	UAU ⎫ Tyr UAC ⎭ ● UAA ⎫ Stop ● UAG ⎭	UGU ⎫ Cys UGC ⎭ ● UGA Stop UGG Trp	**U** **C** **A** **G**
C	CUU ⎫ CUC ⎬ Leu CUA ⎪ CUG ⎭	CCU ⎫ CCC ⎬ Pro CCA ⎪ CCG ⎭	CAU ⎫ His CAC ⎭ CAA ⎫ Gln CAG ⎭	CGU ⎫ CGC ⎬ Arg CGA ⎪ CGG ⎭	**U** **C** **A** **G**
A	AUU ⎫ AUC ⎬ Ile AUA ⎪ ● AUG Met	ACU ⎫ ACC ⎬ Thr ACA ⎪ ACG ⎭	AAU ⎫ Asn AAC ⎭ AAA ⎫ Lys AAG ⎭	AGU ⎫ Ser AGC ⎭ AGA ⎫ Arg AGG ⎭	**U** **C** **A** **G**
G	GUU ⎫ GUC ⎬ Val GUA ⎪ GUG ⎭	GCU ⎫ GCC ⎬ Ala GCA ⎪ GCG ⎭	GAU ⎫ Asp GAC ⎭ GAA ⎫ Glu GAG ⎭	GGU ⎫ GGC ⎬ Gly GGA ⎪ GGG ⎭	**U** **C** **A** **G**

● = Chain-terminating codon
● = Initiation codon

Figure 18-1 The genetic code. The location of the nucleotide in first, second, and third position defines the amino acid encrypted by the code.

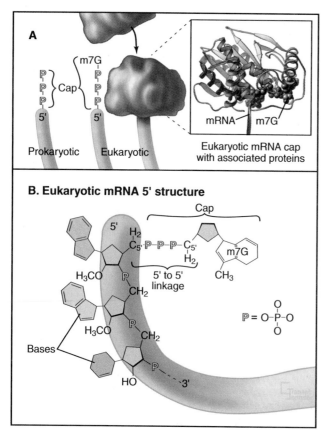

Figure 18-2 *A* and *B,* mRNA cap structures. Prokaryotic mRNAs end with a 5′ triphosphate, whereas eukaryotic mRNAs have a 5′ cap consisting of a methylated base (m7G). This cap binds a protein that protects against degradation by nucleases. (PDB file: 1EJ1.)

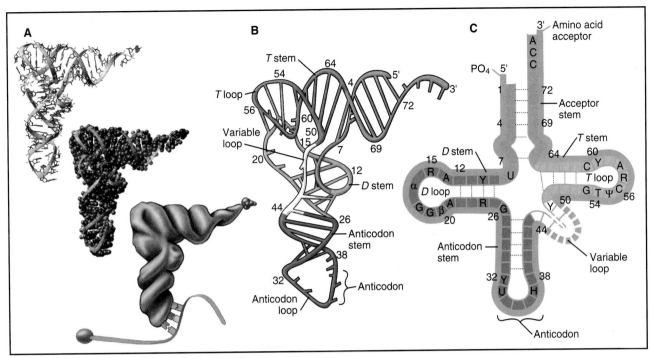

Figure 18-3 Structure of tRNAs. *A,* Ribbon and space-filling models, including base pairing of the anticodon to an mRNA codon. *B,* Backbone model. *C,* Planar model showing stem loops. tRNAs match an amino acid attached at the 3′ end with the mRNA triplet coding for that amino acid. (PDB file: 6TNA)

their corresponding amino acids as they are incorporated into a growing polypeptide (Fig. 18–3; see Chapter 2). One to four different tRNAs are specific for each amino acid, generally reflecting their abundance in proteins. Specialized tRNAs carrying methionine (formylmethionine in bacteria) initiate protein synthesis. Transfer RNAs consist of about 76 nucleotides that base-pair to form four stems and three intervening loops. These elements of secondary structure fold to form an L-shaped molecule stabilized by base pairing. A "decoding" triplet (the **anticodon**) is at one end of the L (the anticodon arm) and the amino acid acceptor site is at the other end of the L (the acceptor arm).

Enzymes called **aminoacyl-tRNA (aa-tRNA) synthetases** catalyze a two-step reaction that couples an amino acid covalently to its cognate tRNA but not to any other tRNA (Fig. 18–4). In the first step, adenosine triphosphate (ATP) and the amino acid react to form a high-energy aminoacyl adenosine monophosphate (AMP) intermediate with release of pyrophosphate. Subsequent hydrolysis of pyrophosphate releases additional energy for the coupling reaction. The second step transfers the amino acid to the 3′ adenine of tRNA, forming an aa-tRNA. This reaction is appropriately called "charging," since the high-energy bond between the amino acid and the tRNA activates the amino acid in preparation for forming a peptide bind

with an amino group in the growing polypeptide chain. Each of the 20 aa-tRNA synthetases couples a particular amino acid to all of its corresponding tRNAs.

The fidelity of protein synthesis depends on near-perfect coupling of amino acids to the appropriate tRNAs. Each synthetase must discriminate among structurally related amino acids and structurally similar tRNAs to select the correct pair. Synthetases recognize three areas of their cognate tRNAs: anticodon; 3′ acceptor stem; and the surface between these sites (see Fig. 18–4). This intimate interaction with only tRNAs for the same amino acid ensures proper recognition. The enzyme must also distinguish the appropriate amino acid. This is accomplished, in several cases, by a "proofreading" mechanism whereby related amino acids are identified and discarded before being linked to the bound tRNA.

Ribosomes

Ribosomes are giant macromolecular machines that bring together an mRNA and aa-tRNAs to synthesize a polypeptide. Base pairing between mRNA codons and tRNA anticodons directs the synthesis of a polypeptide in the order specified by the mRNA codons.

Ribosomes consist of a **small subunit** and a **large subunit** that bind together during translation of an mRNA (Fig. 18–5). Each subunit consists of one or

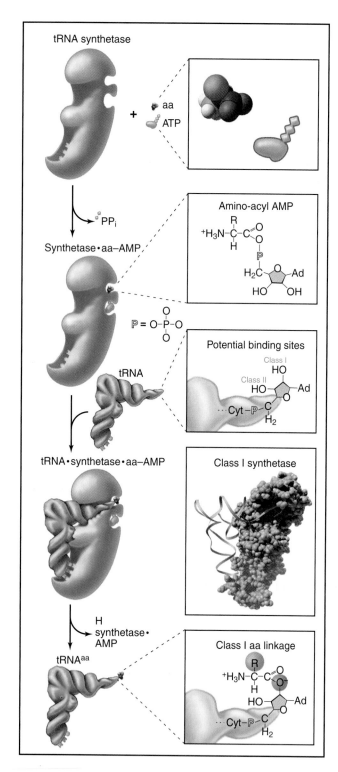

tRNA synthetase

+ aa
  ATP

PP$_i$

Synthetase·aa–AMP

Amino-acyl AMP

tRNA

$$\mathbb{P} = O{-}P{-}O$$

Potential binding sites

tRNA·synthetase·aa–AMP

Class I synthetase

H
synthetase·
AMP

tRNA^{aa}

Class I aa linkage

Figure 18-4 Charging a tRNA with its correct amino acid. tRNA synthetases (shown schematically and as a space-filling atomic model in purple) provide a docking platform for a specific amino acid and its cognate tRNA (shown in orange as a schematic model and as a ribbon model bound to a synthetase). The amino acid is first activated by reaction with ATP. The carboxyl group of the amino acid is coupled to the α-phosphate of AMP with the release of pyrophosphate. The synthetase then transfers the amino acid from the aminoacyl AMP (aa-AMP) to a high-energy ester bond (red disk) with either the 2′ (illustrated here) or 3′ hydroxyl of the adenine at the 3′ end of the tRNA. (PDB file: 1QTQ)

more **ribosomal RNA (rRNA)** molecules and many distinct proteins (Fig. 18–6). High-resolution x-ray structures of a *Eubacteria* small subunit and an *Archaea* large subunit are available. Eubacterial large subunits are similar in models of whole ribosomes made by image processing of electron micrographs. Eukaryotic ribosomes are similar, although they are larger.

Ribosomal RNAs provide the bulk of the mass and the structural core of each ribosomal subunit (Fig. 18–7). The 16S rRNA of the small subunit consists of 1500 bases, most of which are folded into base-paired helices (S refers to the sedimentation coefficient measured in an ultracentrifuge). The large subunit contains two RNAs: 23S rRNA, which consists of 2900 bases; and 5S rRNA, which comprises 121 bases. They are

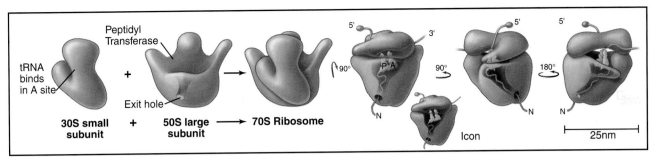

Figure 18-5 Schematic models of the ribosome illustrating overall organization. Two subunits (30S and 50S) form a functional ribosome. An mRNA threads between the subunits in association with the small subunit. tRNAs bind to two sites, designated A site and P site, between the large and small subunits. Codons of the mRNA in the A and P sites on the small subunit specify which aa-tRNAs occupy these sites. The amino acids at the far end of the bound tRNAs are positioned for peptide bond formation by the peptidyl transferase site on the large subunit. The growing polypeptide chain (shown in blue) emerges from a tunnel in the large subunit.

folded into many based-paired helices much as predicted by phylogenetic analysis of sequences (see Fig. 18–6). These helices and their intervening loops pack into a compact structure, as seen in both surface views and cross sections. Although eukaryotic rRNAs differ in size and sequence from prokaryote rRNAs, their predicted secondary structures are similar, and they are expected to fold in the same way. Many features of rRNAs have been conserved throughout evolution, including the surfaces where subunits and elements of RNA structure interact; sites that are required for binding tRNA, mRNA, and protein cofactors; and the residues involved with peptide bond formation.

Ribosomal proteins are generally small (10–30 kD) and basic. They are not related to one another, and (with one exception) there is just one copy of each per ribosome. Most proteins are associated with the surface of the rRNA core of the subunits (see Fig. 18–7). Several proteins extend peptide strands into the core. Small subunit proteins are also bound to the surface of the RNA core, with few of the 21 proteins on the interface with the large subunit.

Decoding of the mRNA and synthesis of the polypeptide take place in the cavity between the subunits. The surfaces of this cavity are generally free of proteins, so that mRNA binding, tRNA binding, and peptide bond formation are carried out largely by RNA. tRNAs move sequentially through three sites shared by the two subunits: the **A site** (aa-tRNA), the **P site** (for peptidyl-tRNA), and the **E site** (for exit). The growing polypeptide chain exits through a tunnel in the RNA core of the large subunit.

The amazing feat of reassembling a functional ribosomal subunit from purified rRNA and proteins from *Escherichia coli* was accomplished more than 25 years ago. The core 16S rRNA folds spontaneously, but efficient assembly depends on adding proteins in

a particular sequence. Ribosome self-assembly requires no additional factors. Details of the assembly pathway are under active investigation.

Soluble Protein Factors

Many soluble proteins participate in protein synthesis. These proteins cycle on and off the ribosome, enhanc-

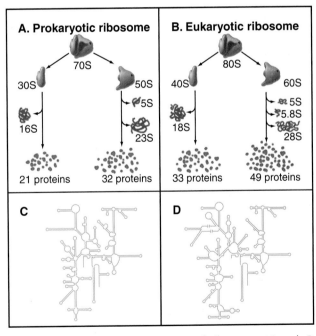

Figure 18-6 Molecular components of ribosomes. *A* and *B,* Schematic inventories of rRNAs and proteins. Prokaryotic and eukaryotic rRNAs and ribosomal proteins differ in size and number but are related by evolution and form similar structures. *C* and *D,* Diagrammatic representations of the secondary structures of prokaryotic 16S rRNA and 18S eukaryotic rRNA illustrate their similarities despite divergent sequences.

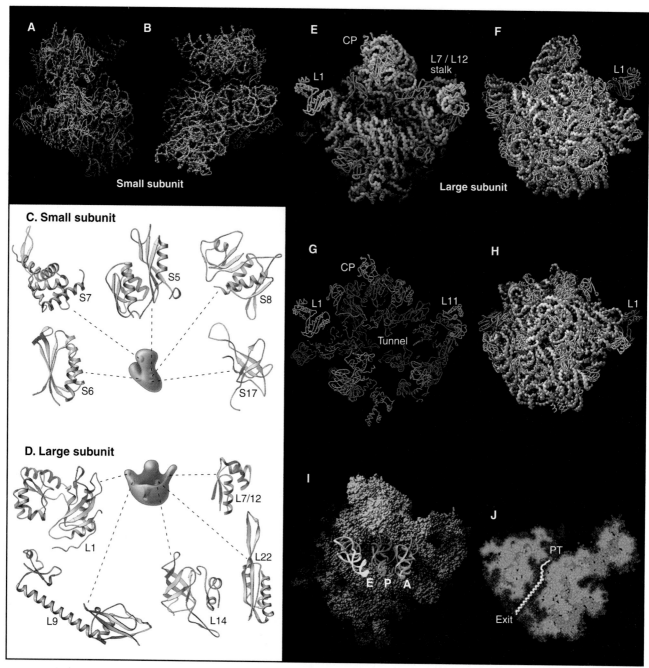

Figure 18-7 Structure of the ribosome. Atomic models show RNA in grey and proteins in gold except in *G,* where various colors are used. *A* and *B,* Two views of the atomic model of the small subunit of *Thermus thermophilus. C* and *D,* Representative structures of individual ribosomal proteins and their locations on the small and large subunits. (PDB file: 1FJF) *E* to *J,* Atomic structure of the large subunit of the ribosome of *Haloarcula marismortui. E,* Crown view from the perspective of the small subunit. *F,* View *C* rotated 180 degrees around a vertical axis. *H,* View *E* rotated 180 degrees around a horizontal axis to show the exit from the nascent polypeptide tunnel, the dark patch in the middle. *I,* Crown view with models of tRNA in the A, P, and E sites. *J,* A cross section shows the tunnel for the nascent polypeptide extending from the peptidyl transferase (PT) site to the exit. (*A* and *B,* Reprinted with permission from Nature. Reference: Wimberly BT, et al: Structure of the 30S ribosomal subunit. Nature 407:327–339, 2000. Copyright 2000, Macmillan Magazines Limited. (*E* to *J,* Adapted from the work of Ban N, et al: The complete atomic structure of the large ribosomal subunit at 2.4Å resolution. Science 289:905–920, 2000; and Nissen P, et al: The structural basis of ribosome activity in peptide bond synthesis. Science 289:920–930, 2000. Copyright 2000, American Association for the Advancement of Science. PDB file: 1FFK.)

ing the rate or fidelity of protein synthesis. The role(s) of these soluble factors are highlighted in the following sections.

Outline of Protein Synthesis

Protein synthesis is divided mechanistically into three steps: initiation, elongation, and termination (Fig. 18–8). Each step utilizes guanosine triphosphatase (GTPase) proteins and their cognate exchange factors to regulate the progress and fidelity of the overall reaction (see Chapter 27 for details on GTPase cycles).

During **initiation,** a complex composed of a small ribosomal subunit and an initiator tRNA (carrying methionine) binds the initiation codon (AUG) of an mRNA. This ternary complex then associates with a large subunit to form a 70S ribosome in bacteria and an 80S ribosome in eukaryotes. Initiation requires many more components in eukaryotes than in prokaryotes, presumably to afford better regulation.

During **elongation,** tRNAs bring amino acids to the ribosome in the order specified by the sequence of codons in the mRNA. The ribosome catalyzes formation of a peptide bond between the amino group of each new amino acid and the carboxyl group at the C-terminus of the growing polypeptide chain and then moves on to the next codon. More than one ribosome is active on most mRNAs, as coding sequences are longer than the 40 to 50 nucleotides associated with a ribosome. For example, the coding sequence for actin, a 43-kD protein, is approximately 1100 nucleotides long. Once a ribosome proceeds about 60 nucleotides beyond the initiation codon, another ribosome-tRNA complex can assemble on the mRNA and start translation. Messenger RNAs with multiple ribosomes are called **polysomes.** This multiple occupancy of mRNAs explains why ribosomes are more abundant than mRNA and how one mRNA molecule guides the synthesis of several copies of its protein product simultaneously.

The final phase is **termination.** At the 3′ end of the coding sequence, the ribosome encounters a termination codon (UAA, UAG, or UGA). At this point, a protein factor (not an aa-tRNA) binds to the mRNA, and the C-terminal amino acid of the polypeptide chain is hydrolyzed from its tRNA, releasing the polypeptide from the ribosome. The ribosomal subunits dissociate and are available to initiate translation of another mRNA.

Translation must proceed at a pace fast enough to supply proteins but slow enough to avoid errors leading to unstable or malfunctioning proteins. Cells balance speed and accuracy during protein synthesis to

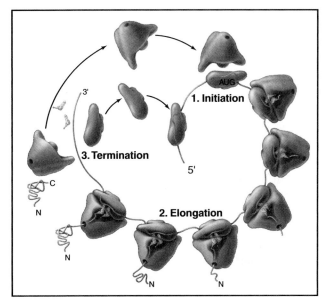

Figure 18-8 Overview of the translation cycle showing six ribosomes on a single mRNA. *1,* Initiation. Initiator tRNA[Met], mRNA, and accessory soluble factors assemble on the small subunit, which then joins with a large subunit. *2,* Elongation. The polypeptide chain is synthesized, in the order specified by the mRNA, in sequential steps by recruitment of new aa-tRNAs that match the mRNA-coding sequence, formation of peptide bonds, and dissociation of free tRNA. *3,* Termination. Specific factors recognize the termination codon and release the nascent polypeptide chain for folding in the cytoplasm.

achieve an error rate of about 1 in 10^4 incorrect amino acids. If greater precision were achieved by slowing the translation reactions, slower cellular growth might be an evolutionary disadvantage. As a result of this compromise, ribosomes add about 20 amino acids per second to a polypeptide at 37°C, so that synthesis of actin (375 amino acids) takes 20 seconds.

All of the components work together to synthesize a protein in a dynamic, sequential reaction. Initiation, elongation, and termination all depend on directed movement of molecular machinery along an mRNA and precise recognition between amino acids, tRNAs, adaptor proteins, and the gene sequence encoded in the mRNA.

Initiation Phase

The goal of initiation is to attach a specialized initiator tRNA carrying methionine (or *N*-formylmethionine, fMet, in bacteria) to both the correct AUG codon in the mRNA and the correct site on the ribosome (Fig. 18–9). In eukaryotes, more than 10 soluble protein factors (eukaryotic **initiation factors,** or eIF) participate in this complex dance. Fewer protein factors (designated IF) participate in prokaryotes. A general theme is that proteins coordinate the recognition and

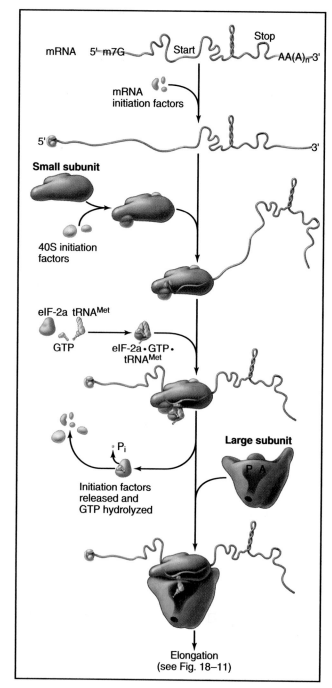

Figure 18-9 Steps in initiation. Cap recognition factors *(blue)* bind mRNA. Other initiation factors *(green)* assemble with mRNA, eIF-2a *(purple, activated with GTP)*, and tRNA^Met on the small ribosomal subunit. This preinitiation complex scans the mRNA for the AUG start codon *(green)*. When it is found, eIF-2a hydrolyzes its bound GTP, initiation factors dissociate, and the small subunit binds a large subunit.

assemble on the 5' cap of the mRNA to promote unwinding or melting of any secondary structure at the 5' end of the mRNA.

Step 2. Formation of preinitiation complex. Independently, initiator Met-tRNA, in association with the GTPase initiation factor eIF-2a (with bound guanosine triphosphate [GTP]), forms a complex with a small ribosomal subunit. This is the only aa-tRNA that binds to the P site on the small subunit.

Step 3. Unwinding and scanning. The mRNA, with its **cap recognition complex,** binds a **preinitiation complex** and begins to unwind any mRNA secondary structure, "scanning" for the correct AUG codon. This activity depends upon ATP hydrolysis and makes the correct AUG codon accessible to base-pair with the initiation codon. The local nucleotide sequence requirements for specifying the correct initiator AUG codon are incompletely understood although eukaryotic mRNAs tend to begin translation at the first AUG codon encountered.

Step 4. Subunit joining. When the preinitiation complex finds the initiation codon, eIF-2a hydrolyzes its bound GTP, and the preinitiation factors dissociate from the small subunit. A large subunit then binds the small subunit with both the mRNA and Met-tRNA correctly positioned for elongation.

Initiation is the most highly regulated step in protein synthesis, and regulation frequently involves phosphorylation of initiation proteins. For example, phosphorylation increases the affinity of eIF-2a for its guanine nucleotide exchange factor (called eIF-2b). Strongly bound exchange factor inhibits general initiation by competing with initiator tRNA for binding eIF-2a. When subjected to stress, cells utilize this phosphorylation step to reduce translation rates that might be detrimental (see Chapter 24). In contrast, phosphorylation of eIF-4F, a protein that recognizes the 5' cap of mRNAs and facilitates initiation, improves its binding to all mRNAs and thereby favors general translation. The 5' caps of particular mRNAs vary in affinity for eIF-4F, probably because of the nearby tertiary structure in the mRNA. Phosphorylation of eIF-4F can also regulate translation of specific mRNAs, since the cellular concentration of eIF-4F is limiting and mRNAs must compete for it. Caps that bind eIF-4F with higher affinity are translated more efficiently.

Elongation Phase

Accurate protein synthesis depends on the fidelity of amino acid coupling to the correct tRNA and of codon-anticodon match-up between mRNA and tRNA. Both reactions occur in two steps, by a mechanism that increases accuracy. Much of the energy invested in protein synthesis is used to achieve this accuracy,

binding of the RNA molecules. In eukaryotic cells, four steps occur in succession:

Step 1. Cap recognition. A complex of four to six factors, including an adenosine triphosphatase (ATPase) with RNA unwinding **(helicase)** activity,

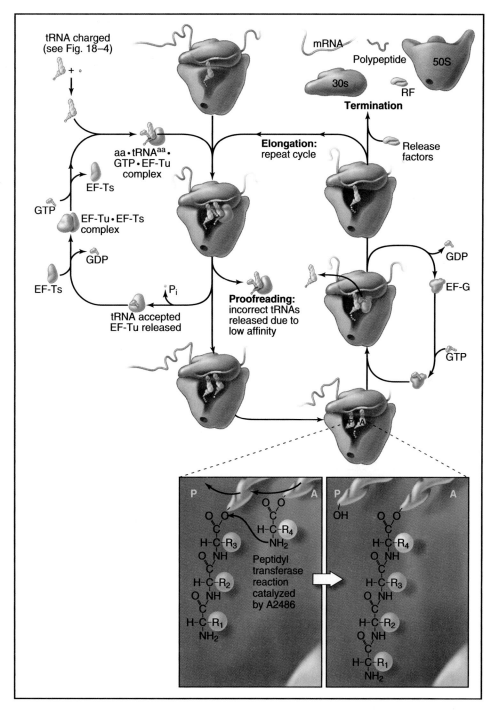

Figure 18-10 Steps in elongation and termination. Starting in the upper left, elongation factor EF-Tu (eEF-1 in eukaryotes) forms a "ternary" complex with GTP and an amino acyl-tRNA^{aa} for delivery of the tRNA^{aa}, matching the mRNA codon in the A site to the ribosome. This ternary complex dissociates rapidly if the anticodon-codon match is incorrect. If the anticodon-codon match is correct, the ternary complex remains bound to the A site long enough for EF-Tu to hydrolyze its bound GTP and dissociate from the tRNA still bound to the A site. The ribosome catalyzes formation of a new peptide bond (inset). EF-G (eEF-2 in eukaryotes) binds the A site transiently after peptide bond formation to facilitate movement of the tRNAs and mRNA through the ribosome. Termination factors (green) recognize termination codons and terminate the polypeptide chain (blue), allowing the mRNA and ribosomal subunits to dissociate. RF, release factors.

and elongation is the most expensive phase of translation in terms of energy expenditure.

With subunits joined to form a 70S or 80S ribosome and an initiator tRNA and mRNA properly in place, repetitive cycles of codon-directed addition of aa-tRNAs can begin (Fig. 18–10). Prokaryotes and eukaryotes share four fundamental steps in each cycle of elongation: (1) binding of a second aa-tRNA at the A site on the ribosome; (2) "proofreading" to ensure that it is the correct aa-tRNA; (3) peptide bond formation;

and (4) translocation, which involves advancing the mRNA by one codon and moving the peptidyl-tRNA from the aa-tRNA (A) site to the peptidyl-tRNA (P) site on the ribosome.

Elongation reactions occur in a cavity between the two ribosomal subunits. mRNA is threaded, codon by codon, between the subunits. aa-tRNAs enter on one side of the interface by binding to the A site; they then shift to the adjacent P site between the subunits and depart empty on the far side. Codon-anticodon recognition takes place at both the A and P sites on the small subunit where the anticodons of the two tRNAs base-pair with mRNA. Peptide bonds form at the other end of the tRNAs, which position the amino acid and peptidyl chain on the A and P sites of the large subunit. The A and P sites are each composed of two half-sites, with half on each ribosomal subunit. Having two half-sites allows ribosomes to maintain contact with one end of each tRNA as they move, step by step, between sites. During elongation, tRNA movements occur independently on the two ribosomal subunits. **Elongation factors** (EF; eEF for eukaryotic elongation factors) and movements of the subunits relative to each other facilitate the movements of the tRNAs. The growing polypeptide exits through a tunnel in the large subunit.

Step 1. aa-tRNA binding. The GTPase eEF-1 (EF-Tu in bacteria; see Fig. 27–8) delivers aa-tRNAs to the A site on the ribosome. eEF-1 with bound GTP has a higher affinity for aa-tRNA than guanosine diphosphate (GDP)–eEF-1. The nucleotide exchange factor eEF-X (EF-Ts in bacteria) promotes the exchange of GDP for GTP to prepare eEF-1 for binding aa-tRNA. Given the abundance of eEF-1, most cellular aa-tRNA is bound to GTP–eEF-1. eEF-1 protects the labile ester bond of the aa-tRNA. The ternary complex of GTP–eEF-1 and aa-tRNA associates only with empty A sites, ensuring that it enters during the correct phase of the elongation cycle.

Step 2. Proofreading. After the complex of GTP–eEF-1 and an aa-tRNA binds to the A site on the ribosome, the tRNA must be checked carefully for correct recognition of the mRNA codon. Correct aa-tRNAs are retained; incorrect aa-tRNAs are rejected. This proofreading process is achieved by a kinetic mechanism using two first-order reactions to ensure accurate translation of mRNA codons into a polypeptide.

The **proofreading reactions** are GTP hydrolysis by eEF-1 and dissociation of GDP–eEF-1 from the ribosome. Peptide bond formation can occur only after these two irreversible reactions are completed. Each reaction takes a few milliseconds. Ribosomes stimulate hydrolysis of GTP bound to eEF-1–aa-tRNA bound to the A site. Hydrolysis rates are identical for correct and incorrect aa-tRNAs. Hydrolysis increases the affinity of the GDP–eEF-1–aa-tRNA for the ribosome.

Correct codon-anticodon pairs are sufficiently stable for the aa-tRNA to remain bound to the ribosome through these two proofreading reactions until the amino acid is incorporated into the growing polypeptide. Incorrect aa-tRNAs have two opportunities to escape before the irreversible formation of a peptide bond. Weak, imperfect codon-anticodon pairs allow incorrect aa-tRNAs to dissociate from the A site during the time required for eEF-1 to hydrolyze GTP and for GDP–eEF-1 to dissociate. This kinetic proofreading mechanism uses internal standards, the rates of two reactions that are not influenced by concentrations or identities of the substrates.

Step 3. Peptidyl transfer. The ribonucleotide base of adenine 2486 of the large subunit rRNA catalyzes the nucleophilic attack of the free amino group of the aa-tRNA in the A site on the esterified carboxyl group of the peptidyl-tRNA in the P site (see Fig. 18–10). Water is eliminated to form a new peptide bond. This is a clear example of RNA catalysis, since the closest protein subunit is >1.8 nm away. The mechanism is similar to the reverse of the cleavage of peptide bonds by proteolytic enzymes like chymotrypsin, and is achieved by a combination of precise orientation of the substrates and stabilization of the transition state (just like protein enzymes). This RNA active site has been highly conserved from *Archaea* to *Eubacteria* and eukaryotes. The idea that RNA catalyzes protein synthesis was difficult to accept, even after the discovery that ribosomes, when stripped of most protein subunits, can form peptide bonds. However, the atomic structures of ribosomes removed all doubt.

Peptide bond formation transfers the polypeptide chain from the tRNA in the P site to the tRNA in the A site (see Fig. 18–10). The aminoacyl arm of the aa-tRNA in the A site swings from the A site on the large subunit toward the P site during peptidyl transfer. The anticodon arm of this charged tRNA remains bound to its codon in the A site of the small subunit.

The antibacterial agent puromycin can disrupt elongation by mimicking a tRNA^{Phe} or tRNA^{Tyr} (Fig. 18–11). Puromycin attacks the esterified carboxyl group of a peptidyl-tRNA in the P site, but, lacking an appropriate acceptor site for further peptidyl transfer reactions, it terminates elongation resulting in premature release of the polypeptide chain from the ribosome.

Step 4. Translocation. Three linked reactions, promoted by elongation factor eEF-2 (and the homologous protein EF-G in bacteria), complete each elongation cycle. EF-2 is another GTPase with domains similar to domains 1 and 2 of EF-Tu plus three domains that mimic the size and shape of a tRNA. Domain 1 binds and hydrolyzes GTP. Domains 3 to 5 target GTP–EF-2 to an empty A site on the ribosome.

Binding of GTP–eEF-2 (or GTP–EF-G) to the site "facilitates" movement of peptidyl-tRNA from the A to the P site on the small subunit with sliding of the mRNA three bases forward in the small subunit. At the same time, deacylated tRNA

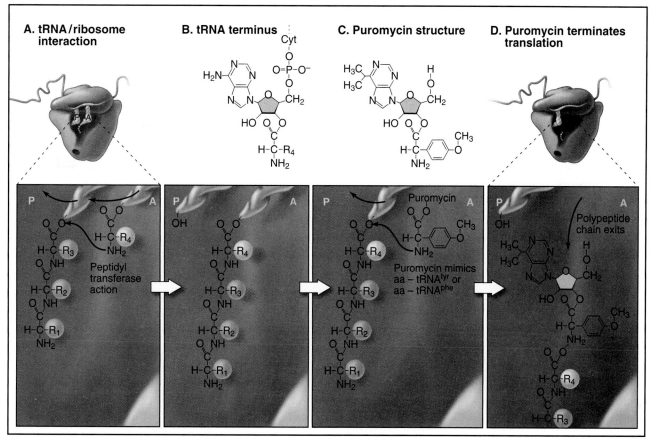

A. tRNA/ribosome interaction

B. tRNA terminus

C. Puromycin structure

D. Puromycin terminates translation

Figure 18–11 Mechanism of the puromycin reaction shown in four steps, *A* to *D*. The antibiotic puromycin mimics the terminus of amino acyl-tRNA^{tyr} or tRNA^{phe}. It is incorporated on the C-terminus of the polypeptide and terminates translation prematurely, as it is not attached to a tRNA and lacks an activated carboxyl group.

is moved out of the P site to the exit (E) site, where it dissociates from the ribosome. These movements can proceed only slowly without eEF-2. Hydrolysis of GTP bound to eEF-2 changes its conformation in a manner yet to be defined and causes it to release from the A site. This opens up the A site for another round of binding an aa-tRNA complexed with a GTP–eEF-1, initiating another round of elongation.

The growing peptide threads through a long tunnel in the large subunit lined with RNA (see Figs. 18–5, 18–7, and 18–8). Inside the ribosome, the polypeptide is fully extended, as the tunnel will not accommodate a folded peptide. The channel accommodates about 40 amino acids; the N-terminus of longer peptides exits from the lower portion of the large subunit.

Termination Phase

The assembly of a protein stops when a termination codon moves into the A site on the small subunit of the ribosome (see Fig. 18–10). A protein called eTF (EF6 in bacteria) binds to this codon and, in a GTP-dependent manner, catalyzes hydrolysis of the peptidyl-tRNA ester at the P site. The completed polypep-

tide chain threads through the ribosome and is released. The large subunit dissociates from the mRNA and the small subunit.

The Role of Chaperones in Protein Folding

Termination is the final step in translation, but just the beginning for a new protein. A polypeptide begins to experience its new environment while still being synthesized. When it is about 40 residues long, its N-terminus emerges from the protected tunnel of the large ribosomal subunit into cytoplasm, where it must fold into a three-dimensional structure (see Chapter 2) and find its correct cellular destination.

The structure of folded proteins and the folding mechanism are both encoded in the amino acid sequence, in most cases making folding spontaneous under suitable conditions. Folding pathways for proteins are fast and tend to follow an energetically favorable route, leading to a stable, low energy state for the final folded structure (Fig. 18–12). This process is more complicated for larger proteins.

Most proteins start folding before the polypeptide is completed, making the process vectorial, beginning

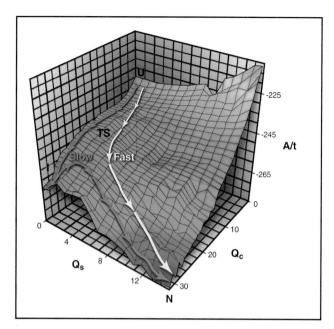

Figure 18-12 Energy considerations in protein folding. As a protein matures from the unfolded state (U) through transitional intermediate states (TS) to the folded state (N), more native-like contacts are formed and the energy of the system decreases. The two paths *(folding trajectories)* illustrate that fast protein folding *(yellow line)* is observed when more native-like contacts are made. When proteins become trapped in partially folded intermediate states, folding is slower *(pink line)* because energy barriers must be overcome. (Adapted from Radford SE, Dobson CM: Computer simulations to human disease: Emerging themes in protein folding. Cell 97:291–298, 1999. Copyright 1999, with permission from Elsevier Science.)

at the N-terminus. Many small proteins fold rapidly in the test tube, but many fail to fold when the polypeptide gets stuck in an incorrect conformation or forms aggregates before completing folding in the protein-rich (200 mg/mL) milieu of the cytoplasm. Mutant proteins are particularly susceptible to these pitfalls. Even newly synthesized native proteins need assistance to overcome local energy minima in intermediate folded states and to avoid irreversible denaturation, aggregation, or destruction by proteolysis.

Two classes of so-called molecular chaperones facilitate folding of newly synthesized and denatured proteins: HSP70s and their regulators; and cylindrical chaperonins. By binding exposed hydrophobic residues of non-native polypeptides, these molecular chaperones inhibit protein aggregation. They release polypeptides in a folding-competent state for attempts at folding. If folding fails, the cycle of binding and release can be repeated.

HSP70s

HSP70s, examples of heat shock proteins, bind a wide range of misfolded proteins and new polypeptide chains as they emerge from ribosomes. They are called heat shock proteins because cells subjected to

stresses, such as elevated temperature, increase the synthesis of these proteins within minutes for protection against denatured proteins. HSP70s are present in prokaryotes and most cellular compartments of eukaryotes. Budding yeasts have genes for 14 HSP70s; vertebrates have more. HSP60 in mitochondria and BiP protein in endoplasmic reticulum perform analogous functions (see Chapter 19).

HSP70s bind hydrophobic peptides of 8 to 13 residues exposed in a wide range of unfolded or incompletely folded polypeptides. Through cycles of peptide binding and release, HSP70s are thought to stabilize partially folded polypeptides and assist in their folding or refolding.

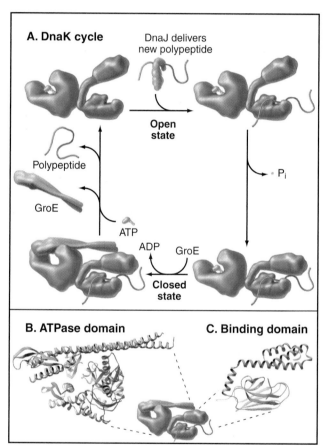

Figure 18-13 HSP70 structure and function. *A,* The HSP70 folding cycle is shown using bacterial DnaK as the example. *B* and *C,* Atomic structures of DnaK *(blue)* and GroE *(green).* An ATPase domain and a peptide-binding domain work together in a cyclical mechanism. DnaJ delivers an unfolded peptide to the ATP-bound open state of DnaK and also promotes ATP hydrolysis. The ADP-bound closed state of DnaK binds the peptide strongly. GroE promotes dissociation of ADP. Rebinding of ATP dissociates GroE and the peptide, which is free to attempt folding. Multiple HSP70 cycles are usually required to complete protein folding. (PDB files: 1DKX and 1DKG. References: Zhu X, Zhao X, Burkholder WF, et al: Structural analysis of substrate binding by the molecular chaperone Dnak. Science 272:1606–1614, 1996. Harrison CJ, Hayer-Hartl M, Hartl F, et al: Crystal structure of the nucleotide exchange factor GrpE bound to the ATPase domain of the molecular chaperone DnaK. Science 276: 431–435, 1997.)

ATP binding and hydrolysis control the affinity of HSP70s for unfolded polypeptides (Fig. 18–13). Bacterial HSP70 (called DnaK) is the prototypical member of the family. It has a peptide-binding domain at the N-terminus connected by a flexible hinge to an ATP-binding domain at the C-terminus. Adenosine diphosphate (ADP) binding favors association of DnaK with an unfolded polypeptide, whereas ATP binding favors release of the polypeptide. A cytosolic protein, DnaJ (HSP40), delivers unfolded proteins to DnaK and promotes their binding by stimulating hydrolysis of ATP bound to DnaK. Another protein, GroE, promotes exchange of ADP for ATP and release of the bound peptide.

A large number of proteins containing "J domains" similar to DnaJ facilitate mammalian HSP70 function, possibly by targeting specific substrates. Mammalian HSP70s have intrinsic nucleotide-exchange activity, so they do not require GroE.

Other HSP70 family members, such as HSP90, stabilize intermediate folding states of important signaling molecules, including steroid-hormone receptors (SHRs) (Fig. 18–14). These receptors bind steroids, including progesterone, glucocorticoids, estrogen, and androgen, in the cytosol and move to the nucleus where they regulate gene expression (see Chapter 14). SHRs first interact with HSP70 and its cofactors, but they are subsequently displaced by HSP90 complex and other folding factors that maintain SHRs in an "open" state, ready for binding hydrophobic steroids. Steroid binding completes the folding of SHR and displaces the HSP90 complex. Active SHR then moves into the nucleus.

Chaperonins

The **chaperonin** family of barrel-shaped particles promotes efficient protein folding (Fig. 18–15). They assist nascent and denatured polypeptides to fold or refold while sequestered in a cylindrical cavity protected from the complex environment of the cytoplasm. Although 85% of newly synthesized proteins fold spontaneously or with the assistance of HSP70s, the remainder require the more isolated folding environment provided by chaperonins. The mechanism of chaperonins is best understood for *E. coli* **GroEL** and its co-chaperonin **GroES.** These assist with folding of nascent polypeptides, which in bacteria occurs largely after translation is complete.

GroEL/GroES complex consists of a cylinder with a central cavity composed of GroEL and a cap structure made of GroES. GroEL forms two rings of seven identical subunits. Mitochondrial (HSP60/HSP10), chloroplast (Cpn60/Cpn10), and eukaryotic chaperonins (TriC) are similar in design, but more elaborate than GroEL/GroES, containing up to eight different gene products. This complexity undoubtedly represents ev-

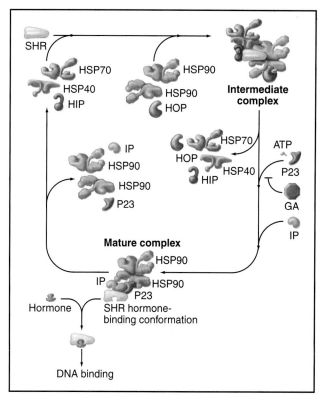

Figure 18-14 Stabilization of ligand-free steroid hormone receptors (SHRs) by HSP70, HSP90, and various accessory factors (HOP, HIP, P23, GA, and IP). Hormone binding releases the chaperones and allows SHR to move to the nucleus. (Reference: Buchner J: Hsp90 & Co.—a holding for folding. Trends Biochem Sci 24:136–142, 1999.)

olutionary diversification for regulation of chaperonin function.

ATP binding and hydrolysis set the tempo for folding cycles. Unfolded polypeptides bind to hydrophobic patches on the inner wall of the GroEL cylinder. Cooperative binding of ATP to each of the subunits in one of the two rings of seven changes their conformation (compare the upper and lower rings in Fig. 18–15*B*), expanding the internal volume by twofold and favoring binding of a heptameric ring of 10-kD GroES subunits. This closes the top of the cylinder and creates a folding cavity for proteins up to about 70 kD. After ATP hydrolysis on the ring surrounding the folding protein and ATP binding to opposite ring of seven GroES, the GroES cap releases and the cage opens. Folded polypeptides escape into the bulk solution, whereas incompletely folded intermediates can rebind GroEL for another attempt at folding.

In bacteria, mitochondria and chloroplast chaperonins related to GroEL/GroES are part of a chaperone "relay." Nascent polypeptides emerging from a ribosome after translocation into an organelle (see Figs. 19–2 and 19–5) first associate with HSP40 and HSP70, which preserve their folding competence and deliver them to the chaperonin complex for final folding. In

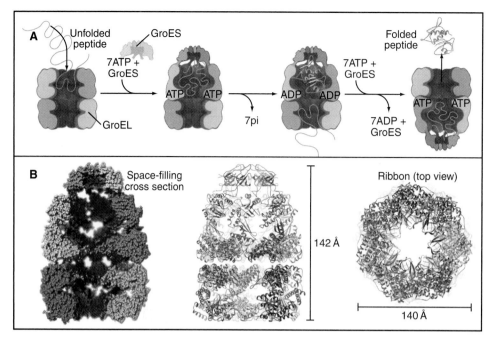

Figure 18-15 Chaperonin-mediated folding by GroEL and GroES. *A*, One folding cycle. *B*, Atomic structure of GroEL with a GroES cap bound to the upper, ATP-bound ring of seven subunits. Unfolded polypeptides bind the rim of an uncapped ring. Cooperative binding of ATP to each of the seven GroEL subunits in one ring changes their conformation, favors GroES binding, and doubles the volume of the central cavity, where the protein folds. Following ATP hydrolysis, binding of ATP and GroES to the lower ring structure dissociates the upper GroES and discharges the folded protein. (*B*, Reprinted with permission from Nature. From the work of Xu Z, Horwich AL, Sigler PB: The crystal structure of the asymmetric GroEL-GroES-(ADP)7 chaperonin complex. Nature 388:741–750, 1997. Copyright 1997, Macmillan Magazines Limited. PDB file: 1AON)

E. coli, it is estimated that up to 30% of total polypeptides utilize the chaperonin system.

Eukaryotic cells have much larger proteins than *E. coli,* many of which are constructed in modular units linked by flexible hinge regions (see Chapter 2). Here, folding is believed to occur largely cotranslationally, utilizing the HSP70/HSP40 system to build individual domains as they emerge from the ribosome. Indeed, the abundance of eukaryotic chaperonins, such as TriC, is low relative to that of GroEL/GroES in *E. coli.* However, the eukaryotic chaperonins may contribute to cotranslational folding by binding and refolding a nascent chain as it emerges from a ribosome, or they may participate in refolding of interacting modular domains. The shift in protein-folding mechanisms from a largely post-translational mechanism in bacteria to a cotranslational mode in eukaryotes reflects the emergence of large modular proteins necessary for the rapid diversification and specialization of eukaryotic cell function.

▌ **Selected Readings**

Clark BFC, Thirup S, Jkeldgaard M, et al: Structural information for explaining the molecular mechanism of protein biosynthesis. FEBS Lett 452:41–46, 1999.

Fedorov AN, Baldwin TO: Cotranslational protein folding. J Biol Chem 272:32715–32718, 1997.

Green R, Noller HF: Ribosomes and translation. Annu Rev Biochem 66:679–716, 1997.

Ibba M, Curnow AW, Soll D: Aminoacyl-tRNA synthesis: Divergent routes to a common goal. Trends Biochem Sci 22:39–42, 1997.

Kisselev LL, Buckingham RH: Translation termination comes of age. Trends Biochem Sci 25:561–566, 2000.

Landry SJ, Georgopoulos C: The ins and outs of a molecular chaperone machine. Trends Biochem Sci 23:138–142, 1998.

Netzer WJ, Hartl FU: Protein folding in the cytosol: Chaperonin-dependent and -independent mechanisms. Trends Biochem Sci 23:68–73, 1998.

Puglisi JD, Blanchard SC, Green R: Approaching translation at atomic resolution. Nature Struct Biol 7:855–861, 2000.

Radford SE, Dobson CM: Computer simulations to human disease: Emerging themes in protein folding. Cell 97:291–298, 1999.

Ramkrishnan V, White SW: Ribosomal structures: Insights into the architecture, machinery and evolution of the ribosome. Trends Biochem Sci 23:208–212, 1998.

Ruddon RW, Bedows E: Assisted protein folding. J Biol Chem 272:3125–3128, 1997.

Thomas PJ, Qu B-H, Pedersen PL: Defective protein folding as a basis of human disease. Trends Biochem Sci 20:456–459, 1995.

chapter 19

POST-TRANSLATIONAL TARGETING OF PROTEINS TO ORGANELLES

Protein synthesis is largely a monopoly of cytoplasmic ribosomes that provide all of the proteins for the nucleus, cytoplasm, peroxisomes, and secretory pathway. Even mitochondria and chloroplasts import most of their proteins from cytoplasm, despite the fact that they originated as Eubacterial endosymbionts and have retained the internal capacity to synthesize proteins. Most of the original Eubacterial genes moved to the nucleus of the eukaryotic host.

Given a common site of synthesis, accurate addressing is essential to direct proteins to their sites of action and to maintain the unique character of each cellular compartment. This is achieved by "zip codes" built into the structure of each protein. Residues in the sequence of each protein—often, but not necessarily, contiguous amino acids—form a signal for targeting.

Targeting signals are both necessary and sufficient to guide proteins to their final destinations. Transplantation of a targeting signal, such as a presequence from a mitochondrial protein, to a cytoplasmic protein reroutes the hybrid protein into the organelle specified by the targeting sequence, mitochondria in this example. Some targeting signals are transient parts of the protein. For example, most mitochondrial proteins are synthesized with N-terminal extensions that guide them to mitochondria and then are removed. Alternatively, signals may be a permanent part of the mature protein, in some cases serving repeatedly to target a mobile protein between different destinations. Permanent nuclear targeting signals can be located at the N-terminus, C-terminus, or even the middle of a protein. Some proteins have more than one targeting signal: a primary code that directs the protein to the target organelle or pathway, and a second signal that

steers the protein to its specific site of residence within the organelle or pathway.

Targeting signals direct proteins to their destination by binding to organelle-specific receptors or using soluble "escort" factors as intermediaries. Next, proteins cross membranes via channels formed by integral membrane proteins. Like ion channels (see Chapter 9), **protein-translocating channels** are gated to prevent indiscriminate transport of cellular constituents when not occupied by a polypeptide. During transit, the polypeptide fits so tightly in the channel that ions do not sneak through. Ions cross membranes via ion channels in a microsecond, whereas polypeptides take tens of seconds to move through translocation channels. Adenosine triphosphate (ATP) hydrolysis or the membrane potential provide the energy to power protein translocation across membranes.

Primary targeting occurs either cotranslationally, coincident with protein synthesis; or post-translationally, after polypeptide synthesis. Chapter 20 covers protein targeting to endoplasmic reticulum where, with a few exceptions, targeting is cotranslational. This chapter covers **post-translational targeting** mechanisms that move proteins across membrane bilayers into mitochondria, chloroplasts, and peroxisomes, and out of bacteria. Eukaryotes also secrete a few proteins directly across the plasma membrane, a nonclassical secretory route. Chapter 16 covers post-translational movements of proteins in and out of the nucleus through a large aqueous channel in the nuclear pore.

Transport of Proteins into Mitochondria

Mitochondrial outer and inner membranes define two spaces, one between the **outer** and **inner membranes (intermembranous space),** and an interior

---

Chapter by William E. Balch and TDP, based on an original draft by Ann L. Hubbard, J. David Castle, and Pat Shipman.

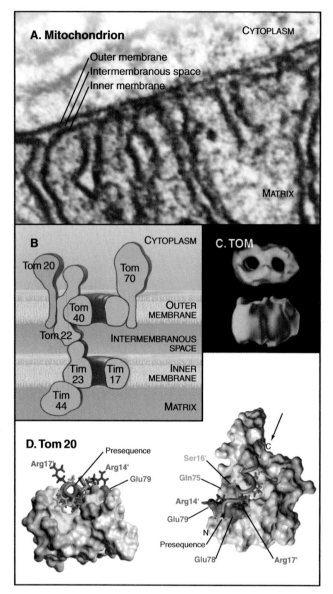

Figure 19–1 Mitochondrial import components. *A,* Electron micrograph of a thin section of a mitochondrion showing outer membrane, inner membrane, and matrix. *B,* Schematic drawing of the mitochondrial import apparatus, including TOM complex in the outer membrane and TIM complex in the inner membrane. *C,* Three-dimensional reconstruction from electron micrographs of TOM core complex, the translocase of the outer mitochondrial membrane. *D,* Atomic structure determined by nuclear magnetic resonance spectroscopy of a presequence peptide bound to a hydrophobic patch on Tom20, a receptor from the mitochondrial outer membrane. The space-filling model of a cytoplasmic domain of Tom20 shows negative *(red)* and positive *(blue)* surface potentials. The presequence forms to two turns of α-helix with two arginines exposed on the surface. N is the N-terminus and C is the C-terminus of the peptide. (*A,* Courtesy of Don W. Fawcett, Harvard Medical School. *C,* From Ahting U, et al: The TOM core complex: The general protein import pore of the outer membrane of mitochondria. J Cell Biol 147:959–968, 1999, by copyright permission of the Rockefeller University Press. *D,* Courtesy of Daisuke Kohda, Kyushu University. From Abe Y, et al: Structural basis of presequence recognition by the mitochondrial protein import receptor Tom20. Cell 100:551–560, 2000. Copyright 2000, with permission from Elsevier Science. PDB file: 1OM2.)

space termed the **matrix** (Fig. 19–1). Each membrane and space has distinct functions and protein compositions. Targeting signals and specific translocation machinery must guide several hundred imported proteins selectively to each compartment. In budding yeast, nuclear genes encode at least 100 proteins for the inner membrane; about 20 for the outer membrane; and about 200 for the intermembranous space and matrix.

Investigators have used yeast genetics and biochemistry to discover and characterize complexes of membrane proteins that allow proteins to enter mitochondria, including the **TOM complex (translocase of the outer mitochrondrial membrane)** and two **TIM complexes (translocase of the inner mitochondrial membrane)** (Figs. 19–2 and 19–3). Although the distinction is not absolute, one TIM is specialized for transport proteins into the matrix and the other is specialized for insertion of integral proteins into the inner membrane. Translocation requires energy and assistance from folding chaperones outside and inside mitochondria.

Step 1: Delivery of Protein to Mitochondria

After synthesis by cytoplasmic ribosomes, most proteins destined for mitochondria bind cytosolic heat shock proteins of the **Hsp70** family. This interaction maintains proteins in unfolded configurations competent for import. Some imported proteins require additional factors, such as mitochrondria-import stimulation factor (MSF) for targeting to the translocation machinery.

Mitochondrial targeting sequences are generally located at the N-termini of precursor polypeptides as contiguous sequences of 10 to 70 amino acids. These targeting motifs are called **presequences** because they are usually removed by proteolytic cleavage in the mitochondrial matrix. Presequences are rich in basic, hydroxylated, and hydrophobic amino acids but share no common sequences. Some mitochondrial targeting sequences are in the middle of polypeptides and are not cleaved after import. Cytochrome *c,* a component of the electron transport chain in the intermembranous space (see Fig. 10–16), has an internal signal for import into mitochondria. Some integral proteins of the inner membrane also have internal signals.

A succession of weak interactions with outer membrane receptors Tom20, Tom22, Tom5, and perhaps Tom70 guide presequences and other target signals to the outer membrane translocon. Initial contact is made between eight residues of the presequence folded into an amphipathic α-helix with a shallow hydrophobic surface groove on Tom20. Arginines on the exposed surface of this helix may then interact with

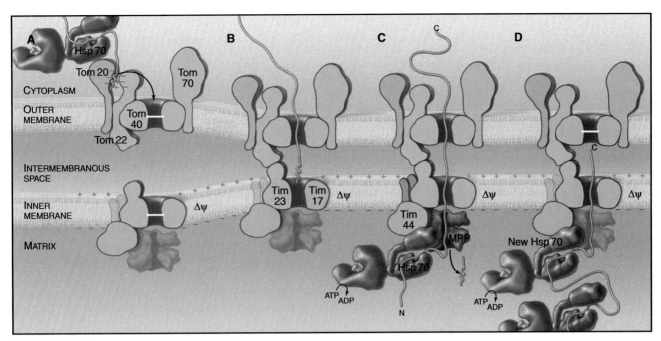

Figure 19-2 Import of matrix proteins into mitochondria. A white bar across a translocase pore indicates that it is closed. *A*, After synthesis on a cytoplasmic ribosome, the polypeptide binds to Hsp70 and the mitochondria targeting presequence associates with Tom20/22. *B*, The basic presequence leads the polypeptide through TOM across the intermembrane space to TIM. *C*, The potential across the inner membrane ($\Delta\Psi$) pulls the presequence through TIM into the matrix, where it is cleaved by the matrix protease MPP. The polypeptide binds matrix Hsp70. *D*, Cycles of Hsp70 binding to the peptide followed by ATP hydrolysis and dissociation of Hsp70 from Tim44 "ratchet" the translocating peptide into the matrix where it folds.

acidic residues on Tom22 (see Fig. 19–1*D*). Other parts of the presequence are thought to interact with Tom40, the translocon itself. Although these associations are weak (K_ds in the micromolar range), collectively, they distinguish mitochondrial presequences from other proteins in the cytoplasm with high fidelity.

Step 2: Translocation Across the Outer Membrane

Outer membrane receptors transfer the polypeptide to the translocon channel composed mainly of Tom40. This integral membrane protein is predicted to span

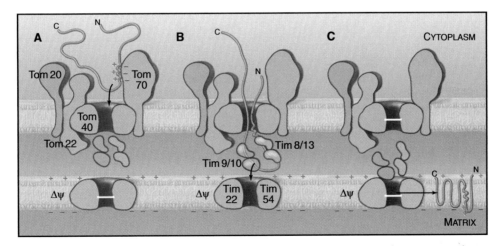

Figure 19-3 Import of the ADP/ATP antiporter ACC and insertion into the inner membrane bilayer. A white bar across a translocase pore indicates that it is closed. *A*, An internal targeting sequence binds the ACC polypeptide to Tom70, which directs it into the TOM channel. *B*, In the intermembranous space, Tim9/10 and Tim8/13 capture the polypeptide and direct it to the TIM22/54 translocon that is used for import of matrix proteins. *C*, TIM22/54, in conjunction with the inner membrane potential ($\Delta\Psi$), promotes insertion of the six transmembrane helices into the inner membrane bilayer.

the bilayer exclusively as β-strands. Electron microscopy has revealed that purified TOM complex has two prominent pores with diameters of approximately 2.0 nm, which is in agreement with the size of the pore as calculated from ion conductance measurements of purified Tom40 inserted into lipid bilayers. Proteins must be largely unfolded to fit through a pore of this size. Like protein-import channels of endoplasmic reticulum (see Chapter 20), TOM channels are likely to be gated, so they close when not occupied by a translocating polypeptide.

Some outer membrane proteins transfer laterally into the bilayer while they are in transit through TOM, whereas porins, among other proteins, enter the intermembranous space, fold, and then insert into the membrane. Some proteins remain in the intermembranous space. Proteins that move on from the intermembranous space use one of two more or less dedicated translocons: either TIM23 for translocation into the matrix, or TIM22 for insertion into the inner membrane.

Step 3A: Translocation Across the Inner Membrane to the Matrix

Proteins destined for the matrix translocate across the inner membrane through a channel formed by the integral membrane proteins Tim23 and Tim17 (see Fig. 19–2). N-terminal presequences of matrix proteins first interact electrostatically with Tom22 and Tim23 in the inner membrane space. These receptors guide the presequence into the translocation channel. Physical interaction of TOM and TIM complexes at junctional regions between the outer and inner membranes may facilitate transfer of matrix proteins across both membranes. The MPP peptidase cleaves off the presequences once they enter the matrix.

Two energy sources—the electrical potential across the inner membrane and ATP hydrolysis by matrix chaperones—drive polypeptides across the inner membrane. The membrane potential (negative inside) pulls positively charged presequences across the membrane. ATP hydrolysis drives cycles of interaction of mitochondrial Hsp70 with translocating polypeptides. One model is that Hsp70 is a molecular "ratchet" that rectifies movements of the polypeptide in the pore, allowing movement forward into the matrix but not backward, so that it eventually ends up as a folded protein in the matrix. Tim44 recruits the ATP-bound Hsp70 to TIM23 channels with an emerging polypeptide. Hsp70 binds the translocating polypeptide, hydrolyzes its bound ATP, and dissociates from Tim44. This allows the polypeptide to slide forward into the matrix, but not backward. If the polypeptide slides forward, another Hsp70 can bind. When Hsp70 dissociates from the polypeptide, the exchange factor mGrp1 rapidly recharges it with ATP, ready for another cycle of binding and release.

Step 3B: Translocation into the Inner Membrane Bilayer

The numerous integral proteins of the inner membrane lack cleaved targeting signals, depending instead on information contained in the intact protein. One example is the most abundant protein of the inner membrane, the adenosine diphosphate (ADP)/ATP antiporter that spans the inner membrane six times (see Fig. 10–15). Its signal sequence is located in the middle of the polypeptide, rather than at the N-terminus like matrix proteins.

When these proteins emerge from TOM into the intermembranous space, they interact with a family of zinc finger proteins called Tim8, Tim9, Tim10, Tim12, and Tim13 (see Fig. 19–3). These "tiny Tims" are required for insertion of proteins into the inner membrane. Complexes of Tim9/10 or Tim8/13 bind polypeptides and deliver them to the inner membrane translocon, perhaps serving as chaperones for these hydrophobic polypeptides to cross the intermembranous space.

The TIM22 translocon used by many inner membrane proteins is a 300-kD complex composed of Tim22 (a homologue of Tom23 and Tom17), Tim54, and Tim18, all different from the TIM23 complex used by most translocating matrix proteins. Insertion of transmembrane segments into the bilayer depends on membrane potential. Inner membrane proteins synthesized in the matrix depend on a protein called Oxa1p, which may be part or all of a third inner membrane translocon similar to bacterial YidC (see later section).

Mitochrondrial Dysfunction and Disease

As expected from the central role of mitochondria in energy metabolism, mitochrondrial dysfunction contributes to a remarkable diversity of human disease (Fig. 19–4), including seizures, strokes, optic atrophy, neuropathy, myopathy, cardiomyopathy, hearing loss, diabetes mellitus, and common age-related disorders, such as Parkinson's and, potentially, Alzheimer's disease. These clinical manifestations arise from mutations in genes for mitochondrial proteins encoded by both mitochondrial DNA (mtDNA) and nuclear DNA. Severe defects in the oxidative electron transport or import pathways are not generally found, presumably because they are lethal. However, a mutation in Tim8 causes a type of deafness. Mild missense mutations compromise selected aspects of mitochondrial function and cause disease. Mitochondria also play a central role in triggering programmed cell death (see Chapter 49).

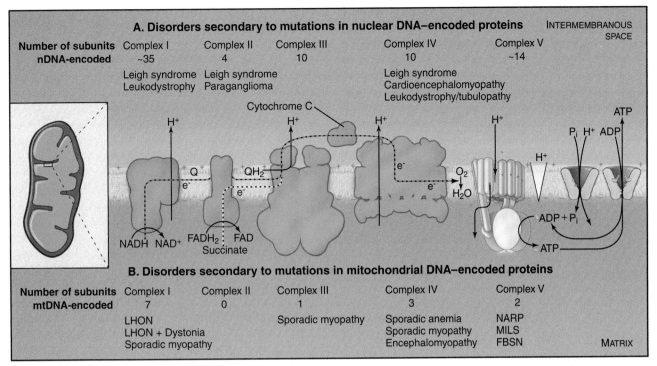

A. Disorders secondary to mutations in nuclear DNA–encoded proteins

Number of subunits nDNA-encoded	Complex I ~35	Complex II 4	Complex III 10	Complex IV 10	Complex V ~14
	Leigh syndrome Leukodystrophy	Leigh syndrome Paraganglioma		Leigh syndrome Cardioencephalomyopathy Leukodystrophy/tubulopathy	

B. Disorders secondary to mutations in mitochondrial DNA–encoded proteins

Number of subunits mtDNA-encoded	Complex I 7	Complex II 0	Complex III 1	Complex IV 3	Complex V 2
	LHON LHON + Dystonia Sporadic myopathy		Sporadic myopathy	Sporadic anemia Sporadic myopathy Encephalomyopathy	NARP MILS FBSN

Figure 19-4 Mutations in both mitochondrial and nuclear genes for mitochondrial proteins cause a variety of diseases by compromising the function of particular mitochondrial subsystems. (See Chapter 10 for details on these components.) LHON, Leber hereditary optic neuropathy; NARP, neurogenic muscle weakness, ataxia, retinitis pigmentosa; MILS, maternally inherited Leigh syndrome; FBSN, familial bilateral striatal necrosis. (Adapted from Schon EA: Mitochondrial genetics and disease. Trends Biochem Sci 25:555–560, 2000.)

Transport of Proteins into Chloroplasts

Nuclear genes encode most chloroplast proteins, which are synthesized on cytoplasmic ribosomes and imported into one of six chloroplast compartments (Figs. 10–17 and 19–5). Although chloroplasts arose from symbiotic Eubacteria like mitochondria, and although both organelles transferred most of their genes to the host cell nucleus, chloroplasts evolved a mechanism of protein import completely distinct from mitochondria. The principles are similar, but the two systems share no common protein subunits. The closest known relatives of any protein component of the chloroplast import machine are found in the ancestors of chloroplasts, photosynthetic cyanobacteria, where they appear to have a role in secretion.

N-terminal signal sequences called **"transit sequences"** target chloroplast proteins to the import machinery in the outer envelope. When added experimentally to the N-terminus of a test protein, transit sequences suffice to guide the test protein into the stroma of chloroplasts. These N-terminal targeting sequences are reminiscent of sequences that target proteins to endoplasmic reticulum and mitochondria, but the sequence determinants of the chloroplast transit sequences are much less well defined. They vary in length from 20 to 120 residues, and the amino acid

sequences have little in common beyond a net positive charge and numerous serines and threonines.

All imported proteins use the same "general import pathway" to cross the inner and outer envelope membranes. The machinery consists of distinct protein complexes in each membrane called **TOC (translocon at the outer envelope membrane of chloroplasts)** and **TIC (translocon at the inner envelope membrane of chloroplasts)** (see Fig. 19–5). These complexes have been identified in biochemical experiments with precursor proteins synthesized in vitro and imported into isolated chloroplasts. Chemical cross-linking of these imported proteins to translocon proteins has allowed identification of subunits that bind the transit sequence and contact imported polypeptides as they cross both membranes. Other subunits account for the requirements for ATP and GTP hydrolysis. Both TOC and a "super complex" of TOC with TIC can be isolated for analysis of their composition. Mutations compromising chloroplast import have only recently started to contribute to an understanding of the process.

The journey of a protein from its site of synthesis in cytoplasm into the stroma is understood in broad outline. Transit sequences target chloroplast preproteins to the outer membrane, where initial interactions do not require the input of energy. Glycolipids in the outer membrane appear to work together with the

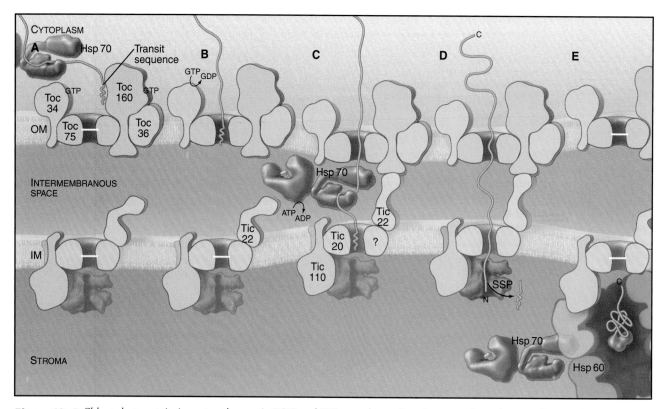

Figure 19–5 Chloroplast protein import pathway via TOC and TIC complexes. Proteins move from the cytoplasm to various chloroplast compartments in five stages. *A,* Energy-independent binding of the transit sequence to outer membrane lipids and proteins, especially Toc160. *B,* Insertion of the transit sequence through the outer membrane pore composed of Toc75 is dependent on GTP hydrolysis by Toc34 and, perhaps, Toc160. *C,* ATP-dependent formation of a translocation intermediate engaged with the TIC complex. *D,* ATP-dependent translocation across the inner membrane through a pore composed in part of Tic20, followed by removal of the N-terminal transit sequence by a stromal protease SPP. *E,* Hsp60 and Hsp70 promote folding of stromal proteins, while other proteins are rerouted to other compartments. (Modified from Chen X, Schnell D: Protein import into chloroplasts. Trends Cell Biol 9:222–227, 1999. Copyright 1999, with permission from Elsevier Science; May T, Soll J: Chloroplast precursor protein translocon. FEBS Lett 452:52–56, 2000.)

Toc160 and Toc75 subunits in binding transit sequences. Then, a step dependent on GTP hydrolysis delivers the transit sequence through a channel in the outer membrane to the inner membrane space. GTP hydrolysis by Toc34 (and, possibly, Toc160) may open the translocation pore or promote binding of TOC to TIC to form a continuous pore across both membranes for translocation into the stroma. The existence of small gene families encoding proteins related to Toc34 and Toc160 suggests that variations of the general import pathway might exist to accommodate the import of distinct classes of chloroplast preproteins. Toc75 is an important part of this protein channel. The pore seems smaller than those in the translocons in endoplasmic reticulum and mitochondria, so it is believed that polypeptides are generally unfolded during transit. But some evidence suggests that small, folded, protein domains can fit through the pore. The composition and properties of the pore across the inner membrane are less well understood, but Tic20 is part of the pore. A signal peptidase cleaves off the transit peptide when it emerges from TIC into the stroma.

ATP hydrolysis in both the intermembranous space and stroma provides energy for translocation of peptides. The subunits catalyzing ATP hydrolysis are thought to be chaperones. Hsp70 chaperones are found in the cytoplasm, intermembranous space, and stroma. An Hsp100 chaperone is associated with the stromal side of TIC. These chaperones are thought to use ATP hydrolysis to promote translocation of the imported protein, as in mitochondria. An **Hsp60 chaperone** similar to GroEL assists with folding in the stroma.

Proteins destined for chloroplast membranes, the inner membrane space, or thylakoid lumen are thought to move through the general import pathway to the stroma and then redistribute to their proper locations. At least four pathways homologous to prokaryotic export pathways (see later section) lead to thylakoid membranes and the thylakoid lumen. One employs a translocon homologous to bacterial SecYE and eukaryotic Sec61p. Like the bacterial export systems, some thylakoid lumen proteins use ATP hydrolysis by a homologue of SecA to power translocation through SecYE. Some lumen proteins with tightly bound redox factors use translocation factors homologous with bacterial Tat proteins to cross the thylakoid membrane while compactly folded. Thylakoid membrane proteins can either insert directly from the stroma or use proteins homologous to those of the signal recognition particle (see Chapter 20) to assist with insertion, perhaps also involving SecYE.

Transport of Proteins into Peroxisomes

Like mitochondria, peroxisomes oxidize lipids and other metabolites although their organization is considerably less elaborate. A single limiting membrane surrounds a matrix containing **oxidative enzymes** (Fig. 19–6). Unlike mitochondria and chloroplasts, peroxisomes lack nucleic acids, and there is no evidence that they arose from an ancient endosymbiont. All peroxisomal proteins are encoded by nuclear genes and translated on cytosolic polyribosomes. Following their synthesis, both soluble peroxisomal enzymes and integral peroxisomal membrane proteins are transported directly from the cytoplasm to the peroxisome.

Two types of targeting signals direct proteins to the peroxisome lumen, or matrix. The type-1 **peroxisomal targeting signal,** or PTS1, is found at the extreme C-terminus of virtually all peroxisomal enzymes. PTS1 is just three amino acids long and it conforms to the consensus sequence of serine-lysine-leucine-COOH, or a conservative variant. For example, alanine or cysteine can substitute at the −3 position, arginine or histidine can function at the penultimate position, and methionine can substitute for the C-terminal leucine. PTS1 has an absolute requirement for the extreme C-terminus, and amidation of the C-terminal carboxylate inactivates the signal. The type-2 peroxisomal targeting signal (PTS2) also targets proteins to the peroxisome matrix, but is found on few proteins (i.e., only four are known in humans, one in yeast). PTS2 is located at or near the N-terminus and has a loose consensus sequence of RLX_5H/QL. Integral peroxisomal membrane proteins lack motifs similar to PTS1 or PTS2 and utilize distinct targeting signals that are as yet poorly understood.

The products of 20 or so *PEX* genes, **peroxins,** recognize newly synthesized peroxisomal proteins, deliver them to peroxisomes, and either translocate them across the membrane or insert them into the peroxisomal membrane (Table 19–1). All of the peroxins have been identified by genetic approaches; their biochemical functions are still under investigation.

Defects in peroxisomal biogenesis cause a spectrum of lethal human diseases known as the **peroxisomal biogenesis disorders**. These diseases include Zellweger syndrome, neonatal adrenoleukodystrophy, infantile Refsum's disease, and rhizomelic chondrodys-

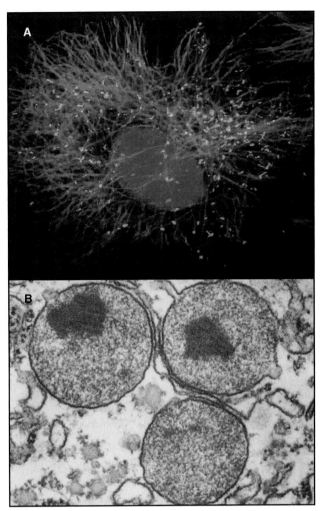

Figure 19-6 Morphology of peroxisomes. *A,* Fluorescence micrographs of a CV1 cell expressing green fluorescent protein fused to PTS1, which labels peroxisomes green. Microtubules are stained red with labeled antibodies and nuclear DNA is stained blue with propidium iodide. *B,* Electron micrograph of a thin section of a tissue culture cell showing three peroxisomes. Peroxisomes have a single bilayer membrane and a dense matrix, including a crystal (in some species) of the enzyme urate oxidase. (*A,* Courtesy of S. Subramani, University of California, San Diego. Reference: Wiemer AC, et al: Visualization of the peroxisomal compartment in living mammalian cells. J Cell Biol: 136:71–80, 1997. *B,* Courtesy of Don W. Fawcett, Harvard Medical School.)

plasia punctata. They are moderately rare, occurring in approximately 1 in 50,000 live births. Most patients with peroxisomal biogenesis disorders display no defect in peroxisome membrane synthesis or import of peroxisomal membrane proteins, but they do have mild-to-severe defects in matrix protein import. However, in rare cases, patients lack peroxisome membranes altogether. Studies of both yeast *pex* mutants and cell lines from patients with peroxisomal biogenesis disorders have provided current models of peroxisome biogenesis.

The best characterized peroxin is PEX5, the import

table 19–1

PEROXIN FEATURES AND KNOWN ROLES*

Peroxin	Features	Functions	Relation to Disease
PEX1	AAA ATPase	Matrix protein import	Mutated in CG1
PEX2	Zinc-binding PMP	Matrix protein import	Mutated in CG10
PEX3	*Orphan PMP*	*Membrane biogenesis*	*Mutated in CG12*
PEX4	UBC	Matrix protein import	?
PEX5	PTS1 receptor	Matrix protein import	Mutated in CG2
PEX6	AAA ATPase	Matrix protein import	Mutated in CG4
PEX7	PTS2 receptor	Matrix protein import	Mutated in CG11
PEX8	PMP	Matrix protein import	?
PEX9	PMP	Matrix protein import	?
PEX10	Zinc-binding PMP	Matrix protein import	Mutated in CG7
PEX11	*PMP*	*Peroxisome division*	?
PEX12	Zinc-binding PMP	Matrix protein import	Mutated in CG3
PEX13	SH3 PMP	Matrix protein import	Mutated in CG13
PEX14	Docking PEX5/7	Matrix protein import	?
PEX15	Orphan PMP	Matrix protein import	?
PEX16	*Orphan PMP*	*Membrane biogenesis*	*Mutated in CG9*
PEX17	Orphan PMP	Matrix protein import	?
PEX18	PEX7 binding	Matrix protein import	?
PEX19	*PMP receptor*	*Membrane biogenesis*	*Mutated in CG14*
PEX20	Thiolase binding	Matrix protein import	?
PEX21	PEX7 binding	Matrix protein import	?
PEX22	PEX4 binding	Matrix protein import	?
PEX23	PMP	Matrix protein import	?

*PEX5 and PEX7 *(underlined)* are import receptors for newly synthesized peroxisomal enzymes. Most other peroxins are also required for matrix enzyme import. Peroxins PEX3, PEX11, PEX16, and PEX19 *(italicized)* are implicated in peroxisome membrane biogenesis rather than matrix protein import. AAA, AAA family of ATPases; CG, complementation group of patients with peroxisomal biogenesis disorders; orphans are novel proteins; PMP, peroxisomal membrane protein; SH3, src-homology-3 domain; UBC, ubiquitin-conjugating enzyme.

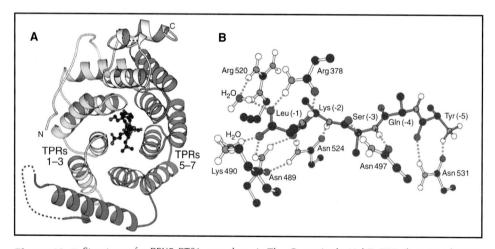

Figure 19–7 Structure of a PEX5-PTS1 complex. *A,* The C-terminal, 40-kD TPR domain of PEX5, shown as a ribbon diagram, surrounds the PTS1 peptide, shown as a stick figure. TPRs 1 to 3 are shown as yellow ribbons, TPRs 5 to 7 are shown as blue ribbons. An α-helical span *(green ribbon)* links the two triplet TPRs at the bottom of this structure; the C-terminal extension *(white ribbons)* also connects the two triplet TPRs. *B,* Detailed view of PEX5-PTS1 interactions between the PTS1 backbone *(red bonds)* and PEX5 side chains *(white bonds)*; the putative hydrogen bonds are shown as dashed green lines. (Courtesy of S.J. Gould, Johns Hopkins Medical School; from Gott GJ, et al: Peroxisomal targeting signal-1 recognition by the TPR domains of human PEX5. Nature Struct Biol 7:1091–1095, 2000. PDB file: 1FCH.)

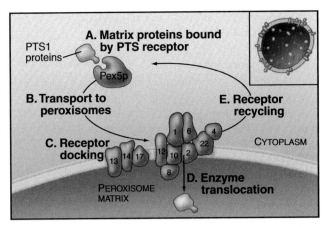

Figure 19-8 *A* to *E,* Model for PTS1 protein import. Matrix enzymes are synthesized by cytoplasmic ribosomes, recognized by the PEX5-PTS1 receptor, and transported to the docking complex on the peroxisome membrane. Interaction with the PEX2/PEX12/PEX10 complex dissociates the ligand from PEX5 and translocates it into the matrix. The PTS1 receptor is recycled. PEX1/PEX6 and PEX4/PEX22 complexes play an important role in PEX5 function before, during, or after matrix protein translocation. (Adapted from a drawing by S.J. Gould, Johns Hopkins Medical School.)

receptor for PTS1-containing enzymes. PEX5 binds PTS1 via its C-terminal tetratricopeptide repeat (TPR) domain. The structure of PEX5 bound to a PTS1 peptide has revealed the chemical basis of PEX5-PTS1 binding, as well as the previously observed sequence constraints of the PTS1 (Fig. 19–7). One class of patients with peroxisomal biogenesis disorder has mutations in *PEX5,* and several such patients have mutations of residues critical for binding PTS1. PEX5 divides its time between the cytoplasm and peroxisome as it delivers newly synthesized peroxisomal enzymes from the cytoplasm to the peroxisome (Fig. 19–8). A similar mode of action is proposed for PEX7, the import receptor for PTS2 proteins. In fact, in higher eukaryotes, PEX5 and PEX7 form a complex and may function as a single, oligomeric import receptor for all peroxisomal matrix proteins.

Both PTS receptors interact with PEX14, a peroxisomal membrane protein that functions as a docking site for receptor-enzyme complexes. However, what happens next in matrix protein import is unclear. The peroxisome membrane contains at least four peroxins, required for translocation, that act downstream of PEX14: PEX12, PEX10, PEX2, and PEX8. These peroxins display a complex set of interactions with one another and with both PEX5 and PEX7, suggesting that the translocation machinery may function like a trapdoor mechanism, with membrane-anchored peroxins forming a pore into which PEX5-enzyme and PEX7-enzyme complexes are inserted. A hypothetical ligand-receptor dissociation factor may then mediate the release of enzymes from their receptors, followed by receptor recycling back to the cytoplasm to initiate another round of import. Many other factors are also

known to be required for matrix protein import; elucidating the mechanism of import will require additional studies of all peroxins.

Import of peroxisomal membrane proteins is less well characterized than matrix protein import. As noted earlier, targeting signals for membrane proteins are ill defined. However, it is known that they are unrelated to PTS1 or PTS2 because membrane protein import occurs normally in cells lacking PEX5 or PEX7. In fact, membrane protein import and peroxisome membrane synthesis occur normally in all *pex* mutants except for those cells that lack PEX3, PEX16, or PEX19. Cells deficient in any of these three peroxins lack detectable peroxisome membranes. The fate of peroxisomal membrane proteins in these cells varies, with most being rapidly degraded and some being mislocalized to other cellular membranes, particularly mitochondria. PEX19 appears to function as an import receptor, or chaperone, for newly synthesized membrane proteins. PEX3 and PEX16 are also postulated to participate in membrane protein import, but these peroxins may participate in some other aspect of peroxisome membrane synthesis.

The mysteries surrounding peroxisomal membrane protein import raise the much debated question of how cells make peroxisome membranes (Fig. 19–9). Until recently, it was thought that peroxisomes arise by the growth and division of preexisting peroxisomes. The discovery of mutant cells lacking peroxisome membranes did not directly challenge this model, but the identification of the mutated gene allowed the experimental synthesis of peroxisomes in the cells lacking preexisting peroxisomes. Specifically, investigators expressed a normal copy of the mutated gene in cells lacking PEX3, PEX16, or PEX19 and observed the restoration of functional peroxisomes. These and other results indicate that peroxisomes may arise by either of two pathways: growth and division of preexisting peroxisomes and de novo synthesis from a yet-to-be-identified preperoxisomal vesicle.

Translocation of Eukaryotic Proteins Across the Plasma Membrane by ABC Transporters

Most proteins secreted by eukaryotic cells travel to the cell surface through the classical secretory pathway, including the endoplasmic reticulum and Golgi apparatus (see Chapters 20 to 22). But, analysis of secretion of a-type mating factor by budding yeast has revealed a novel secretory pathway that targets proteins synthesized in cytoplasm directly to the plasma membrane; a-factor is excised proteolytically from a precursor, prenylated on its C-terminus, and transported across the plasma membrane by an **ABC superfamily transporter** (see Chapter 7). This mechanism has been invoked to explain the secretion of a few mammalian

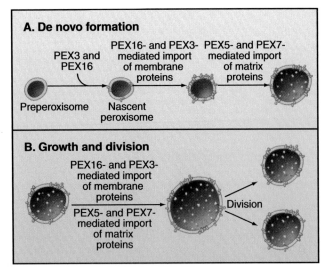

Figure 19-9 Two-pathway model for peroxisome biogenesis. A, Peroxisome synthesis de novo. A "preperoxisomal" vesicle is committed to become a peroxisome by the incorporation of PEX3, PEX16, or both. The presence of PEX3 and/or PEX16 recruits PEX19 and newly synthesized peroxisomal membrane proteins to the preperoxisomal vesicle. The resulting nascent peroxisome acquires the capacity for matrix protein import and becomes a mature peroxisome capable of propagation by the growth and division pathway. B, Growth and division of preexisting peroxisomes. Growth is accomplished by PEX5- and PEX7-mediated uptake of peroxisomal matrix proteins and PEX19-mediated uptake of peroxisomal membrane proteins. Division is catalyzed by PEX11 proteins. (Adapted from a drawing by S.J. Gould, Johns Hopkins Medical School.)

proteins that lack the "signals" required to direct them to the classical secretory pathway. These include some cytokines, fibroblast growth factor, and some blood clotting factors. This is a well-characterized route for secretion of some bacterial proteins.

Targeting to the Cytoplasmic Surface of the Plasma Membrane

Although the mechanisms just described focus on post-translational targeting by translocation across membrane bilayers, a number of proteins are targeted to the cytoplasmic side of the membrane bilayer after being synthesized (see Fig. 6-9). These include many peripheral membrane proteins that bind to cytoplasmic domains of integral membrane proteins or directly to the lipid bilayer. Many proteins are tethered to the bilayer by a covalently attached lipid added as a post-translational modification following synthesis on free cytoplasmic ribosomes.

Lipid modifications on tethered proteins include long-chain, saturated fatty acids and isoprenoids. The saturated fatty acids are either myristate (14 carbons), which is added through amide linkage to amino-terminal glycine residues, or palmitate (16 carbons), which is usually added through thioether linkage to cysteine residues found toward the C-terminus. The isopren-

oids farnesyl (15 carbons) and geranylgeranyl (20 carbons) are added through thioether linkages to cysteine residues located at or near the C-terminus in specific structural motifs. Attachment of a lipid helps to stabilize membrane association, but does not guarantee permanent anchoring to the membrane. Some proteins, such as the catalytic subunit of cyclic AMP–dependent protein kinase, are fatty acylated but mostly soluble in cytoplasm. Other structural signals leading to specific protein interactions are critical in targeting both Src and Ras.

Bacterial Protein Export

Bacteria employ no less than 10 distinct strategies to transport proteins from the cytoplasm across the inner membrane and beyond. Seven of these use a common inner membrane translocon composed of the SecY protein. This section begins with a discussion of six branches of the SecY general secretory pathway and finishes with three novel pathways. This discussion highlights many of the proteins secreted by bacteria that contribute to human disease.

Pathways Dependent on the SecYE Translocon

All the branches of life use translocons to move proteins synthesized in the cytoplasm across membranes: **SecY** in prokaryotes and **Sec61p** in the endoplasmic reticulum of eukaryotic cells (see Chapter 20). Eubacterial SecY spans the membrane 10 times and forms a stable dimer with **SecE,** a protein with a single transmembrane span. These subunits are structural and functional homologues of two Sec61p subunits. Three SecYE dimers assemble a ring-shaped structure with a central pore in the inner membrane, similar to Sec61p (see Fig. 20–3). Deleterious mutations of SecY or SecE compromise translocation of most secreted proteins. Accessory subunits SecG, SecD, SecF, and YajC assist in translocation but are not essential or present in eukaryotes.

Sec B Pathway to the Inner Membrane Translocon

Proteins using the SecB/SecYE pathway are synthesized in the cytoplasm with an N-terminal signal sequence, which is cleaved after translocation across the inner membrane. This is the most abundant class of proteins translocated across the inner membrane, including proteins destined for secretion, the inner membrane, and, in the case of gram-negative bacteria, the periplasm or outer membrane. Even *Bacillus subtilis* (a gram-positive bacterium lacking an outer membrane) has about 300 of these secreted proteins. **Signal sequences** of about 25 residues begin with methionine, followed by a few basic residues, 10 to 15 hydrophobic residues, and a site susceptible to proteolytic cleavage by a signal peptidase. Lipoprotein signal sequences have fewer hydrophobic residues and an invariant cysteine at the cleavage site.

At the time of synthesis, proteins destined for translocation by SecYE bind to **SecB,** a homotetrameric cytoplasmic chaperone that prevents folding and maintains a state competent for translocation (Fig. 19–10). Unlike most other chaperones, SecB does not require ATP hydrolysis for cycles of interaction with substrates. Hsp70 homologues (DnaK) have a secondary role in chaperoning precursors for translocation by SecYE.

On the way to the inner membrane, Sec B, along with its cargo protein, first associates with SecA, a protein that targets the signal sequence to the SecYE translocon. **SecA** is required for translocation of all Eubacterial membrane and secreted proteins with cleavable N-terminal signal sequences but is not present in genomes of Archaea or eukaryotes, despite the fact that they use translocons homologous to SecYE. SecA cycles between cytoplasm, where it regulates its own synthesis by binding its messenger RNA (mRNA), and the inner membrane, where it associates with lipids and SecYE. SecA may also help assemble rings of SecYE subunits.

A system reconstituted from four purified proteins (SecB, SecA, SecY, and SecE), lipids, and ATP can translocate precursor proteins. SecG increases the ac-tivity of reconstituted systems, but its role in vivo is ambiguous. The actual translocation step requires ATP hydrolysis by SecA and is proposed to involve some unprecedented molecular gymnastics. Upon binding ATP, SecA somehow inserts into the inner membrane in association with SecYE. ATP hydrolysis results in SecA retraction from the membrane. One theory is that repeated cycles of ATP binding, insertion, hydrolysis, and deinsertion ratchet the polypeptide across the translocon into the periplasm. The proton gradient across the membrane suffices as the energy source for translocation of the last half of peptides and may also increase the rate of SecA cycle by promoting deinsertion. SecY also "proofreads" the signal sequence associated with SecA, releasing those with defects prior to translocation.

Signal peptidases cleave signal peptides soon after they emerge into periplasm. One of these signal peptidases is very similar to eukaryotic homologues, being anchored to the membrane by two N-terminal transmembrane helices. Several other bacterial signal peptidases have single transmembrane anchors. The signal peptidase dedicated to lipoprotein precursors has four transmembrane segments. It cleaves lipoproteins just before the invariant cysteine. This cysteine is then conjugated to diacylglycerol, which anchors the protein to membranes: the outer surface of the plasma membrane or the outer membrane of gram-negative

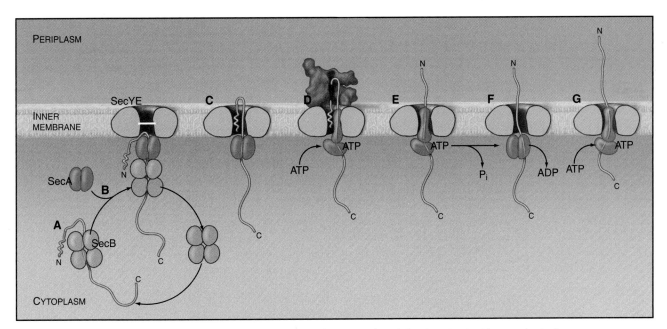

Figure 19–10 Translocation across the bacterial inner membrane mediated by SecYE. *A,* After synthesis by a cytoplasmic ribosome, the polypeptide associates with the SecB chaperone. *B,* SecA binds the presequence and docks on the SecYE translocon. *C,* The presequence inserts into the translocon. *D,* ATP-binding promotes insertion of SecA and the associated polypeptide into the translocon, followed by cleavage of the signal sequence. *E,* The membrane potential drives the polypeptide further across the membrane. *F,* ATP hydrolysis allows retraction of SecA from the translocon. *G,* The SecA cycle is repeated to further translocation. (Modified from Danese PN, Silhavy TJ: Targeting and assembly of periplasmic and outer-membrane proteins in *E. coli.* Annu Rev Genet 32:59–94, 1999, with permission, from the *Annual Review of Genetics,* Vol. 32, © 1998 by Annual Reviews www. AnnualReviews.org.)

bacteria. Signal peptide peptidases rapidly degrade cleaved signal peptides.

Signal Recognition Particle–Cotranslational Pathway to the Inner Membrane Translocon

The **signal recognition particle** (SRP) targets some integral membrane proteins and exported proteins lacking a cleaved signal sequence to the SecYE translocon. In bacteria, this is an alternative to the more common SecB/SecA route to SecYE. In eukaryotes, SRP is on the major pathway for export of proteins into endoplasmic reticulum (see Chapter 20 for a more detailed description of SRP and cotranslational translocation).

Bacterial SRP consists of a small 4.5S RNA called ffs and a protein called Ffh (for "fifty-four homologue," after its eukaryotic counterpart). SRP binds noncleaved signal-anchor sequences as they emerge from the ribosome. This stops translation until SRP docks on the inner membrane with its receptor FtsY and SecYE. Continued translation of the polypeptide drives translocation through the SecYE translocon.

Proteins destined for the inner membrane depend on another protein, YidC, to move laterally out of the SecYE translocon into the lipid bilayer. A subset of inner membrane integral proteins does not require SecYE for insertion. YidC alone suffices for them to incorporate into the bilayer. Homologues of YidC direct proteins into the inner membrane of mitochondria and thylakoid membranes of chloroplasts.

Insertion of Proteins in the Outer Membrane

Outer membrane proteins probably pass through the periplasm before inserting into the outer membrane, although some researchers have theorized that physical connections between inner and outer membranes promote the transfer of outer membrane polypeptides. No specific targeting signals are known for outer membrane proteins, so their localization likely depends on tertiary structure.

Outer membrane porins assemble as follows: the signal sequence is cleaved from unfolded outer membrane precursors as they emerge from the translocon; individual subunits fold on their own or with the assistance of periplasmic chaperones and then associate to form dimers and trimers before, or possibly after, insertion into the outer membrane. Periplasm is an oxidizing environment with a gel-like consistency. Several periplasmic assembly factors participate in protein folding, including enzymes that catalyze the isomerization of proline peptide bonds and oxidation/reduction of cysteine thiol groups.

Outer Membrane Autotransporter Pathway

Some proteins, including secreted proteolytic enzymes and toxins, as well as membrane-anchored adhesins and invasins, hitch a ride to the cell surface on their own outer membrane transporters (Fig. 19–11A). These proteins are fused to a C-terminal "β-domain" thought to be similar to a porin (see Fig. 6–8). The protein uses the SecYE general secretory pathway and inserts into the outer membrane. The N-terminal functional domain then translocates across the outer membrane through its β-domain pore. An outer membrane protease releases toxins and proteases, whereas adhesins that follow this route remain on the surface attached to the β-domain.

Outer Membrane Single Accessory Pathway

Some hemolysins and hemagglutinins move to the periplasm through the SecYE general secretory pathway and then use a single accessory protein to translocate across the outer membrane. The accessory protein is thought to form an outer membrane pore like the β-domain of autotransporters, but there is no sequence homology except with chloroplast outer membrane porins that transport peptides.

Chaperone/Usher Pathway

Gram-negative bacteria use a novel mechanism, downstream of the SecYE general secretory pathway, to transport and assemble pili on their outer surface. These appendages are involved with bacterial pathogenesis, including urinary tract infections. A periplasmic chaperone binds the peptide and promotes folding. The pilus subunit is folded similar to an immunoglobulin (Ig) domain (see Fig. 2–15), but lacking the seventh β-strand. This exposes core hydrophobic residues. The chaperone consists of two immunoglobulin-like domains, one of which donates a strand to complete the immunoglobulin domain of the pilus subunit. The chaperone delivers a pilus subunit to an outer membrane translocon called usher. There, it transfers its bound subunit to the end of a growing chain of pilus subunits, all bound together, head to tail, by strands that complete the seven-strand β-sheet of the adjacent subunit. This growing chain of pilus subunits passes single file through a 2- to 3-nm pore in usher. On the outer surface, the pilus subunits rearrange into a helical pilus. This assembly reaction is thought to provide the energy for translocation. The chaperone prevents premature assembly of the pilus.

Type II Secretion

Bacteria use an alternate route downstream of the general secretory pathway to secrete other toxins and enzymes with cleaved signal sequences. At least a dozen protein subunits participate in this complicated pathway. The pore in the outer membrane is composed of a "secretin," a protein with relatives that also participate in type III secretion, phage biogenesis, and formation of one type of pilus. The secretin pore is a ring of 12 to 14 subunits around a large but gated channel that is 5 to 10 nm in diameter. The mechanism of translocation is not yet well understood.

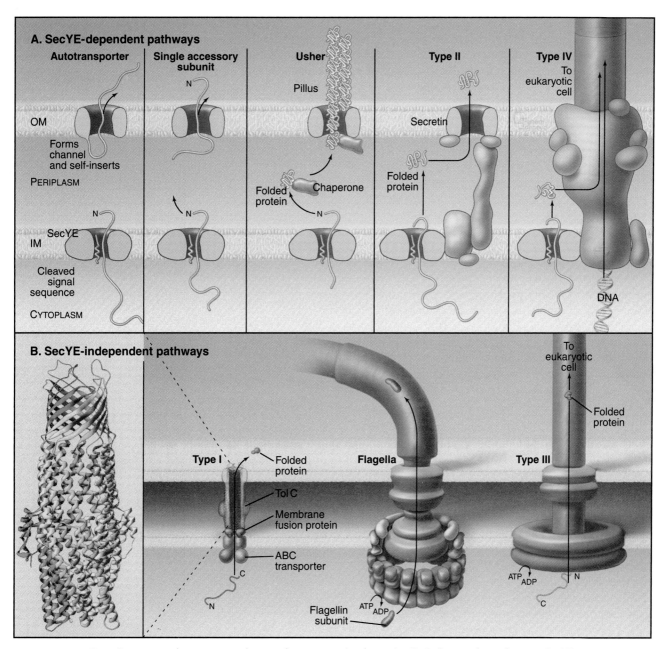

Figure 19-11 Secretion across the outer membrane of gram-negative bacteria. *A,* Pathways dependent on SecYE. The cleaved signal sequence is shown in blue. The β-domain of autotransporters forms a pore for the translocation of part of its own chain, which may remain attached, as shown, or be cleaved for escape from the cell. Single accessory proteins form a pore for secretion of separate proteins. Usher forms a pore for the translocation and assembly of pili. Type II secretion uses a secretin pore for translocation. Type IV secretion employs a large translocon similar to that used by *Agrobacteria* for secretion of DNA. *B,* Pathways independent of SecYE. Type I secretion uses an ABC transporter to cross the inner membrane and additional subunits to cross the periplasm and outer membrane. The inset shows a ribbon model of TolC, one type of translocon that spans the periplasm and outer membrane. Bacterial flagella transport flagellin subunits across both membranes and then through the central channel of the flagellar filaments for incorporation at the growing tip. Type III secretion uses some components similar to the basal body of flagella, as indicated by the colors. IM, inner membrane; OM, outer membrane. (*B,* Reprinted with permission from Nature. Based on Koronakis V, et al: Crystal structure of the bacterial membrane protein TolC central to multidrug efflux and protein export. Nature 405:914–919, 2000. Copyright 2000, Macmillan Magazines Limited. PDB file: 1EK9. *A* and *B,* Drawings based on Thanassi DG, Hultgren SJ: Multiple pathways allow protein secretion across the bacterial outer membrane. Curr Opin Cell Biol 12:420–430, 2000.)

Type IV Secretion

Bacteria secrete a few proteins (such as pertussis toxin by *Borditella pertussis* and a toxin by *Helicobacter pylori*) using an apparatus similar to that used for DNA transfer between two bacteria during conjugation and for DNA injection into plant cells by *Agrobacterium*. DNA is transferred directly from the cytoplasm of the bacterium to the cytoplasm of the other bacterium or plant cell. Secretion of pertussis toxin by this route starts with the general secretory pathway, including a cleaved signal sequence and translocation across the inner membrane by SecYE. Proteins secreted by *Agrobacteria* lack signal sequences.

Pathways Independent of the SecYE Translocon

Type I ABC Transporters

Bacteria use ABC transporters (see Chapter 7) to secrete a small number of toxins (i.e., *Escherichia coli* hemolysin), proteases, and lipases (three in *B. subtilis*). C-terminal signal sequences of 30 to 60 residues target these proteins to the ABC transporter, the only component required for secretion by gram-positive bacteria. Gram-negative bacteria require not only a transporter in the inner membrane, but also two proteins that form a continuous channel across the periplasm and outer membrane (see Fig. 19–11B). A "membrane fusion protein" links the transporter to an outer membrane pore. One example is TolC, a trimeric protein that forms an extraordinary tubular channel across the periplasm and outer membrane. Each TolC subunit contributes four β-strands to a porin-like structure that spans the outer membrane. α-Helical continuations of these β-strands form a tube having an internal diameter of 3.5 nm for transport of proteins across the periplasm. ATP hydrolysis by the ABC transporter provides energy for translocation. TolC conduits engage those ABC transporters with substrates for export and then disengage when translocation is complete. Genes for secreted proteins are generally in the same operon as the export machinery.

Flagellar and Type III Secretion

This pathway uses the same strategy (and some homologous components) as the system that assembles bacterial flagella. The flagellar basal body transports flagellin subunits through a central pore that crosses both membranes (see Fig. 19–11B) and extends the length of the flagellar shaft to the tip where subunits add to the distal end (see Chapter 4). This flagellar pathway transports a few other proteins, including a phospholipase that contributes to the virulence of *Yersinia*, the cause of the black plague.

The type III secretion apparatus allows pathogenic bacteria, such as *Yersinia,* to secrete toxins into the medium or directly into host cells where they disrupt cellular physiology, including formation of pores in target cell membranes. Neither cleaved signal sequences nor SecYE participate. Several signals direct proteins to this pathway. Remarkably, one signal is sequence information in the mRNA for some transported proteins! The other is a protein sequence that binds a chaperone dedicated to targeting toxins to the type III pathway. About 20 different protein subunits form a large translocation apparatus that spans both membranes and the periplasm. The basal body–like structure consists of subunits homologous to flagellar basal bodies, including a cytoplasmic adenosine triphosphatase (ATPase) that provides energy for transport. A secretin forms a pore in the outer membrane, and a rod-shaped projection allows injection of toxins directly into target animal or plant cells.

Double Arginine Pathway

Bacteria direct redox proteins with flavin, FeS, or other cofactors to the periplasm using components first discovered in chloroplasts, where they import similar proteins into the thylakoid lumen. The N-terminal signal peptide for this pathway has a pair of arginines (RR) and an adjacent, large, hydrophobic residue, such as leucine. Translocation of these proteins in *E. coli* requires five Tat proteins homologous to the chloroplast proteins. Gram-positive bacteria have more than a dozen proteins with RR signal peptides as well as genes homologous to the Tat genes. In contrast to the SecYE translocon, even folded proteins appear to pass through the Tat translocon.

■ Selected Readings

Chen X, Schnell DJ: Protein import into chloroplasts. Trends Cell Biol 9:222–227, 1999.

Danese PN, Silhavy TJ: Targeting and assembly of periplasmic and outer-membrane proteins in *E. coli.* Annu Rev Genet 32:59–94, 1999.

Herrmann JM, Neupert W: Protein transport into mitochondria. Curr Opin Microbiol 3:210–214, 2000.

Keegstra K, Cline K: Protein import and routing systems of chloroplasts. Plant Cell 11:557–570, 1999.

Keegstra K, Froehlich JE: Protein import into chloroplasts. Curr Opin Cell Biol 2:471–476, 1999.

Neupert W: Protein import into mitochondria. Annu Rev Biochem 66:863–917, 1997.

Pfanner N: Protein sorting: Recognizing mitochondrial presequences. Curr Biol 10:R412–415, 2000.

Ryan MT, Wagner R, Pfanner N: The transport machinery for the import of preproteins across the outer mitochondrial membrane. Int J Biochem Cell Biol 32:13–21, 2000.

Sacksteder KA, Gould SJ: The genetics of peroxisome biogenesis. Annu Rev Genet 34:623–652, 1999.

Thanassi DG, Hultgren SJ: Multiple pathways allow protein secretion across the bacterial outer membrane. Curr Opin Cell Biol 12:420–430, 2000.

Voos W, Martin H, Krimmer T, Pfanner N: Mechanisms of protein translocation into mitochondria. Biochim Biophys Acta 1422:235–254, 1999.

chapter 20

BIOSYNTHETIC PROCESSES IN THE ENDOPLASMIC RETICULUM AND GOLGI APPARATUS

Cytoplasmic ribosomes synthesize most cellular proteins, which may remain in the cytoplasm or be targeted to particular organelles by signals built into the protein structure. The **endoplasmic reticulum (ER)** is the first stop for all proteins destined for incorporation into the ER itself, the golgi apparatus, later **secretory pathway** organelles, or the plasma membrane or for secretion from the cell. In mammals, most of these proteins are imported into the ER during their synthesis, but in yeast, many enter the ER after translation is complete. Within the ER, chaperones similar to those in cytoplasm and mitochondria assist in folding imported proteins.

From the ER, each protein follows a complex itinerary for delivery to its final destination along the secretory pathway. The first step in this **exocytic pathway** is recruitment of folded proteins into vesicles that bud from the ER, after which these vesicles and their cargo are delivered to the Golgi apparatus. The Golgi apparatus consists of a stack of membrane-bound compartments containing enzymes that can extensively modify a protein. Although morphologically and functionally distinct, the ER and Golgi apparatus are intimately linked to one another through continuous forward and reverse movement of vesicles containing protein and lipid. This pathway is present in all nucleated cells and is highly amplified in cells specialized for secretion, such as pancreas and liver cells.

This chapter describes (1) the mechanisms used to transport proteins into the ER and the modifications made to these proteins by enzymes in the ER and Golgi compartments and (2) the synthesis of lipids by ER. Chapter 21 covers the mechanism of vesicle-mediated transport through the exocytic pathway.

Chapter by William E. Balch and TDP, based on an original draft by Ann L. Hubbard, J. David Castle, and Pat Shipman.

Endoplasmic Reticulum

During the 1950s and 1960s, light and electron microscopy revealed that the ER was a system of membrane-lined channels present in the cytoplasm of all eukaryotic cells (Fig. 20–1). The individual elements of the ER include tubules or flat saccules called **cisternae** (cisterna meaning reservoir) that form a three-dimensional network (a reticulum) stretching from the nuclear envelope to the cell surface. Microtubules and their associated motors generate this extended network by pulling ER membranes out toward the periphery of the cell and then tethering them in place (see Fig. 40–7).

The ER is specialized into three distinctive regions. The **rough ER** is studded with ribosomes on its cytoplasmic surface, defining regions specialized for protein synthesis and folding. Other regions, called **transitional elements,** contain sites where vesicles bud during the export of cargo to the Golgi apparatus (see Chapter 21). The **smooth ER,** composed of other tubular elements lacking ribosomes, is dedicated to enzyme pathways involved in drug metabolism (hepatocytes), steroid synthesis (endocrine cells), or calcium storage (see Chapter 28).

The abundance of ER depends on the specialized functions of particular cells. Cells dedicated to the production, storage, and regulated secretion of proteins are rich in rough ER. One historically important example of an extensive ER labyrinth is the exocrine cell of the pancreas, which produces digestive enzymes for the gut. Experiments on this type of cell first clarified the pathway for synthesis and export of secreted proteins. In such specialized secretory cells, the amount of ER greatly exceeds the surface area of the plasma membrane. For example, in hepatocytes, which are liver cells specialized to secrete serum proteins, the ER

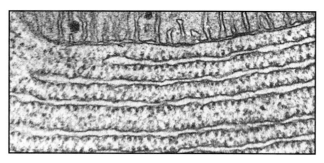

Figure 20–1 Electron micrograph of a thin section of the rough ER and neighboring mitochondrion from pancreas. (A micrograph by Keith R. Porter; courtesy of Don W. Fawcett, Harvard Medical School.)

surface area exceeds the area of plasma membrane by a factor of 30. Similarly, smooth ER is abundant in endocrine cells synthesizing steroid hormones and muscle cells owing to their requirement to store and release Ca^{2+} to control contraction (see Chapter 42).

Translocation into the Endoplasmic Reticulum

Translocation across or insertion into the bilayer of the ER membrane is required for a variety of lipids, proteins, and oligosaccharides that are synthesized on the cytoplasmic side of the membrane. Integral membrane proteins facilitate all of these reactions. Proteins "flip" phospholipids from the cytoplasmic to the luminal (internal) side of the lipid bilayer. Protein-lined channels allow growing polypeptide chains to thread across or insert into the bilayer. Proteins facilitate the transfer of hydrophilic oligosaccharides attached to large lipid carriers across the bilayer.

The orientation of a protein in the bilayer or distribution of a protein to the lumen is established during transfer to the ER and is maintained throughout transit through the exocytic pathway. Thus, domains of transmembrane proteins to be exposed on the cell surface must be inserted into the ER membrane facing the lumen. Similarly, secreted soluble proteins must be translocated into the lumen of the ER. Remarkably, translocation can also run the other way; defective proteins are translocated out of the ER to the cytoplasm for degradation by proteasomes (see Chapter 24).

Coupling of Synthesis to Translocation into the Endoplasmic Reticulum: The Signal Hypothesis

Early studies suggested that proteins are translocated into the ER lumen so rapidly that translocation might occur as the protein is being synthesized. Biochemical assays revealed that proteins known to be delivered to the ER are synthesized as precursors, with extra amino acids at their N-termini that are later removed. These observations formed the basis of what has been called the **signal hypothesis:** (1) an N-terminal extension called the leader or **signal sequence** targets a protein to the ER; (2) an aqueous channel in the ER membrane opens for **translocation** of the protein across the hydrophobic bilayer; and (3) the leader sequence is removed after transfer to the lumen. This hypothesis has been found to be remarkably accurate.

Signal sequences involved in targeting proteins to the ER vary in sequence but are generally 15 to 25 amino acids long. All have an N-terminal region of about 5 residues with 1 or 2 basic amino acids, followed by 10 to 15 uncharged, hydrophobic residues. If fully extended, these sequences would be 8 nm long, exceeding the thickness of the lipid bilayer. These sequences are necessary and sufficient for targeting a protein to the ER, but not to other organelles, such as mitochondria or peroxisomes, which require their own unique targeting signals (see Chapter 19). The addition of an N-terminal ER signal sequence directs most test proteins to the ER.

Cotranslational Translocation into the Endoplasmic Reticulum

Directing a ribosome making a protein with signal sequence to the ER membrane (Fig. 20–2) requires a cytosolic protein–RNA complex, termed the **signal recognition particle (SRP)** (Fig. 20–3). As a signal sequence emerges from a ribosome, the SRP binds both the signal sequence and the ribosome. Interaction of the SRP with the ribosome arrests elongation of the growing polypeptide until the ribosome is positioned over a translocation pore in the ER membrane. The elongated SRP complex may interfere directly with elongation factor or transfer RNA (tRNA) binding to the ribosome (see Chapter 18). SRP also targets the stalled ribosome to a receptor on the ER membrane, which, in turn, transfers the ribosome to a channel called the **translocon** for translocation across the membrane (see Fig. 20–2). Dissociation of the SRP and **SRP receptor** from the ribosome allows protein synthesis to resume, extruding the growing polypeptide into the ER lumen through an aqueous channel in the translocation channel.

Eukaryotic SRP consists of 6 polypeptides and an RNA molecule of 300 nucleotides (see Fig. 20–3). The bacterial homologue is simpler, with but a single protein subunit. The hydrophobic signal sequence binds to a groove, rich in exposed methionines, on the SRP54 protein subunit or the bacterial homologue, Ffh (*fifty-four homologue*). The flexible side chains of me-

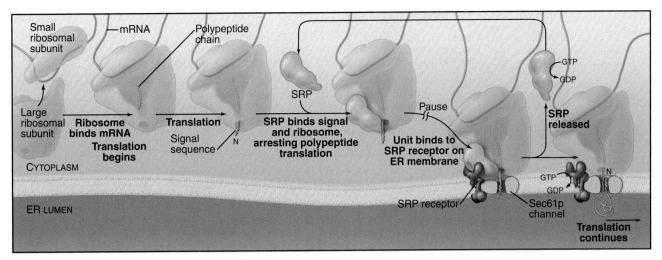

Figure 20–2 Cotranslational translocation pathway from ribosome to ER lumen. Signal recognition particle (SRP) and SRP receptor use a cycle of recruitment and hydrolysis of GTP to control delivery of the ribosome-mRNA complex to the ER translocon. SRP binds a signal sequence emerging from a ribosome and arrests polypeptide translation. SRP also directs the ribosome to the SRP receptor on the ER membrane, where the ribosome docks on the translocon and continues translation. GDP, guanosine diphosphate.

thionine, like bristles of a brush, accommodate the variable shapes of the hydrophobic amino side chains found in different signal sequences. Positive residues at the N-terminus of the signal sequence interact with backbone phosphates of SRP RNA. Signal sequence

binding promotes guanosine triphosphate (GTP) binding to another domain of SRP54/Ffh. The structure of this domain is similar to the Ras family of guanosine triphosphatases (GTPases; see Chapter 27).

The SRP-ribosome complex binds to the ER

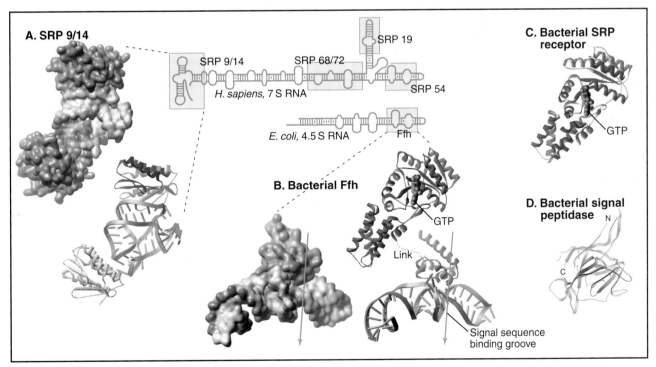

Figure 20–3 Atomic structures of cotranslocation hardware. *A* and *B*, Comparison of bacterial and human signal recognition particles. The diagram shows the base-pairing of human 7S SRP RNA and bacterial 4.5S SRP RNA, with blue boxes indicating protein-binding sites. Atomic structures of elements of the RNA and associated proteins are shown as space-filling and ribbon diagrams. Ffh GTP-binding and N-domains (PDB files: 3NG1; 2NG1), Ffh M-domain bound to RNA (PDB file: 1DUL), RNA (PDB file: 1E9S), SRP9/14 bound to RNA (PDB file: 1E80). *C*, Bacterial SRP receptor subunit FtsY (PDB file: 1fts). *D*, Bacterial signal peptidase (PDB file: 1B12).

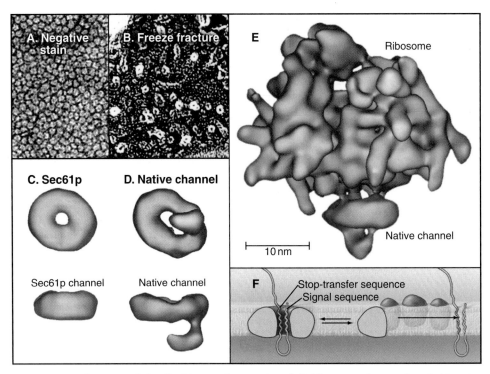

Figure 20-4 Structure of the Sec61p translocon. *A* and *B*, Electron micrographs. *A*, Negative stain of isolated translocons. *B*, Freeze-fracture micrograph of translocons reconstituted in a lipid bilayer. *C* to *E*, Three-dimensional reconstructions from electron micrographs. *C*, Purified, recombinant Sec61 channel. *D*, Native channel isolated from the ER. *E*, A ribosome bound to the Sec61p translocon. *F*, Model for insertion of a polypeptide into the Sec61p translocon and its transfer to the lipid bilayer. This drawing illustrates the hypothesis that the translocon subunits disassemble, at least in part, to allow the polypeptide to enter the bilayer. Alternatively, a gap opens between the subunits. (*A* to *E*, Courtesy of Chris Akey, Boston University. Reference: Menetret J-M, et al: The structure of ribosome-channel complexes engaged in protein translocation. Mol Cell 6:1219–1232, 2000. Copyright 2000, with permission from Elsevier Science.)

through the **SRP receptor** (also called the docking protein), a dimer composed of two different subunits that are associated exclusively with the rough ER in mammalian cells. The bacterial homologue FtsY (see Fig. 20–3*C*) is a component of the inner membrane. The α-subunit of the SRP receptor recognizes SRP54—not the signal sequence—and transfers the ribosome to the translocon. Binding of a signal sequence to the translocon helps to stabilize the interaction. GTP binding to both SRP and SRP receptor is required for these docking reactions (see Fig. 20–2). Interaction of SRP and SRP receptor promotes GTP hydrolysis by both partners and their dissociation from the ribosome. Both SRP and SRP receptor are recycled for further rounds of ribosome docking. This is essential because the number of translocons greatly exceeds the number of SRP receptors. After SRP dissociation, the ribosome resumes polypeptide chain elongation, and translocation across the membrane begins.

Proteins cross the ER membrane through a tightly fitting protein channel called a translocon (Fig. 20–4). Biochemical and genetic approaches have identified the protein components of this translocation pore:

three or four copies of the **Sec61p complex.** This complex is a heterotrimer consisting of Sec61p, an integral protein with 10 transmembrane sequences, and smaller α- and γ-subunits, each with single transmembrane sequences. The homologous bacterial proteins are called SecY, SecE, and SecG. They assemble a similar pore to translocate proteins across the plasma membrane of bacteria (see Chapter 19). During cotranslational import, three or four slender struts anchor the ribosome to the translocon (see Fig. 20–4*E*). The peptide exit site of the ribosome is centered over the pore, but a 1-nm gap exists between them. It is postulated that this gap allows a growing polypeptide to extend laterally between the ribosome and membrane if translocation is blocked. An additional mass associated with the luminal side of native translocons (see Fig. 20–4*D*) is either translocon associated protein (TRAP) or the enzyme oligosaccharyl transferase (see later section). When translocation of the peptide is complete, the ribosome dissociates from the translocon and its pore closes.

Binding of a ribosome and signal sequence to a translocon opens a pore across the membrane estimated to be 4–6 nm in diameter by biophysical criteria, but only 2 nm in reconstructions (see Fig. 20–4C and D). Nevertheless, the pore maintains a tight seal around the translocating peptide, preventing small molecules from entering or leaving the ER lumen. Current evidence suggests that the signal sequence forms a loop in the channel with its N-terminal exposed to the cytoplasm (see Fig. 20–4F).

As the elongating polypeptide chain emerges into the ER lumen, it binds **BiP**, a chaperone related to HSP70 (see Chapter 18). Translation alone is believed to be sufficient to push the polypeptide chain through the translocon, but cycles of **BiP** binding, followed by adenosine triphosphate (ATP) hydrolysis and dissociation, may help to bias the movement of the polypeptide into the lumen but not back out. The **oligosaccharyl transferase** associated with the translocon adds core sugars to the growing chain when an asparagine in an appropriate sequence passes by.

When a peptide grows to about 150 residues, a **signal peptidase** associated with the translocon cleaves off the signal sequence. The ER signal peptidase consists of five subunits ranging from 12 kD to 25 kD. Archaea and a few gram-positive Eubacteria have a similar enzyme complex. Most Eubacteria and eukaryotic organelles (see Figs. 19–2, 19–5, and 19–10) use a structurally unrelated signal peptidase consisting of a single subunit anchored to the membrane to carry out the same cleavage reaction.

Post-Translational Translocation into the Endoplasmic Reticulum

Although fungi have all of the components for cotranslational translocation into the ER, many of their proteins containing typical signal sequences bypass the SRP and enter the ER after their synthesis is complete. This post-translational mode of import relies on cytosolic folding chaperones to maintain the polypeptide in an unfolded state in the cytosol before translocation through the same channel used for cotranslational insertion. The Sec61p translocon recruits a tetrameric Sec62/63 complex to form a receptor-translocation machine that recognizes proteins with appropriate signals for translocation. This strategy is similar to the use of receptors by the TOM complex to import proteins into mitochondria (see Chapter 19). Post-translational translocation into the ER utilizes BiP to promote ratcheting and folding of the protein in the ER lumen.

Targeting of Soluble Secreted Proteins to the Endoplasmic Reticulum

Secreted proteins use the Sec61p translocon to enter the ER lumen (Fig. 20–5A). Signal peptidase cleaves the translocating polypeptide from its signal sequence,

which initially anchors it to the membrane. After signal peptide cleavage, translation continues to push the new N-terminus of the growing polypeptide into the ER lumen. The fate of the cleaved signal peptide is unknown. None has ever been found, so degradation must be very efficient.

Insertion of Integral Proteins into the Endoplasmic Reticulum Membrane

Integration of transmembrane segments into the lipid bilayer is much less well understood than translocation into the ER lumen, so the drawings in Figure 20–5B to E must be considered to be models rather than well-documented mechanisms. In the simplest case (Fig. 20–5B), the C-terminus of a transmembrane protein resides in the cytoplasm upon completion of synthesis (referred to as "type 1" transmembrane protein). Early events involving delivery to the ER using a signal peptide are identical to those in a secreted protein. However, insertion of the hydrophobic transmembrane sequence into the translocon is thought to freeze movement of the growing chain. This hydrophobic stretch functions as a "stop-transfer" signal. Stop-transfer signals are hard to predict from their sequences, and their receptor in the channel is not identified. In contrast to signal sequences, stop-transfer signals are not cleaved. Instead, such transmembrane sequences move laterally out of the channel into the lipid bilayer, anchoring the polypeptide in the membrane. This exit from the translocon is a poorly understood, multistep process involving interaction of the transmembrane sequence with both lipids and translocon proteins. Completion of translation results in a protein with its N-terminus in the lumen and its C-terminus in the cytoplasm. Transmembrane proteins with the opposite orientation (type 2) form if the signal sequence is not cleaved (see Fig. 20–5C). Polytopic proteins that span the membrane multiple times (such as ion channels and carriers) utilize multiple stop-transfer signals (see Fig. 20–5D and E). SRP is probably required to target the first signal sequence to the ER membrane. Thereafter, the dynamics of the channel must accommodate sequences that alternately specify translocation of cytoplasmic loops and then transfer of transmembrane segments to the lipid bilayer.

■ Protein Folding and Oligomerization in the Endoplasmic Reticulum

Together, the tunnel through the large ribosomal subunit and the translocon channel in the ER bilayer shel-

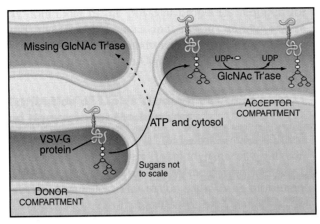

Figure 21–1 Test tube reconstitution of transport from the ER to the Golgi apparatus. Donor ER containing the glycoprotein VSV-G is prepared from mutant cells lacking a golgi glycosylation enzyme. When incubated with an acceptor Golgi stack prepared from normal cells in the presence of cytosol and ATP, vesicles containing VSV-G move from the donor ER to the acceptor Golgi compartment. There, they can be modified by addition of sugar residues by glycosylation enzymes residing in the normal Golgi apparatus. Transfer to the Golgi is measured by following the incorporation of these sugar residues. GlcNAc Tr'ase, N-acetylglycosyl transferase; UDP, uridine diphosphate.

the lysosome and cell surface (see Chapter 22), and those that direct cargo back into the cell through the endocytic pathway (see Chapters 22 and 23).

Vesicle Formation from the Endoplasmic Reticulum

Analysis of Vesicular Transport

Genetic studies in yeast, as well as biochemical methods that include the use of cell-free assays, have contributed to the current understanding of membrane traffic. Cell-free assays detect transfer of cargo between membrane compartments prepared from cell homogenates by taking advantage of the biochemical properties of individual organelles. For example, transport of glycoproteins from the ER (donor compartment) to the Golgi apparatus (acceptor compartment) can be measured by following the processing of their N-linked oligosaccharides, post-translational modifications found only in Golgi compartments (see Chapter 20) (Fig. 21–1).

General Features of Vesicular Traffic

Cargo selection, vesicular budding, and vesicular fusion with the acceptor compartment all occur without leakage of content from the donor or target compartment. Thus, membrane integrity is maintained at all steps of transport. Furthermore, the orientation (called topology) of lipid and protein in the membrane bilayers, established during synthesis in the ER, is main-

tained by vesicular carriers during transport. Thus, one side of the membrane always faces the cytoplasm. The other side starts as the lumen of the ER; remains inside each vesicular compartment; and, in the case of cell surface components, eventually is exposed on the outside of the cell.

Step 1. Cargo Selection Through Sorting Motifs

Every vesicle that buds from a particular membrane compartment incorporates only proteins destined for transport and excludes resident proteins that define the composition of the compartment. Thus, the molecular machinery that generates vesicles must recognize **recruitment signals,** usually a short peptide sequence, on transported cargo proteins. The need to control precisely the composition of intracellular organelles and the plasma membrane makes it unlikely that nonselective mechanisms contribute significantly to vesicular traffic.

Although **sorting motifs** that direct protein trafficking through the endocytic pathway are understood in some detail (see Chapter 23), an understanding of those directing exit from the ER is just beginning to emerge. Analysis of the transport of the vesicular stomatitis virus glycoprotein (VSV-G) has revealed one type of export motif. VSV-G forms a coat on the outside of the viral membrane envelope. It is a type I transmembrane protein with a large domain initially in the lumen of the ER and eventually on the surface of the virus. VSV-G has a short cytoplasmic tail with a key tyrosine (Y) and a **diacidic motif,** aspartic acid-x-glutamic acid (DXE), where x can be any amino acid

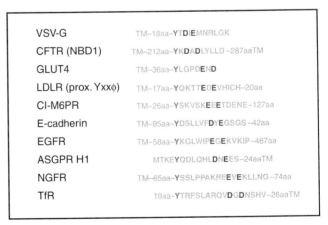

VSV-G	TM–18aa–**Y**TD**I**E**M**NRLGK
CFTR (NBD1)	TM–212aa–**Y**K**D**A**D**LYLLD –287aaTM
GLUT4	TM–36aa–**Y**LG**P**D**E**ND
LDLR (prox. Yxxφ)	TM–17aa–**Y**QKTT**E**D**E**VHICH–20aa
CI-M6PR	TM–26aa–**Y**SKVSK**E**E**E**TDENE–127aa
E-cadherin	TM–95aa–**Y**DSLLVF**D**Y**E**GSGS–42aa
EGFR	TM–58aa–**Y**KGLWIP**E**G**E**KVKIP–467aa
ASGPR H1	MTKE**Y**QDLQHL**D**N**E**ES–24aaTM
NGFR	TM–65aa–**Y**SSLPPAKRE**E**V**E**KLLNG–74aa
TfR	19aa–**Y**TRFSLARQV**D**G**D**NSHV–26aaTM

Figure 21–2 Examples of transmembrane proteins with tyrosine-linked diacidic ER exit codes (acidic-x-acidic) that direct their incorporation into COPII vesicles. ASGPRH1, asialoglycoprotein receptor; CFTR, cystic fibrosis transmembrane regulator; C1-M6PR, mannose 6-phosphate receptor; EGFR, epidermal growth factor receptor; GLUT4, a glucose carrier; LDLR, low density lipoprotein receptor; NGFR, nerve growth factor receptor; TfR, transferrin receptor; vsv-G, vesicular stomatitis virus glycoprotein.

mated to be 4–6 nm in diameter by biophysical criteria, but only 2 nm in reconstructions (see Fig. 20–4C and D). Nevertheless, the pore maintains a tight seal around the translocating peptide, preventing small molecules from entering or leaving the ER lumen. Current evidence suggests that the signal sequence forms a loop in the channel with its N-terminal exposed to the cytoplasm (see Fig. 20–4F).

As the elongating polypeptide chain emerges into the ER lumen, it binds **BiP,** a chaperone related to HSP70 (see Chapter 18). Translation alone is believed to be sufficient to push the polypeptide chain through the translocon, but cycles of **BiP** binding, followed by adenosine triphosphate (ATP) hydrolysis and dissociation, may help to bias the movement of the polypeptide into the lumen but not back out. The **oligosaccharyl transferase** associated with the translocon adds core sugars to the growing chain when an asparagine in an appropriate sequence passes by.

When a peptide grows to about 150 residues, a **signal peptidase** associated with the translocon cleaves off the signal sequence. The ER signal peptidase consists of five subunits ranging from 12 kD to 25 kD. Archaea and a few gram-positive Eubacteria have a similar enzyme complex. Most Eubacteria and eukaryotic organelles (see Figs. 19–2, 19–5, and 19–10) use a structurally unrelated signal peptidase consisting of a single subunit anchored to the membrane to carry out the same cleavage reaction.

Post-Translational Translocation into the Endoplasmic Reticulum

Although fungi have all of the components for cotranslational translocation into the ER, many of their proteins containing typical signal sequences bypass the SRP and enter the ER after their synthesis is complete. This post-translational mode of import relies on cytosolic folding chaperones to maintain the polypeptide in an unfolded state in the cytosol before translocation through the same channel used for cotranslational insertion. The Sec61p translocon recruits a tetrameric Sec62/63 complex to form a receptor-translocation machine that recognizes proteins with appropriate signals for translocation. This strategy is similar to the use of receptors by the TOM complex to import proteins into mitochondria (see Chapter 19). Post-translational translocation into the ER utilizes BiP to promote ratcheting and folding of the protein in the ER lumen.

Targeting of Soluble Secreted Proteins to the Endoplasmic Reticulum

Secreted proteins use the Sec61p translocon to enter the ER lumen (Fig. 20–5A). Signal peptidase cleaves the translocating polypeptide from its signal sequence, which initially anchors it to the membrane. After signal peptide cleavage, translation continues to push the new N-terminus of the growing polypeptide into the ER lumen. The fate of the cleaved signal peptide is unknown. None has ever been found, so degradation must be very efficient.

Insertion of Integral Proteins into the Endoplasmic Reticulum Membrane

Integration of transmembrane segments into the lipid bilayer is much less well understood than translocation into the ER lumen, so the drawings in Figure 20–5B to E must be considered to be models rather than well-documented mechanisms. In the simplest case (Fig. 20–5B), the C-terminus of a transmembrane protein resides in the cytoplasm upon completion of synthesis (referred to as "type 1" transmembrane protein). Early events involving delivery to the ER using a signal peptide are identical to those in a secreted protein. However, insertion of the hydrophobic transmembrane sequence into the translocon is thought to freeze movement of the growing chain. This hydrophobic stretch functions as a "stop-transfer" signal. Stop-transfer signals are hard to predict from their sequences, and their receptor in the channel is not identified. In contrast to signal sequences, stop-transfer signals are not cleaved. Instead, such transmembrane sequences move laterally out of the channel into the lipid bilayer, anchoring the polypeptide in the membrane. This exit from the translocon is a poorly understood, multistep process involving interaction of the transmembrane sequence with both lipids and translocon proteins. Completion of translation results in a protein with its N-terminus in the lumen and its C-terminus in the cytoplasm. Transmembrane proteins with the opposite orientation (type 2) form if the signal sequence is not cleaved (see Fig. 20–5C). Polytopic proteins that span the membrane multiple times (such as ion channels and carriers) utilize multiple stop-transfer signals (see Fig. 20–5D and E). SRP is probably required to target the first signal sequence to the ER membrane. Thereafter, the dynamics of the channel must accommodate sequences that alternately specify translocation of cytoplasmic loops and then transfer of transmembrane segments to the lipid bilayer.

Protein Folding and Oligomerization in the Endoplasmic Reticulum

Together, the tunnel through the large ribosomal subunit and the translocon channel in the ER bilayer shel-

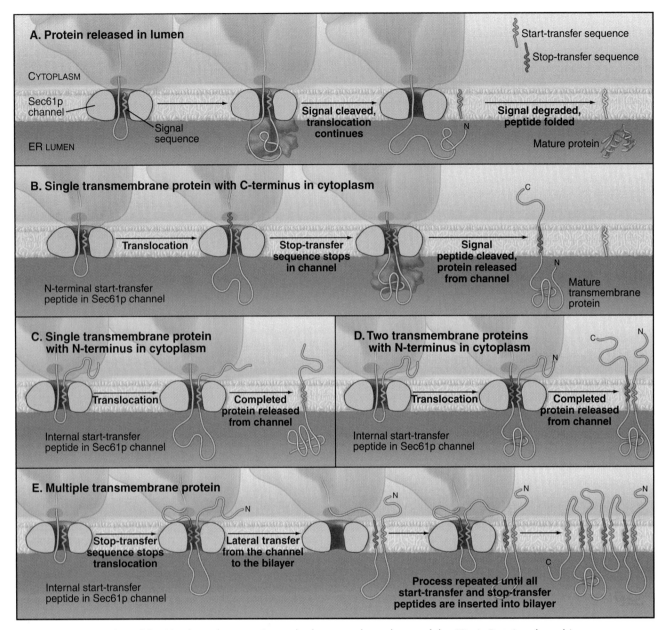

Figure 20–5 Targeting of Sec61p-dependent proteins to the lumen and membrane of the ER. *A,* Protein released in lumen. *B,* Single transmembrane segment with C-terminus in cytoplasm. *C,* Single transmembrane segment with N-terminus in cytoplasm. *D,* Two transmembrane segments. *E,* Multiple transmembrane segments.

ter approximately 70 amino acids of polypeptide. Polypeptide chains longer than 70 amino acids emerge into the ER lumen, where they encounter a wealth of proteins that interact with the nascent polypeptide. They remove the signal sequence, add oligosaccharides, and direct folding, formation of disulfide bonds, and association of oligomers. These reactions begin as soon as a nascent chain enters the lumen, so the modifying factors must reside close to the luminal side of the translocon complex (see Fig. 20–4). The combined activities of these proteins provide quality control to ensure that only functional cargo is exported.

N-Linked Glycosylation

Many secreted and membrane proteins contain covalently attached carbohydrates. Only one type of glycosylation occurs cotranslationally in the ER: the addition of a preformed oligosaccharide complex to asparagine residues. These asparagine or **N-linked oligosaccharides** make polypeptides more hydrophilic, thereby reducing their tendency to aggregate. Moreover, oligosaccharides play an important role in folding by protecting the protein from degradation. Remarkably, they are also utilized by the cell to monitor the progress of

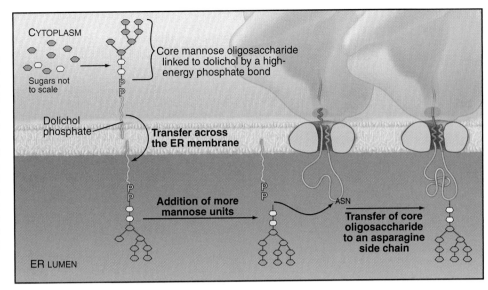

Figure 20-6 Dolichol pathway. A core oligosaccharide consisting of mannose and *N*-acetylglucosamine is synthesized in the cytoplasm, attached through high-energy pyrophosphate bonds to dolichol in the ER membrane. Following transfer across the ER bilayer, the addition of sugars imported into the ER completes the core structure. The oligosaccharide-transferase complex transfers the completed oligosaccharide to the consensus Asn-X-Ser/Thr motif of a nascent chain as it enters the lumen of the ER.

the folding reaction. Furthermore, the great diversity of oligosaccharides found on secreted proteins is crucial for their function outside the cell.

A single, preformed oligosaccharide precursor, composed of 14 sugars, serves as the core for *N*-linked oligosaccharides. This precursor is synthesized in a step-wise fashion while attached to the ER membrane by a **dolichol lipid carrier** (Fig. 20–6). Assembly of the oligosaccharide precursor involves 14 separate transfer reactions, 7 on the cytosolic face of the ER and 7 in the lumen. The mechanism that flips the glycolipid across the bilayer is unknown, but it most likely utilizes a protein channel. The enzyme oligosaccharyltransferase recognizes dolichol and transfers the completed oligosaccharide to appropriate asparagine residues that have emerged a distance of 12 to 14 residues out of the translocon into the ER lumen. Acceptor asparagines are part of the sequence Asn-X-Ser/Thr, where X is any amino acid other than proline. Not all potential acceptor sites are utilized.

Glycosylphosphatidylinositol Anchors

Some type 1 proteins exchange their carboxyl terminal transmembrane segment for an oligosaccharide anchored to the lipid phosphatidylinositol (see Chapter 6, Fig. 20–7). These glycosylphosphatidylinositol (GPI) proteins are transferred to the glycolipid during translation. The protein is cleaved at the luminal face of a stop-transfer signal and transferred to a preformed glycolipid precursor.

Folding of Newly Synthesized Polypeptides

Although a protein may begin to fold as soon as its N-terminus enters the ER lumen, completion of folding and oligomerization (assembly of subunits) occurs after release from the ribosome. Thus, the ER lumen is a highly specialized folding environment. Each polypeptide has a different folding pathway, dictated by its sequence. However, the enzymes assisting in the process are generally the same (Fig. 20–8).

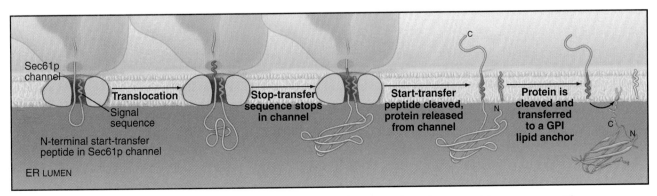

Figure 20-7 Synthesis of a GPI anchor. Certain proteins, such as Thy-1, are cleaved at a special consensus motif during cotranslational insertion into the bilayer. The new C-terminus is then transferred to a glycosylphosphatidylinositol anchor.

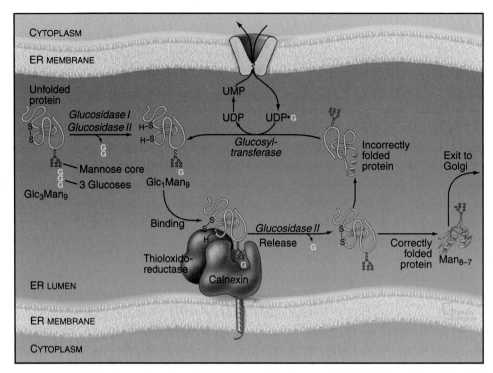

Figure 20-8 Calnexin cycle of protein folding in the lumen of the ER. Glucosidases I and II rapidly remove two of three glucoses from newly synthesized, unfolded glycoprotein. The calnexin-thioloxidoreductase complex binds the monoglucosylated protein. Glucosidase II removes the remaining glucose, releasing the protein. If the released protein is folded, it can exit the ER. If unfolded, it is recognized by glucosyltransferase and reglucosylated so that it reenters the folding cycle until folding is complete or it enters the degradation pathway. Thioloxidoreductases catalyze rearrangements of disulfide bonds during folding. Glc, glucose; man, mannose; UDP, uridine diphosphate; UMP, uridine monophosphate. (Reprinted with permission. Redrawn from Ellgaard L, Molinari M, Helenius A: Setting the standards: Quality control in the secretory pathway. Science 286:1882–1888, 1999. Copyright 1999, American Association for the Advancement of Science.)

In addition to association with BiP during transit through the Sec61p translocon, polypeptides undergoing cotranslational and post-translational folding in the ER lumen associate transiently with one or more classes of chaperone-like proteins. Many of these chaperones are related to adenosine triphosphatase (ATPase) stress proteins that assist with protein folding in the cytoplasm (see Chapter 18). Some ER chaperones are calcium-binding proteins, such as **calnexin,** which monitor folding of glycoproteins containing N-linked oligosaccharides. Calnexin binds nascent glycoproteins through glucose residues on the termini of the oligosaccharide. These glucoses are normally removed by resident **glucosidases** prior to export from the ER. Through repeated cycles of binding and release from calnexin in response to trimming by glucosidases and readdition of these glucose residues by ER **glucosyl transferases,** the chaperone "senses" when the protein is properly folded (see Fig. 20–8). This cycle protects the nascent glycoprotein from premature misfolding and degradation. **Mannosidases,** which are ER proteins that trim mannose residues

from N-linked oligosaccharides, also serve as measuring sticks to mark the completion of protein folding and to target misfolded proteins for degradation.

Proteins entering the exocytic pathway have more **disulfide bonds** than cytosolic proteins. These disulfide bonds stabilize proteins in the oxidizing conditions outside the cell. In contrast to the reducing environment of the cytoplasm, the lumen of the ER is an oxidizing environment that favors disulfide bond formation. Protein disulfide bonds form spontaneously in a test tube exposed to oxygen, but the reaction is faster in the ER owing to catalysis by a family of enzymes called **protein disulfide isomerases (PDIs).** Oxidizing equivalents to form disulfide bonds in the ER are thought to flow from flavin adenine dinucleotide (FAD) through two pairs of cysteines of an ER membrane protein called Ero1p, which oxidizes a pair of cysteines in the active site of protein disulfide isomerase. Protein disulfide isomerase then mediates correct formation of disulfide bonds by forming reversible mixed disulfides with polypeptide substrates until the correct disulfides are formed.

Protein Oligomerization in the Endoplasmic Reticulum

Many polypeptides transferred to the ER are subunits of homo- or hetero-oligomeric protein complexes. Oligomer assembly generally occurs prior to export and also involves chaperones that protect hydrophobic surfaces found at subunit interfaces. Because synthesis of protein subunits occurs on distinct ribosomes and may be unbalanced, additional chaperones may promote subunit interactions and prevent premature export or degradation. For example, they play a critical role in antigen presentation by ensuring that only peptide-loaded major histocompatibility complex (MHC) type I proteins exit the ER (see Chapter 22). They also protect cell surface receptors and other secreted proteins from binding potential substrates that are also imported into the ER. These could trigger premature activation with deleterious consequences on cell metabolism if left unchecked.

Degradation Proteins Misfolded in the Endoplasmic Reticulum

The ER has a highly regulated mechanism to prevent the export of dysfunctional proteins (Fig. 20–9). Improperly folded polypeptides, excess subunits of oligomeric assemblies, or incorrectly assembled oligomers are degraded rather than being exported from the ER. Remarkably, a cytoplasmic enzyme complex called the **proteasome** (see Chapter 24) degrades both luminal and transmembrane proteins. Even more surprising was the discovery that transfer from the ER

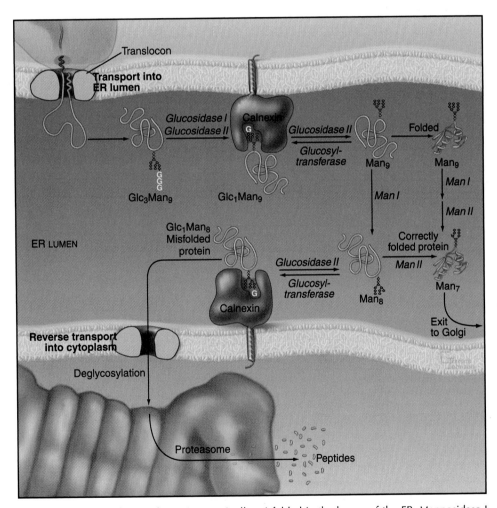

Figure 20–9 Degradation of proteins terminally misfolded in the lumen of the ER. Mannosidase I marks persistently unfolded glycoproteins for degradation by generating an 8-mannose–containing oligosaccharide that is reglucosylated. This poor substrate for glucosidase II remains bound to calnexin and is eventually retrotranslocated out of the ER and degraded by a proteasome. (Redrawn from Liu Y, Choudhury P, Cabral CM, et al: Oligosaccharide modification in the early secretory pathway directs the selection of a misfolded glycoprotein for degradation by the proteasome. J Biol Chem 274:5861–5867, 1999.)

to the cytoplasmic proteasome uses Sec61p, the same translocon used for import. Thus translocon is a two-way road. Transit is differentially regulated to control the fate of proteins in the ER. Viruses, including human immunodeficiency virus, usurp this pathway to promote degradation of components used by the immune system to detect cells infected with viruses, thereby evading destruction of their host cell.

Endoplasmic Reticulum Stress Responses

The folding pathway in the ER is tightly linked to the physiological state of the cell. Conditions that flood the ER with excess protein, or those that result in the accumulation of misfolded protein, trigger two important signaling pathways: the **unfolded protein response** and the **ER overload response.**

Essentially, any condition that exceeds the protein folding capacity of the ER triggers the unfolded protein response: misfolding of mutant proteins, inhibition of ER glycosylation (by tunicamycin), inhibition of disulfide formation (by reducing agents), or even overproduction of normal proteins. To compensate for these events, this stress-induced signaling pathway upregulates genes required to synthesize the entire ER, including folding machinery. In yeast, the unfolded protein response activates more than 300 genes involved with all aspects of ER function, including lipid synthesis, protein translocation, protein folding, glycosylation, and degradation, as well as export to and retrieval from the Golgi apparatus. Developmental

programs may work through the same genetic controls to determine the abundance of ER in differentiated cells, producing, for example, extensive ER in secretory cells, such as plasma cells, liver cells, and pancreatic acinar cells.

The unfolded protein response uses a novel signaling pathway (Fig. 20–10) involving a transmembrane kinase/ribonuclease (Ire1p), a tRNA ligase (Rlg1p), and the messenger RNA (mRNA) for the transcription factor (Hac1p) that activates the genes for ER components. Ire1p is a transmembrane ER protein with a kinase/ribonuclease domain facing the cytoplasm or nucleoplasm. ER overload activates Ire1p by allowing it to dimerize. One possible mechanism is that ER chaperones block dimerization until they are depleted by excess unfolded protein in the lumen. Dimerization activates latent endonuclease activity through autophosphorylation; the kinase domains transphosphorylate each other's activation loops (as in other kinases; see Chapter 27). This is required for subsequent events, but no other substrates for the kinase are known. Instead, kinase activation allows the ribonuclease activity of Ire1p to cleave an intron from the unprocessed mRNA for Hac1p. This intron is not removed by the usual splicing machinery and blocks translation. Rlg1p, a tRNA ligase localized to the inner nuclear envelope, is required to join the two exons created by Ire1p. This processed mRNA is translated to produce Hac1p, a bZip transcription factor (see Chapter 14) that activates expression of its numerous target genes. Note that this splicing mechanism is similar to

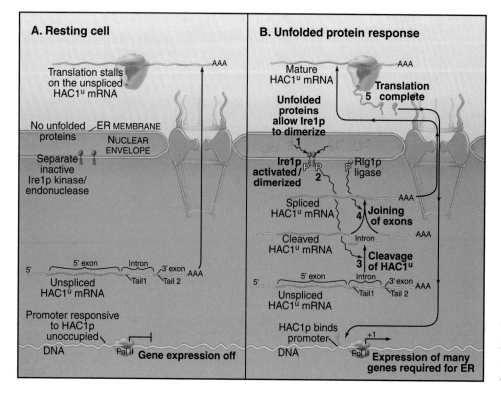

Figure 20–10 Unfolded protein response to stress in the lumen of the ER. *A,* Resting cell. Genes for ER proteins controlled by HAC1p are turned off. *B,* Unfolded protein response. Unfolded proteins accumulating in the ER *(1)* activate Ire1p *(2),* leading to cleavage *(3)* and ligation of *HAC1ᵘ* mRNA *(4)* to generate spliced *HAC1ⁱ* mRNA *(5).* The spliced mRNA is translated to form the protein HAC1p, which up-regulates genes with unfolded protein response elements (UPRE) in the nucleus. (Redrawn and updated from Chapman R, Sidrauski C, Walter P: Intracellular signaling from the endoplasmic reticulum to the nucleus. Annu Rev Cell Dev Biol 14:459–485, 1998, with permission, from the *Annual Review of Cell and Developmental Biology,* Vol. 14, © 1998 by Annual Reviews www.AnnualReviews. org.)

that used for tRNA processing rather than the spliceosome mechanisms that process most mRNAs (see Chapter 15). The unfolded protein response can be turned on and off rapidly because the unprocessed Hac1 mRNA is stable, and because the Hac1p protein is very unstable owing to a protease-sensitive domain.

ER overload response initiates a different signaling pathway involving activation of the transcription factor NF-κB in cytoplasm, leading to expression of genes for cytokines (see Chapter 14), or to apoptosis (see Chapter 49), but none of the genes activated by the unfolded protein response. The response is initiated by accumulation of integral proteins in ER membranes. The primary purpose of this mechanism appears to be defense against viral infection. Enveloped viruses cause the host cells to synthesize viral glycoproteins that accumulate in the ER. This signals the production of cytokines or apoptosis if ER dysfunction is severe.

ER Folding Diseases

Given the central role of the ER in the synthesis of proteins for the entire exocytic (see Chapter 21) and endocytic (see Chapter 23) pathways, as well as secretion, it is not surprising that many inherited diseases are a direct consequence of proteins failing to pass ER quality control. Many metabolic disorders, such as lysosomal storage diseases (see Chapter 24), are a direct consequence of key enzymes failing to be exported from the ER. The most common form of **cystic fibrosis** is due to the inability of cells to export a mutant form of the cystic fibrosis transmembrane regulator (CFTR) to the cell surface where it would normally function as a chloride channel for the respiratory system and pancreas (see Chapter 10). Similarly, inability of the liver to secrete mutated forms of α_1-antitrypsin predisposes individuals to the lung disease emphysema. Mutations in α_1-antitrypsin prevent folding of the protein in the ER, resulting in its degradation. Normally α_1-antitrypsin protects tissues by inhibiting extracellular proteases such as elastase, which is produced by neutrophils. A deficiency of α_1-antitrypsin circulating in the blood allows elastase to destroy lung tissue, leading to emphysema. In severe cases, mutant forms of the protein not only fail to be exported from the ER but also elude degradation pathways, accumulating as insoluble aggregates that induce stress responses and liver failure.

In some conditions, the ER uses the unfolded protein response and the ER overload response to compensate, in part, for mutations in cargo proteins. In congenital **hypothyroidism,** mutant thyroglobulin (the precursor of thyroid hormone) is not exported efficiently from the ER. Excess protein accumulates as insoluble aggregates in the ER. Feedback pathways

trigger massive proliferation of ER in an attempt to produce normal levels of circulating hormone. Similarly, in mild forms of **osteogenesis imperfecta** (see Chapter 34), osteoblasts assemble and secrete defective procollagen chains for bone synthesis, even though the resulting bone tissue is weak. The alternative—complete loss of procollagen by retention and degradation of the mutant procollagen in the ER—would be lethal. Faulty ER quality control has also been suggested to contribute to diseases of the central and peripheral nervous systems, including Alzheimer's disease.

Golgi Function in Biosynthetic Processing

Pioneering studies in the 1960s, using a combination of metabolic labeling with radioactive amino acids and autoradiography, established that newly synthesized secretory proteins are transferred from the ER to Golgi compartments before packaging in secretory granules. This section considers the organization of the Golgi complex and its role in modifying proteins. Chapter 21 covers the mechanism that transports protein through the Golgi apparatus.

Structure and Composition of the Golgi Complex

Although the Golgi complex was first detected by light microscopy in the late 19th century by Camillo Golgi, electron microscopy was necessary to establish that the Golgi complex consists of a set of three or more stacked compartments or cisternae (Fig. 20–11). This stack of membranes typically occupies the perinuclear region of the cell, surrounded by numerous membrane vesicles and tubules. Depending on the cell type, the Golgi apparatus can be a single continuous stack surrounding the nucleus, or, in the case of polarized epithelial cells, a compact group of stacks on one side of the nucleus. Although connections between individual cisternae within a stack are rare, sets of stacks are connected by tubules that appear to link related compartments between each stack. Cells dedicated to protein secretion have the largest Golgi apparatuses. Many lines of evidence demonstrate that the Golgi apparatus is a dynamic structure characterized by constant turnover reflecting the extensive flow of protein and lipid from the ER.

Golgi stacks are highly polarized with respect to the composition of individual cisternae. Cargo from the ER generally enters the *cis* side of the stack proximal to the nucleus. These cisternae consist of branched reticulum called the **cis-Golgi network.** Processed material exits from cisternae found on the *trans* side, consisting of another tubular network, the

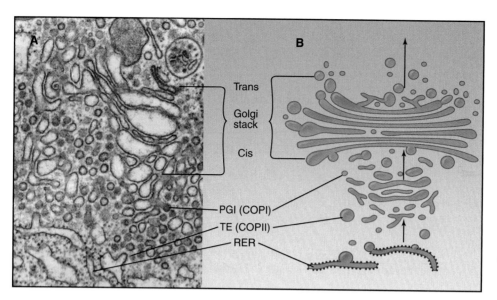

Figure 20–11 Structure of the Golgi complex. *A,* An electron micrograph of a thin section of a pancreatic acinar cell showing the transition between rough endoplasmic reticulum (RER) and Golgi apparatus. TE, tubular element containing vesicle budding structures associated with COPII coats; PGI, pre-Golgi intermediate associated with COPI coats. *B,* Drawing of the Golgi complex. (*A,* Courtesy of George Palade, University of California, San Diego.)

trans-Golgi network (TGN). Each Golgi cisterna contains a different spectrum of processing enzymes. Enzymes that modify *N*-linked oligosaccharides are, for instance, organized along the cis-to-trans axis, reflecting their sequential role in this process. However, compartmentalization of these enzymes is not absolute, suggesting that their location is highly dynamic.

Oligosaccharide Modifications in the Golgi Apparatus

Prior to export from the ER, a polypeptide must be properly folded. In contrast, most functionally important, post-translational modifications that these proteins eventually undergo are incomplete.

Golgi enzymes extensively remodel all of the *N*-linked oligosaccharides that proteins acquire in the ER (Fig. 20–12). Remodeling involves both removal and addition of sugar residues. These **glycosidases** and **glycosyltransferases** are generally integral membrane proteins with active sites in the lumen of the Golgi cisternae. The addition of new sugars to an

oligosaccharide chain requires high-energy sugar-nucleotide precursors that are made in the cytoplasm and transported into the lumen by integral membrane carriers. The distribution of these carriers must be coordinated with that of the transferases mediating modification. The mechanisms that coordinate cargo flow from the ER with processing are still poorly understood.

Golgi enzymes also add oligosaccharides to the hydroxyl groups of serine and threonine residues of selected proteins, such as proteoglycans, heavily glycosylated proteins in secretory granules, and the extracellular matrix (see Chapters 22 and 31). These **O-linked oligosaccharides** can be extensively modified by sulfation and other reactions (see Fig. 31–13).

Proteolytic Processing of Protein Precursors

A number of proteins, particularly peptide hormones, are cleaved into active fragments in the TGN and secretory vesicles. Such proteins are synthesized as large precursors with one or more small hormones embedded in other sequences. One example is a yeast mat-

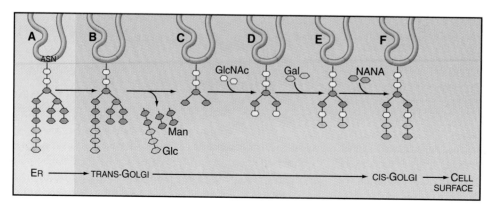

Figure 20–12 Processing of *N*-linked core oligosaccharides in the Golgi apparatus. *A* to *F,* Sequential steps trim the mannose (Man)/glucose (Glc) core and then add *N*-acetylglucosamine (GlcNAc), galactose (Gal), and sialic acid (NANA) to form a variety of complex oligosaccharides, one of which is shown here. ASN, asparagine.

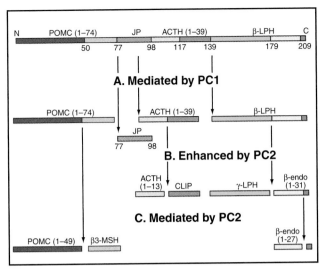

Figure 20-13 Proteolytic processing of pro-opiomelanocortin (POMC) in the secretory granules of pituitary cells. POMC is the precursor of several hormones: melanocyte-stimulating hormone (MSH), adrenocorticotropic hormone (ACTH), β-lipotropin hormone (β-LPH), and β-endorphin (β-endo) hormone. Corticotropes (cells producing ACTH) express PC1, an endoprotease that makes four cleavages. Melanotrophs (cells producing MSH) express an additional endoprotease, PC2, which completes the processing of α-MSH and γ3-MSH, in addition to the other products indicated. (Redrawn from Zhou A, et al: The prohormone convertases PC1 and PC2 mediate distinct endoproteolytic cleavages in a strict temporal order during pro-opiomelanocortin biosynthetic processing. J Biol Chem 268:1763–1769, 1993.)

ing pheromone. Another is pro-opiomelanocortin (POMC), the precursor to no less than six small peptide hormones (Fig. 20–13). Proteolytic enzymes called **prohormone convertases** cleave the precursor proteins into active hormones in the TGN and post-TGN transport intermediates. The mixture of products depends on the prohormone convertases expressed in particular cells. Proteolysis in the TGN also affects the final folding state and activity of many other proteins. Inherited defects in these processing pathways lead to a number of diseases, including hormone insufficiency and a hereditary amyloid disease.

■ Other Functions of the ER and Golgi Apparatus

Lipid Synthesis

The ER and Golgi apparatus make most cellular lipids (see Chapter 6). Synthesis of **phosphoglycerides** alone is an enormous synthetic task. A hepatocyte has about 10^{12} to 10^{13} phosphoglyceride molecules, which are synthesized at a rate of about 10^7 molecules per second. This staggering synthetic rate is essential to meet the ongoing needs of the exocytic pathway and

for the many aspects of cell function that depend on membranes and lipid-signaling molecules.

The ER synthesizes most phosphoglycerides, whereas **sphingolipid** (see Fig. 6–3) synthesis occurs primarily in the Golgi apparatus. Cardiolipin (diphosphatidylglycerol) is synthesized by mitochondria and exclusively found in this compartment. Plasmalogens are phosphoglycerides with one or two alkyl chains attached by an ether linkage rather than fatty acyl chains attached by an ester linkage. Peroxisomes participate in plasmalogen synthesis. These lipids are abundant in nervous tissue, particularly in the myelin membrane that insulates nerve axons.

ER enzymes participating in phosphoglyceride synthesis have their active sites facing the cytoplasm, the site of synthesis of many lipid precursors. Synthesis begins with conjugation of two activated fatty acids to glycerol-3-phosphate to form phosphatidic acid, which can be dephosphorylated to produce diacylglycerol (see Fig. 28–4). Neither phosphatidic acid nor diacylglycerol is a bulk component of membranes; however, they are used in the synthesis of the four major phosphoglycerides: phosphatidylcholine, phosphatidylethanolamine, phosphatidylserine, and phosphatidylinositol (see Fig. 6–2). The most abundant phosphoglycerides—phosphatidylcholine and phosphatidylethanolamine—are produced by comparable reactions of diacylglycerol with the activated head groups, cytidine diphosphate (CDP)–choline and CDP-ethanolamine. Phosphatidylinositol synthesis is a distinct route using inositol and CDP-diacylglycerol produced from phosphatidic acid (see Chapter 28). Phosphatidylserine synthesis (in mammalian cells) is an energy-independent exchange of polar head groups on phosphatidylethanolamine. Head group exchange of phosphoglycerides occurs primarily in the ER, but may also occur in other organelles.

Like other types of biosynthesis carried out in the ER and Golgi complex, phosphoglyceride synthesis creates a topologic problem: synthesis occurs in the cytoplasmic leaflet, restricting membrane growth to that leaflet. These lipids move to the luminal leaflet by the flip-flopping of individual molecules across the bilayer. Flip-flop of phosphoglycerides across the ER bilayer is much faster than in vesicles of pure phosphoglycerides owing to protein translocators called flippases.

Cholesterol Synthesis and Metabolism

Cholesterol is maintained in animal cells by a combination of de novo synthesis in the ER and receptor-mediated endocytosis of lipoprotein particles containing esterified cholesterol (see Chapter 22). Coordinate regulation of these two processes precisely maintains the physiological level of cholesterol in cellular membranes. Peroxisomes may also participate in aspects of cholesterol synthesis and metabolism.

Enzymes in the cytoplasm and ER use 22 sequential steps to synthesize cholesterol from acetate (Fig. 20–14). Cytosolic enzymes catalyze the initial steps using water-soluble molecules to produce **farnesyl-pyrophosphate** (farnesyl-PP) from acetyl coenzyme A (acetyl CoA). An important exception is the step going from 3-hydroxy-3-methylglutaryl CoA (HMG-CoA) to mevalonate. A carefully regulated, integral

membrane protein of the ER (Fig. 20–15), **HMG-CoA reductase,** catalyzes this key step. Enzymes in the ER bilayer catalyze the subsequent condensation of farnesyl-PP to make squalene, and cyclization to cholesterol, progressively less polar molecules. Although the final steps leading to cholesterol take place in the ER, cholesterol is not a resident lipid and is rapidly exported to post-ER membranes, including plasma membrane, where it constitutes up to 50% of the bilayer. Chapter 22 discusses the distribution of cholesterol in the different organelles and current ideas regarding its transport.

Feedback loops sense the cholesterol content of the ER membrane and regulate both the synthesis and degradation of enzymes that synthesize cholesterol (see Fig. 20–15). High cholesterol levels inhibit the synthesis and stimulate the destruction of key synthetic enzymes. A novel transcription factor precursor, steroid regulatory element-binding protein (SREBP), controls the expression of these genes. When cholesterol is abundant, SREBP cleavage-activating protein (SCAP), a partner protein with cholesterol-sensing transmembrane segments, retains SREBP in the ER. When the membrane cholesterol level is low, SCAP and SREBP move to the Golgi apparatus where two successive proteolytic cleavages release the N-terminal domain of SREBP, a basic helix-loop-helix leucine zipper transcription factor, into the cytoplasm. In the nucleus, the transcription factor binds steroid regulatory elements, enhancers for a wide range of genes encoding enzymes that synthesize cholesterol and other lipids, as well as low-density lipoprotein receptors that take up cholesterol from the medium (see Chapter 23). Cholesterol also regulates degradation of HMG-CoA reductase, which has cholesterol-sensing transmembrane domains similar to SCAP. Abundant cholesterol targets HMG-CoA reductase for degradation by the proteolytic pathway that disposes of unfolded proteins through the proteasome (see Fig. 20–9).

Sphingolipid Biosynthesis

Ceremide is the backbone of all sphingolipids (see Fig. 6–3). Its synthesis begins on the cytoplasmic face of ER membranes. Enzymes in the luminal leaflet of the Golgi complex carry out subsequent steps of **sphingolipid** and **glycosphingolipid** synthesis. All types of glycosphingolipids have carbohydrate attached to the terminal hydroxyl group of ceremide facing the lumen of the Golgi apparatus. The number of saccharide residues ranges from 1 to a chain of 20. They are very diverse and have been grouped into families based on the pattern of sugars, the types of linkages between them, and the presence (or absence) of terminal sialic acids. Synthesis of these carbohydrate chains occurs in successive compartments of the Golgi apparatus in a sequence that mimics processing

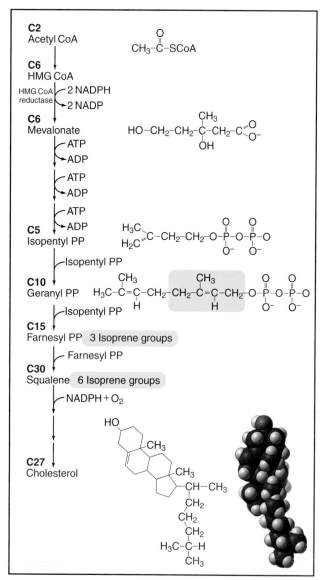

Figure 20–14 Key steps in the biosynthesis of cholesterol from acetyl CoA. Synthesis of mevalonate from 3-hydroxy-3-methyl-glutaryl CoA is closely regulated by controlling the concentration of the enzyme, HMG-CoA reductase, as shown in Figure 20–15. Five-carbon isoprene groups are the building blocks (*yellow*) for making a 10-carbon geranyl-pyrophosphate (PP), a 15-carbon farnesyl-pyrophosphate, and 30-carbon squalene intermediates. Several reactions add a hydroxyl group and join squalene into four rings to make cholesterol. ADP, adenosine diphosphate; NADP, nicotinamide-adenine dinucleotide.

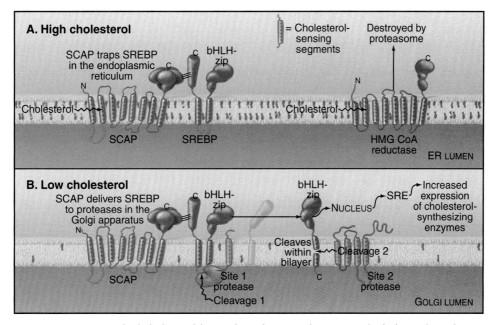

Figure 20–15 Control of cholesterol biosynthesis by proteolysis. *A,* High-cholesterol conditions. Cholesterol-sensing transmembrane segments *(pink)* of SCAP (SREBP cleavage-activating protein) retain intact SREBP in the ER. Similar cholesterol-sensing transmembrane segments of HMG-CoA reductase stimulate its destruction by proteolysis. *B,* Low-cholesterol conditions. SCAP and SREBP move to the Golgi apparatus where the membrane-anchored site 1 serine protease cleaves the loop of SREBP in the lumen. Subsequently, an unusual transmembrane zinc-protease cleaves SREBP at a second site within the bilayer, releasing the basic helix-loop-helix-zip (bHLH-zip) transcription factor. This factor enters the nucleus, where it activates genes for cholesterol biosynthetic enzymes by steroid-responsive elements (SREs). (References: Brown MS, Goldstein JL: A proteolytic pathway that controls the cholesterol content of membranes, cells, and blood. Proc Natl Acad Sci USA 96:11041–11048, 1999, copyright 1999, National Academy of Sciences, U.S.A.; reprinted from Nohturfft A, Yabe D, Goldstein JL, et al: Regulated step in cholesterol feedback localized to budding of SCAP from ER membranes. Cell 102:315–323, 2000. Copyright 2000, with permission from Elsevier Science.)

of *N*-linked oligosaccharides in glycoproteins. Like glycoproteins, glycolipid products retain their topologic distribution in post-Golgi compartments and the plasma membrane.

Lipid Compositions of Organelles and the Cell Surface

Although various organelle membranes contain most classes of lipids, the proportions of these lipids are unique and characteristic for each organelle. This gives each membrane distinct physical properties. Because lipids lack targeting signals and diffuse freely in the plane of bilayers, the distinct lipid composition of each organelle is likely to reflect a complex interplay of factors. These factors include the affinity of lipids for each other, the affinity of particular lipids for hydrophobic transmembrane domains of proteins occupying a particular compartment and giving rise to microdomains, and the length and flexibility of fatty acyl chains in the case of phosphoglycerides.

Differences in lipid composition can be striking. Cardiolipin is restricted locally to its site of synthesis in mitochondria, where it is concentrated in the inner membrane. Phosphatidylcholine and phosphatidylinositol are abundant in the ER, where they are synthesized. Phosphatidylcholine is also abundant in mitochondria, so it must be imported. By contrast, cholesterol is essentially absent from the ER (where it is made), whereas the plasma membrane contains high levels of cholesterol and glycosphingolipids that were made in the Golgi apparatus. Sphingolipids and cholesterol associate in **rafts** (see Fig. 6–7). This probably contributes to their tendency to concentrate in the same membranes. Specific mechanisms ensure that they are transported to and maintained in these membranes.

In addition to the unique lipid compositions of subcellular organelles and the cell surface, within the bilayer of each organelle, lipids are arranged asymmetrically (see Fig. 6–7). Asymmetry is most pronounced for choline-containing lipids, such as phosphatidylcholine and sphingomyelin, which are primarily found in the outer leaflet. Amino-containing phospholipids, including phosphatidylserine and phosphatidylethanolamine, as well as phosphoinositides, are located almost exclusively in the inner leaflet. The reasons for this asymmetry are not known, but **lipid asymmetry** may contribute to the physical properties required for rapid membrane fission and fusion during vesicle transport between compartments of the exocytic and endocytic pathways (see Chapter 21).

Distribution of Lipids Through Vesicular and Nonvesicular Mechanisms

The hydrophobic nature of lipids makes free diffusion between adjacent bilayers thermodynamically unfavorable. Thus, lipids use two other mechanisms to move between organelles. The major pathway is movement through the use of vesicle carriers (see Chapters 21 to 23). In addition, small, soluble **phospholipid exchange proteins** promote movements between membranes. These proteins are specific for particular phospholipids. They catalyze lipid exchange and not net transfer; when the protein delivers a lipid to a target membrane, the protein exchanges that lipid for another one and returns with the second lipid. For example, the phosphatidylinositol/phosphatidylcholine transfer protein senses the lipid composition and regulates lipid synthesis in close conjunction with the phosphatidylcholine biosynthetic enzymes. The importance of lipid transfer by this mechanism is reflected in the essential need for phosphatidylinositol/phosphatidylcholine transfer proteins for transport through the secretory pathway.

Oxidation of Small Molecules

ER enzymes use molecular oxygen to detoxify foreign compounds and hydroxylate endogenous steroids. The ER of hepatocytes and other cells contains a large family of heme-containing membrane proteins, called the **cytochrome P-450 proteins.** P-450 proteins are part of a short electron transfer chain. An ER membrane protein with reductase activity transfers electrons from the reduced form of nicotinamide-adenine dinucleotide phosphate (NADPH) to reduce an oxygen bound to the heme group of cytochrome P-450. Cytochrome P-450 then catalyzes hydroxylation of endogenous steroids, lipid-soluble drugs, and foreign chemicals (xenobiotics) from the environment. It also hydroxylates hydrophobic carcinogenic compounds that concentrate in the ER membrane. Although hydroxylation increases the hydrophilic character of these lipophilic compounds (facilitating their elimination), hydroxylated products may be carcinogenic in some cases.

The more than 40 P-450 proteins have rather broad substrate specificities. Exposure to substrates, such as the drug phenobarbital, can enhance the expression of particular P-450 isoforms up to 70-fold, accompanied by a concomitant increase in membrane lipid biosynthesis, resulting in an enormous expansion of the smooth ER. Studies of the evolution of this gene family suggest that exposure of vertebrates to toxic chemicals in plants may have selected for the diversification of P-450 genes.

Calcium Storage

The ER is the principal site of calcium storage in eukaryotic cells. ATPase pumps in the ER membrane concentrate calcium in the lumen (see Chapters 7 and 28). Calcium is released selectively into the cytoplasm as a second messenger that regulates muscle contraction (see Chapter 42) and many other cellular processes (see Chapter 28).

▍ Selected Readings

Allan BB, Balch WE: Protein sorting by directed maturation of Golgi compartments. Science 285:63–66, 1999.

Aridor M, Balch WE: Integration of endoplasmic reticulum signaling in health and disease. Nature Med 5:745–751, 1999.

Brown MS, Goldstein JL: A proteolytic pathway that controls the cholesterol content of membranes, cells, and blood. Proc Natl Acad Sci USA 96:11041–11048, 1999.

Chapman R, Sidrauski C, Walter P: Intracellular signaling from the endoplasmic reticulum to the nucleus. Annu Rev Cell Dev Biol 14:459–485, 1998.

Ellgaard L, Molinari M, Helenius A: Setting the standards: Quality control in the secretory pathway. Science 286:1882–1888, 1999.

Ellis RJ, Hartl FU: Principles of protein folding in the cellular environment. Curr Opin Struct Biol 9:102–110, 1999.

Frand AR, Cuozzo JW, Kaiser CA: Pathways for protein disulfide bond formation. Trends Cell Biol 10:203–210, 2000.

Johnson AE, van Waes MA: The translocon: A dynamic gateway at the ER membrane. Annu Rev Cell Dev Biol 15:799–842, 1999.

Martoglio B, Dobberstein B: Signal sequences: More than just greasy peptides. Trends Cell Biol 8:410–415, 1998.

Olkkonen VM, Ikonen E: Genetic defects of intracellular membrane transport. N Engl J Med 343:1095–1104, 2000.

Stroud RM, Walter P: Signal sequence recognition and protein targeting. Curr Opin Struct Biol 9:754–759, 1999.

Trombetta ES, Helenius A: Lectins as chaperones in glycoprotein folding. Curr Opin Cell Biol 8:587–592, 1998.

chapter 21

VESICULAR TRAFFIC FROM THE ENDOPLASMIC RETICULUM THROUGH THE GOLGI APPARATUS

Proteins and lipids synthesized in the endoplasmic reticulum (ER) (see Chapter 20) provide the foundation for assembly and function of all compartments comprising the exocytic and endocytic pathways. Cargo moves from the ER through exocytic and endocytic compartments, carried by lipid-bound transport containers that include both small vesicles (60–80 nm in diameter) and elongated membrane tubules. The complexity of the trafficking problem is illustrated by the fact that this process simultaneously moves thousands of different proteins efficiently and precisely between different compartments without a mix-up. Moreover, intracellular transport must be coordinated with the constantly changing needs of cells and tissues in response to the environment and organismal physiology.

Vesicular transport takes place in three steps:

1. *Cargo selection.* Adaptor proteins couple sorting signals on specific cargo molecules to the transport machinery.
2. *Container formation.* Proteins form coat lattices that promote the pinching-off of a part of the donor compartment to form the transport container. A remarkable variety of coat lattices facilitate vesicle formation from different exocytic and endocytic compartments.
3. *Targeting and fusion of the container with the next compartment.* Membrane-associated tethering and fusion proteins direct the delivery of the transport container to the right target compartment.

Large gene families have evolved to route thousands of different proteins to their proper cellular locations. Small guanosine triphosphatases **(GTPases)** regulate all three steps by controlling the assembly and disassembly of transport complexes. (Chapter 27 covers the general principles regarding the structure and mechanisms of GTPases.) In the case of vesicular transport, the cycle of activation through exchange of guanosine diphosphate (GDP) for guanosine triphosphate (GTP) and inactivation by GTP hydrolysis is used to control not only the timing and duration of transport events, but also the fidelity (accuracy) of transport.

Forward transport along the secretory pathway (in an anterograde direction) begins with movement of vesicles from the ER to the compartments constituting the Golgi apparatus. A molecular machine called COPII mediates both cargo selection and assembly of the targeting/fusion components. Because many components involved in anterograde transport are membrane bound, they must be recycled. A different class of vesicles (COPI vesicles) facilitates this retrograde transport pathway. Yeasts use at least 40 to 50 gene products to complete a cycle of budding and fusion of transport containers mediating the anterograde (COPII) and retrograde (COPI) pathways between the ER and the Golgi apparatus. Additional proteins are likely to be required for these transport steps in higher eukaryotes to handle the diversity of specialized compartments in diverse cell types.

This chapter uses transport between the ER and the Golgi apparatus to illustrate the general principles governing vesicular membrane traffic throughout the cell. These other transport processes include movement of cargo from the trans-Golgi compartment to

---

Chapter by William E. Balch, based on an original draft by Ann L. Hubbard, J. David Castle, and Pat Shipman.

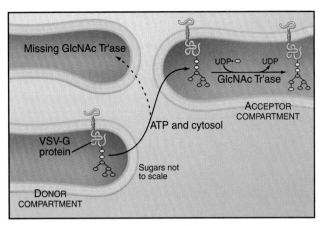

Figure 21-1 Test tube reconstitution of transport from the ER to the Golgi apparatus. Donor ER containing the glycoprotein VSV-G is prepared from mutant cells lacking a golgi glycosylation enzyme. When incubated with an acceptor Golgi stack prepared from normal cells in the presence of cytosol and ATP, vesicles containing VSV-G move from the donor ER to the acceptor Golgi compartment. There, they can be modified by addition of sugar residues by glycosylation enzymes residing in the normal Golgi apparatus. Transfer to the Golgi is measured by following the incorporation of these sugar residues. GlcNAc Tr'ase, N-acetylglycosyl transferase; UDP, uridine diphosphate.

the lysosome and cell surface (see Chapter 22), and those that direct cargo back into the cell through the endocytic pathway (see Chapters 22 and 23).

∎ Vesicle Formation from the Endoplasmic Reticulum

Analysis of Vesicular Transport

Genetic studies in yeast, as well as biochemical methods that include the use of cell-free assays, have contributed to the current understanding of membrane traffic. Cell-free assays detect transfer of cargo between membrane compartments prepared from cell homogenates by taking advantage of the biochemical properties of individual organelles. For example, transport of glycoproteins from the ER (donor compartment) to the Golgi apparatus (acceptor compartment) can be measured by following the processing of their *N*-linked oligosaccharides, post-translational modifications found only in Golgi compartments (see Chapter 20) (Fig. 21–1).

General Features of Vesicular Traffic

Cargo selection, vesicular budding, and vesicular fusion with the acceptor compartment all occur without leakage of content from the donor or target compartment. Thus, membrane integrity is maintained at all steps of transport. Furthermore, the orientation (called topology) of lipid and protein in the membrane bilayers, established during synthesis in the ER, is main-

tained by vesicular carriers during transport. Thus, one side of the membrane always faces the cytoplasm. The other side starts as the lumen of the ER; remains inside each vesicular compartment; and, in the case of cell surface components, eventually is exposed on the outside of the cell.

Step 1. Cargo Selection Through Sorting Motifs

Every vesicle that buds from a particular membrane compartment incorporates only proteins destined for transport and excludes resident proteins that define the composition of the compartment. Thus, the molecular machinery that generates vesicles must recognize **recruitment signals,** usually a short peptide sequence, on transported cargo proteins. The need to control precisely the composition of intracellular organelles and the plasma membrane makes it unlikely that nonselective mechanisms contribute significantly to vesicular traffic.

Although **sorting motifs** that direct protein trafficking through the endocytic pathway are understood in some detail (see Chapter 23), an understanding of those directing exit from the ER is just beginning to emerge. Analysis of the transport of the vesicular stomatitis virus glycoprotein (VSV-G) has revealed one type of export motif. VSV-G forms a coat on the outside of the viral membrane envelope. It is a type I transmembrane protein with a large domain initially in the lumen of the ER and eventually on the surface of the virus. VSV-G has a short cytoplasmic tail with a key tyrosine (Y) and a **diacidic motif,** aspartic acid-x-glutamic acid (DXE), where x can be any amino acid

VSV-G	TM–18aa–**Y**T**D**I**E**MNRLGK
CFTR (NBD1)	TM–212aa–**Y**K**D**A**D**LYLLD –287aaTM
GLUT4	TM–36aa–**Y**LG**PD**E**ND**
LDLR (prox. Yxxφ)	TM–17aa–**Y**QKTT**E**D**E**VHICH–20aa
CI-M6PR	TM–26aa–**Y**SKVSK**E**E**E**TDENE–127aa
E-cadherin	TM–95aa–**Y**DSLLVF**DY**EGSGS –42aa
EGFR	TM–58aa–**Y**KGLWIP**E**G**E**KVKIP–467aa
ASGPR H1	MTKE**Y**Q**D**L**QHLD**NEES–24aaTM
NGFR	TM–65aa–**Y**SSLPPAKR**EE**V**E**KLLNG–74aa
TfR	19aa–**Y**TRFSLARQV**D**G**D**NSHV–26aaTM

Figure 21-2 Examples of transmembrane proteins with tyrosine-linked diacidic ER exit codes (acidic-x-acidic) that direct their incorporation into COPII vesicles. ASGPRH1, asialoglycoprotein receptor; CFTR, cystic fibrosis transmembrane regulator; C1-M6PR, mannose 6-phosphate receptor; EGFR, epidermal growth factor receptor; GLUT4, a glucose carrier; LDLR, low density lipoprotein receptor; NGFR, nerve growth factor receptor; TfR, transferrin receptor; vsv-G, vesicular stomatitis virus glycoprotein.

(Fig. 21–2). Mutation of the aspartic acid and glutamic acid to alanine prevents export. Moreover, transfer of this sorting motif to a protein normally retained in the ER confers efficient export, demonstrating that it is sufficient to direct cargo to the export machinery. Diacidic motifs and tyrosines are present in the cytoplasmic tails of a number of type I transmembrane proteins, including those involved in signal transduction and cholesterol uptake at the cell surface (see Fig. 21–2). Thus, diacidic motifs appear to be a sorting code for one class of proteins. However, many other proteins lack diacidic motifs, so other signals must also direct export. A second group of signals may involve adjacent bulky hydrophobic residues in the cytoplasmic tail of cargo proteins.

How can a common budding machinery recognize different cytoplasmic signals? One possibility is that some budding components have multiple domains that interact with different signals. Alternatively, different sorting signals could engage a common transport machine by utilizing adaptor proteins. Adaptors could function by binding a specific class of cargo through one domain and the vesicular formation machinery through a second, thus serving as a link. One known example for ER export is the protein Rap, which binds low-density-lipoprotein–like receptors (LDL-R) during their biogenesis in the ER. Without Rap, LDL-R cannot exit the ER. Rap not only links LDL-R to the export machinery, but also prevents premature binding of lipoprotein particles that are also synthesized in the ER. Another class of adaptors is needed for export of soluble, secreted cargo molecules initially delivered to the lumen of the ER, as cytoplasmic budding machinery cannot directly detect proteins in the lumen. Here, transmembrane proteins are likely to function as adaptors. One example is the transmembrane protein ERGIC 53/58 that participates in the export of soluble coagulation factors. Individuals lacking ERGIC 53/58 fail to export coagulation factors V and VIII and suffer from a severe bleeding disorder. Although very little is understood at this time about how ER adaptors mediate export, later steps in the secretory and endocytic pathways use well-characterized, multidomain, protein complexes called adaptor proteins (APs) to mediate cargo selection and coat assembly (see Chapter 23).

Exclusion of Resident Cargo

The mechanism that excludes resident ER proteins from export vesicles remains to be clarified. A low level of leakage is dealt with by an efficient retrieval pathway—the COPI machinery (see the following section)—which captures both recycling transport machinery components and escaped resident proteins and returns them to their home base. However, the abundance of ER resident proteins compared to the more limited levels of this recycling machinery suggests that additional mechanisms may operate to en-

sure the general accuracy of ER export. One possibility is that resident ER proteins are tethered to a matrix that is too large to be recruited into a transport container. However, the fact that most resident ER proteins are very mobile within the lumen or the bilayer suggests that this may not contribute significantly to retention. Alternatively, proteins referred to as **fidelity factors** may be involved in protein sorting. Deletion of these abundant proteins leads to a striking increase in the release of ER resident proteins. One possible explanation is that these factors, which actively recycle between the ER and Golgi apparatus, generate a threshold for being recognized efficiently by the export machinery. Those falling below this threshold, such as resident ER proteins, are excluded during vesicular packaging in favor of the fidelity factors. The presence of both adaptors and fidelity factors suggests that both the exocytic and endocytic (see Chapter 23) pathways may consist of a network of signaling cascades that can adjust dynamically to the changing needs of the cell and tissues during development and proliferation, as well as in response to organismal physiology.

Step 2. COPII Vesicular Coat Assembly and Budding from the Endoplasmic Reticulum

Packaging of cargo into transport containers involves the **coat complex II (COPII)** coat machinery (Fig. 21–3). The small GTPase **Sar1** regulates the assembly of the COPII vesicular coat. Like other GTPases (see Chapter 27), Sar1 cycles between an inactive form with bound GDP and an active form with bound GTP. Sar1-GDP is cytoplasmic; Sar1-GTP binds membranes.

Assembly of a COPII coat begins when an ER membrane–associated **guanine nucleotide exchange factor (GEF)**, Sec12, activates Sar1 by promoting exchange of GDP for GTP. A hydrophobic motif at the N-terminus of Sar1 promotes recognition of Sec12. An unknown kinase regulates this step. Active Sar1-GTP then coordinates the recruitment of cargo molecules (through sorting motifs) and a cytosolic protein complex called Sec23/24. Recruitment of Sec23/24 stabilizes activated Sar1, cargo, and other membrane components into a larger protein assembly, the prebudding complex (see Fig. 21–3B). Formation of the prebudding complex is the first committed step in the assembly of the coat. Next, another cytosolic protein complex, Sec13/31, is recruited. This is thought to mediate further coat assembly by linking the cargo containing prebudding complexes into a more extensive molecular lattice, a process that drives membrane invagination to form a bud on the surface of the ER (see Fig. 21–3C). Following unknown steps that trigger reorganization of the lipid bilayer leading to membrane fission, the cargo-containing **COPII-coated transport container** is released into the cyto-

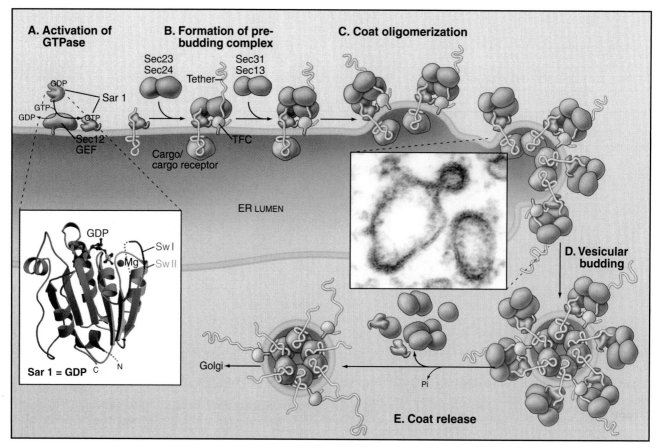

Figure 21–3 COPII vesicle budding from the ER. *A,* Activation of Sar1 to the GTP-bound form by Sec12 GEF. The inset shows a ribbon diagram of Sar1-GDP (PDB file: 1F6B). Sw1 is switch I; SwII is switch II. *B,* Sar1-GTP recruits cargo, vesicular tethering and fusion factors, and the Sec23/24 cytosolic coat component to form the "targeting fusion complex" (TFC). *C,* Prebudding complexes are assembled into a coat lattice through the activity of Sec13/31. *D,* The assembled coat leads to vesicular fission from the ER membrane. *E,* Following fission, the GAP activity of the Sec23/24-Sec13/31 complex returns Sar1 to the inactive GDP-bound form, resulting in disassembly of the coat lattice and release of Sar1, Sec23/24, and Sec13/31 into the cytoplasm. Cargo, tethering factors, and the TFC remain with the vesicle for transport to the Golgi apparatus. The electron micrograph of a thin section illustrates the formation of a typical COPII vesicle when ER membranes are incubated in a test tube with cytosol and ATP. (Courtesy of W. Balch, Scripps Research Institute, La Jolla, CA.)

plasm. Although isolated membranes usually form vesicles having a diameter of 60–80 nm, the COPII coat lattice may be quite flexible, as cells can form much larger tubular structures to accommodate large cargo molecules, such as lipoprotein particles or procollagen (see Chapter 31).

The final step in the budding cycle is to recycle coat components and to prepare the transport container for targeting to the acceptor compartment. Remarkably, uncoating is also triggered by the Sec23/24 complex, as it can function as a **GTPase-activating protein (GAP)** to trigger hydrolysis of GTP bound to Sar1 (see Fig. 21–3*E*). How or when Sec23/24 is converted from a coat assembly factor to a coat disassembly factor is not known, but this step may involve the Sec13/31 complex, the activity of which is sensitive to dephosphorylation and stimulates the GAP activity of Sec23/24. Importantly, coat release exposes targeting components recruited to the vesicle that direct the

vesicle to the acceptor compartment. The observation that receptors found on the cell surface can control cargo selection and budding from the ER suggests that signaling pathways originating outside the cell can control ER function.

Step 3. Vesicular Delivery

Components that direct delivery of a vesicle to the next compartment must be included during the formation of a cargo-containing transport container (see Fig. 21–3). Targeting is a daunting task given the myriad of exocytic and endocytic compartments in the cell. A "targeting complex" functions like a pilot with a specific set of directions to deliver the plane full of passengers to the proper destination. Of course, the destination must also have a unique identity. This identity is conferred by a **"docking complex."** It can recognize the incoming vesicle, thereby serving as a homing device. This process utilizes a complex set of evolutionarily conserved proteins at each step (Figs. 21–4 and 21–5).

Rab GTPases Regulate Assembly of the Delivery System

The **Rab** family of GTPases regulates vesicular delivery (see Fig. 21–4). They function as molecular switches to control the protein-protein interactions that direct the formation of targeting and docking complexes. Rab genes are conserved from yeast to humans, indicating that Rabs control an ancient biochemical process. Mammals express about 60 different Rab proteins to control the diversity of vesicle traffic in various cell types.

Rab proteins are post-translationally modified by two geranylgeranyl lipids at conserved cysteine residues found at their carboxyl termini (see Fig. 21–4). This modification is essential for function and facilitates Rab association with the membrane bilayer. The cysteines are included in a segment of 30 amino acids that vary between Rabs, and they direct each Rab to its correct subcellular location. Targeting and docking complexes assembled by different Rab GTPases generate molecular "zip codes" that specify traffic between compartments.

Rab proteins cycle between the cytoplasm, where they are found in the GDP-bound form, and membranes, where they contain bound GTP. In the cytoplasm, Rab is complexed to a carrier protein, referred to as **guanine nucleotide dissociation inhibitor (GDI),** that prevents exchange of GDP for GTP (see Fig. 21–4). GDI also sequesters the hydrophobic geranylgeranyl groups. During vesicular formation, Rab is recruited to the membrane where a Rab-specific GEF activates it by exchanging GDP for GTP. Activated Rab-GTP recruits the targeting and docking components that facilitate recognition and initiate bilayer fusion. Following fusion, a Rab-specific GAP stimulates GTP hydrolysis, recycling Rab-GDP back to the cytoplasm through binding to GDI. Thus, the **Rab-GTPase cycle** regulates the timing of the assembly and disassembly of multiprotein complexes involved in the trafficking of transport containers. Because each Rab protein functions at a different step of the exocytic and endocytic pathways, these proteins may also serve as fidelity factors for "proofreading" the accuracy of the docking/fusion step, ensuring delivery of cargo to the correct compartment.

Tethering Factors Direct Targeting and Docking of Transport Containers

One of the first steps in Rab function following activation to the GTP-bound form is recruitment of **tethering factors** (see Fig. 21–5). Two different Rab1 complexes participate in transport from the ER to the

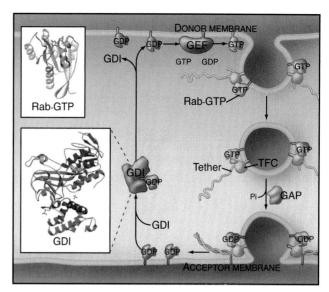

Figure 21–4 Rab-GTPase cycle. Rab GTPases in their GDP-bound form *(purple)* are complexed with GDI in the cytoplasm. Following delivery to the membrane, they are activated by a membrane-associated, Rab-specific GEF. In the GTP-bound form *(pink)*, they recruit tethering factors *(yellow icons)* and fusion factors *(green icons)* that direct the vesicle to the correct target compartment. During or after docking and fusion, Rab GTP is returned to the GDP-bound form by a GAP and recycled to the cytoplasm by GDI. Insets show ribbon diagrams of Rab GTP and GDI (PDB files 3RAB and 1D5T). Pi, inorganic phosphate.

Golgi apparatus. COPII vesicle identity is defined by recruiting the protein p115 to the membrane. The identity of the target compartment, in this case the Golgi apparatus, is established by recruiting GM130/GRASP65 to form the docking complex. These tethering factors are predicted to have long, extended, coil-coiled domains, regions commonly involved in protein recognition, that may serve in the initial recognition between a vesicle and its target. For example, when p115 and GM130/GRASP65 are in close proximity, they bind one another, thereby tethering the vesicle to the Golgi membrane (see Fig. 21–5). Other compartments contain different tethering factors dictated by their associated Rab GTPases.

SNARE Components Direct Late Events Preceding Fusion

Along with tethers, Rab GTPases promote the recruitment of SNAp REceptor **(SNARE)** proteins, which are involved in later steps of vesicular docking and fusion. SNAREs are a family of transmembrane proteins with a cytoplasmic domain containing a coiled-coiled region and small luminal domains (see Fig. 21–5). Members of the SNARE protein family were originally grouped according to whether they were v- or t-SNAREs, referring to whether they conferred function to the vesicle **(v-SNARE)** or target **(t-SNARE)** compartment. For example, synaptobrevin is a v-SNARE

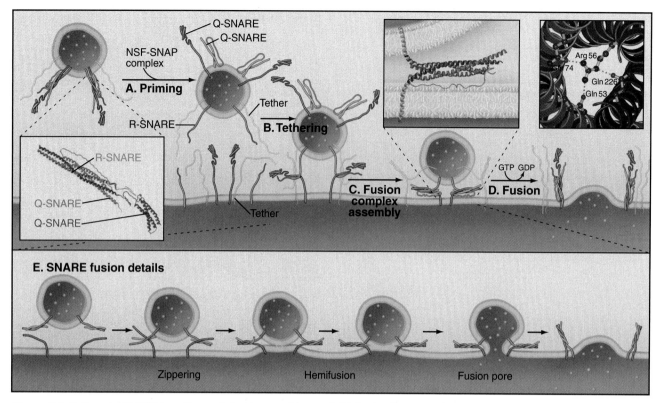

Figure 21-5 Generic SNARE targeting and docking machinery. *A,* Tethering factors and SNARE proteins form cis-SNARE complexes during vesicular formation. The lower left inset shows a ribbon diagram of a SNARE complex of a synaptic vesicle involved in neurotransmitter release involving R-SNARE (synaptobrevin, *blue*) and Q-SNARE (syntaxin, *red*) and SNAP-25 *(green)* SNARE. (PDB file:1SFC) *B* and *C,* Interaction of a vesicle with its target membrane through tethers results in the formation of trans-SNARE pairs involving extensive coiled-coiled regions of the interacting SNARE proteins. The middle inset shows the trans-SNARE pair. The upper right panel is a ribbon diagram looking down the coiled-coil, illustrating the critical Arg (arginine) residue of R-SNAREs that stabilizes interaction with glutamines (Gln) of Q-SNAREs forming the 4-helix bundle in a SNARE complex. *D,* Following trans-SNARE pairing, hydrolysis of GTP bound to Rab (not shown) leads to vesicle fusion. This results in the incorporation of the trans-SNARE pair into the bilayer of the target membrane where it and tethering complexes are disassembled for reuse. *E,* Overview of SNARE-mediated fusion. (*Top right inset,* Adapted from Ossig R, Schmitt HD, et al: Exocytosis requires asymmetry in the central layer of the SNARE complex. EMBO J 22:6000–6010, 2000, by permission of Oxford University Press.)

found on synaptic vesicles involved in neurotransmission, whereas syntaxin 1 is a t-SNARE found on presynaptic densities to which synaptic vesicles fuse to trigger neurotransmitter release (see Fig. 21–5; Chapter 23). Structural analysis shows that the four-helix bundle of SNAREs depends on interactions of an arginine from one helix with glutamines from three other helices (see Fig. 21–5). This requirement suggests an alternate classification of these proteins as either an R-SNARE or a Q-SNARE, based on the presence of these critical arginine (R) or glutamine (Q) residues.

During vesicular formation, a Rab GTPase recruits a unique subset of R- and Q-SNAREs that form a specific complex with one another through their coiled-coiled domains, a process referred to as cis-SNARE pairing (see Fig. 21–5). Members of the SNARE family, like Rabs, are localized to specific subcellular compartments, thus helping to define organelle identity and establish fusion pairs.

Following completion of budding, the cis-SNARE complex is disassembled by a ubiquitous AAA family adenosine triphosphatase (ATPase), **NSF** (for *N*-ethyl maleimide (NEM)–sensitive factor), so named because the sulfhydryl alkylating reagent NEM inactivates NSF and prevents all vesicular transport in the cell. NSF is recruited to the membrane by SNAP proteins. Disassembly of the vesicular cis-SNARE complex by NSF is believed to prime the vesicle for recognition of the target compartment. In order to identify incoming vesicles, the target compartment also forms a cis-SNARE pair.

When two like transport containers encounter each other, they undergo **"homotypic" fusion** through the interaction of identical cis-SNARE pairs. One example is the formation of pre-Golgi intermediates (Fig. 21–6). Frequently, ER export sites are located some distance from the Golgi apparatus in the peripheral cytoplasm. To facilitate transport, COPII vesicles are thought to undergo homotypic fusion to build larger vesicular-tubular structures that are trans-

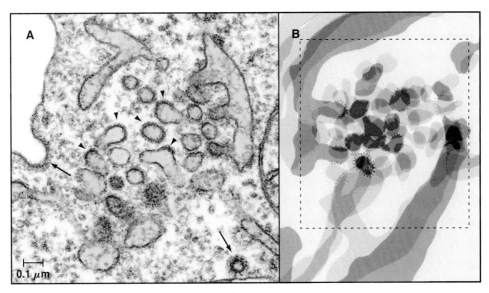

Figure 21-6 Assembly of pre-Golgi intermediates as ER export complexes. COPII vesicles *(blue)* generated at ER export sites undergo homotypic fusion to form pre-Golgi intermediates *(red)* that move en bloc to the central Golgi region. *A,* Electron micrograph of a thin cross section of a typical ER export complex containing a central vesicular-tubular cluster of pre-Golgi intermediates. ER is green, ER-associated buds are blue, pre-Golgi intermediates are red, arrowheads mark COPI coats, arrows mark clathrin-coated vesicles from the plasma membrane. *B,* Reconstruction from four consecutive serial-thin sections illustrating the three-dimensional organization of export complexes demarcated by the box. (From Bannykhl SI, Nishimura N, Balch WE: Getting into the Golgi. Trends Cell Biol 8:21–25, 1998. Copyright 1998, with permission from Elsevier Sciences.)

ported en bloc by a microtubule-dependent process (see Chapters 39 and 40) to the Golgi region.

In contrast, **heterotypic fusion** involves interaction between membranes with different compositions and, therefore, different cis-SNARE pairs, such as fusion of pre-Golgi intermediates with the cis-Golgi cisternae or Golgi-derived recycling vesicles. cis-SNARE proteins associated with the vesicle and target compartment participate in the docking through a process referred to as trans-SNARE pairing (see Fig. 21–5). The highly elongated tethering factors (p115 and GM130/GRASP65, in the case of ER-to-Golgi-apparatus transport) are thought to be critical in bringing the vesicle close enough to the target compartment for trans-SNARE pairing to occur. Tethering and SNARE pairing provide a universal mechanism for directing specific interactions between all intracellular compartments and their transport intermediates.

Step 4. The Mechanism of Bilayer Mixing During Fusion

Following Rab-regulated tethering and trans-SNARE pairing, the events culminating in vesicular fusion require reorganization of the lipid bilayer. Insights into this process have come from a variety of approaches.

Observation of Membrane Fusion in Real-Time

Membrane fusion can be detected by electrophysiological monitoring with a patch clamp (see Fig. 9–13A). Individual secretory granules (see Chapter 23) fusing with the plasma membrane cause the capacitance (a measure of surface area) to increase in a stepwise fashion (Fig. 21–7) owing to addition of membrane from the successive granules to the cell surface. Such electrophysiological studies demonstrate that fusion initially involves generation of a small, unstable pore that may open and close several times (flicker) before it dilates irreversibly and delivers its contents. Proteins comprising the docking/fusion complex and lipids in the pore regulate these flickering events.

Insights from Membrane Fusion Mediated by Viral Proteins

The mechanism used by viruses to invade eukaryotic cells has provided critical insights into the process of membrane fusion. Membrane-enveloped viruses, such as influenza (a major cause of respiratory infections), are internalized by the cell into acidic, endocytic compartments (see Chapter 23). Here, they fuse with the endosome membrane and release their genome into the cytoplasm for replication. Remarkably, the mechanism of fusion requires only one viral membrane glycoprotein, **hemagglutinin,** to carry out the fusion reaction (Fig. 21–8). Electrophysiological measurements show that hemagglutinin-induced fusion is slow relative to the vesicular fusion events, but it exhibits many of the same biophysical characteristics, such as flicker and pore conductance.

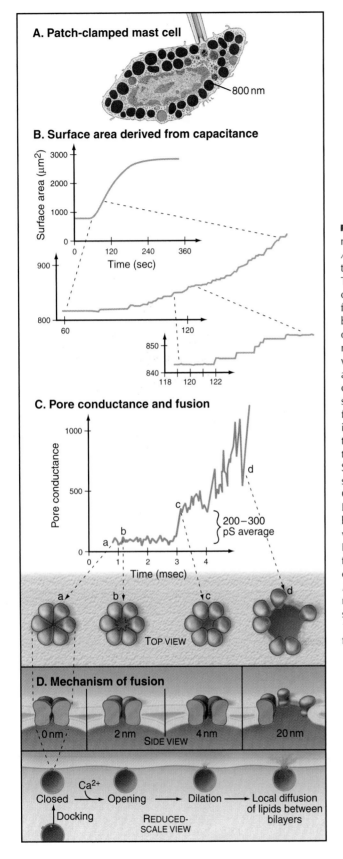

Figure 21-7 Electrophysiological recording of membrane fusion during secretion of mast cells. *A,* Drawing of a mast cell (see Chapter 30) attached to a whole-cell patch-clamp electrode. These cells have numerous secretory granules containing histamine. Extracellular stimuli trigger fusion of these vesicles with the plasma membrane and release of histamine. *B,* Microinjection of a stable analogue of GTP, GTP-γS, into the mast cell triggers fusion of individual granules with the plasma membrane. These fusion events are detected electrophysiologically as incremental changes in capacitance that reflect a change in surface area. *C,* At high-time resolution, rapid fluctuations in conductance can be detected during the fusion of a single vesicle. *D,* Illustration of the postulated molecular events during fusion. (*A* to *D,* References: Almers W, Breckenridge L, Spruce AE: The mechanism of exocytosis during secretion in mast cells. In Armstrong CM, Oxford GS (eds). Secretion and Its Control. New York: Rockefeller University Press, 1989, pp. 270–282, by copyright permission of the Rockefeller University Press. *B* and *C,* Redrawn from Spruce AE, Breckenridge LJ, Lee AK, et al: Properties of the fusion pore that forms during exocytosis of a mast cell secretory vesicle. Neuron 4:643–654, 1990. *D,* Redrawn from Almers W, Tse FW: Transmitter release from synapses: Does a preassembled fusion port initiate exocytosis? Neuron 4:813–818, 1990. *C* and *D,* Copyright 1990, with permission from Elsevier Science.)

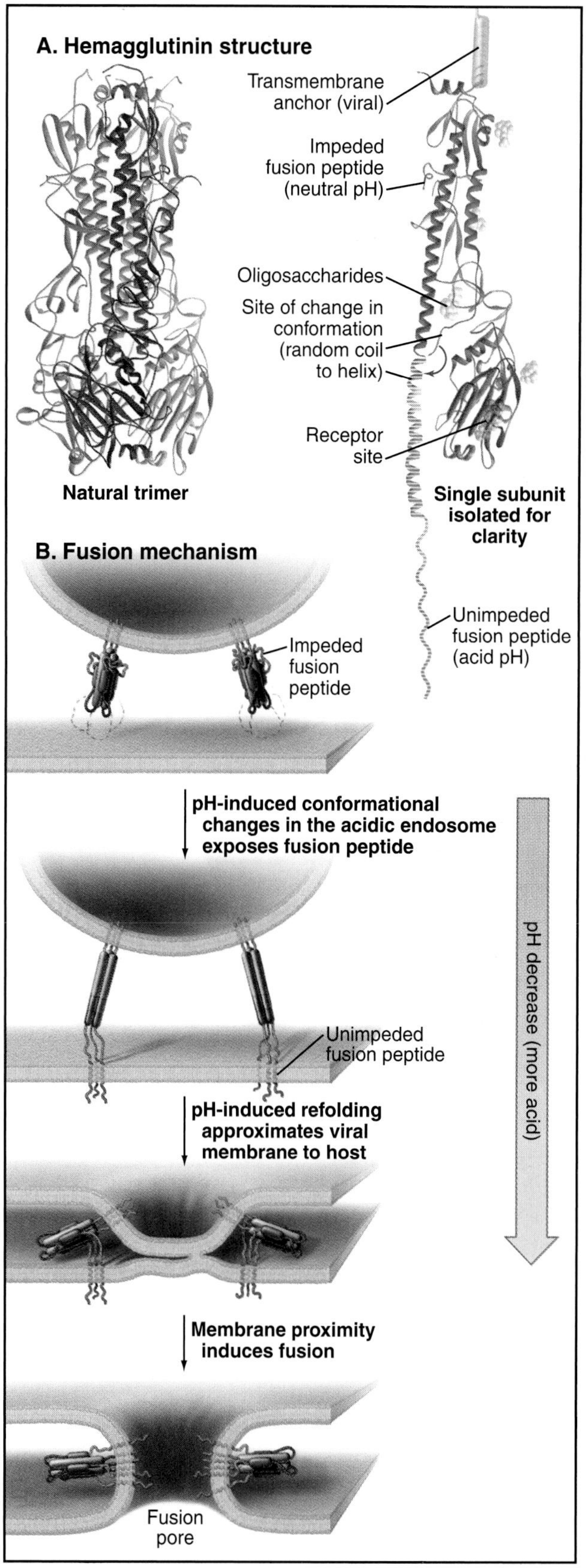

Figure 21-8 Virus-mediated fusion. *A (left),* The influenza virus hemagglutinin molecule is a trimer with the fusogenic peptide *(green)* buried in the core of the structure (PDB file: 4HMG). *A (right),* single subunit from a trimer, comparing the resting and acidic-activated structures. Acid causes a conformational change that releases the fusogenic peptide to interact with a target cell. *B,* Postulated fusion mechanism. The virus first binds sialic acid on the target cell surface. Upon exposure to acid pH (5–6) in the endosome, the trimer disassembles, exposing the fusion peptide that inserts into the lipid bilayer and facilitates bilayer fusion. (Adapted from Armstrong RT, Kushnir AS, White JM: The transmembrane domain of influenza hemagglutinin exhibits a stringent length requirement to support the hemifusion to fusion transition. J Cell Biol 151:425–437, 1998.)

Two key structural features of hemagglutinin are needed for fusion. The first is a nonpolar peptide that inserts into the target membrane. This peptide is normally buried in the structure of the hemagglutinin, which exists as a trimer in the viral coat at neutral pH. Brief exposure to acidic pH (5–6) completely rearranges the molecule, exposing the fusogenic peptide on the surface of the molecule. This peptide is believed to insert into the target bilayer to expedite intimate contact between the bilayers of the virus and the cell. A second feature of hemagglutinin-mediated fusion is that the transmembrane domain that is initially used to form the trimer at a neutral pH forms higher-order complexes with other hemagglutinin molecules upon insertion of the peptide into the bilayer. Following exposure to acid pH, these transmembrane domains build a fusion template that facilitates lipid rearrangements, leading to the assembly of a fusion pore.

None of the proteins that drive intracellular fusion (e.g., SNAREs) undergo folding changes that expose a fusogenic peptide like the viral hemagglutinin. However, trans-SNARE complexes can be embedded in artificial liposomes and will promote their fusion. The roles of the trans-SNARE pair complex and other proteins in the fusion event are being investigated.

■ Transport and Recycling in the Golgi Apparatus

Following export from the ER by COPII vesicles, cargo next appears in pre-Golgi intermediates that are delivered to the Golgi stack. A fundamental issue common to all transport steps is that the integral membrane proteins used to generate and target vesicles to the next compartment must be recycled. For example, during transport from the ER to the Golgi apparatus, SNAREs must be separated from cargo and recycled while the cargo moves forward through the Golgi stack. Moreover, resident proteins that accidentally escape the ER need to be returned.

Recycling of proteins from the Golgi apparatus to the ER is initiated in pre-Golgi intermediates and achieved by the activity of the **coat complex I (COPI;** Fig. 21–9). COPI components are unrelated to COPII coats involved in ER budding. It appears that COPI evolved as a novel solution to balance the forward movement of protein and lipid by forming vesicles that select and concentrate recycling components.

Composition of COPI Coats

The COPI coat found on the cytoplasmic face of pre-Golgi and Golgi compartments is assembled from a preformed hetero-oligomeric protein complex present in the cytoplasm and referred to as **coatomer.** At least six distinct cytosolic polypeptides, ranging in mass from 25 to more than 100 kD, assemble this stable complex. The coat lattice formed by the assembly of multiple coatomer subunits can be readily observed as it forms an electron-dense layer at the rims of Golgi compartments (see Fig. 21–9).

As in the assembly of COPII, COPI coat assembly depends on a small, soluble GTPase—in this case, **Arf1**—to regulate vesicle budding. Together, Arf and **Sar1** GTPases form a family with similar structures distinct from Rab family GTPases, suggesting that they evolved to perform specialized coat assembly functions. Arf proteins have a myristoyl group (see Fig. 6–9B) covalently attached to their N-terminus, rather than C-terminal prenyl groups like Rab GTPases. The myristoyl group is essential for function and facilitates initial attachment of Arf GTPases to the membrane bilayer.

Five different mammalian Arf proteins are believed to regulate COPI vesicle formation at different locales in the exocytic and endocytic pathways. Arf1 is critical for the assembly of COPI on pre-Golgi and early Golgi compartments. Arf1 activation is assisted by Golgi-associated GEFs that contain an evolutionarily conserved domain (referred to as the Sec7 domain). Like COPII, activation of Arf1 to the GTP-bound form leads to the recruitment of recycling cargo, tethering factors, and SNAREs into COPI vesicles (see Fig. 21–9). In addition to its role in COPI coat assembly, Arf1 also regulates the function of phospholipase D, a lipid-metabolizing enzyme, leading to modification of the lipid composition of the Golgi apparatus. Changes in the lipid composition of the Golgi apparatus alter the binding of many other peripheral Golgi-associated proteins, suggesting that both the protein and lipid compositions of COPI vesicles and the Golgi apparatus are tightly regulated to maintain normal function.

The toxic fungal metabolite **brefeldin A** inactivates Golgi-associated Arf1 GEF, thereby preventing Arf1 activation. This not only triggers loss of COPI coats from the Golgi apparatus but somehow also causes the complete collapse of the Golgi apparatus into the ER. This illustrates the vigorous retrograde traffic from the Golgi apparatus to the ER.

During or following completion of COPI coat assembly and vesicular fission, Arf-specific GAPs are believed to initiate coat disassembly (see Fig. 21–9). As GTP hydrolysis is linked to efficient recruitment of recycling cargo into COPI vesicles, Arf-specific GAPs, like the Sec23/24 GAP involved in ER export, may be integral components of the cargo selection machinery. Moreover, the SNARE machinery used in forward transport from the ER to the Golgi apparatus by COPII vesicles also participates in the generation of a novel combination of tethering and cis-SNARE complexes that direct COPI vesicles to the ER. Although this sec-

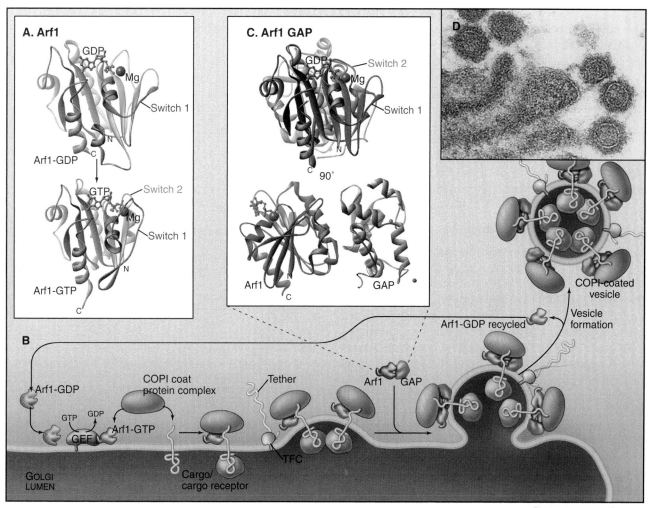

Figure 21-9 COPI-mediated retrograde retrieval from the Golgi apparatus. *A,* Ribbon diagrams of Arf1-GDP (PDB file: 1RRG) and Arf1-GTP (PDB file: 1HFV) showing the different conformations of the switch 1 and switch 2 segments. *B,* Activation of Arf1 to the GTP-bound form by the Sec7 domain of Arf1-specific GEFs results in the coupled recruitment of cargo, vesicle tethering factors, and fusion factors (the "targeting fusion complex" [TFC]) through binding of the cytoplasmic COPI coat complex. During or following fission, Arf1 is returned to the inactive GDP-bound form by the activity of Arf-specific GAPs, resulting in disassembly of the coat lattice and release of Arf1 and the COPI coat complex into the cytoplasm. Cargo, tethering factors, and fusion factors remain with the vesicle for targeting to the next compartment. *C,* Free Arf1 and Arf1 bound to its GAP. *D,* Electron micrograph of a thin section of a typical COPI-coated vesicle budding from the rim of a Golgi stack. (*C,* Courtesy of J. Goldberg, Memorial Sloan Kettering Cancer Center, New York. Reference: Goldberg J: Structural and functional analysis of the ARF1-ARFGAP complex reveals a role for coatomer in GTP hydrolysis. Cell 96:893–902, 1999. *D,* Adapted from Orci L, Perrelet A, Rothman JE: Vesicles on strings: Morphological evidence for processive transport within the Golgi stack. Proc Natl Acad Sci USA 95:2279–2283, 1998.)

tion has focused on the role of the well-characterized COPI retrieval pathway, increasing evidence suggests that COPI-independent recycling pathways also exist.

Signals Involved in Recycling

Incorporation of recycling cargo into COPI vesicles, like exit from the ER, requires a specific sorting motif. Generally, this is a **dilysine motif** in the form Lys-Lys-x-x-COOH (KKxx), where x is any amino acid, although it can also involve two arginine residues for

some proteins. Dilysine motifs are generally found at the cytoplasmic carboxyl terminus of transmembrane proteins. They function in retrieval of proteins from post-ER compartments by interacting with specific subunits of the COPI complex. Moreover, recruitment of proteins bearing the KKxx signal occurs in response to activation of Arf1 to the GTP-bound form.

A recycling signal for soluble (luminal) cargo also has been identified. The resident ER proteins—protein disulfide isomerase (PDI) and Bip—share a common C-terminus sequence: Lys-Asp-Glu-Leu-COOH (**KDEL**).

Bip lacking this sequence is slowly secreted from cells. The addition of KDEL to the carboxyl terminus of a protein that is normally secreted from the cell results in retention in the ER. KDEL-containing proteins that escape the ER are recycled by binding to a novel membrane receptor localized to the *cis* face of the Golgi apparatus (the KDEL receptor). The KDEL receptor, with bound KDEL protein, promotes COPI coat assembly, leading to efficient capture by COPI retrograde vesicles. The KDEL signal is both necessary and sufficient to maintain a molecule in the ER through this rapid **retrieval pathway.**

Movement of Cargo Through the Golgi Stack

The way in which the Golgi apparatus participates in the transport of biosynthetic cargo derived from the ER to the cell surface has been an enigma since its discovery by Camillo Golgi nearly a century ago. Although the Golgi apparatus is clearly composed of a stack of separate compartments with distinct compositions (see Chapter 20), the way that stacks are formed and maintained and the way in which biosynthetic cargo is transferred from stack to stack have not been clarified experimentally. One model proposes that each stack is a stable compartment with its own resident proteins, such as oligosaccharide-processing enzymes. The composition of each compartment is maintained by protein-protein interactions that prevent recruitment of resident proteins (e.g., oligosaccharide-processing enzymes) into vesicles that move biosynthetic cargo forward or recycling SNAREs that move backward through the stack. Another proposal is that COPI vesicles carry biosynthetic cargo forward through use of unknown sorting motifs or adaptor proteins.

An alternative model for Golgi function proposes that the stack is not composed of compartments with a fixed composition, but rather that each compartment is constantly changing in composition. This view emphasizes that the Golgi apparatus is a highly dynamic organelle and maintains itself through a process referred to as cisternal or directed maturation. In this model (see Fig. 21–10), the *cis* or first compartment of the Golgi apparatus is formed by homotypic fusion of pre-Golgi intermediates generated by COPII-coated transport containers exiting the ER. This new *(cis)* compartment is subsequently converted to *medial* and *trans* compartments by retrograde recycling of Golgi apparatus–processing enzymes (Fig. 21–10). The stacked appearance of the Golgi apparatus is, therefore, a consequence of constant input of new membrane from the ER at the *cis* or forming face, and the recycling of components from later compartments in the stack to generate the observed changes in composition in the *cis*-to-*trans* direction (see Chapter 20). The trans-most compartment may be derived, in part,

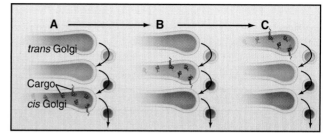

Figure 21–10 Directed-maturation model for transport of cargo through Golgi compartments. *A* to *C* represent successive time intervals showing the location and environment of a cisterna containing a pulse of transmembrane proteins *(red "lollipops")*. At every stage, recycling vesicles move *(curved arrows)* from more mature compartments at the top toward the cis-Golgi compartment at the bottom. The primary colors of the retrograde vesicles illustrate that they contain selected recycling components derived from particular levels of the stack. The gradient of processing enzymes and targeting components across the stack is shown by the mixture of primary colors defining each compartment. *A,* The *cis* compartment containing the pulse of red protein forms by homotypic fusion of vesicles from the ER. This compartment *(purple)* changes composition as it selectively sheds recycling components *(blue)* and receives vesicles containing processing enzymes *(red)* from a more mature cisterna. *B,* The cisterna with the pulse of protein is now in the middle of the stack *(orange)*. *C,* The pulse of protein is now in a trans-Golgi cisterna *(green)*. The Golgi apparatus maintains its structure while cargo is modified as the compartment in which it resides matures from being the *cis* to being the *trans* side of the stack. (Adapted from Allan BB, Balch WE: Protein sorting by directed maturation of Golgi compartments. Science 285:63–66, 1999. Copyright 1999, American Association for the Advancement of Science.)

from the endocytic pathway. Thus, the activity of different coat complexes, COPII in the forward direction directing ER export, and COPI or COPI-independent pathways in the backward direction contribute to balancing the flow of membrane through the early secretory pathway.

Role of the Cytoskeleton in ER-to-Golgi Transport

Molecular motors (see Chapters 39 and 40) assist in the movement of vesicular and tubular cargo containers from peripheral ER export sites to the central Golgi apparatus. These motors move along **microtubule** tracks originating from the microtubule-organizing center located near the Golgi apparatus. Movement of pre-Golgi intermediates toward the Golgi apparatus is mediated by the minus end directed motor, **dynein.** Motors also play a key role in dynamically maintaining the Golgi stack as a functional unit at the center of the cell. Depolymerizing microtubules with agents such as nocodazole results in rapid dispersal of Golgi compartments throughout the cell. The use of microtubules and motors to accelerate the movement of transport containers solved an important traffic problem, as large distances (ranging from micrometers in polarized epithelial cells to meters in the axon) may separate the site of cargo biogenesis in the ER from its final site of residency.

Interruption of Vesicular Traffic During Mitosis

During redistribution of organelles to daughter cells in mitosis, exocytic and endocytic vesicular trafficking is disrupted. Both the ER and Golgi apparatus appear as numerous smaller structures that reassemble upon exit from mitosis. Disassembly of the ER is likely to occur through activation of membrane fission machinery triggering fragmentation. The mechanism of Golgi apparatus disassembly is controversial (see Chapter 47). One model proposes that the Golgi apparatus rapidly collapses back into the ER, similar to the effects of brefeldin A, thus utilizing the ER fragmentation pathway to disassemble. A second model suggests that the Golgi apparatus fragments independently. This occurs in response to both disassembly of the microtubule network and inhibition of COPI vesicular fusion, thereby leading to the accumulation of Golgi-derived vesicles. In either case, reassembly involves the known components of the tethering and SNARE machinery involved in forward transport and a new group of NSF-related factors. Overall, the cycle of assembly and disassembly of exocytic compartments during mitosis is likely to be controlled by cell cycle–dependent kinases and phosphatases that regulate division of the genome (see Chapter 43).

▌ Selected Readings

Allan BB, Balch WE: Protein sorting by directed maturation of Golgi compartments. Science 285:63–66, 1999.

Bannykh S, Nishimura N, Balch WE: Getting into the Golgi. Trends Cell Biol 8:21–25, 1998.

Hauri HP, Kappeler F, Andersson H, Appenzeller C: ERGIC-53 and traffic in the secretory pathway. J Cell Sci 113:587–596, 2000.

Jahn R, Sudhof TC: Membrane fusion and exocytosis. Annu Rev Biochem 68:863–911, 1999.

Skehel JJ, Wiley DC: Receptor binding and membrane fusion in virus entry: The influenza hemagglutinin. Annu Rev Biochem 69:531–569, 2000.

Springer S, Spang A, Schekman R: A primer on vesicle budding. Cell 97:145–148, 1999.

Steyer JA, Almers W: A real-time view of life within 100 nm of the plasma membrane. Nature Rev Mol Cell Biol 2:268–275, 2001.

Waters MG, Pfeffer SR: Membrane tethering in intracellular transport. Curr Opin Cell Biol 11:453–459, 1999.

Wieland F, Harter C: Mechanisms of vesicle formation: Insights from the COP system. Curr Opin Cell Biol 11:440–446, 1999.

Zerial M, McBride H: Rab proteins as membrane organizers. Nature Rev Mol Cell Biol 2:107–117, 2001.

chapter 22

TRANS-GOLGI NETWORK AND BEYOND

The preceding chapters have described how newly synthesized proteins are transported along a biosynthetic assembly line that initiates in the endoplasmic reticulum (ER). Here, proteins fold, form oligomers, and are modified before passing through the Golgi complex for further modification and processing. A "quality-control" checkpoint ensures that exit from the ER and access to the Golgi apparatus is restricted to properly folded and assembled proteins. To a large extent, resident ER proteins are also denied exit, but those that escape are reclaimed by COPI-coated vesicles that mediate recycling prior to and upon arrival at the cis-Golgi apparatus. All newly synthesized proteins that pass inspection proceed through the Golgi complex even if they are not substrates for further processing. But most receive similar sorts of post-translational modifications before being shipped to their individual destinations. Successful passage through the Golgi complex brings the near-final products to the **trans-Golgi network** (TGN), the major distribution center, where they are packaged and sent to different destinations along branching pathways.

This chapter describes the complex organization of the TGN and the distinct intracellular itineraries that emanate from it. The TGN is the first major sorting station along the biosynthetic pathway; therefore, the several mechanisms that operate at the TGN to effect the accurate delivery of divergent cargo to distinct intracellular destinations are considered here in some detail. These mechanisms provide the paradigm for membrane-sorting events at other intracellular locations. Distribution of cargo molecules—either integral membrane proteins or soluble proteins sequestered within the lumen of the TGN—occurs in membrane-

bound containers that maintain the topology of the protein originally established upon translocation into the ER. Although many components of the cargo selection machinery that directs vesicular formation, targeting, and fusion are specific for certain organelles and pathways, the basic mechanisms, described in Chapter 21 for ER-to-Golgi-apparatus trafficking are shared at the TGN and beyond.

Organization of the Trans-Golgi Network

The TGN is an interconnecting network of membranous tubules and associated vesicles located adjacent to the trans-most cisterna of the Golgi apparatus proper. It is recognized as a distinct compartment by its content of resident membrane proteins, such as TGN-38, which are localized at sites distinct from the Golgi markers, such as giantin (Fig. 22–1) or galactosyltransferase. However, it should be noted that the functional boundary between the TGN and the preceding Golgi cisternae is not an abrupt one; there is clear evidence that activities involved in terminal glycosylation (e.g., sialyltransferase) and sulfation spill over from the Golgi into the TGN. Further, experimental evidence has shown that, if exit of cargo from the TGN is impeded, the trans-Golgi cisterna can contribute membrane surface area to the TGN, suggesting that their interrelationship is rather plastic.

The TGN's tubulovesicular organization (Fig. 22–2) is characteristic of sorting compartments, such as ER-Golgi intermediate compartments (see Chapter 21) and sorting endosomes (see Chapter 23). This is the steady-state appearance of a compartment that continuously deploys (and receives) vesicular carriers of various kinds while maintaining the bulk of its membrane in tubules that have relatively little internal volume.

Chapter by Sandra L. Schmid, based on an original draft by Ann L. Hubbard, J. David Castle, and Pat Shipman.

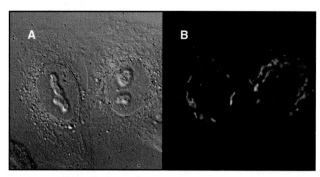

Figure 22-1 Fluorescence micrographs illustrating the morphologic distinction of the Golgi apparatus and the trans-Golgi network (TGN). The cells were stained with a green fluorescent antibody to giantin, a Golgi resident protein, and a red fluorescent antibody to TGN46, a marker of the TGN. *A,* Superimposition of the fluorescence with a differential interference contrast image showing cell outlines, nucleus, and organelles. *B,* Fluorescence micrograph of the same field. The Golgi apparatus and TGN are closely opposed, but resolved. (Courtesy of A. Prescott and S. Ponnambalam, University of Dundee, Scotland.)

Also consistent with its role as a sorting station, budding profiles with morphologically distinct coats are abundant on the TGN (see Fig. 22–2). There is now evidence for at least four different kinds of coats: coats with AP1 and clathrin, coats with AP3- or AP4 that operate independently of clathrin, and caveolin-containing coats (see Chapter 37). A lace-like coat of undefined composition has also been detected in electron micrographs. All are distinct from the COPI- and COPII-containing coats that function in retrograde and anterograde ER-Golgi transport. Each coat presumably packages a specific subset of proteins for delivery to a unique intracellular destination. Whether cytoplasmic coats are required for formation of all types of TGN-derived vesicles, particularly secretion granules, is not known. Moreover, it is not known whether certain (perhaps distinct) coats are needed to maintain the organization and positioning of the TGN itself.

Trafficking Itineraries from the Trans-Golgi Network

Depending on the cell type, the cargo that arrives in the TGN can be distributed, via distinct transport carriers, to several different intracellular locations (Fig. 22–3). Coated vesicles transport hydrolytic enzymes and integral membrane glycoproteins to the lysosome via early or late endosomes, or both. To varying degrees, some lysosomal membrane glycoproteins take the "scenic route," traveling via the plasma membrane before delivery to lysosomes along the endocytic pathway. In polarized cells, integral membrane proteins and secreted molecules can be packaged into distinct vesicles and transported directly to either the apical or basolateral domains of the plasma membrane. Regulated secretory cells, such as endocrine or exocrine cells, and neurons package secretory proteins into large, dense-core granules that accumulate in the cytosol and fuse with the plasma membrane only upon stimulation. The intracellular itinerary taken by each protein depends on **sorting signals** encoded in the polypeptide chain.

Sorting and packaging into distinct classes of transport vesicles occurs by three mechanisms that function alone or in combination:

- *Sorting based on protein motifs* involves the recognition of linear arrays of amino acids and/or carbohydrate molecules by components of the sorting machinery. The cytoplasmic sorting machinery can interact directly with so-called **sorting signals** located on the cytoplasmic domain of membrane proteins, like the recognition of the KKxx motif on the cytoplasmic tail of resident ER proteins by components of the COPI coat (see Chapter 20). Luminal proteins must interact with the cytoplasmic sorting machinery indirectly: for example, KDEL sequences on intraluminal ER resi-

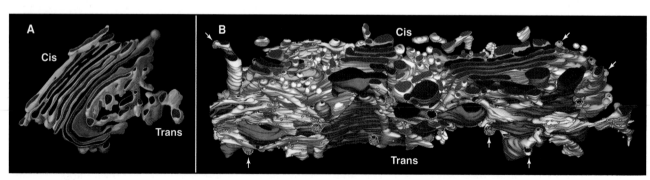

Figure 22-2 Three-dimensional reconstructions of a mammalian Golgi apparatus and TGN generated by tomography of high-voltage electron micrographs of serial thick sections taken at multiple tilt angles. *A,* Simplified view of a Golgi stack and the TGN on the Trans side. *B,* Detailed view showing many small (probably COPI-coated) vesicles *(arrows* on cis side, blue coats) budding from the edges of the cisternae at all levels of the stack. Large clathrin-coated vesicles *(arrows,* on Trans side, yellow coats) can be seen budding only from the TGN *(red).* (Courtesy of M. Landisky, J. R. McIntosh, and K. Howell, University of Colorado, Boulder.)

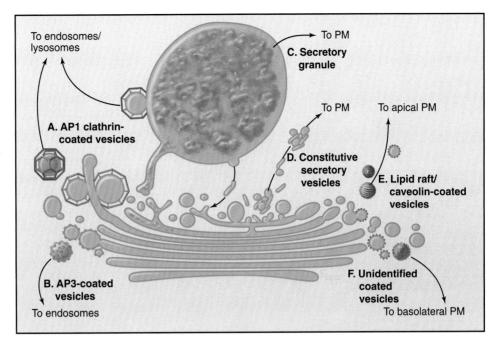

To endosomes/ lysosomes

A. AP1 clathrin- coated vesicles

C. Secretory granule

To PM

To PM

To apical PM

D. Constitutive secretory vesicles

E. Lipid raft/ caveolin-coated vesicles

B. AP3-coated vesicles

To endosomes

F. Unidentified coated vesicles

To basolateral PM

Figure 22-3 Divergence of bio-synthetic/exocytic cargo at the TGN. *A–F,* Cargo destined for secretion or distinct intracellular locations is sorted and pack-aged into distinct transport vesi-cles. The tubular/vesicular ge-ometry of the TGN plays a role in protein sorting. PM, plasma membrane.

dent proteins are recognized by the transmem-brane KDEL receptor whose cytoplasmic tail is, in turn, recognized by the COPI sorting machinery (see Chapter 20).

- *Sorting based on physical properties* is used to package classes of proteins into a transport vesi-cle. For example, membrane proteins that share a propensity for association with a specific lipid species and/or cholesterol are partitioned into subdomains of the membrane, referred to as **lipid rafts** (see Fig. 6–7), that form vesicles targeted to discrete domains on the plasma membrane. The shared tendency of secretory proteins to aggregate in the slightly acidic environment of the TGN fa-cilitates their packaging into large secretory gran-ules that emerge from the TGN, and prevents their inclusion into smaller transport vesicle or tubules.

- *Sorting based on geometric considerations* occurs in proportion to the relative surface-to-volume ra-tio of the transport vesicle or tubule and the sort-ing compartment. Many sorting compartments, such as the TGN, endosomes, and ER-Golgi inter-mediate compartments, have a characteristic tubu-lovesicular structure. Tubular portions of sorting compartments have a high surface-to-volume ratio, whereas vacuolar portions have minimal surface-to-volume ratios. Based on geometric considera-tions alone, luminal content will collect in the vol-ume-rich vacuolar portions of the sorting compartment, whereas membrane-bound content will partition along the tubular portions. Often, the tubular regions of sorting compartments are in-volved in membrane recycling while the vacuolar regions deliver their luminal cargo to the next des-

tination. When coupled to selective mechanisms of retention or exclusion from tubular or vacuolar regions, these geometric considerations can effect efficient sorting.

Proteins often encode more than one sorting mo-tif, which, in combination with the protein's physical properties in distinct intraluminal environments, can dictate a complex intracellular itinerary determined by the hierarchy of interactions and recognition events at distinct intracellular locations. Few, if any, sorting events are 100% effective in a single round. Instead, the complex itineraries traveled by many membrane proteins allow multiple sorting events to be coupled in series to effect overall efficient sorting. In this process, termed **iterative sorting,** the sequential sorting effi-ciencies are cumulative. If sorting is 90% efficient at each stage and there are three sequential stages of sorting, the overall process becomes 99.9% efficient (i.e., the fraction of mis-sorted receptors will be $0.1 \times 0.1 \times 0.1$, or 0.001 after three rounds of sorting). Specific examples of these iterative sorting events and the intracellular itineraries followed by newly synthe-sized proteins as they leave the TGN are presented in the sections that follow.

Lysosomal Biogenesis

Perhaps the best characterized example of motif-based sorting is the delivery of hydrolytic enzymes from the TGN to the lysosome by the **mannose-6-phosphate receptors** (MPRs). Lysosomes are the comprehensive digestive centers of the cell (see Chapter 24), and their

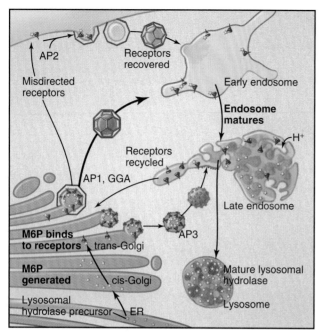

Figure 22–4 Sorting pathways used by mannose 6-phosphate receptors. These receptors carry newly synthesized lysosomal hydrolases from the TGN, via endosomes, to lysosomes, after which they return to the TGN. Receptors mis-sorted to the cell surface are recovered by endocytosis and returned to the pathway in endosomes.

function requires the efficient sorting and delivery of a large and diverse collection of hydrolytic enzymes. MPRs are integral membrane proteins with a single transmembrane domain. The luminal domain binds individual prohydrolase molecules, whereas the cytoplasmic domain encodes sorting motifs that interact with the sorting machinery that directs packaging into

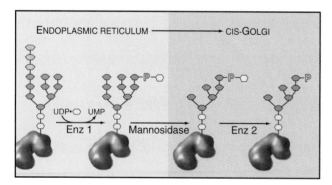

Figure 22–5 Recognition of specific structural motifs on lysosomal hydrolases. Enzyme 1 (UDP-GlcNAc-1-phosphotransferase) transfers a phospho-GlcNAc residue to the oligosaccharide chain as the protein is transported from the ER to the Golgi apparatus. In the cis-Golgi complex, mannosidases trim the mannose core, and enzyme 2 (GlcNAc-1-phosphodiester β-N-acetylglucosaminidase) generates terminal mannose 6-phosphates for recognition by mannose 6-phosphate receptors. UDP, uridine diphosphate; UMP, uridine monophosphate.

carrier vesicles as they leave the TGN destined for endosomes. After MPRs discharge their cargo, other vesicles carry the unoccupied MPRs back from the endosome to the TGN (Fig. 22–4). The two MPRs are distinguished by their size and cation dependence for ligand binding. The 215-kD cation-independent receptor and the 46-kD cation-dependent receptor appear to be functionally redundant with regard to lysosomal biogenesis.

Lysosomal hydrolases are synthesized as enzymatically inactive, higher-molecular-weight precursors, called **prohydrolases.** Importantly, these prohydrolases are glycosylated and, as for other secretory and membrane glycoproteins (see Chapter 20), their N-linked oligosaccharides are processed by the trimming of glucose and mannose residues within the ER. However, upon transport to an early Golgi site, prohydrolases become the unique substrates for two enzymes that act sequentially to generate the lysosomal targeting signal (Fig. 22–5). The first enzyme, uridine diphosphate (UDP)-N-acetylglucosamine (GlcNAc)-1-phosphotransferase, recognizes the prohydrolase through interactions with a patch of noncontiguous amino acid residues located some distance away from the carbohydrate chains on the prohydrolase surface. This enzyme modifies the carbohydrate chains of the

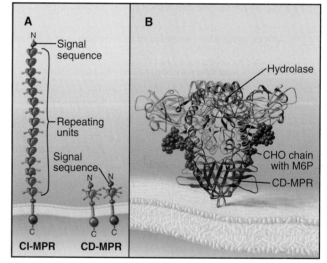

Figure 22–6 Two classes of mammalian mannose 6-phosphate receptors (MPRs). A, The large receptor, consisting of several repeating units, binds ligands independent of cations (CI-MPR). Binding to the small receptor requires cations (CD-MPR). B, Crystal structure of two subunits of the lysosomal hydrolase, β-glucuronidase, bound to the small MPR through interactions with mannose 6-phosphate (M6P) residues and its carbohydrate (CHO) chain (Reference: Olson LJ, Zhang J, Lee YC, et al: Structural basis for recognition of phosphorylated high mannose oligosaccharides by the cation-dependent MPR. J Biol Chem 274:29889–29896, 1999. PDB file: 1C39.)

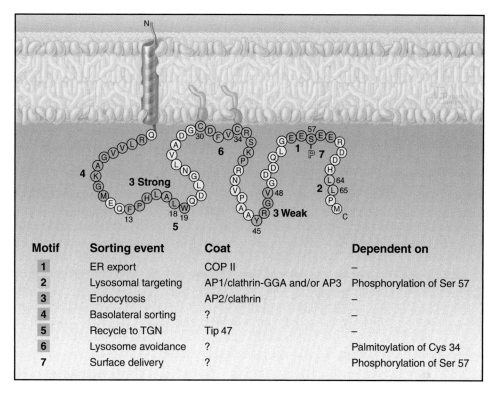

Figure 22-7 Sorting signals in the cytoplasmic domain of MPRs. A hierarchy of sorting signals directs the complex intracellular itinerary. Each signal interacts with specific components of the cargo-selecting and vesicle-forming machinery that direct sorting and targeting decisions. Luminal domains are not shown at the N-terminus.

Motif	Sorting event	Coat	Dependent on
1	ER export	COP II	—
2	Lysosomal targeting	AP1/clathrin-GGA and/or AP3	Phosphorylation of Ser 57
3	Endocytosis	AP2/clathrin	—
4	Basolateral sorting	?	—
5	Recycle to TGN	Tip 47	—
6	Lysosome avoidance	?	Palmitoylation of Cys 34
7	Surface delivery	?	Phosphorylation of Ser 57

prohydrolases by adding GlcNAc phosphate to the 6-position of one or more terminal mannose residues. The second enzyme—GlcNAc-1-phosphodiester β-N-acetylglucosaminidase—then hydrolyzes the GlcNAc-P bond to generate terminal **mannose 6-phosphates,** which are the ligands for sorting.

After reaching the TGN, the mannose 6-phosphate residues bind to the luminal domain of an MPR (Fig. 22–6), which directs their packaging into appropriate transport vesicles. The cation-dependent-MPR is the prototypic sorting receptor, built for efficiency. It provides an excellent example of the hierarchy of sorting signals that operate by backing each other up and ultimately ensuring the efficient intracellular sorting and delivery of potentially harmful hydrolytic enzymes to the lysosome (Fig. 22–7).

Prolysosomal hydrolases captured by the MPR are diverted from the secretory pathway by efficient packaging into clathrin-coated vesicles that bud from the TGN. **Clathrin-coated vesicles** were first discovered in the context of receptor-mediated endocytosis from the plasma membrane; therefore, their structure and function are discussed more extensively in Chapter 23. Their major coat constitutents are **clathrin,** which forms a polyhedral lattice, and heterotetrameric **adapter protein (AP)** complexes, which trigger clathrin assembly on the target membrane (Fig. 22–8). Distinct subunits of the adaptor complexes function to recognize sorting motifs on the cytoplasmic tails of cargo

molecules and to target clathrin assembly onto distinct intracellular membranes. AP2 complexes direct clathrin assembly onto the plasma membrane, whereas AP1 complexes direct clathrin assembly onto the TGN and interact directly with either tyrosine-based or dileucine sorting motifs on the MPR receptor tail. Evidence suggests that the MPR might facilitate the recruitment and assembly of AP1-containing clathrin coat on the TGN

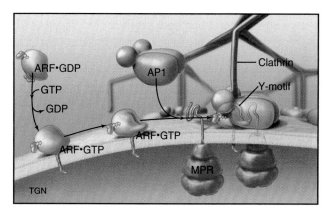

Figure 22-8 Coordination of coat assembly and cargo recruitment at the TGN. An exchange factor activates the small GTPase Arf to bind GTP, which triggers recruitment of AP1 coat constituents to the TGN membrane. AP1, in turn, recruits clathrin to deform the membrane. The MPR is concentrated in the emerging coated vesicle through interactions between a tyrosine-based sorting motif in its cytoplasmic domain and the μ-subunit of AP1.

through direct interaction with the same small guanosine triphosphatase (GTPase)—**Arf1**—that also triggers COPI assembly (see Chapter 20). The assembly of the clathrin-AP1 coat drives receptor clustering and invagination of the TGN membrane to form clathrin-coated transport vesicles. Several lysosomal membrane proteins are also captured in clathrin-coated vesicles by virtue of tyrosine-based sorting motifs within their own cytoplasmic domains.

AP1-containing, clathrin-coated vesicles deliver their cargo of MPR and lysosomal hydrolases to early and/or late endosomes en route to lysosomes (see Fig. 22–4). These recognition and fusion events are mediated by endosome-specific components of the **v-SNARE** and **t-SNARE** families (see Chapter 21) and a **Rab-family GTPase.** The generation of phosphatidylinositol-3-phosphate on endosomal membranes by a phosphatidylinositol-3-kinase is also believed to be important for recruiting components of the fusion machinery to the endosome. A vacuolar proton pump (see Chapter 7) acidifies the lumen of the endosomes and lysosomes to varying degrees, creating a pH gradient from early endosomes (mildly acidic, pH 6–6.5) to late endosomes (pH 5–5.5) to lysosomes (pH 4.5–5). The interior of late endosomes is sufficiently acidic to cause the release of prohydrolases from the MPR into the vacuolar portions of late endosomes. Late endosomes are often referred to as **multivesicular** or **multilamellar bodies** because they contain an elaborate system of intraluminal membranes contiguous with their limiting membrane. Lysosomal membrane glycoproteins localize to the limiting membrane, while sorting motifs within the MPRs localize them to the intraluminal membranes.

A diaromatic motif (FW) in the CD-MPR (Fig. 22–7) is recognized by a cytosolic protein, Tip47, and is required for recycling back to the TGN. Phosphorylation of serine residues activates specific sorting signals on the MPR tail, allowing for recognition by the sorting adaptor PACS-1, which controls cycling between the endosome and the TGN and, perhaps between sorting endosomes and the plasma membrane. However, neither the coat proteins nor the carrier vesicles that recycle MPRs back to the TGN have been identified.

Intracellular sorting steps are never 100% efficient, and, in fact, ~10% of MPR is delivered to the plasma membrane. An endocytic sorting motif in the cytoplasmic tail (see Fig. 22–7) efficiently directs the MPR from the plasma membrane into the endocytic pathway (see Chapter 23) for eventual return from endosomes to the TGN. Additional sorting motifs in the MPR cytoplasmic domain may also ensure its efficient sorting to endosomes. For example, a dileucine motif may be recognized by AP3 complexes to package

MPR into clathrin-independent transport vesicles for targeting directly to late endosomes. Finally, new adaptor molecules called GGAs (Golgi-localized, γ-ear-containing, ARF-binding proteins) have recently been identified. GGAs recognize an acidic cluster in combination with the dileucine motif on the MPR to direct its efficient packaging into transport vesicles. GGAs may work alone or in combination with AP1 to increase the efficiency of sorting into clathrin-coated vesicles.

Currently, it is thought that the vacuolar portion of the late endosome or prelysosome progressively matures into a lysosome. However, fusion events between late endosomes and preexisting lysosomes, as well as among lysosomes themselves, have been documented. The details of these maturation/fusion events are not yet clear. Proteolytic activity within the lysosomes or late endosomes cleaves the prosequences to activate the hydrolases; phosphate groups are removed from the mannose residues; and the mature hydrolases are ready for action.

Lysosomal Storage Diseases

Research on human diseases has provided many insights into lysosome formation. A number of devastating lysosomal storage diseases occur when a patient has mutations in both copies of a gene encoding one of the many lysosomal hydrolases (see Table 24–1). The consequence is that undigested products accumulate in and disrupt the normal function of lysosomes, eventually leading to cell death (see Chapter 24). Death of neurons in the brain leads to mental retardation, and affected patients usually die in childhood.

Landmark studies using cultured cells from patients with lysosomal deficiencies have shown that, if the missing enzymes were provided in the media, they would bind to cell surface MPR and be taken up and delivered to lysosomes via receptor-mediated endocytosis (see Chapter 23). Although it is not feasible to cure these diseases using this strategy, this observation led researchers to identify the mannose 6-phosphate ligand and, subsequently, the MPRs.

Other (rare) patients with **inclusion cell (I-cell) disease,** also known as mucolipidosis type II, produce all of the hydrolases but fail to deliver them to lysosomes. Instead, the hydrolases are secreted, and undegraded substrates accumulate in the hydrolase-deficient lysosomes. The defective enzyme in I-cell disease is GlcNAc-1-phosphotransferase, the initiator of the targeting process for prohydrolases (see Fig. 22–5). Interestingly, lysosomal targeting is defective in many, but not all, cell types from patients with I-cell disease, suggesting the existence of an alternative targeting mechanism.

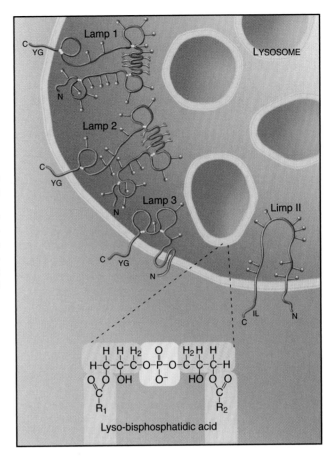

Figure 22-9 Major components of the lysosomal membrane. The schematic drawing shows the transmembrane topology of two related proteins (Lamp 1 and Lamp 2), a bi-span protein (Limp II), and a tetraspan protein (Lamp 3). Each is highly glycosylated, but their functions remain undefined. The unusual lipid species, lyso-bisphosphatidic acid, is highly enriched in the internal membranes of the lysosome and may play a role in restricting the hydrolytic activity of lipases to these membranes.

Lysosomal Membranes

Lysosomal membranes have an unusual phospholipid content that includes cholesterol and a unique lipid with two linked glycerol backbones and two acyl chains, called **lyso-bisphosphatidic acid** (Fig. 22–9). This lipid is highly enriched in the intraluminal membranes of late endosomes and lysosomes and may play a role in creating a lipid subdomain that facilitates protein sorting or lipid turnover, or both. There

is little information regarding the source of this unusual lipid.

Integral membrane proteins are densely concentrated in the lysosomal membrane. Pumps and transporters are present in the lysosomal membrane, but by far, the most abundant proteins are acidic, type I membrane proteins with multiple N-linked oligosaccharide chains (see Fig. 22–9; Table 22–1). Together, these properties are important in maintaining their resistance to degradation by lysosomal proteases. Sorting

table 22-1					
INTEGRAL PROTEIN OF LYSOSOME MEMBRANES					
Lysosomal Constituent	Synonyms/ Homologues	Molecular Weight (kD)	Polypeptide Size	Carbohydrate Content	Lysosomal Sorting Motif
Lamp 1	Limp III (rat) 1gp120 (rat) LEP100 (chicken)	90–120	382–396 aa	55%–65% 17–20 N-linked + O-linked	GY
Lamp 2	Limp IV (rat) 1gp110 (rat)	95–120	380–389	55%–65% 16–17 N-linked + O-linked	GY
Lamp 3	CD63 Limp I	30–55	238	3 N-linked	GY
Limp II	1gp85 (rat)	60–85	478	11 N-linked	IL

motifs, in their often short cytoplasmic C-terminal domains, are recognized by AP1 or AP3 complexes for packaging at the TGN into transport vesicles and targeting to endosomes/lysosomes. A variable proportion of lysosomal membrane glycoproteins are first delivered to the plasma membrane before arrival at lysosomes via the endocytic pathway (see Chapter 23). The extent to which newly synthesized lysosomal membrane glycoproteins travel transiently to the cell surface en route to lysosomes, or proceed more directly to their destination, depends on the protein, but this can be manipulated by varying the amount of protein synthesized. Experimental overexpression of one type of protein leads to the appearance of both this and other lysosomal membrane glycoproteins on the cell surface. This suggests that the different membrane proteins use a common sorting machinery, and that the intracellular sorting capacity can be saturated. Again, the relative strength of interactions between a sorting motif and the sorting machinery is likely to dictate the intracellular itinerary followed by a given membrane protein.

Constitutive Transport from the Trans-Golgi Network to the Plasma Membrane

Secretion is a constitutive activity of most cells, as is the biosynthesis and turnover of resident plasma membrane proteins and lipids. These activities result in a steady stream of both proteins and lipids from the TGN to the cell surface. Removal of retention signals from ER or Golgi proteins leads to the gradual secretion or delivery of these proteins to the plasma membrane. Similarly, although the rate of export from the ER is affected (see Chapter 21), removal of sorting signals from the cytoplasmic domain of integral plasma membrane proteins has little effect on their subsequent delivery from the TGN to the plasma membrane. Thus, it appears that cargo molecules moving from the TGN to the plasma membrane are not selectively packaged and concentrated into constitutively secreted transport vesicles. Consistent with this, no known coat proteins have been identified that function in the formation of these vesicles. Recent studies, using newly synthesized tagged proteins with green fluorescent protein (GFP), have suggested that membrane tubules, rather than small vesicles, carry cargo from the TGN to the plasma membrane. These tubules would have a higher surface-to-volume ratio than vesicles and could account for high rates of transport of bulk membrane markers from the TGN to the plasma membrane. One possibility is that, after selected proteins have been removed from the TGN and diverted to other intracellular destinations, the re-

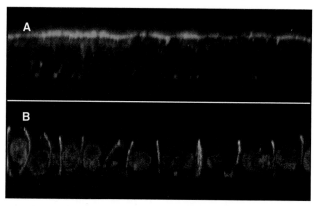

Figure 22-10 Fluorescence micrographs show the restriction of proteins to the apical or basolateral compartments of columnar epithelial cells. Tight junctions (marked with red fluorescence in both *A* and *B*) seal the boundary between these domains. *A,* E-cadherin *(green)* is restricted to the apical plasma membrane. *B,* Syntaxin-3 *(green)* is restricted to the basolateral surface. Cell nuclei are stained red. (Courtesy of T. Weimbs and S. H. Low, Cleveland Clinic Foundation.)

maining TGN is consumed by tubulation and its contents are delivered in bulk to the plasma membrane. New cell-free assays for the formation of these carrier vesicles/tubules from isolated TGN membranes should begin to provide insight into the mechanism of their formation.

In contrast to nonpolarized cells, polarized cells have functionally (and thus compositionally) distinct apical and basolateral domains (Fig. 22-10) separated by tight junctions that cement neighboring cells together and prevent diffusion between the domains (see Chapter 33; Fig. 33-3). Most of our knowledge of membrane sorting in polarized cells has come from studying epithelial cells. As expected, the trafficking complexity increases as destination options increase, and three distinct mechanisms for the polarized sorting of plasma membrane proteins have been revealed (Fig. 22-11). One mechanism involves selective packaging of apically or basolaterally destined proteins into distinct carrier vesicles at the TGN for delivery to the appropriate surface. A second mechanism involves the random delivery of newly synthesized proteins to both surfaces, followed by selective retention or depletion so that, at steady state, they become differentially abundant because they are more stable at one surface than at the other. A third mechanism, exclusively used in hepatocytes, involves delivery of all newly synthesized proteins to the basolateral surface, followed by selective internalization, sorting in the endosomal compartment, and delivery to the apical surface in a process termed **transcytosis.** Most epithelial cells use different combinations of these three mechanisms to generate and maintain cell polarity. Each mechanism is considered in detail in the following paragraphs.

Extensive studies of the direct targeting mechanism have revealed specific **basolateral targeting signals** in the cytoplasmic domains of many proteins. Examples include receptors for low-density lipoprotein, transferrin, MPRs (see Fig. 22–7), and polymeric immunoglobulin receptor. If these signals are abolished through mutagenesis, the proteins proceed to both surfaces of the epithelial cell. Interestingly, these signals are often closely related to and, in some cases, colinear with the tyrosine-based signals that function in receptor-mediated endocytosis and sorting to endosomes (see Chapter 23). In fact, many endocytosis receptors are restricted to either the apical or basolateral domains and, after internalization, are selectively recycled from endosomes back to the appropriate membrane domain. Thus, these sorting signals function both at the TGN and in endosomes (see Fig. 22–11). Like the TGN, endosomes are also decorated with a variety of coats (see Chapter 23) mediating multiple sorting events.

Sorting based on physical properties appears to play a dominant role in sorting directly to the apical surface of polarized epithelial cells. The apical surface of polarized endothelial cells is distinguished from the basolateral surface by its high content of glycosphingolipids. Moreover, many proteins anchored to the membrane by glycophosphatidylinositol (GPI; see Chapter 6) are selectively targeted to the apical surface. The polarized sorting of phospholipids and **GPI-anchored proteins** has given rise to a model (see Fig. 22–11) in which sphingomyelin- and cholesterol-

rich subdomains form **lipid rafts** at the level of the TGN. The unique physical properties of these lipid subdomains render them resistant to detergent solubilization. GPI-anchored proteins, or integral membrane proteins that directly associate with these lipid rafts based on physical properties of their transmembrane domains, are selectively targeted to the apical surface. Indeed, transport vesicles carrying newly synthesized influenza hemagglutinin to the apical surface in polarized Madin-Darby canine kidney (MDCK) cells are detergent insoluble and contain the cholesterol-binding protein, **caveolin,** which may play a role in the assembly and stabilization of lipid rafts.

In some cases, ablation of the basolateral sorting signal by mutagenesis results not in random targeting to both membranes, but to selective delivery at the apical surface. These observations have led to the suggestion that selective sorting to apical membranes might occur through recognition of a widely distributed feature or property common to many membrane proteins. Some evidence suggests that apical sorting can be mediated by a receptor that recognizes carbohydrate moieties on glycoproteins, much like the MPR, but with broader specificity. Clearly, glycoproteins and some GPI-anchored proteins are also targeted to the basolateral surface. In these cases, sorting signals for basolateral targeting are thought to be predominant over apical targeting motifs. The latter are revealed only when the more dominant signal is ablated.

The second sorting mechanism—random delivery followed by selective rearrangements—is particularly relevant to establishing polarity. In this case, uniformly distributed proteins that preexist on a nonpolarized cell will redistribute themselves in a polarized fashion in response to cell-cell contacts that initiate polarization. Often, this occurs by the selective retention of a specific protein at the appropriate surface through intracellular (cytoskeletal) or extracellular (cell-cell or cell-matrix) interactions, or both (see Fig. 22–11). Proteins that are not actively retained on the other cell surface are internalized and degraded in lysosomes. Examples of proteins polarized in this way include Na^+K^+-ATPase (Chapter 7) and the cell adhesion molecule uvomorulin, an immunoglobulin-like cell adhesion molecule (Ig-CAM, see Chapter 32).

A variation of these mechanisms accounts for polarized sorting in hepatocytes and certain intestinal epithelial cells that either lack or have very attenuated vesicular pathways to the apical surfaces. In these cells, apical proteins take an indirect rather than a direct route. They travel basolaterally, together with the basolateral plasma membrane constituents, and are then rapidly internalized and selectively sequestered in endosomes for the second leg of the journey involving transcellular migration or transcytosis (see Fig. 22–11). Post-translational modification of sorting signals or

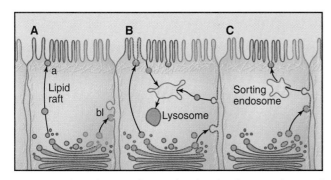

Figure 22–11 Three pathways for the distribution of integral membrane proteins destined for either the apical (a; *red*) or basolateral (bl; *blue*) membranes of polarized epithelial cells. *A,* Direct sorting from the TGN to either the apical or basolateral surface. Apical transport involves inclusion into lipid rafts, whereas proteins destined for direct transport to the basolateral surface carry a cytoplasmic sorting motif for inclusion into specific transport vesicles. *B,* Indirect pathway. Newly synthesized proteins are randomly targeted to both surfaces followed by selective retention and/or selective degradation from one surface or the other, resulting in a polarized distribution. *C,* Indirect pathway in hepatocytes. All newly synthesized proteins are transported to the basolateral surface, followed by retention of basolateral proteins and selective transcytosis of apical proteins to the apical surface.

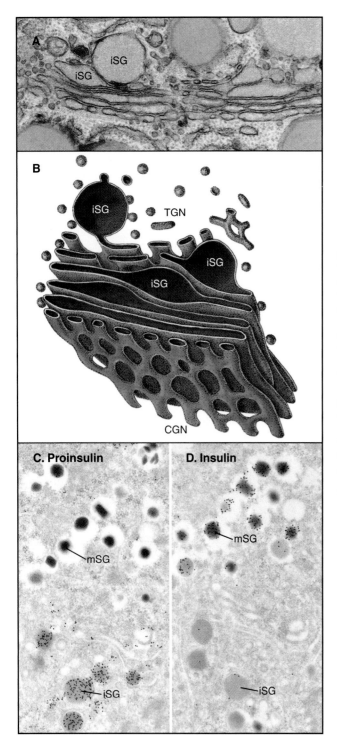

Figure 22-12 Formation of secretory granules. Transmission electron micrograph of a thin section (*A*) and a diagram (*B*) show immature secretory granules (iSG) as they emerge from the TGN. Much of the TGN surface is consumed by forming immature secretory granules. *C* and *D*, Cryo-electron micrographs of frozen sections reacted with gold-labeled antibodies to proinsulin (*C*) or insulin (*D*). Proinsulin is concentrated in immature secretory granules. After processing, insulin is concentrated in mature, dense-core secretory granules (MSG). (*A*, Courtesy of Y. Clermont, McGill University. *B*, Redrawn from Clermont Y, Rambourg A, Hermo L: Trans-Golgi network (TGN) of different cell types: Three-dimensional structural characteristics and variability. Anat Rec 242:289–301, 1995. This material is used by permission of Wiley-Liss, Inc., a subsidiary of John Wiley & Sons, Inc. *C* and *D*, Courtesy of L. Orci, University of Geneva.)

even selective proteolysis at the apical surface ensures the vectorial nature of the transcytotic process.

Regulated Secretory Pathway

An additional major sorting pathway from the TGN occurs in specialized endocrine, exocrine, or neuronal cells that concentrate and package selected proteins in storage granules for eventual mobilization and discharge in response to hormonal or neural stimulation. This is the so-called regulated secretory pathway, which is used for discharging most of the body's polypeptide hormones, enzymes used in the digestive tract, and many other products that are needed intermittently rather than continuously. Far less is known about the sorting mechanisms applied to secretory proteins than about those used for lysosomal hydrolases. This is ironic because electron microscopic studies demonstrated the origin of secretion granules in association with the TGN (Fig. 22–12) well before the existence of mannose 6-phosphate receptors was documented.

Our mechanistic understanding of secretory granule formation and sorting processes is hindered by the apparent lack of a universal sorting signal on all proteins that are destined for inclusion into regulated secretory granules. Instead, secretory granule formation appears to involve physical sorting, selective retention, and geometric considerations. Endocrine or exocrine cells that specialize in regulated secretion are typically highly differentiated and rarely divide, instead committing most of their biosynthetic activity to exported proteins. In these cells, newly synthesized secretory and membrane proteins are captured within the large intraluminal volume and swelling membrane of condensing vacuoles that emerge to form immature secretory granules (see Figs. 22–12 and 22–13). In fact, most or all of the TGN membrane and volume is consumed in the formation of immature secretory granules, and it is impossible to delineate distinct sites where secretory proteins aggregate, where terminal post-translational

modifications of secretory products (e.g., proteolytic processing (see Fig. 20–13) and oligosaccharide sulfation; see Fig. 31–13) take place, or where other TGN activities, like the sorting of lysosomal hydrolases, occur. In fact, each of these activities spills over into immature secretion granules that effectively become a functional extension of the TGN. For example, in β-cells of the endocrine pancreas, lysosomal prohydrolases and plasma membrane proteins are packaged into immature secretory granules and dispatched from there to endosomes, lysosomes, or the plasma membrane. Clathrin-coated vesicles that are often seen in association with maturing granules mediate this remodeling and maturation process (see Fig. 22–13). Sorting signals on errantly packaged proteins mediate their capture into the coated vesicles. In contrast, the large aggregate formed by resident secretory proteins prohibits their inclusion in small vesicles. During maturation, secretory granules lose volume and surface area. Fully mature secretory granules are characterized by highly condensed contents (see Fig. 22–12C and D) and a very low density of integral membrane proteins relative to lipids (as assessed by freeze-fracture analysis.)

Depending on the cell type and secretory process, selective aggregation of secretory proteins may be either homotypic (between like proteins) or heterotypic (between different proteins). A preference for **homotypic aggregation** leads to regional enrichment of a particular protein within the contents of a granule or, in the extreme, to the production of separate granules with different secretory compositions in the same cell. This situation may apply to cells that produce and secrete more than one type of hormone and package them into separate granules. For example, gonadotrophs in the pituitary produce both follicle-stimulating hormone and luteinizing hormone. **Heterotypic aggregation** is characteristic of acinar cells in exocrine glands, like the pancreas, where many different secretory products are intermixed in individual granules. In some cells that produce and store peptide hormones, aggregation involves only selected products of proteolytic processing of hormone precursors. For example, production of **insulin** requires proteolytic enzymes in immature granules that cleave proinsulin at two sites, generating insulin and C-peptide (see Fig. 22–12C and D). Insulin condenses with zinc ion in the granule core, whereas C-peptide is excluded and so accumulates around this core. As a consequence, more C-peptide than insulin is shed into unstimulated secretory pathways that originate from the immature granule. Very tight regulation of insulin secretion is important for controlling the glucose concentration in the blood plasma. This regulation is compromised in certain forms of diabetes.

Some membrane proteins retained during secre-

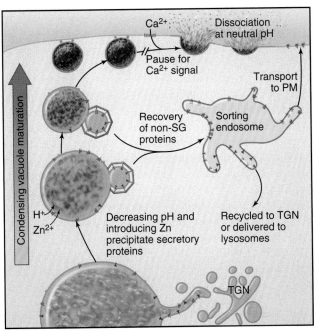

Figure 22–13 Maturation of nascent secretory granules/condensing vacuoles. The vacuolar H⁺-ATPase in the secretory granule (SG) membrane lowers the internal pH. This drives condensation and concentration of the contents. Dense-core, mature secretory granules are stored in the cytoplasm until a Ca^{2+}-mediated signaling event triggers fusion and release of their contents. Proteins inadvertently included in large immature secretory granules emerging from the TGN are captured by clathrin-coated vesicles and recycled to endosomes and the TGN. PM, plasma membrane.

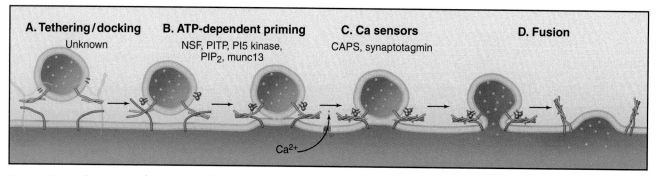

Figure 22–14 Four terminal steps (*A* to *D*) in Ca^{2+}-triggered membrane fusion during regulated secretion. Docking/tethering and fusion are mechanistically similar to other vesicle fusion events (see Fig. 21–5). Additional steps prepare proteins on both the secretory vesicles and plasma membrane to respond rapidly to Ca^{2+} influx, which triggers fusion. NSF, NEM-sensitive factor; PTP, Phosphatidylinositol transfer protein; CAPS, calcium activator protein for secretion; and munc 13 mammalian homologue for *C. elegans* UNC13 (unknown function, critical for Ca^{2+}-triggered fusion of primary vesicles).

tory granule formation have **granule sorting motifs** that direct them specifically to granules. Two well-studied examples are the regulated adhesive glycoprotein, P-selectin (see Chapter 32), and the post-Golgi processing enzymes, PAM (peptide-amidating monooxygenase) and furin (which cleaves proenzymes). The cytoplasmic tails of these transmembrane proteins contain signals that are necessary and sufficient for targeting to regulated secretory granules. These signals may interact in the TGN with some yet-to-be-discovered cytoplasmic coat that is specialized for granule formation. In addition, and perhaps more importantly, these signals mediate the efficient recycling of granule membrane proteins from the plasma membrane back to the TGN after secretion. Again, there is evidence that phosphorylation/dephosphorylation events function to inactivate sorting motifs and differentially control secretion and recycling. Interestingly, soluble forms of PAM are also packaged in secretory vesicles, suggesting that the luminal domain interacts with secretory granule contents for retention.

Regulated Fusion with the Plasma Membrane

All transport vesicles leaving the TGN contain components of the vesicle targeting and fusion machinery (e.g., v-SNARES, members of the synaptobrevin/VAMP family, Rab proteins) required to direct their fusion with the appropriate target organelle containing cognate t-SNARES (members of the syntaxin, SNAP, and Sec1p families) (see Chapter 21). Superimposed on this constitutive machinery for docking and fusion, secretory granules also carry regulatory factors that ensure that fusion takes place only on demand. Regu-

lated fusion has been studied extensively in neurons in the context of synaptic vesicle release, in endocrine cells, and in mast cells. In all cases, **regulated secretion** can be divided into three steps: **docking, priming,** and **fusion** (Fig. 22–14). Docking is the slowest step and is believed to involve interactions of v- and t-SNAREs regulated by the Rab GTPases. In vitro reconstitution studies have suggested a role for a phosphatidylinositol transfer protein, a phosphatidylinositol 5-kinase and phosphatidylinositol 4,5-bisphosphate (PIP$_2$, the product of PI-5 kinase), in priming steps required for regulated secretion in neuroendocrine cells. A cytosolic protein, CAPS (calcium activator protein for secretion), is recruited to the secretory vesicle via interactions with PIP$_2$ and is required for calcium-triggered fusion of dense core secretory granules. In most cases, fusion is triggered by an influx of Ca^{2+}, a process called **calcium-secretion coupling.** Synaptotagmins, part of a family of transmembrane vesicle proteins that also bind calcium and interact with the fusion machinery, are believed to act as clamps, inhibiting fusion until calcium triggers their release.

Diverse signals lead to the calcium influx that triggers fusion. These include ligand activation of G protein–coupled receptors on neuroendocrine cells, activation of immunoglobulin E receptors and kinase cascades in mast cells, and membrane depolarization in neurons (see Fig. 10–8).

Retrospective

The TGN is the initial branch point in the biosynthetic pathway and the primary distribution center serving subsequent destinations. The distribution process is mediated by vesicular carriers and, often, by transmembrane receptors that recruit cargo molecules into these carriers through direct interactions with the cytoplasmic coat machinery. The coats appear to be specific for their site of action and probably for the kind of transport vesicle that they help to form. The intracompartmental ionic environment (pH, divalent cations, etc.) is an essential factor in sorting, both in depositing prohydrolases in the prelysosome and in promoting aggregation of various regulated secretory proteins. Sorting is seldom, if ever, a single-step event. Instead, sorting occurs iteratively, taking advantage of sorting motifs and sorting machinery, as well as physical properties of the cargo and the geometry of the sorting compartment and transport vehicles. The integration of these three sorting mechanisms plays an equally important role in transport along the endocytic pathway (see Chapter 23).

Selected Readings

Bunger AT: Structure of proteins involved in synaptic vesicle fusion in neurons. Ann Rev Biophys Biomolec Struc 30: 157–171, 2001.

Hannah MJ, Schmidt AA, Huttner WB: Synaptic vesicle biogenesis. Ann Rev Cell Devel Biol 15:733–798, 1999.

Ikonen E, Simons K: Protein and lipid sorting for the trans-Golgi network to the plasma membrane in polarized cells. Semin Cell Devel Biol 9:503–509, 1998.

Jahn R, Sudhof TC: Membrane fusion and exocytosis. Ann Rev Biochem 68:863–912, 1999.

Mullins C, Bonifacino JS: The molecular machinery for lysosome biogenesis. BioEssays 23:333–343, 2001.

Robinson MS, Bonifacino JS: Adaptor-related proteins. Curr Opin Cell Biol 13:444–453, 2001.

Tooze SA, Martens, GJ, Huttner WB: Secretory granule biogenesis: rafting to the SNARE. Trends Cell Biol 11:116–122, 2001.

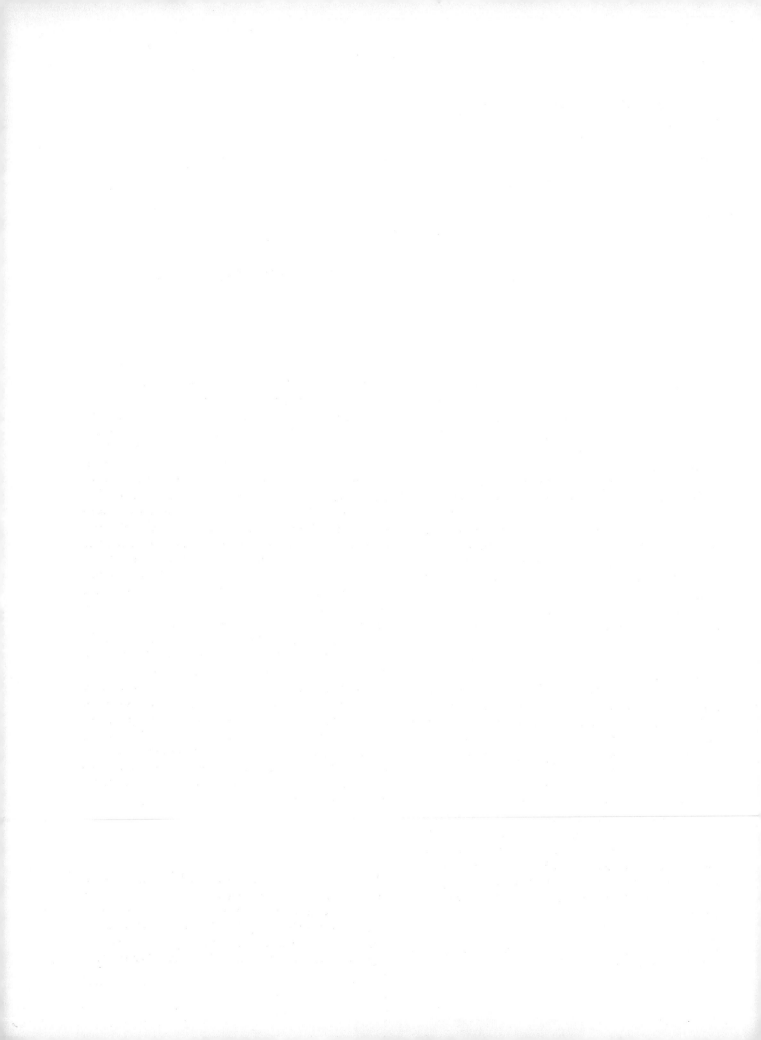

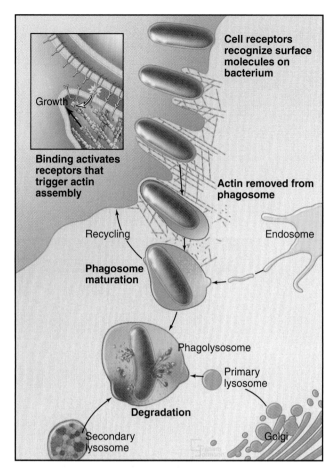

Figure 23-3 Diagram illustrating the molecular mechanism for phagocytosis of a bacterium by a macrophage. Macrophage surface receptors are activated by contact with a bacterium; this triggers actin rearrangements that lead to protrusion of the plasma membrane to engulf the bacterium. The actin filaments encasing the newly formed phagosome depolymerize, and membrane traffic to and from the phagosome leads to its maturation. Hydrolytic enzymes are delivered to the mature phagosome through fusion with primary and secondary lysosomes, and the bacterium is degraded.

opsonins) are continuously distributed, then the zipper closes. But if clumps of teeth are missing (i.e., when opsonin-receptor complexes are not uniformly distributed), the zipper cannot close and complete engulfment cannot occur. Clearly, the assembly and disassembly of actin filaments must be coordinated both spatially and temporally for the particle to be engulfed successfully.

Facilitated by actin-based, unconventional, myosin motors, the particle becomes completely engulfed within a phagocytic vacuole (phagosome) derived from the plasma membrane (see Fig. 23–3). Surrounding actin filaments must disassemble before microtubule-based motors can direct the phagosome deep into the cell for fusion with acidic lysosomes containing active hydrolytic enzymes. The phagosome matures by a series of vesicle fusion and fission reactions that remove plasma membrane–derived proteins and

replace them with the same endosome-specific targeting and fusion machinery used in the biosynthetic pathway (e.g., the small GTPase Rab5 and endosome-specific t- and v-SNARES). This process, termed directed maturation, prepares the phagosome for selective fusion with lysosomes.

Fusion with lysosomes creates a hybrid vacuole called a **phagolysosome** in which the ingested particle is degraded to its constituent amino acids, monosaccharides and disaccharides, lipids, and nucleotides by lysosomal hydrolases. These small products of digestion are transported across the phagolysosomal membrane and may be used by the cell in the synthesis of new molecules. Any undegraded material remains within the lysosome, which is called a **residual body.**

Killing Intracellular Invaders

The invasion of bacteria or protozoa attracts professional phagocytes (see Chapter 30 and Fig. 32–13). Consumed by the phagocytes and within the harsh acidic environment of the **phagolysosome,** the invaders are subjected to a lethal barrage of toxic oxidants generated by the reduced form of nicotinamide-adenine dinucleotide phosphate oxidase within the phagosomal membrane, to proteases and acid hydrolases within the lumen of the phagolysosome, and to small peptides, called **defensins,** that bind to and disrupt microbial membranes. Some pathogens, however, have developed counterstrategies to avoid destruction. Their evasion strategies may include inhibiting fusion between the phagosome and lysosome, resisting the low pH environment of the lysosome, and escaping from the phagolysosome by lysing the surrounding membrane (Table 23–1). An increase in infectious diseases throughout the world has made research on the survival tactics of intracellular pathogens and cellular defenses against them particularly crucial. For example, tuberculosis, which starts with the phagocytosis of the bacteria *Mycobacterium tuberculosis* by macrophages in the lung, is an old disease that has once again become common. The bacillus is now not only resistant to destruction by macrophages, it is also resistant to many antibiotics that were once effective treatments.

Clathrin-Dependent Endocytosis

Clathrin-dependent endocytosisis is used by all eukaryotic cells to obtain essential nutrients, such as iron and cholesterol, and to remove potentially harmful molecules (such as hormones, which are needed acutely but briefly) from the extracellular environment. This process is often more ambiguously referred to as **receptor-mediated endocytosis** because it involves plasma membrane receptors that concentrate ligands

table 23–1

SURVIVAL STRATEGIES FOR INTRACELLULAR PATHOGENS

"Escape"
- Secretion of toxins that disrupt phagosomal membrane *(Shigella flexneri, Listeria monocytogenes, Rickettsia rickettsii)*

"Dodge"
- Entrance through alternative, pathogen-specific pathway *(Salmonella typhimurium, Legionella pneumophila, Chlamydia trachomatis)*
- Inhibition of phagosome-lysosome fusion *(S. typhimurium, Mycobacterium tuberculosis)*
- Inhibition of phagolysosome acidification *(Mycobacterium species)*

"Stand and Fight"
- Low pH-dependent replication *(Coxiella burnetii, S. typhimurium)*
- Enhancement of DNA repair to survive oxidative stress *(S. typhimurium)*
- Protective pathogen-specific virulence factors *(C. burnetii, S. typhimurium)*
- Prevention of the processing and presentation of bacterial antigens *(S. typhimurium)*

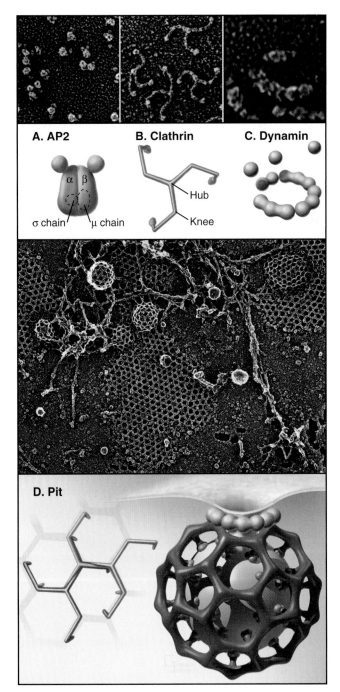

Figure 23–4 Electron micrographs and drawings of the major components of the endocytic clathrin-coated vesicle: AP2 complexes *(A)*, clathrin triskelions *(B)*, and dynamin *(C)*, visualized by platinum shadowing. *D*, Field of coated pits assembled on the cytoplasmic face of the plasma membrane viewed by quick-freeze, deep-etch microscopy. The diagrams are structural models of the major proteins and a model for their coassembly into a coated pit. AP2 complexes interact with docking sites on the membrane and mediate clathrin assembly into a polygonal lattice. Dynamin is targeted to the necks of deeply invaginated coated pits and can self-assemble into ring-like structures that are believed to regulate coated vesicle formation. (Micrographs courtesy of John Heuser, Washington University.)

from the fluid environment onto the surface. Clathrin-dependent endocytosis occurs at specialized patches on the plasma membrane, called coated pits, whose distinctive underlying protein lattice is composed of **clathrin** triskelions and adaptor molecules (see Figs. 23–1*B* and 23–4). Receptor-ligand complexes are concentrated in these small patches, which pinch off, forming **clathrin-coated vesicles** that carry their cargo into the cell. Clathrin-coated vesicles also mediate the retrieval of synaptic vesicle membrane at synapses following neurotransmitter release (see Figs. 10–8 and 10–9).

Components of the Clathrin Coat

Clathrin is utilized for vesicle formation at multiple sites, including the trans-Golgi network (TGN) and endosomes. It consists of three 190-kD heavy chains, each with one of two tightly associated light chains of approximately 30 kD (LCa or LCb). This hexameric complex forms a three-legged structure, termed a triskelion (Fig. 23–4). Clathrin triskelions can self-assemble under special conditions into empty cages. The assembled empty cage is like a soccer ball, with clathrin forming the ribs or seams between adjacent faces. Each rib of the cage incorporates portions of four different triskelions, which are, in turn, arranged in pentagons and hexagons (Fig. 23–5). Clathrin self-assembly is believed to drive curvature of the underly-

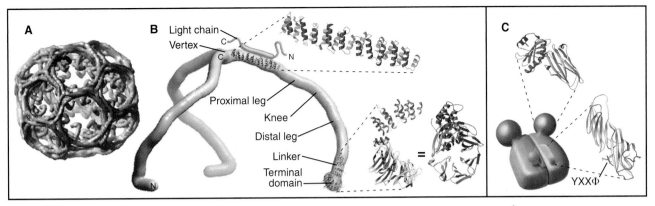

Figure 23-5 *A*, Image reconstruction of clathrin triskelions assembled into a clathrin cage seen at 20 Å resolution. *B*, The extended legs of clathrin triskelions are formed from multiple repeating units consisting of five helix hairpins that give them rigidity. These repeats continue into the linker region, which expands into the N-terminal domain, consisting of a seven-bladed β-propeller similar to a trimeric G protein β-subunit. *C*, High-resolution structures of the C-terminal appendage domain of the AP2 α-adaptin subunit. Accessory proteins required for endocytosis interact with a hydrophobic patch on the β-barrel platform that sits between two α-helices. Consensus YXXΦ internalization motif-containing peptides (stick figure; see text) bind as extended β-strands to a hydrophobic pocket on the μ2-subunit of AP2. (*A*, Courtesy of Corinne Smith, Medical Research Council Laboratory of Molecular Biology, Cambridge, England. *B* and *C*, Courtesy of Frances Brodsky, University of California, San Francisco; Tomas Kirchhausen, Harvard Medical School; and David Owen, Medical Research Council Laboratory of Molecular Biology, Cambridge, England.)

ing membrane and vesicle formation. (See Fig. 4–4 for an explanation of how pentagons and hexagons form closed shells.)

The targeting and transport specificity of the clathrin coat derives from the **adapter** or **assembly protein (AP)** components of the coat. APs are heterotetramers composed of two distinct polypeptides (termed adaptins) of approximately 100 kD, a medium chain (termed μ) of approximately 50 kD, and a small chain (termed σ) of approximately 20 kD. As their name suggests, APs coassemble with clathrin under physiological conditions to form coats that closely resemble those observed on isolated coated vesicles. Four distinct AP complexes—AP1, AP2, AP3, and AP4—have been identified in mammalian cells and/or yeast, and the number may grow. AP1 and AP3 mediate distinct vesicle trafficking events between the TGN and endosome (see Chapter 22) along the biosynthetic pathway. The function of the recently discovered AP4 complex has yet to be established. AP2 functions in endocytic coated vesicle formation from the plasma membrane (see Fig. 23–4). Targeting of AP complexes is mediated, in part, by one of the adaptin subunits; α-adaptin, which is specific to AP2, targets this complex to the plasma membrane, whereas the γ-subunit specific to AP1 targets this complex to the TGN. The other adaptin subunits—β1 for AP1 and β2 for AP2—are closely related and trigger clathrin recruitment and assembly. The β3-subunit of AP3 is more divergent, and, interestingly, AP3 can function in vesicle formation independently of clathrin. The μ-subunits of AP

complexes interact directly with sorting motifs and function to concentrate receptors into coated pits (see Fig. 23–5).

Receptor Clustering into Coated Pits

Clathrin-dependent endocytosis is initiated by the recruitment and assembly of AP2 complexes onto the plasma membrane (Fig. 23–6). Like coat assembly at the endoplasmic reticulum and Golgi, this process is regulated by GTPases (and, perhaps, by phosphorylation and dephosphorylation); however, the mechanisms and molecules involved remain unknown. Similarly, the docking protein for AP2 binding is also unknown, although there is evidence that polyphosphatidylinositol lipids might be involved. Upon recruitment, AP2 complexes cluster and trigger clathrin assembly.

Most but not all endocytic receptors are transmembrane proteins that span the membrane bilayer at least once. So-called **internalization motifs** encoded in the cytoplasmic domains of receptors direct their interaction with the coat machinery. No universal signal is shared by all receptors. The best characterized internalization motif is a short linear sequence of four to six amino acids containing an essential tyrosine residue. The first hints about the nature of the internalization signal came from the study of a patient with familial hypercholesteremia, a defect in cholesterol metabolism that leads to atherosclerosis and early death, usually by the age of 30 years (see Fig. 24–9).

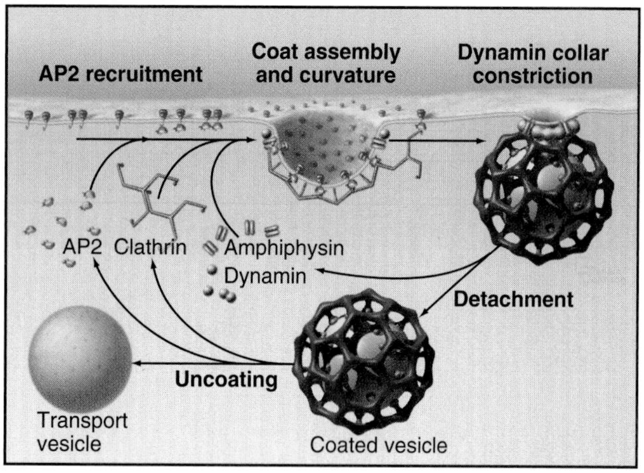

Figure 23-6 Cycle of receptor-mediated endocytosis driven by the clathrin-coated vesicle. AP2 complexes are targeted to docking sites on the plasma membrane and initiate clathrin assembly into a polygonal lattice. Receptors carrying cargo molecules are concentrated in coated pits through interactions between tyrosine-based sorting motifs on their cytoplasmic domains and the clustered μ-subunits of AP2. The GTPase dynamin is targeted to coated pits through interactions with amphiphysin, which also binds AP2 and clathrin and, by mechanisms as yet unknown, regulates membrane invagination and fission to release coated vesicles carrying cargo into the cell. Hsc70 and other uncoating factors disassemble the coat constituents and release the transport vesicles for fusion with endosomes.

In these patients' cells, the plasma membrane receptor for low-density lipoprotein (LDL)—the particle that transports cholesterol through the bloodstream—has a single amino acid substitution (at Tyr 807) in its cytoplasmic tail. This mutation, within the internalization motif, FXNPXY (where X can be any amino acid), severely impairs clustering of the LDL receptor and its subsequent rapid internalization. This short sequence is both necessary and sufficient for efficient endocytosis, as it functions when transplanted onto other transmembrane proteins.

The LDL receptor is one of several constitutively internalized receptors that cluster into coated pits, even in the absence of bound ligand. A second, well-characterized internalization motif, the short sequence YTRF, was identified on the transferrin receptor, a constitutively internalized receptor for the iron-carrying protein, transferrin. A minimum consensus sequence found on several receptors has been identified as YXXϕ (where ϕ is any hydrophobic amino acid, but preferably, an aromatic amino acid). Interestingly, sorting motifs that direct trafficking from the TGN to lysosomes or in polarized cells contain similar sorting motifs with an essential tyrosine residue. Thus, it was not surprising to find that peptides containing these tyrosine-based sorting motifs are recognized by the μ-subunits of both AP1 and AP2 complexes (μ1 and μ2, respectively). A high-resolution structure of the μ2-

subunit has revealed that the YXXϕ-containing peptides bind to the μ chain in an extended conformation (see Fig. 23-5). AP complexes and receptor tails interact with low affinity in vitro, but when clustered on the membrane, the AP complexes are able to concentrate receptors.

Dynamin and Coated Vesicle Budding

Driven by clathrin coat assembly and facilitated by multiple sites of interaction between receptors and coat constituents, the underlying plasma membrane gains curvature, forming a deeply invaginated coated pit (see Fig. 23-6). This process has been reconstituted using isolated membranes and requires adenosine triphosphate (ATP), guanosine triphosphate (GTP), and accessory proteins whose identity and/or function remain unknown. One protein, the GTPase **dynamin,** plays a unique role in vesicle budding. This 100-kD protein is targeted to coated pits and, upon binding GTP, self-assembles into a helical "collar" at the necks of deeply invaginated coated pits. This collar appears to monitor and regulate the processes of coated pit constriction and vesicle release. To function in endocytosis, dynamin must bind the lipid phosphatidylinositol 4,5-bisphosphate. In addition, dynamin recruits another enzyme, **endophilin,** which catalyzes the fatty acylation of lysophosphatidic acid. Thus, for membrane invagination and fission to occur, dynamin may coordinate establishment of localized lipid subdomains in the plasma membrane through localized lipid modifications. It has also been suggested that the dynamin collar plays a direct mechanochemical role in driving membrane fission and vesicle release.

The Uncoating Reaction

Soon after internalization, the vesicle sheds its coat. This reaction serves to recycle the coat components and to free the vesicle for fusion with its target organelle, the endosome. **Hsc70,** a member of the heat shock protein family of chaperones, catalyzes the removal of the clathrin triskelions in vitro. **Auxilin,** which is specifically found on coated vesicles isolated from brain, facilitates hsc70-mediated clathrin release, as does **synaptojanin,** a phosphatidylinositol 5-kinase. Other cytosolic factors are required for AP2 release (see Fig. 23-6). How the uncoating machinery can distinguish a sealed vesicle from a deeply invaginated coated pit is unknown.

Rates of Clathrin-Mediated Endocytosis

A single vertebrate cell has many different types of cell surface receptors present at levels ranging from

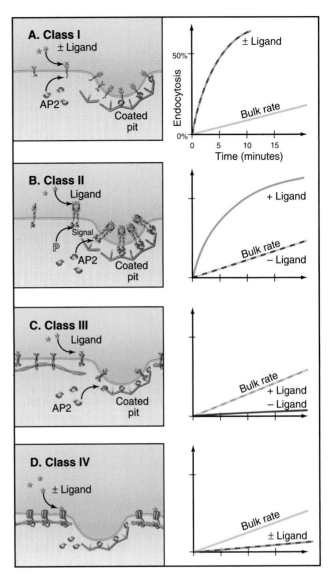

Figure 23-7 Integral membrane proteins on the cell surface fall into four categories with regard to their interactions with the endocytic machinery. *A,* Class I receptors, including receptors for LDL and transferrin, interact constitutively with coat proteins and are concentrated into coated pits with or without bound ligand. They are internalized at rates much faster than bulk membrane. *B,* The internalization signals on class II receptors, typically signaling receptor tyrosine kinases or G protein–coupled receptors, are only activated upon ligand binding. In the absence of ligand, they are internalized at the bulk rate. *C,* Class III receptors are tethered to cytoskeletal elements, which prevents their internalization in the absence of ligands. Ligand binding triggers release of these receptors so that they are now internalized at the bulk rate, unless they also carry internalization motifs that affect their concentration into coated pits. *D,* Class IV proteins, which include resident plasma membrane pumps, are constitutively tethered to cytoskeletal elements and are internalized slowly, if at all.

less than 5000 to more than 500,000 copies, each engaged in the endocytosis of its specific ligand. In general, different receptors can share the same coated pit. Coated pits typically cover 1% to 2% of the plasma membrane surface area and complete the budding process in approximately 1 minute. Therefore, depending on how effectively a receptor–ligand complex is concentrated in coated pits (typically 10- to 20-fold), they can be internalized at rates exceeding 20% to 40% of cell surface receptors per minute.

Receptors interact with the endocytic machinery in four different ways (Fig. 23–7). Nutrient receptors, such as LDL receptors and transferrin receptors, are constitutively concentrated in coated pits, presumably because internalization motifs on their relatively small cytoplasmic tails are always exposed. Signaling receptors, such as those for insulin or epidermal growth factor (EGF), are induced to cluster into coated pits

only by bound ligand. These receptors have very large cytoplasmic domains that include a kinase domain and docking sites for signaling molecules (see Chapters 26 and 29). Although little is known of the structure of the internalization motifs, they may be masked until the ligand binds the external domain of the receptor and autophosphorylation triggers a conformational change to expose the internalization signal. In some cases, receptor-specific accessory molecules are required for targeting to coated pits. Interestingly, the human immunodeficiency virus (HIV) encodes one such accessory molecule that targets class I molecules to coated pits, leading to their internalization and aiding in immunosuppression. A third class of receptors, including the T-cell antigen receptor component, CD4, are tethered on the plasma membrane through interactions with the cytoskeleton. Ligand binding triggers their release, but in the absence of activated internali-

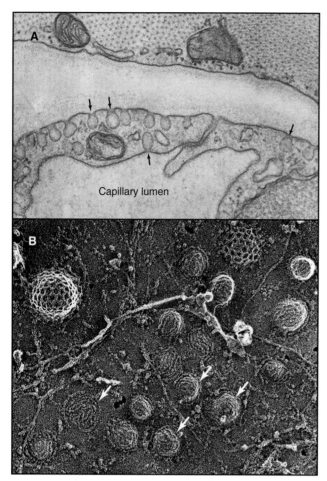

Figure 23-8 *A,* Electron micrograph of a thin section of a muscle capillary showing caveolae ("little caves"), which are abundant in endothelial cells that mediate transcytosis. Arrows show "cave" openings. *B,* Electron micrograph of the inside surface of a fibroblast prepared by quick-freezing, deep-etching, and rotary shadowing. The whorl-like coat on the caveolae formed by self-assembly of caveolin *(white arrows).* Caveolae are typically smaller than clathrin-coated pits shown in the upper left and right. (*A,* Courtesy of D. Fawcett, Harvard Medical School. *B,* Courtesy of John Heuser, Washington University.)

zation motifs, the receptors are randomly captured in budding coated vesicles and internalized at rates of 1% to 2% per minute. Lastly, resident plasma membrane proteins, such as channels, transporters, adhesion molecules, and the like, are tethered at the plasma membrane by interactions with the cytoskeleton or extracellular matrix and are internalized at slower rates than bulk membrane.

Caveolae/Plasmalemmal Vesicles

Plasmalemmal vesicles, or **caveolae,** were the first endocytic vesicles to be recognized by electron microscopy. These small (~50 nm), flask-shaped pits or vesicles make up more than 10% of the surface of endothelial cells (see Figs. 23–1*D* and 23–8) and

were first proposed to mediate transport from the blood across the epithelia to the tissue. Caveolae are also present, albeit less abundantly than in endothelial cells and often with less distinctive morphologic appearance, in virtually all animal cells. They have not been detected in plants or in yeast. Quick-freeze deep-etch electron microscopy first revealed the unique coat material on these vesicles (see Fig. 23–8), and subsequent biochemical studies established that the coat was formed by self-assembly of a 22-kD integral membrane protein called **caveolin.** Caveolin binds cholesterol with high affinity and has a unique topology within the membrane (Fig. 23–9). Caveolae are rich in cholesterol and glycosphingolipids and represent a specialized subset of plasma membrane–associated lipid rafts (see Chapter 22 and Fig. 6–7). Plasma membrane proteins can also be concentrated in caveolae if they are anchored to the extracellular leaflet of the lipid bilayer via glycosylphosphatidylinositol (GPI) anchors or to the intracellular leaflet via fatty acylation. Many signaling molecules (see Chapter 27) fall into these categories and are enriched in caveolae, which can function as highly specialized subdomains to regulate signal transduction.

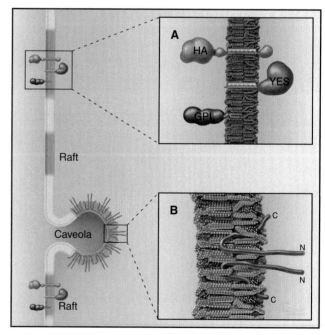

Figure 23–9 Microdomains of the plasma membrane enriched in cholesterol and glycosphingolipids and held together by interactions between lipid head groups and long, saturated acyl-chains. *A,* "Lipid rafts" can exist independently of caveolin. Proteins that are enriched in these lipid rafts include those that are anchored to the outer leaflet by GPI tails or to the inner leaflet by acylation and some integral membrane proteins, depending on the composition of their transmembrane domains. *B,* Caveola. Caveolin *(blue schematic)* binds cholesterol and aids in forming and/or stabilizing these microdomains. HA, influenza virus hemagglutinin; YES, an Src-family tyrosine kinase.

Like clathrin-coated vesicles, caveolae can bud from the plasma membrane to form transport vesicles. Internalization of caveolae is highly regulated and may require dynamin. However, except for endothelial cells, the rates and extents of caveolae-mediated endocytosis are considerably less than those for clathrin-dependent endocytosis, and the physiological significance of caveolae-mediated endocytosis is unclear. In addition to their role in signal transduction and transcytosis, caveolae have been implicated in other processes, including: (1) retrograde trafficking to the endoplasmic reticulum and Golgi; (2) "potocytosis," a specialized endocytic pathway in which caveolae transiently close off, allowing acidification of their lumen and facilitated transport of molecules into the cell; and (3) the maintenance of cellular cholesterol levels through intracellular cholesterol transport and the export of cellular cholesterol to serum lipoproteins. Defining the function(s) and structure of caveolae is an active area of research.

Other Types of Pinocytosis

Cells continuously internalize fluid from their surroundings without concentrating particular molecules. In mammalian cells, fluid-phase endocytosis could be a type of surveillance ("sampling" the environment), but in lower organisms, it plays an essential role in nutrient uptake. Alternatively, or additionally, it could be a mechanism to "wash" the bulk of plasma membrane components by passing them through acidic endosomes to remove nonspecifically adsorbed molecules.

Several types of vesicles have been suggested as entry ports for fluid: clathrin-coated vesicles, macropinocytic vesicles, and poorly characterized non–clathrin-coated vesicles (see Fig. 23–1C). In experiments in which clathrin-coated vesicle endocytosis is inhibited, the volume of clathrin-independent uptake of fluid-phase endocytic tracers varies greatly among cell types. For example, endocytosis is only reduced by approximately 50% in clathrin-deficient yeast, whereas it is almost completely abrogated in clathrin-deficient *Dictyostelium*. In HeLa cells expressing a temperature-sensitive mutant of dynamin, fluid-phase endocytosis is initially inhibited by approximately 50%, but then rapidly recovers to normal levels. This suggests that a process independent of dynamin and clathrin can be up-regulated to compensate for the loss of bulk membrane uptake via clathrin-dependent endocytosis. The mechanisms governing these clathrin-independent endocytic events are unknown.

Macropinocytosis occurs constitutively in some cells, for example, in amoeba (Fig. 23–10), in thyroid cells taking up thryoglobulin, and in dendritic cells,

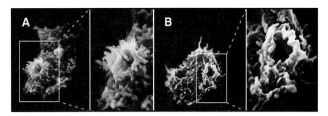

Figure 23-10 *A* and *B*, Scanning electron micrographs of *Acanthamoeba castellanii* showing membrane ruffling and macropinocytosis, the major pathway for nutrient uptake in this organism. (Courtesy of Steve Doberstein, Johns Hopkins Medical School.)

which sample large volumes of extracellular media for immune surveillance. In other mammalian cells, macropinocytosis can be acutely and transiently stimulated with growth factors. This actin-based process accompanies ruffling of membranes, leading to the formation of macropinocytic vesicles that internalize large volumes of fluid (see Fig. 23–1A). Some pathogenic bacteria (e.g., *Salmonella typhimurium*) can trigger macropinocytosis and use this "triggered" phagocytic pathway to invade cells. In this case, the phagosomal membrane is not tightly opposed to the bacterium, as occurs during "zipper" phagocytosis, and the bacterium is internalized in a "spacious" phagosome, avoiding interactions with the endosomal/lysosomal pathway (see Table 23–1).

The Endosomal Compartment and the Endocytic Pathway

Pinocytic vesicles, formed either by clathrin-dependent or clathrin-independent mechanisms, fuse with and deliver their cargo to the **endosomal compartment.** Like the TGN in the biosynthetic pathway, **endosomes** are the major sorting compartments along the endocytic pathway. Consistent with their sorting function, endosomes are structurally pleiomorphic and consist of a collection of vesicles, vacuoles, tubules, and multivesicular bodies (Fig. 23–11). Four classes of endosomes are distinguished based on the kinetics with which they accumulate endocytic tracers, their morphology, localization within the cell, and, most recently, the presence of biochemical markers (Fig. 23–12). Newly internalized proteins are first delivered to so-called **early or sorting endosomes,** which lie near the plasma membrane and appear as an anastomosing network of tubules and vacuoles. Receptors returning to the cell surface accumulate in so-called **recycling endosomes,** which are tubular structures located in the perinuclear Golgi region of the cell. Vacuolar structures or endosome carrier vesicles detach from the early endosome and gradually acquire internal membrane vesicles. These so-called **multivesicular bodies** mature into **late endosomes.** The rela-

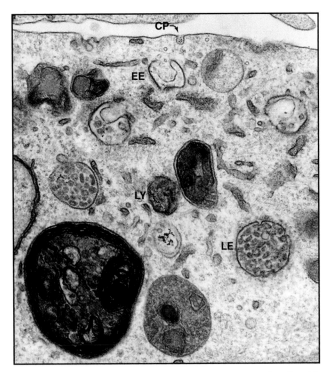

Figure 23-11 Electron micrograph showing internalized gold-conjugated protein being transported through the structurally diverse organelles of the endosomal compartment. The artificial gradient of colors reflects the maturation of early endosomes (EE) to late endosomes (LE) and lysosomes (LY). Gold particles (tiny black dots) are first delivered to early or sorting endosomes *(yellow)* having both tubular and vacuolar regions and few intraluminal membranes. Tubular portions are recycled to the plasma membrane while vacuolar portions undergo maturation. Late endosomes *(light brown)* are vacuolar and contain increasing amounts of intraluminal membrane. Lysosomes *(dark brown)* are very dense organelles, packed with internal vesicles and membrane whorls. CP, coated pit. (Courtesy of Mark Marsh, University College, London.)

tionship among these four endosomal compartments is controversial. Are they each distinct, stable organelles, or do they exist transiently as intermediates in a process of endosomal maturation? Some have suggested that the distinct endosomes represent functional subdomains of a single, interconnected compartment. The answer probably lies somewhere between these extremes.

Endosomal Acidification and Protein Sorting

The endosomal lumen is acidified through the activity of a proton pump, the **vacuolar ATPase** (see Chapter 7 and Fig. 7–5C), which resides in the endosomal membrane. This proton pump produces a membrane potential, so ion channels are also required to acidify the lumen (see Chapter 10). An important element controlling sorting along the endocytic pathway is the pH gradient that extends through the sequential endosomal compartments. The pH in endosomes decreases from approximately 6.5 in early endosomes to approx-

imately 5.0 in late endosomes. Regulation of endosomal pH most likely involves additional ion pumps that either counteract or work with the proton pump, as well as differences in membrane permeability, endosomal volume, and the concentration of the vacuolar ATPase.

The endosomal pH gradient works together with endosomal geometry to affect protein sorting. Interaction of many ligands with their sorting receptors is sensitive to pH. When receptor-ligand complexes reach their threshold pH for dissociation, the ligands are released into the lumen of the endosome, while the receptor remains membrane bound. Soluble ligands accumulate in the volume-rich vacuolar portions of the endosome, whereas receptors accumulate in the membrane-rich tubular portions. Tubules may recycle their content directly back to the plasma membrane or indirectly through the recycling endosome, or they may carry their content back to the TGN, depending on when they detach from endosomes. Vacuolar portions of the endosome undergo directed maturation and eventually fuse with lysosomes delivering their contents for degradation. The pH-dissociation profiles

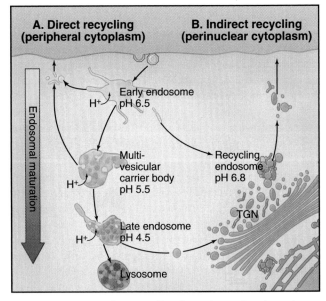

Figure 23-12 Membrane traffic along the endocytic pathway. Internalized cargo and membrane are delivered to tubulovesicular early or sorting endosomes, which are mildly acidic. Most of the membrane, together with receptors, is recycled either by a rapid, direct route or a slower, indirect route through perinuclear recycling endosomes. Ligands released from their receptors in the low pH environment accumulate in the vacuolar portions of early endosomes. During maturation—which involves the accumulation of internal membranes, continued recycling of receptors to the plasma membrane and TGN, delivery of newly synthesized lysosomal hydrolases from the TGN, progressively increasing luminal acidity, and acquisition of targeting and fusion machinery—the late endosome prepares for fusion with primary and secondary lysosomes.

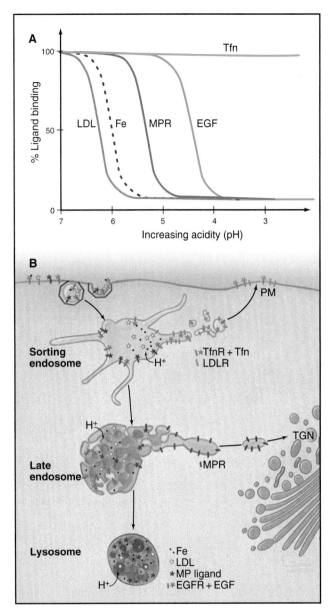

Figure 23-13 Progressive decrease in luminal pH facilitates protein sorting in the endosomal compartment. Interactions of many cargo molecules with their receptors are pH dependent; dissociation places ligands in the luminal space, whereas receptors remain associated with membrane. Geometric considerations, as well as sorting motifs on the receptors, facilitate sorting of membrane from internal volume. Unoccupied receptors whose ligands, such as LDL, have dissociated under the relatively mild acidic conditions encountered in early endosomes are efficiently recycled back to the cell surface. Iron carried by transferin (Tfn) dissociates at a pH of approximately 6, but apoTfn remains bound to and recycles with its receptor. Mannose-6-phosphate receptors (MPRs) carry their ligands to late endosomes before dissociation at lower pH and recycling back to the TGN. EGF remains bound, and both ligand and receptor (EGFR) are delivered to and degraded in lysosomes. PM, plasma membrane.

of ligand-receptor complexes allow researchers to predict where in the endocytic pathway ligands might be separated from their receptors (Fig. 23–13). The pH "signature" of each ligand-receptor system has important implications, as early and late endosomes are usually located in different parts of a cell. For example, hormone stimulation and signal transduction might continue into deeper regions of the cytoplasm if a hormone remained bound to its receptor as the pH dropped. If the endosomal pH gradient changed depending on the cell's physiological state, the action of an internalized hormone would change as well. Likewise, endosomal pH influences receptor dynamics and trafficking patterns. When the pH is perturbed by exposure of tissue culture cells to weak bases, some receptors cannot recycle and, instead, accumulate inside the cell. These perturbations in trafficking can

alter the cell's response to hormonal stimulation; thus, the regulation of endosomal pH can have profound effects on cell physiology.

Receptor Recycling and Endosomes

Bulk membrane is internalized at rates as high as 2% per minute, and nutrient receptors may be internalized at rates exceeding 20% per minute. Therefore, the plasma membrane proteins and receptors, whose lifetimes are typically 20 hours or more, must be recycled efficiently. In fact, more than 90% of all internalized membrane protein (and lipid), as well as approximately 60% to 70% of all internalized fluid, is rapidly returned to the cell surface. Most of this recycling occurs from early endosomes, which have a high surface-to-volume ratio and are enriched in recycling re-

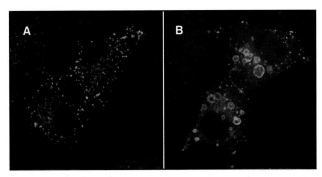

Figure 23-14 Fluorescence micrographs of cultured cells stained with antibodies to Rab5. The early endosomal compartment is greatly expanded in cells overexpressing an activating mutant of Rab5 (Q79L) (*B*) compared to wild-type Rab5 (*A*). (Courtesy of Brian Ceresa, University of Oklahoma.)

ceptors. Recycling is believed to be mediated by tubules that detach and return, either directly (see Fig. 23–13) or indirectly through recycling endosomes (see Fig. 23–12), to the plasma membrane. Receptors destined for delivery to lysosomes remain in the vacuolar portions of these structures. Sorting based on endosomal geometry alone is not sufficient to account for the high efficiencies of recycling of a typical nutrient receptor, which makes at least 100 round trips between endosomes and the plasma membrane without being mistargeted to lysosomes and degraded. Recycling efficiencies are increased both by iterative sorting during maturation of late endosomes (see Fig. 23–12) and by a cytoplasmic sorting machinery that captures receptors for recycling. New methods of imaging sorting endosomes in whole cells have revealed an abundance of coat proteins on their cytoplasmic surface.

A key to efficient recycling is generating a membrane tubule. Where does this excess membrane come from? Part of the answer lies in simple geometric considerations. Because a sphere has the smallest ratio of surface area to volume, when two vesicles of equal diameter fuse with each other to form a larger sphere containing twice the volume, excess membrane is generated. Multiple fusion events generate large amounts of excess membrane. The excess membrane can be removed in the form of tubules, which have a high surface-to-volume ratio. In fact, as many as 30 fusion events are believed to occur while early endosomes execute their sorting functions. These fusion events are controlled by the small GTPase **Rab5** and its effector molecules **EEA1** (early endosome antigen 1) and the t-SNARE protein, syntaxin 13. The lipid phosphatidylinositol 3-phosphate is required to recruit EEA1 to the endosome. Activation or inhibition of Rab5 function leads to an increase or decrease in the size of early endosomes, respectively, and both conditions perturb early endosomal sorting functions (Fig. 23–14). Thus, endosomal structure and function are tightly interrelated.

Recycling efficiencies of receptors can be perturbed experimentally by cross-linking receptors with bivalent antibodies or by perturbing endosomal acidification and preventing the dissociation of receptors from bivalent ligands. Thus, the aggregation state of a receptor can alter its sorting in early endosomes. Physiologically relevant examples of this include ligands, such as antigen-antibody complexes that are composed of multiple copies of immunoglobulin G. These complexes presumably cross-link Fc receptors on the surface of macrophages, prevent their recycling, and instead, cause the aggregated ligand-receptor complexes to be targeted to and degraded in lysosomes. Another example is EGF. EGF binding triggers receptor dimerization, and because EGF does not dissociate until the pH is less than 5.0, the EGF–EGF receptor dimer is targeted for degradation in lysosomes. This process, termed down-regulation (see Chapter 24 and Fig. 24–2), provides the cell with a system for protecting itself (and the larger organism) from an excess of stimulation (see Fig. 29–6).

Late Endosomes and Multivesicular Bodies

After detachment of recycling tubules, the vacuolar portions of early endosomes move along microtubules toward the perinuclear region. The vacuoles begin to accumulate small vesicles and tubules within their lumen by invagination of the limiting membrane. These structures, called **multivesicular bodies,** gradually lose most of the residual plasma membrane markers or recycling receptors that were inadvertently trapped, and they gradually gain lysosomal hydrolases as vesicles are delivered from the TGN along the biosynthetic pathway. Late in this maturation process, multivesicular bodies have a highly complex, intraluminal membrane system, and receptors are segregated into limiting or internal membranes. At this stage, they are called late endosomes. As yet unexplained is the striking observation that the mannose-phosphate receptor that carries lysosomal enzymes to endosomes and then recycles to the TGN prior to delivery to lysosomes is concentrated on the inner membranes. Paradoxically, lysosomal membrane glycoproteins en route to lysosomes are found on the limiting membrane! Multivesicular bodies/late endosomes fuse directly with lysosomes in a process that resembles other intraorganelle fusion events involving organelle-specific v- and t-SNARES, Rab proteins, and NSF (see Chapter 22).

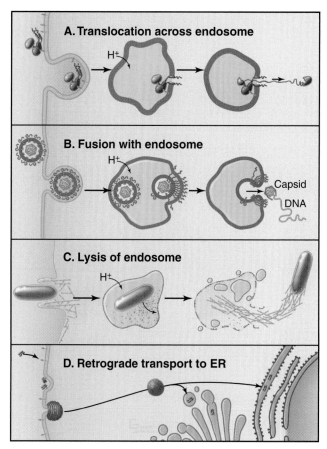

A. Translocation across endosome

H⁺

B. Fusion with endosome

H⁺

Capsid
DNA

C. Lysis of endosome

H⁺

D. Retrograde transport to ER

Figure 23–15 Viruses and toxins have several means to gain entry into the cell. Many viruses and toxins bind to cell surface receptors that are efficiently internalized. *A,* Once in endosomes, pH-dependent conformational changes can trigger the translocation of toxin subunits across the endosomal membrane into the cytosol. *B,* pH-dependent conformational changes can activate fusogenic viral coat proteins to mediate fusion of the viral envelope with the endosomal membrane releasing the nucleocapsid into the cytosol. *C,* Some bacteria secrete toxins after entering the endosome/phagosome; these intercalate into the membrane, creating large pores that disrupt endosomal compartments. *D,* Some toxins enter through alternative endocytic pathways (e.g., through caveolae) and are transported in a retrograde manner back to the endoplasmic reticulum (ER) where they can utilize the cell's translocation machinery—in reverse—to enter the cytoplasm.

Viruses and Protein Toxins As "Opportunistic Endocytic Ligands"

Some enveloped viruses (i.e., those with a membrane bilayer) enter cells by catching a ride on membrane proteins capable of endocytosis. Once inside an endosome, specific viral membrane proteins undergo pH-dependent conformational changes that promote their insertion into and fusion with the organelle membrane. This places the viral nucleocapsid in the cytoplasm where it has access to the cell's synthetic machinery, which it uses to replicate itself (Fig. 23–15*B*).

Both bacteria and plants secrete protein toxins that kill eukaryotic cells efficiently by inhibiting cytosolic functions, such as protein translation. These toxins bind to cell surface "receptors" (either integral proteins or glycolipids) via their B-chains; the toxins are endocytosed, and then the enzymatically active "A-subunit" escapes into the cytoplasm (see Fig. 23–15*A*). Despite their structural similarities, various toxins enter the cytosol from different intracellular compartments, because their requirements for translocation differ. When pH is the trigger, toxins can be translocated directly across the endosomal membrane. Other toxins travel back to the endoplasmic reticulum and use the cell's translocation machinery in reverse to enter the cytoplasm (see Fig. 23–15*D*).

Both clinicians and basic researchers benefit by studying these self-selected "hitchhikers." From them, much can be learned about what properties, sequences, and motifs to look for in endogenous fusogenic proteins. Learning about something as esoteric as the action of a plant toxin may also have medical benefits, as in the treatment of cancer through coupling of the catalytic (A) subunits of toxins to antibodies and targeting of the toxic subunit to malignant cells. These chimeric proteins are called **immunotoxins.** Viruses have evolved efficient mechanisms for delivering their genome into host cells, and so viruses are currently the leading candidates for therapeutic delivery of genes.

Selected Readings

Finlay BB, Cossart P: Exploitation of mammalian host functions by bacterial pathogens. Science 276:718–725, 1997.

Ikonen E: Roles of lipid rafts in membrane transport. Curr Opin Cell Biol 13, 470–477, 2001.

Kirchhausen T: Adaptors for clathrin-mediated traffic. Ann Rev Cell Devel Biol 15:705–732, 1999.

Kirchhausen T: Clathrin. Annu Rev Biochem 69:699–727, 2000.

Lemmo SK, Traub LM: Sorting in the endosomal system in yeast and animal cells. Curr Opin Cell Biol 12:457–466, 2000.

May RC, Machesky LM: Phagocytosis and the actin cytoskeleton. J Cell Sci 114:1061–1077, 2001.

Meresse S, Steele-Mortimer O, Moreno E, et al: Controlling the maturation of pathogen-containing vacuoles: A matter of life and death. Nature Cell Biol 1:E183–E188, 1999.

Mukherjee S, Maxfield FR: Role of membrane organization and membrane domains in endocytic lipid trafficking. Traffic 1:203–211, 2000.

Schmid SL: Clathrin-coated vesicle formation and protein sorting: An integrated process. Annu Rev Biochem 66:511–548, 1997.

Sever S, Damke H, Schmid SL: Garrotes, springs, ratchets and whips: Putting dynamin models to the test. Traffic 1:385–392, 2000.

chapter 24

DEGRADATION OF CELLULAR COMPONENTS

An individual cell can live for weeks, months, years, or even the entire lifetime of the organism, but the cell's constituent proteins, lipids, and RNA turn over continuously. This molecular degradation and replacement serves three functions. Constitutive turnover is a "housekeeping" function that ensures regular replacement of older molecules with newly synthesized ones, or that removes misfolded, mislocalized, or otherwise damaged molecules so that they do not hinder the function of native molecules. Regulated or induced turnover results in rapid degradation of specific target molecules and functions in signal transduction, regulation of the cell cycle, and remodeling of cells and tissues during development. Finally, macroautophagy, a more global mechanism for degradation of cellular proteins or lipids, can be triggered under conditions of starvation, when the cell perceives a shortage of specific raw materials, such as amino acids. This chapter focuses primarily on the elaborate mechanisms governing protein degradation and turnover, as these are the best studied. Lipid turnover is also discussed. Chapter 15 covers RNA turnover.

▌ Characteristics of Constitutive Protein Turnover

The steady-state turnover of body constituents arises from a dynamic flux within which the rates of synthesis and degradation are carefully balanced. The rate of this flux is determined by a pulse-chase experiment. Cells, or whole organisms, are fed a radioactive precursor (e.g., an amino acid) that incorporates into a

"pulse" of newly synthesized molecules. After this labeling period, the radioactive precursor is diluted or flushed out by an excess of unlabeled precursors so that no additional radioactive molecules are synthesized during the "chase" period. Finally, the decrease in radioactivity in the population of molecules is measured over time.

Many studies of constitutive protein degradation have established that the process is random, requires energy, and varies in rate depending on the substrate macromolecule. For example, approximately 40% of total cellular protein in rat liver is degraded every day. The time course follows a single exponential, which provides strong evidence that chance, rather than aging, determines which copies of a specific protein are degraded (see Chapter 3). The rate is usually expressed as a half-life, the time in which half of the molecules are degraded. The intrinsic rate of degradation of a given protein is determined by the sum of many so-called global properties, such as its size, overall charge, thermal instability, flexibility, hydrophobicity, folding, and assembly with other protein subunits (if it is multimeric). Proteins seem to be either long-lived, with half-lives measured in days, or short-lived, with half-lives measured in hours. However, this classification is somewhat arbitrary because there is clearly a continuum of half-lives. Small, basic proteins tend to have longer half-lives than large, acidic proteins, and key enzymes of metabolic pathways usually have very short half-lives. A protein may also have specific sequences or structural motifs that are recognized by the proteolytic machinery. Thus, the rate at which a protein is degraded can be altered either by increasing the activity of its degradative pathway or by exposing a "degradation motif" on the protein to initiate destruction.

Chapter by Sandra L. Schmid, based on an original draft by Ann L. Hubbard, J. David Castle, and Pat Shipman.

Proteolysis: A Compartmentalized Process

Unregulated proteolysis within a cell would clearly be disastrous. Therefore, cells compartmentalize intracellular proteolytic activity in two distinct ways so that access is denied to all but appropriate substrates. **Lysosomes** are membrane-bound proteolytic compartments that sequester **proteases** and provide a low pH environment where these enzymes are optimally active. **Proteasomes** are a second type of compartment for proteolysis. These proteolytic machines are assembled from multiple protein subunits that form a small, cylindrical compartment with the proteolytically active sites sequestered on the inside. The narrow internal diameter of the cylinder and the regulatory complexes that guard the openings allow access only to selected and unfolded polypeptide chains. Intracellular proteolysis depends on specific recognition of protein substrates and their translocation into a proteolytic compartment. Generally speaking, long-lived proteins tend to be degraded by lysosomes, whereas short-lived ones are degraded by proteasomes. The small polypeptide **ubiquitin** is central to targeting molecules for degradation by proteasomes and, at least in some cases, by lysosomes. Ubiquitin is added post-translationally to lysine residues on protein substrates and is recognized by the cellular machinery that targets them for proteolysis. These processes are tightly regulated; thus, energy in the form of adenosine triphosphate (ATP) is required for degradation of proteins, even though hydrolysis of a peptide bond actually releases energy.

■ Degradation in Lysosomes

Lysosomes, the major digestive organelles, contain at least 60 distinct hydrolytic enzymes (see Fig. 23–11 for an electron micrograph). Many lysosomal hydrolases, including proteases, lipases, phospholipases, glycosidases, and nucleases, are soluble glycoproteins that are tagged in the Golgi with mannose-6-phosphate groups on their N-linked oligosaccharides. These sugar residues serve as targeting signals that are recognized by **mannose-6-phosphate receptors** in the trans-Golgi network for diversion to **endosomes** and lysosomes (see Chapter 22). Most lysosomal hydrolases are synthesized as inactive precursors that are activated by proteolysis upon arrival in lysosomes. The low pH of lysosomes, maintained by the vacuolar adenosine triphosphatase (ATPase) proton pump (see

table 24–1
LYSOSOMAL STORAGE DISEASES

Disease(s)	Enzyme Defect	Accumulated Material
Sphingolipidosis GM$_1$ gangliosidosis	β-galactosidase	GM$_1$ ganglioside Glycoproteins
Tay-Sachs disease GM$_2$ gangliosidosis	Hexosaminidase A	GM$_2$ gangliosides
Sandhoff's disease GM$_2$ gangliosidosis	Hexosaminidase A and B	GM$_2$ gangliosides
Krabbe's disease (galactoceramide lipidosis)	Galactosyl ceramid β-galactosidase	Galactocerebrosides
Niemann-Pick disease, types A and B (sphingomyelin lipidosis)	Sphingomyelinase	Sphingomyelin Cholesterol
Gaucher's disease (glucosylceramide lipidosis)	β-glucocerebrosidase	Glucosylceramide
Fabry's disease	α-Galactosidase A	Trihexosylceramide
Glycoprotein storage diseases	α-Fucosidase α-Mannosidase α-Aspartylglucosamine	Glycopeptides Glycolipids Oligosaccharides
Mucopolysaccharidosis (several types)	A-iduronidase Iduronosulfate sulfatase N-acetyl-α-glucosaminidase Heparin sulfatase β-Glucuronidase	Heparin sulfate
Sialidosis	Neuraminidase	Sialyloligosaccharides
Mucolipidosis II (I-cell disease)	UDP-N-acetlyglucosamine (GlcNAc): glycoprotein GlcNAc-1-phosphotransferase	Glycoproteins Glycolipids

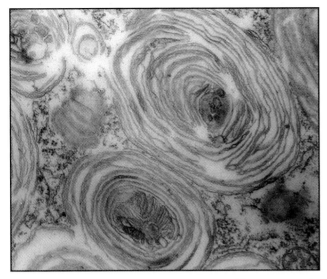

Figure 24-1 Electron micrograph of abnormal lysosomes in the neurons of a patient with GM_1 gangliosidosis. Similar lysosomes, called membranous cytoplasmic bodies, accumulate in the neurons of patients with GM_2 gangliosidosis (Tay-Sachs disease). (Courtesy of Kinuko Suzuki, University of North Carolina, Chapel Hill.)

Fig. 7–5C), is essential for efficient degradation. Most lysosomal enzymes have maximal hydrolytic activity at approximately pH 4 to 5, rather than at the cytoplasmic pH of 6.5 to 7.0. Moreover, the low pH helps to denature most macromolecules, making them more susceptible to degradation. Importantly, the hydrolases themselves are more resistant than most other macromolecules to the harsh environment. Lysosomal enzymes degrade proteins, lipids, and nucleic acids to fragments small enough to be transported across the lysosomal membrane to the cytoplasm, where they are reused to synthesize new macromolecules.

Extracellular particles and solute are delivered to lysosomes via the endocytic pathway for degradation in a process termed **heterophagy** (see Chapter 23). Lysosome-mediated degradation of cellular constituents is generally termed **autophagy.** Studies with specific inhibitors have established that 50% to 70% of cellular protein turnover also occurs in lysosomes, depending on the type of cell and its nutritional state. Delivery of cellular constituents to lysosomes occurs via five distinct mechanisms: endocytosis, **crinophagy, macroautophagy, microautophagy,** and direct translocation from the cytosol. These are all described subsequently. The important role of lysosomes as primary sites for constitutive degradation is reflected in the number (>30) of distinct human lysosomal storage diseases (Table 24–1; see also Chapter 22). Patients with these diseases lack one or more functional lysosomal hydrolases. Consequently, undigested material accumulates in the lysosomes and causes them to swell (Fig. 24–1), ultimately resulting in cell death.

Delivery to Lysosomes via the Endocytic Pathway

Lysosomal degradation of plasma membrane proteins by endocytosis plays an important role in remodeling the plasma membrane in response to cell stimuli. For example, the half-life of the receptor for the epidermal growth factor (EGF) is normally approximately 10 hours. However, when circulating EGF binds, the activated receptor is more efficiently internalized and degraded in lysosomes with a half-time of less than 1 hour. This down-regulates the biologic response (see Fig. 29–9). The complete lysosomal digestion of integral membrane proteins, in particular, signaling receptors with tyrosine kinase activity, requires that they be sequestered into small invaginations that bud inward, forming the intraluminal vesicles or tubules of **multivesicular** bodies (see Fig. 23–12). Multivesicular bodies fuse directly with lysosomes, and the intraluminal vesicles are digested together with their lipid and protein components (Fig. 24–2). Resident lysosomal membrane proteins remain in the limiting membrane, indicating that sequestration into intraluminal vesicles is selective. The invagination of intraluminal vesicles requires lipid modifications, in particular, the formation of phosphatidylinositol-3-phosphate (PI3-P) by PI3-kinase activity. Interestingly, PI3-kinase is activated by several receptor tyrosine kinases (see Chapter 29). Several signaling receptors are also modified with ubiquitin after activation, and, in some cases, ubiquitination is required for receptor **down-regulation** through degradation in lysosomes.

Autophagy

Microautophagy and macroautophagy both describe the consumption of cytoplasmic constituents within lysosomes. Microautophagy occurs as a by-product of the formation of multivesicular bodies (see Fig. 24–2 and Chapter 23). Small volumes of cytoplasm are captured in the intraluminal vesicles and tubules that form by invagination of the endosome or lysosome membrane. The cytoplasmic components are degraded as the vesicles are consumed. Recent studies in yeast suggest the existence of alternative pathways for the selective packaging and delivery of cytosolic proteins to lysosomes. When starved for glucose, the yeast *Saccharomyces cerevisiae* expresses several cytosolic enzymes and membrane transporters required to process more complex sugar substrates. Upon addition of glucose, the yeast switches metabolic pathways and degrades the enzymes it no longer needs. Although membrane-associated transporters are internalized and delivered to the yeast vacuole (the lysosome equivalent) through the formation of multivesicular bodies and microautophagy, unneeded cytosolic enzymes are selectively packaged into small vesicles that deliver

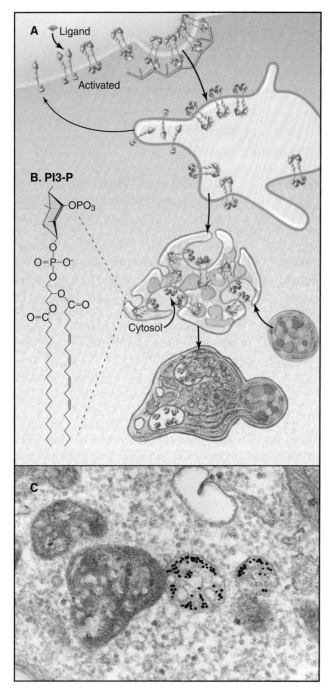

A Ligand
Activated

B. PI3-P

Cytosol

C

Figure 24-2 To limit the time course of EGF stimulation, activated EGF receptors are internalized (A) and delivered to endosomes and sequestered (B) within internal membrane vesicles that accumulate in late endosomes. Invagination of the late endosomal membrane may involve production of the lipid species, PI3-P, by the enzyme PI3-kinase, which is activated by EGF receptors. After fusion with lysosomes, lysosomal proteases and lipases ensure that both the extracellular and cytoplasmic domains of the EGF receptor are degraded, a process termed receptor "down-regulation." Cytosolic proteins are also incorporated into the internal vesicles of multivesicular late endosomes and are degraded in a constitutive process termed microautophagy. C, EM of gold-labeled EGF receptor in multivesicular endosomes fusing with a lysosome. (C, Courtesy of Colin Hopkins, MRC Laboratory, University College, London.)

their contents to the vacuole by fusion. Genetic studies of yeast are unraveling the mechanisms governing these rapidly induced and selective degradation pathways.

Macroautophagy involves the engulfment of large volumes of cytoplasm—including glycogen deposits, ribosomes, and organelles, such as mitochondria and peroxisomes—into an **autophagic vacuole.** The formation of nascent autophagic vacuoles begins when a flattened membrane cisterna encircles a region of cytosol and coalesces to form a double-membrane vesicle (Fig. 24–3). The origin of the smooth membrane cisternae is not certain: some have suggested that it derives from the smooth endoplasmic reticulum (ER), whereas others argue that it derives from the trans-Golgi or endosomal system, as these tubulovesicular membranes would normally contain targeting information for fusion with lysosomes. Late endosomes and lysosomes fuse with the nascent autophagic vacuoles, delivering acid hydrolases into the lumen and forming an **autolysosome** (see Figs. 24–3 and 24–4). Degradation of the inner membrane ensues, followed by degradation of the contents. When digestion is complete, the autolysosome has a characteristically dense core of undegraded material and is referred to as a **residual body.**

The process of formation and degradation of autophagic vacuoles in the liver requires less than 15 minutes. Because large volumes of cytoplasm and entire organelles are destroyed, macroautophagy must be regulated precisely and directly. Although the exact nature of the intracellular messenger that triggers this highly choreographed process is unknown, the signal is thought to be tied to the intracellular levels of particular amino acids, which are, in turn, related to circulating levels of amino acids outside of cells. Amino acids are potent inhibitors of autophagy. Autophagy can also be regulated by circulating peptide hormones, which, upon receptor binding, presumably trigger signaling cascades involving protein phosphorylation. During starvation, circulating levels of glucagon increase and stimulate autophagy in liver cells. Feeding produces the opposite reaction by increasing the levels of insulin, which in turn, decreases autophagy. Diurnal feeding rhythms cause the numbers of autophagic vacuoles to vary along with the fluctuation of essential amino acids in the blood.

The mechanisms governing autophagy are currently unknown, although genetic analysis of yeast suggests that more than 15 gene products are required. The identity of three of these—designated Apg7p, Apg12p, and Apg5p—suggests that a ubiquitin-like system may play a role in directing autophagic degradation. Apg7p is related to ubiquitin-conjugating enzymes (see later section) and catalyzes the covalent attachment of Apg12p, a 186-residue polypeptide, to a membrane-associated substrate, Apg2p. The existence of mammalian homologues to these yeast proteins suggests that this mechanism is conserved. In fact, inhibition of lysosomal hydrolases under conditions of serum starvation leads to the accumulation of ubiquitinated proteins in autolysosomes.

Crinophagy

Fusion of lysosomes directly with secretory vesicles, a process known as crinophagy, results in the degradation of secretory proteins. This process is important in the anterior pituitary, which contains multiple types of regulated secretory cells and intracellular granules that store polypeptide hormones, such as prolactin. When suckling is terminated, and in response to an unknown signal, lysosomes fuse with granules to degrade the prolactin. Crinophagy may also function to remove aged granules containing damaged proteins.

Selective Protein Uptake into Lysosomes

With prolonged starvation, autophagy diminishes, and a selective lysosomal degradative mechanism is initiated. This response may reflect two competing needs: (1) the need to maintain critical levels of key cellular proteins that might otherwise be destroyed through the nonselective process of autophagy; and (2) the

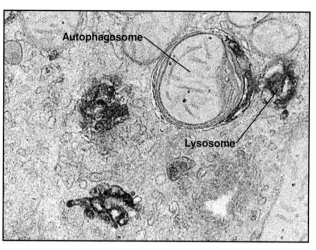

Figure 24-4 Electron micrograph from starved rat liver shows an autophagosome containing a mitochondrion that is fusing directly with a secondary lysosome (Courtesy of William Dunn, University of Florida, Gainesville; reprinted from Dunn WA Jr: Studies on the mechanisms of autophagy: Maturation of the autophagic vacuole. J Cell Biol 110:1935–1945, 1990, by copyright permission of the Rockefeller University Press.)

need to supply amino acids for the synthesis of essential proteins. The 20% to 30% of cytosolic proteins selected for degradation by this mechanism are long-lived and contain structural signals—in particular, the linear sequence KFPRQ—that are recognized by the molecular chaperone, Hsc70, which conducts them to lysosomes. A lysosomal membrane glycoprotein, lgp96 or Lamp2, may function as a receptor for these molecules, and an intralysosomal chaperone, ly-hsc73, seems to be required for translocation across the lysosomal membrane. Although many questions are as yet unanswered, this process is important because it shows that soluble macromolecules can be transported selectively from the cytoplasm into lysosomes.

Degradation by Proteasomes

The proteasome is the second major cellular compartment for proteolysis. Proteasomes are large, cylindrical structures composed of multiple protein subunits and located in both the cytoplasm and nucleoplasm (Fig. 24–5). They are abundant, often accounting for up to 1% of total cellular protein. The several proteolytic active sites in the structure combine to degrade proteins to small peptides. Abnormal and misfolded proteins are substrates of proteasomes, as are many normal, though short-lived, proteins. Proteasomes degrade key substrates in response to signaling cascades or at key transitional stages of the cell cycle. One class of proteasomes processes intracellular antigens for presentation by the immune system.

The proteasome has two major structural components: the core and the cap. The core, referred to as

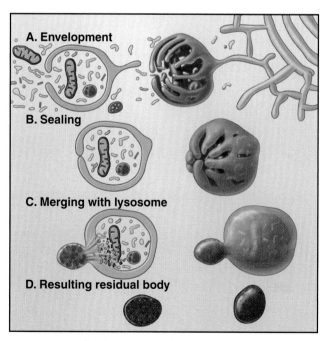

Figure 24-3 The four stages of autophagy. *A,* A membrane cisterna from an as-yet-undefined source envelopes a large region of cytoplasm, including any organelles within this area. *B,* Membrane fusion results in formation of a nascent autophagosome. *C,* The nascent autophagosome fuses directly with a primary or secondary lysosome, which delivers hydrolytic enzymes that degrade the autophagosome contents. *D,* Undigested material remains in electron-dense residual bodies.

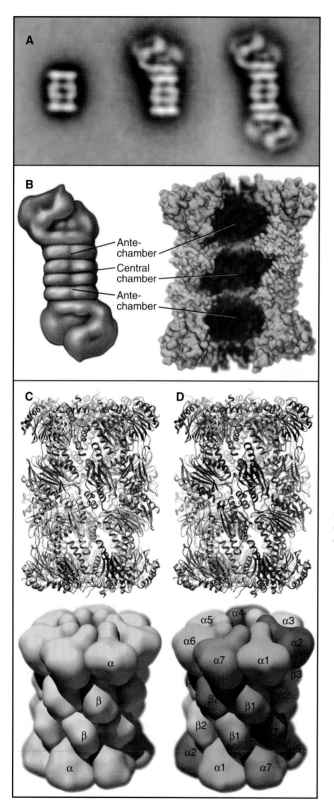

Figure 24–5 Structure of the proteasome. *A,* Electron micrographs of negatively stained 20S proteasomes from bovine red blood cells alone *(left),* or singly *(middle)* or doubly *(right)* capped with PA700, the 19S regulator, to generate the 26S particle. These images were enhanced by computer processing. *B,* Model of the 26S proteasome compared with a space-filling model of the high-resolution crystal structure of the 20S particle on the right. *C* and *D,* Ribbon diagrams and subunit compositions for the 20S proteasomes from *Thermoplasma acidophilum* (*C*) and from *S. cerevisiae* (*D*). Note the conservation of structure from Archaea, to yeast, to mammals. (*A,* Electron micrographs courtesy of Edward P. Gogol, University of Missouri, Kansas City. *C,* PDB file: 1PMA; reference: Lowe J, Stock D, Jap B, et al: Crystal structure of the 20S proteasome from the archaeon T. acidophilum at 3.4 Å resolution. Science 268:533–539, 1995. *D,* PDB file: 1RYP; reference: Groll M, Ditzel L, Lowe J, et al: Structure of 20S proteasome from yeast at 2.4 Å resolution. Nature 386:463–471, 1997.)

the 20S proteasome (named according to its sedimentation coefficient; see Chapter 5) is structurally conserved from bacteria to mammals, although the subunit composition varies. In mammals, the cylindrical 20S core is 15 nm long and 11 nm in diameter, with an overall mass of approximately 700 kD. It is assembled from two copies each of 14 different 25- to 35-kD subunits that can be divided into α-type and β-type groups (see Fig. 24–5*C* and *D*). These subunits are arranged into four seven-membered rings. The α-type subunits form the two outer rings and the β-type subunits form the two inner rings. The central cavity is 5 nm in diameter with four narrow constrictions that form three internal cavities: a central chamber surrounded by the β-subunits and two antechambers at either end of the cylinder (see Fig. 24–5B). The proteolytic active sites on the β-subunits are sequestered in the central chamber. An N-terminal threonine residue on the β-subunits is exposed by autocatalytic proteolysis and serves as the key active site residue for proteolysis. The antibiotic **lactacystin** reacts covalently and selectively with these threonine residues to inactivate the proteasome.

Eukaryotic proteasomes have multiple types of hydrolytic activities that can be ascribed to distinct β-type subunits. In yeast and probably in mammalian proteasomes, the **caspase**-like activity of the β1-subunit cleaves after acidic residues, the trypsin-like activity of the β2-subunit cleaves after basic residues, and the chymotrypsin-like activity of the β5-subunit cleaves after hydrophobic residues (see Chapter 49 for a description of caspases). Other β-type subunits present in the eukaryotic proteasome are apparently not post-translationally processed to mature, catalytically active enzymes. These three activities combine to give the proteasome broad specificity, allowing it to cleave many substrates into diverse cleavage products (Fig. 24–6). It was initially thought that the restricted length (7 to 9 residues) of the final products of proteolysis reflected an "intrinsic molecular ruler," the length of which corresponded to the distance between active sites. However, mutagenesis to selectively inactivate individual β-subunits has no effect on product length, as would be predicted. Thus, the mechanisms restricting peptide length remain unknown.

The noncatalytic α-subunits are presumably involved in translocation of the substrate into the proteolytic chamber. The narrow dimensions of the chamber and constriction points limit access to unfolded polypeptide chains. The 20S proteasome degrades unfolded proteins to small peptides without hydrolyzing ATP. In cells, proteasome function requires ATP hydrolysis, presumably to unfold protein substrates.

In eukaryotes and Archaea, the proteasome is "capped" at one or both ends of the 20S barrel with regulatory complexes to form the 26S proteasome. The type of regulatory complex varies depending on the function of the proteasome. One such complex, called the 19S regulator or PA700, has a mass of approximately 700 kD (see Fig. 24–5A). Several of its subunits are members of the AAA ATPase family (see Chapter 18) and are believed to play a role in the dissociation of target protein oligomers, protein unfolding, and translocation into the central channels. Other subunits are involved in recognition of ubiquitinated proteins and in deubiquitination, a process required to recycle ubiquitin from proteins destined for degradation (see later for more about ubiquitin).

A second regulator complex, the 11S cap or PA28 regulator, is found associated with a subpopulation of the 20S proteasome core, and only in cells of higher vertebrates. This 20S/11S proteasome is induced by the cytokine **γ-interferon** as part of the immune response and is thought to play a specialized role in the ubiquitin-independent cleavage of intracellular antigens (e.g., those derived from an infecting virus) into peptides of uniform length for antigen presentation. It is, therefore, also referred to as the "**immunoproteasome**" (see Fig. 24–5). The 11S cap does not recognize ubiquitinated protein substrates and may play a role as an adapter molecule for the interaction of molecular chaperones with the immunoproteasome. Some of the catalytic β-subunits are also exchanged in the 20S core of the immunoproteasome so that the peptides generated are somewhat longer and better suited for antigen presentation. The immunoproteasome is physically and functionally coupled to a peptide transporter in the ER called the **TAP** (transporter associated with antigen presentation). TAP is composed of two similar subunits, TAP1 and TAP2, which together comprise an **ABC transporter** (see Chapter 7) that mediates the ATP-dependent transport of peptides generated by the proteasome into the ER. In a tightly coupled reaction involving another ER-localized integral membrane protein, tapasin, the translocated peptides are directly loaded onto **class I Major histocompatibility antigen I (MHC) molecules** for transport to the cell surface. On the cell surface, the MHC-peptide complex stimulates T-cells (see Fig. 29–11). To avoid detection by the immune system, some viruses commandeer this pathway and force the translocation of MHC molecules backward through TAP, out of the ER, and into the waiting mouth of the proteasome.

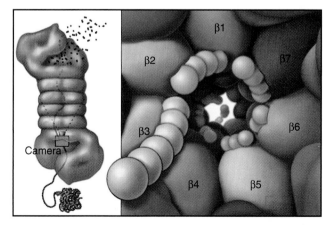

Figure 24-6 Drawing of a polypeptide moving through the central channel of the 20S particle. Note that the distribution of protease sites varies with subunit composition, governing the size of the product peptides.

Ubiquitination Targets Proteins to Proteasomes

The key to regulating degradation by proteasomes is controlling access of molecules into the central proteolytic chamber. The best characterized targeting mechanism involves the reversible, covalent linkage of a small protein, ubiquitin, onto the target protein. Ubiquitination directs the selective and coordinated degradation of abnormally folded proteins and of regulatory proteins, including proteins that control progression through the cell cycle, components of signal transduction systems, and transcriptional regulators. Reversible ubiquitination is also involved in other cellular functions, such as the assembly of ribosomes, proteasomes, and other multimeric complexes, DNA repair, and chromosomal structure. Disruption of the ubiquitination pathway is lethal in yeast.

Ubiquitin is a very abundant and highly conserved 76-residue protein. It has a tightly packed, globular, compact structure from which only the C-terminal 4 amino acids extend (Fig. 24–7). Ubiquitination of protein substrates proceeds through a tightly regulated, elaborate, multistep pathway, which has been elucidated through biochemical purification of mammalian components and in vitro reconstitution of partial reactions. The overall scheme can be subdivided into three stages (Fig. 24–8). The first stage, activation of ubiquitin, is catalyzed by E1, the **ubiquitin-activating enzyme,** and one of several E2 or **ubiquitin-conjugating** (or carrier) **enzymes.** In the first reaction, ubiquitin molecules are linked through their C-terminal glycine residues to a cysteine residue on E1 via a thioester bond. Activated ubiquitin is then transferred

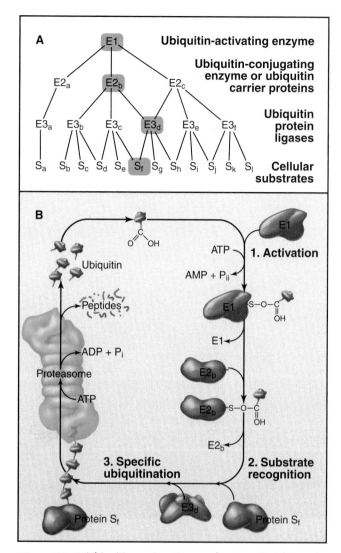

Figure 24–8 Ubiquitin conjugation mechanism. *A,* A hierarchy of ubiquitin-conjugating enzymes and ubiquitin protein ligases work together to recognize and ubiquitinate specific cellular substrates in a highly regulated manner. *B,* The three stages of ubiquitination for one representative set of enzymes. The common enzyme in each pathway is the ubiquitin-activating enzyme (E1). One of several E2 enzymes serves as an intermediate to transfer activated ubiquitin and works with one of several E3 enzymes to recognize the appropriate target protein and to transfer the first ubiquitin molecule. Subsequent polyubiquitination targets the protein for degradation in the proteasome. ADP, adenosine diphosphate; AMP, adenosine monophosphate; P_{ii}, pyrophosphate.

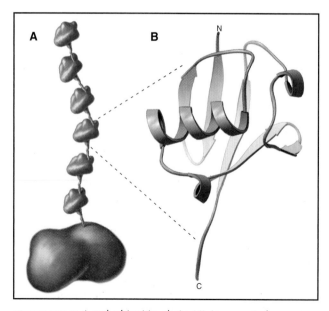

Figure 24–7 A polyubiquitin chain (*A*) is generated on a protein to target it for degradation in the proteasome by sequential conjugation of ubiquitin (*B*), shown in ribbon diagram.

to a cysteine residue on the E2 enzyme. The second stage, substrate recognition, occurs independently and involves one of several E3 enzymes or **ubiquitin ligases.** E3 enzymes constitute a large family of proteins and protein complexes that confer specificity to the ubiquitination reaction. E3 enzymes catalyze the transfer of ubiquitin to the protein substrate from the E2-ubiquitin intermediate either directly or in two steps through an E3-ubiquitin intermediate. Ubiquitination of the protein substrate occurs through an amide

table 24–2
UBIQUITIN/PROTEOSOME TARGETING SYSTEMS

Recognition Determinant	Cellular Substrates	Ubiquitin-Conjugating Enzymes (E2)	Ubiquitin Ligases (E3)
The N-end rule (N-terminal residue F,L,W,Y,R,K,H)	Mislocalized proteins, cell cycle proteins	Ubc2 (Rad6p)	E3α (Ubr1p)
Amphipathic or hydrophobic peptides	α-2 Transcription factor	Ubc6, Ubc7	Unknown
	Misfolded proteins?		
Phosphorylated signals DS*GXXS*	Transcription factors (e.g., IκB, β-catenin)	Several	SCF complexes
PES*T regions	Cell cycle regulators (e.g., cyclins)		
Destruction box R(A/T)(A)L(G)X (I/V)(G/T)(N)	Mitotic cyclins Cell cycle regulators	E2-c (cyclin-specific E2)	APC/c (anaphase-promoting complex/cyclosome)

Note: Asterisk refers to phosphorylation sites on serine residues.

linkage with the ϵ-NH$_4$ group of a lysine residue located in a region of the protein substrate that is relatively unordered (i.e., flexible or mobile) and, therefore, presumably accessible to the E3 enzyme. Additional ubiquitin molecules are then conjugated onto lys48 of preceding ubiquitin to create a **polyubiquitin chain** (see Figs. 24–7 and 24–8). In general, monoubiquitinated proteins are not recognized by the proteasome. Subunits of the proteasome cap structures complete the process by deubiquitinating their substrates as they are fed into the proteolytic central chamber. The released ubiquitin is reutilized.

Motifs That Specify Ubiquitination

The complexity of the ubiquitination pathway provides tight regulation through multiple checkpoints, ensuring that only the appropriate target proteins are recognized, ubiquitinated, and, consequently, degraded. The primary responsibility for substrate selectivity lies with the E3 family of enzymes. These ubiquitin ligases can bind directly to protein substrates or indirectly through adaptor molecules. Although the 13 or more E2 enzymes can interact directly with substrate, in general, they recognize the E3-substrate complex. One E2 enzyme can cooperate with several different E3 enzymes in the ubiquitination reaction (see Fig. 24–8). E2s accept substrates from a single E1 in yeast.

Protein substrates are targeted for ubiquitination and degradation by different determinants, which, in turn, are recognized by different classes of E3 enzymes. Only a few of the rules or motifs governing E3-substrate recognition signals have been identified (Table 24–2) and many more remain to be discov-

ered. The first and simplest signal to be identified is described by the "**N-end rule.**" Through studies of chimeric and fusion proteins in yeast, researchers have found that specific destabilizing amino acids at the N-terminus of a protein are recognized for ubiquitination and subsequent destruction by E3α. Both the destabilizing N-terminal amino acid and a mobile lysine on the substrate are needed for ubiquitination and rapid degradation. The extent to which this simple rule governs proteolysis in vivo remains uncertain, as few proteins naturally encode destabilizing amino acids at their N-terminus and many that do are naturally sequestered within compartments, away from the ubiquitination system and proteasomes. Thus, the N-end rule is thought to play a role in degrading mislocalized proteins—those in the wrong place at the wrong time—rather than in triggering basal or constitutive degradation. One physiological substrate of the N-end rule is the C-terminal fragment of the Scc1 chromosome cohesin molecule that is produced by specific proteolysis at the outset of anaphase (see Chapter 47, Fig. 47–14). Interference with N-end rule degradation of this protein is lethal to the cell, presumably because chromosome segregation is disrupted during mitosis. In addition, the N-end rule becomes a major determinant of proteolysis in different disease states, such as in muscle atrophy.

Amphipathic or hydrophobic stretches of amino acids also function as general recognition determinants for ubiquitination. Although the E3 enzymes involved have not been identified, this pathway is especially prevalent in controlling the degradation of misfolded proteins dislocated from the ER (see Chapter 20). Because hydrophobic surfaces are often buried in a folded protein or at the interface between subunits, exposure of this ubiquitination determinant is thought to assist in targeting misfolded proteins or excess subunits of oligomeric proteins for degradation.

Regulated proteolysis is used in controlling cell cycle progression and transcription activation. In these cases, targeting signals for degradation can be generated by specific phosphorylation events. For example, phosphorylation of a conserved sequence near the N-terminus of several transcription factors or their regulatory subunits generates a determinant recognized by the SCF complex (a family of modular E3 enzymes named for their three core components: *skp1*, *cdc53/cullin*, and an *F*-box-containing protein; see Chapter 43). Phosphorylation of cell cycle proteins containing internal sequences that are rich in proline, glutamine, serine, and threonine (called PEST sequences) can also target these proteins via SCF family E3 enzymes for rapid degradation. A second multi-subunit class of E3 enzymes, designated APC/c (anaphase-promoting complex/cyclosome), recognizes a partially conserved, 9-residue "destruction box" sequence near the N-terminus of several cell cycle regulatory proteins that targets these proteins for degradation. Deletion of the destruction box stabilizes the protein, whereas its transfer to a normally stable protein results in cell cycle–dependent ubiquitination and rapid degradation. In this case, regulation of ubiquitination appears to be at the level of the APC ubiquitin ligase through phosphorylation events and interactions with regulator molecules.

Other Regulated Intracellular Proteolysis

The proteolytic processing of inactive proenzymes or transcription activators into active ones is another form of regulated intracellular proteolysis. One important class of these proteins is the **caspases,** whose initial activation in response to extracellular signals starts an enzyme cascade leading to apoptosis (Chapter 49). In all cases, intracellular proteolysis is tightly regulated through a combination of triggered activation of the protease, specific substrate recognition, and compartmentalization.

Lipid Turnover and Degradation

Distinct pathways exist for the turnover of the three classes of cellular lipids: phosphoglycerides, glycolipids, and cholesterol. Glycolipids, which are restricted to the extracellular leaflet of a lipid bilayer, are degraded primarily in lysosomes, as evidenced from lysosomal storage diseases (see Table 24–2). Sphingomyelin and gangliosides are delivered to lysosomes via vesicular transport and degraded to the level of ceramide, sugars, and fatty acids by a series of lysosomal hydrolases. Recent evidence suggests that the specialized lipidic environment of lysosomal membranes, including the phospholipid species **lysobis-phosphatidic acid,** may play a role in activating spingomyelinases and restricting their hydrolytic activity to intraluminal membranes. Cell surface sphingomyelinases also exist, and their activation triggers production of ceremide, which can function in signal transduction pathways as a second messenger (see Fig. 28–11).

Turnover of phosphoglycerides is much more varied in mechanism and location. Some phosphoglycerides, particularly those found in the outer leaflet of the plasma membrane (and in topologically equivalent surfaces), are degraded to their fatty acid, head group, and glycerol constituents in lysosomes. More frequently, phosphoglyceride degradation is only partial, and the degradative products (e.g., fatty acids, lysophospholipids, and diacylglycerol) are salvaged and reutilized in "short-circuit pathways." In this way, "old" phospholipids are "remodeled," forming new ones with altered properties. These phospholipid remodeling reactions are catalyzed by a variety of **phospholipases** that cleave distinct bonds in the phospholipid to generate distinct products (see Fig. 28–4). Localized lipid remodeling can generate specialized lipid subdomains required for vesicle fusion or fission, or for the selective recruitment of proteins to the membrane. In addition, molecules released from partial degradation of phosphoglycerides, fatty acids, diacylglycerol, and some head groups function as second messengers in signaling cascades (see Chapter 28).

Cholesterol Homeostasis

Cholesterol homeostasis is critical to human health, as evidenced by the number of genetic diseases that are known to result from faulty regulation of cholesterol metabolism (Fig. 24–9). In animal cells, approximately 90% of the free cholesterol is within the plasma membrane. Cholesterol is also the precursor for steroid hormones, which are synthesized in specialized cells but utilized throughout the body for a myriad of essential functions. Finally, cholesterol is the precursor for bile acids, which are synthesized by the liver and transported to the gut, where they aid in the digestion of dietary fat. Unlike virtually all other intracellular molecules, individual cells cannot degrade cholesterol. Instead, cellular levels of cholesterol are regulated by a complex balance of endogenous synthesis, uptake of extracellular cholesterol, and efflux of intracellular cholesterol to vascular fluids. When present in excess, cholesterol accumulates as insoluble plaques in the walls of major blood vessels, contributing to atherosclerosis.

Cholesterol is insoluble and is transported through the body as cholesterol esters packaged in complexes

Figure 24-9 The intracellular processing and regulation of cholesterol biosynthesis. *A,* Dietary cholesterol is delivered to cells in LDL particles. *B,* LDL particles are taken up by clathrin-mediated endocytosis. *C,* Free cholesterol is released in late endosomes/lysosomes and transported to the cell surface or internal membranes, depending, in part, on the activity of NPC-1 (*D*), an integral membrane protein. Excess cholesterol can be acylated by ACAT activity and stored in the cytoplasm as cholesterol esters. ACAT activity is increased by high intracellular cholesterol levels. At the same time, high cholesterol in the membrane decreases new cholesterol synthesis by triggering the proteasome-dependent degradation of the enzyme HMG-CoA reductase. Finally, high cellular cholesterol decreases the uptake of LDL particles and dietary cholesterol by blocking the proteolytic processing of the transcription factor, SREBP, required for LDL-receptor expression (see Fig. 20–15). Genetic defects that perturb steps *A* to *D* required for maintaining the delicate balance of cholesterol homeostasis cause several human diseases. Familial hypercholesterolemia is caused by either a lack of LDL receptor (LDL-R) (*A*), or LDL-R that is defective in endocytic activity (*B*). Wolman disease is a lysosomal storage disease caused by defective lysosomal cholesterol esterase activity; Niemann-Pick disease type C, another lysosomal storage disease, results in defective trafficking of cholesterol out of late endosomes and lysosomes owing to mutations in NPC-1 (*D*).

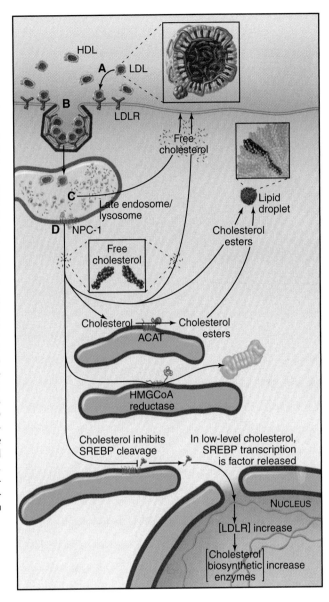

with other lipids and proteins. Dietary cholesterol is packaged in the intestine into particles called chylomicons, which are eventually taken up by the liver, the major site of cholesterol synthesis in mammals. The liver packages dietary and de novo–synthesized cholesterol into **low-density lipoproteins** (LDLs) for transport to other tissues. Peripheral tissues take up LDL particles via receptor-mediated endocytosis and deliver them along the endocytic pathway to lysosomes (see Chapter 23). Some patients with familial hypercholesterolemia have mutations in the LDL receptor, leading to inefficient uptake of extracellular cholesterol and its resulting deposition in arteries. Within the lysosome, cholesterol esters are hydrolyzed (a process defective in patients with Wolman disease), and the bulk of free LDL-derived cholesterol is transported via an as-yet-unidentified cytosolic protein carrier back to the plasma membrane. Importantly, a small portion is also transported to the ER. The recently discovered gene responsible for Niemann-Pick type C disease, a devastating neurodegenerative disease, is a multi-transmembrane domain protein (designated NPC-1) whose activity is somehow required for transport of LDL-derived cholesterol from lysosomes to both the plasma membrane and ER. Cholesterol accumulates in lysosomes of diseased patients, and cholesterol homeostasis is impaired. Interestingly, NPC-1 has a "sterol-sensing domain" common to enzymes regulated by intracellular cholesterol levels, suggesting that its activity is regulated by cholesterol (Fig. 24–10 and 20–15).

Two key enzymes controlling intracellular free cholesterol levels—3-hydroxy-3-methylglutaryl-CoA **(HMG-CoA) reductase,** which catalyzes the initial

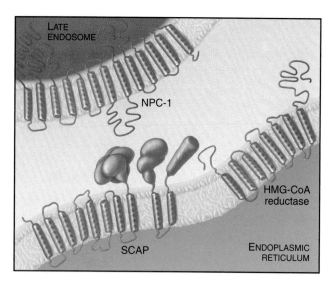

Figure 24-10 Proteins involved in cholesterol trafficking and homeostasis share a common sequence motif, the cholesterol-sensing domain. This is a region of the protein that spans the membrane four times and may be responsive to cholesterol levels in the lipid bilayer in which the protein resides.

step in cholesterol synthesis (see Fig. 20–14) and acyl CoA:cholesterol acyltransferase (ACAT), which catalyzes the esterification of free cholesterol for intracellular storage—are located in the ER. Both enzymes are responsive to cellular pools of cholesterol, the status of which is communicated to the ER through the integrated trafficking of cholesterol between the plasma membrane, lysosomes, and the ER.

The arrival of LDL-derived cholesterol and its accumulation at the ER leads to activation of ACAT, which converts free cholesterol to cholesterol esters for storage. When the levels of free cholesterol (or an oxygenated metabolite of it) increase substantially, secondary responses are activated through sterol-sensing domains in other ER-localized enzymes (see Fig. 20–15). For example, cholesterol triggers the degradation of HMG-CoA reductase through a ubiquitin- and proteasome-dependent pathway. A third sterol-sensing domain protein—SCAP—activates proteolysis of the membrane-bound transcription activator, SREBP, which controls the expression of both HMG-CoA reductase and the LDL receptor. When ER cholesterol is elevated, SCAP activity and, therefore, the production

of SREBP are reduced, lowering the expression levels of LDL receptor and HMG-CoA reductase. This feedback mechanism reduces cholesterol input both from de novo synthesis and from extracellular sources. The intracellular mechanisms for cholesterol homeostasis (see Fig. 24–9) involve coordination of many of the intracellular pathways that have been introduced in this section. These include receptor-mediated endocytosis, trafficking along the endosomal pathway, retrograde transport from endosomes to the ER, and regulation of protein expression by directed, proteasome-mediated degradation and specific intracellular proteolysis.

Selected Readings

Bochtler M, Diitzel L, Groll M, et al: The proteasome. Ann Rev Biophysic Biomolec Struct 28:295–317, 1999.

Bonifacino JS, Weissman AM: Ubiquitin and the control of protein fate in the secretory and endocytic pathways. Ann Rev Cell Devel Biol 14:9–58, 1998.

Brown MS, Goldstein JL: A proteolytic pathway that controls the cholesterol content of membranes, cells, and blood. Proc Natl Acad Sci (USA) 96:11041–11048, 1999.

Deshaies RJ: SCF and Cullin/Ring H2-based ubiquitin ligases. Ann Rev Cell Devel Biol 15:435–468, 1999.

Fineschi B, Miller J: Endosomal proteases and antigen processing. Trends Biochem Sci 22:377–382, 1997.

Lupas A, Flanagan JM, Tamaura T, et al: Self-compartmentalizing proteases. Trends Biochem Sci 22:399–404, 1997.

McGrath ME: Lysosomal cysteine proteases. Ann Rev Biophysic Biomolec Struct 28:181–204, 1999.

Pickart CM: Mechanisms underlying Ubiquitination. Annu Rev Biochem 70:503–534, 2001.

Rechsteiner M, Rogers SW: PEST sequences and regulation by proteolysis. Trends Biochem Sci 21:267–271, 1996.

Simons K, Ikonen E: How cells handle cholesterol. Science 290:1721–1726, 2000.

Teter SA, Klionsky DJ: Transport of proteins to the yeast vacuole: Autophagy, cytoplasm-to-vacuole targeting, and the role of the vacuole in degradation. Semin Cell Dev Biol 11:173–179, 2000.

Varshavsky A: The ubiquitin system. Trends Biochem Sci 22:383–387, 1997.

Villa P, Kaufmann SH, Earnshaw WC: Caspases and caspase inhibitors. Trends Biochem Sci 22:388–392, 1997.

Voges D, Zwickl P, Baumeister W: The 26S proteasome: A molecular machine designed for controlled proteolysis. Ann Rev Biochem 68:1015–1068, 1999.

RECEPTION
AND TRANSDUCTION
OF ENVIRONMENTAL
INFORMATION

chapter 25

INTRODUCTION TO SIGNALING PATHWAYS

Cells tune their activity to adapt to changing environmental conditions. Free living organisms, like yeast and bacteria, respond to changes in temperature, osmotic stress, and nutrients by synthesizing the proteins required to optimize their survival under particular circumstances. Motile cells respond to chemical attractants by migrating up concentration gradients toward the source of the chemical. In animals, the hormone adrenaline (epinephrine) stimulates cellular energy metabolism, and growth factors stimulate cells to duplicate their genomes and divide. Unicellular and multicellular organisms integrate their responses to external stimuli remarkably well as they adapt to ever-changing and sometimes extreme conditions.

Developmentally regulated genetic programs equip each cell type with the molecular hardware required to adapt to remarkably diverse stimuli (Fig. 25–1). These external inputs include purely physical stimuli, such as mechanical force and light; chemicals, including simple gases, amino acids, proteins, nucleotides, steroids, and lipid derivatives; other cells; and the extracellular matrix.

Cells recognize stimuli and transduce their recognition into a response, usually a change in cellular activity. A response typically takes place in several discrete steps (Fig. 25–2). First, a **stimulus** activates a receptor. The stimulus is often a chemical ligand that binds a **receptor.** Second, an active receptor transduces the stimulus into a chemical signal inside the cell, usually a change in concentration of a small messenger molecule or a change in the activity of a messenger protein. This **transduction** step converts one type of signal (stimulus) into another signal (messenger) and commonly amplifies the signal. Third, the intracellular chemical messenger acts upon **effector** systems to modify the behavior of the cell. Integrated input from parallel signaling pathways or feedback loops, or both, usually influences the response at the transduction and effector stages.

Recognition of a stimulus requires physical interaction of the stimulus with a cellular receptor. Usually, the stimulus comes from outside the cell. Most stimuli, like proteins or highly charged biogenic amines, cannot penetrate the plasma membrane, so part of the transduction process involves transfer of information across the plasma membrane. This is accomplished by integral proteins of the plasma membrane, which bind specific ligands and transfer signals across the lipid bilayer. A few stimuli, including light, steroid hormones, and gases, penetrate the plasma membrane and react directly with receptors and effectors inside the cell.

Without exception, receptors are proteins. Although cells bind and respond to thousands of ligands, all known stimuli act through about 20 families of receptors, each coupled to distinct signal transduction mechanisms (Fig. 25–3; see also Chapter 26). Multiple isoforms within each family provide thousands of different receptors with specificity for particular stimuli. For example, of 18,000 genes in the nematode genome, nearly 800 encode receptors with seven transmembrane helices. Presumably, all members of each receptor family arose from a common ancestor and acquired new specificities by multiple rounds of gene duplication and divergent evolution. With few exceptions, the chemical and physical nature of a stimulus cannot be used to predict the type of receptor, the signal transduction mechanism, or the nature of the response.

Energy from interaction with physical and chemical stimuli modifies the structure and activity of receptors. For example, absorption of light alters the structure of the visual receptor rhodopsin, and physical strain opens stretch receptor ion channels. Binding of

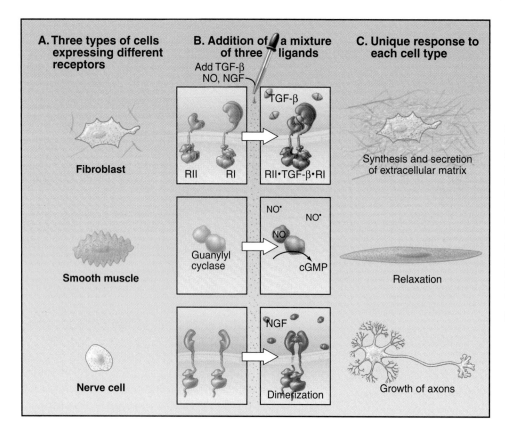

A. Three types of cells expressing different receptors

Fibroblast

Smooth muscle

Nerve cell

B. Addition of a mixture of three ligands

Add TGF-β NO, NGF

RII   RI

TGF-β

RII·TGF-β·RI

Guanylyl cyclase

NO·   NO·

NO

cGMP

NGF

Dimerization

C. Unique response to each cell type

Synthesis and secretion of extracellular matrix

Relaxation

Growth of axons

Figure 25-1 *A* to *C,* Genetically determined protein synthesis equips specialized cells to respond selectively to external signals. A fibroblast, smooth muscle cell, and neuron each have different receptors, so they respond selectively to a mixture of three chemical stimuli: transforming growth factor-β (TGF-β), the gas nitric oxide (NO), and nerve growth factor (NGF). RI and RII are subunits of the TGF-β receptor. cGMP, cyclic guanosine monophosphate.

chemical ligands also alters the structure of receptors, but the details of these changes generally remain to be determined. For example, hormone binding to the extracellular surface of a transmembrane receptor can change its conformation and increase its affinity for cytoplasmic signal-transducing proteins, such as **guanosine triphosphate (GTP)–binding proteins.** Binding the neurotransmitter acetylcholine opens an ion channel in the receptor, leading to depolarization of the plasma membrane (see Chapters 9 and 10). Binding of growth factors promotes dimerization of receptor proteins, activating the enzyme activity of their cytoplasmic domains—**protein kinases** that transfer phosphate from adenosine triphosphate (ATP) to specific amino acids on target proteins (see Chapters 27 and 29).

Considering the diverse information that impinges on cells and the great variety of their responses, a remarkably tiny group of small chemical messengers (see Chapter 28) carries this information by diffusion from one part of the cell to another. These **second messengers** include **Ca^{2+}, cyclic nucleotides,** and **lipids.** A variety of proteins also carry information between receptors and effector systems (see Chapter 27). These signaling proteins are activated by binding a second messenger, like Ca^{2+}, by exchange or hydrolysis of a bound nucleotide, or both, or by **phosphorylation** or **dephosphorylation.** Such proteins often act in cascades, passing a signal from one

to another. For example, a series of kinases can activate one another in turn by phosphorylation. In this way a few "upstream" kinases can activate large numbers of "downstream" kinases, provoking a response that encompasses the entire cell.

Signaling pathways regulate the activity of virtually all cellular processes. Effector systems include transcription factors that control gene expression, regulated secretion apparatus, metabolic enzymes, structural elements and motors of the cytoskeleton, cell surface receptors, cell cycle regulatory proteins, and membrane ion channels. Multiple signaling pathways converge on all of these effector systems. Integration of diverse signals determines cell behavior, whether it secretes or moves, grows, divides, or differentiates.

Understanding signaling pathways is challenging for several reasons. First, cells employ hundreds of distinct signaling pathways, involving hundreds to thousands of different proteins, as the working parts in various mechanisms. The diversity of biological stimuli and receptor systems challenge the memory of student and investigator alike, as it is difficult to match stimuli with signal transduction mechanisms. Second, although the pace of research in this area has been breathtaking, our knowledge about most signaling mechanisms is incomplete. Therefore, important pieces of the puzzle and important connections are missing. New mechanisms are still discovered every year. Third, few signal transduction mechanisms utilize

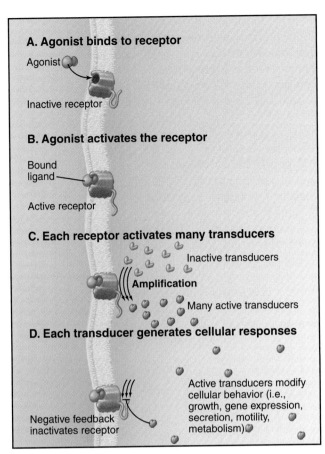

A. Agonist binds to receptor

Agonist

Inactive receptor

B. Agonist activates the receptor

Bound ligand

Active receptor

C. Each receptor activates many transducers

Inactive transducers

Amplification

Many active transducers

D. Each transducer generates cellular responses

Active transducers modify cellular behavior (i.e., growth, gene expression, secretion, motility, metabolism)

Negative feedback inactivates receptor

Figure 25-2 *A* to *D,* The four steps involved in a generic signal transduction pathway.

responses. These **feedback loops** make many signals transient events. Fifth, the response of some pathways depends on both the strength and the temporal pattern of the stimulus. Ultimately, signaling pathways will be understood quantitatively and dynamically as integrated systems, like complex electrical circuits, but this has yet to be achieved in most cases (see Chapter 29).

Given these challenges, this book uses the following strategy to explain how signal transduction mechanisms work. As an introduction and reference, Chapters 26 to 28 explain what is known about the main molecular components: receptors, protein messengers, and second messengers. When studying Chapter 29, which presents detailed accounts of nine well-characterized signal transduction mechanisms, the reader should focus on how the components in each system interact, without being distracted by descriptions of the molecular components. These examples illustrate general principles used by other signaling pathways, which appear elsewhere in the book.

Two main approaches have revealed much about signaling mechanisms: biochemistry/pharmacology and genetic analysis. The biochemical approach generally starts with identification of a naturally occurring or synthetic chemical, such as a hormone, that modifies the activity of an organism, organ, or cell. These compounds are called **agonists.** The general effects of such agonists on cellular metabolism, growth, differentiation, or activity are then described. Characterization of the biological effects of agonists is often aided by the discovery of chemicals that antagonize their action. In many cases, such **antagonists** prove to be useful as drugs, even before the their mechanisms of action are understood. Aspirin is just one example (see Chapter 28). To define the mechanism linking the stimulating chemical to the modification of cellular activity, it is necessary to find and characterize the receptor that binds the chemical and then to trace the biochemical steps from receptor to effectors. The affin-

simple linear pathways from a stimulus to a change in behavior. Rather, most pathways branch and converge multiple times, making it possible for information from several inputs to influence each effector system. This provides for integration of regulatory mechanisms but makes it difficult to predict how information flows through a system or even to determine all of the possibilities. Fourth, most pathways have positive or negative feedback loops that can either augment or inhibit

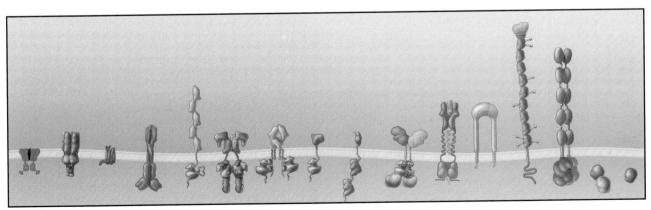

Figure 25-3 Overview of the structures of sixteen families of receptors to preview the molecular diversity. Scale drawings are based, when available, on atomic structures. Details are found in Figure 26–1 and the following chapters.

ity of a receptor for agonists and antagonists frequently provides an assay to isolate the receptor by biochemical fractionation of cells. Once a model mechanism has been defined for a particular class of receptors, the primary structure of a new receptor usually reveals (by homology with known receptors) the type of transduction mechanism and suggests the sorts of molecules that lie between the receptor and the effector systems in the cell. Thus, each newly discovered receptor can be classified quickly into one of the groups listed in Table 26–1.

The genetic approach involves identification and characterization of mutants that affect the flow of information through a signaling pathway. By collecting enough mutants and testing for a hierarchy of effects, investigators can usually define the flow of information through a pathway. By cloning and sequencing the mutated genes, one can identify the proteins involved. By now, many newly discovered proteins are found to be homologues of known signaling proteins, but before the pathways were well characterized, many components were initially discovered by this ap-

proach. Because one need make no assumptions about the nature of the biochemical hardware or how the components are connected, completely novel molecules emerge from genetic screens just as easily as familiar ones. One particularly fruitful genetic approach has been to analyze genes that predispose individuals to cancer or that cause naturally occurring heritable diseases in humans, mice, or other species. Many proteins responsible for regulating cell growth and proliferation cause cancer when constitutively activated by mutations. Inactivating mutations in other signaling proteins cause disorders of growth and development or endocrine diseases.

To understand the dynamics of a signaling system, one really needs to know all of the converging and diverging pathways and how the rates of the various reactions depend on the intensity and pattern of the stimuli. This has only been achieved for one signaling system—bacterial chemotaxis (see Chapter 29)—but our understanding of some other systems, including olfaction (smell) and phototransduction (vision), is progressing rapidly.

chapter 26

PLASMA MEMBRANE RECEPTORS

Cells use about 20 different families of receptor proteins (Fig. 26–1) to detect and respond to a myriad of incoming chemical and physical stimuli (Table 26–1). Most receptors are plasma membrane proteins that interact with their **ligands** or are stimulated by physical events on the cell surface. A few chemical stimuli, including steroid hormones and the gas nitric oxide, cross the plasma membrane and bind receptors inside the cell.

Gene duplication and divergent evolution within each family have produced genes for multiple **receptor isoforms** that interact with different ligands. Selective expression of certain receptors and their associated cytoplasmic transduction machinery allows differentiated cells to respond specifically to particular ligands, but not others (see Fig. 25–1). Fortunately, the mechanisms of the best characterized receptors usually apply to the rest of their family. Thus, learning about a few examples provides a working knowledge of many related receptors.

Members of each family of receptors share one or more structurally homologous domains. In some families, the members share both ligand-binding and signal-transducing strategies (seven-helix, G protein–coupled receptors; cytokine receptors). Members of other families share either a similar ligand-binding structure (tumor necrosis factor [TNF] receptor family) or a common signal-transducing method (receptor tyrosine kinases), but differ in other respects. In families that share a common scaffold to bind similar ligands, amino acid substitutions on this scaffold allow different family members to recognize their specific ligands.

One cannot predict the type of receptor, signal transduction mechanism, or nature of the response from the chemical and physical nature of a stimulus (see Table 26–1). Although proteins and peptides are the only known ligands for receptor kinases and kinase-linked receptors, proteins and peptides also stimulate some seven-helix receptors and guanylyl cyclase receptors. A particularly wide range of stimuli activate seven-helix receptors, including photons, amino acids, nucleotides, biogenic amines, lipids, peptides, proteins, and hundreds of different organic molecules. Some ligands bind distinct receptors on different cells. For example, acetylcholine activates muscle contraction by opening a ligand-gated ion channel. It also binds seven-helix receptors on other cells, activating signaling pathways mediated by guanosine triphosphate (GTP)–binding proteins. Some ligands with similar names bind to different types of receptors. For example, several interleukins (IL-2 through IL-6) bind to cytokine receptors, but IL-1 activates a sphingomyelinase-linked receptor and IL-8 binds a seven-helix, G protein–coupled receptor (see later discussion).

Determination of how receptors transfer energy from ligand binding across the plasma membrane to activate cytoplasmic signals remains the subject of intense experimentation. Two different strategies have been proposed. Ligand binding may cause a conformational change in the receptor that propagates across to the membrane to alter the structure of the part of the receptor in the cytoplasm. Seven-helix receptors use this strategy. Ligand binding also induces a conformational change in preformed dimers of cytokine receptors. Alternatively, ligand binding may cluster inactive receptor subunits diffusing in the plane of the membrane. Dimerization of receptor tyrosine kinases by ligands brings the cytoplasmic kinase domains of the partners close enough together to phosphorylate and activate each other.

Most signal-transducing pathways include one or more enzymes. In some receptor families, an enzyme is part of the receptor protein itself (receptor tyrosine kinases), but in others, the receptor interacts with a separate cytoplasmic enzyme (trimeric G proteins, cytoplasmic protein kinases).

This chapter covers eight families of well-characterized receptors that transfer signals across the plasma membrane. Other chapters describe additional receptor families: Chapter 9, ligand-gated and voltage-gated ion channels; Chapter 14, nuclear receptors for steroids and other ligands; Chapter 27, receptors with protein-phosphatase activity; Chapter 28, cytoplasmic nitric oxide receptors with guanylyl cyclase activity; Chapter 29, two-component receptors and tyrosine kinase–linked receptors; and Chapter 32, cell adhesion receptors, including integrins, cadherins, and selectins.

Seven-Helix Receptors

Members of the largest family of plasma membrane receptors are built from a serpentine arrangement of seven transmembrane α helices. These diverse receptors use **trimeric GTP-binding proteins** (see Chapter 27) to relay signals to effector proteins inside cells. Seven-helix receptors are found in slime molds, so the genes for these proteins originated in early eukaryotes more than 1 billion years ago. Four percent of the genes of the nematode *Caenorhabditis elegans* (790) encode seven-helix receptors, the largest family of proteins in the organism. In mammals, olfactory cells alone use 500 to 1000 different seven-helix receptors to discriminate odorant molecules (see Chapter 29). Other cells are estimated to express another 500 seven-helix receptors to respond to light, amino acids, peptide and protein hormones, catecholamines, and lipids. These receptors are targets of a very large proportion of medically useful drugs with known targets (see Table 26–1).

Seven hydrophobic sequences traverse the plasma membrane as α helices (Fig. 26–2), similar to bacteriorhodopsin (see Fig. 6–10). Comparative analysis of amino acid sequences suggests that all seven-helix receptors have the same arrangement of helices. For example, the minimum length of sequences connecting the helices is only compatible with the helices being arranged sequentially from I to VII in a serpentine fashion as they cross the lipid bilayer. The N-terminus is outside the cell and varies from 5 to nearly 600 residues. Some of the larger N-terminal domains participate in ligand binding. The C-terminal segment of the polypeptide is in the cytoplasm and varies in length from 12 to more than 350 residues.

Binding a soluble chemical ligand is the usual way in which seven-helix receptors are activated, but some

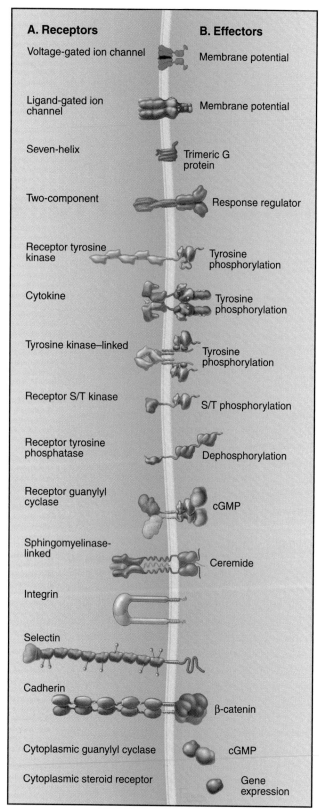

A. Receptors

Voltage-gated ion channel

Ligand-gated ion channel

Seven-helix

Two-component

Receptor tyrosine kinase

Cytokine

Tyrosine kinase–linked

Receptor S/T kinase

Receptor tyrosine phosphatase

Receptor guanylyl cyclase

Sphingomyelinase-linked

Integrin

Selectin

Cadherin

Cytoplasmic guanylyl cyclase

Cytoplasmic steroid receptor

B. Effectors

Membrane potential

Membrane potential

Trimeric G protein

Response regulator

Tyrosine phosphorylation

Tyrosine phosphorylation

Tyrosine phosphorylation

S/T phosphorylation

Dephosphorylation

cGMP

Ceremide

β-catenin

cGMP

Gene expression

Figure 26–1 *A* and *B*, Sixteen classes of receptors with signal transduction mechanisms. S/T, serine/threonine.

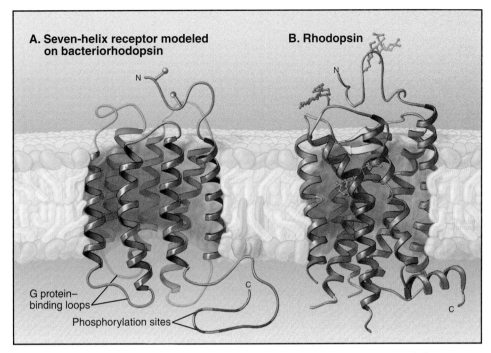

Figure 26-2 Structure of seven-helix receptors. *A,* Model of the generic seven-helix receptor, used throughout this text. The structure is based on the atomic structure of bacteriorhodopsin and the amino acid sequence of a typical vertebrate seven-helix receptor. Seven hydrophobic segments cross the membrane as α-helices. Oligosaccharides are blue. The C-terminal cytoplasmic tail is anchored to the lipid bilayer by two fatty acids covalently bound to a pair of adjacent cysteines. *B,* Atomic structure of bovine rhodopsin, the receptor for photons in the retina. Covalently bound retinal pigment is green. Oligosaccharides on extracellular loops are blue. (Reference: Palczewski K, et al: Crystal structure of rhodopsin: A G protein-coupled receptor. Science 289:739–745, 2000; PDB file: 1F88)

interesting variations can occur. Biochemical and mutagenetic experiments support the idea that most small ligands bind in a central pocket among the extracellular ends of the helices. Residues lining this pocket are highly variable between receptors, providing specificity for each receptor to bind a particular ligand. The light-absorbing pigment, **11-*cis* retinal,** of the photoreceptor protein **rhodopsin** is the best characterized. This "ligand" is unusual in that it is bound covalently to the receptor (Fig. 26–2*B*) and is activated by absorbing a photon (see Chapter 29). In other respects, it is a good model for other ligands (Fig. 26–3). **Neurotransmitters,** like norepinephrine, and drugs also bind between the helices about one third of the way across the membrane. Peptide hormones bind deep in the helical pocket, but probably also interact with residues more exposed on the cell surface. The blood-clotting enzyme, thrombin, activates its receptor on platelets by proteolysis of the receptor rather than by direct binding. The N-terminal peptide cleaved from the receptor dissociates and activates other receptors; what is left of the truncated N-terminus binds its own receptor and activates it. Receptors for some large ligands (pituitary glycoprotein hormones, such as lu-

teinizing hormone, follicle-stimulating hormone, and thyroid-stimulating hormone) and some small ligands (glutamate, γ-aminobutyric acid, calcium) bind with high affinity to extracellular N-terminal domains of their seven-helix receptor. This ligand–N-terminus complex then stimulates the transmembrane domain of the receptor.

Seven-helix receptors exist in an equilibrium between two conformations: a **resting state** and an **activated state** with the ability to catalyze the exchange of nucleotide bound to trimeric G proteins (see Fig. 26–3). Without bound ligand, the resting state is strongly favored. Ligand binding to the receptor (or the isomerization of retinal after absorbing light) initiates signal transduction by shifting the equilibrium to the active state. Activation involves movement of at least two transmembrane helices, but the structural details of this conformational change are not yet well defined. In any event, activation must rearrange the cytoplasmic ends of the helices and the loops connecting them to create a binding site for a target G protein. Active receptors can interact successively with more than 100 G proteins, causing them to dissociate their bound guanosine diphosphate (GDP) (see Chap-

table 26-1

RECEPTORS AND LIGANDS

Classes of Receptors Activators	Nature of Activation	Examples of Biological Function
Voltage-gated ion channels → membrane depolarization or repolarization		
Voltage-gated potassium channel	Electrical	Membrane repolarization
Voltage gated sodium channel	Electrical	Action potential
Ligand-gated ion channels → changes in membrane permeability		
Acetylcholine (nicotinic)	Biogenic amine	Action potential
Adenosine triphosphate	Nucleotide	Change in membrane potential
Glutamate (N-methyl-D-aspartate)	Amino acid	Change in membrane potential
Glutamate (non–N-methyl-D-aspartate)	Amino acid	Change in membrane potential
Glycine	Amino acid	Change in membrane potential
Serotonin	Biogenic amine	Change in membrane potential
Seven-helix receptors → trimeric G proteins → diverse responses		
Acetylcholine (muscarinic)	Biogenic amine	Slows heart; stimulates intestinal secretion
Adrencorticotropic hormone	Peptide	Stimulates adrenal cortisol production
Adenosine	Nucleoside	Dilates blood vessels
Angiotensin II	Peptide	Stimulates aldosterone secretion; contracts smooth muscle
Bradykinin	Protein	Stimulates intestinal secretion
Calcitonin	Protein	Inhibits calcium resorption from bone
Cholecystokinin	Peptide	Stimulates intestinal secretion
Complement (C5a, C3a)	Protein	Leukocyte chemoattractant
Dopamine	Biogenic amine	Neurotransmitter; inhibits prolactin secretion
Eicosanoids (prostaglandins)	Lipid	Promotes platelet aggregation
Endothelins	Protein	Vasoconstriction
Epinephrine	Biogenic amine	Glycogenolysis; increases cardiac contractility
F-met-leu-phe	Peptide	Leukocyte chemotaxis
Follicle-stimulating hormone	Protein	Growth of ovarian follicle
γ-aminobutyric acid	Amino acid	Inhibitory neurotransmitter; stimulates intestinal secretion
Glucagon	Peptide	Glycogenolysis; stimulates intestinal secretion
Glutamate	Amino acid	Modulates synaptic transmission
Growth hormone–releasing factor	Peptide	Stimulates secretion of growth hormone
Histamine	Amino acid	Allergic responses; vasodilation; stimulates secretion
Interleukin, IL-8	Protein	Chemotaxis of leukocytes
Leutinizing hormone	Protein	Steroid production by ovarian granulosa cells
Light → rhodopsin	Photon	Vision
Lysophosphatidic acid	Lipid	Fibroblast proliferation, neurite retraction
Melanocyte-stimulating hormone	Protein	Melanin synthesis
Neurokinins (substance P)	Peptide	Stimulates gastrointestinal and pancreatic secretion; neurotransmitter
Norepinephrine	Biogenic amine	Smooth muscle relaxation
Odorants	Organics	Olfaction
Opioids	Alkaloids	Alters mood
Oxytocin	Peptide	Contraction of uterus
Parathyroid hormone	Protein	Bone calcium resorption
Peptide-releasing factors	Protein	Secretion of pituitary hormones
Platelet-activating factor	Lipid	Platelet activation
Serotonin	Biogenic amine	Stimulates intestinal secretion
Somatostatin	Peptide	Inhibits secretion of growth hormone, insulin, and glucagon
Thrombin	Protein	Activates platelets
Thyroid-stimulating hormone	Protein	Thyroid hormone secretion
Vasoactive intestinal peptide	Peptide	Stimulates intestinal secretion

table 26-1

RECEPTORS AND LIGANDS *Continued*

Classes of Receptors Activators	Nature of Activation	Examples of Biological Function
Vasopressin	Peptide	Regulates the permeability of the renal tubule to water
Wingless (Wnt)	Protein	Modulates gene expression
Two-Component systems: Receptor/histidine kinase → response regulator → diverse responses		
Aspartate	Amino acid	Controls flagellar motor and chemotaxis
Osmotic pressure	Physical	Regulates gene expression
Receptor tyrosine kinase → ras, MAP kinase, PLC, PI3 kinase		
Epidermal growth factor	Protein	Epithelial cell proliferation and differentiation
Fibroblast growth factor-α	Protein	Mesoderm differentiation; fibroblast mitogen
Fibroblast growth factor-β	Protein	Fibroblast mitogen
Hepatocyte growth factor (scatter factor)	Protein	Epithelial cell mitogenesis, motility
Insulin	Protein	Glucose uptake; cell growth
Insulin-like growth factor I	Protein	General body growth
Macrophage colony- stimulating factor	Protein	Growth and differentiation of monocytes
Neurotrophins (nerve growth)	Protein	Neural growth; neuron survival
Platelet-derived growth factor	Protein	Smooth muscle, fibroblast, glial growth and differentiation
Steel ligand	Protein	Development of melanocytes, germ cells
Transforming growth factor-α	Protein	Differentiation of connective tissue
Vascular endothelial cell growth factor	Protein	Endothelial cell growth
Cytokine receptors → JAK kinase → STAT transcription factors → gene expression		
Ciliary neurotrophic factor	Protein	Survival/differentiation of neurons and glial cells
Erythropoietin	Protein	Growth and differentiation of red cell precursors
Granulocyte (colony- stimulating factor)	Protein	Growth and differentiation of granulocyte precursors
Granulocyte-monocyte (colony-stimulating factor)	Protein	Growth and differentiation of leukocyte precursors
Growth hormone	Protein	Cell growth and differentiation of somatic cells
Interleukin, IL-2	Protein	Growth factor for lymphocytes
Interleukin, IL-3	Protein	Growth factor for hematopoietic stem cells
Interleukin, IL-4	Protein	Regulates gene expression
Interleukin, IL-5	Protein	Regulates gene expression
Interleukin, IL-6	Protein	Regulates gene expression
Interferon α/β	Protein	Regulates gene expression
Interferon γ	Protein	Macrophage and lymphocyte gene expression
Prolactin	Protein	Stimulates milk synthesis
Tyrosine kinase–linked receptors → cytoplasmic tyrosine kinase → gene expression		
MHC-peptide complex → T- cell receptor	Protein	Growth and differentiation of T lymphocytes
Antigens → B-cell receptor	Various	Growth and differentiation of B lymphocytes
Receptor serine/threonine kinase → Smad transcription factors → control of gene expression		
Activin	Peptide	Mesoderm development
Bone morphogenetic protein	Protein	Mesoderm development
Inhibins	Protein	Inhibition of gonadal stromal mitogenesis
Transforming growth factor-β	Protein	Growth arrest, mesoderm development
Membrane guanylyl cyclase receptors → cGMP → regulation of kinases and channels		
Atrial natriuretic peptide	Peptide	Vasodilation; sodium excretion; intestinal secretion
Heat-stable endotoxin, guanylin		Unknown
Sea urchin egg peptides	Peptide	Fertilization
Sphingomyelinase-linked receptors → ceremide-activated kinases → gene expression		
Interleukin, IL-1	Protein	Inflammation, wound healing
Tumor necrosis factor	Protein	Inflammation, tumor cell death

Table continued on following page

table 26–1

RECEPTORS AND LIGANDS *Continued*

Classes of Receptors Activators	Nature of Activation	Examples of Biological Function
Integrins → nonreceptor tyrosine kinases → diverse responses		
Fibronectin, other matrix proteins	Protein	Cell motility, gene expression
Selectins		
Mucins	Glycoproteins	Cell adhesion
Cadherins		
Like cadherins on another cell	Protein	Contact inhibition
Notch		
Delta	Cell surface protein	Cell fate determination
Cytoplasmic guanylyl cyclase receptors → cGMP → kinases, cGMP-gated channels		
Nitric oxide	Gas	Smooth muscle relaxation
Cytoplasmic steroid receptors → active transcription factor → gene expression		
Retinoic acid	Organic	Cell growth and differentiation
Steroid hormones	Steroids	Cell growth and differentiation
Thyroid hormone	Amino acid	Cell growth and differentiation

ter 27). Replacement of GDP with GTP activates the G proteins, enabling them to stimulate target effector proteins. Multiple interactions at each step usually amplify the signal. For example, absorption of a single photon by one rhodopsin activates several trimeric G proteins, each of which activates an enzyme that breaks down many cyclic guanosine monophosphate (cGMP) molecules. The decrease in cGMP concentration closes many cGMP-gated ion channels and changes the membrane potential. This **cascade** of three successive intermolecular interactions is very fast, taking less than 10 msec (see Chapter 29 for details).

If extracellular stimulation is sustained, most signaling systems turn down their response. The literature variously calls this **adaptation,** attenuation, desensitization, tachyphylaxis, or tolerance. For example, rhodopsin and odorant receptors turn off within a second of continuous stimulation. This allows one to dis-

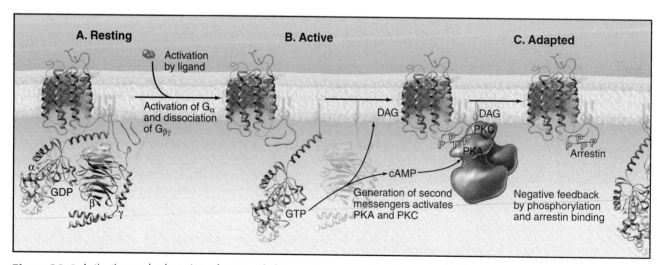

Figure 26–3 Activation and adaptation of a seven-helix receptor: *A,* resting; *B,* active; *C,* adapted. Ligand binding shifts the equilibrium from the resting conformation toward the active conformation. Active receptor promotes dissociation of GDP from the α-subunit of multiple trimeric G proteins, allowing GTP to bind. Typically, this dissociates G_α from $G_{\beta\gamma}$, each of which activate downstream effectors that produce, for example, the second messengers cAMP and diacylglycerol (DAG). cAMP and DAG activate PKA and PKC, which phosphorylate active receptors on their C-terminus. This attracts arrestin, putting the receptor into the inactive adapted state. PKA, protein kinase A; PKC, protein kinase C.

tinguish rapidly changing visual information and concentrations of odors.

Phosphorylation of the C-terminal tail inactivates many types of seven-helix receptors. Two different strategies, sometimes acting on the same receptor, provide this **negative feedback** (see Fig. 26–3). One strategy is for **second messengers** produced in response to receptor activation to stimulate general protein kinases (including cyclic adenosine monophosphate [cAMP], protein kinase A [PKA], and protein kinase C [PKC]; see Chapter 27), which phosphorylate the activated receptor. Phosphorylation inhibits the receptor. This mechanism allows for crosstalk between receptors, as activation of one class of receptors can inactivate other types of receptors. The second strategy involves a class of protein kinases specific for the receptors themselves. They are called **G protein–coupled receptor kinases,** or GRKs. Several isoforms exist, some expressed in specific cells, some more generally. These kinases phosphorylate multiple serines or threonines on the C-terminal cytoplasmic tail of active (but not inactive) receptors. Phosphorylation promotes the binding of a regulatory protein called **arrestin,** which inactivates the receptor by blocking interaction of the receptor with trimeric G proteins. Arrestin binding to some seven-helix receptors promotes their removal from the plasma membrane by endocytosis, a longer-term mechanism that turns down the response of a cell to continuous stimulation. Chapter 29 covers some dramatic examples of receptor adaptation by GRKs and second-messenger kinases.

Most seven-helix receptors require ligand binding to shift to the active state, but mutations can render a seven-helix receptor constitutively active without ligand. Such activating mutations can cause human diseases (Table 26–2). Examples of these include particu-

lar rhodopsin mutations that cause night blindness or degeneration of photoreceptor cells; mutations in the receptor of luteinizing hormone that cause precocious male puberty; and mutations in a calcium receptor that cause dysfunction of the parathyroid gland. The physiology of these activating mutations is complicated owing to efforts of the cells to compensate for the continually active receptors, using feedback mechanisms to turn down the receptor.

Receptor Tyrosine Kinases

Many polypeptide growth factors activate cells by binding plasma membrane receptors with cytoplasmic protein tyrosine kinase activity (Fig. 26–4). This group of receptors consists of 13 families with more than one member and 6 other single receptors with distinct structural features. Most of these receptor subunits consist of a single polypeptide chain. The insulin receptor family is more complicated (see Chapter 29). The domain structure of the ligand-binding extracellular parts of these receptors is quite varied. A single segment (presumed to be an α helix) crosses the lipid bilayer and allows receptor subunits to diffuse laterally in the plane of the membrane. Ligand binding causes two subunits to form a dimer and stimulates transphosphorylation of the partner subunit. This activates the receptor kinase, which phosphorylates and activates effector proteins that control cellular proliferation and differentiation (see Chapter 29).

Receptor tyrosine kinases bind a variety of growth factors. For example, **epidermal growth factor** (EGF) stimulates proliferation and differentiation of epithelial cells. **Platelet-derived growth factor** (PDGF) stimulates growth of smooth muscle cells, glial cells, and fibroblasts. Some of these ligands and their receptors were discovered by biochemical purification of factors that stimulate cell growth and differentiation. EGF was discovered with a bioassay, as it causes the eyelids of newborn mice to open prematurely. Some receptors, like erbB (the EGF receptor), were discovered during the search for cancer-causing oncogenes. Still others were discovered by studying mutations in flies or worms that affect development. The *Drosophila sevenless* gene encodes a receptor tyrosine kinase related to insulin receptor. Mutations in the *sevenless* gene result in failure to develop the number 7 photoreceptor cell in the fly's eye. Biochemistry has provided much information about mechanisms of action, whereas genetics has confirmed physiological functions and has helped to establish the order of events along these signaling pathways (see Chapter 29).

The extracellular ligand-binding parts of the various receptor tyrosine kinases consist of domains with familiar folds, such as immunoglobulin and fibronectin

table 26–2

SEVEN-HELIX RECEPTORS AND DISEASE

Defective Receptor	Disease Phenotype
Parathyroid Ca^{2+} sensor	Hyperparathyroidism; failure to respond to high levels of serum Ca^{2+}
Luteinizing hormone receptor	Precocious puberty
Vasopressin receptor	Nephrogenic diabetes insipidus; failure of kidneys to resorb water
Adrenocorticotropic hormone receptor	Glucocorticoid deficiency; failure to make glucocorticoids
Cone cell opsin	Color blindness; no response to certain wavelengths
Rhodopsin	Retinitis pigmentosa; retinal degeneration

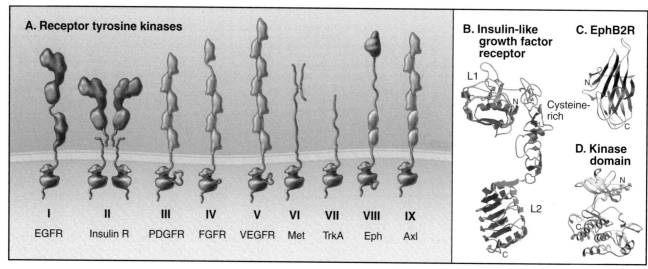

Figure 26-4 Receptor tyrosine kinases. *A,* Drawing of the domain architecture of nine families of receptor (R) tyrosine kinases. *B* to *D,* Ribbon models of atomic structures of the domains of receptor tyrosine kinases. *B,* Extracellular part of the insulin-like growth factor receptor. A cysteine-rich domain connects two similar β-helical domains. These three domains are thought to surround the ligand. *C,* The globular domain of the EphB2 receptor is a β sandwich with a ligand-binding site that includes the exposed loop on the front of this model. *D,* The cytoplasmic kinase domain from the insulin receptor is similar to most known kinases. A C-terminal tail (not shown) contains the tyrosine phosphorylation sites. Atomic structures are also available for FGFR and VEGFR with bound ligands. Axl, receptor for the growth factor Gas6; EGFR, epidermal growth factor receptor; EphR, receptor for ephrin, membrane-bound ligands in the nervous system, the largest class of receptor tyrosine kinases; FGFR, fibroblast growth factor receptor; Met, receptor for hepatocyte growth factor; PDGFR, platelet-derived growth factor receptor; TrkA, receptor for nerve growth factor; VEGFR, vascular endothelial growth factor. (*A,* Adapted from Hubbard SR, Till JH: Protein tyrosine kinase structure and function. Annu Rev Biochem 69:373–398, 2000. With permission, from the *Annual Review of Biochemistry,* Vol. 69, © 2000 by Annual Reviews www.AnnualReviews.org. *B* to *D,* Reprinted with permission from Nature. *B,* Reference: Garrett TP, et al: Crystal structure of the first three domains of the type-1 insulin-like growth factor receptor. Nature 394:395–399, 1998. PDB file: 1IGR. *C,* Reference: Himanen JP, et al: Crystal structure of the ligand-binding domain of the receptor tyrosine kinase EphB2. Nature 396:486–491, 1998; PDB file: 1NUK. *B* and *C,* Copyright 1998, Macmillan Magazines Limited. *D,* Reference: Hubbard SR, et al: Crystal structure of the tyrosine kinase domain of the human insulin receptor. Nature 372:746–754, 1994. Copyright 1994, Macmillan Magazines Limited. PDB file: 1IRK.)

III domains (see Figs. 2–15 and 26–4*A*). Receptors for insulin-like growth factor and EGF have two β-helical domains connected by a cysteine-rich domain (see Fig. 26–4*B*). These three domains are thought to wrap around the ligand. The globular ligand-binding domain of Eph receptors is folded into a β-strand "jelly roll," with the likely ligand-binding site on one concave surface (see Fig. 26–4*C*).

The common feature of these receptors is a cytoplasmic protein kinase domain specific for tyrosine phosphorylation (see Fig. 26–4*D*). These domains are folded like other protein kinases (see Chapter 27). Some have 15 to 100 residues inserted in the kinase domain, and all have extensions at the C-terminus (see Fig. 26–4*A*). These inserts and extensions include a number of tyrosine residues that are transphosphorylated in active, dimerized receptors, creating phosphotyrosine-binding sites for downstream adapter and effector proteins (Fig. 26–5; see Chapters 27 and 29).

Ligand binding to dimeric receptors activates receptor tyrosine kinases (see Fig. 26–5) either by

changing the conformation of a preformed dimer, by bringing together receptor dimers from a pool of subunits diffusing in the plane of the membrane, or by a combination of these effects. **Induced dimerization** is the accepted mechanism. On the other hand, insulin receptors are held together in stable dimers by a disulfide bond, so insulin binding is likely to induce a change in the orientation of the subunits, including the cytoplasmic kinase domains (see Fig. 29–7). Even for receptors without disulfide bonds between subunits, some preformed dimers appear to have an increased affinity for ligands and may be responsible for signaling. Some growth factors, such as PDGF, are dimeric, so it is easy to imagine how they could interact with two receptor proteins on the surface of the cell.

Receptor activation either by dimerization or by a conformational change is thought to bring together two kinase domains in the cytoplasm. Juxtaposition allows each kinase to phosphorylate its partner kinase on specific tyrosine residues (see Fig. 26–5). The most

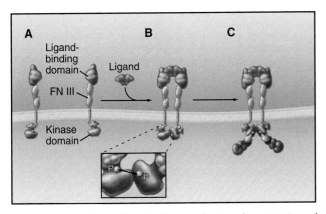

Figure 26–5 Subunit dimerization mechanism for activation of a receptor tyrosine kinase. *A,* Ligand binding brings together two receptor subunits. Alternatively, ligand might change the conformation of a preformed subunit dimer. *B,* Proximity of the kinase domains allows transphosphorylation of the neighboring subunit. *C,* Effector and adaptor proteins with SH2 domains bind to particular phosphotyrosine residues on the receptor. FN III, fibronectin III domain.

important initial phosphorylation event is phosphorylation of one or more tyrosines in the **activation loop** of the catalytic domain, which flips the catalytic domain into an active conformation (see Fig. 27–3*D*). Then the active kinase phosphorylates additional tyrosine residues on the receptor and effector proteins.

The phosphotyrosines on the kinase insert and C-terminal extension sequences act as ligands for a number of downstream effector and adapter proteins. This third step of signal transduction depends on small protein domains called **SH2** and **PTB** domains that recognize phosphotyrosine residues. (Chapter 27 provides additional details on SH2 and PTB domains.) Each SH2 domain binds preferentially to certain phosphotyrosine sites by virtue of a pocket that binds phosphotyrosine, as well as interactions with side chains of one or more residues at positions +1 to +6 C-terminal to the phosphotyrosine (see Fig. 27–11). For example, each of five phosphotyrosines of the PDGF receptor favors binding of different effector or adapter proteins.

Receptor tyrosine kinases activate effector proteins in two different ways. First, binding of effector protein to a receptor phosphotyrosine favors phosphorylation by the receptor kinase. In the case of the effector protein **phospholipase Cγ₁**, tyrosine phosphorylation both activates its catalytic activity and dissociates the enzyme from its phosphotyrosine-binding site, allowing it to move to its site of action on the membrane. Second, the close proximity of the effectors to the membrane when bound to the receptor may, by itself, promote activity by bringing these effector proteins near their substrates. This may apply to **phosphoinositide-3-kinase,** which acts upon lipid substrates in the membrane bilayer, as well as a guanosine triphos-

phatase (GTPase)–activating protein, **Ras-GAP,** which acts on the small G protein Ras, which is anchored to the membrane bilayer (see Fig. 29–6).

Mutations in receptor tyrosine kinases cause human disease. Mutations in EGF receptor cause cancer (see Chapter 29). Activating mutations in one of the receptors for fibroblast growth factor lead to a variety of congenital abnormalities of the skeleton, such as a form of dwarfism and fusion of the sutures between the bones of the skull. Some of these mutations activate by promoting receptor dimerization through disulfide bonds or association of transmembrane helices. Others change ligand specificity.

Cytokine Receptors

Cytokines are a diverse family of polypeptide hormones and growth factors that regulate many cellular process. Although they differ in detail, all cytokines are four-helix bundles. Pituitary **growth hormone** controls body growth and development; receptor mutations cause one type of dwarfism. **Erythropoietin** regulates the proliferation and differentiation of red blood cell precursors (see Chapter 30); receptor mutations can cause excess red blood cell production. **Interleukins** modulate cells of the immune system; receptor mutations can cause immunodeficiency.

Cytokine receptors consist of either two identical subunits, or two or three different subunits (Fig. 26–6). All have two extracellular fibronectin III domains that bind ligand (see Fig. 26–6*B*). A single polypeptide segment, presumed to be an α helix, crosses the membrane. Cytoplasmic domains lack enzyme activity but bind one of several protein tyrosine kinases called **JAKs** (see Fig. 26–6*A*).

Ligand binding activates cytokine receptors, either by bringing together separate subunits or by changing the conformation of preformed dimers (Fig. 26–7). Binding of erythropoietin to the extracellular domain of its receptor positions the transmembrane segments close together (see Fig. 26–6*B*), which is suitable for bringing together two JAK kinases bound to the cytoplasmic domains. This proximity allows JAKs to activate each other by transphosphorylation. Active JAKs then phosphorylate selected members of a family of transcription factors called **STATs**, which migrate to the nucleus to regulate gene expression (see Fig. 29–10).

The structure of inactive, ligand-free receptors is less certain. Individual cytokine receptor subunits may be dissociated and diffuse in the plane of the membrane. On the other hand, erythropoietin receptor without ligand can be crystallized as a dimer with transmembrane domains that are far apart (see Fig. 26–6*C*). This separation of transmembrane segments (and cytoplasmic domains) could explain the lack of

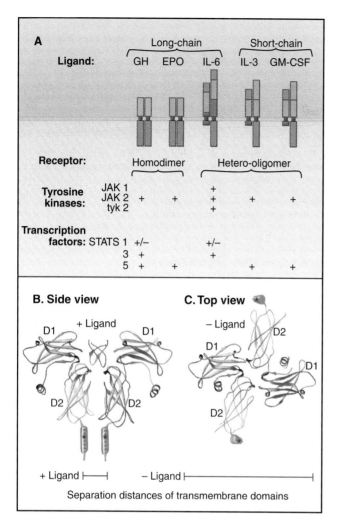

Separation distances of transmembrane domains

Receptor Serine/Threonine Kinases

A third class of growth factor receptors consists of a pair of different subunits, each with a cytoplasmic serine/threonine kinase domain. When brought together by their dimeric protein ligands, the two subunits cooperate to activate cytoplasmic transcription factors, called **Smads,** that regulate genes required to control cellular proliferation and differentiation (Figs. 26–8, 26–9, and 29–10).

Ligands for receptor serine/threonine kinases are dimeric proteins, including **transforming growth factor-β (TGF-β), inhibins, activin,** and **bone morphogenetic proteins.** These growth factors are particularly important during embryonic development. For example, the local concentration of activin strongly influences the differentiation of early embryonic cells into primitive germ layers. Bone morphogenetic proteins influence differentiation of many cells, including osteoblasts, which lay down bone matrix. Activin was discovered as a releasing factor for pituitary follicle-stimulating hormone, but is also active during embryonic development. TGF-β has two distinct effects. First, it inhibits proliferation of most adult cells. Mice with null mutations of one of their three TGF-β genes die of inflammation in multiple organs caused by excessive proliferation of lymphocytes. Second, TGF-β stimulates production of extracellular matrix, including

Figure 26–6 Cytokine receptors. *A,* Drawing of the domain architecture and coupled signaling components of selected cytokine receptors. EPO, erythropoietin; GH, growth hormone; GM-CSF, granulocyte-monocyte colony-stimulating factor; IL, interleukin; *B* and *C,* Atomic structures of erythropoietin receptors. *B,* Side view of a receptor with a synthetic ligand called EMP1 *(green). C,* Top view of a receptor without ligand. D1 and D2 are the fibronectin III domains. The pink helices are models of the transmembrane segments. Pink bars indicate the separation of transmembrane segments. Association of erythropoietin and growth hormone with their receptors is remarkable, as a single, small, asymmetrical protein ligand binds between two identical receptor subunits using *different sites* on each receptor subunit! (*A,* Adapted from Wells JA, de Vos AM: Hematopoietic receptor complexes. Annu Rev Biochem 65:609–634, 1996. With permission, from the *Annual Review of Biochemistry,* Vol. 65, © 1996 by Annual Reviews www.AnnualReview.org. *B* and *C,* PDB files: 1EBP, 1ERN; based on the work of Livnah O, et al: Crystallographic evidence for preformed dimers of erythropoietin receptor before ligand activation. Science 283:987–990, 1999. Copyright 1999, American Association for the Advancement of Science.)

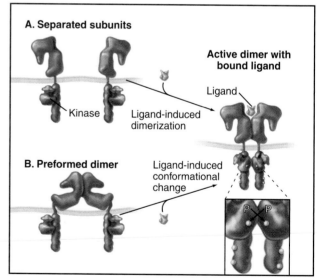

Figure 26–7 Cytokine receptor activation models. *A,* Ligand-induced dimerization of separate subunits. *B,* Ligand-induced conformational change in a preformed dimer. In either case, proximity of the cytoplasmic domains allows associated JAK tyrosine kinases to activate each other by transphosphorylation. (Based on the work of Remy I, et al: Erythropoietin receptor activation by a ligand-induced conformational change. Science 283:990–993, 1999.)

activity of ligand-free dimers. A conformational change in a preformed dimer would explain how erythropoietin can activate cells even with low concentrations of receptors on the cell surface.

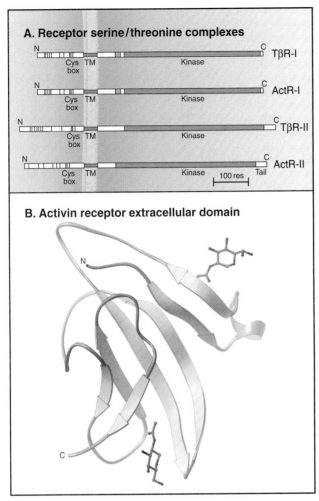

Figure 26-8 Receptor serine/threonine kinases. *A*, Drawing of domain architecture. *B*, Ribbon diagram of the atomic model of the ligand-binding domain of the activin receptor type II, which is similar to a three-finger snake toxin. (Reference: Greenwald J, et al: Three-finger toxin fold for the extracellular ligand-binding domain of the type II activin receptor serine kinase. Nature Struct Biol 6:18–22, 1999; PDB file: 1bte) TM, transmembrane domain.

domains are folded similarly to neurotoxins secreted by snakes (see Fig. 26–8*B*). Single transmembrane sequences link these ligand-binding domains to cytoplasmic domains with serine/threonine kinase activity. Signal transduction requires the kinase activities of both subunits.

Empty receptors are thought to exist as monomers or homodimers in the plasma membrane. Ligands first bind receptor II and then add receptor I, forming a complex with at least four receptor subunits. Once juxtaposed, the constitutively active receptor II kinase phosphorylates the cytoplasmic domain of receptor I on serine and threonine residues. This activates receptor I kinase, which phosphorylates cytoplasmic transcription factors called Smads. Phosphorylated Smads move to the nucleus, where they cooperate with other transcription factors to regulate gene expression (see Fig. 29–10).

In addition to these transducing receptors, cells have a greater abundance of another TGF-β–binding protein on the plasma membrane that lacks signal transduction activity. This large proteoglycan is anchored to the plasma membrane by a single transmembrane sequence linked to a small cytoplasmic domain without any features that implicate it in signaling. It may concentrate TGFβ on the cell surface.

collagen, proteoglycans, and adhesive glycoproteins (see Chapter 31). These proteins are essential for the development of organs. Inappropriate expression of TGF-β may provide a link between inflammation and the pathologic fibrosis that scars diseased organs. Overproduction of extracellular matrix is a common feature of many chronic inflammatory diseases. On the other hand, loss of TGF-β receptors during progression of some tumors makes them unresponsive to growth inhibition by TGF-β and contributes, in part, to their ability to replicate autonomously.

Signal-transducing serine/threonine kinase receptors are composed of two types of subunits called receptor I and receptor II, present on the cell surface in small numbers. Small, extracellular, ligand-binding

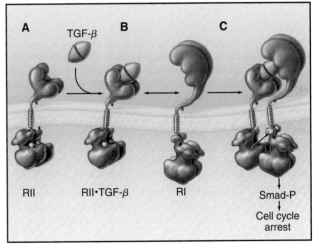

Figure 26-9 *A* to *C*, Mechanism of receptor serine/threonine kinase activation. Ligand binds a type II receptor (RII), which is followed by association with a type I receptor (RI) and formation of a multimeric (probably tetrameric) receptor complex. In this complex, the type II receptor phosphorylates and activates the type I receptor, which in turn phosphorylates a cytoplasmic transcription factor called Smad. Phosphorylated Smad (Smad-P) binds Smad4 and moves to the nucleus to activate particular genes. TGF, transforming growth factor. (Adapted from Massague J: TGF-β signal transduction. Annu Rev Biochem 67:753–792, 1998. With permission, from the *Annual Review of Biochemistry*, Vol. 67, © 1998 by Annual Reviews www.AnnualReview.org.)

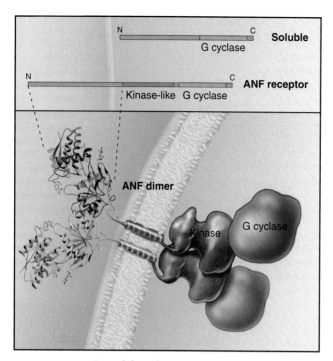

Figure 26-10 Guanylyl cyclase (G-cyclase) receptors. *Upper panel,* Comparison of the domain architecture of the transmembrane atrial natriuretic factor (ANF) receptor and the cytoplasmic nitric oxide receptor. *Lower panel,* Atomic model of ANF receptor. (Reprinted with permission from Nature. Reference: van den Akker F, et al: Structure of the dimerized hormone-binding domain of a guanylyl-cyclase-coupled receptor. Nature 406:101–104, 2000. Copyright 2000, Macmillan Magazines Limited. PDB file: 1DP4.)

Guanylyl Cyclase Receptors

Animals have a family of cell surface receptors (Fig. 26–10) with intracellular domains that catalyze the formation of $3'-5'$-**cGMP** from GTP. Vertebrates have at least seven isoforms; nematode worms have more than 25. The gases **nitric oxide** and carbon monoxide activate related cytoplasmic enzymes that participate in additional signal transduction pathways. (Chapter 28 covers the enzyme mechanisms in detail.) Regardless of its enzymatic origin, cGMP regulates the same targets: **cGMP-gated ion channels** (see Fig. 9–9), **cGMP-stimulated protein kinases** (see Fig. 27–4), and **cyclic nucleotide phosphodiesterases** (see Chapter 28) that contain an allosteric regulatory site for cGMP.

All known ligands for guanylyl cyclase receptors are peptides, although the ligands for four of the vertebrate receptors are not known. Most insights regarding function have come from knowledge about ligands, tissue distribution of receptors, and receptor gene disruptions, as highly specific inhibitors of the cell surface guanylyl cyclases are not available.

Guanylyl cyclase receptors are homodimers with novel, ligand-binding extracellular domains (see Fig. 29–10). The first cytoplasmic domain resembles a protein kinase but appears to be enzymatically inactive. The second cytoplasmic domain is the guanylyl cyclase, closely related structurally to both cytoplasmic guanylyl cyclases and adenylyl cyclases (see Fig. 28–2). The enzymatically inactive kinase domain is not required for basal cyclase activity, but is required for the ligand-binding signal to stimulate guanylyl cyclase activity.

Guanylyl cyclase receptor A (GC-A) binds **atrial natriuretic factor,** a polypeptide hormone secreted mainly by the heart to control blood pressure. It stimulates excretion of salt and water by the kidney and dilates blood vessels. Mice with null mutations for GC-A have high blood pressure and enlarged hearts and fail to respond when overloaded with fluid and salt administered intravenously. Intestinal guanylyl cyclase receptor C (GC-C) binds bacterial **enterotoxin,** the mediator of fluid secretion in bacterial dysentery. The bacterial toxin mimics endogenous peptides of unknown function, which are secreted by various tissues, but principally by the intestine. Mice with null mutations for GC-C are completely resistant to enterotoxin but have no apparent physiological defects. Guanylyl cyclase receptors E and F (GC-E, GC-F) are restricted to the eye; a null mutation for GC-E results in loss of cone visual receptor cells. Guanylyl cyclase receptor D is restricted to olfactory neuroepithelium. Sea urchin spermatozoa use a guanylyl cyclase receptor to respond to peptides secreted by eggs.

Tumor Necrosis Factor Receptor Family

Tumor necrosis factor (TNF) and its receptor are the models for a diverse and vital group of cell-signaling partners (Fig. 26–11). Lymphocytes produce three isoforms of TNF (also called lymphotoxin and cachectin). Many functions have been ascribed to these lymphokines, including protection from bacterial infections, induction of hemorrhagic necrosis of human tumors, mediation of wasting in chronic disease, and production of shock and inflammation. Mice with a genetic deletion of the lymphotoxin-α gene have no lymph nodes, so TNF participates in the development of the immune system. Other ligands (**nerve growth factor** and **Fas-ligand**) use receptors related to the TNF receptor to regulate cell proliferation and death (see Chapter 49).

Human cells express two types of TNF receptors that bind the same ligands but generate different responses. The two receptors have similar ligand-binding domains coupled by single transmembrane segments to different cytoplasmic domains. In the absence of ligand, individual receptor subunits are presumed to diffuse independently in the plane of the membrane. The extracellular part of these receptors consists of 4 similar repeats of about 40 amino acids, each with 6 conserved cysteines (see Fig. 26–11*B*). The cysteines form three disulfide bridges, arranged like the rungs of a ladder, to stabilize these small domains.

The atomic structure of TNF bound to the extracellular part of its receptor has provided extraordinary insights about how the receptor works. The cysteine-rich domains of the receptor form long, flexible, molecular prongs that grasp the trimeric ligand. Other receptors with cysteine-rich domains are thought to bind their multimeric ligands similarly. For example,

the atomic structures of TNF receptors α and β are similar despite only 33% sequence identity of the polypeptides.

Three finger-like receptors cooperate to grasp one trimeric TNF molecule by binding along the interfaces between TNF subunits. Interaction is stabilized by both hydrophobic and hydrophilic interactions. Association of the receptor prongs with the tapered TNF molecule brings the C-terminal ends of the extracellular domains of three receptors close together near the surface of the membrane. This juxtaposes both transmembrane and cytoplasmic domains of the three receptor subunits.

TNF receptor appears to be coupled to a plasma membrane phospholipase that hydrolyzes sphingomyelin, producing the second messenger **ceremide** (see Fig. 28–11). Little is known about how ligand binding activates this enzyme, but the structure of the receptor-ligand complex suggests that clustering may be involved. Other receptors employing linear arrays of cysteine-rich subdomains, like the TNF receptor, also bind to multimeric ligands, so receptor activation by clustering of their different cytoplasmic signal transduction domains may be a general theme. Chapter 49 presents an example in which Fas ligand triggers cell death by activating a cascade of intracellular proteolysis.

TNF receptors also bind a number of adaptor proteins that recruit protein kinases to the active receptor. In many cases these kinases ultimately bring about activation of the transcription factor NF-κB, producing alterations in gene expression.

Notch Receptors

Components of the Delta/Notch signaling pathway have been identified by analysis of mutations affecting early development in flies and nematodes. Ligands are transmembrane proteins called **Delta** in flies and vertebrates and LAG-2 in worms. These ligands and **Notch receptors** regulate cellular fates during early embryonic development. Typically, cells expressing Delta interact with Notch receptors on adjacent cells to force the neighboring cells to chose a different fate than their own. The actual outcome depends on the context; in each tissue, Delta/Notch signals are integrated with the actions of other signaling pathways. As a general point, Delta/Notch signals tend to reinforce differences between cells in a particular tissue. For example, Delta on the earliest neurons directs adjacent cells to other fates. Defects in Delta or Notch result in excess neurons. The original literature on this subject is challenging, because homologous components may have different names from species to species.

Genetic analysis has established that Delta/Notch

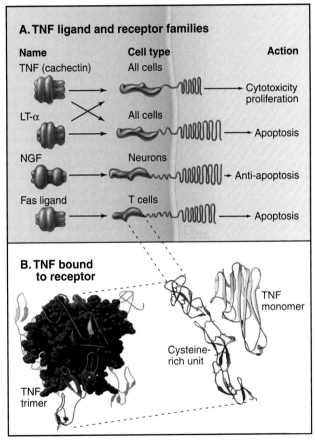

Figure 26–11 Tumor necrosis factor (TNF) receptor family. *A,* Domain architecture of a sample of members from the TNF receptor family. LT-α, lymphotoxin-α; NGF, nerve growth factor. Fas and Fas ligand are presented in Chapter 49. *B,* Atomic model of TNF bound to its receptor. TNF is a trimer of three identical β sandwich subunits arranged in a pear-like structure. The four extracellular cysteine-rich domains of the receptor grasp TNF-like prongs. (*A,* Adapted from Beutler B, vanHuffel C: Unraveling function in the TNF ligand and receptor family. Science 264:667–668, 1994. Copyright 1994, American Association for the Advancement of Science. *B,* Reference: Banner DW, et al: Crystal structure of the soluble human 55 kD TNF receptor-human TNF beta complex: Implications for TNF receptor activation. Cell 73:431–445, 1993. Copyright 1993, with permission from Elsevier Science. PDB file: 1TNR.)

signaling is vital for animal development, but less is known about the mechanisms than the other receptors presented in this chapter. Some Delta is active as a cell surface protein that interacts locally with adjacent cells, but a matrix metalloproteinase (see Chapter 31) cleaves some Delta from the membrane, allowing it to act at a distance from its cell of origin. Certain receptors, called Notch (flies, vertebrates) and Lin-12 (worms), consist of several extracellular EGF-like domains, a single transmembrane span, and an intracellular region that lacks any known enzyme activity. Notch is synthesized as a single polypeptide chain and is cleaved once before transport to the plasma membrane. The two polypeptides remain covalently associated, presumably by a disulfide bond. Cells carrying Delta activate Notch receptors on adjacent cells and activate transcription of certain genes. The mechanism is incompletely understood, but it involves a transcription factor called CSL and proteolytic cleavage of the intracellular domain of the receptor, small amounts of which may move into the nucleus.

Hedgehog Receptors

Genetic studies of *Drosophila* development have revealed a novel class of protein ligands, called **hedgehog,** and two membrane proteins, called **patched** and **smoothened,** that are required for signal transduction. Patched is a novel protein with about 12 transmembrane segments, whereas smoothened is an unusual seven-helix receptor. In flies, this signaling system is essential (along with the **Wnt** system; see Chapter 32) for establishing cellular fates, including boundaries between segments of the embryo. Homologues of these proteins have similar functions in vertebrates and regulate cellular differentiation in many tissues, including the nervous system. Mutations in one of three known mammalian hedgehog genes (sonic hedgehog) cause widespread developmental defects that range from mild to grotesque, including a single eye in the middle of the face. Mutations in the gene for patched cause basal cell carcinoma of the skin, the most common cancer in fair-skinned people.

Every aspect of this novel signaling pathway has established new principles. A signal sequence guides hedgehog protein into the secretory pathway, but before it reaches the cell surface, the protein cleaves itself in two pieces. This autocatalytic mechanism also adds a molecule of cholesterol to the new C-terminus of the first half of the protein, the domain with signaling activity. The latter half is required for the cleavage reaction. **Covalently bound cholesterol** anchors the signaling domain to the cell surface by inserting into the lipid bilayer. This was the first example of cholesterol being used for a post-translational modification

of a protein. Some hedgehog protein is secreted and interacts with distant cells. Patched is thought to be the receptor for hedgehog, although this needs further experimental verification. In the absence of hedgehog, patched inhibits the seven-helix receptor smoothened. In contrast to other seven-helix receptors, smoothened is constitutively active. It initiates an uncharacterized signaling pathway that results in the synthesis of several proteins, including a transcription factor called Gli1, an oncogene originally discovered in brain tumors. Hedgehog turns on this pathway by inhibiting patched, which releases smoothened to be active. Smoothened is a proto-oncogene; activating mutations prevent its inhibition by patched and cause skin tumors. Although this pathway is still incompletely understood, it is instructive, as few of its features were anticipated from lessons learned from better characterized receptors.

Selected Readings

Artavanis-Tsakonas S, Rand MD, Lake RJ: Notch signaling: Cell fate control and signal integration in development. Science 284:770–776, 1999.

Bray D: Signaling complexes: Biophysical constraints on intracellular communication. Annu Rev Biophys Biomol Struct 27:59–75, 1998.

Burke D, Wilkes D, Blundell TL, Malcolm S: Fibroblast growth factor receptors: Lessons from the genes. Trends Biochem Sci 23:59–62, 1998.

Hackel PO, Zwick E, Prenzel N, Ullrich A: Epidermal growth factor receptors: Critical mediators of multiple receptor pathways. Curr Opin Cell Biol 11:184–189, 1999.

Heldin C-H, Miyazono K, ten Dijke P: TGF-β signaling from cell membrane to nucleus through Smad proteins. Nature 390:465–471, 1997.

Hubbard SR, Till JH: Protein tyrosine kinase structure and function. Annu Rev Biochem 69:373–398, 2000.

Kimble J, Henderson S, Crittenden S: Notch/Lin-12 signaling: Transduction by regulated protein slicing. Trends Biochem Sci 23:353–357, 1998.

Massague J: TGF-β signal transduction. Annu Rev Biochem 67:753–792, 1998.

Murone M, Rosenthal A, de Sauvage FJ: Sonic hedgehog signaling by the Patched-Smoothened receptor complex. Curr Biology 9:76–84, 1999.

Naismith JH, Sprang SR: Modularity in the TNF-receptor family. Trends Biochem Sci 23:74–79, 1998.

Pitcher JA, Freedman NJ, Lefkowitz RJ: G protein-coupled receptor kinases. Annu Rev Biochem 67:653–692, 1998.

Rao VR, Oprian DD: Activating mutations of rhodopsin and other G protein-coupled receptors. Annu Rev Biophys Biomol Struct 25:287–314, 1996.

Wells JA, de Vos AM: Hematopoietic receptor complexes. Annu Rev Biochem 65:609–634, 1996.

Seven-helix receptor web site: available from ⟨http://swift.embl.heidelberg.de/7tm/⟩.

chapter 27

PROTEIN HARDWARE FOR SIGNALING

This chapter introduces cytoplasmic proteins that are widely used for signal transduction, including protein kinases, protein phosphatases, guanosine triphosphatases (GTPases), and adapter proteins. Remarkably, both kinases and GTPases use the same strategy to operate molecular switches that carry information through signaling cascades: the simple addition and removal of inorganic phosphate. Protein kinases add, and phosphatases remove, phosphate groups on specific protein targets. GTPases bind guanosine triphosphate (GTP) and hydrolyze it to guanosine diphosphate (GDP). In both cases, the presence or absence of a single phosphate group can switch a protein between active and inactive conformations. Because the addition and removal of phosphate is reversible, both types of switches can be used as molecular timers that cycle on and off at tempos determined by the intrinsic properties of the switch and its environment. GTPases are active with bound GTP and switch off when they hydrolyze GTP to GDP. Similarly, phosphorylation activates many proteins, although in some cases, phosphorylation turns proteins off rather than on.

In all of these examples, a single protein acts as a simple binary switch. Turning a series of such molecular switches on and off carries information through a **signaling cascade**. The concept is simple in theory but often complicated in practice, as elaborated in Chapter 29, because many signaling pathways use both GTPases and kinases, and many use a series of different kinases. Cascades of switches can amplify and sharpen the cellular response to stimuli. Furthermore, few signaling pathways are linear; instead, most branch and intersect, allowing cells to integrate information from multiple receptors and to control multiple effector systems simultaneously.

Enzymes along signaling pathways (including kinases) often act as amplifiers. Turning on the binary switch of one enzyme molecule usually produces many product molecules, each of which, in turn, may continue to propagate and amplify the original signal by activating downstream molecules.

Protein Phosphorylation

Reversible phosphorylation is the most common post-translational modification of proteins and regulates the activity of one or more proteins along most signaling pathways considered in this book. Among other things, phosphorylation controls metabolic enzymes, cell motility, membrane channels, assembly of the nucleus, and cell cycle progression. Sometimes, phosphorylation turns a process on, sometimes off. In either case, both the addition of a phosphate by a **protein kinase** and its removal by a **protein phosphatase** are required to achieve regulation.

For historical and practical reasons, it has been easier to study protein kinases than protein phosphatases, so most research and accounts of regulation by phosphorylation emphasize kinases. Furthermore, many have assumed incorrectly that phosphatases are constitutively active, leading to a lack of interest in the role of protein phosphatases in signaling reactions. Nevertheless, readers should not forget that this is a two-way street; the next section considers protein phosphatases.

In eukaryotes, more than 99% of cellular phosphorylation occurs on **serine** and **threonine** residues, but phosphorylation of **tyrosine** residues is essential for regulating many cellular processes (Fig. 27–1). Eubacteria and Archaea use histidine and aspartate phosphorylation for signaling (see Chapter 29). Phosphorylation of **histidine** and **aspartate** appears to be less important in eukaryotes, but important signaling pro-

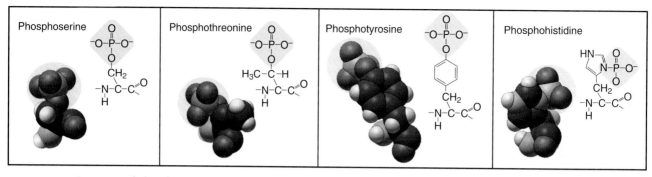

Figure 27–1 Structures of phosphoamino acids. In addition to the N1 nitrogen illustrated, histidine is often phosphorylated on N3 at the upper left.

cesses using these phosphoamino acids may have escaped detection because they are more difficult to assay than other phosphorylated residues.

Effects of Phosphorylation on Protein Structure and Function

Although only a small chemical group, the addition of a phosphate to the side chain of a single amino acid can profoundly change the activity of a protein. Phosphate groups can induce conformational changes or alter interactions with substrates or other molecules in several ways.

- *Steric interference.* Phosphorylation can alter the affinity of a protein for one or more of its ligands. Phosphorylation inhibits the metabolic enzyme isocitrate dehydrogenase by blocking substrate binding to the active site (Fig. 27–2). Both direct steric hindrance and electrostatic repulsion between the negatively charged phosphate and the negatively charged substrate prevent substrate binding. Phosphorylation can also inhibit protein assembly reactions, such as the polymerization of intermediate filaments (see Chapter 38) and binding of ADF/cofilin proteins to actin monomers and filaments (see Chapter 36).
- *Conformational change.* Phosphorylation activates tyrosine kinases by inducing a dramatic change in a polypeptide loop that blocks the substrate bind-

ing site of the inactive enzyme (Fig. 27–3D). Phosphorylation of the metabolic enzyme glycogen phosphorylase produces a conformational change that activates the enzyme. The unphosphorylated, inactive enzyme has an open conformation. Phosphorylation of serine 14 provides negative charges that stabilize the compact, active conformation.
- *Creation of binding sites.* Reversible phosphorylation controls interactions between partner proteins that require a phosphorylated residue to complete a binding site. SH2 (Src homology) and some PTB domains require a phosphotyrosine on their protein ligands. A phosphoserine is required on protein ligands for binding 14-3-3 domains, some WW domains, and some FHA domains (see later section for details).

Protein Kinases

Genes for protein kinases are remarkably abundant: 116 in budding yeast (second only to transcription factor genes); 409 in nematode worms (second only to seven-helix receptor genes); and more than 800 in vertebrates. Phylogenetic analyses of sequences have established that genes for the catalytic domains of virtually all eukaryotic **serine/threonine/tyrosine kinases** had a common evolutionary origin and branched into about a dozen families early in evolution (Table 27–1). These related catalytic domains (Fig. 27–3) are joined to additional polypeptides that participate in regulation or localization of the enzyme (see Fig. 27–4). Few exceptions to this common origin exist. Genes for **histidine kinases** had a separate origin in prokaryotes, and the catalytic domain has a different fold than eukaryotic serine/threonine/tyrosine kinases. The first example of the second novel class was a threonine kinase, from the slime mold *Dictyostelium* that phosphorylated myosin II heavy chain. Related proteins from mammals and *Caenorhabditis elegans* phosphorylate protein synthesis elongation factor eEF-2. Yeasts lack these novel kinases, which appear to favor as substrates threonines in α helices.

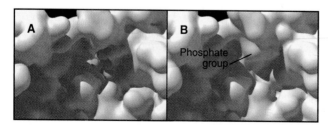

Figure 27–2 Phosphorylation blocks substrate binding to isocitrate dehydrogenase. *A,* Surface representation with isocitrate *(blue)* bound to the active site. *B,* Phosphorylation of serine 113 *(yellow)* blocks isocitrate binding. (PDB files: 3ICD and 4ICD.)

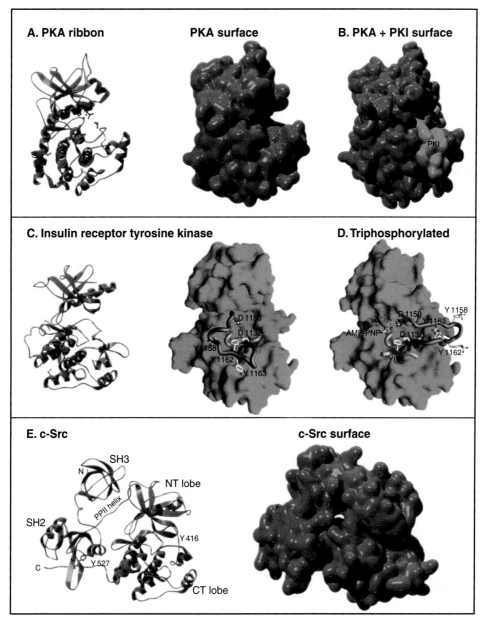

Figure 27-3 Protein kinase structures. *A,* Ribbon diagram and space-filling model of cAMP-dependent protein kinase with nonhydrolyzable ATP analogue *(red)* bound to the active site. The adenine base of the ATP fits into a hydrophobic cleft formed by β sheets lining the interface of the two lobes. The phosphates bind to conserved residues in loops connecting the β-strands. (PDB file: 1CPK.) *B,* Space-filling model of PKA with bound inhibitory peptide PKI. The location of this inhibitory peptide revealed the binding site for protein substrates. (PDB file: 1FMO.) *C,* Insulin receptor tyrosine kinase. Ribbon diagram and space-filling model with the catalytic loop in orange and the activation loop in green. (PDB file: 1IRK.) *D,* Space-filling model of insulin receptor tyrosine kinase triphosphorylated on the activation loop. This rearranges the activation loop, allowing substrates *(pink with a white tyrosine side chain)* access to the active site. AMP-PNP is a nonhydrolyzable analogue of ATP with nitrogen bridging the β- and γ-phosphates. (PDB: 1IR3.) *E,* Ribbon diagram and space-filling models of c-Src. When tyrosine-527 is phosphorylated, the SH2 domain binds intramolecularly to the C-terminus, locking the kinase in an inactive conformation. The N-terminal SH3 binds intramolecularly to a proline-rich sequence (PPII helix) connecting the SH2 and kinase domains. NT and CT are the N- and C-terminal lobes of the kinase domain. (*C* and *D,* Space-filling models courtesy of Steven Hubbard, New York University.)

table 27–1

FAMILIES OF PROTEIN KINASES

Family	Substrates	Bacterial Genes	Yeast Genes	Worm Genes	Examples	Regulation	Targets/Regulated Functions
AGC	S, T	0	17	30	PKA	cAMP	Metabolic enzymes, TFs, ion channels
					PKB	PI3K, PDKs	GSK3/Metabolism, survival
					PKC	Calcium, lipids	Receptor tyrosine kinases, ion channels, TFs
					PKG	cGMP	IP$_3$R, CFTR, VASP
					RSK	MAPK, PDKs	Ribosome/Synthesis of translation machinery
					GRK	G proteins	7-Helix receptor down-regulation
CaMK	S, T	0	16	31	CaMK	Ca^{2+}, calmodulin	Synaptic transmission, cytoskeleton, TFs
					AMP-PK	AMP	Fatty acid, cholesterol synthesis
					MLCK	Calcium, calmodulin	Myosin/Contraction
CMGC	S, T (Y)	0	21	41	CDK	Phosphorylation	Many/Cell cycle
					MAPK	Phosphorylation	TFs/Proliferation
					GSK3	PKB	Glycogen metabolism, survival
					Clk-related	?	MAP kinase pathway, RNA splicing
Raf	S, T	0	0	2	MAPKKK	Ras	MAPKK/Proliferation
STE11/20	S, T	0	10	17	MAPKKK	Phosphorylation	MAPKK/Proliferation
					PAK	Small GTPases	LIMK/Cytoskeleton
STE7/MEK	S, T, Y	0	8	9	MAPKK	MAPKKK	MAPK/Proliferation
Casein kinases	S, T (Y)	0	7	86	CK-I, CK-II	?	Numerous circadian clocks, Wnt signaling, chromatin
Polo	S, T	0	1	3	hPLK-1, Cdc5	Phosphorylation	Several/Mitosis, cytokinesis
Receptor S/T kinases	S, T	0	1	3	TGF-βR	TGF-β	Smads/Differentiation
Tyrosine kinases	Y	0	0	68	Src family, JAK, Fak, Abl, Syk	Phosphorylation	Many/Proliferation, lymphocyte activation, actin cytoskeleton, cell adhesion
Receptor tyrosine kinases	Y	0	0	23	GF receptors	Growth factors	Proliferation, cytoskeleton
Dual specificity	S, Y	0	4	3	wee1	Phosphorylation	Cdc2/Cell cycle
Histidine kinases*	H	0 to >30	2	0	Tar	Osmolarity (yeast)	Bacterial chemotaxis, gene expression
Phosphatidylinositol (PI) kinases	Inositol	0	10	10	PI kinases	SH2 targeting	Phosphoinositides, proteins/Proliferation

*Number of histidine kinases in prokaryotes. *Bacteria: Bacillus substilis* (37); *Escherichia coli* (7); *Borrelia burgdorferi*—Lyme disease spirochaete (2); *Myobacterium tuberculosis* (14) also has 11 eukaryotic serine/threonine kinase genes, likely derived by lateral gene transfer from eukaryotic hosts. *Archaea: Methanococcus jannaschii* (0); *Aquifex aecolicus* (0); *Archaeoglobus fulgidus* (3). AMP-PK, adenosine monophosphate (AMP)–activated protein kinase; CaMK, calmodulin activated protein kinase; CDK, cyclin-dependent kinase; CFTR, cystic fibrosis transmembrane regulator; CK, casein kinase; Clk, Cdc-like kinase; GF, growth factor; GRK, G protein–coupled receptor kinase; GSK, glycogen synthase kinase; hPLK-1, human polo-like kinase; IP$_3$R, inositol trisphosphate receptor, a Ca^{2+} release channel; LIMK, LIM-kinase; MAPK, mitogen-activated protein kinase (also called ERK, for extracellular signal–regulated kinase); MAPKK, MAPK kinase (also called MEK): MAPKKK, MAPK kinase kinase; MLCK, myosin light chain kinase; PAK, p21 (small GTPase)-activated kinase; PDK, 3-phosphoinositide–dependent protein kinase; PKA, cyclic AMP–dependent protein kinase; PKB, protein kinase B (also called Akt); PKC, calcium-dependent protein kinase; PKG, cyclic GMP–dependent protein kinase; polo, a *Drosophila* gene; Raf, cellular homologue of retroviral oncogene; RSK, ribosomal subunit 6 kinase; STE7, 11, 20, budding yeast genes; TFs, transcription factors; VASP, vasodilator-stimulated phosphoprotein; wee1, fission yeast gene.
Unclassified kinases: NimA; GCN2 (translational control); LIM-kinase; Mos; Pim (proto-oncogene–activated)
Yeast-specific: BUB1; ELM; Ran; NPR

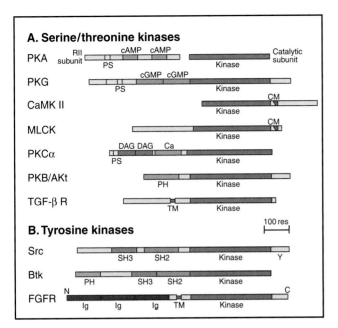

Figure 27-4 *A* and *B*, Protein kinase domain architecture. See Table 27-1 for definitions of the kinase names. B+k, Bruton tyrosine kinase; Ca, calcium-binding site; cAMP and cGMP, cyclic nucleotide binding sites. CM, calmodulin-binding site; DAG, diacylglycerol-binding site; FGFR, Fibroblast growth factor receptor; Ig, immunoglobulin domains; PH, pleckstrin homology domain; PS, pseudosubstrate sequences; SH2 and SH3, Src-homology domains; TM, transmembrane domain.

Most families of kinases are represented in animals, but yeast lack several families (see Table 27–1), including tyrosine kinases. It is argued that these kinases appeared in animals after their divergence from fungi, but fungi may have lost some kinase genes as their genomes became more specialized. More knowledge regarding genomes of protozoa and algae will answer this question. Fungi have some phosphotyrosine by virtue of two families of kinases that phosphorylate tyrosine in addition to serine and threonine. (They have three protein tyrosine phosphatases to reverse these reactions.) On the other hand, fungi have several families of kinases not found in animals. Prokaryotes have been thought to lack eukaryotic-type serine/threonine/tyrosine kinases, except for a few such genes acquired by bacteria by lateral transfer of genes from eukaryotes. On the other hand, a few uncharacterized gene sequences in bacteria and Archaea suggest an ancient origin for these genes.

Protein kinases catalyze the transfer of the γ-phosphate from adenosine triphosphate (ATP) (or rarely, guanosine triphosphate [GTP]) to amino acid side chains of proteins. Many vertebrate protein kinases phosphorylate either serine or threonine. Others phosphorylate tyrosine. A few phosphorylate serine, threonine, *and* tyrosine. **Lipid kinases** have a catalytic domain related to typical protein kinases. They phosphorylate either inositol phospholipids or a few pro-

teins, several of which are involved with cell cycle control (see Chapter 46).

The catalytic domain of protein kinases consists of about 260 residues in two lobes surrounding the ATP-binding pocket (see Fig. 27–3). Despite extensive sequence divergence, all of these enzymes have a similar polypeptide fold with conserved residues at critical positions required for catalysis. Although tyrosine kinases are easy to distinguish from serine/threonine kinases on the basis of amino acid sequence alone, the mechanism for selecting tyrosine versus serine/threonine is not yet clear from the atomic structures.

Each kinase has a restricted range of protein substrates, so that activation of a particular protein kinase changes the phosphorylation and activity of a discrete set of proteins. Substrate specificity is achieved by selective binding of substrates to a groove that positions the acceptor amino acid at the active site, as well as secondary sites. "**Pseudosubstrates**" (part of the kinase itself or a separate subunit) inhibit kinases by binding to the substrate groove (see Fig. 27–3B). Typically, all substrates that bind a particular kinase have similar residues surrounding the target serine, threonine, or tyrosine, allowing each substrate to interact with the same complementary residues on the kinase. Targeting of kinases to particular parts of cells also limits the range of proteins phosphorylated.

Additional peptide sequences flank the catalytic domain of most kinases and serve many functions (see Fig. 27–4). Pseudosubstrates regulate kinase activity. Adapter domains, such as SH2, SH3, and pleckstrin homology domains, target kinases to specific sites in the cell (see later section and Chapter 29). The Src-homology domains (SH2 and SH3) were first recognized in Src, the first oncogene to be characterized (see Fig. 27–3E and Box 29–1). Transmembrane segments anchor receptor kinases to membranes. Receptor tyrosine kinases usually have additional residues inserted in the kinase domain and at the C-terminus. Phosphorylation of tyrosines in these inserts creates binding sites for effector proteins carrying SH2 domains.

Regulation of Protein Kinases

Each kinase has its own regulatory mechanism, but most involve one or more of three strategies: (1) reversible phosphorylation; (2) interactions with intrinsic peptides or extrinsic subunits that may themselves be targets for second messengers or regulatory proteins; and (3) targeting to specific cellular locations, such as the nucleus, plasma membrane, or cytoskeleton, enhancing interaction with specific substrates.

Phosphorylation

Phosphorylation can either activate or inhibit protein kinases. In some cases, a kinase of the same type carries out the phosphorylation, but often, another type of kinase is responsible. When linked in series, different types of kinases, form a signaling cascade that often amplifies and sharpens the response to a stimulus. Most sections of this book, particularly Chapter 29, covers examples of **kinase cascades.**

- *Activation loop phosphorylation.* Phosphorylation of three tyrosines on an **activation loop** near the active site activates insulin receptor kinase (see Fig. 27–3D). Phosphorylation dramatically refolds the activation loop, allowing access of substrates. It also rotates the two domains of the kinase, bringing together the residues required to form the catalytic active site. Activation loop phosphorylation also turns on many other kinases including other receptor tyrosine kinases, Src-family tyrosine kinases (see Fig. 27–3E and Box 29–1), mitogen-activated protein (MAP) kinases, cyclin-dependent kinases, and calcium-calmodulin–dependent kinases.

- *Inhibitory phosphorylation.* Phosphorylation of myosin light chain kinase (by protein kinase A [PKA]) reduces its affinity for its protein substrate, and phosphorylation of platelet-derived growth factor (PDGF) receptor tyrosine kinase (by protein kinase C [PKC]) inhibits its activity. Phosphorylation of a C-terminal tyrosine inhibits Src-family tyrosine kinases (see Fig. 27–3E). Intramolecular binding of this phosphotyrosine to an SH2 domain at the N-terminus traps the kinase in an inactive conformation. Cyclin-dependent cell cycle kinases can also be inhibited by phosphorylation (see Chapter 43).

Regulation of Substrate Binding

Peptides intrinsic to the kinase or part of a separate protein can inhibit kinases by competing with protein substrates for binding to the enzyme (see Fig. 27–3B).

- *Autoinhibition.* Pseudosubstrate sequences (PSs) built into myosin light chain kinase, calmodulin activated kinase (CaMK), PKC, and protein kinase G (PKG) bind to and block the substrate sites (see Fig. 27–4). These autoinhibitory peptides mimic the protein substrate but lack a phosphorylatable residue. **Ca²⁺-calmodulin** activates myosin light chain kinase and CaMK by binding to a helical segment of their inhibitory peptides immediately adjacent to the pseudosubstrate site. This displaces the inhibitory peptide from the kinase and allows substrates to bind. Cyclic guanosine monophosphate (cGMP) binding to PKG displaces the autoinhibitory peptide from the catalytic domain, activating the enzyme.

- *Extrinsic regulation by inhibitory subunits.* Separate **regulatory (R) subunits** inhibit PKA by blocking the protein substrate site (see Fig. 27–4). The RI subunit is not phosphorylated as it has

alanine, rather than serine, at the phosphorylation site. The RII subunit has a serine at the phosphorylation site. It is phosphorylated but does not dissociate from the catalytic subunit like phosphorylated substrates. Cyclic adenosine monophosphate (**cAMP**) regulates the affinity of the regulatory subunits for the catalytic subunit. In resting cells, the regulatory subunit is free of cAMP and binds the catalytic subunit with high affinity. With a rise in cAMP concentration (see Chapter 28), cAMP binds the regulatory subunit, dissociates it from the catalytic subunit, and allows substrates access to the active site.

- *Extrinsic regulation by activating subunits.* Regulatory subunits can also activate protein kinases. Regulatory subunits called **cyclins** bind and contribute to activating cyclin-dependent cell cycle kinases, **Cdks** (see Chapter 43).

- *Dual or triple regulation.* Multiple factors regulate most kinases. Both interaction of calcium-calmodulin with an intrinsic pseudosubstrate and activation loop phosphorylation activate CaMK. Both inhibitory and activating phosphorylation, as well as cyclins, regulate **cyclin-dependent kinases**.

Targeting

Several mechanisms target kinases to specific cellular locations, bringing the enzyme close to particular substrates and contributing to specificity. This helps explain how kinases with rather broad specificity can have specific effects in particular target cells.

- The intracellular location of PKA is determined by both its RI and RII subunits and a family of **A kinase–anchoring proteins (AKAPs)**. When the cAMP concentration is low, regulatory subunits bind and inhibit PKA. RII subunits also bind to AKAPs, which target the inhibited PKA catalytic subunit variously to centrosomes, actin filaments, microtubules, endoplasmic reticulum, peroxisomes, mitochondria, and plasma membrane. Some AKAPs bind other protein kinases such as PKC and phosphatases (PP2B), as well as RII subunits of PKA. An increase in cAMP releases active PKA in close proximity to particular substrates. Once freed from RI or RII subunits by cAMP, the PKA catalytic subunit can also migrate into the nucleus where a different array of substrates is available and gene transcription can be regulated. The inhibitory protein PKI is capable of capturing the catalytic subunit in the nucleus, thereby targeting it for transport from the nucleus back to the cytoplasm. Similar to AKAPs, the inner centromere protein, INCENP, binds and targets the aurora-B kinase to various structures during cell division: centromeres early in mitosis, and the central spindle and cleavage furrow late in mitosis (see Chapter 47).

- **Pleckstrin homology (PH)** domains (see later section) and lipid tags target kinases to lipid bilayers. **PKB/Akt** has a pleckstrin homology domain that targets it to membrane polyphosphoinositides. This lipid interaction opens up sites on the catalytic domain for phosphorylation and activation by PDK1, another kinase with a pleckstrin homology domain. An N-terminal myristic acid anchors Src tyrosine kinase to the plasma membrane.
- Phosphorylation can induce the MAP kinase ERK2 to form homodimers, which somehow trigger movement into the nucleus where they regulate gene expression.
- A scaffolding protein called STE5, first identified in yeast, brings together three protein kinases that form part of the cascade of kinases that activate MAP kinases (see Chapter 29).

Kinases and Disease

Constitutive activation of some kinases—for example, the receptor tyrosine kinase RET in endocrine cancers and cyclin-dependent kinase CDK4 in melanoma—predisposes individuals to cancer. Most patients with chronic myelogenous leukemia have a gene rearrangment that produces a fusion between the protein bcr and c-abl, a nonreceptor tyrosine kinase. The constitutively active fusion protein is essential for cancerous transformation of white blood cell precursors. A selective inhibitor of bcr-abl kinase activity kills myelogenous leukemia cells and has shown promise in clinical treatment of the disease. Inactivation of the serine/threonine kinase LKB1 causes Peutz-Jeghers syndrome with predisposition to various cancers.

Protein Phosphatases

Eukaryotes have several families of protein phosphatases that remove phosphate from amino acid side chains (Table 27–2 and Fig. 27–5). Like protein kinases, most protein phosphatases are active toward either phosphoserine/threonine or phosphotyrosine, although a few dual specificity phosphatases can dephosphorylate all three residues. Members of each subfamily of phosphatases have similar structures but

table 27-2
PROTEIN PHOSPHATASES

Catalytic Subunit	Regulatory Elements	Inhibitors	Regulated Functions
Serine-Threonine Phosphatases			
PPP Family			
PP1C subfamily = catalytic subunit + regulatory subunit	>15 regulatory subunits that target and regulate catalytic subunit	Okadaic acid Microcystin	Glycogen metabolism, muscle contraction, cell cycle, mRNA splicing
PP2A subfamily = catalytic subunit + 65-kD A subunit + B subunit	B subunits target and regulate core enzyme	Okadaic acid Microcystin	MAP kinase pathway, metabolism, cell cycle
PP2B (calcineurin) = catalytic A subunit + one of two B subunits	Calcium-calmodulin activates by binding autoinhibitory peptide	Cyclosporin-cyclophilin FK506-FKBP	T-lymphocyte activation, brain NMDA receptor signaling
PPM Family			
PP2C	Integral N- or C-terminal peptides	Unsaturated fatty acids	Antagonism of stress-activated kinases
Protein Tyrosine Phosphatases			
PTP Family			
Cytosolic PTPs (PTP1B, SHP1, SHP2)	SH2 and other domains target to substrates	Vanadate	Various signaling pathways
Transmembrane PTPs (CD45, RPTPμ, RPTPα)	Homodimerization may inhibit activity	Vanadate	Lymphocyte activation
Dual-specificity Family (MAP kinase phosphatases, etc.)			MAP kinase pathway
Cdc25 Family	Polo kinase, Chk1 kinase, phosphatases	Sulfirein, coscinosulfate	Cell cycle
Low-molecular-weight (Acid phosphatases)	Located in lysosomes	—	Unknown

mRNA, messenger RNA; NMDA, *N*-methyl-**D**-aspartate.

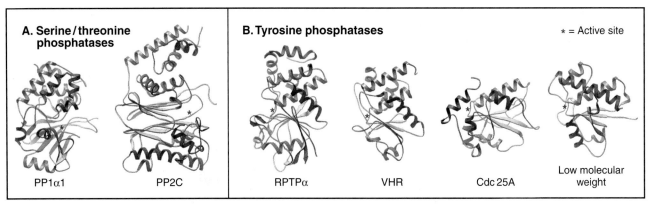

Figure 27-5 Protein phosphatase structures. Ribbon diagrams with a red asterisk marking the active sites. *A,* Serine/threonine phosphatases: PP1α1 (PDB file: 1FJM) and PP2C (PDB file: 1A6O). *B,* Four families of protein tyrosine phosphatases: receptor tyrosine phosphatase RPTPα (PDB file: 1YFO); dual-specificity phosphatase VHR (PDB file: 1VHR); Cdc25A (PDB file: 1c25); and low-molecular-weight phosphatase (PDB file: 1PNT).

often carry out diverse functions depending upon their association with an array of accessory subunits that regulate enzyme activity and also target catalytic subunits to particular substrates or parts of the cell. Phosphatases have been said to have broader substrate specificity than protein kinases, but this conclusion was based on experiments with isolated catalytic subunits under artificial laboratory conditions. Ongoing research is adding novel members to the inventory of phosphatases. Polypeptide sequences flanking catalytic domains, as well as accessory subunits, participate in regulation and localization of the enzymes (Fig. 27–6).

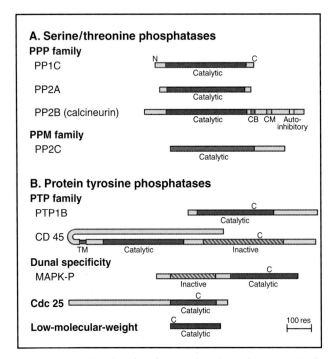

Figure 27-6 Protein phosphatase domain architecture. Scale linear models. *A,* Serine/threonine phosphatases. *B,* Protein tyrosine phosphatases. CB, calcium binding; CM, calmodulin-binding; TM, transmembrane segment. The five different catalytic domain folds are coded with different colors.

PPP Family of Phosphates

Members of the PPP family of **serine/threonine phosphatases** are found in Eubacteria, Archaea and in all tissues of eukaryotes. PP1 and PP2A are two of the most evolutionarily conserved of all enzymes. All three PPP subfamilies (see Fig. 27–6A) share the same catalytic fold with a two-metal ion cluster (Fe^{2+} and Zn^{2+} in vivo) in the active site (see Fig. 27–5A). Diverse regulatory subunits restrict the substrates for **PP1** and **PP2A** by targeting catalytic subunits to specific sites in the cell. In many cases, the substrate specificity in vivo is not yet known, but a few examples have been thoroughly studied.

M subunits target the 38-kD catalytic subunit of PP1 to myosin, restrict reactivity with other substrates, and regulate phosphatase activity. G subunits target PP1 to glycogen particles, where it sits poised to dephosphorylate two metabolic enzymes, glycogen phosphorylase, and glycogen synthase (see Fig. 29–3). Dephosphorylation inactivates phosphorylase, turning off glycogen breakdown, and activates glycogen synthase, an example of reciprocal regulation. The hormone adrenaline regulates PP1, acting through PKA. When PKA phosphorylates the G subunit, this reduces its affinity for PP1 and releases PP1 from the glycogen particle, allowing glycogen breakdown.

The serine/threonine phosphatase PP2A usually associates with two other subunits: a 65-kD scaffold subunit and a "B" subunit from diverse families. PP2A dephosphorylates many substrates, including kinases in the MAP kinase cascade (see Chapter 29). The inhibitors okadaic acid (a polyketide from dinoflagellates) and microcystin (a cyclic peptide from cyanobacteria) block access of substrates to the active site of PP2A.

Protein phosphatase 2B, also known as **calcineurin,** is the only cytoplasmic phosphatase regulated by Ca^{2+}. It couples Ca^{2+} signals to protein dephosphorylation. Among several substrates, the transcription factor **NF-AT** (nuclear factor–activated T cells) is the best known. Activation of T-cell receptors on T lymphocytes releases Ca^{2+} in the cytoplasm and turns on PP2B. Dephosphorylation of NF-AT permits its import into the nucleus, where it turns on the expression of several lymphocyte growth factors, including interleukin-2 (see Fig. 29–8). The importance of PP2B in the immune response was revealed, in part, because it is the indirect target of two potent drugs that inhibit the immune rejection of transplanted organs. These drugs—**cyclosporin** and **FK506**—bind to two different small proteins: **cyclophilin** and **FK-binding protein**. Both drug-protein complexes bind similar sites on PP2B and inhibit the phosphatase by directly blocking the active site. This prevents gene expression by NF-AT in response to Ca^{2+} and suppresses the immune response.

PP2B consists of two subunits. The A subunit forms the phosphatase active site, including the Fe^{2+} and Zn^{2+} ions that are essential for enzyme activity. The B subunit is similar to calmodulin (see Chapter 28) in that it binds one Ca^{2+} tightly but does not participate in the response to Ca^{2+}. At low concentrations of Ca^{2+}, a C-terminal autoinhibitory segment of the A subunit blocks its own active site. A transient increase in cytoplasmic Ca^{2+} activates PP2B by first binding to calmodulin. Calcium-calmodulin then binds the autoinhibitory segment and displaces it from the active site.

PPM Family of Phosphates

The large family of PPM serine/threonine phosphatases can be found in bacteria, plants, fungi, and animals. The sequence for the core catalytic domain is incorporated into a variety of genes that encode various N- and C-terminal peptides that confer specificity on the enzyme activity. PPMs are unrelated to PPPs in structure (PP2C in Fig. 27–5), but both have two metal ions in the active site (Mg^{2+} for PPM), and both catalyze the same phosphomonoester hydrolytic reaction. This is thought to be a rare example of **convergent evolution** toward similar active sites. PPM substrates include stress-activated kinases and mitochondrial dehydrogenases.

Protein Tyrosine Phosphatase Family

Protein tyrosine phosphatases (PTPs) generate considerable interest, as they participate in lymphocytic activation and regulation of cell proliferation by reversing the action of protein tyrosine kinases. But tyrosine dephosphorylation can also activate important enzymes, such as the Src tyrosine kinase (see Fig. 27–3*E*) and cyclin-dependent protein kinases (see Chapter 43).

The four families of PTPs represent a remarkable evolutionary tale. All bind phosphotyrosine in a narrow but deep pocket, transfer the phosphate to the sulfur atom of a cysteine in the sequence Cys-x-x-x-x-x-Arg, and release the phosphate in the rate-limiting step, when water attacks the phosphocysteine intermediate. Nevertheless, sequence analysis and atomic structures (see Fig. 27–5*B*) have shown that this is another case of **convergent evolution** from three different ancestors. PTPs and dual-specificity phosphatases, such as VHR, have similar three-dimensional structures derived from a common ancestor, whereas Cdc25 and low-molecular-weight tyrosine phosphatases have different folds. Initial impressions suggested that PTPs had broad substrate specificity, but as the inventory of these enzymes expanded, additional examples of high specificity emerged. As in the case of protein kinases, localization has an important influence on specificity. For example, a transmembrane segment anchoring a PTP such as CD45 (see Fig. 27–6) to the plasma membrane can enhance its access to some substrates and restrict its access to other substrates.

PTP Subfamily

The PTP catalytic domain of about 230 residues is encoded by a large number of genes, some of which produce cytoplasmic proteins and others of which have transmembrane and extracellular domains that may bind extracellular ligands (see Fig. 27–6 and Table 27–2). PTPs favor phosphotyrosine as a substrate by a factor of 10^5 over phosphoserine or phosphothreonine.

Many cytoplasmic PTPs are bound to cellular partners. Adapter domains, such as SH2 domains, bind the phosphatases SHP-1 and -2 to phosphotyrosines. C-terminal hydrophobic residues bind the phosphatase PTP1B to the endoplasmic reticulum. A sequence homologous with red blood cell protein 4.1 may target the phosphatase PTP H1 to the actin cytoskeleton. Targeting to substrates and phosphorylation is thought to regulate the activity and specificity of PTPs.

Transmembrane PTPs have a variety of extracellular domains linked by a single transmembrane segment to one or two PTP catalytic domains in the cytoplasm (see Fig. 27–6). The membrane proximal PTP domain has phosphatase activity. In most cases, the second PTP domain is inactive, so it may be regulatory. Extracellular domains are attractive candidates as receptors, and some have been implicated in cellular adhesion. Certain *Drosophila* PTPs are required for nerve processes to find their pathways to their target during embryonic development, but their extracellular ligands are not known. No extracellular ligand has been shown to regulate phosphatase activity.

CD45, the best characterized transmembrane PTP, constitutes a remarkable 10% of the plasma membrane protein in white blood cells. CD45 is required for antigens to activate B and T lymphocytes. Cells lacking CD45 fail to release intracellular Ca^{2+}, secrete lymphokines, or proliferate in response to antigen stimu-

table 27-3

PARALLELS AMONG GUANOSINE TRIPHOSPHATE–BINDING PROTEINS

Family	Bacterial Genes	Yeast Genes	Worm Genes	Functions	GDP Dissociation Inhibitors	Receptors	GTP Exchange Factors	GTPase-Activating Factors	Direct Effectors
Small GTPases									
Arf	0	6	11	Vesicular formation		Cargo molecules?	Sec-7/ARNO		Coat proteins
Rab	0	10	24	Vesicle targeting and fusion	Rab-GDI				Docking and fusion factors
Ran	0	2	2	Nuclear transport, mitotic spindle			Ran-GDF1, RCC1	RanBP1, RanGAP1	Importin β
Ras	0	4	8	Transduction of growth factor signals		Receptor tyrosine kinases	SOS	Ras-GAP	Raf
Rho	0	7	10	Regulation of actin cytoskeleton	Rho-GDI	Receptor tyrosine kinases, seven-helix	Dbl/PH-GEFs	Rho-GAP	p65 PAK, Rho kinase, WASp
Sar	0	1	3	Vesicular formation		Cargo molecules?	Sec12	Sec23	Coat proteins
Trimeric G Proteins	0	2	20	Transduction of a wide variety of signals	Gβγ	Seven-helix receptors	Seven-helix receptors	Effector proteins, RGS proteins	Many enzymes, channels
Elongation factors									
EF-Tu/ EF1α	1–2	4	5	Protein synthesis			EF-Ts/EF1β	Ribosome	
EF-G/ EF2	1–2	5	4	Protein synthesis			—	Ribosome	
RF1,2/ eRF	1–2	1	1– 12						
Dynamin	0	2	1–3	Endocytosis	?		Not required?	Intrinsic GAP domain	Membrane fission factors
Translocation GTPases	0	2	?	Translocation of polypeptides into endoplasmic reticulum			Nascent polypeptide chains	SRP receptor	Sec 61 translocon

GEFs, guanine nucleotide exchange factors.

lation. It is thought that the CD45 phosphatase activates one or more Src-family tyrosine kinases associated with the T-cell receptor by dephosphorylating inhibitory phosphotyrosine residues (see Fig. 27–3E and Chapter 29).

Dual-Specificity Subfamily

The dual-specificity family of phosphatases prefers phosphotyrosine as a substrate, but owing to the fact that its substrate binding site is shallower than that of a PTP, it can also dephosphorylate serine and threonine at about 1% that rate. The most interesting members of this group, the MKPs, inactivate **MAP kinases** by dephosphorylating both phosphotyrosine and phosphothreonine residues (see Fig. 29–6).

Cdc25 Subfamily

In terms of substrate specificity and biological function, Cdc25 is one of the best characterized tyrosine phosphatase families (see Chapter 43). Cdc25s remove inhibitory phosphates from an adjacent threonine and tyrosine on the master cell cycle kinases Cdk1 and Cdk2, releasing these key enzymes to promote cell cycle progression. This is another example of a phosphatase having a positive effect on a biological process. Cdc25 itself is activated by serine/threonine phosphorylation during the cell cycle.

Genetically Inactive Protein Tyrosine Phosphatases

A number of genes encode PTP-like sequences with substitutions for one of the key catalytic residues in the active site. The C-terminal PTP domain of transmembrane PTPs is one example, but more are being discovered. Their functions are not clearly established, but because they bind but do not hydrolyze phosphotyrosine, they may serve as adapters to bind proteins with phosphotyrosines.

Cooperation Between Kinases and Phosphatases

Research has uncovered protein phosphatases that are stably associated with their substrate proteins. One example is the dual-specificity MAP kinase phosphatase-3 (MPK-3) bound to ERK2, one of the MAP kinases. Another is PP2A bound to calmodulin-dependent protein kinase IV. In both cases, this close association is thought to provide a built-in mechanism to terminate the activation of these kinases. Upstream kinases activated by growth factors (for ERK2) or Ca^{2+} (for CaMKIV) turn on these target kinases, which remain active only transiently owing to their dephosphorylation by their associated phosphatases. These have been called self-correcting signal complexes, but more broadly speaking, this is an example of a biological timer.

Pharmacologic Agents for Studying Protein Kinases and Phosphatases

Inhibitors of protein kinases and protein phosphatases (see Table 27–2) are widely used to explore the biological functions of these enzymes. Few, if any, of these inhibitors are entirely specific for one protein kinase or phosphatase. Given that the families of these proteins are so large, caution is required in interpreting experiments with these agents. Nevertheless, some inhibitors of tyrosine kinases are active against Src and are being tested clinically as anti-cancer drugs. Development of specific inhibitors of protein phosphatases is challenging owing to the chemistry of the dephosphorylation reactions and the fact that the enzymes have similar active sites.

Guanosine Triphosphate–Binding Proteins

Eukaryotic cells use GTP-binding proteins (called **GTPases** or **G proteins**) to regulate a host of functions ranging from transduction of signals from plasma membrane receptors to regulation of the cytoskeleton, membrane traffic, nuclear transport, and protein synthesis (Table 27–3). All of these proteins share a homologous core domain that binds a guanine nucleotide (Fig. 27–7) and use a common enzymatic cycle of GTP binding, hydrolysis, and product dissociation to switch the protein on and off (Fig. 27–8). Note that not all GTP-binding proteins are related. Tubulin, the microtubule subunit (see Chapter 37), and related bacterial proteins also bind and hydrolyze GTP but have a completely different fold than the GTPases considered here.

The conformation of a GTPase depends on whether GTP or GDP is bound. The GTP-bound conformation is active, as it interacts with and stimulates effector proteins. The GDP conformation is inactive because it does not bind effectors. GTP hydrolysis and phosphate dissociation switch GTPases from the active to the inactive state. Thus, the presence or absence of the γ-phosphate of GTP turns these molecular switches on and off. Most GTPases bind guanine nucleotides with high affinity and hydrolyze GTP slowly. They accumulate in the inactive GDP state unless receptors or other accessory proteins catalyze dissociation of GDP, making it possible for GTP to rebind and activate the protein. GTPases then remain active until they hydrolyze GTP. In many cases, binding to effector proteins or regulatory proteins accelerates this inactivation step.

Although GTPase superfamily members differ in many ways, their GTP switches are similar, making it possible to draw parallels between the specific acces-

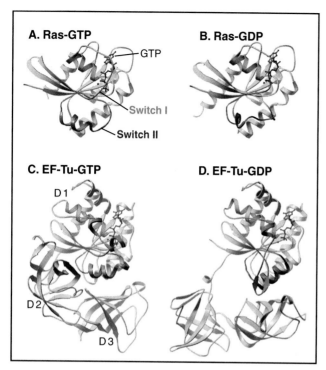

Figure 27-7 GTPase atomic structures. Ribbon models with ball-and-stick models of bound nucleotides. Switch I is green and switch II is red. *A,* Ras-GTP (PDB file: 121P). *B,* Ras-GDP (PDB file: 1Q21). *C,* EF-Tu-GTP (PDB file: 1EFT). *D,* EF-Tu-GDP (PDB file: 1TUI). GTP hydrolysis and phosphate dissociation cause major changes in the conformations of the switch loops of both proteins and of the orientation of the D2 and D3 domains of EF-Tu.

21 and 22), nuclear transport (see Chapter 16), or assembly of the mitotic spindle (see Chapter 47). Specific regulatory proteins and effectors interact with each family (and, frequently, each specific isoform) of small GTPases to accomplish these tasks. Most small GTPases require extrinsic **GTPase-activating proteins (GAPs)** to stimulate the GTP hydrolysis that turns them off.

- *Trimeric GTPases* (also called G proteins). These GTP-binding proteins transduce signals received from **seven-helix receptors** for hormones, light, and odors to a variety of effector proteins, including enzymes and ion channels. Trimeric G proteins have three subunits (see Fig. 27–9). **Gα** subunits have a GTP-binding domain similar to small GTPases plus a second domain that helps to trap the bound nucleotide more tightly. **Gβ** and **Gγ** subunits bind tightly to each other and reversibly to Gα. Seven-helix receptors activate trimeric G proteins by promoting dissociation of GDP bound to an inactive trimeric protein. GTP binding changes the conformation of Gα and dissociates Gβγ. This generates two signals, as both Gα and Gβγ can engage downstream effector proteins.

- *Elongation factors.* These GTPases act as timers to ensure the fidelity of protein synthesis (see Chapter 18). **Elongation factor Tu (EF-Tu)** consists of a GTP-binding domain like a small GTPase and two accessory domains hinged to the GTPase core

sory proteins that regulate their GTPase cycles (see Table 27–3). Most GTPases have intrinsic domains or extrinsic partner proteins that inhibit GDP dissociation, stimulate GDP dissociation, stimulate GTP hydrolysis, or bind either the activated GTP-bound form (downstream effectors) or the inactive GDP-bound form (upstream activators).

Genes for GTPases are ancient, as all known forms of life use GTPases to regulate protein synthesis. Gene duplication and divergence have created 10 families of GTPases in eukaryotes (see Table 27–3). Further evolution has produced multiple isoforms within these families to provide more specificity. Proteins in these families share a similar GTP-binding core but use diverse intrinsic or extrinsic protein modules to regulate the GTPase cycle. Each GTPase also interacts with its own particular partner proteins. Here are the main families of GTPases.

- *Small GTPases.* The six families of small GTPases consist of a single domain of about 200 residues (see Ras in Fig. 27–7A). Particular GTPases transfer signals from cell surface receptors that regulate cell growth (see Chapter 29) or the actin cytoskeleton and cell polarity (see Chapters 36 and 41). Others control vesicular trafficking (see Chapters

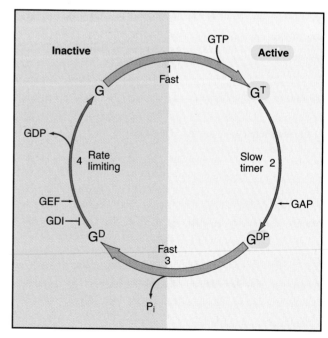

Figure 27-8 Generic GTPase cycle. The size of the arrows indicates the relative rates of the reactions. GAP, GTPase activating protein; G^D, GTPase with bound GDP; GDI, guanine nucleotide dissociation inhibitor; G^{DP}, GTPase with bound GDP and inorganic phosphate; GEF, guanine nucleotide exchange factor G^T, GTPase with bound GTP.

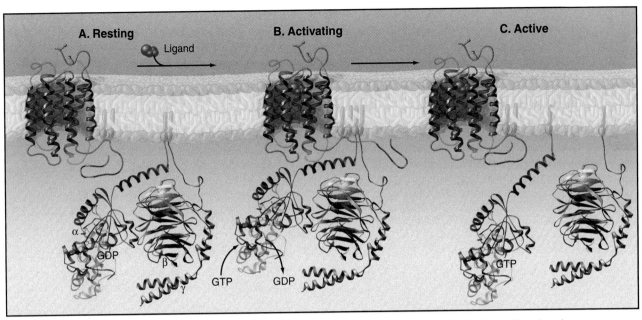

Figure 27–9 Atomic models of a seven-helix receptor and trimeric G protein. *A,* Resting state lacking a ligand and with the trimeric G protein in its inactive GDP-Gαβγ state. Both Gα and Gγ are anchored to the lipid bilayer. *B,* Ligand binding activates the receptor, which catalyzes the exchange of GDP for GTP on Gα. *C,* Active Gα and Gβγ dissociate from each other and the receptor and are available to interact with effector proteins.

(see Figs. 18–10 and 27–7*C*). GTP EF-Tu binds and delivers aminoacyl-tRNAs (transfer RNAs) to the A site of a ribosome. If the tRNA anticodon matches the mRNA codon at the A site, it remains bound long enough for GTP to be hydrolyzed. This releases EF-Tu from the ribosome and allows the correct amino acid to be added to the growing polypeptide chain. The accessory factor EF-Ts is the GDP exchange factor for this system.

• *Dynamin-related GTPases.* These large GTP-binding proteins have an N-terminal GTP-binding domain and a C-terminal domain that stimulates the hydrolysis of bound GTP and allows self-assembly into spiral polymers. Dynamin, the prototypical family member, also contains domains that bind membrane lipids and that target it to the plasma membrane where it participates in endocytosis (see Chapter 23). Other dynamin family members regulate vacuolar trafficking in yeast and maintain the structure of mitochondria in yeast, worms, and vertebrates.

Trimeric G proteins and some small GTPases are anchored to membrane bilayers by **covalently attached lipids.** These hydrophobic chains are required for activity. The low affinity of these lipid tails for the bilayer is augmented by direct interactions of the proteins with phospholipids or with other membrane proteins. Gα subunits of trimeric G proteins are modified with an N-terminal myristic fatty acid (Fig. 27–9). A prenyl group (see Chapter 6) on the C-terminus of Gγ anchors Gβγ subunits to the bilayer. Some membrane-associated small GTPases (Ras and some Rho and Rab

proteins) are modified with a C-15 or C-20 prenyl chain on a C-terminal cysteine. Arfs are myristoylated, but other small GTPases, like Ran, are not modified and are soluble in the cytoplasm. Even membrane-associated GTPases may cycle into the cytoplasm when their lipid tails turn over or when they bind cytoplasmic regulatory proteins such as **Rho-GDI** (Rho-guanine nucleotide dissociation inhibitor). Rab, Arf, and Sar GTPases also recycle through the cytoplasm as they direct vesicular traffic from one compartment to another. Membrane association can be regulated either by interactions with accessory proteins (in the case of Rab) or through guanine nucleotide–dependent conformational changes (in the case of Arf and Sar).

Structure of the GTPase Core

All GTPases share a core GTP-binding domain with a minimum of about 200 residues (see Fig. 27–7). The basic architecture of this domain was maintained during the evolutionary divergence of the various GTPases, despite the fact that about 80% of the residues in this core differ between the major classes. The common GTP-binding domain consists of a six-stranded β sheet sandwiched between five α helices. GTP binds in a shallow groove formed largely by loops at the ends of elements of secondary structure. A network of hydrogen bonds between the protein and guanine base, ribose, triphosphate, and Mg^{2+} anchor the nucleotide.

Small 20-kD GTPases such as Ras (see Fig. 27–7*A* and *B*) consist simply of this GTP-binding core domain. The 39- to 45-kD Gα subunits of trimeric G proteins have an additional domain consisting of a bundle of α helices hinged to the core domain by two strands (see Fig. 27–9). This helical domain covers the GTP binding site. EF-Tu and dynamin have additional domains required for intermolecular interactions (see Fig. 27–7C and D).

The Basic Guanosine Triphosphatase Cycle

All GTPases use the same enzyme cycle, which involves four simple steps (see Fig. 27–8).

1. *GTP binding.* Binding of GTP is fast and is favored over GDP because the cytoplasmic concentration of GTP (about 1 mM) is 10 times greater than that of GDP. GTP binding activates GTPases by changing the conformation of three segments of the polypeptide chain called switch-I, -II, and -III. Folding of these three loops around the γ phosphate of GTP creates a binding site for a particular effector protein, such as an enzyme (see Fig. 27–7).
2. *GTP hydrolysis.* GTP hydrolysis is irreversible and intrinsically slow, occurring with half-times measured in tens of seconds to hours, depending on the GTPase.
3. *Inorganic phosphate dissociation.* Dissociation of inorganic phosphate is fast and reverses the conformational change of the three switch loops. This inactivates GTPases by dismantling the binding site for effector proteins.
4. *GDP dissociation.* GDP dissociation is typically the slowest (rate-limiting) step in the GTPase cycle. GDP-bound GTPases do not bind or activate effectors.

On their own, GTPases accumulate in the inactive GDP state. GTP cannot bind until GDP dissociates. Most GTPases depend on other proteins, called **guanine nucleotide exchange factors** (GEF), to accelerate the rate-limiting dissociation of GDP (see Table 27–3). Although unrelated in structure, guanine nucleotide exchange factors have similar mechanisms. They distort the P loop, the part of the nucleotide binding site that interacts with the β phosphate, allowing GDP to escape, and then bind tightly to nucleotide-free GTPase. Most GTPases also depend on other proteins or intrinsic accessory domains to stimulate GTP hydrolysis and terminate activation. The details differ for small GTPases and trimeric G proteins.

Small Guanosine Triphosphatases

Four classes of small GTPases—Rab, Arf, Sar, and Ran—act as switches for intracellular traffic of membrane vesicles and of cargo moving into and out of the nucleus. All of these proteins are explained in detail in other chapters. The other two families of small GTPases, Ras and Rho, participate in transduction of stimuli received by cell surface receptors and are introduced here.

Ras is the prototypical small GTPase. Normally, Ras is part of a signal transduction pathway coupling growth factor receptor tyrosine kinases to the control of gene expression and cellular proliferation (see Figs. 29–6 and 29–7). In quiescent cells, Ras accumulates in the inactive GDP form. Stimulation of growth factor receptors attracts SOS, the Ras nucleotide exchange factor, to the membrane where it activates Ras by exchanging GDP for GTP. Ras-GTP then activates a cascade of protein kinases that ultimately control gene expression. Ras has low intrinsic GTPase activity (rate = 0.005 s^{-1}; half-time = 140 seconds) that is not affected by binding effector proteins. An accessory protein called **Ras-GAP** stimulates GTPase activity 10^5-fold by providing a crucial arginine for the active site. This inactivates Ras until SOS again stimulates dissociation of GDP. Mutations that inhibit GTP hydrolysis, are oncogenic (cause cancer), because without GTP hydrolysis, Ras is continually active and stimulates cellular growth.

The Rho family consists of a number of isoforms with specialized functions, including Rho itself, Rac, and Cdc42. All appear to regulate the actin cytoskeleton and cellular growth. An accessory protein called Rho-GDI (guanine nucleotide dissociation inhibitor) retards nucleotide dissociation and traps these GTPases in the inactive GDP state. Rho-GDI is useful experimentally, but its physiological function is not clear. Stimulation of certain seven-helix receptors and receptor tyrosine kinases activates Rho-GTPases. The link from the receptors is uncertain, but it activates a group of GDP exchange factors that catalyze the exchange of GDP for GTP. Activated Rho-family proteins stimulate kinases (such as **PAK [p21-activated kinase]** and Rho-kinase), which mediate downstream effects on the actin cytoskeleton. For example, Rho-kinase activates myosin II by phosphorylating the regulatory light chain and inhibiting the light chain phosphatase (see Chapter 42). Activated Cdc42 binds **Wiskott-Aldrich syndrome protein (WASp),** a protein that regulates actin filament nucleation (see Chapters 36 and 41). WASp is defective in Wiskott-Aldrich syndrome, an inherited human disease characterized by a deficiency in blood cell function.

Trimeric G Proteins

Subunit Diversity

Trimeric G proteins consist of three subunits called Gα, Gβ, and Gγ (see Fig. 27–9). The complete genome of the nematode *C. elegans* has genes for 20 Gα, 2 Gβ, and 2 Gγ subunits. Sixteen of the Gα

le 27-4

:CEPTORS AND EFFECTORS FOR G-PROTEIN ISOFORMS

mily (No. of Human Members)	Receptors	Effectors
$G_i\alpha$ (7)	α-Adrenergic amines, acetylcholine, chemokines, various neurotransmitters, tastants	Inhibits adenylyl cyclase, opens potassium channels, closes calcium channels
$G_q\alpha$ (5)	α-Adrenergic amines, acetylcholine, various neurotransmitters	Activates phospholipase Cβ to produce IP_3, which releases Ca^{2+}
$G_s\alpha$ (3)	β-Adrenergic amines, hormones (corticotropin, glucagon, parathyroid, thyrotropin, others)	Stimulates adenylyl cyclase to produce cAMP, receptor kinase
$G_t\alpha$ (2)	Rhodopsin, which absorbs light	Activates cGMP phosphodiesterase to break down cGMP, receptor kinase
$G_{13}\alpha$ (2)	Thrombin and others	Rho and others
$G_{olf}\alpha$	Odorant receptors	Activates adenylyl cyclase, receptor kinase

proteins are used in a few chemosensory cells. The others are used by many cell types. Yeasts have genes for just two Gα proteins, one of which participates in responses to sex pheromones. Mammals are known to have genes for 16 Gα, 6 Gβ, and 12 Gγ subunits, and more are likely to be revealed by completion of genome sequences. Alternative splicing of Gα mRNAs creates additional diversity. If the known subunits were combined in all possible ways, mammals could make more than 1000 different trimeric G proteins. However, only a restricted number of combinations have been detected, and no one knows the full range of the physiological combinations. Given the more than 1000 types of seven-helix receptors that activate these trimeric G proteins, the potential physiological diversity is staggering.

Each type of seven-helix receptor is linked to a particular trimeric G protein, which, in turn, acts downstream on a limited variety of effectors, including ion channels, kinases, and enzymes that produce second messengers (Table 27-4). Seven-helix receptor diversity far exceeds known trimeric G protein diversity, so many receptors use the same G proteins to transduce signals. For example, the hundreds of different odorant receptors in the nose are all thought to activate G$_{olf}\alpha$ (see Fig. 29-1).

Structure of Trimeric G Proteins

The GTPase core of Gα is linked to a helical domain that covers the GTP-binding site. Gβ is a torus-shaped molecule composed of seven modules, each folded into an antiparallel β sheet (see Fig. 27-9). These so-called **WD repeats** are found in many proteins but are best characterized in Gβ. Loops on one face of the torus interact with Gα, whereas those on the other interact with Gγ. The small Gγ subunit associates surprisingly tightly with Gβ through an N-terminal helical coiled-coil and other interactions. A C-20 prenyl group on a C-terminal cysteine of most Gγ subunits anchors G$\beta\gamma$ to a membrane bilayer. An

N-terminal fatty acid, usually myristate, anchors Gα independently to lipid bilayers. Some Gα subunits have an additional palmitic acid anchor on a reactive cysteine. Tight interaction of G$\beta\gamma$ with Gα-GDP blocks effector interaction sites on both partners.

Guanosine Triphosphatase Cycle

Seven-helix receptors activate trimeric G proteins by catalyzing exchange of GDP for GTP on the Gα subunit. This dissociates the Gα from G$\beta\gamma$, allowing each to activate effector proteins. Some effector proteins and a family of **RGS proteins** (regulators of G-protein signaling) promote GTP hydrolysis, returning Gα to the inactive GDP state, which reassociates with G$\beta\gamma$. It is convenient to think about this process as two cycles: a GTPase cycle coupled to a subunit cycle (Fig. 27-10).

The rate of GDP dissociation from trimeric G proteins is near zero (half-life ~ 10-60 minutes) unless they bind an activated seven-helix receptor. Activated seven-helix receptors increase the rate of GDP dissociation by many orders of magnitude, allowing GTP to exchange for GDP on a millisecond-to-second time scale, even fast enough for vision (see Fig. 29-2)! Evidence suggests that activated receptors bind Gα on the opposite side from GDP. Receptor binding to both Gα and G$\beta\gamma$ triggers a conformational change that propagates across Gα to weaken bonds with GDP. The cleft between the Gα domains must open transiently to release GDP and accept a GTP from solution.

Gα refolds around GTP in a significantly different conformation than around GDP. This conformational change is the physical manifestation of the transfer of a signal from an activated receptor to Gα. GTP draws the three switch loops together around the γ phosphate in a conformation that favors dissociation of G$\beta\gamma$ and association with effector proteins.

Like all GTPases, the duration of the signal carried by trimeric G proteins depends on the rate of GTP

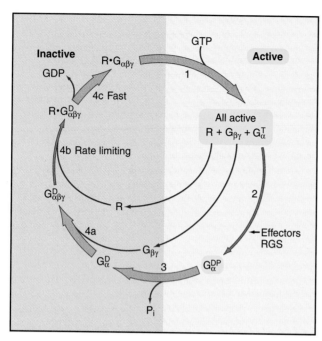

Figure 27–10 GTPase cycle and subunit cycle of a trimeric G protein. The size of the arrows indicates the relative rates of the reactions around the outer circle. GTP (T), GDP-P_i (DP), and GDP (D) bound to $G\alpha$ are indicated as superscripts. R is a seven-helix receptor. Regulators of G protein signaling (RGS) and some effector proteins stimulate GTP hydrolysis.

hydrolysis. The half-time of about 10–20 seconds is adequate for prolonged activation of a target protein. Trimeric G proteins hydrolyze GTP faster than small GTPases by virtue of a strategically placed arginine (on a linker to the helical domain) that promotes the hydrolysis of the terminal phosphate of the GTP. Thus, the helical domain acts both as an intrinsic inhibitor of GDP dissociation and as an activator of GTP hydrolysis, similar to two separate regulators of small GTPases (GDI and GAP). When the two domains are produced separately in the laboratory, the nucleotide-binding core domain binds GTP and activates effectors but does not hydrolyze GTP rapidly unless it is recombined with the separate helical domain containing the critical arginine.

Both effector proteins and extrinsic GTPase activators, called RGS proteins, stimulate GTP hydrolysis and terminate the signal. For example, $G_q\alpha$-GTP binds and stimulates phospholipase Cβ, which produces two second messengers, inositol 1,4,5-triphosphate (IP_3) and diacylglycerol (see Chapter 28). At the same time, phospholipase Cβ accelerates the GTPase of $G_q\alpha$, providing feedback to turn off the signal. G proteins regulate some physiological processes that require a rapid response, such as the heart rate ($G_i\alpha$) and vision ($G_t\alpha$). In these cases, a family of 20 or more RGS proteins stimulates GTPase activity of G proteins about 100-fold, yielding half-times of less than 1 second. These RGS proteins work by stabilizing the transition state. Some RGS proteins also have a Rho–guanine

nucleotide exchange factor domain, so they may connect seven-helix receptors and trimeric G proteins to the Rho family of small GTPases.

Subunit Cycle

GTP binding, hydrolysis, and dissociation drive not only the GTPase cycle, but also a linked subunit cycle (see Fig. 27–10). $G\alpha$ cycles both $G\beta\gamma$ and the receptor on and off as it traverses its GTPase cycle. The conformational change in $G\alpha$ that is induced by GTP binding affects all of its molecular interactions. GTP binding reduces the affinity of $G\alpha$ for both its receptor and associated $G\beta\gamma$ subunits, so all three molecular partners separate on the cytoplasmic face of the membrane (see Fig. 27–9). Once dissociated, the receptor, $G\alpha$, and $G\beta\gamma$ are all free to interact with other partners (see Table 27–4). The conformation of $G\beta\gamma$ is the same whether bound to $G\alpha$ or free, so its activation by dissociating from $G\beta\gamma$ is attributable simply to unmasking of effector binding sites. $G\beta\gamma$ is not a passive partner in these linked cycles, as it must be bound to $G\alpha$-GDP before activated membrane receptors can trigger dissociation of GDP. In addition to activating membrane targets, such as ion channels, $G\beta\gamma$ provides a membrane anchor to enhance the interaction of cytoplasmic effectors (such as receptor kinases) with membrane targets (receptors).

The properties of the linked GTPase and subunit cycles allow activation of a single receptor to generate a large signal. Although most seven-helix receptors are active only briefly (owing to rapid ligand dissociation and rapid inactivation [see Chapter 28]), they can turn on multiple G proteins, each with a longer lifetime. Slow GTP hydrolysis by $G\alpha$ subunits allows ample time for these G proteins to activate downstream effector proteins. Because these effectors are typically enzymes or channels, they amplify the signal in a short time.

Mechanisms of Effector Activation

Both $G\alpha$ and $G\beta\gamma$ subunits participate in signaling by interacting with downstream effector proteins. In some cases, $G\alpha$ and $G\beta\gamma$ subunits act individually; in other cases, they may act synergistically and even antagonistically. The two following examples, elaborated upon in Chapter 29, illustrate how G proteins activate effector proteins.

In the eye, when the seven-helix photoreceptor, rhodopsin, absorbs a photon, the G protein $G_t\alpha$ (also called transducin) relays and amplifies a signal (see Fig. 29–2). Each activated rhodopsin generates about 500 $G_t\alpha$-GTPs, which bind an inhibitory subunit of the enzyme cGMP phosphodiesterase. This stimulates the activity of the phosphodiesterase, which lowers the cytoplasmic concentration of cGMP and closes an ion channel. The signal is transient, because both an RGS protein and the inhibitory subunit itself promote the hydrolysis of GTP bound to $G_t\alpha$. Inactive $G_t\alpha$-GDP dissociates from the inhibitory subunit, terminating the signal that flowed through $G_t\alpha$ to the enzyme.

In the heart, the β-adrenergic receptor activates $G_s\alpha$, releasing both $G_s\alpha$-GTP and $G\beta\gamma$ to bind effector proteins (see Fig. 29–3). During its 10-second lifetime, $G_s\alpha$-GTP binds and stimulates the enzyme adenylyl cyclase to produce the second messenger, cAMP. $G\beta\gamma$ assists in receptor inactivation by binding β-ARK, the kinase that phosphorylates and turns off the β-adrenergic receptor, terminating the signal.

Trimeric G Proteins in Disease

Both abnormal activation or inactivation of G proteins can cause disease (Table 27–5). Mutations interfering with GTP hydrolysis cause $G\alpha$ to accumulate in the GTP state and persistently activate downstream effectors. For example, mutations in arginine or glutamine residues of $G\alpha$ that are crucial for GTP hydrolysis can cause tumors by prolonging the activation of pathways responsible for cell proliferation. Similarly, a protein toxin produced by the cholera bacterium causes diarrhea by enzymatically modifying $G_s\alpha$. **Cholera toxin** catalyzes the addition of an adenosine diphosphate (ADP)–ribose to the arginine required for GTPase activity. Activated $G_s\alpha$-GTP accumulates, prolonging activation of adenylyl cyclase and producing high levels of cAMP, which stimulates salt and water secretion into the intestine.

On the other hand, **pertussis toxin** (an enzyme secreted by the whooping cough bacterium) adds ADP-ribose to cysteine-347 of $G_i\alpha$ or corresponding residues in other $G\alpha$ subunits. This inhibits the interaction of the trimeric G protein with activated receptors, so the trimeric G protein accumulates at the inactive GDP stage in its cycle. The consequence is an increase in airway irritability. Similarly, *Clostridium botulinus* C3 toxin ADP-ribosylates and inhibits Rho-GTPases, whereas a *Clostridium difficile* toxin uses uridine diphosphate (UDP)–glucose to glucosylate and turn off the whole class of Rho proteins.

Experimental Tools

Site-directed mutations, especially those that constitutively activate GTPases (by inhibiting GTP hydrolysis) or inactivate GTPases, have been the most powerful tools for investigating GTPase functions in live cells. For biochemical experiments, slowly hydrolyzed analogues of GTP, such as GTPγS (with a sulfur substituted for one of the γ-phosphate oxygens), are used to activate GTPases. Similarly, aluminum fluoride and beryllium fluoride bind very tightly in place of the hydrolyzed γ phosphate, keeping $G\alpha$ in an active GDP-P_i state similar to GDP. The fungal metabolite brefeldin A blocks nucleotide exchange on some Arfs catalyzed by guanine nucleotide exchange factors. This disrupts membrane traffic between the Golgi complex and the endoplasmic reticulum (see Chapter 21).

Molecular Recognition by Adapter Domains

During the characterization of signaling pathways, several patterns of amino acid sequence appeared repeatedly in different proteins, such as Src (see Figs. 27–3E and 27–4B). These turned out to be compactly folded domains (Fig. 27–11) that are incorporated into

---

table 27–5

GUANOSINE TRIPHOSPHATASES AND DISEASE

Disease	GTPase	Mechanism
Excess Signal		
Cholera	$G_s\alpha$	Cholera toxin ADP-ribosylation of R201 inhibits GTP hydrolysis in intestinal epithelium.
Pituitary and thyroid adenomas	$G_s\alpha$	Somatic point mutations of R201 or Q227 inhibit GTP hydrolysis; constitutive activity mimics signal from hormones that stimulate proliferation and secretion by these glands.
Various cancers	Ras	Point mutations inhibit GTP hydrolysis, generating persistent stimulation of signals for cell proliferation.
Deficient Signal		
Whooping cough	$G_i\alpha$	Pertussis toxin ADP-ribosylation of $G_i\alpha$ C347 in the bronchial epithelium blocks receptor activation; connection to coughing not established.
Night blindness	$G_t\alpha$	Germ line point mutation in G38.
Pseudohypoparathyroidism type Ia	$G_s\alpha$	Point mutations result in loss of $G_s\alpha$ or may block its activation by receptors.

(Adapted from Farfel Z, Bourne HR, Iiri T: The expanding spectrum of G protein diseases. N Engl J Med 340:1012–1020, 1999.)
C, cysteine; G, glycine; Q, glutamine; R, arginine.

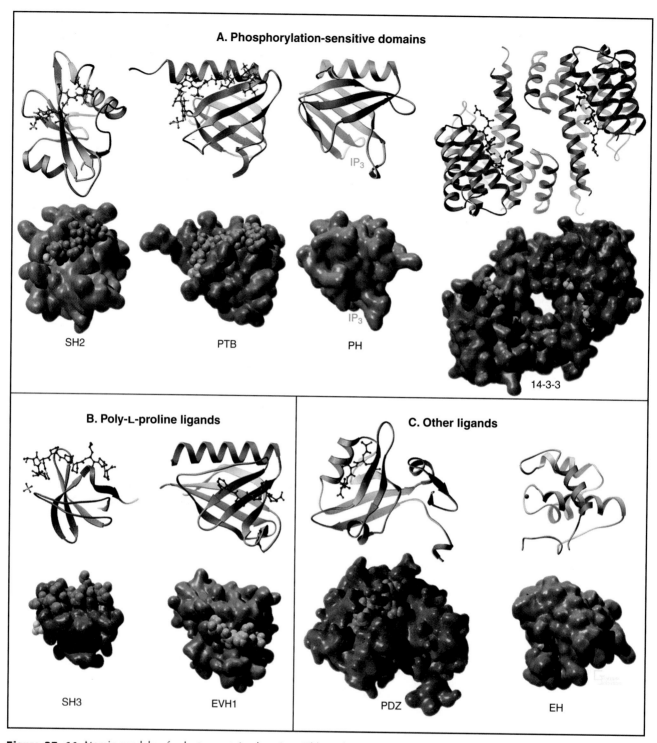

A. Phosphorylation-sensitive domains

SH2   PTB   PH   14-3-3

B. Poly-L-proline ligands

SH3   EVH1

C. Other ligands

PDZ   EH

Figure 27-11 Atomic models of adapter protein domains. Ribbon diagrams show their architecture, whereas the surface renderings show how ligands bind. *A*, Domains with phosphorylation-sensitive interactions. *B*, Domains with poly-L-proline ligands. *C*, Domains with other ligands. SH2 (PDB file: 1HCS), PTB (PDB file: 1IRS), PH (PDB file: 1DYN), 14-3-3 (PDB file: 1A38). SH3 (PDB file: 1ABO) and EVH1 (PDB file: 1EVH). PDZ (PDB file: 1BEQ) and EH (PDB file: 1EH2).

a variety of proteins (Fig. 27–12), including many not involved with signaling. These domains mediate interactions of proteins with each other and with membrane lipids (Table 27–6).

The names of adapter domains have no functional significance. They generally came from the proteins where they were originally recognized. For example, **Src homology (SH)** domains were first recognized in the Src tyrosine kinase (see Fig. 27–3E). SH1 is the tyrosine kinase domain, SH2 domain binds phosphotyrosine peptides, and SH3 binds polyproline type II helices.

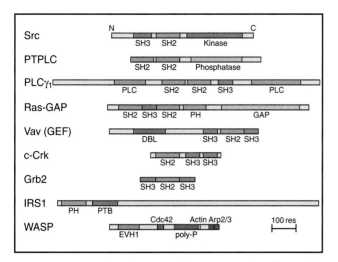

Figure 27-12 Scale drawings of proteins with adapter domains. Src, cytoplasmic tyrosine kinase; PTPLC, protein tyrosine phosphatase; PLC, phospholipase C; Ras-GAP, Ras GTPase activating protein; Vav, a guanine nucleotide exchange protein; c-Crk and Grbz, multi-domain adapter proteins; IRS1, insulin receptor substrate; WASP, Wiskott-Aldrich syndrome protein; SH, Src-homology; PH, pleckstrin homology; GAP, GTPase activating; DBL, a guanine nucleotide exchange factor domain; PTB, protein tyrosine binding domain; poly-P, polyproline. Actin and Arp2/3 indicate binding sites for actin monomers and Arp2/3 complex. Cdc42, a Rho-family GTPase; EVH1, Ena-Vasp homology 1 domain.

Other sections of this text, particularly Chapter 29, provide detailed examples of how adapter domains function. This section provides an overview of their structure and ligand-binding properties. The following points apply to adapter proteins in general.

• Adapter domains mediate interactions required to assemble proteins into multimolecular functional units that typically carry out a series of reactions. To facilitate these interactions, many signaling proteins have more than one adapter domain or ligand for adapter domains, or both. In signal transduction, these physical associations make transmission from receptors to effectors increasingly reliable, more like a solid-phase machine than one that relies solely on diffusion and random associations. Mutations in experimental organisms and the occurrence of human diseases have verified the importance of adapter domains for many pathways. Interactions mediated by adaptor domains complement the organizing activities of anchoring proteins, such as STE5 and AKAPs (see earlier section).

• All members of each family of adapters have similar structures (and common evolutionary origins) but differ in their affinity for a range of similar ligands. For example, all SH2 domains bind peptides with a sequence phosphotyrosine-X-X-hydrophobic residue. All require phosphotyrosine but differ in their affinity for peptides depending on the hydrophobic residue and the intervening residues. This lock-and-key strategy creates specificity with lots of particular combinations, as in real locks and keys. Although lacking in sequence similarity, three of these domains—PH, PTB, and EVH1—have similar folds (see Fig. 27-11) and may have had a common ancestor. Nevertheless, their ligands are quite distinct from each other and bind to different sites on the commonly folded domains.

• Some interactions depend on reversible covalent modifications of ligands: tyrosine phosphorylation for SH2 and some PTB domains; serine phosphorylation for some 14-3-3 and WW domains; and 3-phosphorylation of inositol for some PH do-

table 27-6

ADAPTER DOMAINS

Domain Name	Size (Residues)	Consensus Ligands	Example of Proteins with Domain
EH (Eps15 homology)	95	S/T-N-P-F-Φ	Clathrin adapter proteins, synaptojanin I
EVH1 (Ena-VASP homology)	110	D/E-Φ-P-P-P-P	WASp, VASP, Ena
PH (Pleckstrin homology)	100	PIP_2, PIP_3	Kinases, scaffolds, GEFs, GAPs, PLCδ, dynamin
PDZ	100	-x-x-S/T-x-V-COOH -x-x-Φ-x-Φ-COOH	Scaffolds for channels and transduction enzymes
PTB (phosphotyrosine binding)	125	-Φ-x-N-P-x-pY-	IRS1, Shc scaffold proteins
SH2 (Src homology 2)	100	-pY-x-x-Φ-	Transduction enzymes and scaffold proteins
SH3 (Src homology 3)	60	(+) -R/K-x-x-P-x-x-P- (−) -x-P-x-x-P-x-R/K-	Tyrosine kinases, phosphatases, Grb2, PLCγ, spectrin, myosin I
WW	38–40	-P-P-x-Y-	Peptidyl prolyl isomerase, ubiquitin ligase
14-3-3	250	-R-S-X-pS-x-P-	14-3-3 isoforms

Φ, hydrophobic residue; COOH, C-terminus; Ena, enabled gene; GAP, GTPase-activating protein; GEF, guanine nucleotide exchange factor; Grb2, adapter protein; IRS1, insulin receptor substrate 1; PLC, phospholipase C; pS, phosphoserine; pY, phosphotyrosine; Shc, receptor tyrosine kinase substrate; VASP, vasodilator-stimulated phosphoprotein, WASp, Wiskott-Aldrich syndrome protein; (−), minus orientation; (+), plus orientation.

mains. This allows networks using these adapters to assemble and disassemble in response to signals that modulate phosphorylation.

- Many interactions of adapter domains with their ligands are tenuous, so associations are reversible on a time scale of seconds, allowing rearrangements in response to signals. Frequent dissociations are also required for covalent modifications, such as dephosphorylation.

Phosphorylation-Sensitive Adapters

SH2 Domains

SH2 domains bind short peptide sequences that begin with a phosphotyrosine. Like a two-pronged plug, these peptides insert into two cavities in the SH2 socket. Phosphotyrosine is one prong. It is the key residue, as it provides most of the binding energy by virtue of an extensive network of hydrogen bonds between the phosphate and its deep binding pocket. A phosphate on the tyrosine increases the affinity of a peptide for its partner SH2 domain by orders of magnitude. This allows reversible phosphorylation to control interactions between SH2 domains and their ligands. This switching mechanism is used in growth factor signaling and lymphocyte activation (see Figs. 29–6 to 29–9). The second prong is a hydrophobic side chain of the third residue C-terminal from phosphotyrosine. It inserts into a hydrophobic cavity on the surface of the SH2 domain. The size of this side chain is a major determinant of binding specificity. Two residues between these plug residues straddle the β sheet of the SH2 with their side chains exposed to solvent.

SH2 interactions with target peptides and proteins are relatively weak, with K_ds in the range of 0.1–1 μM. This allows for rapid exchange of partners and dephosphorylation of phosphotyrosine. Nevertheless, these interactions appear to be specific, with each SH2 domain engaging a limited number of target phosphoproteins. SH2 domains target several signal transduction enzymes to receptor tyrosine kinases (see Fig. 29–6) as the first step in propagating signals to effectors, including second messengers and transcription factors. Intramolecular binding of the Src SH2 to a C-terminal phosphotyrosine regulates the catalytic activity of the enzyme (see Fig. 27–3E).

PTB Domains

Most phosphotyrosine binding (PTB) domains require a phosphotyrosine at the C-terminal end of the peptide ligand. Hydrophobic residues preceding phosphotyrosine in the sequence contribute to binding specificity. The bound peptide is hydrogen-bonded onto the edge of a β sheet, and phosphotyrosine interacts with basic residues. PTB domains target adapter proteins to phosphotyrosines on receptor tyro-

sine kinases, such as insulin receptor (see Fig. 29–7). In a few cases, PTB domains bind unphosphorylated peptide ligands. Note that the fold of PTB domains and their mode of interaction with ligand peptides have nothing in common with SH2 domains.

14-3-3 Proteins

Vertebrates have at least seven genes for 14-3-3 subunits that assemble into homodimers or heterodimers. Protein ligands with an appropriate sequence and a central phosphoserine bind each subunit with sub-micromolar affinity. Peptides with two appropriate sequences bind much tighter. 14-3-3 proteins regulate protein kinases, including the Ras-activated kinase Raf (see Fig. 29–6) and cellular death pathways (see Chapter 49). During interphase, a 14-3-3 protein inhibits the cell cycle phosphatase Cdc25, when it is phosphorylated on a serine (see Chapter 47).

WW Domains

These tiny adapter domains are found in more than 100 proteins. They bind certain phosphoserine or phosphothreonine peptides. These phosphorylation-dependent interactions regulate Cdc25 and ubiquitin-mediated protein destruction.

PH Domains

Dozens of proteins have a domain of about 100 residues similar to one first recognized in **pleckstrin,** the major substrate for protein kinase C in platelets. PH domains have a common framework—a compact, seven-strand β-barrel—but they vary in sequence, especially in the loops connecting these strands. PH domains bind **polyphosphoinositides:** PH domains of dynamin and phospholipase Cδ prefer phosphatidylinositol (PI) (4,5) P_2 (PIP$_2$), whereas the PH domain of Bruton's tyrosine kinase (Btk) favors PI(3,4,5)P$_3$ (PIP$_3$), binding at a different site. These interactions target proteins with PH domains to membrane bilayers rich in PIP$_2$ and PIP$_3$ and make these membrane interactions responsive to the activities of phosphoinositide kinases (see Chapter 28). PH-domain proteins include kinases (PKB/Akt, PDK1), signaling scaffolding proteins (insulin receptor substrate 1 [IRS1]; see Fig. 29–7), enzymes (phospholipase Cγ1; see Chapter 28), and guanine nucleotide exchange factors. Mutations in the PH domain of the tyrosine kinase, Btk, reduce affinity for PI(3,4,5)P$_3$ and cause a failure of B-lymphocyte development (see Chapter 30), resulting in immunodeficiency due to a lack of antibodies.

Adapters with Proline-Rich Ligands

SH3 Domains

SH3 domains bind proline-rich peptides on the surface of specific target proteins. SH3 domains in adapter protein Grb2 (see Fig. 27–12) help to assemble signaling complexes that link activated growth factor receptors to the nucleotide exchange protein for Ras (see Fig. 29–6). SH3 domains are also found in tyrosine kinases and cytoskeletal proteins, including myosin I, spectrin, and cortactin. Ligand peptides form a left-handed, **type II polyproline helix** that repeats every three residues. All of these interactions depend on both hydrophobic contacts of prolines with conserved aromatic residues in a shallow groove on the SH3 domain, as well as hydrogen bonds contributed by ligand peptide carbonyl oxygens. Depending on the SH3 domain, the peptide can be oriented in either direction. Residues flanking the central proline helix contribute to binding specificity. Even optimal peptide ligands bind with relatively low affinity (K_ds in the micromolar range), so they exchange rapidly. When incorporated into proteins, type II poly-L-proline helices with appropriate sequences bind somewhat more tightly owing to secondary interactions.

EVH1 Domains

EVH1 domains are found in WASp and other proteins that respond to signals and help to initiate actin polymerization. EVH1 domains are folded like PH and PTB domains, but they bind type II proline-rich helices in a groove that is occupied by an α helix intrinsic to some PH domains. This site also differs from that for phosphotyrosine peptides on PTB domains. Thus, a common scaffold has diverged to form three completely different binding sites!

Other Adapter Domains

PDZ Domains

PDZ domains are found in one to seven copies in scaffolding proteins that cluster together ion channels and signal transduction proteins at synapses and in photoreceptors. PDZ domains bind specific sequence motifs, most commonly, ones found at the very C-terminus of proteins, and less commonly, at the end of β hairpin structures. PDZ domains bind their ligands, in a manner reminiscent of PTB domains, by incorporating them through hydrogen bonds as an extra strand in a β sheet.

EH Domains

EH domains are small and comprise a bundle of four α helices that bind peptides with the sequence asparagine-proline-phenylalanine. Flanking residues contribute to specificity. The best characterized EH-mediated interactions are involved with endocytosis.

▌ Selected Readings

Abergel C, Chavrier P, Claverie J-M: Triple association of CDC25-, Dbl- and Sec7-related domains in mammalian guanine-nucleotide exchange factors. Trends Biochem Sci 23:472–473, 1998.

Barford D: Molecular mechanisms of the protein serine/threonine phosphatases. Trends Biochem Sci 21:407–412, 1996.

Barford D, Das AK, Egloff M-P: Structure and mechanism of protein phosphatases: Insights into catalysis and regulation. Annu Rev Biophys Biomolec Struct 27:133–164, 1998.

Berman DM, Gilman AG: Mammalian RGS proteins: Barbarians at the gate. J Biol Chem 273:1269–1272, 1998.

Bos JL: A target for phosphoinositide 3-kinase:Akt/PKB. Trends Biochem Sci 20:441–442, 1995.

Brown GC, Hoek JB, Kholodenko BN: Why do protein kinase cascades have more than one level? Trends Biochem Sci 22:288, 1997.

Cherfils J, Chardin P: GEFs: Structural basis of their activation of small GTP-binding proteins. Trends Biochem Sci 24:306–311, 1999.

Cohen PTW: Novel serine/threonine phosphatases: Variety is the spice of life. Trends Biochem Sci 22:245–250, 1997.

Dell'Acqua ML, Scott JD: Protein kinase A anchoring. J Biol Chem 272:12881–12884, 1997.

Dohlman H, Thorner J: RGS proteins and signaling by heterotrimeric G proteins. J Biol Chem 272:3871–3874, 1997.

Farfel Z, Bourne HR, Iiri T: The expanding spectrum of G protein diseases. N Engl J Med 340:1012–1020, 1999.

Fauman EB, Saper MA: Structure and function of the protein tyrosine phosphatases. Trends Biochem Sci 21:413–417, 1996.

Ferrell JE: How responses get more switch-like as you move down a protein kinase cascade. Trends Biochem Sci 22:288–289, 1997.

Gutkind JS: The pathways connecting G protein–coupled receptors to the nucleus through divergent mitogen-activated protein kinase cascades. J Biol Chem 273:1839–1842, 1998.

Hamm H: The many faces of G protein signaling. J Biol Chem 273:669–672, 1998.

Hanks SK, Hunter T: The eukaryotic protein kinase superfamily: Kinase (catalytic) domain structure and classification. FASEB J 9:576–596, 1995.

Hubbard SR, Till JH: Protein tyrosine kinase structure and function. Annu Rev Biochem 69:373–398, 2000.

Hunter T, Plowman GD: The protein kinases of budding yeast: Six score and more. Trends Biochem Sci 22:18–21, 1997.

Iiri T, Farfel Z, Bourne HR: G-protein diseases furnish a model for the turn-on switch. Nature 394:35–38, 1998.

Klee CB, Ren H, Wang X: Regulation of calmodulin-stimulated protein phosphatase, calcineurin. J Biol Chem 273:13367–13370, 1998.

Kuriyan J, Cowburn D: Modular peptide recognition domains in eukaryotic signaling. Annu Rev Biophys Biomolec Struct 26:259–288, 1997.

Lohmann SM, Vaandrager AB, Smolenski A, et al: Distinct functions of cGMP-dependent protein kinases. Trends Biochem Sci 22:307–312, 1997.

Mackay DJG, Hall A: Rho GTPases. J Biol Chem 273:20685–20688, 1998.

Marate BM, Downward J: PKB/Akt: Connecting phosphoinositide 3-kinase to cell survival and beyond. Trends Biochem Sci 22:355–358, 1997.

Pawson T, Scott JD: Signaling through scaffold, anchoring and adaptor proteins. Science 278:2075–2080, 1997.

Peles E, Schlessinger J, Grumet M: Multiligand interactions with receptor-like protein tyrosine phosphatase β: Implications for intercellular signaling. Trends Biochem Sci 23:121–124, 1998.

Rizo J, Sudhof TC: C2 domains, structure and function of a universal Ca^{2+}-binding domain. J Biol Chem 273:15879–15882, 1998.

Ryazanov AG, Pavur KS, Dorovkov MV: Alpha-kinases: A new class of protein kinases with a novel catalytic domain. Curr Biol 9:R43–R45, 1999.

Saras J, Heldin C-H: PDZ domains bind carboxy-terminal sequences of target proteins. Trends Biochem Sci 21:455–457, 1996.

Scheffzek K, Ahmadian MR, Wittinghofer A: GTPase activating proteins: Helping hands to complement an active site. Trends Biochem Sci 23:257–262, 1998.

Songyang Z, Cantley LC: Recognition and specificity in protein tyrosine kinase-mediated signalling. Trends Biochem Sci 20:470–475, 1995.

Sprang SR: G-protein mechanisms: Insights from structural analysis. Annu Rev Biochem 66:639–678, 1997.

Thomas SM, Brugge JS: Cellular functions regulated by SRC family kinases. Annu Rev Cell Devel Biol 13:513–610, 1998.

Ui M, et al: Wortmanin as a probe for PI3K. Trends Biochem Sci 20:303–306, 1995.

Vanhaesebroek B, Leevrs SJ, Panayotou G, Waterfield MD: Phosphoinositide 3-kinases: A conserved family of signal transducers. Trends Biochem Sci 22:267–272, 1997.

Whitmarsh AJ, Davis RJ: Structural organization of MAP-kinase signaling modulues by scaffold proteins in yeast and mammals. Trends Biochem Sci 23:481–490, 1998.

Williams JC, Wierenga RK, Saraste M: Insights into Src kinase functions: Structural comparisons. Trends Biochem Sci 23:179–184, 1998.

Wishart MJ, Dixon JE: Gathering STYK: Phosphatase-like form predicts functions for unique protein-interaction domains. Trends Biochem Sci 23:301–306, 1998.

Wittinghoffer A, Nassar N: How Ras-related proteins talk to their effectors. Trends Biochem Sci 21:488–491, 1996.

chapter 28

SECOND MESSENGERS

This chapter considers the remarkable variety of small molecules that carry signals inside the living cell. These second messengers are chemically diverse, ranging from hydrophobic lipids confined to membrane bilayers, to an inorganic ion (Ca^{2+}), to nucleotides (cyclic adenosine monophosphate [cAMP], cyclic guanosine monophosphate [cGMP]) to a gas (nitric oxide). The messages carried by these molecules are encoded by their concentrations. In the simplest case, a rise or fall in the concentration of the second messenger conveys a signal from its source to its target. In other cases, the signal depends on the rate or frequency of the fluctuations in the concentration of the second messenger. Generally, the concentration of a second messenger is determined by its rate of synthesis and degradation by specific enzymes. These enzymes can switch on and off rapidly, allowing them to modulate the concentration of second messengers on a millisecond time scale. In the case of Ca^{2+}, the cytoplasmic concentration is determined by channels that release the ion from membrane stores and by pumps that remove it from cytoplasm.

The physical state of second messengers has important consequences. Lipid-derived second messengers reach different targets in the cell depending on whether they are more soluble in the lipid bilayer or in water. Similarly, Ca^{2+} only acts locally in cytoplasm, which contains a high concentration of binding sites that impede its free diffusion. On the other hand, cyclic nucleotides act globally because they diffuse rapidly throughout the cytoplasm.

The complexity of the signaling pathways is determined by the number of sources and the number of targets of each second messenger. Generally, multiple signal sources and multiple second-messenger targets generate more complexity than one can fully appreciate. This chapter deals with this complexity only in

passing. Chapter 29 considers a few model systems where it is possible to understand how signals are integrated and transduced.

This chapter discusses second messengers in four sections: cyclic nucleotides, lipid-derived messengers, calcium, and nitric oxide. None of these topics is really independent of the others, as second messengers are parts of integrated signaling systems. For example, nitric oxide controls the production of cGMP, and inositol triphosphate derived from a membrane lipid controls the release of Ca^{2+} into cytoplasm.

Cyclic Nucleotides

Two cyclic nucleoside monophosphates—adenosine $3',5'$-cyclic monophosphate **(cAMP)** and guanosine $3',5'$-cyclic monophosphate **(cGMP)**—are employed as second messengers (Fig. 28–1). Both act by binding reversibly to specific target proteins. Enzymes that produce and degrade cyclic nucleotides determine the concentrations of the messengers available to bind targets. These enzymes turn over their substrates rapidly, so they can amplify signals massively on a millisecond time scale, under the control of diverse signaling pathways (see Fig. 28–1 and Chapter 29). Cyclases make cyclic nucleotides in a single step from the corresponding nucleoside triphosphate, adenosine triphosphate (ATP) or guanosine triphosphate (GTP). They are counteracted by soluble cytoplasmic phosphodiesterases that degrade cAMP and cGMP to inactive nucleoside $5'$-monophosphates.

Cyclic nucleotides diffuse in the cytoplasm at about the same rate as in free solution, activating a modest repertoire of downstream targets, including **protein kinases** (see Chapter 27 and Fig. 27–4), **cyclic nucleotide–gated ion channels** (see Fig. 9–9),

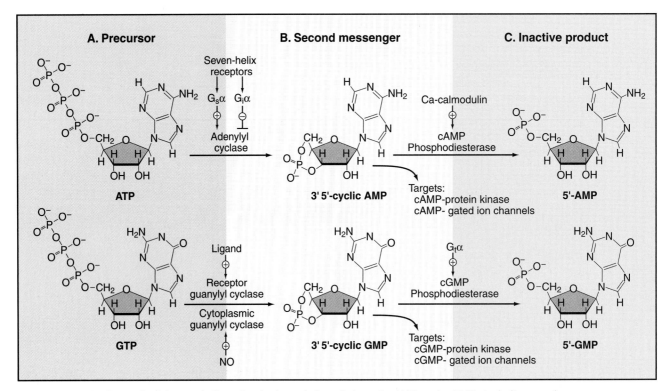

Figure 28–1 Cyclic nucleotide metabolism. Synthesis and degradation of cAMP and cGMP, including regulatory inputs and targets. $G_s\alpha$, $G_i\alpha$, and $G_t\alpha$ are trimeric GTPase α-subunits (see Chapter 27). Ca, calcium; NO, nitric oxide.

and one class of nucleotide exchange factors for small guanosine triphosphatases (GTPases). The domains of these target proteins that bind cAMP or cGMP are homologous and are related to the cAMP-binding domain of bacterial CAP, a transcription factor. Thus the components of this system are quite ancient.

Vertebrate **adenylyl cyclases,** the enzymes that synthesize cAMP, are large transmembrane proteins with two homologous catalytic domains in the cytoplasm (Fig. 28–2). These cytoplasmic domains can be produced separately as soluble proteins and recombined to make fully active enzyme. Both domains are necessary because the active site lies at the interface of the two domains. Transmembrane segments anchor the enzyme to the plasma membrane, but their function is not understood. Generally, the concentration of adenylyl cyclases is very low.

Vertebrates produce at least 10 adenylyl cyclases with similar enzyme activities but diverse and often multiple regulatory mechanisms that act synergistically. GTP-**$G_s\alpha$,** the GTPase subunit of a trimeric G protein, activates all known adenylyl cyclases. It binds far from the active site (see Fig. 28–2) but causes a conformational change that stimulates activity. Ca^{2+}-calmodulin or protein kinase C (PKC) activates some adenylyl cyclases. GTP-**$G_i\alpha$,** the GTPase subunit of another trimeric G protein, or protein kinase A (PKA) inhibits some cyclases. $G\beta\gamma$ subunits of trimeric G proteins

activate some adenylyl cyclases but inhibit others. These diverse regulatory mechanisms allow adenylyl cyclases to integrate a variety of input signals. The diterpene **forskolin** from the *Coleus* plant activates all adenylyl cyclases. Forskolin is very useful experimentally for manipulating the cAMP concentration in cells, and it was essential in the initial purification of the enzyme by affinity chromatography.

The cAMP concentration in resting cells is so low, on the order of 10^{-8} M, that it does not bind the regulatory (RII) subunit of PKA or cAMP-gated channels. Stimulation of appropriate receptors (such as the seven-helix β-adrenergic receptor, see Chapter 29) increases the cytoplasmic cAMP concentration more than 100-fold, enough to saturate the PKA regulatory subunits (Fig. 28–3). This activates the PKA catalytic subunit and affects its distribution in the cell (e.g., moving into the nucleus to activate the transcription factor CREBP, cyclic nucleotide regulatory element binding protein [see Fig. 14–19]).

Outside the animal kingdom, cAMP has many functions. In bacteria, cAMP controls gene expression in response to nutritional conditions. The cellular slime mold *Dictyostelium* uses cAMP as an extracellular signal, acting through a seven-helix receptor, for its social interactions. A series of since retracted papers suggested that plants use cAMP as a second messenger, but this remains an open question.

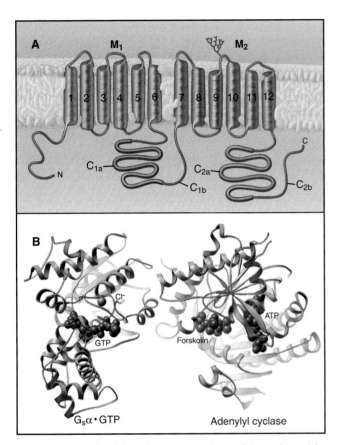

Figure 28-2 Adenylyl cyclase. *A,* Topology of the polypeptide. The C_{1a} and C_{2a} regions fold together to form the active enzyme. *B,* Atomic structure of the catalytic domains of adenylyl cyclase associated with $G_s\alpha$. ATP is bound to the active site. (Reference: Tesmer JJ, et al: Crystal structure of the catalytic domains of adenylyl cyclase in a complex with $G_s\alpha$ GTPγS. Science 278: 1907–1916, 1997. Copyright 1997, American Association for the Advancement of Science. PDB file: 1CJK.)

Guanylyl cyclases are dimeric enzymes very similar to adenylyl cyclases. In fact, mutation of just two residues can convert a guanylyl cyclase to an adenylyl cyclase. Vertebrates express two types of guanylyl cyclase: a soluble, heterodimeric enzyme found in cytoplasm and a family of transmembrane receptors with cytoplasmic cyclase domains (see Fig. 26–10). Nitric oxide and carbon monoxide activate the cytoplasmic enzyme by binding a heme group in a regulatory domain (see later section).

■ Lipid-Derived Second Messengers

The membrane lipids, phosphoglycerides, and sphingolipids (see Chapter 6), are not only structural components, forming barriers between the cell and the extracellular space and between internal organelle compartments, but they also participate in a wide range of signaling mechanisms. A growing list of intra-

cellular and extracellular second messengers are derived from lipids, and more will undoubtedly be identified in the future.

Three membrane lipids are the primary source of these signaling molecules (Fig. 28–4).

1. **Phosphatidylinositol** and its various phosphorylated derivatives, discussed later, are minor lipids of the cytoplasmic leaflet of the plasma membrane and some organelle membranes.
2. **Phosphatidylcholine** is a major membrane phosphoglyceride found in both leaflets of the plasma membrane and organelle membranes.
3. **Sphingomyelin,** the major membrane sphingolipid, is concentrated in the outer leaflet of the plasma membrane.

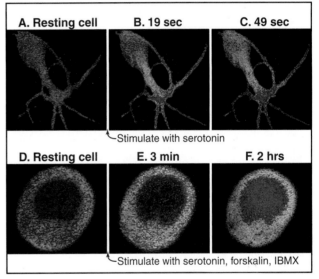

Figure 28-3 Images of cAMP transients in cultured *Aplysia* sensory neurons. Neurons were injected with protein kinase A (PKA) labeled on the catalytic subunit with fluorescein and on the regulatory subunit with rhodamine. Fluorescence energy transfer between the dyes on the two subunits provides an assay for cAMP, which dissociates the subunits and reduces energy transfer. Fluorescent dyes also allow detection of the subunits inside the neuron. *Top row*: A, Free cAMP in the resting cell is <50 nM *(blue)*. B and C, Stimulation with serotonin activates adenylyl cyclase and increases cytoplasmic cAMP to the micromolar range *(red)*, especially within fine processes with a high surface-to-volume ratio. Images 120 μm wide were taken just inside the cell near the cover slip. *Bottom row*: D, Another resting neuron imaged at the level of the nucleus. At the low resting level of cAMP, <50 nM *(blue)* labeled PKA is excluded from the nucleus. E, Stimulation with serotonin, plus forskolin (to stimulate adenylyl cyclase) and isobutylmethylxanthine (IBMX) (to inhibit cAMP breakdown), raises the concentration of cAMP around the nucleus *(yellow)*. F, Two hours later, the free catalytic subunit of PKA *(pink)* accumulates in the nucleus. (Courtesy of R.Y. Tsien, University of California, San Diego. Reference: Bacskai BJ, et al: Spatially resolved dynamics of cAMP and protein kinase A in *Aplysia* neurons. Science 260: 222–226, 1993. Copyright 1993, American Association for the Advancement of Science.)

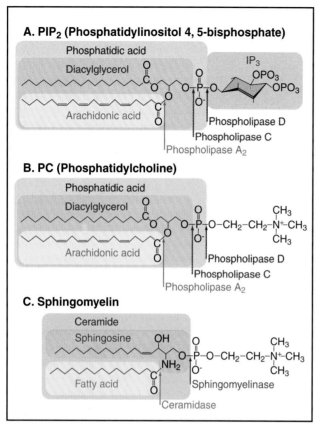

A. PIP₂ (Phosphatidylinositol 4, 5-bisphosphate)

B. PC (Phosphatidylcholine)

C. Sphingomyelin

Figure 28-4 *A* to *C*, Production of lipid second messengers by enzymatic attacks on PIP₂ (phosphatidylinositol 4,5-bisphosphate), PC (phosphatidylcholine), and sphingomyelin. Second messengers are named and surrounded by colored boxes.

Enzyme Reactions That Produce Lipid Second Messengers

Just three kinds of enzymes—phospholipases, lipid kinases, and lipid phosphatases—produce most lipid-derived second messengers. Remarkably, essentially all conceivable products produced by these enzymes from the three parent lipids participate in signaling reactions, either directly or indirectly. In most cases, the second messengers produced by these reactions partition between the aqueous phase of the cytoplasm (products designated by *italics* in this section) and the hydrophobic phase of the membrane bilayer (products designated by ***bold italics*** in this section). In the following paragraphs, the details of the various enzymatic reactions and the structures of the lipid derivatives are less important than the broader principle that cells use the full range of chemical diversity in their membrane lipids to create chemical signals that regulate cellular activities.

Three types of enzyme reactions generate lipid second messengers:

1. Different **phospholipases** cleave the four ester bonds of phosphoglycerides (see Fig. 28–4). Corresponding enzymes attack the two ester bonds

and single amide bond of sphingomyelin. Cells have three main intracellular phospholipases. **Phospholipase A2** (PLA2) removes the C2 fatty acid, yielding a *free fatty acid,* which partitions into the cytoplasm with the aid of fatty acid–binding proteins, and a ***lysophosphoglyceride***. The corresponding ceramidase removes the fatty acid from sphingomyelin. When **phospholipase C** (PLC) cleaves the phosphorylated head group (such as *inositol 1,4,5-triphosphate [IP₃]*) from a phosphoglyceride, it leaves behind ***diacylglycerol*** (***DAG***) in the membrane bilayer. The corresponding sphingomyelinase leaves behind ***ceramide*** in the membrane bilayer. **Phospholipase D** (PLD) cleaves the polar head group from phosphoglycerides, producing ***phosphatidic acid*** that remains in the bilayer. (Note that the phospholipase A1 that cleaves the ester bond linking the fatty acid to the C1 position on the glycerol is not yet known to participate in signaling and is shown in Fig. 28–4.)

2. **Lipid kinases** add phosphate groups to diacylglycerol to make ***phosphatidic acid*** and to phosphatidylinositol to make a variety of polyphosphoinositides, including ***phosphatidylinositol 4-phosphate*** (***PIP***), ***phosphatidylinositol 4,5-biphosphate*** (***PIP₂***), and ***phosphatidylinositol 3,4,5-triphosphate*** (***PIP₃***). PIP₂ is a substrate for a family of phosphoinositide-specific phospholipase Cs that produce the important signaling molecules ***DAG*** and *IP₃*.

3. **Lipid phosphatases** remove phosphate from phosphatidic acid (another way to make ***DAG***) and phosphates from inositol head groups.

Cells also contain transferases that add or exchange head groups or fatty acids on membrane phosphoglyerides. For example, transferases add choline (as the nucleotide conjugate cytidine diphosphate (CDP)–choline) to DAG to make phosphatidylcholine). In the case of phosphatidylinositol, the head group is provided by the dephosphorylation of IP₃ to inositol, which is recombined enzymatically with a CDP conjugate of DAG to make phosphatidylinositol. These enzymes are essential for lipid biosynthesis, but have not been implicated in signaling processes.

Cells produce some lipid second messengers by the successive action of two or more enzymes. For example, the cell can make ***DAG*** in two steps from phosphatidylcholine by the successive action of PLD to make phosphatidic acid, followed by dephosphorylation by phosphatidic acid phosphatase. *Lysophosphatidic acid* is made from phosphatidylcholine by PLD and PLA2. The production of a huge family of fatty acid derivatives called eicosanoids is initiated by the liberation of the fatty acid arachidonic acid from phosphatidylcholine by PLA2. Cyclooxygenases and lipoxygenases then modify arachidonic acid to make *prosta-glandins, thromboxanes,* and *leukotrienes,* which diffuse *out* of the cell to interact with cell surface receptors.

Agonists and Receptors

Most major signaling pathways (see Chapter 29) stimulate enzymes that produce lipid second messengers. Transduction mechanisms include G protein–coupled seven-helix receptors, cytokine receptors, and growth factor receptors. Some pathways activate enzymes directly; receptor tyrosine kinases bind and activate certain **phosphatidylinositol phospholipase Cs** (PI-PLCs) directly. Activation of another PI-PLC by seven-helix receptors is only one step removed, mediated by an activated G protein. Other enzymes that produce lipid second messengers are activated indirectly. For example, PKC activates one isoform of phospholipase D. This PKC is itself activated by DAG or other second messengers downstream from G protein–coupled receptors or receptor tyrosine kinases. Thus, many agonists (the molecules that activate receptors) have the potential to generate lipid second messengers, provided that the target cell expresses the appropriate enzymes.

Targets of Lipid Second Messengers

Downstream targets of the lipid second messengers are also diverse, but can be generalized to some extent into three categories (Fig. 28–5).

1. Most lipid second messengers derived from phosphoglycerides and retained in the membrane bi-layer exert their physiological effects on one of the PKC isozymes (see the following section). Ceramide is also retained in the bilayer where it activates another protein kinase and a protein phosphatase (see later section). Phosphatidic acid activates a lipid kinase, PI5 kinase, which phosphorylates phosphatidylinositol.

2. IP$_3$ and sphingosine-1-phosphate use different mechanisms to release Ca^{2+} from vesicular stores in the cytoplasm (see the discussion of Ca^{2+} later in this chapter). Choline is also generated from phosphatidylcholine during the production of phosphatidic acid, but it has no known signaling activity.

3. All water-soluble lipid second messengers containing or derived from fatty acids (platelet-activating factor [PAF], lysophosphatidic acid [LPA], eicosanoids) somehow escape from the cell and bind to G protein–coupled, seven-helix receptors on the surface of target cells.

With so much potential for information transfer (multiple agonists, multiple membrane transduction mechanisms, multiple lipid second messengers, and multiple downstream targets), where is the specificity in these systems? Do all cells respond in all possible ways? The answer is no, and the explanation is that the protein hardware required for these reactions is selectively expressed in differentiated cells and carefully localized at particular sites in cells, such as the plasma membrane, nucleus, or cytoskeleton. In addition, targeting of PKC isozymes to particular cellular compartments ensures that only selected substrates are phosphorylated in response to lipid second messenger production. Thus, each cell takes a limited number of

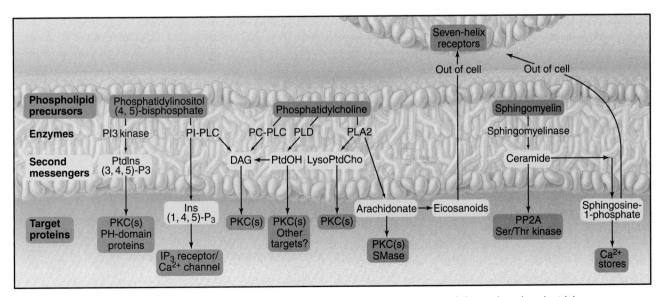

Figure 28-5 Generation of lipid second messengers and their cellular targets. LysoPtdCho is lysophosphatidyl choline; PKC is protein kinase C; PP2A is protein phosphatase 2A; PtdIns (3,4,5)-P$_3$ is PIP$_3$; PtdOH is phosphatidic acid; SMase is sphingomyelinase. (Adapted from Liscovitch M, Cantley LC. Lipid second messengers. Cell 77:329–334, 1994. Copyright 1994, with permission from Elsevier Science.)

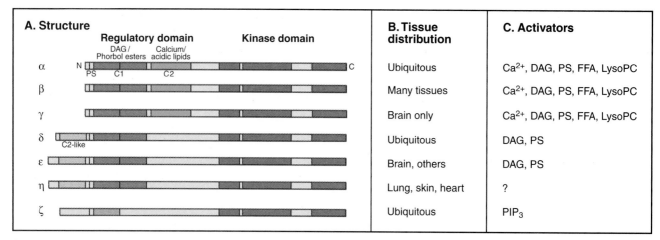

Figure 28-6 Protein kinase C (PKC) family. *A,* Domain organization of PKC isozymes with ligand-binding sites. PS indicates the pseudosubstrate sequence that binds to and inhibits the kinase catalytic site. *B,* Tissue distribution. *C,* Activators. DAG, diacylglycerol; PS, phosphatidylserine; FFA, free fatty acid, LysoPC, lysophosphatidylcholine; PIP_3 is phosphatidylinositol 3,4,5-trisphosphate.

items from the lipid second messenger menu and uses them to produce a selective, customized response to each agonist.

Lipid second messengers participate in many processes considered in greater detail elsewhere in the book. For example, regulated secretion (see Chapter 22) in response to an agonist binding a seven-helix or tyrosine kinase receptor requires a transient Ca^{2+} signal in the cytoplasm. The Ca^{2+} is released from the membrane stores by IP_3, which is produced by the action of a PI-PLC on PIP_2. IP_3-mediated Ca^{2+} release from the endoplasmic reticulum also controls smooth muscle contraction (see Chapter 42).

Protein Kinase C

Many lipid second messengers, including DAG, PIP_3, arachidonic acid, phosphatidic acid, and lysophosphatidylcholine activate one or more of the 10 protein kinase C (PKC) isozymes expressed by vertebrate cells (Fig. 28–6). The existence of multiple PKC isozymes provides a selective response to various lipid second messengers. Some, but not all, PKC isozymes also require Ca^{2+} for activation. Sphingosine may inhibit some PKC isozymes.

PKCs have a standard protein kinase catalytic domain (see Chapter 27) and distinctive N-terminal regulatory domains. A **pseudosubstrate sequence** near the N-terminus binds intramolecularly to the active site and inhibits activity by blocking substrate binding. Pseudosubstrates have alanine at the phosphorylation site instead of serine like substrates.

Lipid second messengers activate PKC by binding C1 regions and dissociating the pseudosubstrate from the active site. **Phorbol esters,** pharmacological acti-

vators of PKC that promote tumor formation, bind PKC in a similar fashion. Binding DAG or phorbol esters also requires phosphoglycerides, such as phosphatidylserine. Ca^{2+}-dependent PKC isozymes have C2 regions that mediate binding to phospholipids in the presence of Ca^{2+}.

Activated PKCs have many potential targets in cells and have been implicated in the regulation of cellular activities ranging from gene expression to cell motility to the generation of lipid second messengers. PKC isozymes differ in their activity toward protein substrates. Localization of various PKC isozymes to different parts of the cell may provide additional specificity. Proteins called **RACKs** (*r*eceptors for *a*ctivated *C* *k*inases) bind C2 regions and target PKC isozymes to the plasma membrane, cytoskeleton, or nucleus.

PKCs can provide either positive or negative feedback to the signaling mechanisms that turn them on. PKC activates PLD and PLA2 and provides positive feedback, because those enzymes produce more DAG to sustain the activation of PKC. On the other hand, PKC provides negative feedback when activated by growth factor receptors and PI-PLCγ1 via DAG. PKC phosphorylates and inhibits both growth factor receptors and PI-PLCγ1. PKC also phosphorylates and inhibits PI-PLCβ, generating negative feedback after activation of seven-helix receptors. Negative feedback makes both of these signaling events transient.

Phosphoinositide Signaling Pathways

Although minor in terms of mass in biological membranes, phosphoinositides are major players in signaling (Fig. 28–7). The parent compound, phosphatidylinositol (PI), is a phosphoglyceride with a cyclohexanol head group called inositol. Specific lipid kinases phosphorylate the 4 and 5 hydroxyl groups of phosphatidylinositol to form PI(4-)P and PI(4,5-)P$_2$, usually referred to simply as PIP and PIP$_2$.

PIP$_2$ is a substrate for a family of receptor-controlled PI-PLCs that cleave off the phosphorylated head group, producing two potent second messengers: IP$_3$ and DAG. Water-soluble IP$_3$ activates calcium release channels in the endoplasmic reticulum (see later section) and lipid-soluble DAG activates PKC. In contrast to Ca^{2+}, which diffuses slowly and acts locally, IP$_3$ diffuses rapidly through cytoplasm, triggering Ca^{2+} release. DAG is confined to membranes, but diffuses laterally to bind and activate PKC. Both IP$_3$ and DAG are inactivated enzymatically. DAG is inactivated by phosphorylation to make phosphatidic acid, a second messenger in its own right, but also an intermediate in the resynthesis of phosphoinositides. IP$_3$ is dephosphorylated to inositol, which is inactive as a second messenger. LiCl inhibits the final step, dephosphorylation of inositol-1-phosphate. Remarkably, Li$^+$ is clinically useful as a treatment for manic depressive psychosis, presumably by interfering with phosphoinositide signaling in the brain. In some tissues IP$_3$ is inactivated by phosphorylation to inositol 1,3,4,5-tetrakisphosphate (IP$_4$).

Vertebrates use 10 classes of PI-PLCs to provide tissue-specific coupling of various receptors to the production of IP$_3$ and DAG. PI-PLCγ1, expressed in brain, is activated by tyrosine phosphorylation when its SH2 domains binds a tyrosine-phosphorylated receptor tyrosine kinase (see Chapters 26, 27, and 29) Another isozyme, PI-PLCβ, is activated by the α subunit of the trimeric G protein, G$_q\alpha$ (see Chapters 27 and 29).

When a PI-PLC hydrolyzes PIP$_2$, phosphatidylinositol-4 kinase and phosphatidylinositol-5 kinase respond to replace the pool of PIP$_2$ at the expense of membrane phosphatidylinositol. This generates a transient flux of lipid molecules from phosphatidylinositol to PIP to PIP$_2$ to DAG. On a longer time scale, phosphatidylinositol is replaced by synthesis from phosphatidic acid and inositol.

Receptor tyrosine kinases activate another family of lipid kinases, **PI-3 kinases,** which phosphorylate the 3-hydroxyl group of PI, PIP, and PIP$_2$. The products are PI(3-)P, PI(3,4-)P$_2$ and PI(3,4,5-)P$_3$. PI(3,4,5-)P$_3$ is not a substrate for the PI-PLCs that transduce cell surface events, but it activates some PKC isozymes and binds some pleckstrin homology (PH) domains, anchoring those proteins to the lipid bilayer. One example is protein kinase B **(PKB/Akt)** that participates in insulin signaling (see Fig. 29-7). A steroid-like molecule called **wortmannin** inhibits PI-3 kinase relatively specifically and is used to investigate the physiological roles of PIP$_3$.

Phosphatidylcholine Signaling Pathways

Phosphatidylcholine is not only a major structural lipid of the plasma membrane, but it is also an important source of DAG and a large family of other signaling molecules (see Fig. 28-5). In response to agonist stimulation, cells produce two waves of DAG (Fig. 28-8). Within seconds, PI-PLCs activated by seven-helix or tyrosine kinase receptors produce the first wave of DAG from PIP$_2$. Then, over a period of minutes, a second wave of DAG is derived from phosphatidylcholine, either directly by a PC-PLC or in two steps by PLD (to remove choline) and a phosphatidic acid phosphatase (to remove the phosphate from the phosphatidic acid intermediate). The first wave of DAG may contribute to the second wave, as PKC activates one PLD isoform. Ca^{2+} produced in the first wave may also activate PLD.

Phosphatidylcholine is also the main source of fatty acid–derived second messengers. PLA2 releases **arachidonic acid** (AA), a C20 unsaturated fatty acid

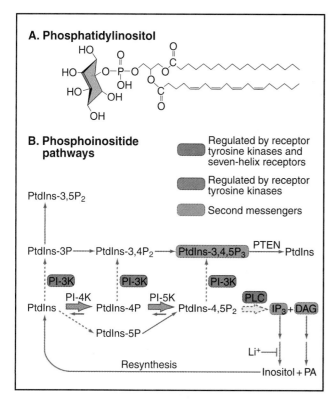

Figure 28-7 *A* and *B,* Synthesis and turnover of phosphoinositides. Enzymes regulated by receptor tyrosine kinases and seven-helix receptors are indicated in purple. Enzymes regulated by receptor tyrosine kinases are indicated in blue. Second messengers are indicated in green. PA, phosphatidic acid; PI-3k is phosphatidylinositol 3 kinase; PI-4k is phosphatidylinositol 4 kinase; PI-5k is phosphatidylinositol 5 kinase; PtdIns, phosphatidylinositol; PTEN, phosphatase and tensin homologue deleted on chromosome ten (a tumor supressor).

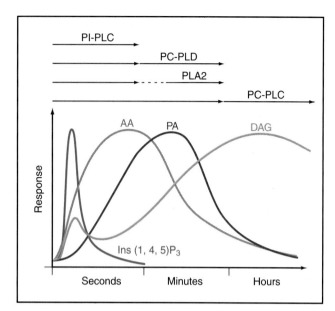

Figure 28-8 Time course of lipid second messengers produced by various phospholipases following activation of receptor tyrosine kinases or seven-helix receptors. AA, arachidonic acid; DAG, diacylglycerol; PA, phosphatidic acid; PC, phosphatidylcholine; PI, phosphatidylinositol.

found predominantly at the C2 position of phosphoglycerides. Arachidonic acid activates some PKC isozymes and, together with DAG, provides positive feedback to PLA2 and PLD to sustain the production of arachidonic acid and DAG.

Lipid-Derived Second Messengers for Intercellular Communication

Cells produce an amazing array of bioactive compounds from phosphatidylcholine and arachidonic acid, forming a distinct group of second messengers that escape from the cell and mediate their effects by binding to cell surface receptors on the cell of origin or neighboring cells. Thus, these compounds are locally active hormones. This sets them apart from classical second messengers, which (with the exception of nitric oxide) act inside the cell of origin. All of the compounds presented here activate target cells by binding G protein–coupled, seven-helix receptors. Vertebrates make a particularly rich variety of these lipid-derived signaling molecules, but even slime molds and algae use some of the same compounds for communication.

Eicosanoids are a diverse family of arachidonic acid metabolites, including **prostaglandins, thromboxanes, leukotrienes,** and **lipoxins** (Figs. 28–9 and 28–10). They augment normal physiological responses to agonists and are important medically as mediators of inflammation. Depending on the particular receptor and G protein, eicosanoids selectively activate or inhibit the synthesis of cAMP, release Ca^{2+},

activate PKC, or regulate ion channels. Biological consequences are diverse, depending on the specific eicosanoid and target cell. For example, platelets initially activated by the blood-clotting protein, thrombin, produce thromboxane A_2, which diffuses locally to promote irreversible platelet aggregation and blood vessel constriction. This secondary response, mediated by the eicosanoid, reinforces the initial response to thrombin and ensures that a clot forms with minimal loss of blood. Unfortunately, sensitive, positive feed-

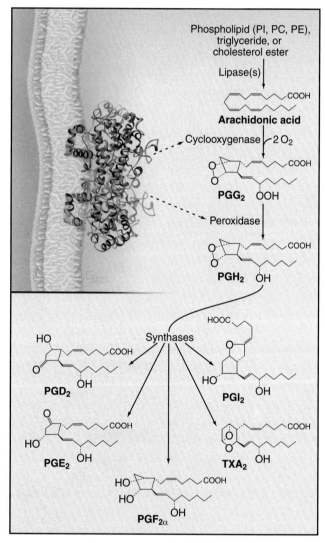

Figure 28-9 Pathway of prostaglandin (PG) synthesis. Cyclooxygenase-1 (ribbon diagram) is a homodimer bound to the surface of a lipid bilayer by hydrophobic membrane-binding helices. This enzyme has two active sites that convert arachidonic acid to prostaglandin H_2. A hydrophobic channel 2.5 nm long leads from the bilayer to the active sites. Nonsteroidal anti-inflammatory drugs compete with arachidonic acid for binding to the cyclooxygenase active site, and aspirin covalently modifies serine 530 in the active site. Specific prostaglandin synthases convert prostaglandin H_2 into various products. PC, phosphatidylcholine; PE, phosphatidyl ethanolamine; PI, phosphatidylinositol; TXA_2, thromboxane A. (PDB file: 1 CQE.)

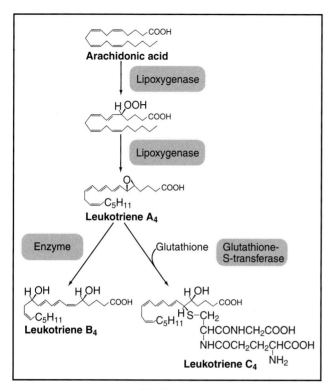

Figure 28-10 Pathways of leukotriene synthesis.

back through thromboxane A_2 can contribute to the pathological formation of clots in vital blood vessels and cause heart attacks and strokes. On the other hand, prostaglandin E_1 inhibits platelet activation. Other functions of eicosanoids include: (1) prostacyclin produced by endothelial cells dilates blood vessels and inhibits interaction of platelets with the vessel wall; (2) tissue injury provokes synthesis of prostaglandins E_2 and I_2, which mediate inflammation locally by dilating blood vessels, sensitizing pain receptors, and causing fever; and (3) leukotrienes also mediate inflammatory responses in injured tissues.

Prostaglandins and thromboxanes are synthesized from arachidonic acid by pairs of enzymes, the first being generic and the second being specific for a particular product (see Fig. 28–9). Typically, differentiated cells express primarily one second-step enzyme and thus produce only one of these local hormones.

The first enzyme, **prostaglandin H synthetase (cyclooxygenase),** has two active sites that catalyze successive reactions that convert arachidonic acid into prostaglandin G_2 and then into prostaglandin H_2. Most cells express cyclooxygenase-1 constitutively as a housekeeping enzyme. Inflammatory stimuli induce expression of **cyclooxygenase-2,** a nearly identical enzyme. Cyclooxygenases are anchored to the inner surface of the membranes of the endoplasmic reticulum and nuclear envelope.

Second-tier enzymes are specific prostaglandin synthetases that convert prostaglandin H into various prostaglandin and thromboxane products. Physiological responses to these products depend upon selective expression of specific seven-helix receptors that provide a customized response to each eicosanoid. For example, prostaglandin F_{2a} prepares pregnant mammals for delivery. Thromboxane A_2 from activated platelets causes constriction of smooth muscle by binding to a receptor coupled to the trimeric G protein $G_q\alpha$. This G protein triggers production of IP_3, release of Ca^{2+}, and contraction of smooth muscle (see Chapter 42). Other prostaglandins participate in inflammation, including pain and fever.

Nonsteroidal anti-inflammatory drugs, including aspirin and ibuprofen, target both cyclooxygenase isozymes. Most of these drugs competitively inhibit arachidonic acid binding to both enzymes, but aspirin covalently and irreversibly acetylates a serine residue in their active sites. Either way, these drugs inhibit the synthesis of all prostaglandins and thromboxanes. Inhibition of thromboxane A_2 synthesis by platelets reduces platelet aggregation and clotting in blood vessels of the heart and brain, accounting for the ability of aspirin to reduce the incidence of heart attacks and strokes. Low doses of aspirin are selective and effective for platelets, as platelets lack the capacity for protein synthesis to replace inactivated enzyme. Aspirin also protects against colon cancer. High doses of aspirin and other nonsteroidal anti-inflammatory drugs reduce inflammation, pain, and fever by inhibiting the synthesis of other eicosanoids, but this is not without side effects, including gastrointestinal bleeding. New drugs that selectively inhibit cyclooxygenase-2 allow treatment of inflammation without the gastrointestinal side effects caused by inhibition of cyclooxygenase-1.

Leukotrienes and lipoxins are synthesized by enzymes, called **lipoxygenases,** by the addition of oxygen to specific double bonds of arachidonic acid (see Fig. 28–10). The first biologically active product, leukotriene A_4, can be further modified by the addition and subsequent trimming of glutathione to yield a variety of active leukotrienes. Leukotrienes are potent mediators of inflammatory reactions, including constriction of blood vessels, leakage of plasma from small vessels, and attraction of white blood cells into connective tissue. These effects, together with constriction of the respiratory tract, contribute to the symptoms of asthma. Lipoxins are another family of mediators active upon blood vessels. They are formed by the addition of oxygen to both the C-5 and C-15 positions of arachidonic acid. Drugs that inhibit lipoxygenases would be valuable for the treatment of inflammatory diseases.

Phosphatidylcholine is also the starting point for production of two other water-soluble, intercellular, second messengers: **lysophosphatidic acid (LPA)** and **platelet-activating factor (PAF).** Activated platelets and injured fibroblasts produce LPA from phosphatidylcholine by the action of the phospholipases PLD and PLA2 (see Fig. 28–4). A variety of cells synthesize PAF in two steps, using PLA2 to remove the C2 fatty acid from phosphatidylcholine molecules with an ether-bonded fatty alcohol (rather than an ester-bonded fatty acid) on the C1 position and a second enzyme to acetylate the C2 hydroxyl group. LPA and PAF escape cells and stimulate target cells by binding to seven-helix receptors. Depending on their signaling hardware, cells respond to LPA in different ways: activation of the PLC/IP$_3$ mechanism releases intracellular Ca^{2+} in some cells; activation of a mitogen-activated protein (MAP) kinase pathway (see Chapter 29) stimulates some cells to divide; and activation of Rho-family small GTPases stimulates formation of actin bundles in cultured cells (see Chapter 36). As expected from its name, PAF activates platelets, but it also modifies the behavior of other blood cells, inhibits heart contractions and stimulates contraction of the uterus.

Endocannabinoids are fatty acid amides that bind and activate the seven-helix receptors that also respond to (-)-Δ^9-tetrahydrocannabinal, the active ingredient in marijuana. Many tissues, including the brain, synthesize the classic endocannabinoid, *N*-arachidonoyl-ethanolamine, from ethanolamine and arachidonic acid. The physiological functions of these intriguing compounds are not well characterized, but may be diverse, as class 1 cannabinoid receptors are found in many tissues, including brain. Lymphocytes express related receptors. Another lipid amide, oleamide (*cis*-9,10-octadecenoamide), induces sleep in mammals, but does not bind cannabinoid receptors.

Sphingomyelin/Ceramide Signaling Pathways

Activation of plasma membrane receptors for **tumor necrosis factor (TNF)** and **interleukin-2 (IL-2)** (Fig. 26–11) stimulates formation of the lipid-soluble second messenger **ceramide** from sphingomyelin (Fig. 28–11). Sphingomyelin consists of a sphingosine base esterified to a fatty acid through an amide bond and to phosphorylcholine (see Fig. 28–4). It is concentrated in the external leaflet of the plasma membrane. Ligand binding to TNF or IL-2 receptors activates a plasma membrane **sphingomyelinase** (a specialized PLC) that removes phosphorylcholine from sphingomyelin, producing ceramide. Ceramide flips across the lipid bilayer to the cytoplasmic surface and activates a plasma membrane, proline-directed, serine/threonine protein kinase. Target proteins have the sequence X-Ser/Thr-Pro-X and include epidermal growth factor (EGF) receptor and Raf kinase. Downstream events include activation of MAP kinase, which activates transcription factors and other effectors (see Fig. 29–6). Ceramide also activates a protein phosphatase 2A.

Sphingosine and ***sphingosine-1-phosphate*** are produced from sphingomyelin by a succession of enzymatic reactions (see Fig. 28–4). Ceramidase removes the fatty acid, and sphingomyelinase removes the phosphorylcholine head group to form sphingosine. Then sphingosine kinase adds phosphate to C1 to make sphingosine-1-phosphate. Growth factor signaling pathways may regulate this lipid kinase. Sphingosine-1-phosphate escapes from cells and activates seven-helix receptors to release Ca^{2+}. The biological effects of sphingosine are also incompletely defined, but they include the inhibition of PKC and of chemotactic cell motility.

Crosstalk

Interaction (crosstalk) among lipid second messenger pathways is a common feature that is thought to contribute to integration of signals from different agonists. Consequently, it is difficult to define distinct linear pathways from an agonist to an individual effector through lipid second messengers. The following are some examples of crosstalk using the various enzymes defined in Fig. 28–4.

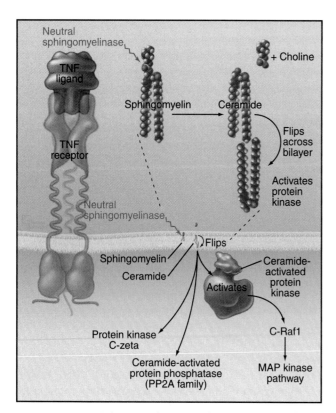

Figure 28-11 Sphingomyelin/ceramide signaling pathway. Stimulation of the tumor necrosis factor (TNF) receptor activates a neutral sphingomyelinase which cleaves choline from sphingomyelin. Ceramide flips across the bilayer and activates a cytoplasmic kinase, as well as PKC-ζ and a protein phosphatase.

1. Two pathways may modulate each other. PI-PLCs produce DAG, which activates PKC, which phosphorylates and activates PLA2 and PLD. These activated enzymes produce additional lipid second messengers (arachidonic acid and phosphatidic acid) to amplify and diversify the initial response.
2. Two pathways may converge on the same target. Arachidonic acid (produced by activated PLA2) and DAG (produced by either a PI-PLC or PLD and phosphatidic acid phosphatase) synergistically activate some PKC isozymes.
3. A messenger from one pathway can be converted to a messenger on a second pathway. DAG and phosphatidic acid are readily interconverted by the appropriate kinase and phosphatase.

Calcium

Overview of Calcium Regulation

Calcium ion, Ca^{2+}, is a versatile second messenger that regulates many processes, including synaptic transmission, fertilization, secretion, muscle contraction, and cytokinesis. All eukaryotes (but not prokaryotes) use Ca^{2+} signals. Nature probably chose Ca^{2+} for signaling by default. Because cells depend on phosphate for energy metabolism (ATP), nucleic acid structure, and many other functions, and because calcium phosphate precipitates, early cells needed a mechanism to extrude Ca^{2+} from cytoplasm. Cells use the resulting Ca^{2+} gradient between cytoplasm and ocean water (or extracellular space in animals) to drive tiny pulses of Ca^{2+} into cytoplasm for signaling. This movement of Ca^{2+} between compartments via ion channels is very fast.

In contrast to all other second messengers, which are synthesized and metabolized, Ca^{2+} levels are controlled by release into and removal from the cytoplasm (Fig. 28–12). ATP-driven **Ca^{2+} pumps** of the plasma membrane and endoplasmic reticulum keep cytoplasmic Ca^{2+} levels low (about 0.1 μM in resting cells) and generate a 10,000-fold concentration gradient across these membranes. A remarkable variety of stimuli, operating through many different receptors (Table 28–1), open **calcium channels** in the plasma membrane or endoplasmic reticulum, allowing a concentrated puff of Ca^{2+}, called a Ca^{2+} transient, to enter

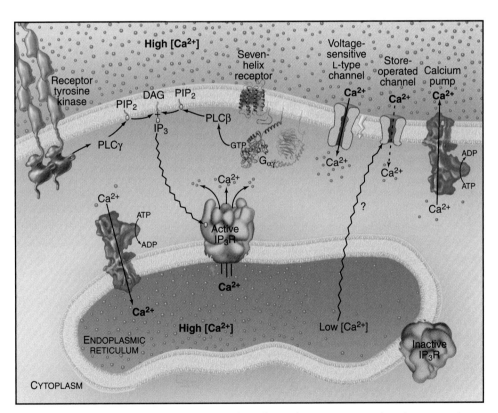

Figure 28–12 Pathways of Ca^{2+} release and uptake. Calcium pumps in the plasma membrane and endoplasmic reticulum membrane use ATP hydrolysis to pump Ca^{2+} out of the cytoplasm. A variety of receptors activate phospholipase C (PLC) isozymes to produce IP_3 from PIP_2. IP_3 diffuses to the endoplasmic reticulum where it opens IP_3 receptors (IP_3R), releasing Ca^{2+} from the lumen into cytoplasm. Voltage-sensitive L-type calcium channels respond to membrane depolarization by admitting extracellular Ca^{2+}. Depletion of Ca^{2+} stores in the endoplasmic reticulum activates Trp-class plasma membrane calcium channels, which admit extracellular Ca^{2+} to replenish stores.

table 28–1
STIMULI FOR Ca²⁺ SIGNALS

Stimulus	Receptor Class	Second Messenger	Cells
Action potentials	Voltage-sensitive Ca^{2+} channels	None	Nerve, muscle
ATP	Ligand-gated plasma membrane channels	None	Smooth muscle
Peptide growth factors	Receptor tyrosine kinases	IP_3	Many cells
Antigens	T-cell receptor, tyrosine kinases	IP_3	Lymphocytes
Peptide hormones	G protein–coupled receptors	IP_3	Endocrine cells
Neurotransmitters	G protein–coupled receptors	IP_3	Neurons
Light	Rhodopsin, G proteins	IP_3	Photoreceptors

the cytoplasm. Peak cytoplasmic Ca^{2+} concentrations in stimulated cells are in the micromolar range. The duration of Ca^{2+} signals may range from milliseconds to minutes depending on the duration of the stimulus, the type of release channel, the rate of Ca^{2+} pumping out of cytoplasm, and the rates of binding and dissociation on target proteins. Ca^{2+} levels can rise locally, flood the whole cytoplasm, or travel in waves across a cell.

Ca^{2+} signals differ from other second messages because they work locally rather than globally in cytoplasm. Although Ca^{2+} is a small ion with a large diffusion coefficient in water, diffusion through cytoplasm is very slow owing to efficient sequestering mechanisms and abundant Ca^{2+}-binding proteins, estimated to be 300 μM. Thus, only about 1 in 100 Ca^{2+} ions is free to diffuse in cytoplasm; the other 99 are bound. At a concentration of 0.1 μM in the cytoplasm of resting cell, the half-time for a free Ca^{2+} ion is about 30 μs and its range of diffusion is only about 0.1 μm. Although Ca^{2+} pours through release channels at a rate of 10^6 per second, it does not spread, but acts locally. Ca^{2+}, when bound to a protein messenger like **calmodulin,** has a wider range of about 5 μm.

Cellular responses to Ca^{2+} signals depend on the repertoire of Ca^{2+}-sensitive proteins and effector systems available (Table 28–2). Some Ca^{2+}-binding proteins carry out effector functions directly, such as **Ca²⁺-activated ion channels,** whereas others initiate a cascade of downstream reactions. For example, Ca^{2+} binding to calmodulin has no direct consequence, but Ca^{2+}-calmodulin interacts with more than a dozen effector proteins, including protein kinases and adenylyl cyclase, which act, in turn, on diverse substrates.

The following sections consider each component that regulates Ca^{2+} signals: pumps that clear Ca^{2+} from cytoplasm, Ca^{2+} storage compartments, membrane channels that release Ca^{2+} into cytoplasm, stimuli that open these channels, and effector proteins that mediate the effects of Ca^{2+} signals.

Removal of Ca²⁺ from Cytoplasm

The best characterized Ca^{2+} storage compartment is the **sarcoplasmic reticulum** of striated muscle (see Chapter 42), a specialized smooth endoplasmic reticulum with remarkably high concentrations of the classic calcium-ATPase pump and ryanodine receptor calcium channels (Table 28–3). These proteins give sarcoplasmic reticulum a great capacity to handle rapid Ca^{2+} transients that control muscle contraction. Other cells use similar mechanisms, but are endowed more modestly with these calcium-handling proteins. Mitochondria sequester Ca^{2+} using carriers driven by the electrochemical potential across the inner membrane. Although their Ca^{2+} content is high, mitochondria do not participate in signal transduction by regulated release of Ca^{2+} into cytoplasm.

Pumps

ATP-driven calcium pumps of the plasma membrane and endoplasmic reticulum remove Ca^{2+} from cytoplasm (see Fig. 7–7). They move Ca^{2+} out of cytoplasm against a concentration gradient of about 10^4, hydrolyzing one ATP for each Ca^{2+} transferred from the cytoplasm out of the cell or into the endoplasmic reticulum storage compartment (see Fig. 7–8). Cytoplasmic Ca^{2+} activates calcium pumps until the Ca^{2+} in the cytoplasm falls to about 0.1 μM, the resting level. Three different genes and alternative splicing produce at least five different calcium-ATPase pumps. In heart, the activity of the calcium-ATPase is modulated by **phospholamban,** a 6-kD integral membrane protein of the sarcoplasmic reticulum. Phosphorylation by PKA and calmodulin-activated (CaM) kinase dissociates phospholamban from the calcium pump, stimulating its activity.

Sequestering Proteins

Proteins in the lumen of the endoplasmic reticulum bind much of the Ca^{2+}, but their low affinity

table 28–2
EXAMPLES OF Ca²⁺ REGULATED PROTEINS

Protein	Binding Site	Function
First Order Proteins That Bind Ca²⁺ Directly		
Membrane proteins		
Annexins	Novel	Promote membrane interactions
Ca²⁺-activated Cl⁻ channels	Novel	Participate in secretion
Ca²⁺-activated K⁺ channels	Novel	Control membrane excitability
IP₃ receptor	Novel	Calcium-release channel; activated and inhibited by Ca²⁺
Ryanodine receptor	Novel	Calcium-release channel, activated and inhibited by Ca²⁺
Synaptotagmin	Novel	A synaptic vesicle Ca²⁺ sensor
Enzymes		
Calmodulin-domain protein kinases	EF hand	Plant protein kinases
Calpain	EF hand	Calcium-dependent protease
Protein kinase C, some isozymes	Novel	Multifunctional protein kinases activated by Ca²⁺
Cytoskeletal proteins		
α-actinin (some isoforms)	EF hand	Actin filament cross-linking protein
Centrin/caltractin	EF hand	Ca²⁺-sensitive contractile fibers
Gelsolin, villin	Novel	Actin filament severing and capping proteins
Molluscan myosin light chains	EF hand	Regulate muscle contraction; activated by Ca²⁺
Troponin C	EF hand	Ca²⁺-activated regulator striated muscle contraction
Calcium-binding proteins		
Calbindin, D9, D28	EF hand	Cytoplasmic Ca²⁺ buffer
Calmodulin	EF hand	Ca²⁺-activated regulator of many proteins
Calretinin	EF hand	Activates guanylyl cyclase
Parvalbumin	EF hand	Cytoplasmic Ca²⁺ buffer
Recoverin	EF hand	Regulates visual phototransduction
Second-Order Proteins Activated by Calcium-Calmodulin		
Membrane proteins		
Adenylyl cyclase (some isoforms)		Produces cAMP
Ca²⁺-dependent Na⁺ channels		Na⁺ currents
cGMP-gated cation channels		Phototransduction
Plasma membrane Ca²⁺-ATPase pumps		Clears cytoplasm of Ca²⁺
Enzymes		
Calcineurin		Protein phosphatase 2B
CaM kinase (several isozymes)		Multifunctional protein kinase
cAMP phosphodiesterase		Degrades cAMP
IP₃ kinase		Phosphorylates IP₃
Myosin light chain kinase		Activates smooth muscle and cytoplasmic myosin
NAD kinase		Phosphorylates NAD
Nitric oxide synthetase		Makes Nitric oxide
Phosphorylase kinase		Phosphorylates phosphorylase
Cytoskeletal proteins		
MARCKS		Actin filament cross-linking protein

EF hand is the abbreviation for the Ca²⁺ binding site in calmodium consisting of α-helices E and F.

ensures that bound and free Ca^{2+} are in a rapid equilibrium, providing free Ca^{2+} for release when membrane channels open. **Calsequestrin** is a major Ca^{2+}-binding protein of the sarcoplasmic reticulum. In nonmuscle cells, the endoplasmic reticulum lumen sometimes contains calsequestrin, but more commonly, it contains **calreticulin,** a 47-kD protein with a low affinity ($K_d = 250~\mu M$) but high capacity (25

moles) for Ca^{2+}. (Calreticulin is the Ro/SS autoantigen in the autoimmune disease called Sjögren's syndrome.)

Refilling Endoplasmic Reticulum
Repeated stimulation can deplete Ca^{2+} from intracellular stores, because some released Ca^{2+} is pumped out of the cell by plasma membrane pumps. Endoplasmic reticulum stores can also be depleted experi-

table 28–3

MOLECULAR COMPONENTS OF THE CALCIUM-SEQUESTERING COMPARTMENTS

Cell Type	Calcium Pump	Sequestering Proteins	Release Channel
Skeletal muscle	SR Calcium ATPase	Calsequestrin	Ryanodine receptor
Smooth muscle	Calcium ATPase	Calreticulin > calsequestrin	IP$_3$ receptor and ryanodine receptor
Nonmuscle cells	One of 5 Calcium ATPases	Calreticulin > calsequestrin	IP$_3$ receptor and/or ryanodine receptor

mentally by **thapsigargin.** Thapsigargin, a lactone isolated from plants, inhibits most known endoplasmic reticulum calcium pumps. It depletes Ca^{2+} stores by blocking the reuptake of any Ca^{2+} released by membrane channels or by depletion through leak channels.

In both cases, the cell replenishes the stores by admitting extracellular Ca^{2+} through low-conductance channels of the Trp family (see Fig. 28–12). This is called **store-operated calcium entry.** Some types of Trp channels respond to IP$_3$. Other types respond to low Ca^{2+} in the endoplasmic reticulum without mediation by IP$_3$.

Calcium-Release Channels

Voltage-gated and agonist-gated channels in the plasma membrane (Table 28–4; see Fig. 28–12) admit Ca^{2+} into the cytoplasm from outside. Chapter 9 explains in detail how the membrane potential or agonists open these channels. Voltage-gated channels are essential in excitable cells like muscles and neurons. Owing to automatic inactivation, these channels produce brief, self-limited Ca^{2+} pulses.

Two types of agonist-gated channels—called IP$_3$ receptors and ryanodine receptors—release Ca^{2+} from endoplasmic reticulum. Each is regulated in different ways, allowing diverse stimuli to trigger the release of Ca^{2+}. In excitable cells, plasma membrane calcium channels trigger ryanodine-receptor channels to release Ca^{2+} from the endoplasmic reticulum. In nonexcitable cells, stimulation of either seven-helix receptors or receptor tyrosine kinases produces IP$_3$, which triggers IP$_3$ receptors to release Ca^{2+} from the endoplasmic reticulum. Skeletal muscle uses ryanodine re-

table 28–4

CALCIUM-RELEASE CHANNELS

Type	Distribution	Control	Features
Plasma membrane channels			
ATP-activated channel	Smooth muscle	Extracellular ATP	
cAMP-activated channel	Sperm	Cytoplasmic cAMP	
L-channel	Skeletal and cardiac muscle, brain, other non-muscle cells	Voltage	Excitation-contraction coupling, defective in muscular dysgenesis High threshold, dihydropyridine (DHP)-sensitive, regulated by PKA
N-channel	Neurons, endocrine cells	Voltage	Neurotransmitter release, G protein–modulated High threshold, conotoxin-sensitive
P-channel	Purkinje neurons	Voltage	Insensitive to dihydropyridine and cono-toxin
T-channel		Voltage	Low threshold
Endoplasmic reticulum Ca-channels			
IP$_3$ receptors	Smooth muscle, other cells	IP$_3$, Ca^{2+}	Heparin-sensitive
Ryanodine receptors			Ryanodine-sensitive Ca^{2+} release
Type I	Skeletal muscle	DHP-receptor, Ca^{2+}	Ca^{2+} release stimulates contraction
Type II	Cardiac muscle, other cells	Ca^{2+}, cADP-ribose	Ca^{2+} release stimulates contraction
Type III	Smooth muscle, other cells	Ca^{2+}, cADP-ribose	Ca^{2+} release stimulates contraction

ceptors, whereas smooth-muscle and nonmuscle cells have both types of release channels. Two types of experiments have suggested that release channels are segregated in different parts of the endoplasmic reticulum in some (but not all) smooth-muscle and nonmuscle cells. In one experiment, isolated membrane vesicles released only part of their Ca^{2+} when either type of release channels was stimulated (all would come out if both channels were in each vesicle). In another experiment, immunostaining revealed IP_3 receptors and ryanodine receptors concentrated in different parts of the endoplasmic reticulum.

Nicotinic acid adenine dinucleotide phosphate, a metabolic product of β-NADP (nicotinamide-adenine dinucleotide phosphate), also releases Ca^{2+} from internal stores. The receptor is not yet known, but initial evidence is consistent with the hypothesis that Ca^{2+} released by nicotinic acid adenine dinucleotide phosphate activates Ca^{2+} release by IP_3 receptors and ryanodine receptors that have been sensitized by their ligands.

Inositol 1,4,5-Trisphosphate Receptor Calcium Channels

IP_3 receptors respond to IP_3 by releasing Ca^{2+} from the endoplasmic reticulum. Several signal transduction pathways generate IP_3 from PIP_2 (see earlier section). IP_3 receptors are giant tetramers of 313-kD polypeptides (Fig. 28–13). The large, cytoplasmic N-terminal domain of each subunit binds IP_3 with submicromolar affinity. Six C-terminal transmembrane segments form a calcium channel thought to be related structurally to other cation channels. Tetrameric IP_3 receptors have four IP_3-binding sites; IP_3 must bind at least two, and perhaps as many as four, of these sites to open the channel. Three genes and alternative splicing produce a variety of IP_3 receptors expressed in various cells and developmental stages.

Cytoplasmic IP_3 and Ca^{2+} cooperate to open and close the channel, with IP_3 setting the sensitivity of the channel to Ca^{2+} (Fig. 28–14). Channels respond rapidly, because binding and dissociation of both ligands occurs quickly ($k_+ = 33\ \mu M^{-1}s^{-1}$, $k_- = 6\ s^{-1}$ for IP_3). Type I and type II IP_3 receptors respond to Ca^{2+} with a bell-shaped concentration dependence. Below 0.1 μM and above 100 μM of Ca^{2+}, the channel is generally closed. Calmodulin probably mediates these long-lasting inhibitory effects of Ca^{2+}. The maximum probability for a channel to be open is at about 0.3 μM cytoplasmic Ca^{2+}. High concentrations of Ca^{2+} compete with IP_3 for binding the channel. When IP_3 activates a channel, Ca^{2+} release provides rapid *positive feedback* as its local cytoplasmic concentration rises into the micromolar range, stimulating channel opening and slow *negative feedback* as the local Ca^{2+} con-

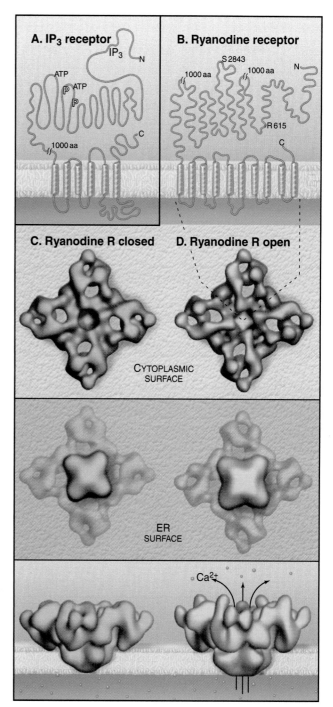

Figure 28–13 Calcium release channels. *A*, IP_3 receptor (R)– channel domain organization. One segment of 1000 residues is omitted. *B*, Ryanodine receptor–channel domain organization. The cytoplasmic domain is far too large to depict to scale in this space, so two segments of 1000 residues are omitted. The number of transmembrane segments is not firmly established. Mutation of R615 causes malignant hyperthermia. S2843 is phosphorylated. *C* and *D*, Three-dimensional reconstructions of electron micrographs of ryanodine receptors in the closed and open conformations. (Reference: Sharma MR, et al: Three-dimensional structure of ryanodine receptor isoform three in two conformational states as visualized by cryoelectron microscopy. J Biol Chem 275:9485–9491, 2000.)

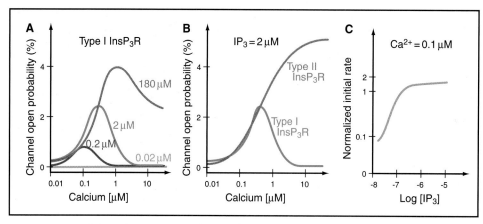

Figure 28-14 Gating of IP$_3$ receptor (InsP$_3$R) calcium release channels. *A*, Dependence of channel open probability of type I receptors on the concentrations of IP$_3$ (concentrations given next to each curve) and Ca^{2+}. *B*, Comparison of the dependence of open probability of type I and type III receptors on the concentration of Ca^{2+} at a fixed concentration of 2 μM IP$_3$. Note that high concentrations of Ca^{2+} inhibit type I receptors but not type III receptors. *C*, Dependence of open probability of type I receptors on the concentration of IP$_3$ at a fixed concentration of 0.1 μM Ca^{2+}. (*A*, Reference: Kaftan EJ, et al: InsP$_3$ and calcium interact to increase the dynamic range of InsP$_3$ receptor-dependent calcium signaling. J Gen Physiol 110:529–538, 1997, by copyright permission of the Rockefeller University Press. *B*, Reprinted with permission from Nature. Reference: Hagar RE, et al: Type III InsP$_3$ receptor channel stays open in the presence of increased calcium. Nature 396:81–84, 1998. Copyright 1998, Macmillan Magazines Limited. *C*, Reference: Hirota J, et al: Kinetics of calcium release by IP$_3$ receptor in reconstituted lipid vesicles. J Biol Chem 270:19046–19051, 1995.)

centration climbs higher. The result is a short, self-limited pulse of Ca^{2+} release in response to a modest change in IP$_3$ concentration. Type III IP$_3$ receptors are different; Ca^{2+} activates them, but high Ca^{2+} concentrations do not compete with IP$_3$ or inhibit calcium release. This lack of negative feedback (or very slow feedback) allows cells with these IP$_3$ receptors to produce a large, global pulse of Ca^{2+} that can ultimately drain endoplasmic reticulum stores.

High concentrations of Ca^{2+} in the endoplasmic reticulum lumen sensitize receptors to IP$_3$. Phosphorylation by PKA, PKC, and CaM kinase can increase or decrease the sensitivity to IP$_3$. IP$_3$ receptors are highly selective for inositol 1,4,5-triphosphate and do not bind related inositol phosphates.

Ryanodine Receptor Calcium Channels

Ryanodine receptors release Ca^{2+} from the endoplasmic reticulum to trigger contraction of striated muscles. The name comes from the high affinity of the channel for a plant alkaloid called ryanodine, which can activate or block Ca^{2+} release, depending upon its concentration and the target tissue. Ryanodine has no physiological function, but the name has stuck because binding of radioactive ryanodine was the key assay for isolating the protein. Purified protein was reconstituted into phospholipid bilayers and shown to function identically to the calcium channels in isolated endoplasmic reticulum.

Ryanodine receptors are homotetramers of 565-kD subunits with a massive cytoplasmic domain and 6 to

10 putative transmembrane segments near the C-terminus that form the Ca^{2+} channel (see Fig. 28–13*B*). Three ryanodine receptor genes encode homologous proteins that are about 60% identical and expressed in different cells (see Table 28–4). Ryanodine receptors are the sole release channels in striated muscles. In smooth muscle and nonmuscle cells, ryanodine receptors play a supporting role to IP$_3$ receptor calcium-release channels.

The three isoforms respond to different activators: cytoplasmic Ca^{2+}, **cyclic ADP-ribose,** and physical contact with activated **L-type calcium channels.** Like IP$_3$ receptors, all ryanodine receptors are activated by Ca^{2+} with a bell-shaped concentration dependence. This calcium-induced Ca^{2+} release allows activation to spread locally and transiently from one ryanodine receptor to the next.

Cyclic adenosine diphosphate (cADP)–ribose sets the Ca^{2+} sensitivity of ryanodine receptors, just as IP$_3$ does for its receptor. At low concentrations of cADP-ribose, high levels of cytoplasmic Ca^{2+} are required to open the channel, whereas at high concentrations of cADP-ribose, even resting Ca^{2+} concentrations open the channel. A single enzymatic step produces cADP-ribose from the metabolite nicotinamide adenine dinucleotide, NAD$^+$. cGMP regulates **ADP-ribosyl cyclase,** presumably through a cGMP-dependent protein kinase. cADP-ribose has been implicated in the Ca^{2+} transient that triggers secretion of insulin from pancreatic β cells in response to glucose. In fertilization of echinoderm eggs, cADP-ribose releases Ca^{2+} through

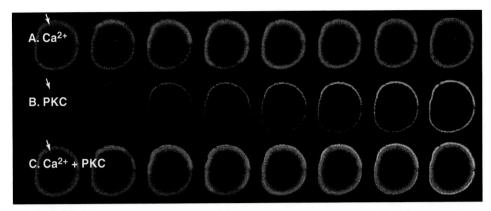

Figure 28-15 *A to C*, Wave of Ca²⁺ release and PKC activation spreading from the site of artificial activation of a *Xenopus* egg. *A*, Ca²⁺ signal; *B*, PKC activation; *C*, superimposition of the two signals. The egg was injected with calcium red (a fluorescent dye sensitive to the concentration of Ca²⁺) and a fusion protein, consisting of green fluorescent protein and PKC, which produces green fluorescence when PKC is activated. The egg was activated by a needle prick *(arrows)* and imaged at intervals of 20 seconds. A wave of Ca²⁺ (more intense red) precedes a wave of active PKC *(green)* from the site of activation. (Courtesy of Carolyn Larabell, Lawrence Berkeley Laboratory.)

endoplasmic reticulum ryanodine receptors in parallel with IP₃-mediated Ca²⁺ release. Vertebrate eggs depend entirely on the IP₃ release mechanism (Fig. 28–15).

Phosphorylation, caffeine, nanomolar ryanodine and the general anesthetic halothane also stimulate ryanodine receptor activity. Caffeine is used to test for ryanodine receptors in isolated membrane fractions and to activate sperm in fertility tests. Phosphorylation of ryanodine receptors by PKA increases channel activity and may contribute to the effects of β-adrenergic receptor stimulation on the heart (see Fig. 10–12). FKBP, a protein that binds the immunosuppressant drug FK506, binds ryanodine receptors in heart and skeletal muscle (and IP₃ receptors as well). This interaction suppresses spontaneous channel openings. Deletion of the mouse FKBP gene causes an enlarged heart. Micromolar ryanodine, the local anesthetic procaine, and calmodulin all inhibit Ca²⁺ release by ryanodine receptors.

Point mutations in the nRyR1 ryanodine receptor gene (expressed in skeletal muscle) cause **malignant hyperthermia** in humans and pigs. The human form is autosomal dominant with an incidence of about 1 in 50,000. Mutant ryanodine receptors are unusually sensitive to activation by anesthetics, which trigger Ca²⁺ release, sustained skeletal muscle contraction, and pathological heat generation. If not treated promptly, the fever can be lethal. The pig mutation is autosomal recessive, and stress can trigger lethal attacks.

Calcium Dynamics in Cells

Methods to visualize Ca²⁺ concentrations inside living cells have revealed an amazing temporal and spatial complexity of Ca²⁺ signals. The original calcium sensor was a jellyfish protein called **aequorin,** which emits light when it binds Ca²⁺. An evolving series of **Ca²⁺-sensitive fluorescent dyes** (Fura-2, calcium green, calcium red, Fluo-3) have largely replaced aequorin and made possible the observations in the following paragraphs. Even newer calcium sensors, constructed as fusion proteins of calmodulin and mutants of green fluorescent protein, offer considerable advantages, including targeting to particular cellular compartments and the ability to adjust the response range widely by mutating the Ca²⁺-binding site.

Voltage-dependent calcium channels in excitable cells like neurons and striated muscles respond rapidly (<1 msec) to an action potential to admit extracellular Ca²⁺. At chemical synapses, this produces a brief, anatomically confined Ca²⁺ pulse that triggers the release of synaptic vesicles (see Fig. 10–8). In striated muscles, each action potential causes a transient, global increase in cytoplasmic Ca²⁺ lasting tens of milliseconds (Fig. 42–15). The details differ in skeletal and cardiac muscle, but the elementary events are similar. Voltage-sensitive L-type calcium channels in T tubules (invaginations of the plasma membrane; see Chapter 42) activate one or a few ryanodine receptor channels in the adjacent endoplasmic reticulum through direct physical interaction in skeletal muscle and through Ca²⁺ release in heart. Ca²⁺ released by these ryanodine receptors triggers Ca²⁺ release from nearby ryanodine receptors, generating a local pulse of Ca²⁺ called a **calcium spark.** Because T tubules penetrate throughout the muscle cytoplasm, thousands of these sparks are produced simultaneously, yielding a transient global spike in Ca²⁺. The brief duration of the excitatory signal and the robust Ca²⁺ pumping activity of the endoplasmic reticulum limit the duration of the signal.

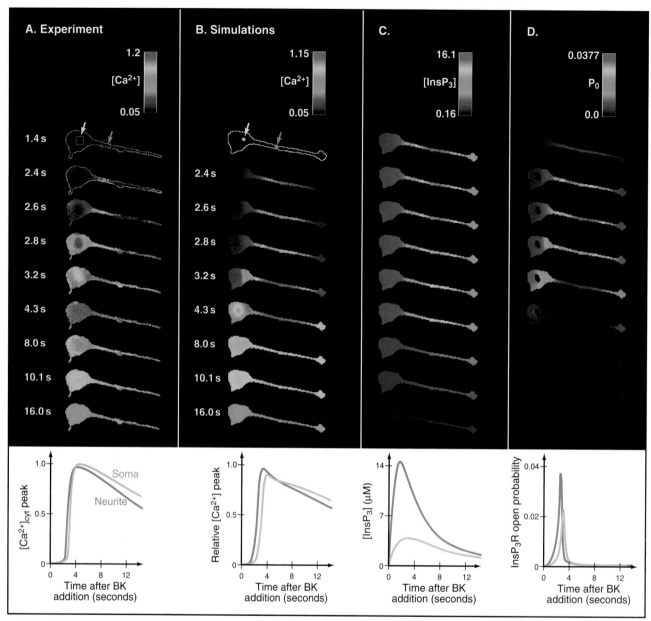

Figure 28-16 Wave of Ca²⁺ released in the cytoplasm of a cultured neuroblastoma cell stimulated at time zero with bradykinin and followed at intervals for 16 seconds. False colors indicate Ca²⁺ concentration or modeled IP₃ concentration or modeled open probability of IP₃ receptor channels. The model was made with Virtual Cell software taking into account measured local concentrations of IP₃ receptors and their biochemical properties. Graphs show the time course of various parameters in the neurite and cell body. *A,* Experimental data with Ca²⁺ (micromolar) measured with the intracellular indicator calcium green. *B,* Model of the local cytoplasmic Ca²⁺ concentration (micromolar). *C,* Model of the local cytoplasmic IP₃ concentration (micromolar). *D,* Model of the open probability of IP₃ receptor channels. InsP3, IP₃. (Courtesy of L. Loew, University of Connecticut. References: Fink CC, et al: Morphological control of IP₃-dependent signals. J Cell Biol 147:929–935, 1999; by copyright permission of The Rockefeller University Press. Fink CC, et al: An image-based model of calcium waves in differentiated neuroblastoma cells. Biophys J 79:163–183, 2000.)

Nonexcitable cells generally rely on slower, receptor-mediated production of IP₃ to produce transient changes in cytoplasmic Ca²⁺. For example, activation of a frog egg at one point by entry of a sperm or artificial activation by pricking with a needle (Fig. 28–15) results in a self-propagating wave of cytoplasmic Ca²⁺ that spreads slowly around the cell. This pro-

duces a wave of secretion and activation of downstream effectors, such as PKC.

Many cells with type I and II IP₃ receptors respond to a constant agonist stimulation with transient bursts or spikes of cytoplasmic Ca²⁺ (Fig. 28–16). The agonist concentration sets the level of cytoplasmic IP₃ (and, possibly, cADP-ribose), which determines the sensitivity of release channels to cytoplasmic Ca^{2+}. A region of a cell with a high density of the most sensitive channels then initiates Ca^{2+} bursts at a focus. The resulting Ca^{2+} transient often spreads through the cytoplasm as a planar or spiral wave driven locally by calcium-induced Ca^{2+} release from either ryanodine receptors or IP_3 receptors. Such transients are self-limited locally, because cytoplasmic Ca^{2+} concentrations exceeding 0.5 μM inhibit both IP_3 receptors and ryanodine receptors. This negative feedback closes release channels and allows Ca^{2+} pumps to clear the cytoplasm of Ca^{2+}. Release channels recover slowly from this negative feedback, creating an interval between spikes. In this way the cell decodes the concentration of agonist as the frequency of Ca^{2+} pulses. Colliding waves annihilate each other owing to negative feedback by high concentrations of Ca^{2+} or local depletion of Ca^{2+} stores. A different response to continuous agonist stimulation occurs in cells with type III IP_3 receptors, which respond to agonists with a large burst of Ca^{2+} that fills the entire cytoplasm for seconds owing to their lack of negative feedback by high Ca^{2+}.

Participation of multiple second messengers and channel types can produce complex responses to stimulation. For example, agonists, such as acetylcholine or cholecystokinin, employ Ca^{2+} to stimulate polarized epithelial cells of the pancreas to secrete digestive enzymes. Ca^{2+} spikes begin at the apex of these polarized cells owing to a high concentration of IP_3 receptors. With a strong stimulus, a Ca^{2+} wave spreads from the apex throughout the cell. The frequency of these spikes depends on agonist concentration. Pathways from these agonists appear to be initiated by nicotinic acid adenine dinucleotide phosphate. Downstream of this, IP_3 and cADP-ribose and their receptors in the endoplasmic reticulum set the sensitivity of the release mechanisms to cytoplasmic Ca^{2+}.

Ca²⁺ Targets

The diversity of targets for Ca^{2+} (see Table 28–2) emphasizes the widespread and complex effects of this second messenger. The response to a Ca^{2+} signal depends upon the available targets, as well as modulating effects of parallel signaling pathways. Some proteins bind Ca^{2+} directly, including Ca^{2+}-activated plasma membrane channels for K^+ and Cl^-, troponin-C in striated muscles, synaptotagmin (a Ca^{2+}-sensing synaptic vesicle protein), and calpain (a Ca^{2+}-activated protease). Ca^{2+} activates many other proteins indirectly by first binding and activating calmodulin. Some calmodulin targets, like CaM kinase II, act on a number of different substrates, greatly amplifying the effect of Ca^{2+}.

Owing to the oscillatory, transient nature of Ca^{2+} signals, some cellular responses may depend on the

frequency of Ca^{2+} spikes. At least one target protein, CaM kinase II, can decode frequency information into a prolonged adjustment in its level of activity.

■ Nitric Oxide

Nitric oxide is a free radical gas (NO·) that provides cells with a unique way to transmit signals. It diffuses rapidly through membranes, allowing the signal to spread from cell to cell rather than being confined to the cytoplasm of a single cell like other second messengers. Nitric oxide has long been known as a mildly toxic air pollutant, so it was not surprising to find that nitric oxide that is produced by macrophages contributes to the killing of microorganisms and tumor cells. On the other hand, it was surprising to learn in the late 1980s that nitric oxide is a diffusible messenger from endothelial cells lining blood vessels that relaxes smooth muscle in the walls of arteries and also that it acts as an unconventional neurotransmitter in both the central and peripheral nervous systems. Carbon monoxide (CO) may be another gaseous intercellular second messenger under some circumstances.

Nitric oxide is not a single chemical species. NO· is only one of several readily interconvertible redox states of nitrogen monoxide, including nitrosonium (NO^+) and nitroxyl (NO^-) ions. Although nitric oxide is stable in water, it reacts readily with oxygen and has a half-life of only a few seconds in the body. Consequently, nitric oxide must be produced continuously to provide a sustained effect. Much nitric oxide is inactivated by binding to the heme of hemoglobin. Nitric oxide is eventually metabolized to nitrate and nitrite and excreted from the body. Note that the stable anesthetic gas nitrous oxide, N_2O or laughing gas, is not part of this family of nitrogen monoxides.

An enzyme, **nitric oxide synthase,** produces nitric oxide by converting L-arginine and molecular oxygen into citrulline and nitric oxide (Fig. 28–17). NADPH provides reducing equivalents for the reaction. Nitric oxide synthase (NOS) is really two enzymes in one. The N-terminal oxidase domain has a

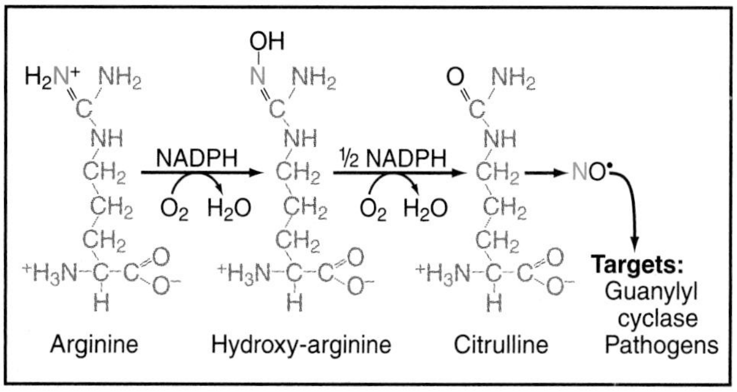

Figure 28–17 Synthesis of nitric oxide (NO·).

heme group that participates directly in oxidation of arginine. The C-terminal reductase domain supplies electrons to the oxidase domain. NOS depends on an extraordinary number of cofactors to handle the electron transfers required to produce nitric oxide: heme and tetrahydrobiopterin bound to the oxidase domain; and flavin adenine dinucleotide, flavin mononucleotide, and NADPH in the reductase domain.

Vertebrates express three NOS isozymes selectively in various tissues. Inducible NOS (iNOS) is found in macrophages, liver, and fibroblasts. Macrophages produce iNOS only when stimulated by endotoxin, interferon-γ, or other factors. Endothelial NOS (eNOS) is also made by some neurons. Neuronal NOS (nNOS) is made by about 1% of neurons in the cerebral cortex, as well as skeletal muscle and epithelial cells. eNOS and nNOS are produced constitutively. eNOS is targeted to membranes by N-terminal myristoylation and palmitoylation. nNOS associates with the plasma membrane dystrophin complex in skeletal muscle and is one of the components lost from the membrane in patients with muscular dystrophy.

Ca^{2+}-calmodulin and phosphorylation regulate NOS activity independently. Ca^{2+}-calmodulin activates NOS by binding a short regulatory sequence between the two enzyme domains. Ca^{2+} signals activate NOS in most tissues, although macrophage iNOS binds Ca^{2+}-calmodulin so tightly that it is permanently activated. Protein kinase B/Akt, the kinase activated by PIP_3 (see Chapter 27 and an earlier section in this chapter), phosphorylates and activates eNOS.

The main target for the low concentrations of nitric oxide used for signaling is guanylyl cyclase, the enzyme that makes cGMP. Nitric oxide binds tightly to iron in the heme group of guanylyl cyclase, causing a conformational change that activates the enzyme. Nitric oxide has been reported to affect other proteins either through binding or covalent modification, but the physiological significance of these effects is less well characterized. Macrophages produce concentrations of nitric oxide high enough to kill microorganisms directly. The nitric oxide combines with superoxide anion (O_2^-) to form peroxynitrite ($OONO^-$), which rapidly breaks down into $OH^.$ and $NO_2^.$, both very toxic oxidants that kill ingested microorganisms. Plants also produce nitric oxide as part of their defense mechanism against pathogens.

Nitric oxide from three different sources regulates blood flow and blood pressure in response to local physiological demands. During exercise, the repeated release of Ca^{2+} that stimulates skeletal muscle contraction (see Chapter 42) also binds calmodulin and activates NOS to produce nitric oxide. Nitric oxide diffuses out of the skeletal muscle and into smooth muscle cells surrounding nearby blood vessels. Nitric oxide relaxes smooth muscle by activating cGMP pro-duction and lowering the internal Ca^{2+} level through incompletely understood mechanisms. This increases local blood flow to supply oxygen and nutrients. Endothelial cells lining the inside of blood vessels also use nitric oxide to regulate vascular smooth muscle. Mechanical shear stress from blood flow continuously stimulates endothelial cell phosphatidylinositol-3 kinase to produce PIP_3, which stimulates PKB/Akt to phosphorylate and activate NOS. This provides a sustained, long-term signal to relax vascular smooth muscle. Acutely, hormones like acetylcholine and bradykinin can stimulate endothelial cells to produce nitric oxide by causing Ca^{2+} release from endoplasmic reticulum. Mice lacking eNOS have high blood pressure.

Mono- and di-N^G-methylated arginines strongly inhibit NOS and thus have been used experimentally to reveal many biological functions of nitric oxide. Inhibition of NOS inhibits killing of bacteria by macrophages. Similarly, inhibition of endothelial nitric oxide production causes vascular smooth muscle cells to contract, raising blood pressure and demonstrating a constitutive role for nitric oxide in relaxing these cells. Nitric oxide produced by autonomic nerves causes erection of the penis by stimulating the production of cGMP and relaxing vascular smooth muscle cells. The drug sildenafil (Viagra) is used to treat impotence as it inhibits the phosphodiesterase that breaks down cGMP. Other autonomic nerves use nitric oxide to control the smooth muscle cells in the walls of the intestines. Nitric oxide is the active metabolite of nitroglycerin, a drug widely used to relieve the pains (angina pectoris) associated with compromised blood flow in the heart. It dilates coronary arteries and improves circulation. In addition to regulating cerebral blood flow, nitric oxide produced by nerve cells in the brain may contribute to certain types of learning by reinforcing the release of neurotransmitters. (See Fig. 10–10 for a discussion of long-term potentiation.)

▌ Selected Readings

Berridge MJ, Bootman MD, Lipp P: Calcium—A life and death signal. Nature 395:645–648, 1998.

Clapham DE: Calcium signaling. Cell 80:259–268, 1995.

Crivici A, ad Ikura M: Molecular and structural basis of target recognition by calmodulin. Annu Rev Biophys Biomol Struct 24:85–116, 1995.

DiMarzo V: Review: 'Endocannabinaoids' and other fatty acid derivatives with cannabimimetic properties. Biochim Biophys Acta 1392:153–175, 1998.

Fruman DA, Meyers RE, Cantley LC: Phosphoinositide kinases. Annu Rev Biochem 67:481–508, 1998.

Gaffney BJ: Lipoxygenases: Structural principles and spectroscopy. Annu Rev Biophys Biomol Struct 25:431–459, 1996.

Gallione A, White A: Ca^{++} release induced by cyclic ADP-ribose. Trends Cell Biol 4:431–436, 1995.

Hodgkin MN, Pettitt TR, Martin A, et al.: Diacylglycerols and phosphatidates: Which molecular species are intracellular messengers? Trends Biochem Sci 23:200–204, 1998.

Houslay MD, Milligan G: Tailoring cAMP-signaling responses through isoform multiplicity. Trends Biochem Sci 22:217–224, 1997.

Ikura M: Calcium binding and conformational response in EF-hand proteins. Trends Biochem Sci 21:14–17, 1996.

Leevers SJ, Vanhaesebroeck B, Waterfield MD: Signaling through phosphoinositide 3-kinases: The lipids take centre stage. Curr Opin Cell Biol 219–225, 1999.

MacLennan DH, Rice WJ, Green NM: The mechanism of Ca^{2+} transport by the sarco(endo)plasmic reticulum Ca^{2+}-ATPases. J Biol Chem 272:28815–28818, 1997.

Mayer B, Hemmens B: Biosynthesis and action of nitric oxide in mammalian cells. Trends Biochem Sci 22:477–481, 1997.

Meldolesi J, Pozzan T: The endoplasmic reticulum Ca^{2+} store: A view from the lumen. Trends Biochem Sci 23:10–14, 1998.

Niggli E: Localized intracellular calcium signaling in muscle: Calcium sparks and calcium quarks. Annu Rev Physiol 61:311–335, 1998.

Rhee SG, Bae YS: Regulation of phosphoinositide-specific phospholipase C isozymes. J Biol Chem 272:15045–15048, 1997.

Rios E, Stern MD: Calcium in close quarters: Microdomain feedback in excitation-contraction coupling and other cell biological phenomena. Annu Rev Biophys Biomol Struct 26:47–82, 1997.

Smith WL, DeWitt DL, Garavito RM: Cyclooxygenases: Structural, cellular and molecular biology. Annu Rev Biochem 69:145–182, 2000.

Wolfe MM, Lichtenstein DR, Singh G: Gastrointestinal toxicity of nonsteroidal antiinflammatory drugs. N Engl J Med 340:1888–1899, 1999.

chapter 29

INTEGRATION OF SIGNALS

This chapter outlines how a variety of well-characterized signal transduction mechanisms work at the molecular level. These examples illustrate diverse mechanisms, but common strategies, for carrying information about changing environmental conditions into cells and for eliciting adaptive responses. Chapters 26 to 28 describe the molecular hardware used in these pathways. Here, the focus is on the flow of information, including examples of branching and converging pathways. For each pathway, the key events are reception of the stimulus, transfer of the stimulus into the cell, amplification of a cytoplasmic signal, and modulation of effector systems over time. Few signaling pathways operate in isolation; physiological responses usually depend on the integration of pathways.

Although each of the pathways illustrated here is the best characterized of its kind, none is yet fully understood. Generally, gaps exist in our knowledge about one or more aspects: the full inventory of the components, concentrations of molecules, the organization of the system in cells, and rates of reactions that transfer signals. This is expected, as most pathways are complicated and investigators have only recently learned their basic properties. Moreover, very few pathways are currently amenable to quantitative analysis of their dynamics in live cells. Continued investigations should refine the schemes presented in the following sections, particularly with respect to how each operates as an integrated system. The chapter concludes with bacterial two-component phosphotransfer systems. These signaling pathways use different molecular components but the same strategies as the eukaryotic systems that are covered first.

Signal Transduction by G Protein–Coupled, Seven-Helix Transmembrane Receptors

The first three signaling pathways use seven-helix receptors coupled to trimeric G proteins. Two highly specialized sensory systems—olfactory and visual reception—are particularly well characterized because their outputs are electrophysiological events that can be monitored at the level of single cells and single membrane ion channels on a rapid time scale. On a millisecond time scale, these two sensory transducers amplify minute stimuli to produce changes in the membrane potential that initiate a signal to the central nervous system. The response of cells to the hormone epinephrine through the β-adrenergic receptor provides an interesting contrast to these rapidly responding sensory systems. Although many of the protein components are similar, the response is slower and much more global, affecting cellular metabolism and responsiveness as a whole.

Sensory Perception in the Olfactory System

Metazoan sensory systems detect external stimuli with extremely high sensitivity and specificity. The chemosensory processes of smell and taste have evolved into highly specialized biochemical and electrophysiological pathways that connect individuals with their environment. Of these two sensory modalities, olfaction is more sensitive, allowing humans to detect **odorants** at concentrations of a few parts per trillion in air and to distinguish among more than 10,000 different odorants. Most volatile chemicals with molecular weights of less than 1000 are perceived to have some odor. The olfactory system shares features with many systems that eukaryotes use for communication, including external pheromone signals of yeast and insects, as well as internal hormonal signals, like adrenaline, that circulate in the blood between organs of higher organisms.

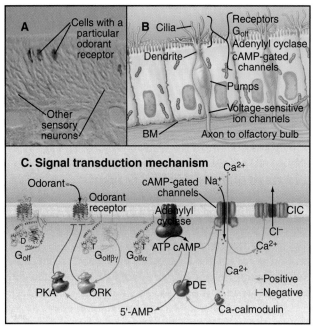

Figure 29-1 Olfaction. *A*, Light micrograph of a section of sensory epithelium from the nasal passage of a mouse after staining *(brown)* for one olfactory receptor mRNA. Note that only few cells express this gene. *B*, Drawing of the sensory epithelium highlighting one olfactory sensory neuron and the signal-transducing proteins concentrated in three parts of the cell. *C*, Signal transduction mechanism. An odorant molecule binds a specific seven-helix plasma membrane receptor and changes its conformation. The activated receptor catalyzes the exchange of GDP for GTP on multiple trimeric G proteins, causing dissociation of $G_{olf}\alpha$ from $G\beta\gamma$. $G_{olf}\alpha$-GTP activates adenylyl cyclase to produce multiple cAMPs. cAMP binds to and opens cyclic nucleotide–gated ion channels in the plasma membrane, depolarizing the plasma membrane. Ca^{2+} admitted by the cAMP-gated channel opens chloride channels (ClC), which augment membrane depolarization. Membrane depolarization triggers an action potential that travels along the axon to secondary neurons in the brain. Multiple negative feedback loops *(red)* terminate stimulation. cAMP activates PKA, and $G\beta\gamma$ activates odorant receptor kinase (ORK), both of which phosphorylate and inhibit the receptor. Ca^{2+} binds calmodulin, which inhibits the cAMP-gated channel and activates phosphodiesterase (PDE) to break down cAMP. BM, basement membrane. (*A*, From Ressler KJ, Sullivan SL, Buck LB: A zonal organization of odorant receptor gene expression in the olfactory epithelium. Cell 73:597–609, 1993.)

Odorant Binding to Mucus Carrier Proteins

The initial step in olfaction is binding of volatile odorant compounds to proteins highly concentrated in the mucus that bathes the sensory tissue in the nasal cavity. A family of **odorant-binding proteins** solubilize odorants and increase their concentration in mucus. Similar proteins, present in the hemolymph of moths and other insects, bind pheromones and play a role in the chemoreception in those organisms. Odorant-binding proteins typically have low affinities for their ligands, so odorants exchange rapidly on and off their binding proteins in the mucus. When they dissociate they can interact with receptor proteins located on specialized cilia of the olfactory neurons.

Overview of the Transduction Mechanism

Specific odorants are detected by **olfactory sensory neurons** located in the nasal epithelium (Fig. 29–1) and signaled to the brain by action potentials. The signal transduction mechanism in the sensory neurons is initiated by odorant binding to plasma membrane seven-helix receptors coupled to trimeric G proteins. Reception and transduction of stimuli takes place in five steps:

1. Odorant binding changes the conformation of its plasma membrane receptor.
2. Activated receptor catalyzes the exchange of guanosine diphosphate (GDP) for guanosine triphosphate (GTP) on multiple trimeric G proteins, causing the dissociation of $G_{olf}\alpha$ from $G\beta\gamma$. This is the first stage of amplification.
3. Each $G_{olf}\alpha$ activates adenylyl cyclase to produce many molecules of cyclic adenosine monophosphate (cAMP). The cytoplasmic cAMP concentration peaks in less than 100 msec. This is the second stage of amplification.
4. cAMP binds to and opens cyclic nucleotide-gated ion channels, depolarizing the plasma membrane.
5. Membrane depolarization opens voltage-gated ion channels, triggering an action potential (a self-propagating wave of membrane depolarization; see Chapter 10) that moves along the axon of the sensory neuron to secondary neurons in the brain.

As one can appreciate from everyday experience, olfactory signal transduction is very sensitive but adapts quickly to the continued presence of an odorant. An understanding of each step in the sensory transduction and adaptation pathways helps to explain how animals can discriminate so many different odors.

Molecular Anatomy of the Sensory Neuron

The sensory neurons are located within a neuroepithelium (see Fig. 29–1*A*) that is analogous to the sensory epithelia in the visual and auditory systems. (Neurons in an epithelium may seem odd, but the reader should recall that the entire central nervous system derives from the embryonic ectoderm.) Olfactory neurons are unique among neurons in their ability to replace themselves every 60 days throughout adult life from neuroblast-like precursor cells that lie near the base of the epithelium. Direct exposure of these sensory cells to the environment may explain the requirement for this special self-renewing property. If protected from viruses and environmental toxins, the turnover of sensory neurons is slower. Loss of olfactory function with age results, in part, from a decreased ability to maintain this neuronal replacement process.

When the neuronal progenitors mature, they migrate into the more apical regions of the epithelium, extending apical processes comparable to the dendrites of other neurons. Approximately 12 **sensory cilia** sprout from these dendritic processes, and **axons** project from the base of the neuron to their targets, secondary neurons, in the **olfactory bulb** at the front of the brain.

Olfactory neurons have three specialized zones. Apical sensory cilia are specialized for responding to particular extracellular odorants. High concentrations of four proteins in the ciliary membrane—one or more specific odorant receptors, G_{olf}, type III adenylyl cyclase, and cyclic nucleotide-gated ion channels—allow extracellular odorants to control the membrane potential. The cell body contains the nucleus, protein-synthesizing machinery, and plasma membrane pumps and channels that set the resting electrical potential of the plasma membrane. Depolarizing currents, initially generated in the cilia, spread to the cell body and initiate action potentials at the transition from cell body to axonal process. Voltage-gated ion channels in the axon generate action potentials to propagate the signal to the central nervous system.

Odorant Receptors

The olfactory system detects a wide range of ligands present at low concentrations in mucus, so it was postulated that odorant receptors comprise a family of related proteins, all activating one or a small number of messenger pathways. This was confirmed by molecular cloning of a large family of complementary DNAs (see Chapter 5 for more on cDNAs) from the olfactory epithelium that encode seven-helix transmembrane receptors (see Chapter 27) and demonstration that these proteins are highly concentrated in cilia of olfactory neurons. The sequences of these receptors are most divergent in the transmembrane spans, the presumed odorant-binding sites. Experimental expression of an odorant receptor in non-neuronal cells allows the cells to respond to a specific odorant. It is estimated that mice have 1000 odorant receptor genes, humans have 500, and fish have 100. A limited number of olfactory neurons express any given receptor (see Fig. 29–1*A*), with each sensory neuron expressing as few as a single type of receptor. In all, at least 1000 cells in the olfactory epithelium of a mouse express each receptor.

Odorant binding changes the conformation of the receptor, allowing it to catalyze the exchange of nucleotide on trimeric G proteins associated with the cytoplasmic face of the plasma membrane. Like the visual system, in which single photons can generate a small current, activation of a single odorant receptor may generate a signal sufficient to elicit an action potential.

G-Protein Relay

Activated receptors catalyze the rapid exchange of GDP for GTP on a specialized isoform of trimeric G protein called G_{olf}. This isoform is expressed in olfactory neurons and is concentrated in sensory cilia. In less than 100 msec, an activated receptor can produce 10 to 100 activated GTP-$G_{olf}\alpha$ molecules, which then dissociate from their $G\beta\gamma$ subunits. This second step in olfactory signal transduction provides significant amplification of the original signal and allows the diverse range of ligands and their receptors to converge on a common intracellular signaling pathway. Note that the encoding of the chemical identity of the stimulus depends simply on which cells respond, not on the firing pattern of the neuron or other complex encoding of the signal itself.

Production of cAMP

In the third step, GTP-$G_{olf}\alpha$ binds to and activates a specialized olfactory isozyme of **adenylyl cyclase.** During activation, each enzyme generates nearly 100 cAMP molecules. By 75 msec after stimulation, the concentration of cAMP inside the cilium peaks at >10 μM, returning to baseline within 500 msec. This dramatic fluctuation in cAMP concentration is made possible by the high surface-to-volume ratio of cilia, which ensures that membrane-associated signaling components interact rapidly and that the cAMP they produce is confined within a small volume. The cAMP transient is short-lived owing to hydrolysis by a **phosphodiesterase** with a high turnover rate but relatively low affinity for cAMP. The cAMP transient is considerably faster than the following step, which it triggers.

Action Potential Generation by Cyclic Nucleotide-Gated Channels

In the fourth step, cAMP binds to **cyclic nucleotide-gated ion channels** that open to admit ions that depolarize the plasma membrane. These channels are highly concentrated in the ciliary membranes (>2000 per μm²) compared with those in the cell body (6 per μm²). Binding of at least two cAMP molecules increases the probability that the channel is open from near 0 to about 0.65. Because the probability is not 1.0, individual activated channels flicker open and closed on a millisecond time scale. Together the ensemble of many activated channels admits enough Na⁺ and Ca²⁺ to depolarize the membrane. Additional current is carried by Ca²⁺-activated chloride channels. These channels are highly concentrated in the ciliary membrane and dissipate the charge imbalance that occurs when the positive ions enter the cell (see Chapters 9 and 10 for details). The lag of 200–500 msec between binding of the odorant and peak membrane depolarization is attributable to the relatively slow binding of cAMP to the channel. The role of cAMP in olfaction is distinctly different than in most other tissues where most of the effects of cAMP can be accounted for by the activation of protein kinase A (PKA; see Chapter 28). The role of cAMP in olfactory signaling has been established by experiments on isolated olfactory neurons, in which the effect of odorants, membrane-permeant cyclic nucleotide analogues, and phosphodiesterase inhibitors has been explored.

Depolarization of the ciliary membrane initiates an action potential by activating voltage-gated sodium channels (see Fig. 10–6) in the cell body. The action potential propagates along the axon to a chemical synapse with the second neuron in the pathway, located in the olfactory bulb of the brain.

Adaptation

Desensitization—the waning of perceived odorant intensity despite its continued presence—results from a combination of central and peripheral processes. Peripheral processes contributing to adaptation include modulation of each step in the signaling pathway following odorant binding (see Fig. 29–1C). At the molecular level, this adaptation is reflected in the transient nature of G-protein activation, the self-limited increase in cAMP, and the limited duration of the membrane depolarization, all of which occur with constant exposure to odorant. Importantly, the sequential nature of many of these feedback circuits implies that they have intrinsic delays and, therefore, serve not only to alter the magnitude of the response but also to alter its time course.

G protein–coupled receptors are desensitized by protein kinases that phosphorylate the receptor and by proteins called **arrestins** that bind phosphorylated receptors (see Fig. 26–3). These modifications inhibit the interaction of activated receptors with G proteins

and provide negative feedback at the first stage of signal amplification. Negative feedback is coupled to receptor stimulation, because the **olfactory receptor kinase** is brought to the plasma membrane by binding the G$\beta\gamma$ subunits released by receptor-induced G-protein dissociation.

Cyclic nucleotide–gated channels are permeable to both Na⁺ and Ca²⁺; Ca²⁺ binds calmodulin, and the complex provides negative feedback at two levels. Calcium-calmodulin activates the cAMP phosphodiesterase that rapidly converts cAMP to 5′-AMP. Calcium-calmodulin also binds to the cyclic nucleotide–activated channel, reducing its affinity for cAMP by 10-fold. This reduces the probability of the channel opening at less than saturating cyclic nucleotide concentrations and may accelerate the otherwise slow dissociation of cAMP from the channel. These two effects of Ca²⁺ serve to alter the responsiveness of the cell to initial odorant exposure, shape the time course of the response, extend the dynamic range over which the cell can respond, and make a cell transiently refractory to additional stimulation.

Photon Detection by the Vertebrate Retina

Overview of Visual Signal Processing

Photons are energetic but unconventional agonists. They are very small, move very fast, and penetrate most biochemical materials. These properties create a formidable challenge for detecting photons and transducing their properties (intensity and wavelength) into a signal that can be transmitted to the brain. Nevertheless, vertebrate photoreceptor cells capture single photons and convert this energy into a highly amplified electrical response (Fig. 29–2). This is the best understood eukaryotic sensory process because the system is amenable to sophisticated biophysical, biochemical, and physiological analysis. Single-cell organisms use similar mechanisms to respond to light (see Fig. 41–14).

Vertebrate **photoreceptor cells** are neurons located in a two-dimensional array in the retina, an epithelium inside the eye. The cornea and lens of the eye form an inverted real image of the outside world on the retina, so that the intensity of the light across the field of view is encoded by geographically separate photoreceptor cells. Photoreceptor cells lie at the base of a complex neural processing system. Having detected the rate of photon stimulation at a particular place in the visual field, photoreceptor neurons communicate this information to higher levels of the visual system. Initial processing of the information takes

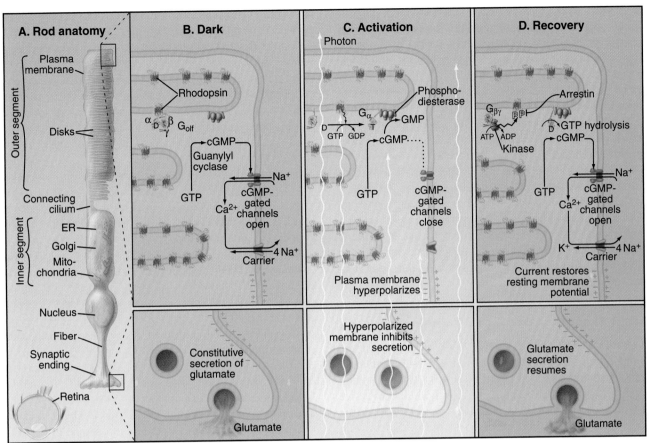

Figure 29–2 Vertebrate visual transduction. *A*, Drawing of a rod cell. Disks in the outer segment are rich in rhodopsin. *B* to *D*, Drawings of small portions of an outer segment (*upper panels*) and the synaptic terminal of a rod cell (*lower panels*) in three physiological states. Active components are highlighted by bright colors. *B*, Resting cell in the dark. Constitutive production of cGMP keeps a subset of the plasma membrane cGMP-gated channels open most of the time, allowing an influx of Na$^+$ and Ca^{2+}. At the resting membrane potential, the synaptic terminal constitutively secretes the neurotransmitter glutamate. Ca^{2+} leaves the outer segment via a sodium/calcium exchange carrier in the outer segment, whereas Na$^+$ leaves the cell via a sodium pump in the plasma membrane of the inner segment. *C*, Absorption of a photon activates one rhodopsin, allowing it to catalyze the exchange of GTP for GDP bound on many molecules of transducin (G$_T$). This dissociates G$_T\alpha$ from G$\beta\gamma$. Each G$_T\alpha$-GTP binds and activates one molecule of phosphodiesterase (attached to the disk membrane by N-terminal isoprenyl groups), which rapidly converts cGMP to GMP. As the concentration of free cGMP declines, the cGMP-gated channels close, leading to hyperpolarization of the plasma membrane. This inhibits glutamate secretion at the synaptic body. *D*, Recovery is initiated when rhodopsin kinase phosphorylates activated rhodopsin. Binding of arrestin to phosphorylated rhodopsin prevents further activation of G$_T$. Phosphodiesterase stimulates hydrolysis of GTP bound to G$_T$, returning G$_T$ to the inactive G$_T\alpha$-GDP state. Synthesis of cGMP by guanylyl cyclase returns the cytoplasmic concentration of cGMP to resting levels and opens the cGMP-gated channels. Constitutive secretion of glutamate resumes.

place in the retina, where secondary and tertiary neurons take input from multiple photoreceptors to derive local information regarding image contrast, as well as color and intensity. Neuroscience texts present more detailed information on higher levels of visual processing in the retina and brain.

The response of photoreceptor cells depends on the intensity of the light, that is, the flux of photons. Vertebrate retinas detect light with intensities that range over 10 orders of magnitude. **Rod photoreceptors** (see Fig. 29–2*A*) detect low levels of light from about 0.01 photons per μm^2 per second (dim stars) to

10 per μm^2 per second, but do not discriminate light of different colors. **Cone photoreceptors** (cones) respond to more intense light, up to about 10^9 photons per μm^2 per second (full sunlight). Three classes of cones with chromophores sensitive to different wavelengths of light allow humans to encode wavelength and color vision to operate.

Rods and cones have three specialized regions with different molecular components and functions. The nucleus and the organelles in the **inner segment** maintain the cell's structure and metabolism. A vestigial cilium connects the inner segment to the **outer**

segment, which consists of a stack of internal membrane **disks** containing the photoreceptor protein, rhodopsin, surrounded by the plasma membrane. Disks form by invagination and pinching off of flattened sacks of plasma membrane. Rhodopsin synthesized in the cell body is transported to the plasma membrane along the secretory pathway and segregated into disk membranes. The lumen of the disks corresponds topologically to the lumen of the endoplasmic reticulum or the extracellular space. Other components of the signaling cascade also concentrate in the outer segment. G-protein subunits and phosphodiesterase associate with the cytoplasmic face of the disk membrane via covalent lipid groups. cGMP-gated channels are components of the plasma membrane. Vesicles in the synaptic terminal are filled with glutamate, the transmitter that activates the next neuron in the visual circuit.

Light Absorption and Signal Transduction

Vertebrate visual systems use a G protein–coupled, signal transduction cascade (see Fig. 29–2) similar to that used for olfaction and hormones, but employing isoforms of most of the protein components exclusive to photoreceptor cells. Absorption of light reduces the release of synaptic transmitter on to the next neuron in the pathway. Signals flow through the system as follows:

1. A chromophore bound to a seven-helix receptor absorbs light and changes the conformation of the receptor.
2. Active receptor catalyzes the exchange of GDP for GTP on a trimeric G protein.
3. G proteins activate an enzyme, cGMP phosphodiesterase.
4. Phosphodiesterase rapidly reduces the cytoplasmic concentration of cGMP.
5. The reduction in cytoplasmic cGMP closes cGMP-gated cation channels, hyperpolarizing the plasma membrane.
6. The change in membrane potential reduces the rate of transmitter release at the synapse between the photoreceptor cell and the next neuron in the visual circuit.
7. Feedback loops operate at every level in this signal transduction pathway, turning off the response to a flash of light.

The following sections explain how these reactions achieve their spectacular sensitivity in rods. Cones operate similarly, but with lower sensitivity.

Rhodopsin

Rhodopsin, the photoreceptor protein of rods, is a seven-helix, G protein–coupled receptor with a light-absorbing chromophore, **11-cis retinal,** covalently attached to lysine 296 through a protonated Schiff base (see Fig. 26–2B). Although 11-cis retinal is bound to a site in the bundle of transmembrane helices similar to sites where ligands bind other seven-helix receptors, this form of rhodopsin is inactive with respect to catalyzing nucleotide exchange on its trimeric G protein. Thus, rhodopsin is a seven-helix receptor with a covalently attached, but inactive, ligand. The photoreceptors of color-sensitive cone cells are also seven-helix receptors with distinct visual pigments.

The ability of rods to detect single photons depends on two favorable properties. First, the noise level is very low owing to the stability of the 11-cis retinal. In vertebrate rods, less than 1 molecule in 4×10^{10} isomerizes spontaneously every second so the background level of activated rhodopsin is very low, even with 10^8 molecules of rhodopsin per cell. Thus, one does not see spots of light in the dark. Second, rods absorb photons very efficiently. This is achieved by the high concentration of rhodopsin in disks and by stacking thousands of disks on top of each other in the direction of incoming photons. The concentration of rhodopsin in the disk membranes is remarkably high; it constitutes 90% of the disk membrane protein and 45% of the disk membrane mass. About half of the photons that traverse the outer segment are absorbed, and about two thirds of absorbed photons produce an electrical change in the plasma membrane.

Absorption of light initiates the signal transduction pathway. Picoseconds after the 11-cis retinal chromophore absorbs a photon, the energy isomerizes it to **all-trans retinal.** This initiates a cascade of intramolecular reactions that activates rhodopsin by changing its conformation. **Metarhodopsin II,** the stable active conformation, has rearranged cytoplasmic loops that catalyze nucleotide exchange on **transducin,** its trimeric G-protein partner (see Fig. 27–9). The signal initiated by absorption of light is amplified by two successive enzymatic reactions and by the closing of ion channels. Following activation, rhodopsin is inactivated by hydrolysis of the Schiff base linking all-trans retinal to the protein and dissociation of the chromophore. Rhodopsin is regenerated by binding a fresh molecule of 11-cis retinal, derived from vitamin A.

The Positive Arm of the Signal Cascade

Metarhodopsin II catalyzes the exchange of GDP for GTP on the α subunit of transducin, which then dissociates its $\beta\gamma$ subunits. Each metarhodopsin II produces hundreds of activated transducins in a fraction of a second, nearly as fast as the molecules collide while they diffuse in the plane of the disk bilayer. Nucleotide exchange on transducin is rate-limiting in the whole transduction cascade, even with a 10^7 acceleration by metarhodopsin II.

Transducin α-GTP activates **phosphodiesterase** by binding its two inhibitory γ subunits. This step does not amplify, but frees the catalytic α and β subunits of phosphodiesterase to break down cGMP to GMP at a high rate. Active phosphodiesterase amplifies the signal by reducing the concentration of cGMP. The cytoplasmic concentration of cGMP depends largely on its rate of destruction by light-activated phosphodiesterase, as it is made continuously by **guanylyl cyclase.**

Diffusion of cGMP carries the signal from the disk membrane to the plasma membrane. As the concentration of cGMP decreases, **cGMP-gated cation channels** in the plasma membrane close. These channels (see Fig. 9–9) are very sensitive to the concentration of cGMP. Binding of four cGMPs opens a channel, whereas the loss of one cGMP closes a channel. Closure of cGMP-gated channels hyperpolarizes the membrane and inhibits glutamate release at the synapse.

Amplification in this pathway is spectacular. Within 1 second after absorption of a single photon, rhodopsin activates 1000 transducins and a similar number of phosphodiesterases, which break down 50,000 cGMPs. This closes hundreds of cGMP-gated channels, each of which blocks the entry of more than 10,000 cations.

The electrical circuit that responds to the signal has the following features. In the dark, the resting cGMP concentration in the outer segment produces a steady-state "dark current" arising from the 1% of channels that are open at any time. This inward current is balanced by an outward current that flows through potassium channels in the inner segment. The concentrations of Na^+, which would otherwise accumulate in the cell, and K^+, which would otherwise be depleted, are maintained by a sodium/potassium pump in the inner segment. Ca^{2+} entering the outer segment through cGMP-gated channels is extruded by an exchange carrier in the outer segment's plasma membrane. This carrier exchanges Ca^{2+} and K^+ for Na^+.

When the cGMP concentration declines in response to absorption of a photon, the open probability of the cGMP-gated channels decreases, on a millisecond time scale, along with the cation current into the outer segment, hyperpolarizing the plasma membrane. The cytoplasmic Ca^{2+} concentration also declines from about 300 nM to 50 nM. The magnitude of the response depends on the number of photons absorbed and the size of the amplified signal.

Like the cyclic nucleotide–gated channel of olfactory neurons, the photoreceptor channel is largely blocked in the presence of physiological levels of extracellular Ca^{2+}. This affords two useful properties to the system. First, it reduces the burden on pumps that must maintain the ionic gradients in the cell. Second, by reducing the current carried by each channel and opening more channels, an improved signal-to-noise ratio is achieved. For example, if only two channels were responsible for the dark current, the statistical opening or closing of one channel would create large fluctuations in the current. If the same amount of current were carried by 100 partially blocked channels, then opening or closing of one additional channel has a modest effect on total current.

Recovery and Adaptation

After a dim flash of light, the decreased cytoplasmic cGMP concentration and the plasma membrane hyperpolarization are short-lived, on the order of 2 seconds in rods, briefer in cones. Rods reset the signaling pathway by inhibiting metarhodopsin II, inactivating transducin α-GTP, and activating the synthesis of cGMP.

- **Rhodopsin kinase,** associated with the disk membrane by a C-terminal farnesyl group, phosphorylates several residues near the C-terminus of metarhodopsin II. Like other seven-helix receptor kinases, rhodopsin kinase is only active toward the activated form of the receptor. Phosphorylation of rhodopsin reduces its ability to activate transducin. Binding of a second protein, **arrestin,** to phosphorylated rhodopsin prevents further production of transducin α-GTP.
- GTP hydrolysis dissipates the light-activated burst in transducin α-GTP. The low GTPase activity of transducin is activated by association with phosphodiesterase and by an **RGS protein** (regulator of G protein signaling; see Chapter 27), inactivating transducin in less than 1 second. Dissociation of transducin α-GDP from phosphodiesterase inhibitory subunits terminates cGMP breakdown.
- The reduction in cytoplasmic Ca^{2+} that accompanies closure of cGMP-gated cation channels stimulates the guanylyl cyclase that restores the cGMP concentration. This opens the cation channels and returns the membrane potential to the resting level.

Regulation of Metabolism Through the β-Adrenergic Receptor

Epinephrine, a catecholamine also called adrenaline (see Fig. 29–3), is secreted by the neuroendocrine cells of the adrenal gland and other tissues when an animal is startled, stressed, or otherwise needs to respond vigorously. **Norepinephrine,** a closely related catecholamine, is secreted by sympathetic neurons, including those that regulate the contractility of the

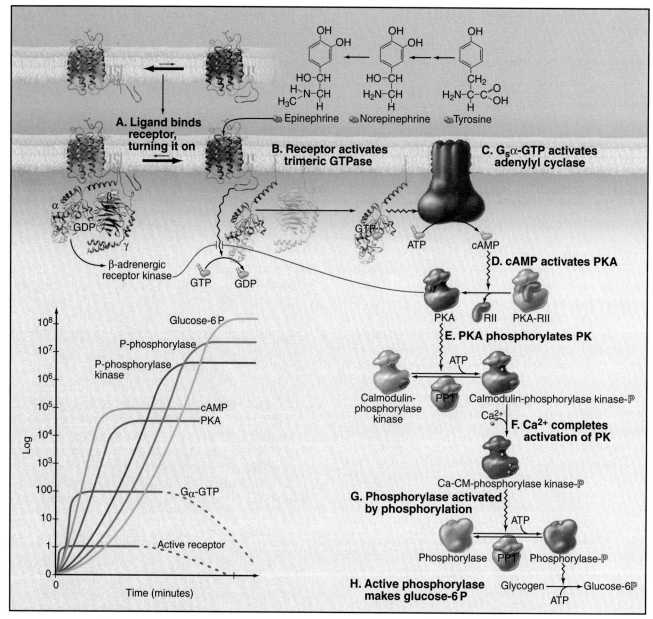

Figure 29–3 β-adrenergic signaling mechanism. Active components are shown in bright colors. *Upper right,* Pathway of epinephrine synthesis. *Lower left,* Time course of the amplification of the signal by the catalytic cascade of signal-transducing enzymes. *A,* Epinephrine binds the seven-helix β-adrenergic receptor, shifting its equilibrium to the active conformation. *B,* Active receptor catalyzes the exchange of GDP for GTP on $G_s\alpha$, dissociating $G_s\alpha$-GTP from $G\beta\gamma$. *C,* $G_s\alpha$-GTP activates adenylyl cyclase, which produces multiple cAMPs. *D,* cAMP activates protein kinase A (PKA) by dissociating the regulatory subunit, RII (not shown to scale). *E,* PKA phosphorylates and partially activates multiple molecules of phosphorylase kinase (PK). *F,* Ca^{2+} binds to calmodulin (CM) associated with phosphorylase kinase, completing activation. *G,* Phosphorylase kinase phosphorylates and activates phosphorylase. *H,* Phosphorylase catalyzes the conversion of glycogen to glucose–6 phosphate. Negative feedback loops (*red*) terminate stimulation. cAMP activates PKA and $G\beta\gamma$ activates β-adrenergic receptor kinase, both of which phosphorylate and inhibit the receptor from catalyzing nucleotide exchange. PP1, protein phosphatase 1.

heart. These hormones flow through the blood and stimulate cells of many types throughout the body to heighten their metabolic activity. These catecholamines stimulate many cells, including skeletal muscle and liver, to break down glycogen to glucose to provide energy. Smooth muscle cells of arteries relax to facilitate blood flow. Norepinephrine stimulates heart cells to contract more frequently and with greater force. The variety of physiological responses depends on selective expression of a family of nine **adrenergic receptors** and their associated signaling hardware in particular differentiated cells (Table 29–1).

table 29–1

table 29–1
FOUR EXAMPLES OF ADRENERGIC RECEPTORS AND PHYSIOLOGICAL RESPONSES

Receptor	Tissue	Signaling Pathway	Responses
α_1	Smooth muscle, blood vessels	G_q, PLC-β, IP$_3$, Ca^{2+}, MLCK	Contraction
	Smooth muscle, GI tract	G_q	Relaxation
	Liver	G_q	Glycogenolysis
α_2	Smooth muscle, blood vessels	G_i, Ca^{2+}	Contraction
	Pancreatic islets	G_i, inhibit A-cyclase, K$^+$ channel open	Secretion inhibition
β_1	Heart	G_s, A-cyclase, cAMP, PKA, phospholamban	Increased contraction
β_2	Liver	G_s, A-cyclase, cAMP, PKA, phosphorylase	Glycogenolysis
	Skeletal muscle	G_s, A-cyclase, cAMP, PKA, phosphorylase	Glycogenolysis

GI, gastrointestinal; MLCK, myosin light chain kinase; PLC-β, phospholipase C-β.

Epinephrine binding to the β-adrenergic receptor is the classic example of a pathway utilizing a seven-helix receptor (see Chapter 26), a trimeric G protein (see Chapter 27), and adenylyl cyclase (see Chapter 28) to produce the second messenger, cAMP. cAMP mediates a wide variety of cellular responses by activating PKA (see Chapter 26), which changes the activity of many different cellular proteins by phosphorylation. Specialized cells vary in their responses because they express different targets for PKA. Heart PKA responds to epinephrine by phosphorylating phospholamban, a small membrane protein that regulates the Ca^{2+} pump of the smooth endoplasmic reticulum (see Chapter 42). Smooth muscle PKA phosphorylates and inhibits myosin light chain kinase, preventing it from initiating contraction (see Chapter 42). Liver PKA activates enzymes that break down glycogen, releasing glucose into the circulation.

This section explains how β-adrenergic receptors regulate the production of glucose-6 phosphate from glycogen (see Fig. 29–3). As with vision and olfaction, the response to epinephrine is sensitive, highly amplified, and subject to negative feedback control. Five stages of amplification along the seven-step pathway allow binding of a single molecule of epinephrine to a receptor to activate millions of enzyme molecules that produce many million molecules of glucose-6 phosphate.

1. Epinephrine binds to a β-adrenergic receptor and traps it in its active conformation. The resting system is on the verge of activation because the ligand-free receptor is in a rapid equilibrium between activated and unactivated states. Even without agonist, a small fraction of receptors is active at any given time. Experimentally increasing the total concentration of receptors (and therefore the concentration of spontaneously active receptors) can maximally activate downstream pathways, even in the absence of agonists.

2. Each activated receptor catalyzes the exchange of GDP for GTP on many molecules of the trimeric protein **G$_s$**, causing the dissociation of the G$_s\alpha$ and G$\beta\gamma$ subunits. This amplifies the signal up to 100-fold. The G protein subunits remain attached to the membrane by their lipid anchors, but go their separate ways to activate different targets. This is the first branchpoint in the pathway.

3. The GTP-G$_s\alpha$ binds and activates **adenylyl cyclase,** an integral membrane protein (see Fig. 28–2), which produces many molecules of cAMP. This is the second stage of amplification.

4. cAMP activates **PKA** by binding and dissociating the inhibitory RII subunit (see Chapter 27). Activation of PKA mediates most effects of cAMP, but cAMP may also activate cyclic nucleotide–gated ion channels in some cells.

5. Each activated PKA amplifies the signal by phosphorylating many substrate molecules, including **phosphorylase kinase.** This protein kinase is regulated synergistically by phosphorylation and Ca^{2+}, which binds to calmodulin, one of the subunits of the enzyme. The enzyme requires Ca^{2+} for activity, but phosphorylation by PKA reduces the Ca^{2+} requirement, so that the kinase is active even at resting (0.1 μM) Ca^{2+} concentrations. On the other hand, high cytoplasmic Ca^{2+} concentrations alone, as during muscle contraction, can activate phosphorylase kinase without phosphorylation. PKA also inhibits protein phosphatase 1 (PP1), which dephosphorylates phosphorylase kinase.

6. Each activated phosphorylase kinase further amplifies the signal by phosphorylating many molecules of the enzyme **phosphorylase b,** turning on their enzyme activity. PKA enhances this phosphorylation step by inhibiting protein phosphatase 1, which dephosphorylates phosphorylase.

7. Each activated phosphorylase molecule (called phosphorylase a) removes many glucose subunits from glycogen, one at a time. This fifth stage of amplification produces glucose-1-phosphate,

which can enter the glycolytic pathway of the cell or, in the case of liver, can be dephosphorylated and released into the bloodstream to provide an energy source for other cells in the body.

The positive response to epinephrine is transient owing to reactions that counterbalance the positive arm of the pathway, even in the continued presence of epinephrine. First, each activating reaction is reversible, either spontaneously or after being catalyzed by specific enzymes. Second, the system has several negative feedback loops.

Activating steps are reversed in several different ways. Epinephrine dissociates rapidly from receptors, so if the plasma concentration of epinephrine declines, the β-receptor equilibrium shifts promptly toward the inactive state. Activated GTP-$G_s\alpha$ hydrolyzes its bound nucleotide slowly, at a rate of about 0.05 s^{-1}. GDP-$G_s\alpha$ then rebinds $G\beta\gamma$, returning the complex to its inactive state. cAMP is degraded to 5'AMP by a phosphodiesterase, an enzyme activated by Ca^{2+}-calmodulin. This allows signaling pathways that release Ca^{2+} (see Chapter 28) to modulate the β-adrenergic pathway. Protein phosphatase 1 turns off both phosphorylase kinase and phosphorylase by removal of activating phosphates.

The negative feedback loops operate on a range of time scales. $G\gamma$ is anchored to the membrane lipid bilayer by a C-terminal C-20 geranylgeranyl group, so $G\beta\gamma$ subunits released from $G_s\alpha$ provide a membrane-binding site for cytoplasmic β-**adrenergic receptor kinase** (βARK). Over seconds to minutes, membrane-associated βARK phosphorylates serines in the C-terminal cytoplasmic tail of active receptors. β-**arrestin** binding to phosphorylated receptors has two negative effects: it blocks interactions of the active receptor with G proteins, and, on a time scale of many minutes, its interaction with clathrin mediates removal of receptors from the cell surface by endocytosis. Prolonged stimulation results in receptor degradation. Active PKA produced by the pathway independently, phosphorylates the receptor with the same negative consequences as βARK phosphorylation.

In addition to these effects on glucose metabolism, active β-adrenergic receptors produce at least two other signals. $G\beta\gamma$ subunits activate calcium channels in some cells. This Ca^{2+} can augment glycogen breakdown at the phosphorylase kinase step. In addition to its negative effects, β-arrestin binding to phosphorylated receptors can initiate a positive signal, activation of the mitogen-activated protein (MAP) kinase pathway (see later section). β-arrestin serves as a membrane-anchoring site for the cytoplasmic tyrosine kinase, c-Src, which initiates signaling to the MAP kinase cascade.

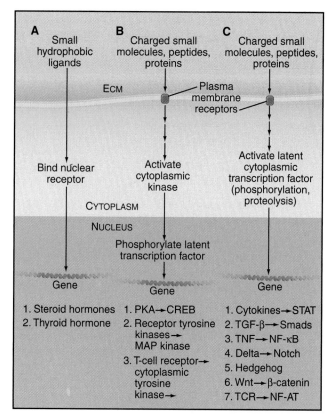

Figure 29-4 The three signaling pathways by which extracellular ligands influence gene expression. *A*, Nuclear receptor pathway for small hydrophobic ligands that penetrate the plasma membrane. (See Fig. 14–19*A* for an example.) *B*, Pathways employing a plasma membrane receptor and a cytoplasmic protein kinase that enters the nucleus to activate a latent transcription factor. (See Fig. 14–9*B* for the PKA pathway, Fig. 29–6 for a receptor tyrosine kinase pathway, and Fig. 29–8 for a cytoplasmic tyrosine kinase pathway.) *C*, Pathways employing a plasma membrane receptor and activating a latent transcription factor in the cytoplasm. The list includes six known pathways of this type. See Fig. 29–8 for NF-AT, Fig. 29–9 for a STAT pathway, Fig. 29–10 for a Smad pathway, Fig. 14–19*C* for the NF-κB pathway, Chapter 26 for the Notch and Hedgehog pathways, and Fig. 32–8 for the β-catenin pathway. CREB, cAMP response element–binding protein; ECM, extracellular matrix; TCR, T cell receptor; TNF, tumor necrosis factor.

Signaling Pathways Influencing Gene Expression

The following sections present signaling several pathways that regulate gene expression. The fact that numerous specific examples have been investigated makes it challenging to discern general principles. Fortunately, only a modest number of underlying mechanisms seem to have appeared during evolution, such that all of the known pathways fall into just a few categories (Fig. 29–4).

Small hydrophobic ligands that penetrate the plasma membrane, such as steroids and thyroid hormone, bind nuclear receptors in the cytoplasm. Ligand-bound receptors enter the nucleus and, in combination with other proteins, activate transcription of specific genes (see Fig. 14–19).

Ligands that cannot penetrate the plasma membrane, including small charged molecules, peptides, and proteins, activate plasma membrane receptors. These receptors relay the signal to the nucleus using one of two general strategies:

1. Some plasma membrane receptors turn on cytoplasmic protein kinases that enter the nucleus, where they activate latent transcription factors by phosphorylation. These **mobile kinases** include PKA (see Fig. 14–19) and MAP kinase, used by many receptors to carry signals to the nucleus (see Figs. 29–5 to 29–8).

2. Other plasma membrane receptors activate latent transcription factors in the cytoplasm, generally by phosphorylation or proteolysis. These activated transcription factors then enter the nucleus. The seven known pathways use **mobile transcription factors** called NF-AT (see Fig. 29–8), STATs (see Fig. 29–9), Smads (see Fig. 29–10), NF-κB (see Fig. 14–19), Notch (see Chapter 26), Hedgehog (see Chapter 26), and β-catenin (Fig. 32–8). Activated transcription factors produced by either strategy cooperate with other nuclear proteins to regulate the expression of specific genes.

MAP Kinase Pathways to the Nucleus

Cascades of three protein kinases terminating in a **MAP kinase** (mitogen-activated protein kinase) relay signals from diverse stimuli and receptors to the nucleus (Fig. 29–5). The first kinase activates the second kinase by phosphorylating serine residues. The second kinase has dual specificity and activates MAP kinase by phosphorylating both a tyrosine and a serine residue in the activation loop (Fig. 27–3D). Active MAP kinase enters the nucleus and phosphorylates transcription factors, which regulate gene expression. Key targets include genes that control the cell cycle either by turning it on or off, depending on the system. MAP kinases also regulate the synthesis of nucleotides required for making RNA and DNA.

Inputs come from a variety of cell surface receptors. The example just presented explained how β-arrestin couples inactivated seven-helix β-adrenergic receptors to an MAP kinase pathway. Budding yeast activate MAP kinase pathways in two ways. Mating pheromones bind seven-helix receptors that release Gβγ subunits of trimeric G proteins, which activate the first kinase in the cascade. On the other hand, osmotic shock activates a two-component receptor (see Fig. 29–11) upstream of another MAP kinase pathway that regulates the synthesis of glycerol, which

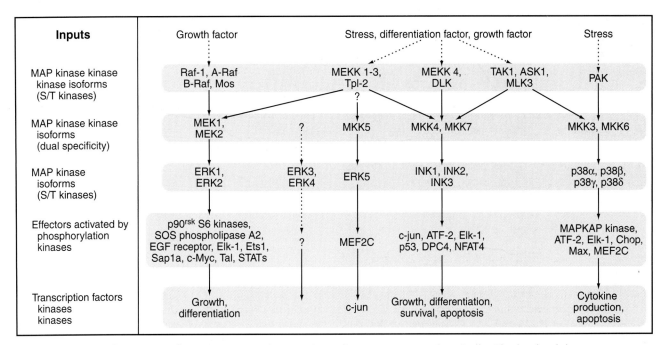

Figure 29–5 Five distinct MAP kinase (MAPK) pathways. The pathways are arranged vertically. The levels of the pathways are arranged horizontally. Dual specificity protein kinases phosphorylate S/T and Y residues. (Adapted from Garrington TP, Johnson GL: Organization and regulation of mitogen-activated protein kinase signaling pathways. Curr Opin Cell Biol 11:211–218, 1999, with permission from Elsevier Science.) PIP₂, phosphatidyl (4,5)-biphosphate.

is used to adjust cytoplasmic osmolarity. The following sections explain how receptor tyrosine kinases, such as growth factor receptors (see Fig. 29–6) and insulin receptors (see Fig. 29–7), use the small guanosine triphosphatase (GTPase), Ras, to activate **MAP kinase cascades.** Engagement of T lymphocytes with antigen-presenting cells activates a cytoplasmic nonreceptor tyrosine kinase, ZAP-70 (ζ chain–associated protein) that triggers the same pathway through Ras to MAP kinase (see Fig. 29–8). Other nonreceptor tyrosine kinases (in parentheses following) couple many other receptors to Ras and MAP kinase, including interleukin-2 (Lck), interleukin-3 (Lyn), and granulocyte-macrophage (GM)-colony-stimulating factor (Lyn). Employing Ras as an intermediate in multiple pathways allows cells to integrate mitogenic signals from diverse stimuli, which can act together to control cell growth.

Animal cells have five distinct MAP kinase cascades with particular isoforms of the three kinases linked in series and leading to different effectors (see Fig. 29–5). The kinases comprising these pathways are expressed selectively in various cells and tissues. Crosstalk between the pathways in cells that express multiple kinases blurs their distinction to some extent.

Because the net result of triggering any of these pathways is activation of a MAP kinase, one might ask why the mechanism is so complicated. Why use a cascade with sequential activation rather than having a receptor tyrosine kinase activate MAP kinase directly? Cascades provide opportunities to integrate inputs from converging pathways and to amplify a signal. One striking example of amplification by an MAP kinase cascade is the switch-like response of frog oocytes to the hormone progesterone. These oocytes are arrested in the G2 stage of the cell cycle until progesterone activates a MAP kinase cascade consisting of Mos, MEK1, and the MAP kinase ERK 2. The fact that both MEK1 and MAP kinase require two independent phosphorylation events for activation results in an all-or-nothing switch, with all of the cell's MAP kinase doubly phosphorylated and active, or all of it unphosphorylated and inactive. Consequently, a marginal stimulus turns some cells on strongly and others not at all, rather than producing a graded response in all of the cells. Experimental evidence for signal amplification by MAP kinase cascades is generally lacking in other cells.

In yeast and mammals, two or three of the kinases in a particular MAP kinase pathway may be anchored to a common **scaffolding protein.** Physical association of the enzymes may facilitate transfer of the signal and may insulate an anchored pathway from parallel pathways. On the other hand, binding a series of kinases to the same scaffold presumably precludes amplification, so more work is being done to understand the physiological significance of these scaffolds.

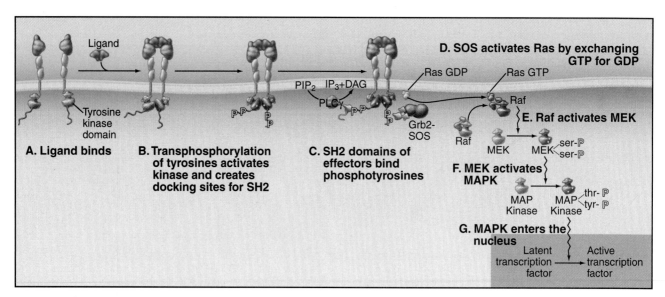

Figure 29–6 Growth factor receptor tyrosine kinase signaling pathway through MAP kinase. Active components are shown in bright colors. *A,* Ligand binding brings together the tyrosine kinase domains of two receptor subunits. *B,* Transphosphorylation activates the kinases and creates specific docking sites for effector proteins with SH2 domains. *C,* Phospholipase Cγ (PLCγ) binds one phosphotyrosine and is activated by phosphorylation to break down phosphatidyl 4,5-bisphosphate-(PIP$_2$) into diacylglycerol (DAG) and IP$_3$. *D,* A complex of the adapter protein Grb2 and the nucleotide exchange factor SOS binds another phosphotyrosine and catalyzes the exchange of GDP for GTP on the membrane-associated small GTPase Ras. Ras-GTP attracts the cytoplasmic serine/threonine kinase Raf to the plasma membrane. *E,* Raf phosphorylates and activates the dual-function kinase MEK. *F,* MEK phosphorylates and activates MAP kinase (MAPK). *G,* MAP kinase enters the nucleus and activates latent transcription factors.

Growth Factor Receptor Tyrosine Kinase Pathway Through Ras to MAP Kinase

Protein and polypeptide **growth factors** control the behavior of cells, including expression of genes required for growth and development. For example, the protein **epidermal growth factor** (EGF) controls proliferation and differentiation of epithelial cells in vertebrates. **Platelet-derived growth factor** (PDGF) stimulates the proliferation of connective tissue cells required to heal wounds (see Fig. 34–11). Similar proteins specify the differentiation of cells in fly eyes and the reproductive tract of nematode worms. Mutations that constitutively activate proteins along this pathway contribute to the development of many human tumors by driving cellular proliferation (see Chapter 44).

Growth factor signaling pathways transfer information through at least eight different protein molecules (Fig. 29–6). Conservation of the main features of the mechanism in vertebrates, worm, and flies has made it possible to piece together the main principles of this exceedingly complex pathway by pooling information from different systems. Genetic tests in flies, worms, and yeast have identified the components and established the order of their interactions. Many components were identified independently as **oncogenes** and by biochemical isolation and reconstitution of individual steps. The universality of the molecular mechanism was established by comparing the primary structures and activities of the proteins; it was confirmed by showing that components from diverse species can substitute for each other in vivo. Information flows from growth factors to the nucleus as follows:

1. Growth factors, such as EGF and PDGF, bind to the extracellular domain of their receptors.
2. Ligand binding causes two receptor subunits to dimerize, allowing each to **transphosphorylate** specific tyrosine residues on the **activation loops** of the cytoplasmic domain of its partner (see Fig. 27–3D). This turns on kinase activity and leads to phosphorylation of other tyrosines on the cytoplasmic domains of the receptor.
3. The newly created **phosphotyrosines** are specific binding sites for SH2 domains of several downstream effectors, including **phospholipase Cγ1**, phosphatidylinositol 3(**PI-3**)-**kinase** and a preformed complex of the adapter protein **Grb2** with **SOS**. Amino acids flanking each phosphotyrosine create specific binding sites for each type of SH2 domain. Grb2 and SOS continue the signaling pathways to the nucleus. Grb2 consists of three Src homology domains: SH3/SH2/SH3 (see Fig. 2–15). The SH2 domain binds tyrosine phos-

phorylated growth factor receptors. The SH3 domains anchor proline-rich sequences (PPPVPPRR) of SOS. The gene for SOS protein got its name—*son of sevenless*—as a downstream component of the *sevenless* growth factor receptor gene required for the development of photoreceptor cell number seven in the fly eye.

4. When brought to the plasma membrane, SOS catalyzes the activation of the small GTPase, **Ras,** by exchanging GDP for GTP. Association of Grb2-SOS with the receptor raises its local concentration near Ras, which is anchored nearby to the bilayer by its farnesyl group. This proximity appears to be all that is required, as experimental targeting of SOS to the plasma membrane by other means also activates Ras.
5. Ras-GTP triggers a MAP-kinase cascade by providing a binding site on the membrane for **Raf-1,** a serine/threonine kinase (a MAP kinase kinase kinase). Interaction with Ras-GTP, and possibly other factors, activates Raf-1.
6. Active Raf-1 phosphorylates and activates the dual-function protein kinase **MEK** (a MAP kinase kinase).
7. MEK activates MAP kinase by phosphorylating both threonine and tyrosine residues on the activation loop.
8. Active MAP kinase enters the nucleus, where it phosphorylates and activates several transcription factors (see Fig. 29–5). These transcription factors control the expression of the genes required to drive the cell through the cell cycle (see Chapter 44).

The pathway has at least two other branches initiated by other signaling proteins that associate with phosphotyrosine on the receptor. Binding of phospholipase Cγ1 to the receptor results in its activation by phosphorylation. Active phospholipase Cγ1 produces inositol 1,4,5-triphosphate (IP$_3$) (with release of Ca^{2+} from intracellular stores) and diacylglycerol (DAG) (resulting in activation of protein kinase C [PKC]). PI-3 kinase, stimulated by interaction with a phosphorylated receptor, produces polyphosphoinositides, which activate other isoforms of PKC, as well as protein kinase B **(PKB/Akt).** These pathways mediate the acute effects of EGF stimulation, including actin-based membrane ruffling. PKC also provides negative feedback by phosphorylating growth factor receptors on a serine residue that tends to inactivate them.

Growth factor pathways are double-edged swords. They are essential for normal growth and development, but malfunctions cause disease by inappropriate cellular proliferation. One example is the release of PDGF at the sites of blood vessel injury, where it stimulates proliferation of smooth muscle cells, an early event in the development of **arteriosclerosis.**

Many components of growth factor signaling pathways were discovered during the search for genes that cause cancer. The genes were first identified in cancer-causing viruses as oncogenes responsible for transforming cells in tissue culture. Subsequently, homologues of these genes were found in the normal vertebrate genome, and mutations in these genes were found in human cancers. The products of the normal genes were recognized as components of the growth factor signaling pathway, and the mutant proteins were shown to be constitutively active, so that they produced a continuous positive signal for growth even in the absence of external stimuli (see Chapter 44). For example, the *sis* oncogene is a retroviral homologue of PDGF, the *erbB* oncogene is a homologue of the EGF receptor, and the *raf* oncogene is part of the MAP kinase cascade. As J. Marx put it, "growth pathways are liberally paved with oncogene products."*

Mutations in the Ras gene are widespread in human cancers. For example, point mutations resulting in substitution of valine for glycine-12 constitutively activate Ras by reducing its GTPase activity about 10-fold. This results in an increase in the concentration of active Ras-GTP, sending positive signals for growth down the pathway in the absence of external stimuli.

Ras can sustain an activating signal for some time, as its intrinsic rate of GTP hydrolysis is very low $(0.005 \ s^{-1})$. In contrast to some other G proteins, the GTPase activity is not stimulated by its downstream effector, Raf-1. Active Ras is normally inactivated by a GTPase-activating protein **(Ras-GAP)** that also binds to the receptor and stimulates GTP hydrolysis. Inactivating mutations of GAPs such as NF1 (the gene causing neurofibromatosis, the so-called elephant man disease) predisposes individuals to malignant disease by prolonging the lifetime of activated Ras-GTP.

Although the general features of these vital signaling pathways leading from the cell surface through Ras and MAP kinase to nuclear transcription factors are clear, much more quantitative information is required to understand how they work on a system level. Only then will it be possible to appreciate how much the signal is amplified at each step and how signals are integrated as parts of networks rather than simple linear pathways.

Insulin Pathways to GLUT4 and MAP Kinase

The **insulin receptor tyrosine kinase** not only stimulates the MAP kinase cascade, but it also triggers the

*Marx J: Forging a path to the nucleus. Science 260:1588–1590, 1993.

acute response of muscle and adipose cells to the elevation of blood glucose following a meal (Fig. 29–7). High blood glucose levels stimulate β cells in the islets of Langerhans in the pancreas to secrete insulin, a small protein hormone. Insulin receptors are found on many cells, particularly muscle and fat cells. The insulin receptor is a stable dimer of two identical subunits, each consisting of two polypeptides covalently linked by a disulfide bond. One polypeptide forms the insulin-binding extracellular domain. The other has a single transmembrane helix connected to a cytoplasmic tyrosine kinase domain. Insulin binding changes the conformation of the extracellular domains in a way that brings together the tyrosine kinase domains on the other side of the membrane. The juxtaposed kinases phosphorylate each other's activation loop, thus stimulating kinase activity (see Fig. 27–3D). The kinases propagate the signal by phosphorylating adapter proteins called **IRS (insulin receptor substrates**, isoforms 1–4), **SHC** (for SH2 and collagen-like), and **Cbl.** Each plays a distinct role in the ensuing response. This strategy differs from growth factor receptors, which use phosphotyrosine on the receptor itself to dock SH2-domain effector enzymes. Note that neither the insulin receptor nor IRS1 bind phospholipase Cγ1 or Ras-GAP as do tyrosine-phosphorylated growth factor receptors.

The best known effects of insulin are to stimulate glucose uptake from blood (particularly into skeletal muscle and white fat) and synthesis of glycogen, protein, and lipid. Glucose uptake is accomplished by the glucose carrier, **GLUT4** (see Chapter 8). Resting cells store GLUT4 in the membranes of cytoplasmic vesicles. Insulin stimulates fusion of these vesicles with the plasma membrane, making GLUT4 available to transport glucose into the cell. This membrane fusion event requires two separate signals, both of which are downstream from the insulin receptor. Binding of PI-3 kinase to a particular phosphotyrosine on IRS initiates one signal. PI-3 kinase synthesizes PIP$_3$, which activates the protein kinases PKB/Akt, PKCλ, and PKCζ. Phosphorylation of the adapter protein Cbl initiates the second signal. Cbl activates a nucleotide exchange protein **(guanine nucleotide exchange factor** [GEF]), which activates the small GTPase **TC10.** The three kinases and TC10-GTP cooperate to promote fusion of GLUT4 vesicles with the plasma membrane. Activation of PKB is also thought to initiate another pathway that stimulates the conversion of glucose to its storage form, glycogen. PKB phosphorylates glycogen synthase kinase (GSK) 3. This inhibits GSK3 and results in activation of **glycogen synthase** (the enzyme that makes glycogen) because active GSK3 inhibits glycogen synthase by phosphorylation. Insulin activation of protein phosphatase 1 may also contribute to glycogen synthesis by dephosphorylating glycogen synthase.

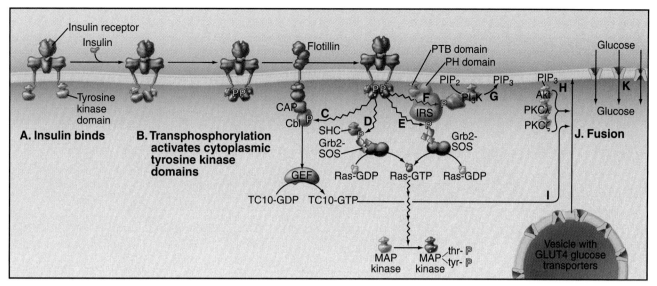

Figure 29-7 Insulin signaling pathways in an adipose cell. Active components are shown in bright colors. *A,* Insulin binds the preformed dimeric receptor, bringing together the tyrosine kinase domains in the cytoplasm. *B,* The tyrosine kinase domains activate each other by transphosphorylation of activation loops (see Fig. 27–3*D*). Receptor kinases then phosphorylate a variety of downstream targets: *C,* the adapter protein Cbl, which activates a nucleotide exchange protein (GEF), which activates the small GTPase TC10; *D,* the adapter protein SHC, which binds Grb2-SOS and slowly initiates the MAP kinase pathway; *E,* the adapter protein IRS, which binds Grb2-SOS and rapidly initiates the MAP kinase pathway; and *F,* another IRS phosphotyrosine binds phosphatidylinositol 3-kinase (PI3K). *G,* PI3K phosphorylates PIP$_2$ to make PIP$_3$. *H,* PIP$_3$ binds and activates several protein kinases: Akt (PKB), PKCλ, and PKCζ. *I,* These kinases, together with activated TC10, stimulate fusion (*J*) of vesicles carrying the glucose transporter, GLUT4 with the plasma membrane. *K,* GLUT4 transports glucose into the cell. CAP binds Cbl to the plasma membrane protein flotillin. The PTB domain of IRS binds phosphotyrosine, and the PH domain binds PIP$_3$.

Insulin is also a growth factor for some cells, acting through the Ras/MAP kinase pathway to nuclear transcription factors. The signaling circuit to Ras has two arms acting on different time scales. The fast pathway, acting within seconds, is through tyrosine phosphorylation of IRS, which binds Grb2-SOS and initiates the MAP kinase pathway. The slow arm, acting over a period of minutes, is through phosphorylation of SHC, which binds larger quantities of Grb2-SOS and slowly initiates a sustained response of the MAP kinase pathway. Other protein hormones, notably, insulin-like growth factor 1, have similar receptors and use IRS1 to channel growth-promoting signals to the nucleus.

T-lymphocyte Pathways through Nonreceptor Tyrosine Kinases

Some signaling pathways that control cellular growth and differentiation operate through **cytoplasmic protein tyrosine kinases** separate from the plasma membrane receptors. The best-characterized pathways control the development and activation of lymphocytes in the immune system. **T lymphocytes** are the example in this section. T lymphocytes defend against intracellular pathogens, such as viruses, and assist B lymphocytes in producing antibodies (Fig. 30–9).

T cells are activated during interactions of cell surface receptors (TCRs) and accessory proteins with peptide antigens bound to histocompatibility proteins on the surface of an antigen-presenting cell (Fig. 29–8). Some interactions of T cells with the antigen-presenting cells are generic; others are specific. These interactions on the surface of the T lymphocyte trigger a network of interactions among protein tyrosine kinases, adapter proteins, and effector proteins on the inner surface of the plasma membrane. Tyrosine phosphorylation of multiple membrane and cytoplasmic proteins activates two separate pathways to the nucleus. One involves a Ca^{2+}-regulated protein serine/threonine phosphatase that leads to the activation of transcription factors. Another activates transcription factors via the Ras/MAP kinase pathway.

The **T-cell antigen receptor** is a complex of eight transmembrane polypeptides (see Fig. 29–8*A*). The α and β chains, each with two extracellular immunoglobulin-like domains, provide antigen-binding specificity. Similar to antibodies, one of these immunoglobulin domains is constant and one is variable in sequence. The genes for T-cell receptors are assembled from separate parts, similar to the rearrangement of antibody genes. Genomic sequences for variable domains are spliced together randomly in developing lymphocytic cells from a panel of sequences, each encoding a small part of the protein. This combinato-

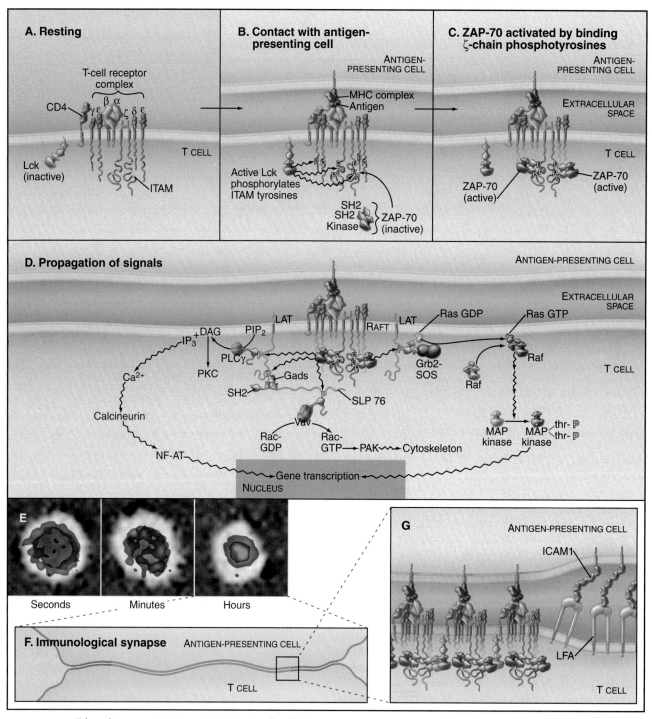

Figure 29-8 T-lymphocyte activation. *A,* Resting T cell with inactive nonreceptor tyrosine kinase Lck and the T-cell receptor complex (TCR) with unphosphorylated cytoplasmic phosphorylation sites (ITAMs). *B,* An encounter with an antigen-presenting cell with an MHC-antigenic peptide complex complementary to the particular TCR initiates signaling. Active Lck phosphorylates various ITAMs. *C,* The nonreceptor tyrosine kinase ZAP-70 is activated by binding via its two SH2 domains to phosphorylated ITAMs on the zeta chains. *D,* Active ZAP-70 phosphorylates various targets, including the transmembrane protein LAT and the adapter protein SLP76, which then propagate the signal. Phospholipase Cγ binds a LAT phosphotyrosine and produces IP$_3$ and DAG. IP$_3$ releases Ca^{2+} from vesicular stores. Ca^{2+} activates calcineurin (protein phosphatase 2B), which activates the latent transcription factor NF-AT. Vav, the nucleotide exchange factor of the small GTPase Rac, is activated by binding to SLP76. Grb2-SOS binds another phosphorylated ITAM and initiates the MAP kinase cascade. *E,* Micrographs of the time course of the interaction of a T cell with an artificial membrane mimicking a specific antigen-presenting cell. Each image is a superimposition interference reflection micrograph showing the closeness of contact as shades of gray (with white being closest apposition) and a fluorescence micrograph showing TCRs in green and ICAM1 in red. The stable arrangement of ICAM1 around concentrated TCRs is called an immunological synapse. *F* and *G,* Drawings of an immunological synapse with a central zone of TCRs bound to MHC complexes and peripheral ICAM1 bound to the integrin LFA. Gads is an adapter protein; RAFT is a lipid raft. (*E,* Courtesy of M. Dustin, New York University)

rial strategy creates a diversity of T-cell antigen receptors, with one type expressed on any given T cell. Variable sequences of α and β chains provide binding sites for a wide range of different peptide antigens bound to proteins, collectively termed the **major histocompatibility complex (MHC)** antigens, and presented on the surface of cells. These peptides are fragments of viral proteins or other foreign matter that have been degraded inside the cell, inserted into compatible MHC molecules during their assembly in the endoplasmic reticulum, and transported to the cell surface. Assembly of T-cell receptors in the endoplasmic reticulum requires six additional transmembrane polypeptides, each with one or more short sequence motifs, called **immunoreceptor tyrosine activation motifs (ITAMs)** in their cytoplasmic domains.

The expression of a single type of α and β chains provides individual T cells with specificity for a particular peptide. Although T-cell antigen receptors bind specifically, their affinity for the complex of peptide and MHC is low (K_d in the range of 10 μM). Given the small number (hundreds) of unique MHC-peptide complexes found on the target cell surface, this low affinity would not be sufficient for a lymphocyte to form a stable complex with an antigen-presenting cell. Accessory proteins called coreceptors, such as **CD4** (the human immunodeficiency virus [HIV] receptor) and **CD8** (see Fig. 32–3), bind directly to any MHC protein and reinforce interaction of the two cells.

Two classes of protein tyrosine kinases are required to transmit a signal from the engaged TCR to effector systems. The first class of kinases, including **Lck** and Fyn, are relatives of the product of Src (see Fig. 27–3E), the first oncogene to be characterized (Box 29–1). These tyrosine kinases are anchored to the plasma membrane by a myristolated N-terminal glycine and inhibited by phosphorylation of a tyrosine near the C-terminus (see Fig. 27–3E). This tyrosine is phosphorylated by a kinase, Csk, and dephosphorylated by the transmembrane protein tyrosine phosphatase, **CD45**. Apparently, CD45 keeps Lck partially dephosphorylated and, therefore, partially active in resting lymphocytes. **ZAP-70** is the most important of the second class of protein tyrosine kinases. Two SH2 domains allow ZAP-70 (zeta associated protein-70kD) to bind tyrosine-phosphorylated ITAMs on ζ chains.

Physical contact of a T lymphocyte with an **antigen-presenting** cell carrying an MHC-peptide specific for its T-cell receptor generates multiple signals as follows:

1. Engagement of TCRs leads to activation of Lck by phosphorylation of its activation loop. The mechanism is still under investigation.
2. Active Lck phosphorylates ITAMs on the several TCR accessory chains.

box 29–1

Src FAMILY OF PROTEIN TYROSINE KINASES

The founding member of the Src family of protein tyrosine kinases has a prominent place in modern biology. During the 1920s, Peyton Rous discovered the first cancer-causing virus, in a mesodermal cancer of chickens called a sarcoma. Later, the Rous sarcoma virus was found to be a retrovirus with an RNA genome. By comparing similar viruses that did not cause cancer, investigators learned that one gene, named *src*, is responsible for transforming cells into cancer cells. Finally, a gene very similar to *src* was found in normal chicken cells. The cellular protein product, c-Src, is a carefully regulated protein tyrosine kinase that participates in the control of cellular proliferation and differentiation. Mutations in the gene for viral *src*, *v-src*, activate its protein product constitutively, driving cells to proliferate and contributing to the development of cancer.

The family of Src-like proteins recognized in vertebrates shares a common structure (see Fig. 27–3E). Five functionally distinct segments are recognized in the sequences. An N-terminal myristic acid anchors the protein to the plasma membrane. Without this modification, the protein is inactive. The next domains are the founding examples of Src homology domains SH3 and SH2 (see Fig. 27–11), which bind proline-rich peptides and peptides containing a phosphorylated tyrosine respectively. The kinase domain is followed by a tyrosine near the C-terminus. Phosphorylation of this tyrosine and its intramolecular binding to the SH2 domain lock the kinase in an inactive conformation. Dephosphorylation of the C-terminal tyrosine and phosphorylation of the activation loop activate the kinase.

Expression of c-Src is highest in brain and platelets, but a null mutation in mice produces relatively few defects, except in bones where a failure of osteoclasts to remodel bone leads to overgrowth, a condition call osteopetrosis (see Chapter 34).

3. ZAP-70 is activated by binding phosphorylated ITAMs.
4. Active ZAP-70 phosphorylates various targets, including the transmembrane protein LAT and the adapter protein SLP76, which then propagate the signal along several branches.
5. Signals reach the nucleus by two pathways. First, phospholipase Cγ1 is activated by binding a phosphotyrosine on LAT and by tyrosine phosphorylation. Active phospholipase Cγ1 produces IP$_3$ and DAG. Release of Ca^{2+} from vesicular stores by IP$_3$ activates **calcineurin** (protein phos-

phatase 2B), which activates the latent transcription factor **NF-AT**. Second, Grb2-SOS binds another phosphotyrosine on LAT and initiates the MAP kinase cascade by activating Ras. The events to this point appear to take place in lipid rafts.

6. The signal reaches the cytoskeleton via Vav, the nucleotide exchange factor of the small GTPase Rac. Vav is activated by binding a phosphotyrosine on the adapter protein SLP76. Rac-GTP activates p21-activated protein kinase (PAK), which stimulates assembly of actin filaments (see Chapter 36).

Massive rearrangement of TCRs and adhesion proteins in the interface between the T cell and the antigen-presenting cells is required to sustain the signal to the T-cell nucleus. This rearrangement can be followed in real time by fluorescence microscopy (see Fig. 29–8E). When a T cell initially contacts an antigen-presenting cell, TCRs spread around the periphery of a region of contact mediated by immunoglobulin-cellular adhesion molecules (ICAMs) on the antigen-presenting cell and integrins (LFA) on the T cell. With time, these zones reverse positions, yielding a stable **"immunological synapse"** with the plasma membranes of the two cells in close contact in a central region where TCRs are bound to MHC-peptides. This zone is surrounded by a ring of adhesion molecules (see Fig. 29–8F and G). The concentrated assembly of engaged TCRs generates a long-term signal to the nucleus.

The best available **immunosuppressive drugs** used in human organ transplantation block lymphocyte proliferation by inhibiting calcineurin, the phosphatase that activates NF-AT. When given within 1 hour of the stimulus, these drugs completely block T-cell activation, but they have little effect after several hours once the genetic program has been initiated. **Cyclosporin** and FK506 bind to separate cytoplasmic proteins, cyclophilin, and FK-binding protein. Both of these drug-protein complexes bind calcineurin and inhibit phosphatase activity. Considering that many cells express calcineurin, the effects of these drugs on lymphocytes is amazingly specific, with relatively few side effects. Specificity arises from the low concentration of calcineurin in lymphocytes: only 10,000 molecules in T cells compared with 300,000 in other cells. Hence, low concentrations of inhibitor can selectively block calcineurin in T lymphocytes. Cyclosporin is an agent that has made human heart and liver transplantation feasible.

The response to T-cell receptor activation depends upon the particular state of differentiation of the T cell that encounters its partner antigenic peptide. Stimulation causes some T cells to secrete toxic peptides that kill the antigen-presenting cell, others to synthesize and secrete lymphokines (immune system hormones), others to proliferate and differentiate, and yet others to commit to apoptosis.

Cytokine Receptor, JAK/STAT Pathways

A large number of polypeptide hormones and growth factors (collectively called **cytokines;** see Fig. 26–6) stimulate cells by binding plasma membrane receptors that lack intrinsic enzymatic activity. The receptors are linked to the activation of **signal transducers and activators of transcription (STATs)**—mobile, cytoplasmic transcription factors—by the **JAK** family of protein tyrosine kinases (see explanation of acronym that follows). The three-component relay from cytokine receptor to JAK to STAT is the most direct signal transduction pathway for extracellular growth factors to the nucleus (Fig. 29–9).

Two families of cytokine receptors (see Fig. 26–6) bind and activate a member of the JAK family protein tyrosine kinases. These kinases were originally given the lighthearted name "*just another kinase*" (JAK). In view of their pivotal role between diverse receptors and transcription factors, the more pretentious name *Janus kinase* (for the Greek god who opens doors) has been suggested. Some cytokine receptors bind a single type of JAK; others are promiscuous. JAKs are massive compared with many other kinases. The active kinase domain is located near the C-terminus next to a kinase-like domain that lacks key residues required for kinase activity. In their N-terminal halves, most JAKs share several short regions of sequence homology with each other. The N-terminal half and kinase-like domain mediate association of JAKs with activated receptors.

The seven members of the STAT family are controlled by tyrosine phosphorylation and cellular targeting. Cytoplasmic STATs cannot enter the nucleus until they are phosphorylated on a conserved tyrosine located near the C-terminus. The atomic structure of a STAT dimer bound to DNA has revealed how phosphorylation allows reciprocal interaction of the key phosphotyrosine with an SH2 domain on the partner STAT. Active dimers can then enter the nucleus and bind to specific promoter sequences. The signal moves from the cytokine receptor to the nucleus as follows:

1. Ligand binding to the extracellular domain of a cytokine receptor rearranges the extracellular domains and brings the cytoplasmic domains close together. Atomic structures of the extracellular domain of the human erythropoietin receptor (see Fig. 26–6) with and without ligand suggests that the inactive receptor dimer is preformed in the membrane.

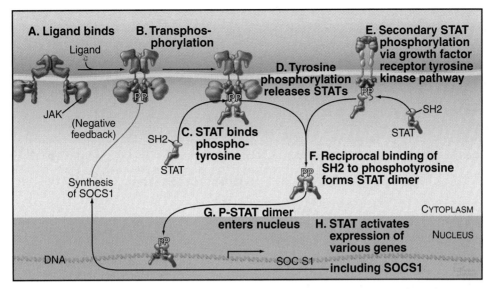

Figure 29-9 Cytokine JAK/STAT signaling pathway. *A,* Cytokine binds a preformed receptor dimer (see Fig. 26–7), bringing together the cytoplasmic domains with a bound tyrosine kinase, JAK. *B,* JAKs activate each other by transphosphorylation and then phosphorylate the tyrosines on the receptor. *C,* The SH2 domain of the latent transcription factor STAT binds a receptor phosphotyrosine. *D,* JAK phosphorylates the STATs, which then dissociate from the receptor. *E,* Growth factor receptor tyrosine kinases can also activate STATs. *F,* The STATs form an active dimer by reciprocal SH2-phosphotyrosine interactions. *G,* The STAT dimer enters the nucleus. *H,* The STAT dimer activates the expression of various genes. One of these genes encodes SOCS1, which creates negative feedback by inhibiting further STAT activation.

2. Juxtaposition of the cytoplasmic domains allows the associated JAKs to activate each other by transphosphorylation. JAKs also phosphorylate tyrosines on the cytoplasmic tails of the receptors.

3. When the SH2 domain of the latent transcription factor STAT binds a receptor phosphotyrosine, JAK phosphorylates the STAT.

4. Phosphorylated STAT dissociates from the receptor and forms an active dimer by reciprocal interactions between the SH2 domain of one partner and a phosphotyrosine of the other partner.

5. Active STAT dimers enter the nucleus and activate expression of various genes.

6. A slowly acting, negative feedback loop limits the duration of the response. One of the genes expressed in response to STAT encodes SOCS1. Once synthesized, the SOCS1 protein inhibits further STAT activation by interaction with the cytokine receptor.

Active STAT dimers are either homodimers or heterodimers of two different STATs. A variety of STATs, with some unique and some common subunits, bind regulatory sites on the family of genes required to activate the target cells. Selective expression of cytokine receptors, JAKs, and STATs in specific target cells and selective activation of specific STATs by each JAK explain why different cell types respond uniquely to various cytokines. The products of genes controlled by STATs are generally used for differentiated cellular functions rather than for control of proliferation. Accordingly, JAKs and STATs are not known to be proto-oncogenes, like so many components in the growth factor signaling pathways.

The three-component pathway from a cytokine receptor to JAK to activated STAT is appealing in its simplicity, but in reality, the response may be complicated by converging signals from growth factor receptors and a diverging pathway to Ras. EGF- and PDGF-receptors can phosphorylate and activate STATs. This provides a second input to STAT-responsive genes. Further, some cytokine receptors may activate the Ras pathway through Shc and Grb2-SOS.

Serine/Threonine Kinase Receptor Pathways Through Smads

Three families of dimeric polypeptide growth factors, **activins, bone morphogenetic proteins,** and **transforming growth factor-β (TGF-β)** (see Chapter 26) specify developmental fates during embryogenesis and control cellular differentiation in adults. All activate a short pathway consisting of **receptor serine/threonine kinases** and a family of at least 10 different mobile transcription factors called **Smads.** The receptors consist of two types of subunits (called RI and RII) that are activated by ligand binding and transphosphorylation (see Fig. 26–9). Active receptors

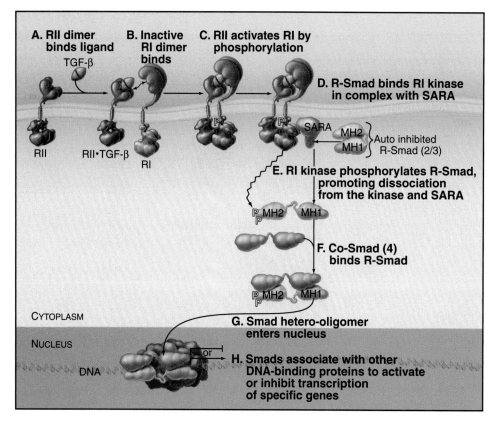

A. RII dimer binds ligand

TGF-β

RII

B. Inactive RI dimer binds

RII·TGF-β

RI

C. RII activates RI by phosphorylation

D. R-Smad binds RI kinase in complex with SARA

SARA

MH2
MH1 } Auto inhibited R-Smad (2/3)

E. RI kinase phosphorylates R-Smad, promoting dissociation from the kinase and SARA

MH2   MH1

F. Co-Smad (4) binds R-Smad

MH2   MH1

CYTOPLASM

G. Smad hetero-oligomer enters nucleus

NUCLEUS

DNA

or

H. Smads associate with other DNA-binding proteins to activate or inhibit transcription of specific genes

Figure 29–10 TGF-β/Smad signaling pathway. *A,* TGF-β binds a dimer of RII receptors. *B,* This is followed by association with a dimer of RI receptors. *C,* RII phosphorylates and activates RI. *D,* An autoinhibited R-Smad binds RI in a complex with the adapter SARA. *E,* RI kinase phosphorylates R-Smad, which promotes dissociation. *F,* Co-Smad binds to R-Smad. *G,* The Smad heterodimer enters the nucleus. *H,* The Smad heterodimer associates with other DNA-binding proteins to activate or inhibit transcription of specific genes.

phosphorylate regulated Smads (R-Smads), such as Smad2 and Smad3. These phosphorylated R-Smads form active heterodimers with Smad4, called a co-Smad because it is not subjected to phosphorylation itself. Other Smads regulate these pathways by inhibiting phosphorylation of R-Smads. After activation of a receptor, information is transmitted to the nucleus as follows (Fig. 29–10):

1. An autoinhibited R-Smad binds an activated RI receptor in a complex with an adapter protein called SARA.
2. Active RI receptor kinase phosphorylates the R-Smad.
3. Phosphorylated R-Smad dissociates from RI and binds co-Smad4.
4. The R-Smad/co-Smad heterodimer enters the nucleus and associates with other DNA binding proteins to activate or inhibit transcription of specific genes.

The Smad pathway activated by TGF-β regulates cellular proliferation and differentiation of many cell types, including epithelial and hematopoietic cells. TGF-β stimulation stops the cell cycle in G1 by promoting expression of negative regulators of cyclin-dependent kinases (see Chapter 44). Homozygous mutations in genes for the components of their TGF pathway cause death of mice during embryonic development. Mutations in the genes for TGF-β receptors

or Smads appear in up to 50% of some types of human tumors. Mutations in an accessory receptor for TGF-β (endoglin) cause malformed blood vessels in the human disease hereditary hemorrhagic telangiectasia.

Two-Component Phosphotransfer Systems

Prokaryotes, fungi, and plants transduce stimuli ranging from nutrients to osmotic pressure using signaling systems consisting of as few as two proteins, a receptor-linked histidine kinase, and a "response regulator" activated by phosphorylation of an aspartic acid (Box 29–2; Fig. 29–11*D*). Such "two-component" systems from bacteria are the only signaling pathways in which the atomic structures of all the components are known and the dynamics of information transfer are reasonably well understood. Extensive collections of mutants in these pathways and sensitive single-cell assays for responses, such as flagellar rotation, provide tools for rigorous tests of concepts derived from biochemical experiments on isolated components.

For years, two-component systems appeared to be restricted to prokaryotes, but response regulators eventually were discovered in yeast and plants. Eubacteria have genes for up to 70 response regulators with 32 response regulators and 30 histidine kinases in

Escherichia coli. Archaea have genes for up to 24 response regulators. The slime mold *Dictyostelium* has more than 10 histidine kinases, whereas fungi have just one or two of these systems. Plants use a two-component system to regulate fruit ripening in response to the gas ethylene.

Bacterial Chemotaxis

The two-component system regulating bacterial chemotaxis (Fig. 29–12) is the best understood signaling pathway of any kind. *E. coli* cells use five types of plasma membrane receptors to sense a variety of different chemicals. These receptors are also called methyl-accepting chemotaxis proteins as they are regulated by methylation. The most abundant, with about 2000 copies per cell, is Tar (see Fig. 29–11*A* and *B*), the receptor for the nutrients aspartic acid (D) and maltose, protons (as part of pH sensing), temperature, and the repellent nickel. Tar is concentrated at one end of the cell (see Fig. 29–12*A*). Clustering facilitates interactions between receptor molecules, but this polarized distribution has nothing to do with sensing the direction of chemical gradients.

The chemotactic signaling system guides swimming bacteria toward attractive chemicals and away from repellents in a biased random walk. Environmental chemicals influence the behavior of the cell by biasing the direction that the rotary flagellar motor turns (see Figs. 41–19 and 41–20 for details on the motor itself). In its default mode, the motor turns counterclockwise and the bacterium swims smoothly in a more or less linear path. When the flagella turn the other way, the bacterium tumbles about in one place. A **tumble** allows a bacterium to reorient its direction randomly, so that when it resumes **smooth swimming**, it usually heads off in a new direction. In the absence of chemoattractants, bacteria swim for about 0.9 seconds and then tumble for about 0.1 seconds, allowing for random reorientations every second.

A gradient of chemical attractant promotes the length of runs up the gradient by suppressing tumbling (see Fig. 29–12*D*). A two-component signaling pathway controls the frequency of tumbling. The degree of saturation of the flagellar motor with the response regulator CheY determines which way it rotates.

Ligand-free Tar stimulates the phosphorylation of the associated histidine kinase CheA. ("Che" refers to a gene required for chemotaxis, as most of these components were discovered by mutagenesis. (A lowercase "p" represents the shorthand for phosphorylation in these bacterial systems.) CheAp activates the response regulator, CheY, by transferring phosphate from histidine to D57 of CheY. CheYp has a higher affinity for the flagellar motor than CheY, and ligand-free receptor maintains an equilibrium with the rotors partially saturated with CheYp. With several bound CheYps, the motor reverses from its free-running, counterclockwise state about 10% of the time, inducing a brief tumble about once per second.

Information about aspartate in the environment flows rapidly through the pathway as changes in the *concentrations* of the phosphorylated species CheAp and CheYp. A key point is that Tar with bound aspartate, Tar-D, does not activate histidine phosphorylation of CheA. Hence asparate binding to Tar reduces the saturation of the flagellar motors with CheYp and the frequency of tumbles.

For the cell to respond to aspartate on a subsecond time scale, an accessory protein, **CheZ,** is required to increase the rate of CheYp dephosphorylation more than 100-fold from its slow spontaneous rate of 0.03 s^{-1}. Given this fast dissipation of CheYp, maintenance of a tumbling rate of about 1 s^{-1}, in the absence of an attractant, requires constant flow of phosphate from ATP to CheAp to CheYp (Fig. 29–13*A*). (In most other two-component pathways, dephosphorylation of the response regulator is much slower, allowing responses over a period of minutes rather than milliseconds.) The following sections examine chemotaxis on the system level, starting with the response to a rapid change in concentration of aspartate.

Temporal Sensing of Gradients

Bacteria are too small and move too fast to detect a spatial gradient directly. Instead, they sense the gradient as a *change in concentration of attractant or repellent as a function of time*. When a bacterium swims up a gradient of chemoattractant, the concentration of attractant increases with time and the signaling mechanism suppresses tumbling. This biases movement toward the attractant. When a cell swims down the gradient, tumbling is more frequent.

A sudden increase in the concentration of aspartate yields a smooth swimming response within 200 msec due to rapid re-equilibration of the concentrations of all of the cytoplasmic signaling components (see Fig. 29–13*B*). Aspartate binds Tar and inhibits autophosphorylation of CheA. Because CheYp has a half-life <100 msec, the concentrations of CheAp and CheYp decrease rapidly. CheYp dissociates from the flagellar motor and the motor persists in the counterclockwise, smooth swimming direction. If the concentration change with time is due to a gradient of aspartate, the bacterium tends to swim steadily up the gradient toward the source.

The opposite sequence of events takes place if a bacterium swims down a gradient of aspartate. The fraction of Tar with bound aspartate declines, CheAp and CheYp concentrations rise, and tumbling is more frequent, providing opportunities to reorient and swim back up the gradient.

box 29–2

TWO-COMPONENT SIGNALING

Two-component receptors may include either a cytoplasmic histidine kinase domain (see Fig. 29–11C) or they may bind a separate histidine kinase, like the aspartate chemotactic receptor **Tar** (Fig. 29–11B). Tar consists of two identical subunits. Three of these dimers are thought to be anchored at their bases in the cytoplasm (see Fig. 29–11B). Binding of aspartic acid between the extracellular domains of two subunits changes their orientation by a few degrees. Transmission of this conformational change across the membrane alters the activity of **CheA,** a histidine kinase associated with the most distal cytoplasmic domains of the receptor.

Histidine kinases have a conserved catalytic domain of about 350 residues that is structurally unrelated to eukaryotic serine/threonine/tyrosine kinases. Another domain allows them to form homodimers. Histidine kinases are incorporated into a wide variety of proteins, including transmembrane receptors (see Fig. 29–11C) and cytoplasmic proteins with a variety of accessory domains such as CheA (see Fig. 29–11B). The catalytic domain transfers the γ-phosphate from ATP to just one substrate, a histidine residue of its homodimeric partner. This histidine is usually located in the dimerization domain.

All **response regulators** have a domain of about 120 residues folded like **CheY** (see Figs. 3–11 and 29–11B). Transfer of phosphate from the phosphohistidine of a kinase to an invariant aspartic acid changes the conformation of the response regulator. Most response regulators are larger than CheY, having C-terminal effector domains like CheB (see Fig. 29–11B) and OmpR (see Fig. 29–11C). Many effector domains, including OmpR, bind DNA and regulate transcription of specific genes when the response regulator is activated by aspartate phosphorylation. Other response regulators are included as a domain of the histidine kinase itself.

Reversible phosphorylation transfers information through two-component systems. The mechanism differs fundamentally from eukaryotic kinase cascades, which transfer phosphate from ATP to serine, threonine, or tyrosine, forming phosphoesters at every step. By contrast, two-component systems first transfer a phosphate from ATP to a protein histidine. The first component then donates this high-energy phosphate to an aspartic acid on a response regulator (RR):

$$\text{ATP} + \text{kinase-his} \rightleftharpoons \text{ADP} + \text{kinase-his}\sim\text{P}$$
$$\text{kinase-his}\sim\text{P} + \text{RR-asp} \rightleftharpoons \text{kinase-his} + \text{RR*-asp}\sim\text{P}$$
$$\text{RR*-asp}\sim\text{P} + \text{H}_2\text{O} \rightleftharpoons \text{RR-asp} + \text{phosphate}$$

The high-energy his~P phosphoramidate bond is unstable, and the phosphate is readily transferred to the side chain of an aspartic acid of the response regulator.

Phosphorylation activates response regulators (RR*) by changing their conformation. Details differ depending on the response regulator. In the case of OmpR, phosphorylation relieves autoinhibition of the DNA binding domain (see Fig. 29–11C). Phosphorylation of CheY reveals a binding site for the flagellar rotor. The signal dissipates by dephosphorylation of the response regulator, either by autocatalysis or stimulation by accessory proteins. Lifetimes of the high-energy aspartic acylphosphate vary from seconds to hours.

A minimal two-component system, such as a bacterial osmoregulatory pathway (see Fig. 29–11C) consists of a dimeric plasma membrane receptor with a cytoplasmic histidine kinase domain and a cytoplasmic response regulator protein. Signal transduction is carried out in four steps. A change in osmolarity alters the conformation of the receptor, activating the kinase activity of its cytoplasmic domain. The kinase phosphorylates a histidine residue on the other subunit of the dimeric receptor. This phosphate is transferred from the receptor to an aspartic acid side chain of the response regulator protein OmpR. Phosphorylation changes the conformation of the response regulator domain of OmpR, allowing its DNA-binding domain to activate the expression of certain genes.

box 29–2

TWO-COMPONENT SIGNALING *Continued*

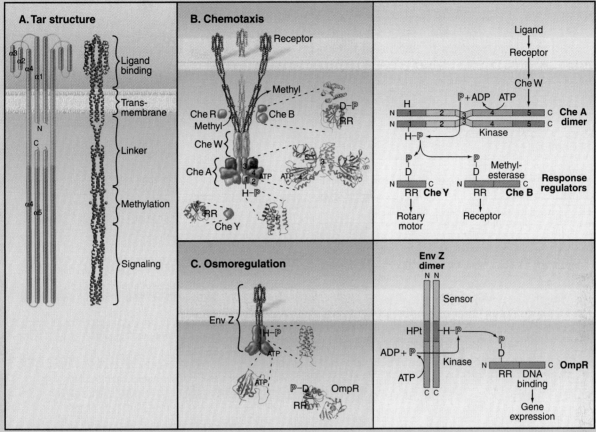

Figure 29–11 Two-component bacterial signaling systems. *A*, Atomic model of the aspartate receptor, Tar. The atomic structures of the extracellular and cytoplasmic domains were determined by x-ray crystallography. The transmembrane α-helices are models based on the primary structure. The two polypeptides are shown in red and blue. Each polypeptide starts in the cytoplasm and passes twice through the lipid bilayer. *B*, Bacterial chemotaxis. Scale models of the molecular components and pathway of information transfer. The domains shown on the right are color coded in the molecular models on the left. An accessory protein, CheW, facilitates binding of the histidine kinase CheA to the aspartate receptor, Tar. CheY and CheB are response regulators. CheR is a methyl transferase. *C*, Bacterial osmoregulation. The histidine kinase forms the cytoplasmic domain of the receptor. OmpR is the response regulator with a DNA-binding domain. Scale models of the molecules *(left)* and pathway of information transfer *(right)*. (*A*, Modified from material provided courtesy of S. H. Kim, University of California, Berkeley; Reference: Kim KK, Yokata H, Kim SH: Four helical-bundle structure of the cytoplasmic domain of a serine chemotaxis receptor. Nature 400:787–792, 1999; PDB file: 1QU7. *B* and *C*, Based on material supplied courtesy of A. M. Stock, HHMI and Robert Wood Johnson Medical School; Reference: Stock AM, Robinson WL, Goudreau PN: Two-component signal transduction. Annu Rev Biochem 69:183–215, 2000.)

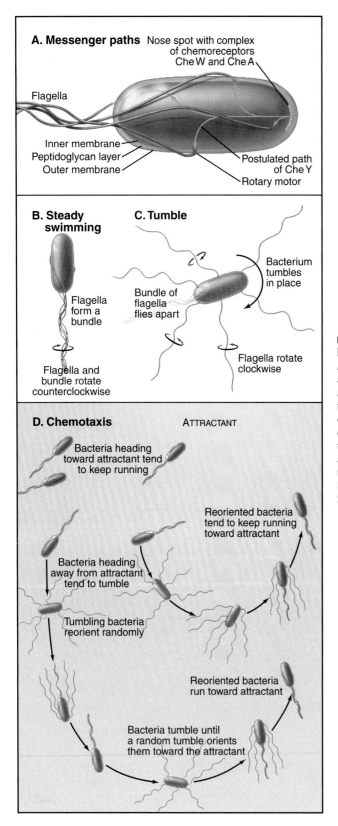

Figure 29-12 Motility of bacteria is determined by the direction of rotation of their flagella. *A*, Arrangement of signal transduction components and flagella in *Escherichia coli*. *B*, Flagella that are rotating counterclockwise (viewed from the tip of the flagella) form a bundle that pushes the cell smoothly forward. *C*, When flagella rotate clockwise, the bundle flies apart and the cell tumbles in place. *D*, An attractive chemical biases movement toward its source by modulating the frequency of runs and tumbles. (*A*, Reference: Parkinson JS, Blair DF. Does *E. coli* have a nose? Science 257:1702, 1993.)

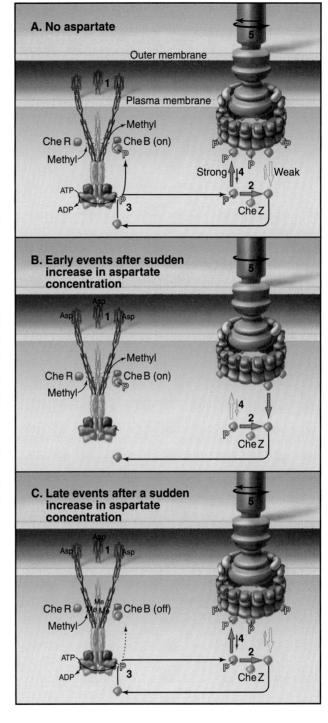

Figure 29-13 Signaling during bacterial chemotaxis. *A,* Absence of aspartate. (1) Ligand-free Tar allows (3) CheA to phosphorylate CheY and CheB. (2) Constant dephosphorylation of CheYp drives a cycle of phosphorylation. (4) The steady-state concentration of CheYp keeps the motor partially saturated. (5) The partially saturated motor turns counterclockwise 90% of the time (runs, *thick arrow*) and clockwise 10% of the time (tumbles, *thin arrow*). *B,* Rapid response to the presence of aspartate. (1) Aspartate binding turns off Tar. (2) Constant dephosphorylation depletes CheYp on a time scale of tens of milliseconds. (4) CheYp dissociates from the motor. (5) The motor, without CheYp, rotates counterclockwise, so the bacterium runs continuously. *C,* Slower, adaptive response to the presence of aspartate. (1) Inactive CheA stops phosphorylating CheB, allowing dephosphorylation of CheBp on a time scale of seconds. This inactivates CheB, allowing net methylation of Tar by CheR. (2) Even with bound aspartate, methylated Tar is partially active, allowing phosphorylation of CheA. (3) CheY is phosphorylated. (4) CheYp rebinds the motor. (5) The flagella turns clockwise part of the time, causing occasional tumbles.

Adaptation

After a step change in aspartate, bacteria respond quickly with smooth swimming, but within tens of seconds to minutes, they return to their normal pattern of intermittent tumbling. In fact, the steady-state tumbling frequency is independent of the concentration of aspartate. This remarkable capacity to adapt is accomplished by a negative feedback loop provided by reversible **methylation** of the receptor (see Fig.

29–13*C*). Methylated Tar has a somewhat lower affinity for aspartate than Tar, but Me-Tar with bound aspartate is more effective at stimulating CheA phosphorylation than Tar with bound aspartate.

Two relatively slow enzymes determine the level of Tar methylation (see Fig. 29–11*B*). **CheR** adds methyls to four glutamic acid residues on each receptor polypeptide, whereas **CheB** removes them. CheR is constitutively active, but sensitive to the overall metabolic state of the cell, as it depends on the concentration of S-adenosyl methionine, a methyl donor used in many metabolic reactions.

A variable rate of demethylation determines the level of Tar methylation. CheB methylesterase is a response regulator activated by phosphorylation by CheAp. CheB is autoinhibited by its response regulator domain blocking the active site. Phosphorylation displaces the response regulator domain from the active site, making CheBp much more active than CheB.

Adaptation occurs because aspartate binding to Tar activates two different pathways *on different time scales*. On a *millisecond* time scale, the concentrations of both CheAp and CheYp decline, CheYp dissociates from the motor, and the cell swims smoothly. The rapid reduction in CheAp also reduces the concentration of CheBp, but on a *second* time scale, as the rate of CheBp dephosphorylation is only 0.1 s^{-1}. The slow decline in CheBp gradually reduces methylesterase activity and results in a higher level of Tar methylation. This, in turn, allows the receptor, still saturated with aspartate, to reactivate CheA phosphorylation. Remarkably, the cell returns exactly to its prestimulus frequencies of runs and tumbles. This **robust adaptation** mechanism is an integral feedback system, just like a thermostat on a heater. Both methylation and demethylation are sensitive to the conformation of the receptor, so another level of complexity contributes to the capacity of the system to adapt.

Extended Range of Response

An amazing feature of this system is its ability to respond with fast changes in flagellar rotation and slow adaptation to changes in aspartate concentration of *just a few percentage points* over a range of five orders of magnitude! Clearly, a simple bimolecular reaction of aspartate with Tar cannot change the fractional saturation of Tar over such an extended range of concentrations. This extended range of sensitivity is valuable for the survival of the bacterium and must depend on some sort of amplification at the level of the receptor. The mechanism is not proven, but an attractive proposal is that aspartate binding to one Tar activates many surrounding Tars in the receptor clusters at the end of the cell.

Bacterial chemotaxis illustrates some of the classical features of signaling pathways, including high sensitivity secondary to amplification at the level of CheA phosphorylation, negative feedback through methylation of Tar, and branching networks that respond on different time scales to the same stimulus. The mechanism has been tested thoroughly by mutating all of the signaling components and observing the consequences. For example, loss of either CheA or CheY results in smooth running bacteria. Cells without CheZ

respond slowly to a change in aspartate. Loss of CheR and CheB results in bacteria that respond to signals over a limited range of concentration but are unable to adapt to them.

▌ Selected Readings

Armitage JP: Bacterial tactic responses. Adv Microb Physiol 41:229–289, 1999.

Attisano L, Wrana JL: Smads as transcriptional co-modulators. Curr Opin Cell Biol 12:235–243, 2000.

Blobe GC, Shiemann WP, Lodish HF: Role of transforming growth factor β in human disease. N Engl J Med 342:1350–1358, 2000.

Burack WR, Shaw AS: Signal transduction: Hanging on a scaffold. Curr Opin Cell Biol 12:211–216, 2000.

Darnell JE: STATs and gene regulation. Science 277:1630–1635, 1977.

Garrington TP, Johnson GL: Organization and regulation of mitogen-activated protein kinase signaling pathways. Curr Opin Cell Biol 11:211–218, 1999.

Grakoui A, Bromley SK, Sumen C, et al: The immunological synapse: A molecular machine controlling T cell activation. Science 285:221–226, 1999.

Ihle JN: The Stat family in cytokine signaling. Curr Opin Cell Biol 13:211–217, 2001.

Insel PA: Adrenergic receptors—Evolving concepts and clinical implications. N Engl J Med 334:580–585, 1996.

Kane LP, Lin J, Weiss A: Signal transduction by the TCR for antigen. Curr Opin Immunol 12:242–249, 2000.

Mombaerts P: Seven-transmembrane proteins as odorant and chemosensory receptors. Science 286:707–711, 1999. (See also related articles in same issue.)

Myung PS, Boerthe NJ, Koretzky GA: Adapter proteins in lymphocyte antigen-receptor signaling. Curr Opin Immunol 12:256–266, 2000.

Ottensmeyer FP, Beniac DR, Luo R Z-T, Yip C: Mechanism of transmembrane signaling: Insulin binding and the insulin receptor. Biochemistry 39:12103–12112, 2000.

Palczewski K, Kumasaka T, Hori T, et al: Crystal structure of rhodopsin: A G protein–coupled receptor. Science 289:739–745, 2000.

Pitcher JA, Freedman NJ, Lefkowitz RJ: G protein–coupled receptor kinases. Annu Rev Biochem 67:653–692, 1998.

Rieke F, Baylor DA: Single photon detection by rod cells of the retina. Rev Mod Physics 70:1027–1036, 1998.

Stock AM, Robinson VL, Goudreau PN: Two-component signal transduction. Annu Rev Biochem 69:183–215, 2000.

Whitehead JP, Clark SF, Urso B, James DE: Signalling through the insulin receptor. Curr Opin Cell Biol 12:222–228, 2000.

Whitmarsh AJ, Davis RJ: Structural organization of MAP-kinase signaling modules by scaffold proteins in yeast and mammals. Trends Biochem Sci 23:481–485, 1998.

Wilkinson MG, Millar JBA: Control of the eukaryotic cell cycle by MAP kinase signaling pathways. FASEB J 14:2147–2157, 2000.

CELLULAR INTERACTIONS AND THE EXTRACELLULAR MATRIX

chapter 30

CELLS OF THE
EXTRACELLULAR MATRIX

Most cells, even unicellular organisms, require molecular mechanisms to adhere to other cells and objects that they encounter in their environments. Unicellular algae and yeast adhere to each other during mating. Amoebae and white blood cells bind microorganisms that they engulf by phagocytosis (see Chapter 23). Slime mold amoebae adhere to each other as they develop into fruiting bodies. Platelets adhere to each other during the repair of damage to small blood vessels and blood clotting. Epithelial cells bind tightly to the underlying extracellular matrix, as well as to each other, to form semipermeable barriers between compartments in organs of higher organisms (see Chapter 33). Nerve cells establish complex interactions with other nerve cells and muscle cells to receive and transmit nerve impulses (see Chapter 10). Muscle cells apply force to each other and the extracellular matrix when they contract (see Chapter 42).

Remarkably, much of cellular adhesion is explained by just a few classes of cellular adhesion molecules, membrane glycoproteins that make specific interactions with complementary proteins on the surface of target cells. Each class is represented by numerous isoforms. Expression of a limited repertoire of adhesion protein isoforms allows differentiated cells of multicellular organisms to establish specific interactions with appropriate partner cells while avoiding inappropriate interactions with other cells.

Cells in tissues of multicellular organisms also interact with an extracellular matrix composed of fibrous proteins, linker proteins, and complex polysaccharides. Connective tissue fibroblasts, epithelial cells, muscle cells, and neurons secrete collagen fibrils, elastic fibers, adhesion proteins, and complex polysaccharides that constitute this extracellular matrix (Fig. 30–1). In the simplest case, a thin layer of matrix, called the basal lamina, surrounds muscle cells and provides

a sort of rug beneath epithelia (see Chapter 31). Basal laminae are so inconspicuous that they are difficult to detect by light microscopy. On the other hand, tendons, ligaments, and some layers of the intestinal wall are largely composed of massive collagen fibrils with relatively few cells. Cellulose-based cell walls of plants, algae, and fungi serve an equivalent purpose in supporting their cells and tissues.

The abundance, organization, and proportions of macromolecular components determine the mechanical properties of the extracellular matrix (Fig. 30–2): skin and blood vessels are resilient because of numerous elastic fibers; tendons have great tensile strength owing to collagen; and bone is incompressible and rigid because of its calcified collagen matrix. Extracellular matrix supports specialized and relatively defenseless epithelial, neuronal, and muscle cells in various organs. On the level of gross anatomy, cells and fibers form fascia, tendons, cartilages, and bones that support the organs of the body.

The extracellular matrix also provides an arena for cellular defense systems. Specialized "professional" phagocytic cells and immune system cells roam connective tissue to find foreign cells and other matter in organs throughout the body. Connective tissue also provides avenues for communication and supply within the body. Both the circulatory system and the peripheral nervous system run through connective tissue compartments of each organ. The vascular system transports phagocytic and immune system cells to sites where they are needed for defense.

This chapter introduces the cells found in the extracellular matrix of animals. The following chapters cover the molecules of the extracellular matrix and the membrane adhesion proteins that enable cells to bind to each other and to the extracellular matrix. Chapters 32 to 34 illustrate how these molecules are used dur-

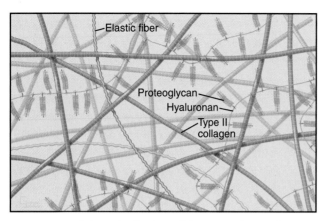

Figure 30-1 Schematic drawing of the major classes of macromolecules in the extracellular matrix: collagen fibrils, elastic fibrils, hyaluronan (a polysaccharide), and proteoglycans (proteins with polysaccharide side chains).

ing embryonic development, formation of epithelia, assembly of specialized forms of connective tissue, wound healing, and blood clotting.

▍ Two Classes of Connective Tissue Cells

A remarkable variety of specialized cells populate the connective tissues of multicellular organisms. These cells manufacture extracellular matrix, defend against infection, and maintain energy stores in the form of lipid (Fig. 30–3). Some of these cells arise in connec-

tive tissue and remain there. They are called **indigenous cells**. The origins of the remaining cells are more complicated as they arise elsewhere, travel transiently through blood and lymph, and enter connective tissue as needed. These cells are known as **immigrants**.

Indigenous Connective Tissue Cells

Primitive Mesenchymal Cells

Primitive mesenchymal cells are undifferentiated, multipotential stem cells that proliferate and differentiate (see Fig. 30–3) to give rise to all of the indigenous cells of connective tissue (fibroblasts, fat cells, mast cells, chondrocytes, and osteoblasts). Small numbers of these inconspicuous precursor cells hide along the small blood vessels but cannot be identified by light microscopy. By electron microscopy (Fig. 30–4B), they resemble fibroblasts, but with minimal organelles of the secretory pathway.

Fibroblasts

Fibroblasts are the connective tissue workhorses, synthesizing and secreting most of the macromolecules of the extracellular matrix (Fig. 30–4). Accordingly, mature fibroblasts have abundant rough endoplasmic reticulum and a large Golgi apparatus. They are generally spindle-shaped, with an oval, flattened nucleus. The migratory patterns of the fibroblasts determine the patterns of collagen fibrils in tissues. In response to tissue damage, fibroblasts proliferate and

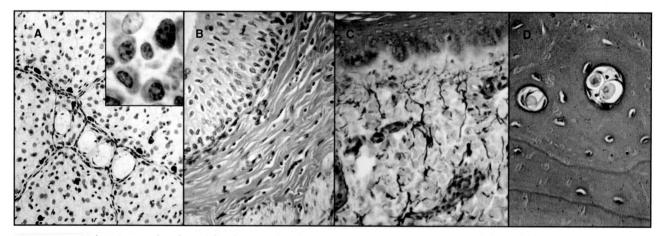

Figure 30-2 Light micrographs of specialized connective tissues. *A*, Loose connective tissue with limited fibers and many cells. Darkly staining mast cells are found along the small blood vessels. The clear ovals are fat cells. The inset shows several plasma cells and one eosinophil with bright red cytoplasmic granules. *B*, Dense connective tissue from the wall of the urethra. Transitional epithelium fills the upper left quadrant. The dense connective tissue consists of wavy fibers of collagen, stained pink, and fibroblasts, identifiable by their purple nuclei. Smooth muscle fills the lower right corner. *C*, Elastic connective tissue in the skin contrasted with a special purple stain for elastic fibrils. Collagen is stained yellow. Stratified squamous epithelium is at the top. *D*, Bone with a few osteocytes embedded in the solid extracellular matrix of calcified collagen. The bone matrix is stained pink. The nuclei of osteocytes are purple. Haversian canals contain small blood vessels. (Micrographs courtesy of D. W. Fawcett, Harvard Medical School.)

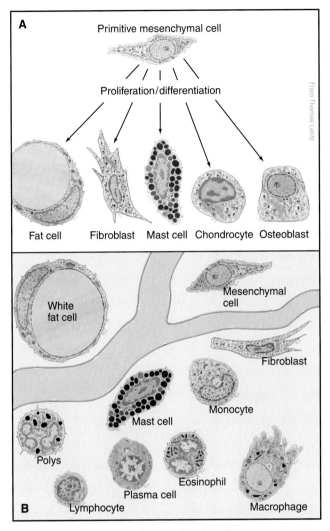

Figure 30–3 Connective tissue cells. *A,* Indigenous connective tissue cells all originate from a stem cell called a primitive mesenchymal cell. *B,* Schematic diagram of connective tissue near a small blood vessel showing indigenous cells in blue and immigrant cells in green. Polys, polymorphonuclear leukocytes.

migrate into the wound where they synthesize new matrix to restore the integrity of the tissue (see Fig. 34–11).

Mast Cells

Mast cells are secretory cells that mediate "immediate hypersensitivity" reactions by secreting histamine-containing granules in response to insect bites or exposure to allergens, as occurs in hay fever. Mast cells distribute along blood vessels in connective tissue (Fig. 30–5). The large, abundant **granules** contain, by mass, 30% heparin–basic protein complex, 10% **histamine,** and 35% basic proteins, including proteases. A variety of stimuli can induce secretion of the granule contents. The most specific stimulus operates through plasma membrane receptors for immuno-

globulins of the **immunoglobulin E (IgE)** class. These receptors bind a random selection of soluble IgEs that the immune system has made in response to exposure to allergens. When the same antigen binds to IgE on a mast cell surface, the receptors aggregate, triggering a cytoplasmic Ca^{+2} pulse (see Chapter 28) and fusion of granules with the plasma membrane (see Chapter 23). Mechanical trauma, radiant energy (heat, x-rays), and toxins or venoms are less specific stimuli but can have the same result. Outside the cell, the carrier proteins release heparin and histamine. Histamine binds to cellular receptors, causing blood vessels to leak plasma, smooth muscle to contract, and itching sensations to occur. This results in the congestion and constriction of the respiratory tract in allergic

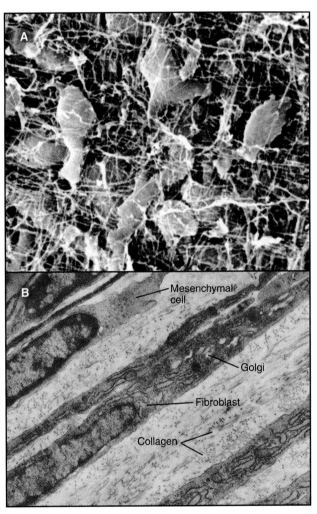

Figure 30–4 Fibroblasts. *A,* Scanning electron micrograph of fibroblasts migrating through collagen fibrils. *B,* Transmission electron micrograph of a thin section of a fibroblast illustrating the abundant organelles of the secretory pathway (endoplasmic reticulum and Golgi apparatus) and extracellular collagen fibrils. A primitive mesenchymal cell is shown in the upper left. (*A,* Courtesy of E. D. Hay, Harvard Medical School. *B,* Courtesy of D. W. Fawcett, Harvard Medical School.)

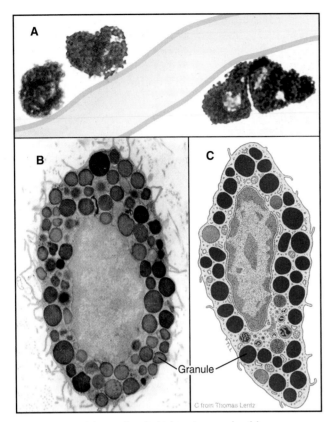

Figure 30–5 Mast cells. *A,* Light micrograph of loose connective tissue, stained with toluidine blue, illustrating mast cells scattered along a blood vessel (drawn in to enhance the contrast). Large mast cell granules stain intensely purple with basic thiazine dyes like toluidine blue. *B,* Transmission electron micrograph of a thin section of a mast cell. *C,* Drawing of a mast cell. (*A* and *B,* Courtesy of D. W. Fawcett, Harvard Medical School. *C,* Modified from T. Lentz, Yale Medical School.)

reactions and swelling of the skin after an insect bite. Secreted fibrinolysin and heparin inhibit blood clotting.

White Fat Cells

Fat cells (**adipocytes**) distributed in connective tissue beneath the skin and in the mesentery of vertebrates store lipids as a dynamic energy reserve. These round cells vary in diameter depending on the size of their single, large, **lipid droplet** (Fig. 30–6). Intermediate filaments and endoplasmic reticulum separate the lipid droplet from the thin rim of cytoplasm. These metabolically active cells take up fatty acids and glycerol from blood after a meal and synthesize **triglycerides** (see Chapter 6) for storage in the lipid droplet. During fasting, these triglycerides are hydrolyzed and the fatty acids are released back into the blood to provide energy for other organs. These metabolic reactions are controlled by hormones. Fat cells also secrete a regulatory hormone called **leptin,** which binds receptors in the brain that modulate appetite. Defects in this receptor lead to obesity.

Brown Fat Cells

Brown fat cells derive their color from numerous mitochondria, which they use to generate heat in response to cold or (in lean rodents) to excess food intake. Cytochromes make mitochondria brown. Fat is

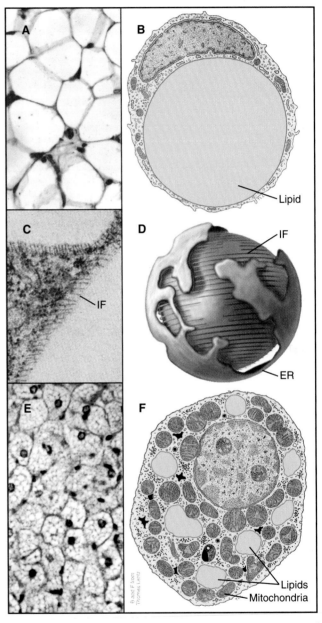

Figure 30–6 Fat cells. *A,* Light micrograph of a section of white fat cells stained with hematoxylin and eosin. *B,* Drawing of a white adipose cell. *C,* Transmission electron micrograph of a thin section of the edge of a lipid droplet showing the circumferential sheath of vimentin intermediate filaments (IF) (see Chapter 38). *D,* Interpretive drawing of a lipid droplet with its associated filaments (IF, intermediate filament) and endoplasmic reticulum (ER). *E,* Light micrograph of a section of brown fat. *F,* Drawing of a brown fat cell. (*A, C,* and *E,* Courtesy of D. W. Fawcett, Harvard Medical School. *B* and *F,* Modified from T. Lentz, Yale Medical School. *D,* Modified from Werner Franke, University of Heidelberg.)

stored in multiple, small droplets (see Fig. 30–6). Brown fat is less abundant than white fat, being concentrated in connective tissue between the scapulae in mammals. Newborn humans have more brown fat than adults in order to generate heat during the adjustment to a new environment after birth. Hibernating animals use brown fat to raise their temperatures when emerging from hibernation.

Brown fat cells generate heat by short-circuiting the proton gradient that is usually used to generate adenosine triphosphate (ATP) in mitochondria (see Fig. 10–16). Stimulation of β-adrenergic receptors (see Fig. 29–3) activates the expression of an "uncoupling protein," which inserts into the inner mitochondrial membrane. This protein dissipates the proton electrochemical gradient across the inner membrane. The energy is lost as heat rather than being used to synthesize ATP. **Thermogenesis** may be an "energy buffer" that, when defective, contributes to obesity.

Immigrant Connective Tissue Cells and Other Cells of the Blood

Origins of Blood Cells

The blood of vertebrates contains a variety of cells, each with a specialized function (Fig. 30–7; Table 30–1). For example, red blood cells transport oxygen, platelets repair damage to blood vessels, and white blood cells defend against infections.

All blood cells derive ultimately from **pleuripotential stem cells** (see Fig. 30–7). After purification, these stem cells can restore the production of all blood cells in mice that have been irradiated to destroy their own blood cell precursors. These stem cells are also responsible for restoring blood cell production following human bone marrow transplantation. Proliferation and differentiation of the progeny of pleuripotential stem cells produce mature blood cells. At several stages in each line of cells, precursors undergo irreversible differentiation that commits them to remain in a particular lineage. For example, committed erythroid stem cells give rise to mature red blood cells through division and further differentiation, but not to white blood cells. Platelets, red cells, granulocytes, and monocytes develop in bone marrow. Lymphocytes develop in lymphoid tissues (thymus, spleen, and lymph nodes).

Minute quantities of specific glycoprotein **growth factors** control the balance between self-renewal and proliferation at each stage of development, starting with pleuripotential stem cells. Feedback mechanisms control production of these growth factors. For example, the oxygen level in the kidney controls the synthesis of **erythropoietin**, the growth factor for the red blood cell series. Deficient oxygenation caused by low levels of red blood cells, poor blood circulation in

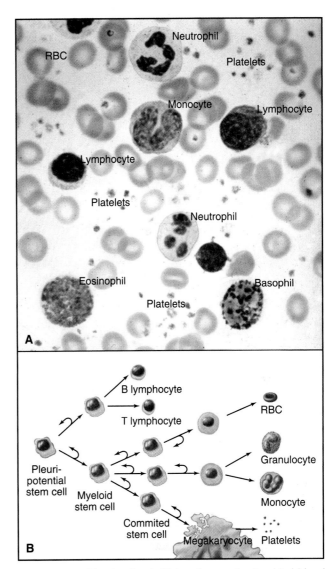

Figure 30-7 Blood cells. *A,* Light micrograph of a dried blood smear prepared with Wright's stain. *B,* Family tree of blood cells showing the developmental relationships of the various lineages. Looping-back arrows indicate renewal of the cell type. Forward-oriented arrows indicate differentiation and proliferation. RBC, red blood cell. (*A,* Courtesy of J.-P. Revel, California Institute of Technology.)

the kidney, or high altitude stimulates secretion of erythropoietin, which increases red blood cell production. (See Fig. 29–9 for the erythropoietin signaling pathway.) If an increased concentration of red blood cells compensates for the cause of poor oxygenation, as when one travels to a high altitude, synthesis of erythropoietin returns to basal levels.

Destruction of stem cells (e.g., by drugs like chloramphenicol) leads to **aplastic anemia,** a condition in which few blood cells are produced owing to a lack of precursors. On the other hand, mutations altering the growth control (see Chapters 44–46) of a stem cell give rise to monoclonal proliferative disorders, such as **leukemia.** In chronic myelogenous leukemia, the progeny of a single mutated white blood cell precur-

table 30–1
BLOOD CELLS (AS SEEN ON A STAINED SMEAR OF BLOOD)

Type	Concentration	Features
Platelets	300,000/μL	Anucleate; 2–3 μm wide; purple granules
Erythrocytes	~5 × 10^6/μL	7-μm; diameter biconcave disks; no nucleus; pink cytoplasm
Neutrophils	~60% of total WBCs	10–12 μm wide; multilobed nucleus; many unstained granules; few azurophilic granules
Eosinophils	~2% of total WBCs	Bilobed nucleus; numerous, large, refractile, pink-stained granules; ~12 μm wide
Basophils	~0.5% of total WBCs	Lobed nucleus; large, blue-stained granules; ~10 μm wide
Lymphocytes	~30% of total WBCs	Small, round, intensely stained nucleus; some small azurophilic granules; variable amount of clear blue cytoplasm, so they may be classified as either small (~7–8 μm wide), medium, or large
Monocytes	~5% of total WBCs	Up to 17 μm wide; large, indented nucleus and gray-blue cytoplasm with a few azurophilic granules

WBCs, white blood cells

sor proliferate unchecked, crowding out and inhibiting the production of other blood cells, leading to anemia and platelet deficiency. Affected individuals are prone to infection because the immature white blood cells are ineffective phagocytes. Uncontrolled proliferation of a clone of red blood cell precursors causes a similar condition, characterized by excess red cells, called **polycythemia vera.**

Erythrocytes (Red Blood Cells)

Red blood cells (see Figs. 6–6 and 30–7) contain more than 300 mg/mL of hemoglobin to carry oxygen from the lungs to tissues and carbon dioxide from tissues to the lungs. These highly specialized cells discard their nuclei and organelles late in their development. A resilient, spectrin-actin membrane cytoskeleton (see Fig. 6–10) maintains the biconcave shape even as the cell is heavily distorted every time it passes through a small capillary. The elasticity of the membrane skeleton allows it to snap back. After circulating in blood for 120 days, erythrocytes abruptly become senescent, and phagocytes in the spleen, liver, and bone marrow remove them from the blood. The biochemical basis of this precise cellular aging and clearance is still being investigated.

In **hereditary spherocytosis** (and other hemolytic anemias), the membrane cytoskeleton loses its resiliency as a result of mutations, causing deficiencies or molecular defects of spectrin or other component proteins. These defective cells are easily damaged and lose some membrane and contents, eventually becoming smaller and rounder than normal. Many different mutations of the globin genes decrease the stability or oxygen-carrying capacity of hemoglobin. In **sickle cell disease,** hemoglobin S is prone to assemble into tubular polymers that distort the cell and clog up the circulation.

Granulocytes and Monocytes

Monocytes and the three granulocytes (neutrophils, eosinophils, and basophils) originate from a common stem cell in bone marrow and share a number of physiological features. Through differentiation, each also acquires unique functions that are emphasized in the following sections. Like lymphocytes, all of these cells participate in host defense; however, they all also contribute to inflammation. Also like lymphocytes, all are motile and are attracted to sites of infection or inflammation by (in humans) a family of about 40 small proteins called **chemokines.** The chemokines are secreted by tissue cells and leukocytes at sites of infection or inflammation. Chemokines were discovered in many different settings and given diverse names (IL-8, RANTES, eotaxin, MCP-1, and so on) that are not indicative of their similar structures and that bear no relation to the family of 14 different chemokine receptors expressed selectively by lymphocytes, monocytes, and granulocytes. **Chemokine receptors** are seven-helix transmembrane proteins coupled to trimeric G proteins (see Chapters 26 and 27). They fall into three families: CXCR1 through 5, CCR1 through 8, and CX$_3$CR1.

Neutrophils

Neutrophils, variously known as polymorphonuclear leukocytes or "polys," are the main phagocytes in blood. They have a multilobed nucleus and two types of granules (Fig. 30–8). Specific granules contain lysozyme and alkaline phosphatase. They do not stain with either the basic or acidic dyes used for blood smears, so these cells are called neutrophils. Azurophilic granules are true lysosomes and are present in lesser numbers than specific granules. Neutrophils have copious glycogen but few mitochondria, so they rely on glycolysis for ATP synthesis in poorly

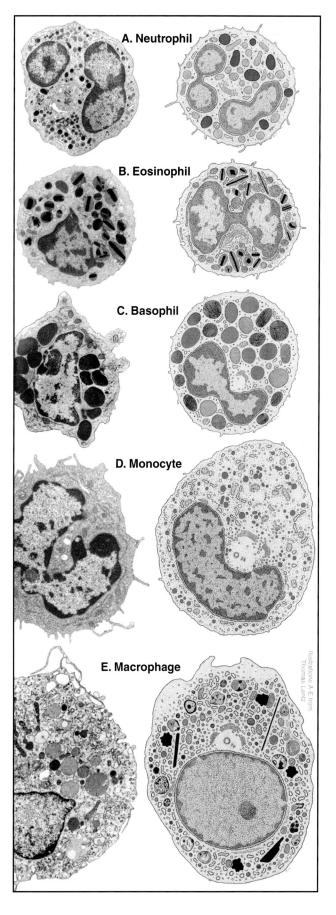

Figure 30-8 White blood cells. Transmission electron micrographs of thin sections of each cell and interpretive drawings with lysosomes shown in brown. *A*, A neutrophil showing the multilobed nucleus and the two classes of granules. *B*, An eosinophil showing the bilobed nucleus and the large, specific granules containing a darkly stained crystalloid. *C*, Basophil with large specific granules colored blue. D, Blood monocyte. *E*, Macrophage grown in tissue culture. (Micrographs courtesy of D. W. Fawcett, Harvard Medical School; drawings modified from T. Lentz, Yale Medical School.)

oxygenated wounds. They are among the most motile cells in the body.

Human bone marrow produces about 80 g of neutrophils each day. In response to infection or injury, a circulating factor controls the release of neutrophils from a bone marrow storage pool. Neutrophils spend about 10 hours in blood, alternating between a circulating pool and a so-called marginated pool adherent to endothelial cells, chiefly in the lung. Exercise and epinephrine release marginated neutrophils into the circulating pool; smoking increases the marginated pool. Neutrophils leave the blood by receptor-mediated attachment to endothelial cells and then crawling between endothelial cells into the connective tissue (see Fig. 32–13), where they perish after a day or two of phagocytosis.

Neutrophils are humans' first line of defense against bacterial infection, as they are highly specialized for the ingestion and destruction of bacteria. Bacterial products, especially N-formylated peptides, attract neutrophils by binding plasma membrane receptors and stimulating locomotion toward the bacteria. Chapter 23 provides details regarding the recognition, ingestion, and destruction of bacteria. The production of superoxide (O_2^-) radicals not only contributes to the killing of injested bacteria, but also damages the neutrophil. Genetic defects in the enzymes that produce superoxide cause chronic granulomatous disease, a serious human disease because neutrophils cannot kill ingested bacteria.

Eosinophils

Eosinophils are distinguishable in blood smears as cells with a bilobed nucleus and large specific granules that stain brightly with eosin (see Fig. 30–7). Specific granules contain a cationic protein, a ribonuclease and peroxidase, in addition to a crystalloid of a basic protein (see Fig. 30–8). Like neutrophils, eosinophils are transient in blood, making their way to connective tissue where they survive for about 2 weeks. Chemotactic factors generated by the complement system, basophils, some tumors, parasites, and bacteria all attract eosinophils. Many of the same factors attract other leukocytes, but particular chemokines are specialized for eosinophils. Eosinophils accumulate in blood and tissues in response to parasitic infections. Eosinophils bind parasites and lyse them, like killer lymphocytes (see later discussion), by secreting a cationic protein that forms pores in their membrane. Production of superoxide and hydrogen peroxide also contributes to killing. Excess eosinophils in some allergic disorders can contribute to inflammation.

Basophils

Basophils are the least abundant and most obscure granulocytes. They look much like neutrophils but have a bilobed nucleus and large, basophilic-specific granules containing heparin, serotonin, and all of the blood histamine (see Fig. 30–7). Basophils are weak phagocytes. Like mast cells, they have cell surface receptors that bind IgE and release the vasoactive agents stored in their granules when antigens bind to these bound immunoglobulins. Basophils and mast cells have many common features, but they appear to have different origins. Basophils arise from bone marrow stem cells, whereas mast cells are derived from connective tissue mesenchymal cells. Humans have both circulating basophils and tissue mast cells, but this is not universal. Mice have mast cells but no basophils. Turtles have basophils but no mast cells.

Lymphocytes and Plasma Cells: The Immune System

In response to infection, lymphocytes in the immune systems of vertebrates produce two kinds of responses: humoral and cellular. **B lymphocytes** produce the humoral response by secreting **antibodies,** proteins that diffuse freely in the blood, and extracellular fluids. Two types of T lymphocytes mediate the cellular arm of the immune response. **Cytotoxic T lymphocytes** or killer T cells destroy cells infected with viruses, whereas **helper T cells** assist in regulating other lymphocytes. These responses protect against infection, but fail in acquired immunodeficiency syndrome (AIDS) when the human immunodeficiency virus (HIV) kills helper T cells. A blood smear reveals lymphocytes of various sizes and shapes (see Fig. 30–7), but not their remarkable heterogeneity at the molecular level (Fig. 30–9).

Antibodies produced by B cells provide chemical defense against viruses, bacteria, and toxins. Antibodies, or immunoglobulins, are an incredibly diverse family of proteins, each with a unique binding site that can accommodate one of hundreds of thousands of different ligands termed antigens (see Fig. 2–15). Antigens include proteins, polysaccharides, nucleic acids, lipids, and small organic molecules that are biologically or chemically manufactured. Antibody binding can mark an antigen for phagocytosis or neutralize its toxicity.

The huge repertoire of antigen-binding sites present in the collection of antibodies that circulate in a single individual arises through **DNA rearrangement** and facilitated mutations. This remarkable process was exploited during evolution specifically for the use of the immune system. Each immunoglobulin is composed of four polypeptide chains—two identical heavy chains and two identical light chains—each encoded by different genes (see Fig. 2–15). Light chains and heavy chains both contribute to the antigen-binding site. In vertebrate genomes, immunoglobulin genes exist in segments aligned along a chromosome. Several of these gene segments must be combined in

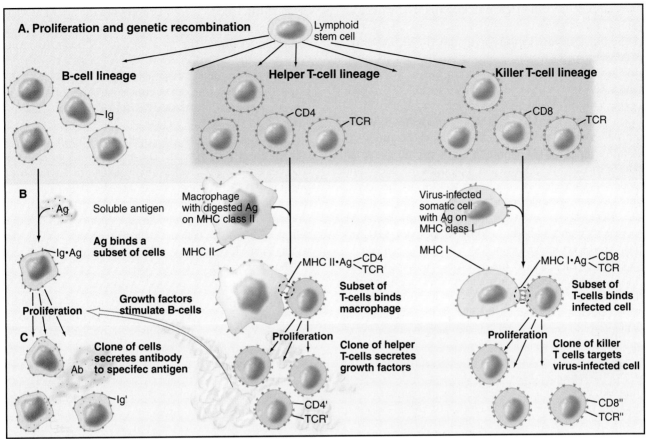

Figure 30-9 The immune response by three classes of lymphocytes through three parallel steps. *A,* Genetic recombination produces populations of cells with a wide variety of antigen specificities provided by cell surface immunoglobulins (Ig) or T-cell receptors (TCR). *B,* The binding of specific antigens (Ag) to surface immunoglobulins or T-cell receptors selects a subset of the cells. *C,* Proliferation of clones of the selected cells yields many cells specialized to produce antibody (Ab) to soluble antigens, secretion of growth factors by helper T cells in response to ingested and degraded antigens, or killing of virus-infected cells identifiable by the viral peptides on their surface. The helper and killer T cells use a common set of T cell receptors and are guided to the appropriate target cells by the CD4 and CD8 accessory molecules. See Figure 29–8 for details on T-lymphocyte activation.

the proper order to make a full-length antibody gene. Some of these gene segments encode the framework of the antibody protein, which is essentially identical within each class of antibodies. Other gene segments, present in many variations, encode the part of the polypeptide chain that forms the antigen-binding site.

During B cell maturation, **recombination enzymes** (RAG1 and RAG2) assemble immunoglobulin gene segments into one unique full-length gene for a heavy chain and one for a light chain. As a result of random gene arrangements, each B cell makes and displays on its surface one type of antibody. The process is precise in that the right number of segments is always chosen to make a heavy chain or a light chain, but it is also random in that any one of the variable segments may be chosen. The resulting antibody contains two identical but unique antigen-binding sites. Because the gene segments can be assembled in many different combinations, because most any heavy chain can assemble with most any light chain and because pre-B cells go through a period of controlled muta-

genesis of their immunoglobulin genes, an enormous number of antigen-binding specificities results from this random process of gene assembly and mutation. In principle, about 3000 different light chains and 60,000 heavy chains can combine to produce about 100 million different antibodies. In fact, it is possible experimentally to induce a mouse to make an antibody specific for almost any naturally occurring or synthetic chemical.

Infection by a pathogen results in the production of antibodies that bind to the pathogen but not to any of the individual's own molecules. This response comes from activation and proliferation of pre-existing B cells with the capacity to make antibodies to molecules of the pathogen. Activation requires a chance encounter of particular B cells with the pathogen and results in maturation of the cell into a factory for secreting antibodies. Alternate splicing of messenger RNA (mRNA; see Fig. 15–9) directs the same antibody to either the plasma membrane or secretory pathway. The activated cells also divide to increase their numbers, a process called **clonal expansion,** which amplifies the production of antibody specific for the pathogen. The final progeny of the B-cell response is a **plasma cell,** which is highly specialized to secrete one specific antibody. In addition, some B cells activated by the pathogen become so-called **memory cells.** These long-lived cells display a particular antibody on their surface and stand ready to mount an amplified response upon subsequent exposure to the same antigen. This immunologic memory explains why exposure to a particular pathogen or vaccination against a pathogen results in protection, in the form of antibodies, for many years.

Specialized, mature B lymphocytes and plasma cells secrete different antibody isoforms or isotypes. **IgG** isotypes, produced in lymph nodes and spleen, circulate in blood and tissue fluids. **IgA** isotypes, produced by lymphoid nodules in the respiratory and gastrointestinal tracts and by mammary glands, are first taken up and then secreted by epithelial cells of these organs. IgE isotypes bind to receptors on the surface of mast cells and basophils (see earlier discussion).

T lymphocytes provide cellular responses to pathogens. Cytotoxic T cells execute tumor cells and virus-infected cells. Helper T cells stimulate antibody production by B cells. The specificity of these responses is provided by variable cell surface receptors called **T-cell receptors** (see Fig. 29–8). A set of segmented genes analogous to immunoglobulin genes encode T-cell receptors. In contrast to antibodies, T-cell receptors do not bind free antigens, but rather recognize peptide antigens displayed on the surface of target cells complexed to proteins called **major histocompatibility complex (MHC)** antigens. These highly variable MHC proteins are responsible for the rejection of tissue grafts from nonidentical individuals.

The two types of MHC proteins—class I and class II—acquire their antigenic peptides differently. All somatic cells produce class I MHC proteins. If infected by a virus, a cell's cytoplasmic proteosomes degrade some viral proteins to peptides (see Chapter 24), which ABC transporters (TAP1, 2) move from the cytoplasm (see Chapter 7) into the endoplasmic reticulum. In the lumen of the ER, peptides insert into the binding site of compatible class I molecules and move to the plasma membrane. In contrast, macrophages and other so-called **antigen-presenting cells** of the immune system such as **dendritic cells** ingest foreign matter and degrade it in endosomes and lysosomes. Peptide fragments bind to class II proteins in endosomes and thence move to the cell surface of these antigen-presenting cells.

T lymphocytes patrol the body, inspecting the surface of other cells. A chance encounter with a cell displaying a peptide-MHC complex complementary to its T-cell receptor stimulates the T cell (see Fig. 29–8). The response is proliferation and expansion of a clone of identical T cells. Accessory membrane proteins CD4 and CD8 on the T-cell surface cooperate with T-cell receptors to direct the two types of T cells to target cells with the appropriate MHC proteins. T-cell receptors provide antigen specificity. Immature T-cells express both CD4 and CD8, but lose one of them as they mature into cytotoxic (CD8$^+$) or helper (CD4$^+$) T cells.

CD8-positive cytotoxic T cells are specialized to kill cells infected with viruses. The presence of virus inside is revealed by MHC class I proteins displaying vital peptides on the surface of the infected cell. CD8 binds to a constant region of MHC class I proteins carrying viral peptides. During intimate encounters with a target cell, a cytotoxic T cell uses three weapons to kill the target. First, T cells carry a ligand for the Fas receptor on the target, which stimulates apoptosis of the target cell (see Chapter 49). Second, activated T cells secrete **perforin,** a protein that inserts into the plasma membrane of the target cell, forming large (10 nm) pores that leak cytoplasmic contents and ultimately lyse the cell. Third, T cells secrete toxic enzymes that enter target cells through the plasma membrane pores.

CD4 binds a constant part of the MHC class II protein and targets helper T cells to cells presenting ingested antigens. The progeny of stimulated helper T cells secrete growth factors (lymphokines or interleukins) in the vicinity of B cells with the foreign antigen bound to immunoglobulins on their surface. Helper T cells are required for B cells to make antibodies against most antigens. This explains how **HIV** causes AIDS. The virus uses CD4 as a receptor to infect and eventually kill helper T cells. Loss of helper T cells severely limits the capacity of B cells and cytotoxic T cells (which also require T-cell help) to mount antibody and cellular responses to microorganisms. Infections that the immune system normally dispatches with ease then become life-threatening. Genetic defects cause a wide variety of **immunodeficiency diseases.** For example, defects in Bruton tyrosine kinase result in failure to produce B cells. Remarkably, humans lacking function of the metabolic enzyme adenosine deaminase have no B cells or T cells but are otherwise normal. Deficiencies of many specialized lymphocyte proteins (cytokine receptors, interleukin receptors, Lck tyrosine kinase, ZAP-70 tyrosine kinase, RAG1 or RAG2, TAP1 or TAP2) lead to immunodeficiencies.

Monocytes and Macrophages

Monocytes are precursors of tissue macrophages that circulate in the blood. These large cells have an indented nucleus and a small number of azurophilic granules (see Figs. 26–7 and 26–8). Monocytes develop in bone marrow from the same committed stem cells that produce granulocytes. Monocytes circulate in the blood for about 3 days until they enter connective tissues to differentiate into tissue-specific macrophages. Their progeny include **osteoclasts** that remodel bone (see Fig. 34–6), spleen macrophages that remove aged red blood cells, and liver macrophages, called Kupffer cells, that line the venous sinuses.

After blood monocytes enter the connective tissue, growth factors, including lymphokines secreted by lymphocytes, stimulate their differentiation into macrophages. They enlarge and amplify their machinery for locomotion, phagocytosis, and killing of microorganisms and tumor cells (see Fig. 30–8). These "professional phagocytes" may divide and survive for months in the connective tissue, where they ingest foreign material, participate in the immune response, and secrete growth factors that influence other cells.

The primary function of macrophages is **phagocytosis** (see Chapter 23) of microorganisms, senile cells (old red blood cells), cellular debris, and foreign material. Macrophages have plasma membrane receptors for antibodies that mark targets as foreign and facilitate their ingestion. Primary lysosomes fuse with phagosomes to degrade the contents. Eventually, the cytoplasm fills with secondary lysosomes containing the remains of injested material. Macrophages generally follow neutrophils to wounds or infections, where they clean up debris, including the remains of neutrophils that perish secondary to oxidative damage as they kill injested microorganisms. When confronted with large foreign bodies, macrophages can fuse together to form **giant cells.** Multinucleate, bone-eating cells called osteoclasts form in this way (see Chapter 34). No challenge is too great. Giant multinucleated microphages will even try to ingest a Petri dish if it is coated with antibody.

Macrophages participate in the immune response by degrading ingested protein antigens and presenting fragments on their surface bound to MHC class II proteins (see Fig. 30–9). This complex activates helper T lymphocytes carrying the appropriate T-cell receptors. The activated T cells then proliferate and secrete growth factors that stimulate B lymphocytes to produce antibody. Macrophages also secrete a variety of factors involved with host defense and inflammation. These include interleukin-1, transforming growth factor-α, transforming growth factor-β, platelet-derived growth factor, and a series of important proteins called chemokines. The chemokines are essential for attracting cells of the immune system to sites of inflammation. These factors stimulate the proliferation of the cells required to heal wounds (see Chapter 34).

Platelets

Platelets are small, anucleate, cellular fragments that contribute to blood clotting and repair minor defects in the sheet of endothelial cells that lines blood vessels. A long coiled microtubule presses out against the plasma membrane, like a spring, to maintain their disk shape (Fig. 30–10). The most prominent organelles are two types of membrane-bound granules containing stores of adenosine diphosphate (ADP), serotonin, fibrinogen, thrombospondin (a large, adhesive glycoprotein), and a potent hormone called **platelet-**

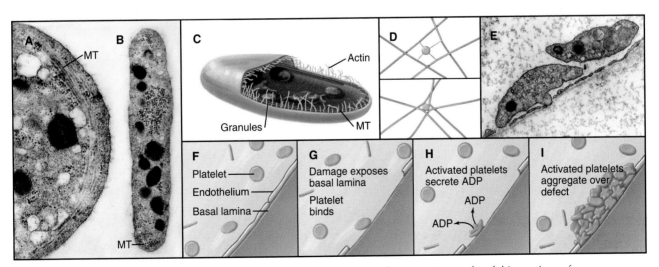

Figure 30–10 Platelets and their role in hemostasis. *A* and *B*, Transmission electron micrographs of thin sections of platelets. *C*, Interpretive drawing showing the circumferential band of microtubules (MT), actin filaments in the cortex, and granules in the cytoplasm. *D*, Role of platelets in blood clot retraction. Filopodia grasp strands of fibrin in a blood clot (*upper*) and pull them together (*lower*). *E*, Electron micrograph of a thin section showing platelets adhering to each other and one adhering to the basal lamina through a small defect in the endothelium. *F* to *I*, Stages in the repair of a defect in the endothelial lining of a blood vessel. *F*, Circulating platelets do not bind to normal endothelial cells. *G*, Damage to the endothelium exposes the basal lamina, and a platelet binds to the collagen. *H*, Collagen activates the platelet to secrete ADP, which activates passing platelets. *I*, Activated platelets bind together, covering the defect in the endothelium. (*A* and *B*, Courtesy of O. Behnke, University of Copenhagen.)

derived growth factor (PDGF). PDGF has a role in wound healing but also contributes to atherosclerosis by stimulating the abnormal proliferation of smooth muscle cells in the walls of damaged arteries.

Platelets bud from precursor cells—giant polyploid cells in the bone marrow called **megakaryocytes. Thrombopoietin,** a growth factor related to erythropoietin, controls platelet production. The liver and kidneys secrete thrombopoietin at a constant rate. Platelets appear to remove thrombopoietin from the circulation, so the blood concentration of thrombopoietin available to stimulate megakaryocyte maturation and platelet budding is inversely related to the platelet concentration. This provides a feedback loop to stimulate platelet production if the platelet supply is low.

Like red blood cells, platelets are confined to the vasculature. Two pools freely exchange with each other: about two thirds of the total platelets circulate, whereas one third of the platelets are stored in the blood vessels of the spleen. The stored pool may increase when the spleen is enlarged, decreasing the platelet count in the blood. The life span of platelets in the blood is about 10 days. It is not clear whether they are destroyed by random utilization or become senile and are then removed.

Platelets control bleeding in two ways. First, platelets are required for **blood clotting.** They contribute a protein (factor VIII) to the cascade of proteolytic reactions that culminate in the cleavage of plasma fibrinogen to form fibrin, which polymerizes to form a blood clot. The fibrin gel stops the flow of blood from damaged blood vessels. Platelets also bind to fibrin strands in the clot and cause the clot to contract. This may help to close the defect in a damaged blood vessel.

Second, platelets repair defects in the endothelial cell lining of blood vessels that are produced by the mild trauma of daily existence. Platelets bind to collagen in the basal lamina when it is exposed by damage to the endothelium. This triggers one of the best understood examples of regulated cellular adhesion (see Fig. 32–14). Activated platelets aggregate, extend actin-containing filopodia, and secrete the contents of their granules. This fills in the endothelial defect as the ADP and thrombospondin activate and aggregate additional platelets.

Patients with defective platelets or reduced circulating platelets (a complication of bone marrow disease and cancer chemotherapy) bruise easily owing to unrepaired damage in small blood vessels, and may even bleed spontaneously. Conversely, hyperactive platelets may initiate pathologic clots in the blood vessels of the heart, causing heart attacks.

Selected Readings

Baggiolini M: Chemokines and leukocyte traffic. Nature 392: 565–568, 1998.

Banchereau J and Steinman RM: Dendritic cells and the control of immunity. Nature 392:245–252, 1998.

Buckley RH: Primary immunodeficiency diseases due to defects in lymphocytes. New Engl J Med 343:1313–1324, 2000.

Delves PJ, Roitt IM: The immune system. New Engl J Med 343:37–49, 108–117, 2000.

Kaufmann SHE: Cell-mediated immunity: Dealing a blow to pathogens. Curr Biol 9:R97–99, 1999.

Kaushansky K: Thrombopoietin. N Engl J Med 339:746–754, 1998.

Klein J, Sato A: The HLA system. New Engl J Med 343:702–709, 782–786, 2000.

Lanzavecchia A, Sallusto F: Dynamics of T lymphocyte responses: Intermediates, effectors and memory cells. Science 290:92–97, 2000.

Lekstrom-Himes JA, Gallin JI: Immunodeficiency diseases caused by defects in phagocytes. New Engl J Med 343: 1703–1714, 2000.

Rothenberg ME: Esosinophilia. N Engl J Med 338:1592–1600, 1998.

van Andrian UH, Mackay CR: T-cell function and migration. New Engl J Med 343:1020–1034, 2000.

chapter 31

EXTRACELLULAR MATRIX MOLECULES

Although the extracellular matrix is composed of only five classes of macromolecules—collagens, elastin, proteoglycans, hyaluronan, and adhesive glycoproteins—it can take on a rich variety of different forms with vastly different mechanical properties. This is possible for two reasons. First, each of these classes of macromolecule comes in a number of variants (encoded by different genes or produced by alternative splicing), each with distinctive properties. Second, the cells that constitute the extracellular matrix are versatile with respect to secreting different proportions of these isoforms in different geometrical arrangements. As a result, the extracellular matrix in different tissues is adapted to particular functional requirements, which are as different as tendons, blood vessel walls, cartilage, bone, the vitreous body of the eye, and subcutaneous fat. Beyond providing mechanical support, the extracellular matrix also strongly influences embryonic development, provides pathways for cellular migration, and sequesters important growth factors. This chapter introduces the macromolecules of the extracellular matrix.

Collagen

The collagen family is the most abundant class of proteins in the human body. It is also one of the most versatile. Collagens form a wide range of different structures with remarkable mechanical properties. Weight for weight, fibrous collagens are as strong as steel. Their name, which comes from the Greek words for "glue" and "birth," reflects the long-known adhesive properties of denatured collagen extracted from animal tissues.

The defining feature of collagens is a rod-shaped domain composed of a **triple helix** of polypeptides (Fig. 31–1). Each polypeptide folds into a left-handed helix that repeats every third residue with the side chains on the outside. Three of these helices associate to form a triple helix that may be up to 420 nm long. The triple helical domains have a repeating amino acid sequence: glycine-X-Y, where X is most often proline and Y is most often hydroxyproline. The small glycine residues allow tight contact between the polypeptides in the core of the triple helix. Larger residues, even alanine, interfere with packing. Poly-L-proline has a strong tendency to form a left-handed helix like individual collagen chains, but does not form a triple helix owing to steric interference. The triple helix is most stable if all X residues are proline and all Y residues are hydroxyproline, but other residues at some of these positions are essential for collagen to assemble higher-order structures. (Despite their name (α chains) the collagen polypeptides do not form α helices!)

The collagen family is remarkably diverse. Humans have about 100 genes with collagen triple repeats, and more than 20 specialized collagen proteins have been characterized (Table 31–1; Fig. 31–2).

Other proteins, including the extracellular enzyme acetylcholine esterase and some cell surface receptors, have similar triple helical domains, but are not classified as collagens. To be a collagen, a protein must also form fibrils or other assemblies in the extracellular matrix. Nematodes, which lack connective tissue, seem to have lost the genes for fibrillar collagens, but have elaborated a family of 160 genes for collagens that form their cuticle.

Collagen biochemistry is challenging because many tissue collagens are insoluble owing to covalent cross-linking between proteins. Historic purification protocols began with proteolytic digestion to liberate protease-resistant triple helical fragments. An alterna-

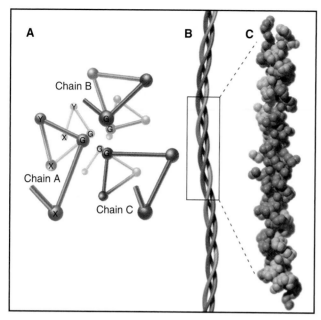

Figure 31–1 Collagen triple helix. *A,* End-on view of three left-handed polyproline type II helices with glycines (G) in the core. *B,* Longitudinal view of the strands of a triple helix. *C,* Space-filling model of the structure of a short collagen triple helix. (*A,* Redrawn from van der Rest M, Garrone A: Collagen family of proteins. FASEB J 5:2814–2823, 1991. *C,* PDB file: 1bkv.)

tive biochemical approach has been to isolate intact collagens produced by cells in tissue culture.

The size and shape of collagens vary according to function. Collagens are named numerically (type I, type II, and so on) in the order of their discovery, a nomenclature that bears no relationship to their function. Table 31–1 groups collagens according to function. Polypeptides are called **α chains,** and Roman numerals in their names correspond to their type number. Some collagens are homotrimers of three identical α chains. Others are heterotrimers of two or three different α chains. Some chains [α1(II)] are used in more than one type of collagen.

Fibrillar Collagens

Triple helical rod-shaped collagen molecules about 300 nm long self-associate to form banded fibrils (see Fig. 31–2). Collagen fibrils provide tensile strength to tendons, ligaments, bones, and dense connective tissue, thus reinforcing most organs. They also form the scaffolding for cartilage and the vitreous body in the eye. Fibrillar collagens are widespread in nature and have been highly conserved during evolution, so the homologues from sponges to vertebrates are similar. Each fibrillar collagen can form homopolymers in vitro, but in vivo, most form heteropolymers with at least one other type of fibrillar collagen (see Table 31–1). This mix of the fibrillar collagen subunits is

one factor that regulates the size of collagen fibers. Proteoglycans also participate (see Table 31–2).

The biosynthesis and assembly of fibrillar collagens involve a remarkable number of post-translational modifications, including several rounds of precise proteolytic cleavage, glycosylation, catalyzed folding, and chemical cross-linking (see Fig. 31–4). The final product is a smooth fibril with staggered molecules cross-linked to their neighbors. These strong but flexible collagen fibrils reinforce all the tissues of the body, where they form a variety of higher-order structures. Loose connective tissue (Fig. 31–3) has an open network of individual fibrils or small bundles of fibrils that support the cells (see Fig. 30–2*A*). In many tissues, the fibrils of type I and associated collagens aggregate to form the so-called collagen fibers visible with light microscopy (see Fig. 31–3*A*). In extreme cases, such as with tendons, the extracellular matrix consists almost exclusively of tightly packed, parallel bundles of collagen fibers. Layers of orthogonal collagen fibers make the transparent cornea through which one sees (Fig. 31–3*C*). In bone, type I collagen fibrils form regular layers reinforced by calcium phosphate crystals (see Chapter 34). In cartilage and the vitreous body of the eye, type II collagen fibrils trap glycosaminoglycans and proteoglycans, which retain enough water for the matrix to resist compression (see Chapter 34) and, in the case of the eye, to provide an optically clear path for light.

Biosynthesis and Assembly of Fibrillar Collagens

All fibrillar collagens are likely to be produced by similar mechanisms, but type I collagen has been studied the most extensively. Type I collagen is synthesized and secreted by fibroblasts using the exocytic pathway employed for other secretory proteins (see Chapters 18 and 22), but the biosynthesis of collagen is noteworthy for the extensive number of processing steps required to prepare the protein for assembly in the extracellular matrix.

Large genes with 42 exons encode the α chains of type I collagen. In the triple helical domain, all the exons are derived by duplication and divergence from a primordial exon of 54 bp coding for 18 amino acids or 6 turns of polyproline helix. About half consist of 54 bp; a few with 45 bp have lost one Gly-X-Y; the rest are 108 (2 × 54) or 162 (3 × 54) bp. Distinctive exons encode the N- and C-terminal globular domains.

The initial transcript, referred to as **preprocollagen,** translocates into the rough endoplasmic reticulum, where intracellular processing begins (Fig. 31–4). First, removal of the N-terminal signal sequence yields **procollagen** with unfolded α chains with N- and C-terminal nonhelical propeptides. Second, enzymes hydroxylate some prolines and lysines. Third, enzymes add sugars (gal-glu or gal) to the delta-carbon of some

table 31–1

COLLAGEN FAMILIES

Type	Chains	Assembly	Interactions	Distribution	Diseases
Fibrillar collagens					
I	$[\alpha1(I)]2\ \alpha2(I)$	Fibrils	Self; types III and V collagen; types XII and XIV collagen	Bone Tendons, ligaments Skin, dentin	Mutated in osteogenesis imperfecta Mutated in Ehlers-Danlos syndrome type VII Kniest dysplasia, Stickler's syndrome
II	$[\alpha1(II)]3$	Fibrils	Self; type IX and XI collagen	Hyaline cartilage, vitreous body	Mutated in spondyloepiphyseal dysplasia, hypochondrogenesis, achondrogenesis, Kniest dysplasia, Stickler's syndrome
III	$[\alpha1(III)]3$	Fibrils	Self; type I collagen	Skin, blood vessels	Mutated in Ehlers-Danlos syndrome type IV
V	$[\alpha1(V)]2\ \alpha2(V)$	Fibrils	Self; type I collagen	Fetal membranes, skin, bone	
	$\alpha1(V)\ \alpha2(V)\ \alpha3(V)$	Fibrils		Placenta, synovial membranes	
XI	$\alpha1(XI)\ \alpha2(XI)\ \alpha1(II)$	Fibrils	Self; type II collagen	Hyaline cartilage	Mutated in some Stickler's syndrome
Sheet-forming collagens					
IV	$[\alpha1(IV)]2\ \alpha2(IV)$	Nets	Self; perlecan laminin, nidogen, integrins	Basement membranes	Autoantigen in Goodpasture's syndrome $\alpha3(IV)$, $\alpha4(IV)$, $\alpha5(IV)$ mutated in Alport's nephritis
VIII	$[\alpha1(VIII)]?\ [\alpha2(VIII)]?$	Hexagonal net	Self	Descemet's membrane (cornea)	
X	$[\alpha1(X)]3$	?	?	Hypertrophic cartilage	Mutated in Schmid metaphyseal chondrodysplasia
Connecting and anchoring collagens					
VI	$\alpha1(VI)\ \alpha2(VI)\ \alpha3(VI)$	Beaded fibrils	Self; type IV collagen	Vessels, skin, intervertebral disk	Mutated in Bethlem myopathy
VII	$[\alpha1(VII)]3$	Anchoring fibril	Self; type IV collagen	Epidermal-dermal junction	Mutated in dystrophic epidermolysis bullosa
IX	$\alpha1(IX)\ \alpha2(IX)\ \alpha3(IX)$	Linker	Covalent GAG; type II collagen	Hyaline cartilage, vitreous body	Mutated in multiple epiphyseal dysplasia
XII	$[\alpha1(XII)]3$	?Linker	GAG; ?type I collagen	Embryonic tendon, skin	
XIV	$[\alpha1(XIV)]3$	?Linker	GAG; ?type I collagen	Fetal tendon, skin	
XVIII	$[\alpha1(XVIII)]3$	?Linker	GAG	Basal lamina	
Transmembrane					
XIII	$[\alpha1(XIII)]3$	Transmembrane			
XVII	$[\alpha1(XVII)]3$	Transmembrane	Hemidesmosomes, basal lamina	Epidermal-dermal junction	Mutated in blistering conditions; antigen in bullous pemphigoid

lysines, by a mechanism distinct from the typical glycosylation of asparagine or serine.

A novel mechanism initiates the folding of collagen in the endoplasmic reticulum: the **C-terminal propeptides** of three α chains form a globular structure stabilized by cysteines linked in disulfide bonds. An enzyme, protein **disulfide isomerase,** catalyzes the formation of these disulfides. Formation of this globular domain has three important consequences. First, it ensures the correct selection of α chains (two

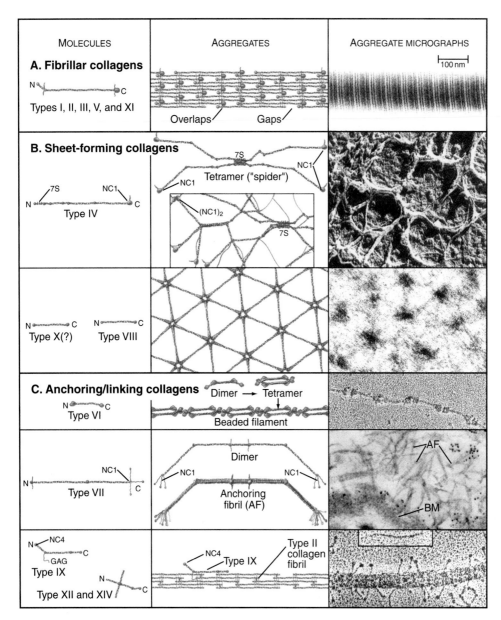

Figure 31–2 *A* to *C*, Comparison of major collagen families. Scale drawings and micrographs of collagen molecules and their assembly into higher-order structures. AF, anchoring fibrils; BM, basement membrane. (Redrawn from van der Rest M, Garrone A: Collagen family of proteins. FASEB J 5:2814–2823, 1991.)

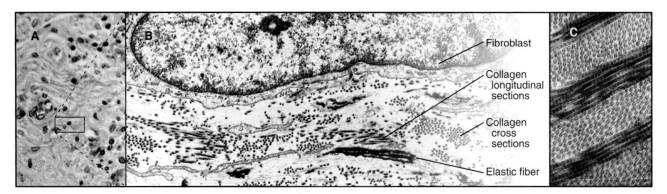

Figure 31–3 Micrographs of collagen fibrils in connective tissues. *A*, Collagen fibrils (*pink*) in the dense connective tissue of the dermis. *B*, Electron micrograph of a thin section of a fibroblast, collagen fibrils, and elastic fibers. *C*, Orthogonal layers of collagen fibrils in the cornea of the eye. (*A*, Courtesy of D. W. Fawcett, Harvard Medical School. *B*, Courtesy of J. Rosenbloom, University of Pennsylvania. *C*, Courtesy of E. D. Hay, Harvard Medical School.)

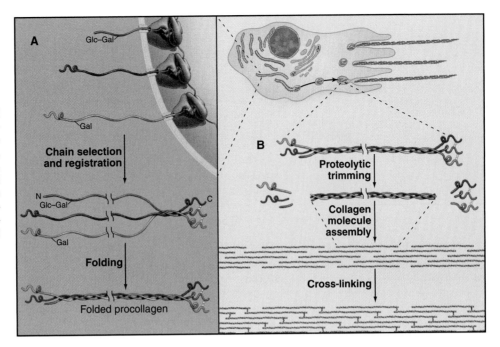

Figure 31-4 Biosynthesis and assembly of fibrillar collagen illustrating details covered in the text. A, Translation of α chains, chain registration, and folding. B, Secretion, assembly, and cross-linking. (Redrawn from Prokop DJ: Mutations in collagen genes as a cause of connective tissue diseases. N Engl J Med 326:540–546, 1992.)

α 1 chains and one α 2 chain in the case of type I collagen). Second, it aligns the three polypeptides with their first Gly-X-Y repeats in register, ensuring that the triple helix will form with all three chains in phase. Third, the globular propeptides prevent assembly of procollagen into fibrils during transit through the secretory pathway. Given their repeating Gly-X-Y structure, separated collagen chains without propeptides are indiscriminating with respect to association with other chains. For example, gelatin is simply a mixture of collagen chains without propeptides. Boiling dissociates the chains from each other. When cooled, the chains randomly associate *out of register* at random positions along their lengths, forming a branching network that solidifies into the gel used in food preparation.

Following selection and registration of the three α chains, the helical rod domains zip together, beginning at the C-terminus. Correct folding of the triple helix requires all-*trans* peptide bonds. Because proline forms *cis* and *trans* peptide bonds randomly, the slow isomerization of *cis* prolyl-peptide bonds to *trans* limits the rate of triple helix folding in vitro. The rapid rate of folding of the triple helix in vivo suggests that the enzyme **prolyl-peptide isomerase** catalyzes the propagation of the triple helix. The resulting rod-shaped, triple-helix glycoprotein is called procollagen.

Procollagen passes through the Golgi apparatus and moves in vesicles to the cell surface, where it is secreted. Some cells have specialized collagen assembly sites (see Fig. 31–4). Like ships laying down communication cables on the ocean floor, movements of fibroblasts through tissues help determine the arrangement of the collagen fibrils (see Fig. 31–3C).

Outside the cell, proteolytic enzymes—procollagen proteases—cleave the propeptides from the triple helical domain, forming the mature collagen molecule (formerly called tropocollagen). Relieved of its inhibitory propeptides, collagen self-assembles into fibrils by a classical entropy-driven process (Fig. 31–5). Adjacent collagen molecules are staggered by 67 nm, so a 35-nm gap is required between the ends of the collagen molecules (five staggers at 67 nm = 335 nm = one molecular length of 300 nm + a 35-nm gap).

Weak, noncovalent bonds between collagen molecules specify the self-assembly of fibrils but provide little tensile strength, so **covalent cross-linking** is required for reinforcement. For most fibrillar collagens, the enzyme **lysyl oxidase** catalyzes the formation of covalent bonds between the ends of collagen molecules (see Figs. 31–4 and 31–6). The enzyme oxidizes

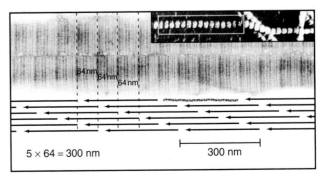

Figure 31-5 Structure of collagen fibrils. Electron micrographs and drawing of molecular packing. (Micrographs courtesy of Alan Hodges, Marine Biological Laboratory, Woods Hole, MA.)

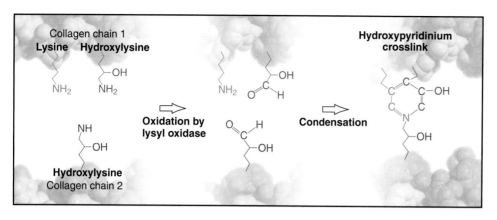

Figure 31-6 Covalent cross-linking of collagen molecules. After lysyl oxidase oxidizes hydroxylysine side chains, the aldehydes condense with each other and a lysine to form two- and three-membered (shown) crosslinks between adjacent collagen molecules.

the ϵ amino groups of selected lysines and hydroxylysines to aldehydes. These aldehydes react spontaneously with nearby lysine and hydroxylysine side chains to form a variety of covalent crosslinks between two or three polypeptides. Disulfide bonds, rather than modified lysine side chains, cross-link type III collagen fibrils. Covalent bonds between the inextensible triple helices give mature collagen fibrils their great tensile strength.

Point mutations or deletions in collagen genes, or deficiencies of the several enzymes that process collagen (lysyl hydroxylase, lysyl oxidase, or procollagen proteases), all can cause defective collagen fibrils (see Table 31–1). These defects cause a remarkable variety of deforming and even lethal human diseases: brittle bones (osteogenesis imperfecta), fragile cartilage (several forms of dwarfism) and weak connective tissue (Ehlers-Danlos syndrome). Chapter 34 covers these diseases in more detail.

Sheet-Forming Collagens

A second group of collagens polymerizes into sheets rather than fibrils (Fig. 31–2). These sheets surround organs, epithelia, or even whole animals. Six different human genes for type IV collagen encode proteins that form net-like polymers that assemble into the **basal lamina** beneath epithelia (Fig. 31–7) and around muscle and nerve cells. The concluding section of this chapter provides details about basal lamina structure, function, and diseases. Hexagonal nets of type VIII collagen form a special basement membrane (Descemet's membrane) under the endothelium of the cornea. Related collagens form the cuticle of earthworms and the organic skeleton of sponges.

Linking Collagens

Connecting and anchoring collagens (see Fig. 31–2) link fibrillar and sheet-forming collagens to other structures. The type VII collagen homotrimer has an exceptionally long triple-helix domain with nonhelical domains projecting at the N-terminus of each chain (see Fig. 31–2). Type VII molecules self-associate tail to tail to form antiparallel dimers. In the process, a protease removes the C-terminal globular domain. Several dimers associate laterally to form so-called **anchoring fibrils** that link type IV collagen of the basal lamina of stratified epithelia to plaques in the underlying connective tissue (see Fig. 31–7). Mutations in type VII collagen cause both the dominant and recessive forms of a severe blistering disease, dystrophic **epidermolysis bullosa.** In heterozygotes, mutated chains interfere with the assembly of anchoring fibrils by normal type VII collagen chains. Without anchoring fibrils, the basal lamina adheres weakly to the connective tissue matrix. Even mild physical trauma to the

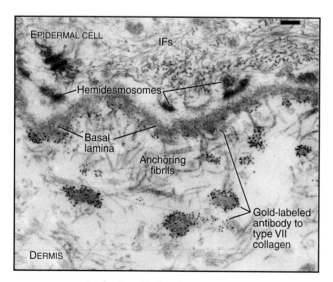

Figure 31-7 Anchoring fibrils of type VII collagen. Electron micrograph of a thin section of human skin reacted with a gold-labeled antibody to the C-terminal domain of type VII collagen. *Top to bottom,* Basal epithelial cell with keratin intermediate filaments (IFs) attached to hemidesmosomes, which link to the basal lamina. Short fibrils of type VII collagen link the basal lamina to plaques in the dermis. Both ends of these bipolar fibrils (see Fig. 31–2) are labeled with gold. Bar is 0.1 μm. (Courtesy of D. R. Keene, Portland Shriners Hospital.)

skin causes the epithelium to pull away from the connective tissue, forming a blister. Chapter 38 describes related diseases caused by mutations in intermediate filaments.

Type IX collagen links glycosaminoglycans to type II collagen fibrils (see Fig. 31–2). This collagen heterotrimer has a serine modified with a glycosaminoglycan chain of variable length. Type IX collagens do not polymerize, but they associate laterally with type II collagen fibrils. The N-terminal helical segment and associated glycosaminoglycan project from the surface of the type II collagen fibril. In the vitreous body of the eye, these polysaccharides fill most of the extracellular space.

▌ Elastic Fibers

In contrast to inextensible collagen fibrils, elastic fibers are similar to rubber. They are found throughout the body but are prominent in the connective tissue of skin (see Fig. 30–2), the walls of arteries (Fig. 31–8) and the lung. They recoil passively after tissues are stretched. Every time the heart beats, pressurized blood flows into and stretches the large arteries. Energy stored in elastic fibers pushes blood through the circulation between heart beats.

Elastic fibers are a composite material: a network of **fibrillin microfibrils** is embedded in an amorphous core of cross-linked **elastin,** which makes up 90% of the organic mass (Fig. 31–9). Fibroblasts produce both components. Loose bundles of microfibrils initiate assembly. Elastin subunits assemble between the microfibrils and become covalently cross-linked.

Fibrillin forms the 10-nm microfibrils. Two fibrillin genes encode similar, thread-like proteins consisting of a tandem array of domains (Fig. 31–10). Fibrillin-1 and fibrillin-2 are both components of microfibrils, along with several glycoproteins. The structure and assembly of microfibrils are still being investigated. Intermolecular disulfide bonds contribute to their insolubility. Microfibrils are also found in the basal lamina.

Elastin subunits are a family of closely related 60-

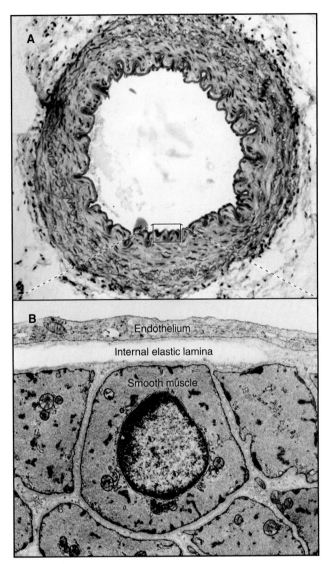

Figure 31–8 Elastic fibers in the wall of a small artery. *A,* Light micrograph of a cross section prepared with a special red stain to visualize elastic fibers. The boxed area includes the internal elastic lamina between the endothelial cells lining the lumen and the underlying smooth muscle cells. *B,* Electron micrograph of a longitudinal thin section illustrating the internal elastic lamina. In such standard preparations, elastic fibers stain poorly and appear amorphous except for occasional 10-nm microfibrils on the surface. (Courtesy of Don W. Fawcett, Harvard Medical School.)

Figure 31–9 Electron micrographs of developing elastic fibers from a fetal calf. *A,* Longitudinal section. *B,* Cross section. Fibrillin microfibrils form a scaffolding for elastin, which stains darkly in this preparation. (Courtesy of J. Rosenbloom, University of Pennsylvania.)

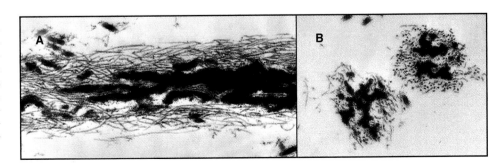

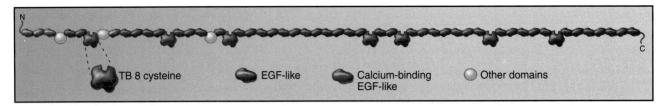

Figure 31–10 Domain organization of human fibrillin. A tandem array of independently folded domains, including 47 epidermal growth factor (EGF)-like domains, forms a linear molecule. (Redrawn from Rosenbloom J, et al: Extracellular matrix 4: The elastic fiber. FASEB J 7:1208–1218, 1993.)

kD proteins called **tropoelastins,** the products of alternative splicing from a single elastin gene. They have long sequences rich in hydrophobic residues interrupted by short sequences with pairs of lysines separated by two or three small amino acids (Fig. 31–11). Lysine-rich sequences are thought to form α helices with pairs of lysines adjacent on the surface.

As tropoelastin assembles on the surface of elastic fibers, lysyl oxidase oxidizes paired lysines of tropoelastin to aldehydes. Oxidized lysines condense into a **desmosine** ring that covalently cross-links tropoelastin molecules to each other (see Fig. 31–11). The four-way crosslinks, involving pairs of lysines from two tropoelastin molecules, are unique to elastin. The

same enzyme catalyzes the cross-linking of collagen, but it forms only two- and three-way crosslinks.

Elastic fibers are similar to rubber except that elastic fibers require water as a lubricant. Hydrophobic segments between the crosslinks are thought to form extensible random coils that account for the elastic properties of the fibril (Fig. 31–12). A difference in entropy of the polypeptide in the contracted and stretched states is thought to be the physical basis for the elasticity. The birefringence of elastic fibers increases when they are stretched, presumably as a result of alignment of polypeptide chains. Stretched fibers store energy owing to ordering (low entropy) of the polypeptide chains. Fibers shorten when the resis-

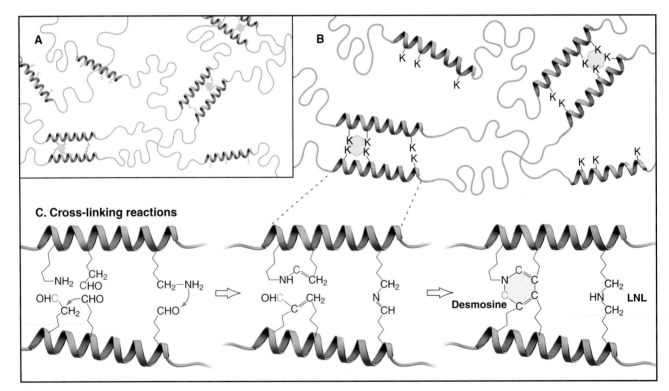

Figure 31–11 Elastin polypeptides and cross-linking reactions. *A,* Lysine-rich helical domains separate random chains rich in hydrophobic residues. *B* and *C,* Lysyl oxidase converts lysine amino groups to aldehydes, which react with other lysines to form simple linear crosslinks or six-membered rings linking two polypeptides. If the peptide bonds are hydrolyzed experimentally (not shown here), the linear crosslink is released as leucyl-norleucine (LNL) and the six-membered crosslink is released as the amino acid desmosine. (Redrawn from Rosenbloom J, et al: Extracellular matrix 4: The elastic fiber. FASEB J 7:1208–1218, 1993.)

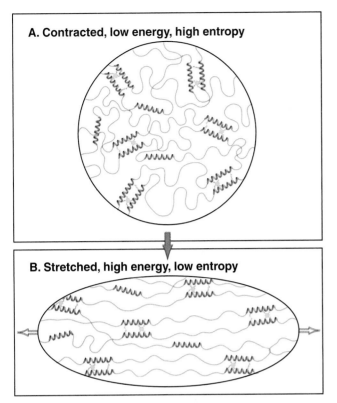

A. Contracted, low energy, high entropy

B. Stretched, high energy, low entropy

Figure 31-12 *A* and *B,* Physical model of elastin elasticity. Elastin polypeptides form a continuous, covalently bonded network. Application of force stretches the chains between the crosslinks. This is a low-entropy, high-energy state. Reduced force allows the chains to contract into a more disordered, higher-entropy state with lower energy. (Redrawn from Rosenbloom J, et al: Extracellular matrix 4: The elastic fiber. FASEB J 7:1208–1218, 1993.)

tance is reduced, because the polypeptide chains return to their disordered, lower-energy, higher-entropy state. Unfolding of fibrillin domains may contribute to the elasticity similar to titin in muscle cells (see Fig. 42–7), but this has not been studied.

Only embryonic and juvenile fibroblasts synthesize elastic fibers, which turn over slowly, if at all, in adults. Consequently, adults must make do with the elastic fibers formed during adolescence. Fortunately, these fibers are amazingly resilient. Arterial elastic fibers withstand more than 2 billion cycles of stretching and recoil during a human life. Many tissues become less elastic with age, particularly the skin (see Fig. 30–2), which is subjected to damage from ultraviolet irradiation. Compare, for example, how readily the skin of a baby recoils from stretching compared with that of an aged person. The loss of elastic fibers in skin is responsible for wrinkles.

Collagens are found across the phylogenetic tree, but only vertebrates are known to produce elastin. Invertebrates evolved two completely different elastic proteins. Mollusks have elastic fibers composed of the protein abductin. Insects use another protein, called resilin, to make elastic fibers.

Marfan syndrome, the disease caused by dominant mutations in the fibrillin-1 gene, illustrates the physiological functions of elastic fibers. Elastic fibers of patients with Marfan syndrome are poorly formed, accounting for most of the pathologic changes observed. Most dangerously, weakness of elastic fibers in the aorta leads to an enlargement of the vessel called an aneurysm, which is prone to rupture, with fatal consequences. Prophylactic replacement of the aorta with a synthetic graft and medical treatment with β-blockers (see Chapter 29) allow patients a nearly normal life span. In some patients, a floppy mitral valve in the heart causes regurgitation of blood from the left ventricle back into the left atrium. Weak elastic fibers that suspend the lens of the eye result in dislocation of the lens and impaired vision. Weak elastic fibers result in lax joints and curvature of the spine. Most affected patients are tall, with long limbs and fingers, but the connection of these features to fibrillin is not known. The manifestations of the disease are quite variable, even within one family, for reasons that are not understood. Mutations in fibrillin-2 cause congenital contractural arachnodactyly, a disease characterized by joint stiffness. New fibrillin mutations arise spontaneously, and most families tested have different mutations, including both point mutations and deletions. All patients are heterozygotes. Most of the known fibrillin-1 mutations make the protein unstable and susceptible to proteolysis. Other point mutations interfere with folding.

Dominant mutations in the elastin gene cause a human disease called cutis laxa. The skin and other tissues of patients with this disease lack resilience.

Glycosaminoglycans and Proteoglycans

Glycosaminoglycans (GAGs; formerly called mucopolysaccharides) are long polysaccharides made up of repeating disaccharide units, usually a hexuronic acid and a hexosamine (Fig. 31–13). With one important exception—hyaluronan—GAGs are synthesized as covalent, post-translational modifications of proteins called proteoglycans. This family of proteins is large and heterogeneous with respect to structure and function. Bound GAGs are their only common feature. Thus, classifying them together makes little more sense than, for example, grouping all phosphorylated proteins together. Nevertheless, some general principles regarding their chemistry and synthesis make it convenient to consider them as a group.

Many cells, including all vertebrate cells, synthesize proteoglycans. Most are secreted into the extracel-

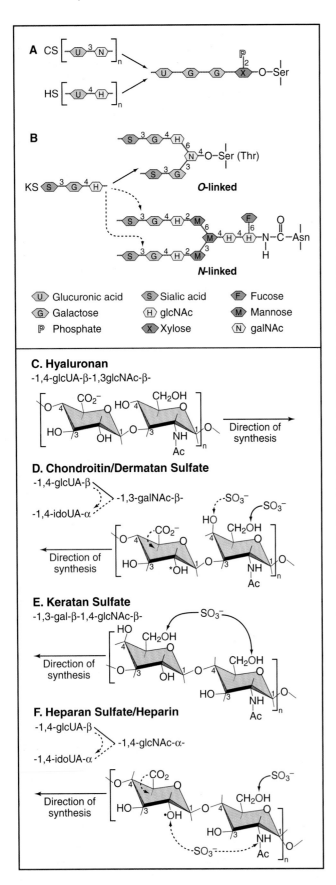

C. Hyaluronan

-1,4-glcUA-β-1,3glcNAc-β-

D. Chondroitin/Dermatan Sulfate

-1,4-glcUA-β
-1,3-galNAc-β-
-1,4-idoUA-α

E. Keratan Sulfate

-1,3-gal-β-1,4-glcNAc-β-

F. Heparan Sulfate/Heparin

-1,4-glcUA-β
-1,4-glcNAc-α-
-1,4-idoUA-α

Figure 31-13 Synthesis of glycosaminoglycans. *A* and *B*, Three short oligosaccharides link GAGs (*left*) to proteoglycan core proteins (*right*). *A*, A tetrasaccharide anchors chondroitin sulfate (CS), dermatan sulfate, and heparan sulfate (HS) to serine residues. *B*, Two different, branched oligosaccharides link keratan sulfate (KS) to either serine or asparagine. *C* to *F*, Four parent polymers and postsynthetic modifications. *C*, Hyaluronan [D-glucuronic acid β (1 → 3) D-N-acetylglucosamine β (1 → 4)]$_n$ ($n \leq 25{,}000$) is not modified postsynthetically. *D*, Chondroitin sulfate and dermatan sulfate are synthesized as [D-glucuronic acid β (1 → 3) D-N-acetylgalactosamine β (1 → 4)]$_n$ (n usually <250) and then modified. Random N-acetylgalactosamines are sulfated. In dermatan sulfate, D-glucuronic acids are epimerized to iduronic acid. *E*, Keratan sulfate is synthesized as [D-galactose β (1 → 4) D-N-acetylglucosamine β (1 → 3)]$_n$ (n usually = 20–40) and then modified by sulfation. *F*, Heparan sulfate/heparin is synthesized as [D-glucuronic acid β (1 → 4) D-N-acetylglucosamine α (1 → 40)]$_n$ (n usually <100) and then modified by sulfation and by epimerization of D-glucuronic acid to iduronic acid. galNAc, N-acetylgalactosamine; glcNAc, N-acetylglucosamine. (Redrawn from Wright TN, Heinegard DK, Hascall VC: Proteoglycans, structure and function. In Hay ED (ed): Cell Biology of the Extracellular Matrix, 2nd ed. New York, Plenum Press, 1991, pp. 45–78.)

lular matrix where they are major constituents of cartilage, loose connective tissue, and basement membranes. Mast cells package the proteoglycan serglycin, along with other molecules in secretory granules. A few proteoglycans, including syndecan and CD44, are plasma membrane proteins with their GAGs exposed on the cell surface.

Of the known GAGs, **hyaluronan** (formerly called hyaluronic acid) is exceptional in two regards. First, enzymes on the cell surface synthesize the alternating polymer of [D-glucuronic acid β (1 → 3) D-N-acetyl glucosamine β (1 → 4)]$_n$ (see Fig. 31–13). Other GAGs are post-translational modifications of a core protein. Second, hyaluronan is *not* modified post-synthetically like all other GAGs. The linear polymer, often exceeding 20,000 disaccharide repeats (a length >20 μm) is released into the extracellular space.

In contrast to proteins, nucleic acids, and even N-linked oligosaccharides, which are precisely determined macromolecular structures, the GAG chains of proteoglycans are variable both in length and in the sequence of the sugar groups. Given their large size, these properties might make them hopelessly complicated. Fortunately, the mechanism of GAG synthesis (see Fig. 31–13) provides a simple explanation for their highly variable structures. There are four steps:

1. Ribosomes associated with the endoplasmic reticulum synthesize the **core protein,** which enters the secretory pathway.
2. In compartments between the endoplasmic reticulum and the trans-Golgi apparatus, **glycosyltransferases** initiate GAG synthesis by adding one of three different, short, *link oligosaccharides* to serine or asparagine residues of the core proteins (see Fig. 31–13*A–B*). The structural clues identifying these sites are not understood, as they do not have a common sequence motif. A tetrasaccharide attached to serine anchors dermatan sulfate, chondroitin sulfate, and heparan sulfate. Branched oligosaccharides anchor keratan sulfate to serine or asparagine.
3. In the trans-Golgi network, other glycosyltransferases elongate the polysaccharide by adding, sequentially, *two alternating sugars* to the growing chain (see Fig. 31–13*D–F*). Only three primary products are made. All are homogeneous, linear structures, each with one pair of alternating sugars.
4. A few enzymes *randomly* modify these homogeneous alternating sugar polymers by adding sulfate to specific hydroxyl or amino groups, or isomerizing specific carbons to convert the D-glucuronic acid to its epimer L-iduronic acid (see Fig. 31–13*D–F*). The variable length of the polymers and the random nature of the modifications make the final products heterogeneous.

The nomenclature for proteoglycans is in flux, so the literature is confused by references to specific proteoglycans by different names. The old nomenclature was based on the identity of the GAGs bound to the protein. For example, the major proteoglycan found in basement membranes was called heparan sulfate proteoglycan. This nomenclature is imprecise, as more than one type of proteoglycan carries heparan sulfate. Once the core proteins were identified and sequenced, it was reasonable to develop a nomenclature based on these core proteins. Consequently, the basement membrane proteoglycan is now known as perlecan, the name of its core protein. The weakness of this system is that the protein name reveals nothing about the associated GAGs. This information is important because various cells add different GAGs to the same core protein or can modify the same GAG in different ways.

Cells secrete many proteoglycans into the extracellular matrix, but they retain some types on the plasma membrane through transmembrane polypeptides or a glycosylphosphatidylinositol anchor (Table 31–2 and Fig. 31–14). The core proteins vary in size from 100 to 4000 amino acids. Many are modular, consisting of familiar structural domains: EGF, complement regulatory protein, leucine-rich repeats, or lectin. The aggrecan polypeptide includes a sequence, similar to link protein, another protein that attaches it to hyaluronan. Three collagens are proteoglycans: types IX and XII have chondroitin sulfate chains, and type XVII has heparin sulfate chains. Type XVII is a ubiquitous component of the basal lamina. An 18-kD fragment from the C-terminus of the core protein has been isolated as a suppressor of blood vessel formation and tumor growth, and has been given the name endostatin.

The number of GAGs attached to the core protein varies from one (decorin) to more than 200 (aggrecan) (see Fig. 31–14). A particular core protein can have identical (fibroglycan, glypican, versican) or different (aggrecan, serglycin, syndecan) GAGs. Specialized cell types can add different GAGs to the same core protein.

Determining the functions of specific proteoglycans has been challenging. Many hypotheses are based on the physical properties of the molecules and their sites of expression, rather than on direct experiments. Given their physical properties and distribution among the fibrous elements of the extracellular matrix, proteoglycans and hyaluronan are thought to be elastic space-fillers. Each hydrophilic disaccharide unit bears a carboxyl or sulfate group, or both, so GAGs are highly charged polyanions that extend themselves by electrostatic repulsion in solution and attract up to 50 g of water per gram of proteoglycan. The largest GAG—hyaluronan—occupies a vast volume. A single hydrated molecule of 25,000 kD occupies a volume

table 31–2

PROTEOGLYCANS

Name	Core Protein	Glycosaminoglycans	Expression	Functions
Secreted proteoglycans				
Aggrecan	One-gene, 250-kD protein with link protein, EGF, lectin and complement regulatory domains	100–150 keratin sulfate chains >150 chondroitin sulfate chains	Cartilage	Binds hyaluronan and link protein; hydrates and fills the ECM; no known diseases
Biglycan	One-gene, 38-kD protein	2 chondroitin sulfate or dermatan sulfate chains	Developing mesenchyme (muscle, bone, cartilage) and epithelia	Associated with cell surfaces; no known ligands or functions
Decorin	One-gene, 38-kD protein	1 chondroitin sulfate or dermatan sulfate chain	Connective tissue fibroblasts	Binds collagen fibrils and modifies their assembly
Fibromodulin	One-gene, 43-kD protein	4 asparagine-linked keratin sulfate chains	Cartilage, skin, tendon	Binds collagen I and II; reduces size of collagen fibrils
Perlecan	One-gene, 400-kD protein	3 heparan sulfate chains of 30–60 kD	All cells making basement membranes (epithelia, muscle, peripheral nerve)	Self-associates; binds laminin in basal-lamina; binds basic fibroblast growth factor
Serglycin	One-gene, 12-kD protein; 24 serine-glycine repeats	Chondroitin sulfate or heparin chains	White blood cells	Binds histamine in secretory granules
Versican	One-gene, 260-kD protein with link-protein, GAG attachment, 2 EGF, lectin and complement regulatory domains	12–15 chondroitin sulfate chains *N*- and *O*-linked oligosaccharide chains	Fibroblasts; ? other cells	May bind hyaluronan; functions unknown
Membrane-associated proteoglycans				
Fibroglycan	One-gene, integral membrane protein of 20 kD	Heparan sulfate chains	Fibroblasts	Binds collagen I and fibronectin; cell adhesion to ECM
Glypican	62-kD protein with glycosyl phosphatidylinositol anchor to membrane on C-terminus	4 heparan sulfate chains	Lung, skin, epithelia, endothelium, smooth muscle	Binds fibronectin, collagen I, and anti-thrombin III; cell adhesion to ECM
Syndecan	One-gene, integral membrane protein of 33 kD	Variable number of heparan sulfate and chondroitin sulfate chains depending on cell type	Embryonic epithelia and mesenchyme, developmentally regulated in adult lymphocytes	Binds fibronectin; collagen I, III, and V; thrombospondin; basic fibroblast growth factor; cell adhesion to ECM

ECM, extracellular matrix.

similar to that of a small organelle with a diameter of 200 nm. Retention of water by hyaluronan and **aggrecan**-keratan sulfate/chondroitin sulfate proteoglycan is essential in cartilage (see Fig. 34–3). In the extracellular matrix of other tissues, networks of densely charged hyaluronan restrict water flow, limit diffusion of solutes (especially macromolecules), and impede the passage of microorganisms. Hyaluronan and proteoglycans also act as lubricants in joint cavities and as an optically transparent, space-filling medium in the vitreous body of the eye.

The tissue- and age-specific distributions of secreted proteoglycans suggest that they may have more subtle functions as well. They can promote or inhibit

Figure 31-14 *A* to *F,* Scale drawings of a variety of proteoglycans. Core proteins are purple and pink and the glycosaminoglycans are color-coded. Proteins were named according to the following: aggrecan aggregates along hyaluronan; decorin decorates collagen fibrils; perlecan resembles a string of pearls; serglycin has 24 ser-gly repeats; syndecan (syndein = link) links cells to the matrix; glypican has a glycosyl-phosphatidylinositol (GPI) membrane anchor. CS, chondroitin sulfate; DS, dermatan sulfate; HS, heparan sulfate; Hep, heparin; KS, keratan sulfate. (Redrawn from Wright TN, Heinegard DK, Hascall VC: Proteoglycans, structure and function. In Hay ED (ed): Cell Biology of the Extracellular Matrix, 2nd ed. New York, Plenum Press, 1991, pp. 45–78.)

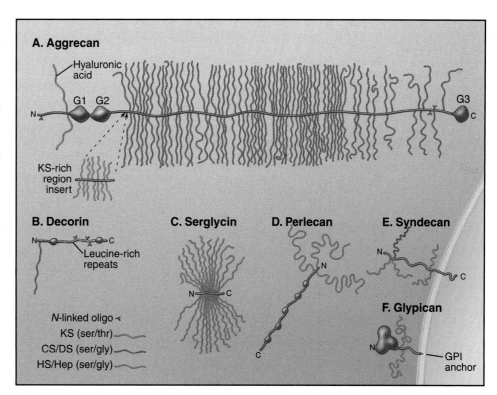

cell motility or adhesion. Decorin and fibromodulin both regulate assembly of collagen fibrils. Expression of several proteoglycans at specific times during embryonic development and wound healing suggests that they may provide signals for organizing connective tissue fibers and cells.

Transmembrane proteoglycans can link cells to fibronectin and connective tissue collagens. **Syndecan** provides a particularly clear example. Lymphocytes express syndecan twice: early in their maturation when they adhere to matrix fibers in the bone marrow, and later, when, as mature plasma cells, they adhere to the matrix of lymph nodes. In between, syndecan expression is lower while the lymphocytes circulate in the blood.

Many polypeptide growth factors (including acidic fibroblast growth factor, basic fibroblast growth factor, platelet-derived growth factor, and transforming growth factor-β) bind to proteoglycans in the extracellular matrix. This allows the matrix to concentrate circulating growth factors at specific locations and to release them locally over a period of time. This timed-release mechanism is potentially important in controlling many aspects of embryonic development and integrating the stimulation of target cells over a period of time.

The well-known anticoagulant effects of heparin and heparan sulfate are attributable to their ability to bind both thrombin (the proteolytic enzyme that converts fibrinogen to fibrin) and a thrombin inhibitory protein. This promotes interaction of the inhibitor with thrombin and inactivates the clotting cascade. A short sequence of six modified sugars has the anticoagulant activity.

Adhesive Glycoproteins

In principle, the fibrous and gelatinous macromolecules of the extracellular matrix and the constituent cells could all stick to each other through relatively nonspecific interactions; however, the available evidence suggests that specific molecular interactions mediate virtually all of the interactions required to organize the matrix and the associated cells. Most interactions are between proteins. Some are between proteins and sugars. Although some of these interactions are direct (with some cell surface receptors binding collagen directly), adapters called adhesive glycoproteins mediate many of the interactions (Table 31–3).

Investigators originally identified adhesive glycoproteins in biochemical assays for factors that favor particular interactions, such as the adherence of cells to a matrix component. Subsequent work has revealed that adhesive glycoproteins are more than molecular glue; they also provide cells with signals required for the development and repair of tissues. Cells receive these signals when they bind to the matrix components. Chapter 32 focuses on their receptors.

table 31–3

ADHESIVE GLYCOPROTEINS

Name(s)	Composition	Expression	Ligands	Functions and Diseases
Agrin	One-gene, 205-kD protein with cysteine-rich, EGF, and Kazal protease inhibitor domains	Secreted by motor neurons into the basal lamina of the neuromuscular junction	?Acetylcholine receptor	Aggregates acetylcholine receptors
Fibrinogen	2 × 67 kD Aα chains, 2 × 56 kD Bβ chains, and 2 × 47 kD γ chains, all joined by interchain disulfide bonds; N-linked CHO on Bβ and γ chains	Secreted into blood by hepatocytes	Platelet integrin GPIIb/GPIIIa	Thrombin cleaves fibrinogen peptides, releasing fibrin, which polymerizes into fibrils stabilized by covalent cross-linking by transglutaminase; deficiency or defects cause bleeding
Fibronectin	One gene; alternative splicing generates isoforms of 235–270 kD; dimers are disulfide-bonded; 12 FN-I, 2 FN-II, and 15–17 FN-III domains; N- and O-linked CHO	Many tissues; increased with wounding	Fibrin, heparin, cells via integrins, collagen	Assembles fibrils in ECM; promotes cellular adhesion to ECM and migration
Fibulin	One gene; alternative splicing generates monomeric isoforms of 566, 601, and 683 residues with 9 EGF and 3 complement-like domains; N- and O-linked CHO	Fibroblasts; present in plasma and some basement membranes	Ca^{2+}, fibronectin, fibrinogen	Assembles fibrils
HB-GAM (heparin-binding, growth-associated molecule)	136 residues, 5 internal disulfide bonds	Brain, uterus, intestine, kidney, muscle, lung, skin	Heparin	?Neuronal differentiation
Laminin	1 × 200–400 kD A chain 1 × 200 kD B1 chain 1 × 200 kD B2 chain, several isoforms of each; poly-N-acetyl galactosamine	Epithelium, endothelium, smooth and striated muscle, peripheral nerve, myotendinous junction	Six integrins, nidogen, perlecan heparan sulfate proteoglycan, collagen IV, α-dystroglycan	Self-associates into network in basement membrane linked to collagen IV network by nidogen; promotes cell adhesion and migration
Laminin-binding protein Mac-2)	Soluble S-type monomeric lectin of 29–35 kD	Macrophages, epithelia, fibroblast, trophoblast, cancer cells	Poly-N-acetyl galactosamine on laminin	?
Link protein	One gene; alternative splicing generates isoforms of 41, 46, and 51 kD with two 4-cysteine and one immunoglobulin domains; CHO content variable	Cartilage	Aggrecan and hyaluron	Links aggrecan to hyaluronan
Mucins	Heterogeneous secreted and transmembrane glycoproteins	Gastrointestinal tract, salivary glands	Selectins	Lubricates mucous membranes

table 31-3

ADHESIVE GLYCOPROTEINS *Continued*

Name(s)	Composition	Expression	Ligands	Functions and Diseases
Nidogen (entactin)	One-gene, 148-kD monomeric protein with 8 EGF and 2 EF hand domains; *N*- and *O*-linked CHO	Basement membranes of epithelia, muscles, and nerves	Laminin ($K_d = 1$ nM), collagen IV, Ca^{2+}	Links collagen IV to laminin in basement membrane
Osteopontin (secreted phosphoprotein)	Monomer of ~300 residues, phosphorylated, *N*- and *O*-linked CHO, including sialic acid	Bone, milk, kidney, uterus, ovary	?Vitronectin receptor; ?hydroxyapatite	Promotes cell adhesion to ECM, including osteoclasts to bone
Restrictin	3 × 180 kD chains linked by disulfide bonds; each has 1 cystine-rich, EGF, 9 FN-III and 1 fibrinogen-like domains	A limited number of neurons in embryonic nervous systems	Cells, receptor unknown	?Cell adhesion
SPARC ("secreted protein rich in cysteine"); osteonectin	One-gene; 32-kD monomer	Bone, skin, connective tissue	Collagens III and V, Ca^{2+}, hydroxyapatite, cells	?Wound healing, development
Tenascin (cytotactin)	One gene; alternate splicing generates 190, 200, and 230 kD isoforms with 14 EGF, 8–11 FN-III, and fibrinogen-like domains; 6 chains linked by disulfides	Embryonic mesenchyme; adult perichondrium, periosteum, tendon, ligament, myotendinous junction, wounds	Integrins, Ig-CAMs, proteoglycans	Unknown; normal development in mice with null mutation
Thromobospondin	420-kD protein with procollagen, EGF, and complement-like domains	Platelets, fibroblasts, embryonic heart, muscle, bone, brain	Integrin $\alpha v\beta 3$, CD36 cell surface receptor, syndecan, Ca^{2+}	Platelet aggregation; stimulates proliferation of smooth muscle; inhibits proliferation of endothelium
Vitronectin	One-gene, 75-kD protein with *N*-linked CHO, phosphorylated, sulfated	Secreted by liver into blood	Integrin $\alpha V\beta 3$, heparin, glass, plastic	Promotes cell adhesion, inactivates heparin, stabilizes plasminogen activator inhibitor
von Willebrand's factor	One-gene, 2050-residue protein that forms head to head and tail to tail disulfide-linked oligomers, *N*- and *O*-linked CHO	Endothelium, platelets	Factor VIII, heparin, collagen, platelet integrin GPIIb/GPIIIa	Promotes adhesion of platelets to collagen and each other; required to control bleeding; deficiency causes most common congenital blood clotting abnormality

CHO, oligosaccharide chains; EF, hand calcium binding motif of calmodulin family

Adhesive glycoproteins provide specific molecular interactions in the matrix by binding to cells, matrix macromolecules, or both (see Table 31–3). Adhesive proteins with multiple binding sites for cell surface receptors link cells together. For example, fibrinogen aggregates platelets during blood clotting (see Fig. 32–14). Adhesive proteins with binding sites for both cells and matrix molecules link cells to the extracellular matrix. For instance, fibronectin mediates the attachment of cells to fibrin and collagen. A third group of adhesive proteins with multiple binding sites for matrix macromolecules link them together. For example, nidogen attaches laminin to collagen and link protein attaches aggrecan-proteoglycan to hyaluronan.

Given the variety of tasks, it is not surprising that this family of adhesive proteins is quite diverse in terms of structure and function. In fact, diversity exists beyond the named proteins (see Table 31–3), as multiple genes or, more commonly, alternative splicing of the product of a single gene (see Fig. 15–9), generate a number of isoforms of most of the named proteins. These isoforms are generally expressed in specific tissues at predictable times during development, suggesting specific functions. In fact, isoforms can have different receptor-binding specificity.

Fortunately, consideration of the structures of these large proteins is simplified because many are constructed from a series of compact modules (see Table 31–3 and Fig. 2–15). Adhesive glycoproteins use complement-like, cysteine-rich, EF-hand, EGF, fibronectin I (FN-I), fibronectin II (FN-II), fibronectin III (FN-III), fibrinogen, immunoglobulin, and lectin domains. In the few cases studied, adjacent domains appear to interact relatively rigidly. Duplication and recombination of the coding sequences for the domains produced the genes for these large proteins during evolution. In addition to the domains, each of these proteins also contains a significant fraction of unique sequences.

Most adhesive glycoproteins that interact with cells bind to heterodimeric transmembrane receptors called **integrins** (see Chapter 32). Remarkably, the integrin-binding sites of many adhesive proteins include the simple tripeptide arginine-glycine-aspartic acid (**RGD**) (see Fig. 31–15).

Designing direct tests for the biological functions of adhesive glycoproteins is challenging. First, many different molecules contribute to the integrity of the matrix and its associated cells, so some may have overlapping functions. Second, biochemical characterization of the interactions of giant matrix macromolecules is much more difficult than for smaller soluble molecules. Initial hypotheses were based on the identification of binding partners and the time and place of expression of each protein. Later, antibodies or peptides were used to disrupt specific molecular interactions in live organisms. Disruption of the genes for specific proteins or their receptors provides the most definitive data, and the consequences can be surprising. Some phenotypes are milder than expected from earlier studies. These results argue that the adhesive glycoproteins function as a complementary system with partially overlapping functions. Two examples illustrate what we know about adhesive glycoproteins.

Fibronectin

Fibronectins are large proteins consisting of two polypeptides of about 235 kD linked by disulfide bonds near their C-termini (Fig. 31–15). In electron micrographs, fibronectin appears as a V-shaped pair of long, flexible rods connected at one end. In solution, the molecule is probably more compact. Each polypeptide is a linear array of three types of domains called FN-I, FN-II, and FN-III. All three types of fibronectin domains consist of antiparallel β strands with conserved residues in their hydrophobic cores. Two disulfide bonds stabilize FN-I and FN-II domains, whereas FN-III domains have no disulfide bonds. FN-I and FN-II domains consist of about 45 residues; FN-III domains are twice as large. FN-I and FN-II domains are present in a few other proteins, whereas the human genome contains about 170 genes with FN-III domains, including proteins in the extracellular matrix

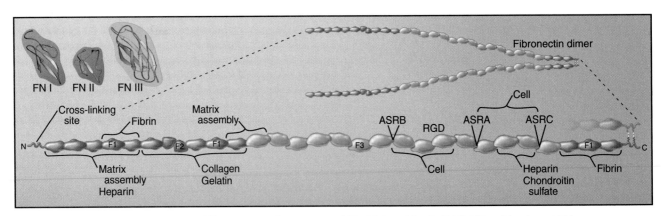

Figure 31–15 Domain organization of fibronectin. A linear array of FN-I (45 residues), FN-II (45 residues), and FN-III (90 residues) domains forms a rod-shaped subunit. Disulfide bonds near the C-termini covalently link two identical subunits in the dimeric molecule. Ligand-binding sites are indicated. The FN-III domain 10 contains the RGD sequence that binds cell surface integrins. Binding sites for fibrin, collagen, and glycosaminoglycans are indicated. Alternative splicing at sites ASRB, ASRA, and ASRC creates different isoforms. (Reference: Potts JR, Campbell ID: Fibronectin structure and assembly. Curr Opin Cell Biol 6:648–655, 1994. Copyright 1994, with permission from Elsevier Science. PDB files: FN7, 1PDC, 1FNA.)

(see Table 31–3), on the cell surface (human growth hormone receptor; see Fig. 26–6), and inside cells (titin; see Fig. 42–7).

Fibronectin binds a variety of ligands, including cell surface receptors, collagen, proteoglycans, and fibrin (another adhesive protein). Thus, it contributes to adhesion of cells to the extracellular matrix and may also cross-link matrix molecules. Investigators have identified the ligand-binding sites in the various domains by isolating proteolytic fragments and by expressing fibronectin fragments (see Fig. 31–15). The RGD sequence that contributes to the integrin-binding site of fibronectin is located on an exposed loop of FN-III domain 10. The variably spliced V domain included in plasma fibronectin has a second integrin-binding site. Chapter 32 provides additional details on integrins.

Two pools of fibronectin have different distributions and solubility properties. *Tissue fibronectin* forms insoluble fibrils in connective tissues throughout the body, especially in embryos and healing wounds. Fibroblasts use an integrin-dependent process to assemble fibronectin dimers into fibrillar aggregates large enough to visualize by light microscopy (Fig. 31–16). The structure of these microscopic fibrils is not known. Denaturing agents and disulfide reduction are required to solubilize these fibrils. Disulfide bonds between the two subunits of fibronectin are also essential to form this continuous protein network, so fibronectin with deletions from the C-terminus cannot assemble into fibrils. Although difficult to study because of their large size and insolubility, fibronectin fibrils seem to bind cells more efficiently than soluble fibronectin, and may have additional activities important for biological functions.

Soluble *plasma fibronectin* dimers circulate in the body fluids. The protein differs from tissue fibronectin as a result of alternate splicing of the mRNA. In blood clots, the enzyme transglutaminase covalently couples plasma fibronectin to fibrin, forming a provisional matrix for wound repair (see Fig. 34–11).

Given its ligand-binding and assembly properties, together with its expression in vertebrate embryos even before their implantation in the uterus, fibronectin appears to contribute to the extracellular matrix in early embryos. A collagen-based matrix replaces this primordial matrix as the embryo matures. Furthermore, embryonic cells, such as neural crest cells (precursors of pigment cells, sympathetic neurons, and adrenal medullary cells), migrate along tracks in the extracellular, fibronectin-rich matrix. Antibodies or fibronectin fragments that interfere with the adhesion of cells to fibronectin inhibit neural crest cell migration, gastrulation, and the formation of many embryonic structures derived from mesenchymal cells. Consequently, it was

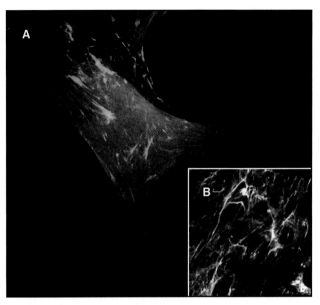

Figure 31–16 Fluorescence micrographs of fibronectin networks in tissue culture. *A*, This fibroblast expressed fibronectin-YFP (fibronectin fused to yellow fluorescent protein, appearing yellow-green) and moesin-CFP (moesin fused to cyan fluorescent protein, appearing red). The fibronectin assembled an extracellular network. Moesin is associated with actin filaments in stress fibers. *B*, Lower magnification of a fibronectin network. (Courtesy of T. Ohashi and H. P. Erickson, Duke University.)

thought that fibronectin might provide cellular adhesion sites required for these movements.

Thus, it was predicted that deletion of the single fibronectin gene in mice would be lethal owing to devastating effects very early in embryogenesis. It is true that homozygous null mutant mice die during embryogenesis as a result of failure to form mesodermal structures, including the notochord, muscles, heart, and blood vessels. However, the surprise was how far the embryos developed without fibronectin. In fact, up to about day 8 (when the basic body plan is already determined), the embryos appeared to be almost normal. (Mice with null mutations in the main fibronectin receptor, integrin α5, were found to have similar but slightly milder defects.) One interpretation is that fibronectin and its receptor are less important for early development than anticipated. Changes in the expression of other adhesive glycoproteins or receptors may compensate for the fibronectin defects during the first few days of development.

Tenascin

Tenascin, a giant protein with six arms (Fig. 31–17), is expressed in many embryonic tissues, wounds, and tumors. However, its physiological function is in question because mice with a disrupted tenascin-C gene

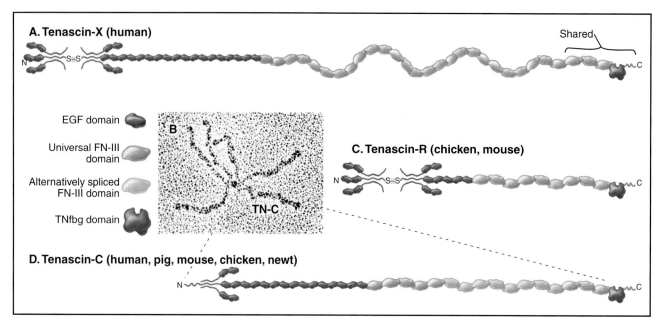

Figure 31-17 Domain organization of the three isoforms of tenascin and an electron micrograph (*B*) of tenascin-C. TNFbg, fibrinogen-like domain. *A,* Tenascin-X. *C,* Tenascin-R. *D,* Tenascin-C. Each of these tenascin molecules has 6 identical chains. One is shown in its entirety. Five chains are represented only by their v-terminal Z EGF domains (*A, C*) or just two of the other five chains (*D*). (Courtesy of H. P. Erickson, Duke University.)

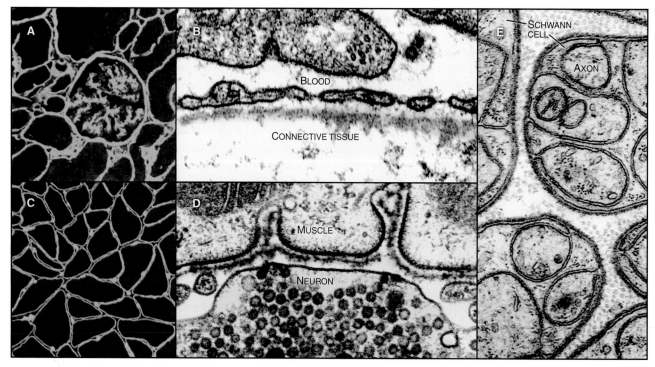

Figure 31-18 Micrographs of the basal lamina. *A* and *C,* Fluorescence micrographs of tissue sections stained with fluorescent antibodies to type IV collagen, a major component of basal laminae. *A,* Kidney with basal laminae around the tubules and blood vessels, including those of the glomerulus in the center. *C,* Skeletal muscle with basal laminae around the muscle cells. *B, D,* and *E,* Electron micrographs of thin sections showing basal laminae (*pink*). *B,* Endothelial cell lining a blood vessel with a platelet in the lumen. *D,* Neuromuscular junction. *E,* Unmyelinated nerve with numerous axons (*yellow*) surrounded by invaginations of Schwann cells (*blue*). (*A* and *C,* From Odermatt BF, et al: Monoclonal antibody to human type IV collagen. Proc Natl Acad Sci USA 81:7343–7347, 1984. *B* and *E,* Courtesy of Don W. Fawcett, Harvard Medical School; *D,* Courtesy of J. Heuser, Washington University.)

appear normal. This observation shocked investigators working on tenascin, because the precise expression of tenascin-C in particular embryonic tissues had suggested that it must have a role in development. On the other hand, vertebrates have four tenascin genes, so the four isoforms may have overlapping functions, with tenascin-R, tenascin-X, or tenacin-Y compensating for the loss of tenascin-C. However, expression of the four isoforms hardly overlaps, so some tissues must develop normally with little tenascin.

Tenascin is modular protein, consisting of an N-terminal self-association domain, a number of EGF and FN-III domains, and a C-terminal domain similar to part of fibrinogen. The last three FN-III domains and the fibrinogen-like domains are similar in all four isoforms, whereas the number of EGF and FN-III domains differ. Three subunits self-associate, through a triple helical coiled-coil. Disulfides covalently link two of these three-chain units to make the six-armed molecule. All vertebrates express tenascin, but it has not yet been found in an invertebrate.

The biochemical activities of tenascin have been difficult to define, perhaps reflecting a misunderstanding about its function. Tenascins bind to cells via integrins, cell surface proteoglycans, and receptors of the immunoglobulin-superfamily, but the significance of these interactions is unclear. Depending upon the cell and the experimental situation, tenascin can promote or inhibit adhesion of cells to culture dishes. Efforts to implicate tenascin as a growth factor are also controversial. Despite this ambiguity, it is impressive that vertebrates have maintained the tenascin genes over hundreds of millions of years since they diverged from each other. Further experimentation is required to understand the selective advantage provided by tenascins.

▌ The Basal Lamina

The basal lamina, a thin, planar assembly of extracellular matrix proteins, supports all epithelia, muscle cells, and nerve cells outside the central nervous system (Fig. 31–18). This two-dimensional network of protein polymers forms a continuous rug under epithelia and a sleeve around muscle and nerve cells. In addition, basal laminae are semipermeable filters for macromolecules, a particularly important role that they play in the formation of urine in the kidney. The genes for basal lamina components are very ancient, having arisen in early metazoans.

In electron micrographs of thin sections of tissues prepared by chemical fixation, the basal lamina is a homogenous, finely fibrillar material separated from the adjacent cell by a clear gap (see Fig. 31–18D). This gap is not present when the tissue is prepared by rapid freezing, so it may be an artifact. This would

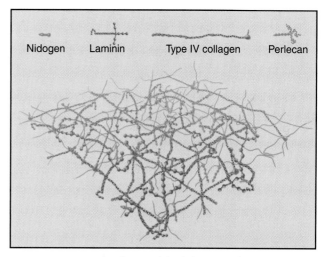

Figure 31–19 Molecular model of the basal lamina showing the sizes and shapes of the component molecules and their postulated three-dimensional arrangement in the basal lamina. (Redrawn from Yurchenco P, et al: Laminin forms an independent network in basement membranes. J Cell Biol 117:1119, 1992, by copyright permission of the Rockefeller University Press.)

reconcile biochemical evidence that plasma membrane proteins connect cells directly to the basal lamina. In some tissues, fine type VII collagen fibrils connect the lamina to underlying connective tissue. The basal lamina and associated collagen fibrils form the "basement membrane" observed in histological preparations of epithelia. A basal lamina alone cannot be seen by light microscopy without special labels, such as those used in Figure 31–18.

Basal laminae vary to some extent in molecular composition among tissues and during embryonic development, but most consist of an intermeshed network of two protein polymers formed by **type IV collagen** and **laminin** (Fig. 31–19). Collagen IV self-assembles into a branching two-dimensional network (see Fig. 31–2). Independently, laminins self-assemble into continuous, two-dimensional networks through noncovalent interactions of their short arms. In early embryos, the laminin network can form first, with type IV collagen added later. Tissues express different isoforms of collagen IV and laminin, accounting for the localized pathology in patients with genetic defects in one of these proteins or autoantibodies directed against a particular isoform.

Additional proteins reinforce the double-polymer scaffold. A rod-shaped protein known as nidogen (also called entactin) cross-links laminin to type IV collagen, stabilizing the association of the two protein scaffolds. **Perlecan,** a heparan sulfate proteoglycan, provides additional crosslinks, as it binds to itself in addition to laminin, nidogen, and collagen IV. These crosslinks help to determine the porosity of basal lamina and thus the size of molecules that can filter through it.

Epithelial and muscle cells synthesize and secrete the components of basal lamina, which self-assemble immediately adjacent to the cell. Membrane receptors for laminin and collagen IV, including integrins and **dystroglycan** (see Fig. 32–12), presumably concentrate these proteins at the plasma membrane and restrict their coassembly near to the cell surface. Mouse embryos lacking dystroglycan die early in development owing to failure to make basal lamina. In embryos, two different cells can cooperate to produce a basal lamina. For example, epithelial cells make laminin and mesenchymal cells make nidogen for the same basal lamina.

The interwoven network of protein fibers provides the physical basis for the two main functions of the basal lamina: physical support and selective permeability. The basal lamina is a physical scaffold to anchor epithelial, muscle, and nerve cells. In epithelia, all of the basal cells attach to the underlying basal lamina. The basal lamina, in turn, is anchored to the underlying connective tissue. Thus, forces applied to an exposed epithelial surface, like skin, are transmitted through the basal lamina to connective tissue. Similarly, all epithelial cells in tubular structures, such as blood vessels and glands, adhere to a cylindrical basal lamina that contributes to the integrity of the tube. In muscle, the basal lamina around each cell transmits the contractile forces between cells and to tendons.

The fibrous network in the basal lamina also acts as a filter for macromolecules and a permeability barrier for cellular migration. In kidney, a basal lamina sandwiched between two epithelial cells filters the blood plasma to initiate the formation of urine. The molecular weight threshold for the filter is about 60 kD, so many serum proteins are retained in the blood, whereas salt and water pass into the excretory tubules. The high charge of basal lamina proteoglycans contributes to filtering by electrostatic repulsion. Basal laminae also confine epithelial cells to their natural compartment. If neoplastic transformation occurs in an epithelium, the basal lamina prevents the spread of the tumor into the connective tissue and beyond, at least until the cancer cells develop the matrix metalloproteinases (see later section) required to break it down.

Several genetic defects and autoimmune diseases cause defects in the basal lamina (Table 31–4). These diseases are remarkably specific for particular organs, in part because expression of several basal lamina components is restricted to one or a few tissues. For example, owing to expression of a particular collagen IV isoform, the kidney is affected more than other tissues in Alport's and Goodpasture's syndromes, whereas one blistering skin disease results from a mutation in a laminin that is confined to the skin. The major basement membrane type IV collagen consists of 2 α1(IV) chains and 1 α2(IV) chains, but restricted tissues express four additional type IV collagen chains; remarkably, each has been implicated in human disease. (No human mutations in the two major type IV collagen genes have been observed, presumably because they have a dominant lethal phenotype during embryogenesis, as observed in *Drosophila*.) Patients with Alport's X-linked familial nephritis all have mutations in the α5(IV) collagen gene. More than 200 different point mutations and deletions are known. Other patients with autosomally inherited Alport's syndrome have mutations in their α3(IV) or α4(IV) collagen genes. The defects in the type IV collagens caused by these mutations disrupt the basement membranes that form the blood filtration barrier in the glomerulus of the kidney, causing progressive kidney failure that is usually fatal in males. These mutations also cause defects in the eye and ear, presumably because these are other places where the α5(IV) collagen gene is expressed. In Goodpasture's syndrome, the immune system produces autoantibodies to the C-terminal 36 amino acids of the α3(IV) collagen chain. These antibodies bind to basement membranes in the kidney and lung, causing inflammation that leads to kidney failure and bleeding in the lungs. The protein sequence eliciting autoantibody production is normally buried in the folded C-terminal domain of the collagen molecule and may be exposed during bacterial infection or exposure to organic solvents, common predisposing events in this syndrome. Deletions in the

table 31–4		
INHERITED DISEASES OR MUTANT PHENOTYPES OF BASAL LAMINA COMPONENTS		
Protein Subunit	**Distribution**	**Disease or Mutant Phenotype**
Collagen α3IV	Many tissues	Human autoantibodies cause Goodpasture's syndrome of renal failure.
Collagen α5IV	Kidney, muscle	Human mutation causes Alport's syndrome of renal failure.
Laminin α1	Many tissues	Fly null mutation is lethal during embryogenesis.
Laminin α2	Muscle, heart	Mouse dy mutation causes muscular dystrophy.
Laminin γ2	Epidermis	Human mutation causes Herlitz's junctional epidermolysis bullosa.
Perlecan	Many tissues	Worm unc-52 mutation disrupts myofilament attachment to membrane.

$\alpha5(IV)$ and $\alpha6(IV)$ collagen genes can also cause benign smooth muscle tumors of the esophagus.

Matrix Metalloproteinases

Many physiological processes depend on the controlled degradation of the extracellular matrix. Examples of this degradation process include tissue remodeling during embryogenesis (e.g., the resorption of a tadpole tail); wound healing; involution (massive shrinkage secondary to loss of cells and extracellular matrix) of the uterus after childbirth; shedding of the uterine endometrium during menstruation; and invasion of the uterine wall by the embryonic trophoblast during implantation. Conversely, uncontrolled destruction of the extracellular matrix contributes to the pathologic effects of degenerative diseases, such as emphysema and arthritis, and to tumor cell invasion and metastasis. A group of about 20 homologous metalloproteinases appear to account for both the physiological and pathological degradation of the extracellular matrix.

Matrix metalloproteinases (MMPs) share a 180-residue zinc-protease domain (Fig. 31–20) similar to bacterial thermolysin. Gelatinases have three FN-II domains inserted into the sequence of the catalytic domain. All have an N-terminal signal sequence and are processed through the secretory pathway. Between the signal sequence and the catalytic domain, all MMPs have an **autoinhibitory propeptide,** including a conserved cysteine that binds to the zinc ion in the catalytic site. Proteolytic cleavage and dissociation of the propeptide activate the enzyme. A C-terminal transmembrane domain anchors MMP-14 (and related MMP-15, -16, and -17) to the plasma membrane. All other MMPs are secreted. Most MMPs have a C-terminal regulatory domain that influences the substrate specificity of the catalytic domain.

After secretion, inactive pro-MMPs bind to cell surface receptors where they are activated and carried to specific substrates in the extracellular matrix by movements of the cell. Propeptide cleavage activates MMPs on the cell surface. Membrane-anchored MMP-14 directly activates MMP-2, which then degrades basement membrane collagen and other substrates.

Secreted proteins called **tissue inhibitors of metalloproteinases** (TIMPs) bind tightly to the active site of MMPs, inhibiting their activity. The atomic structure of a TIMP bound to an MMP has provided a valuable starting point for designing drugs to inhibit particular MMPs for use in the treatment of human diseases.

Growth factors, cytokines, and the extracellular matrix itself control the production and activation of these proteolytic enzymes, restricting their activity to

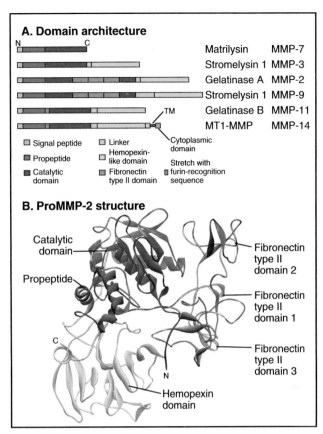

A. Domain architecture

Matrilysin	MMP-7
Stromelysin 1	MMP-3
Gelatinase A	MMP-2
Stromelysin 1	MMP-9
Gelatinase B	MMP-11
MT1-MMP	MMP-14

Signal peptide Linker
Propeptide Hemopexin-like domain
Catalytic domain Fibronectin type II domain
Cytoplasmic domain
Stretch with furin-recognition sequence

B. ProMMP-2 structure

Catalytic domain
Propeptide
Fibronectin type II domain 2
Fibronectin type II domain 1
Fibronectin type II domain 3
Hemopexin domain

Figure 31–20 Matrix metalloproteinase (MMP) structures. *A,* Domain organization of MMP isoforms. All have an N-terminal cleaved signal sequence, a propeptide that binds to the active site and inhibits the protease activity, and a catalytic domain. Gelatinases have FN-II domains inserted in the catalytic domain. Matrilysin lacks the C-terminal domain. MMP-14 has a transmembrane segment near its C-terminus. *B,* Atomic structure of MMP-2 showing the arrangement of the domains and the propeptide occupying the active site. (PDB file: 1CK7.)

sites of physiological tissue breakdown, such as the involuting uterus. On the other hand, many tumor cells constitutively express active MMPs. This is correlated with their ability to break through basement membranes and invade normal tissues. MMP inhibitors can stem the growth of some experimental tumors. Mice survive null mutations in any one of several MMPs tested, but the loss of an MMP may alter the mice's susceptibility to disease dramatically. Mice without MMP-12 (macrophage elastase) are resistant to cigarette smoke, which causes emphysema in normal mice. Without MMP-12, smoke fails to stimulate elastin degeneration, which weakens lung tissue and mediates inflammation.

A related class of about 20 proteases called ADAMs (*a d*isintegrin *a*nd *m*etalloproteinase) are anchored to the plasma membrane by a single transmembrane sequence. Like other metalloproteinases, they are inhibited by TIMPs. ADAMs cleave and release extracellular domains of cell surface proteins, some of which are important informational molecules (e.g., tumor necrosis factor [TNF]-α; transforming growth factor [TGF]-α). ADAM-17 null mutations are lethal during embryogenesis owing to a lack of TGF-α or other ligands for EGF receptors.

▌ Selected Readings

Basebaum CB, Werb Z: Focalized proteolysis: Spatial and temporal regulation of extracellular matrix degradation at the cell surface. Curr Opin Cell Biol 8:731–738, 1996.

Baum J, Brodsky B: Folding of peptide models of collagen and misfolding in disease. Curr Opin Struct Biol 9:122–128, 1999.

Bernfield M, Götte M, Park PW, et al: Functions of cell surface heparan sulfate proteoglycans. Annu. Rev Biochem 68:729–777, 1999.

Burgeson RE, Christiano AM: The dermal-epidermal junction. Curr Opin Cell Biol 9:651–658, 1997.

Hutter H, Vogel BE, Plenefisch JD, et al: Conservation and novelty in the evolution of cell adhesion and extracellular matrix genes. Science 287:989–994, 2000.

Izzo RV: Matrix proteoglycans: From molecular design to cellular function. Annu Rev Biochem 67:609–652, 1998.

Kreis T, Vale R, (eds): Guidebook to the Extracellular Matrix and Adhesion Proteins, 2nd ed. Oxford and New York: Oxford University Press, 1999.

Perrimon N, Bernfield M: Specificities of heparan sulphate proteoglycans in developmental processes. Nature 404: 725–728, 2000.

Ricard-Blum S, Dublet B, van der Rest M: Unconventional Collagens Types VI, VII, VIII, IX, XIV, XVI and XIX. Oxford: Oxford University Press, 2000.

Rosenbloom J, Abrams WR, Mecham R: Extracellular matrix 4: The elastic fiber. FASEB J 7:1208–1218, 1993.

Schwarzbauer JE, Sechler JL: Fibronectin fibrillogenesis: A paradigm for extracellular matrix assembly. Curr Opin Cell Biol 11:622–627, 1999.

Shapiro SD: Matrix metalloproteinase degradation of extracellular matrix: Biological consequences. Curr Opin Cell Biol 9:602–608, 1998.

Timpl R: Macromolecular organization of basement membranes. Curr Opin Cell Biol 8:618–624, 1996.

van der Rest M, Garrone A: Collagen family of proteins. FASEB J 5:2814–2823, 1991.

Vrhovski B, Weiss AS: Biochemistry of tropoelastin. Eur J Biochem 258:1–18, 1998.

Yurchenco PD, O'Rear JJ: Basal lamina assembly. Curr Opin Cell Biol 6:674–681, 1994.

chapter 32

CELLULAR ADHESION

All cells interact with molecules in their environment, in many cases using cell surface adhesion proteins to bind these molecules. Multicellular organisms are particularly dependent upon adhesion of cells to each other and the extracellular matrix. During development, a carefully regulated program of cell-cell and cell-matrix interactions specifies the architecture of each tissue and organ. Some adhesive interactions are stable. Muscle cells must adhere firmly to each other and to the connective tissue of tendons to transmit force to the skeleton (see Chapter 42). Skin cells must also bind tightly to each other and the underlying connective tissue to resist abrasion. On the other hand, some cellular interactions are transient and delicate. At sites of inflammation, leukocytes bind transiently to the endothelial cells lining small blood vessels and then migrate into connective tissue.

How is all this achieved? Do differentiated cells each have novel adhesion systems, or can some general principles simplify the understanding of these complicated processes? The answer, thankfully, is that cells use a relatively small repertoire of adhesion mechanisms to interact with matrix molecules and other cells. Variations on these themes allow cells to form the highly specific interactions required for embryonic development, maintenance of organ structure, and migrations of cells of our defense systems. One could not have made this claim about general mechanisms in 1980.

The conceptual breakthrough came when comparisons of amino acid sequences showed that most adhesion proteins fall into four large families (Figure 32–1). Each family is distinctive. The existence of these families and the modular construction of the proteins resulted from duplication of ancestral genes and their subsequent divergence during evolution, giving rise to

adhesion proteins with many different specificities. Common properties within each family allowed the appreciation of general mechanisms to emerge from characterizing a few examples. Several important adhesion proteins fall outside the four major families, and additional families may emerge from continued research.

Learning about adhesion proteins is challenging, in part, because their names arose historically rather than logically. The original names provide few clues about the family or function of the proteins. Many have more than one name. Related proteins can have completely different names. Tables 32–1 through 32–6 may help the reader keep straight the classification of these families of adhesion proteins. Many adhesion proteins are named CD followed by a number. This stands for "clusters of differentiation," a nomenclature used to classify cell surface antigens recognized by monoclonal antibodies, independent of any knowledge about the structure or function of the antigen. Hence, adhesion proteins in the immunoglobulin–cell adhesion molecule family **(Ig-CAM)**, as well as the **integrin, selectin,** and **mucin** families all have CD numbers.

This chapter first highlights some general features of adhesion proteins and then introduces the major families. While learning about these molecules, the reader should not lose track of an important point: these receptors rarely act alone. Rather, they usually function as parts of multicomponent systems. Two examples at the end of the chapter illustrate the cooperation required for leukocytes to respond to inflammation and for platelets to repair damage to blood vessels. Chapters on specialized connective tissues (see Chapter 34) and cell motility (see Chapter 41) provide more examples of cellular adhesion.

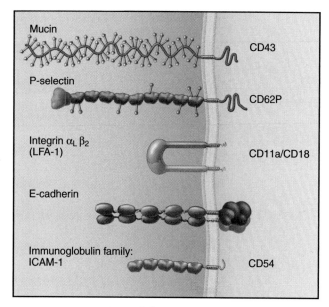

Figure 32–1 Drawings of the major classes of adhesion proteins. Mucins display multiple carbohydrates for interactions with other cells. Selectins have a Ca²⁺-dependent lectin (carbohydrate-binding) domain (*green*), an EGF-like domain (*blue*), and a variable number of complement regulatory domains (*red*). Integrins are heterodimers of α and β subunits that establish a wide range of specificities for matrix molecules by pairwise combinations of 1 of 16 α chains and 1 of 8 β chains. Cadherins have five or more extracellular CAD domains (*red*) that typically bind the same class of cadherin on a neighboring cell. Ca²⁺ stabilizes the interaction of neighboring CAD domains. Ig-CAMs have one or more extracellular domains folded like an immunoglobulin domain. CD numbers refer to the names of representative adhesion molecules based on the "clusters of differentiation" nomenclature (see text). Single transmembrane segments attach all of these receptors to the plasma membrane. Adapter proteins link the cytoplasmic tails of most adhesion proteins to the actin cytoskeleton or, in the case of specialized cadherins and integrins, to intermediate filaments. (Redrawn from van der Merwe PA, Barclay AN: Transient intercellular adhesion: The importance of weak protein-protein interactions. Trends Cell Biol 19:354–358, 1994. Copyright 1994, with permission from Elsevier Science.)

▌General Principles of Cellular Adhesion

First Principle of Adhesion

Cells define their capacity for adhesive interactions by selectively expressing plasma membrane receptors (cell adhesion molecules or CAMs) with limited ligand-binding activity. Generally, expression of the proper mix of receptors is part of the genetically determined program that led to the differentiation of the cell. In some cases, extracellular stimuli control expression of adhesion receptors. For example, endothelial cells produce E-selectin only when stimulated by inflammatory hormones or endotoxin.

Second Principle of Adhesion

Many adhesion proteins bind one main ligand, and many ligands bind a single type of receptor (see Tables 32–1 through 32–6). If this one-to-one pairing were the rule, adhesion would be simple indeed. However, many exceptions exist, particularly in the integrin family of receptors (see Table 32–4). These receptors generally bind more than one ligand, and some ligands, like fibronectin, bind more than one integrin. One can generalize about the ligands for the several families of cell adhesion molecules.

- **Cadherins** strongly prefer to bind themselves, so they promote the adhesion of like cells. These **homotypic interactions** (association of like receptors on two cells) require Ca²⁺.
- Selectins bind anionic polysaccharides like those on mucins. Generally, such interactions bind together two different types of cells.
- Most Ig-CAMs bind other cell surface adhesion proteins. These **heterotypic interactions** (association of unlike receptors on two cells) may occur between the same or different cell types.
- Integrins stand apart because they bind a variety of ligands: matrix macromolecules, such as fibronectin and laminin (see Chapter 31), soluble proteins, like fibrinogen in blood, and adhesion proteins on the surface of other cells, including Ig-CAMs and one cadherin.

Third Principle of Adhesion

Cells modulate adhesion by controlling the surface density, state of aggregation, and state of activation of their adhesion receptors. Surface density reflects not only the level of synthesis, but also the partitioning of adhesion molecules between the plasma membrane and intracellular storage compartments. For example, endothelial cells express P-selectin constitutively, but store it in membranes of cytoplasmic vesicles. When the cell is activated by inflammatory cytokines, these vesicles fuse with the plasma membrane, exposing P-selectin on the cell surface, where it binds white blood cells. The importance of surface density is illustrated by an experiment in which cells expressing different levels of the same cadherin are mixed together. Over time, they sort out from each other, with the more adherent cells forming a cluster, surrounded by the less adherent cells (Fig. 32–2). Such differential expression of cadherin determines the position of the oocyte in *Drosophila* egg follicles. Intracellular signals control the activity of integrins. A variety of extracellular stimuli activate intracellular signaling pathways in lymphocytes, platelets, and other cells, which enhance or inhibit the ligand binding of integrins already lo-

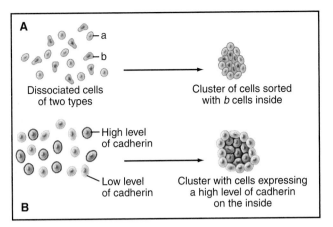

Figure 32-2 Two experiments on sorting of embryonic cells. *A*, When cells from different tissues are dissociated and mixed together, they spontaneously sort themselves into two layers, with the more adherent cells inside the less adherent cells. *B*, Cells with high concentrations of cadherin sort inside less adherent cells. (Based on the work of M. Steinberg, Princeton University.)

cated on the cell surface. The cytoplasmic domains of integrins are likely to mediate this activation. Integrin activation also regulates cellular interactions during development.

Fourth Principle of Adhesion

The rates of ligand binding and dissociation are important determinants of cellular adhesion. Quantitative data on this point are limited, but many cell surface adhesion proteins (including members of the Ig-CAM, integrin, and selectin families) bind their ligands weakly compared with other specific macromolecular interactions, such as the interaction of antigens and antibodies, hormones and receptors, or transcription factors and DNA. The measured dissociation equilibrium constants for these adhesion receptors are in the range of 1 to 100 μM, reflecting high rate constants (>1 s^{-1}) for dissociation of ligand. In some cases, this makes good biological sense. Rapidly reversible interactions allow white blood cells to roll along the endothelium of blood vessels. Transient adhesion also allows fibroblasts to migrate through connective tissue. On the other hand, weak interactions do not make sense for stable cellular interactions in epithelia or muscle. Homotypic interactions of cadherins may be stronger, but have not been characterized quantitatively. Strength may also be found in numbers, with multiple weak interactions between clustered adhesion proteins cooperating to stabilize adherens junctions and desmosomes. The combined strength of these bonds is said to increase the "avidity" of the interaction.

Fifth Principle of Adhesion

Many adhesion receptors, including cadherins and integrins, interact with the cytoskeleton inside the cell. Adapter proteins link cadherins and integrins to actin filaments in many cells and to intermediate filaments in other cells. These interactions provide mechanical continuity from cell to cell in muscles and epithelia, allowing them to transmit forces and resist mechanical disruption. Less is known about cytoskeletal associations of other types of receptors.

Sixth Principle of Adhesion

Association of ligands with adhesion receptors can activate intracellular signal transduction pathways leading to changes in gene expression, cellular differentiation, secretion, motility, receptor activation, and cell division. Signaling through adhesion receptors allows cells to respond appropriately to physical interactions with the surrounding matrix or cells. Compared with other signal transduction pathways (see Chapter 29), our understanding of the molecular mechanisms is still incomplete.

▌ Identification and Characterization of Adhesion Receptors

The ability of mixed populations of cells to sort into homogeneous aggregates has revealed that cells have mechanisms designed to bind like cells together. Similar assays have shown that cells also bind matrix macromolecules, such as fibronectin, laminin, collagen, and proteoglycans. Direct biochemical isolation of the responsible adhesion molecules was challenging initially, but it progressed rapidly once it was possible to produce monoclonal antibodies that inhibit adhesion. These antibodies provided assays for purification of the adhesion protein and cloning of its cDNA. With a few examples in hand, the cloning of cDNAs for additional family members was relatively straightforward.

Steady progress is being made to determine the atomic structures of adhesion receptors. Their modular construction makes it possible to isolate proteolytic fragments or to express one or more domains of recombinant protein suitable for crystallization or nuclear magnetic resonance (NMR) analysis. Given the sequence homologies within each family, the structure of many extracellular domains can now be approximated from the atomic structures of a few examples. Much less is known about the atomic structures of the cytoplasmic domains of most adhesion receptors.

Insights about the functions of adhesion receptors have usually come in several steps. Localization of a protein on specific cells frequently provides the first clues. Typically, each protein is restricted to a subset of cells or to a specific time during embryonic development, or both. Next, investigators use specific antibodies to test for the participation of the adhesion protein in cellular interactions in vitro or in developing embryos. Blistering skin diseases called pemphigus dramatically illustrate the serious consequences when pathological autoantibodies disrupt adhesion between skin cells expressing the antigen (see later section). High-level expression of either the extracellular or intracellular domain of an adhesion receptor can produce a dominant negative phenotype by competing for extracellular or intracellular binding sites for that receptor. Finally, both human genetic diseases and experimental genetic knockouts produce defects caused by the absence of adhesion proteins. In leukocyte adhesion deficiency, white blood cells lack the β_2 integrin that is required to form receptors for Ig-CAMs on the surface of the endothelial cells that line blood vessels. These white blood cells fail to bind to blood vessel walls or to migrate into connective tissue at sites of infection. Similarly, patients with a bleeding disorder called Bernard-Soulier syndrome lack one of the adhesion receptors for von Willebrand factor, a protein that activates platelet aggregation. Loss of cadherins contributes to the spread of cancer. Experimental deletion of specific integrins is lethal in both vertebrates and invertebrates.

Immunoglobulin Family of Cell Adhesion Molecules

The members of the large Ig-CAM family (for which hundreds of genes have been identified) have 1 to 7 extracellular domains, similar to immunoglobulin domains, anchored to the plasma membrane by a single, hydrophobic transmembrane sequence (Fig. 32–3; Table 32–1). In most cases, the identification of immunoglobulin domains is based on sequence comparisons, but atomic structures have confirmed the antibody-like fold of the extracellular domains of several lymphocyte adhesion proteins (T-cell receptor, CD2, CD4, and CD8), as well as ICAMs, ligands for leukocyte integrins. These compact Ig domains consist of 90 to 115 residues folded into 7 to 9 β strands in 2 sheets, usually stabilized by an intramolecular disulfide bond. The N- and C-termini are at opposite ends of these domains, which is convenient for forming linear arrays of immunoglobulin domains.

Some Ig-CAMs consist of a single polypeptide, but others are multimeric, with two (CD8) or four (T-cell

receptor [TCR]) subunits. Other features of these receptors are variable. Those in the nervous system have three or four fibronectin III (FN-III) domains between the immunoglobulin domains and the membrane anchor. FN-III domains (see Chapters 2 and 31) are also a sandwich of seven β strands, but are thought to have arisen separately during evolution. The C-terminal cytoplasmic tails of these receptors vary in sequence and binding sites. The cytoplasmic domains of the lymphocyte accessory receptors CD4 and CD8 bind protein tyrosine kinases required for cellular activation (see Fig. 29–8). The cytoplasmic domains of the neuronal Ig-CAMs bind ankyrin, a protein that links the spectrin-actin membrane skeleton to integral membrane proteins (see Fig. 6–10), but this connection to the actin cytoskeleton may not be a general feature of Ig-CAMs.

Differentiated metazoan cells express Ig-CAMs selectively, especially during embryonic development, when they may contribute to the specificity of cellular interactions required to form the organs. Neurons and glial cells express specific Ig-CAMs that guide the growth of neurites and promote the formation of myelin sheaths. In adults, interaction of endothelial cell ICAM-1 with a white blood cell integrin is essential for adhesion and movement of the leukocytes into the connective tissue at sites of inflammation (see Example 1).

Like other cell adhesion proteins, Ig-CAMs partici-

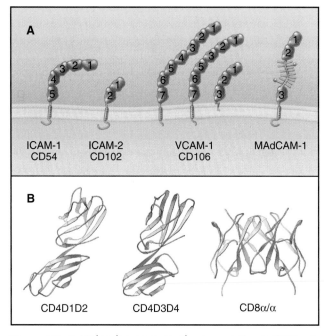

Figure 32–3 Molecular structure of representative Ig-CAMs. *A*, Domain maps. *B*, Ribbon diagrams of the lymphocyte coreceptors CD4 (domains 1 and 2 on the left and 3 and 4 on the right) and CD8. (*A*, Reference: Springer T: Traffic signals for lymphocyte and leukocyte emigration: The multi-step paradigm. Cell 76:301–314, 1994; PDB files: 3CD4, 1CID, and 1CD8.)

table 32–1

CELL ADHESION MOLECULES: IMMUNOGLOBULIN FAMILY (HUNDREDS KNOWN)

Examples	Structure	Extracellular Ligands	Intracellular Ligands	Expression	Functions
CD2*	2 Ig-1 TM	LFA-3 (CD58)		T cells	T-cell activation
CD4*	4 Ig-1 TM	Class II MHC	Lck	T cells, macrophages	T-cell coreceptor
CD8*	Dimer: 1 Ig-1 TM	Class I MHC	Lck	Cytotoxic; other T cells	T-cell coreceptor
C-CAM	4 Ig-1 TM	Self		Liver, intestine, WBCs	Cell adhesion
F11 (contactin)	6 Ig-4 FN-II-1 TM	?		Neurons	Neurite fasciculation
ICAM-1*	5 Ig-1 TM	LFA-1, MAC-1		Epithelia, WBCs	WBC adhesion
ICAM-2	2 Ig-1 TM			Endothelium, WBCs	
L1 (Ng-CAM) [mouse]	6 Ig-3 FN-III-1 TM	Self	Ankyrin	Neurons, Schwann cells	Adhesion
LFA-3 (CD58)	2 Ig-1 TM or GPI anchor	CD2		WBCs, epithelia, fibroblasts	Adhesion
MAG	5 Ig-1 TM	Neurons		Glial cells	Myelin formation
NCAM	5 Ig-3 FN-III-1 TM	Self		Neurons, other cells	Adhesion
Neurofascin [chick]	6 Ig-4 FN-III-1 TM	?Self	Ankyrin	Neurites	Bundling neurites
PECAM-1 (CD31)	6 Ig-1 TM	?Self		Platelets, endothelium, myeloid cells	Adhesion
TAG-1	6 Ig-4 FN-III-GPI anchor	?Self		Neurons	? Adhesion
VCAM-1	7 Ig-1 TM	WBC α_4 integrin		Endothelium (regulated)	WBC/endothelium adhesion

*, partial atomic structure; CAM, cell adhesion molecule; CD, cellular differentiation antigen; FNIII, fibronectin-III domain; GPI, glycosylphosphatidylinositol; ICAM, intercellular adhesion molecule; Ig, immunoglobulin domain; Lck, nonreceptor tyrosine kinase; LFA, lymphocyte function associated antigen; MAG, myelin associated glycoprotein; MHC, major histocompatibility complex; NCAM, neural cell adhesion molecule; PECAM, platelet/endothelial cell adhesion molecule; TAG, transient axonal glycoprotein; TM, transmembrane domain; VCAM, vascular cell adhesion molecule; WBC, white blood cells.

pate in signaling processes. Best understood are interactions of lymphocytes with antigen-presenting cells during immune responses. Ig-CAMs reinforce the interaction of antigen-specific T-cell receptors with major histocompatibility complex (MHC) molecules carrying appropriate antigens on other cells (see Fig. 29–8). Although individual interactions are weak, the combination of specific (T-cell receptor) and nonspecific (CD2 and CD4) interactions with the target cell is sufficient to initiate signaling. Another example is RAGE, which binds the matrix protein amphoterin and signals through the mitogen-activated protein (MAP) kinase pathway (see Chapter 29) during the outgrowth of embryonic neurites. Some tumor cells use this RAGE signaling pathway when they invade normal tissues.

Cadherin Family of Adhesion Receptors

More than 80 cadherins contribute to the Ca^{2+}-dependent associations that most vertebrate cells (and some invertebrate cells) use to form organs. Their name derives from "calcium (Ca)-dependent adhesion" protein. Cadherins link epithelial and muscle cells to their neighbors, especially at specialized adhesive junctions called **adherens junctions** and **desmosomes** (Fig. 32–4 and Fig. 33–7). Interactions of the cytoplasmic domains of cadherins with actin filaments or intermediate filaments reinforce these junctions and maintain the physical integrity of tissues. Contacts mediated by cadherins also influence cellular growth and migration, including suppression of growth and invasion of tumors, as well as formation of synapses in the nervous system. Table 32–2 lists a few cadherins.

Several properties set cadherins apart from other adhesion proteins: (1) cadherins do not interact with the extracellular matrix; (2) interactions with like cadherins on the surfaces of other cells are strongly favored over other interactions (i.e., E-cadherin on one cell binds to E-cadherin on another cell, not to other cadherins); and (3) this homophilic binding requires calcium. The rare exceptions to homophilic binding are interesting. Some lymphocytes use integrins to bind E-cadherin on gut epithelial cells. N-cadherins bind and stimulate fibroblast growth factor receptors on nerve cells to stimulate growth of their axons.

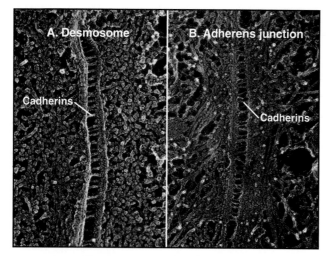

Figure 32-4 Electron micrographs of rod-like cadherins connecting the plasma membranes of adjacent cells. Intestinal epithelial cells were prepared by rapid freezing, freeze-fracture, deep etching, and rotary shadowing. *A*, Desmosome with associated intermediate filaments in the cytoplasm. *B*, Adherens junction with associated actin filaments. (Courtesy of N. Hirokawa, University of Tokyo. Reference: Hirokawa N, Heuser J. Quick-freeze, deep-etch visualization of the cytoskeleton beneath surface differentiations of intestinal epithelial cells. J Cell Biol 91:399–409, 1981.)

The structural hallmark of the cadherin family is the **CAD domain** of about 115 residues (Figs. 32–5 and 32–6). The so-called "classic" cadherins have five extracellular CAD domains. Typically, a single hydrophobic sequence, presumed to be an α helix, spans the plasma membrane, but T-cadherin has a glycophosphatidylinositol (GPI) anchor (see Chapter 6). Cytoplasmic domains vary in size, sequence, and binding sites for associated proteins. The proto-oncogene, RET, is a cadherin with a cytoplasmic tyrosine kinase domain.

Atomic structures of the N-terminal domains of E- and N-cadherin provide a model for all CAD domains (see Fig. 32–6). The sandwich of seven β strands is similar to immunoglobulin and FN-III domains, but the limited sequence homology suggests independent origins and convergent evolution. N- and C-termini are on opposite ends of the CAD domain. Ca^{2+} bound to three sites between adjacent domains links them together into the rigid rod that is observed by electron microscopy. Without Ca^{2+}, the domains rotate freely around their linker peptides.

Two types of interactions between N-terminal CAD1 domains are required for pairs of identical cadherins to link two cells together (see Fig. 32–6). Parallel interactions associate two cadherins side by side on the same cell. These dimers are the right size to account for the rod-like connections at adherens junctions and desmosomes (see Fig. 32–4). Antiparallel interactions found in crystals of N-cadherin CAD1 are proposed to bind a pair of cadherins on partner cells. Together, these interactions are thought to create an interlocking molecular zipper to bind cells together.

Intercellular adhesion depends on the interaction of cadherins with the cytoskeleton. Adapter proteins

table 32-2

CELL ADHESION MOLECULES: CADHERIN FAMILY (>80 KNOWN)

Examples	Structure	Extracellular Ligands	Me²⁺	Intracellular Ligands	Expression	Functions
Desmocollin-1, -2, -3	5 CAD-1 TM-1 CB-5 repeats	Self	Cal	Plakoglobulin, IF	Epithelia	Desmosomes
Desmocollin-1, -2, -3	5 CAD-1 TM-1 CB	Self	Cal	Plakoglobulin, IF	Epithelia, heart	Desmosomes
E-cadherin* (uvomorulin)	5 CAD-1 TM-1 CB	Self	Cal	Catenins, actin	Epithelia, others	Adherens junctions
LCAM	5 CAD-1 TM-1 CB	Self	Cal	Catenins, actin	Liver, others	Intercellular adhesion
N-cadherin*	5 CAD-1 TM-1 CB	Self	Cal	Catenins, actin	Neurons, muscle, endothelium	Intercellular adhesion
P-cadherin	5 CAD-1 TM-1 CB	Self	Cal	Catenins, actin	Placenta, epithelia	Intercellular adhesion
RET proto-oncogene	5 CAD-1 TM-tyrosine kinase	Self	Cal	None	Endocrine glands, neurons	Intercellular adhesion
T-cadherin	5 CAD-GPI anchor	Self	Cal	None	Early embroys, neurons	Intercellular adhesion
Protocadherins	7 CAD-1 TM-Fyn binding	Self	Cal	Fyn tyrosine kinase	Neurons	Synapse formation

*, partial atomic structure; CAD, cadherin extracellular repeat; CB, catenin binding; GPI, glycosylphosphatidylinositol; IF, intermediate filament; LCAM, liver CAM; Me²⁺, divalent cation dependence; TM, transmembrane domain.

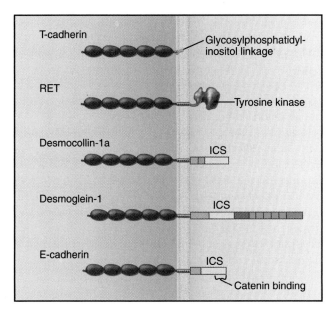

Figure 32–5 Domain maps of a variety of cadherins, all with five extracellular CAD domains but differing in their membrane anchors or cytoplasmic domains. Four are anchored by a single transmembrane segment; one is anchored by a GPI tail. One has a cytoplasmic tyrosine kinase domain; three have cytoplasmic domains that interact with actin filaments (E-cadherin) or intermediate filaments (desmocollin and desmoglein) via catenin adapters. ICS, catenin binding domain.

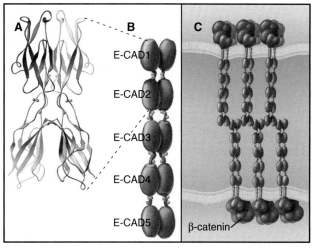

Figure 32–6 Atomic structure and proposed adhesion mechanism of cadherins. *A*, Ribbon diagram of the atomic structure of a side-by-side dimer of E-cadherin CAD domains 1 and 2. Three Ca^{2+} ions (*blue*) stabilize the intramolecular interaction of each CAD1 with CAD2. *B*, Five CAD domains stack end to end to form the rod-shaped extracellular domain of classical cadherins. These extracellular domains form lateral dimers through interaction of CAD1 domains. *C*, A model for cadherin links between adjacent cells based on interactions of CAD1 domains in crystals of N-cadherin. (*A*, Reference: Pertz O, Bozic D, Koch AW, et al: A new crystal structure, Ca^{2+} dependence and mutational analysis reveal molecular details of E-cadherin homoassociation. EMBO J 18:1738–1747, 1999; PDB file: 1FF5. *C*, Reference: Shapiro L, Fannon AM, Kwong PD, et al: Structural basis of cell-cell adhesion by cadherins. Nature 374:327–337, 1995.)

called catenins link the cytoplasmic tails of classic cadherins to actin (Fig. 32–6*C*). The cytoplasmic tail is disordered when free, but it binds along the entire length of **β-catenin,** a long, twisted helix of 36 short α-helices. **α-catenin** links β-catenin to actin filaments. A related protein, vinculin, helps to link integrins to actin filaments (see Fig. 32–10). Vinculin itself or other proteins may reinforce the link between cadherins and actin. Desmosomal cadherins, called desmocolins and desmogleins, have more complicated cytoplasmic domains that interact with proteins called plakoglobin and desmoplakin. Desmoplakin links the cadherins to keratin intermediate filaments (see Fig. 33–7). These associations of cadherins with the cytoskeleton contribute to adhesion by stabilizing the physical links between cells.

Carefully controlled expression of specific cadherins at appropriate times and places is the key to their ability to guide the sorting of various cell types that arise during development and to stabilize the architecture of organs. Most cells express more than one cadherin. Specialized cells typically express characteristic cadherins, such as osteoblast (OB-cadherin), kidney (K-cadherin), and muscle cadherin (M-cadherin). Cells with matching cadherins bind together and exclude cells that do not share those cadherins (or other appropriate adhesion receptors).

Cells in the nervous system express not only clas-

sic N-cadherin, but also a large family of more than 50 **protocadherins.** Each protocadherin has a unique extracellular domain consisting of seven CAD domains encoded by a single exon. These novel regions are spliced to a common cytoplasmic domain that binds signaling molecules, such as the nonreceptor tyrosine kinase Fyn, rather than catenins. Selective expression of protocadherins, alone or with N-cadherin, is thought to contribute to the specificity of synaptic connections in the central nervous system.

Differential expression of cadherins is particularly evident during embryonic development (Fig. 32–7). Initially, the egg and all cells of early embryos express several different cadherins. As soon as the embryo forms its three germ layers, the ectoderm on the outside surface expresses E-cadherin. In its absence, embryos die. Subsequently, when ectoderm folds inward to form the neural tube, the cells switch to expressing N-cadherin. Experimental expression of mutant cadherins confirms the physiological significance of these changes in cadherin expression. For example, embryos that overexpress E-cadherin lacking the essential cytoplasmic domain initiate development normally but fail eventually because of deficient adhesion in the ectoderm.

Cadherins and catenins participate in transduction

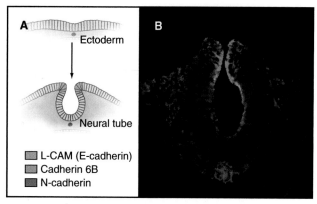

Figure 32-7 Restricted expression of cadherins during embryonic formation of the neural tube. *A*, Drawing of the distribution of three cadherins before and after the neural tube forms. *B*, Fluorescent antibody staining reveals the selective expression of cadherin 6B (*green*) and N-cadherin (*red*) in the neural tube of a developing chick embryo. (Courtesy of M. Takeichi, Kyoto University.)

of extracellular signals that control cell proliferation, migration, and differentiation. Cadherins contribute to the signal for **"contact inhibition"** of growth and motility produced when epithelial cells interact. Within a few seconds after epithelial cells contact each other, adherens junctions form. They suppress proliferation of normal cells and inhibit the spread of cancer cells that arise due to somatic mutations. Loss of E-cadherin can be a key event in the transition from benign to invasive malignant tumors. Expression of E-cadherin can often correct this defect in adhesion in tissue culture cells. Genetic defects in E-cadherin predispose individuals to stomach cancer. The *Drosophila* tumor suppressor gene *fat* encodes a membrane protein with many extracellular CAD domains. The oncogenic tyrosine kinase, Src (see Chapter 27), phosphorylates both E-cadherin and β-catenin. This is associated with loss of adhesion of epithelial cells, suggesting one way that transformation might alter cellular adhesion. Most fibroblasts lack cadherins and must therefore use another mechanism for contact inhibition.

The mechanism of signal transduction is clearer in the unusual case of the **RET proto-oncogene,** with its cytoplasmic tyrosine kinase (see Fig. 32–5). Oncogenic point mutations in the CAD domain or tyrosine kinase of RET cause dominantly inherited cancers of the endocrine glands. These mutations cause constitutive dimerization of the receptor or activation of the tyrosine kinase, or both, leading to neoplastic transformation. On the other hand, if RET is disabled by mutations, autonomic nerves in the wall of the intestines fail to develop, causing severe dysfunction in mice and in humans with **Hirschsprung's disease.**

β-Catenin participates in an unusual pathway that regulates gene expression (Fig. 32–8). The pathway

was discovered in *Drosophilia* as part of the mechanism that determines the polarity of segments in early embryonic development. Vertebrates have a similar pathway. Most β-catenin is bound to cadherins, but a second pool exchanges between a cytoplasmic protein complex and the nucleus. Nuclear β-catenin recruits transcription factors to regulate gene expression. In resting cells, cytoplasmic β-catenin turns over rapidly, with little entering the nucleus. Degradation is controlled by a cytoplasmic complex that includes the product of the **APC** gene (defective in patients with familial **a**denomatous **p**olyposis **c**oli, giving rise to multiple precancerous polyps in the large intestine) and glycogen synthase kinase **(GSK),** a protein kinase that phosphorylates β-catenin. Phosphorylated β-catenin is ubiquinated and degraded by proteosomes. Loss of APC or mutations in the phosphorylation site on β-catenin result in excess free β-catenin that enters the nucleus. Extracellular signaling proteins called **Wnts** (from the original *Drosophila* gene Wingless) activate the β-catenin gene expression pathway. Wnts bind seven-helix receptors in the plasma membrane. Several steps downstream, the Wnt signal inhibits GSK. Inhibition of GSK stops β-catenin proteolysis and raises the concentration of β-catenin free to enter the nucleus.

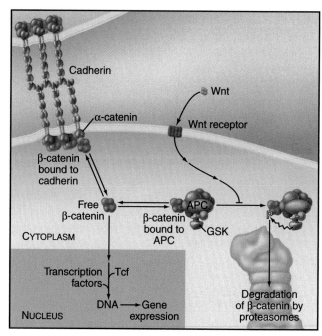

Figure 32-8 Participation of β-catenin in gene expression. Free β-catenin is in equilibrium with binding sites on cadherins and APC and may also enter the nucleus, where it combines with Tcf/LEF-1 transcription factors to regulate gene expression. The concentration of free β-catenin is determined by its rate of degradation: GSK phosphorylates β-catenin bound to APC, triggering its degradation. Extracellular Wnt acts through a seven-helix receptor to promote gene expression by blocking the degradation of β-catenin through inhibition of GSK.

table 32–3

CELL ADHESION MOLECULES: INTEGRIN FAMILY (24 KNOWN)

Examples	Structure	Extracellular Ligands	Me²⁺	Intracellular Ligands	Expression	Functions
Fibronectin receptors	$\alpha_5\beta_1$, others	Fibronectin	Cal	Talin, paxillin	Fibroblasts, other cells	Cell-matrix adhesion
GPIIb/GPIIIa	αIIbβ_3	Fibrinogen, von Willebrand	Cal	Talin, paxillin	Platelets	Platelet aggregation
Laminin receptor	$\alpha_6\beta_1$, $\alpha_7\beta_1$	Laminin	Yes	Talin, paxillin	Epithelia, muscle	Cell-matrix adhesion
LFA-1* (CD11/CD18)	αLβ_2	Ig-CAM-1, -2, -3	Mg	Talin, paxillin	All WBCs	WBC/endothelium adhesion
MAC-1*	αMβ_2	Ig-CAM-1, fibrinogen	Yes	Talin, paxillin	WBCs except lymphocytes	WBC/endothelium adhesion
Vitronectin receptor*	αVβ_3	Vitronectin, fibronectin	Cal	Talin, paxillin	Endothelium, smooth muscle, others	
VLA-4*	$\alpha_2\beta_1$	Collagen, laminin	Mg	Talin, paxillin	WBCs, epithelium, endothelium	WBC/matrix adhesion

*, partial atomic structure; CD, cellular differentiation antigen; GP, glycoprotein; ICAM, intercellular adhesion molecule; LFA, lymphocyte function associated antigen; Me²⁺, divalent cation dependence; VLA, very late antigen; WBC, white blood cell.

Integrin Family of Adhesion Receptors

Integrins are the main cellular receptors for the extracellular matrix (Table 32–3), and they also bind a few selected adhesion molecules on other cells. Integrins are also signal transduction receptors, relaying information about adhesive ligands to control cell growth and structure. Integrins allow fibroblasts and white blood cells to adhere to fibronectin and collagen as they move through the extracellular matrix. Integrins bind epithelial and muscle cells to laminin in the basal lamina, providing the physical attachments necessary to transmit internal forces to the matrix and to resist external forces. When defects in small blood vessels need repair, integrins allow platelets to adhere to basement membrane collagen and to each other via plasma fibrinogen. Mouse sperm bind integrins on the egg membrane during fertilization. Other integrins cooperate with adhesion receptors of the Ig-CAM, mucin, and selectin families to facilitate the adhesion of white blood cells to endothelial cells at sites of inflammation. Some tissues supplement integrins with structurally distinct matrix adhesion proteins, such as muscle dystroglycans and platelet GP1b-IX. Together, these interactions are essential for the development and tissue integrity of multicellular organisms. Most null mutations of integrin genes produce obvious phenotypes, including human diseases.

Three features set integrins apart from the adhesion proteins that bind cell surface ligands. First, about one third of matrix ligands for integrins involve the sequence motif arginine-glycine-aspartic acid (**RGD**) or other simple sequences. Other ligands use a critical oxygenated residue other than aspartic acid. Second, extracellular stimuli, acting through intracellular signaling pathways, regulate the affinity of integrins for their ligands. Third, integrins are more promiscuous than most adhesion receptors, as they tend to bind to several protein ligands, and many matrix molecules bind to more than one integrin. Fibronectin binds to at least nine different integrins, and both laminin and von Willebrand's factor bind at least five different integrins. This promiscuity may reflect common motifs, such as RGD, in otherwise unrelated ligands. Multiple integrins with overlapping ligand-binding activity provide cells with diverse pathways to activate different signaling pathways.

Integrins are heterodimers of two transmembrane polypeptides called α and β chains, which both contribute to ligand-binding specificity (Fig. 32–9). This allows vertebrate cells to use a combinatorial strategy to establish their integrin repertoire. They selectively express a subset of 18 different α chains and 8 β chains (Table 32–4). These chains combine to form at least 24 different kinds of dimers, each with different ligand-binding specificity. Alternative splicing also adds to the diversity of integrin isoforms. Since both α and β subunits contribute to ligand binding, combining all of the known gene products has the potential to generate 128 different dimers with unique specificities. Additional combinations of α and β chains and new ligands for known integrins are likely to exist.

With the exception of red blood cells, integrins are present in the plasma membranes of most animal cells, even sponges and corals from phyla that

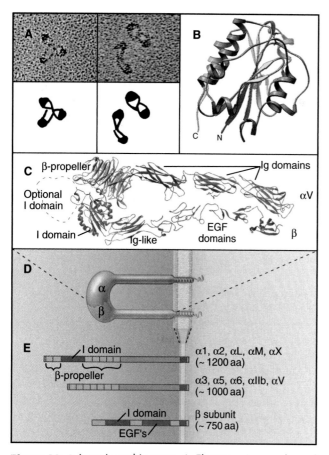

Figure 32-9 Integrin architecture. *A,* Electron micrographs and interpretative drawings of isolated integrin molecules. *B,* Ribbon model of the I-domain from integrin α_L with the bound divalent cation (manganese in this experiment, shown in red) at the top. The incomplete coordination shell of this divalent cation is completed by oxygens from the side chains of ligands, such as the aspartic acid in RGD peptides. *C,* Model of integrin $\alpha V\beta 3$ based on an atomic structure of the extracellular domain. The I-domain is inserted into the sequence of an immunoglobulin-like domain. *D,* Integrin icon used throughout this book. *E,* Domain models of integrin polypeptides. Both α-chains and β-chains have single transmembrane segments and cytoplasmic tails that vary in length. All β-chains and some α-chains have an I-domain *(red)* that binds a divalent cation and participates in ligand binding. The seven blades of the α-chain beta-propeller domains are shown in orange. The α-chain I-domain, if present, is inserted between the second and third of the seven blades of its propeller domain. (*A,* From Nermut MV, et al: Electron microscopy and structural model of human fibronectin receptor. EMBO J 7:4093–4099, 1988. *B,* Courtesy of D. Leahy, Johns Hopkins Medical School; PDB file: 1LFA. *C,* Based on an atomic model, PDB file: 1JV2. Reference: Xiong JP, Stehle T, Diefenbach B, et al: Crystal structure of the extracellular segment of integrin $\alpha V\beta 3$. Science 294:339–345, 2001. *E,* Redrawn from Kuhn K, Eble J: The structural basis of integrin-ligand interactions. Trends Cell Biol 4:256–261, 1994. Copyright 1994, with permission from Elsevier Science.)

branched early in evolution. Many vertebrate cells express β_1 and β_3 integrins for adhesion to the extracellular matrix. Only white blood cells express β_2 integrins, which they use to bind to other cells, especially

the endothelial cells lining the vessel walls. Only platelets express α_{IIb} integrins, important receptors for soluble adhesive ligands in plasma, such as fibrinogen.

The integrin heterodimer consists of two transmembrane polypeptides called alpha- and beta-chains (see Fig. 32–9). Two stalks elevate the large ligand-binding region of the dimer about 16 nm above the membrane. The stalks of the two chains are constructed of different domains. The stalk of the α-chain consists of three domains folded similar to immunoglobulins, whereas the stalk of the β chain has four EGF-like domains and a novel domain. All integrin β-chains and a subset of integrin α-chains have an I-domain (inserted domain) with a bound divalent cation that interacts with acidic residues of ligands. All α-chains have an N-terminal beta propeller domain similar to a Gβ subunit of a trimeric G protein (see Fig. 26–9). Interaction of the α-chain propeller domain with the β-chain I-domain holds the integrin dimer together, remarkably like the interaction between Gα and Gβ subunits of trimeric G proteins. Ligands bind to both the I-domains and the beta propeller. Single transmembrane segments anchor both integrin chains to the cell. Short ($\alpha \leq 77$ residues; $\beta = 40-60$ residues, except $\beta_4 = 1000$ residues) C-terminal cytoplasmic tails contribute to efficient heterodimer assembly. Tail sequences of homologous chains are conserved between species, and several have important roles in signal transduction (see later discussion).

Both α and β chains participate in binding at least two sites on ligands. Integrin $\alpha_5\beta_1$ binds two sites on fibronectin: an RGD sequence on a surface loop of FN-III domain 10, and a secondary site on the adjacent FN-III domain 9 (see Fig. 31–15). Neither site is sufficient for binding, so simple RGD peptides can dissociate fibronectin. Integrin binding sites of some ligands are on separate polypeptide chains. The RDD binding site for integrin $\alpha_1\beta_1$ on type IV collagen is on three different polypeptide chains of the triple helix.

Integrins generally have a low affinity for their extracellular ligands. The micromolar K_d of integrin $\alpha_5\beta_1$ and fibronectin makes the interaction dynamic. Rapid association and dissociation allow cells to adjust their grip on fibronectin in the matrix as they move through connective tissue. Nonadhesive RGD proteins, such as tenascin, may also reduce the duration of these interactions by competing with fibronectin and other ligands for binding integrins.

Cytoplasmic tails of integrins interact with a remarkable variety of signaling and structural proteins (Fig. 32–10). These interactions are best understood at **focal contacts,** specialized sites where integrins cluster together to transduce transmembrane signals and link actin filaments to the extracellular matrix. The adapter proteins **talin** and **vinculin** link the cytoplas-

table 32–4

INTEGRIN HETERODIMERS AND THEIR LIGANDS

	β₁	β₂	β₃	β₄	β₅	β₆	β₇	β₈
α₁	*Col-I, Col-IV, Lam*	ICAM-1, -2, -3						Tenscn, FN, VN
α₂	*Col-I, Col-IV, EV-1, FN, Lam*							
α₃	*Col-I,* Epil, FN, *Lam*							
α₄	FN, Invasins, V-CAMs						FN, ACAM-1, VCAMs	
α₅	FN							
α₆	*Lam,* sperm			? *Lam*				
α₇	*Lam*							
α₈	vWF							
α₉	vWF							
αIIb			Bor b, Col-VI, deCol, Disin, FN, Fibgn, Thrbn, VN, vWf					
α_L		ICAMs						
α_M		ICAMs, Fx-X, Fibgn, iC3b						
α_V	FN, VN, Fibgn		deCol, Tenscn, Disint, FN, Fibgn, Ostpn, Thrbn, VN, vWF		Tat, VN	Tenscn, FN		vWF
α_X		Fibgn, iC3b						

Known combinations of integrin α and β chains and their ligand binding specificities. Underlined entries are RGD-dependent; *italicized* entries are conformation-dependent. Ligand abbreviations: Bor b, *Borrelia burgdorferi;* Col-I, collagen I; Col-IV, collagen IV; Col-VI, collagen VI; deCol, denatured collagen; Disint, disintegrins; epil, epiligrin; EV-I, echovirus I; Fibgn, fibrinogen; FN, fibronectin; Fx-X, factor X; iC3b, complement fragment 3b; ICAM (-1, -2, -3), intercellular adhesion molecule; Lam, laminin; Ostpn, osteopontin; Tat, human immunodeficiency virus (HIV) Tat protein; tenscn, tenascin; thrbn, thrombospondin; VN, vitronectin; vWB, von Willebrand factor.

mic domains of β integrins to actin filaments at the ends of stress fibers. **Paxillin** links integrins to signaling proteins, forming a scaffold for Src family tyrosine kinases (see Chapter 27) and **focal adhesion kinase** (a novel tyrosine kinase lacking SH2 and SH3 domains).

Integrin binding to matrix ligands initiates signals that modify cellular adhesion, locomotion, and gene expression. The responses depend upon the particular integrin and cell, but include the following:

1. Within seconds, cytoplasmic tyrosine kinases phosphorylate several focal adhesion proteins, including paxillin, tensin, and focal adhesion kinase.
2. Within a minute, some cells raise their cytoplasmic Ca²⁺ concentration high enough to initiate many calcium-dependent processes (see Chapter 28).
3. Over a period of minutes, cells in culture spread out on ligand-coated surfaces, rearrange their cytoskeleton, and begin to move (see Chapter 41). Integrins cluster together in small "focal complexes" at their leading edge that grow into mature focal contacts, also called "focal adhesions," which anchor actin filament stress fibers to the cell membrane. Contraction of stress fibers applies tension to the focal contacts, which remain stationary as the cell advances past them. A Ca²⁺-mediated signal inactivates obsolete attachments at the rear of the cell. The adhesiveness of a cell for its substrate (a function of integrin density on

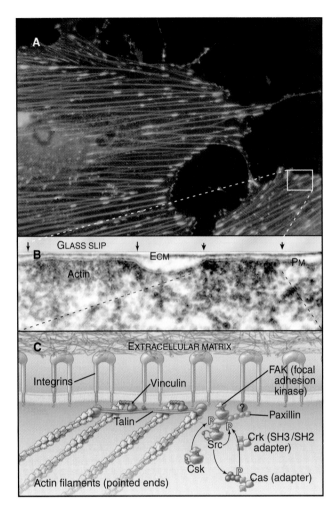

Figure 32–10 Focal contacts of epithelial cells with the extracellular matrix (ECM). *A,* Fluorescence micrograph of parts of two vertebrate tissue culture cells with focal contacts labeled with a fluorescent antibody to phosphotyrosine (*orange*). Actin filament stress fibers are stained green with phalloidin. *B,* Electron micrograph of a thin section of two focal contacts showing fine connections to the extracellular matrix deposited on the surface of the glass coverslip and cross sections of actin filaments in the cytoplasm. This HeLa cell was grown on a glass coverslip, fixed, and cut perpendicular to the substrate. *C,* Drawing of the interactions of some of the proteins concentrated on the cytoplasmic face of the membrane at focal contacts. For clarity, the actin filament interactions (*left*) are shown separately from some signaling proteins (*right*). The short cytoplasmic domains of β-integrins interact with talin. Vinculin interacts with membrane phospholipids, actin filaments, and talin. An unidentified (?) protein links the adapter protein paxillin to integrins. Paxillin anchors tyrosine kinases (FAK and Src) and, after phosphorylation, the adapter proteins Crk and Cas. (*A,* Courtesy of K. Burridge, University of North Carolina, Chapel Hill. *B,* Courtesy of Pamela Maupin, Johns Hopkins University. Reference: Maupin P, Pollard TD: Improved preservation and staining of HeLa cell actin filaments. J Cell Biol 96:51–62, 1983, by copyright permission of the Rockefeller University Press. *C,* References: Turner C: Paxillin and focal adhesion signaling. Nature Cell Biol 2:E231–E236, 2000; Critchley DR: Focal adhesions—The cytoskeletal connection. Curr Opin Cell Biol 12:133–139, 2000. Copyright 2000, with permission from Elsevier Science.)

the cell, ligand density on the substratum, and their affinity) determines the rate of movement. The maximum rate occurs at intermediate adhesiveness. Rapid association and dissociation of integrins on matrix ligands allows cells to rearrange their hold on the matrix as they move. Rho-family GTPases regulating actin assembly and contraction (see Chapter 41) coordinate protrusion of the leading edge and withdrawal of the tail.

4. In an hour, the pH of the cytoplasm rises owing to the activation of an Na^+/H^+ antiporter (see Chapter 8).

5. After several hours, activation of the Ras/MAP kinase pathway (see Chapter 29) turns on the expression of selected genes. In the long term, these changes in gene expression contribute to cellular differentiation during development. Other stimuli operating through different receptors can activate most of these cellular responses. Integrins allow cells to include the extracellular matrix as an input that affects their behavior.

Transduction of the matrix-binding signals depends on aggregation of integrins and on the actin cytoskeleton, but the mechanism is incompletely understood. As in other signaling systems (see Chapters 26 and 29), physical aggregation of integrin receptors may activate associated kinases by bringing them close enough together to transphosphorylate each other. Simply clustering integrins with extracellular bivalent antibodies concentrates focal adhesion kinase inside the membrane. This is followed by tyrosine phosphorylation and accumulation of other signaling proteins. Aggregation of integrins by multivalent ligands activates additional cytoplasmic proteins and stimulates assembly of the actin cytoskeleton. Focal adhesion kinase is postulated to have a central role in transducing these signals. Mouse mutants lacking focal adhesion kinase die during development but, surprisingly, their cells assemble focal contacts with high levels of tyrosine-phosphorylated proteins.

Several types of integrins associate laterally, in the plane of the bilayer, with other transmembrane proteins. The best characterized of the latter is CD47 (integrin-associated protein), an Ig-CAM with five transmembrane segments. Binding of the adhesive glycoprotein, thrombospondin, to the extracellular immunoglobulin-like domain of CD47 generates a transmembrane signal through trimeric G proteins that contributes to neutrophil and platelet activation.

Integrins also participate in the decision of cells to undergo apoptosis, programmed cell death (see Chapter 49). Normal epithelial cells require anchorage to the basal lamina by β_4 integrins to grow and divide. When forced to live in suspension or when dissociated from the matrix by RGD peptides, these cells arrest in the G1 phase of the cell cycle (see Chapter 44) and eventually undergo apoptosis. Anchorage by other adhesion proteins will not substitute for integrins. Loss of contact with the basal lamina may contribute to the terminal differentiation and death of cells in the upper levels of stratified epithelia, like skin (see Figs. 38–6 and 43–1). Epithelial cancers typically lose this integrin-mediated, anchorage-dependence for growth, one of the normal limitations to uncontrolled proliferation in inappropriate locations.

Integrins not only participate in signal transduction, but are also controlled by three different mechanisms, operating in different time domains.

1. Cells fine-tune their interactions with the matrix on a fast timescale by regulating the activity of cell surface integrins. Integrins on white blood cells (see Example 1 at the end of the chapter) and platelets (See Example 2) require activation by an intracellular signal before binding their ligands. This "inside-out" activation mechanism must be remarkable because intracellular signals acting on cytoplasmic tails change the conformation of the ligand-binding sites located 18 nm away on the other side of the plasma membrane.
2. In minutes, some cells mobilize a reserve pool of integrins stored in cytoplasmic vesicles. For example, chemoattractants stimulate white blood cells to fuse storage vesicles containing $\alpha_M\beta_2$ integrins with the plasma membrane (see Example 1).
3. Over hours or days, developmental programs establish the basic integrin repertoire. Growth factors like transforming growth factor-β (TGF-β; see Chapter 26) also influence integrin expression by differentiated cells.

Experiments with neutralizing antibodies and competitive peptides provided initial clues about the functions of integrins, but genetic diseases and experimental gene disruptions provide more definitive answers. For example, RGD peptides and integrin antibodies inhibit cell migration and embryonic development by competing with fibronectin. Like null mutations in fibronectin (see Chapter 31), homozygous disruption of the integrin α_4 or α_5 genes is lethal during development. Cells lacking these integrins can form focal contacts in vitro, but fibronectin receptors using other α subunits cannot substitute for α_5 in vivo. Dysfunction of β_2 integrins is not lethal, but patients are highly susceptible to infections owing to defects in the emigration of white blood cells from the blood at sites of infection (see Example 1). Melanoma tumor cells with a deficiency of $\alpha_4\beta_1$ integrin have an increased tendency to invade other tissues unless the missing integrin is replaced.

Snake venoms contain small, monomeric RGD proteins that inhibit blood clotting by competing with fibrinogen for binding the integrins that activated platelets use for aggregation. These "disintegrins" are potential inhibitors of the pathological thrombosis that contributes to heart attacks and strokes. Both small molecule and antibody antagonists for integrins are now used as clinical treatments for heart attacks and stroke.

Selectin Family of Adhesion Receptors

White blood cells and platelets use selectins to interact with vascular endothelial cells. In lymph nodes or at sites of inflammation, selectins snare circulating white blood cells, allowing them to roll over the surface of endothelial cells and eventually to exit the blood (see Example 1). Selectins (Table 32–5) may be important in other systems, but little is known about them outside the vasculature.

The defining feature of selectins is a calcium-dependent lectin domain (Fig. 32–11) that binds O-linked sulfated oligosaccharides containing sialic acid and fucose. The lectin domain sits at the end of a rod-shaped projection that is anchored to the plasma membrane by a single transmembrane sequence.

Natural ligands for selectins are mucin-like glycoproteins expressed on endothelial and white blood cells. Selective binding to mucins requires selectins to interact with both the oligosaccharide and mucin protein. The lectin domains bind mucin oligosaccharides, but the affinity is low (millimolar K_ds), and they do not discriminate among oligosaccharides. For example, all three selectins bind the tetrasaccharide chains of red blood cell glycolipids (the sialyl Lewis-x and sialyl Lewis-a blood group antigens), but they are not natural ligands. Interaction with the mucin protein is less well understood, but one or more sulfated tyrosine residues on the leukocyte mucin called PSGL-1 participate in binding P-selectin.

Bonds between selectins and their mucin ligands have high tensile strength, but form and dissociate rapidly. Consequently, only a few selectin-mucin bonds are required to tether white blood cells to the endothelium, whereas the lifetime of the bonds is brief enough to allow the blood flow to propel the cells with a rolling motion over the surface of the endothelium (see Example 1).

table 32–5

CELL ADHESION MOLECULES: SELECTIN FAMILY (LEC-CAM)

Examples	Structure	Extracellular Ligands	Me²⁺	Expression	Functions
E-selectin* (CD62E, ELA)	Lectin-EGF-6 CR-1 TM	L-selectin	Cal	Endothelium (regulated)	WBC-endothelium adhesion
L-selectin (CD62L, gp90M)	Lectin-EGF-2 CR-1 TM	E-selectin, mucins	Cal	Lymphocytes, other WBCs	WBC-endothelium adhesion
P-selectin (CD62P, GMP-14)	Lectin-EGF-9 CR-1 TM	Mucins	Cal	Endothelium, platelets	WBC-endothelium adhesion

*, partial atomic structure; CD, cellular differentiation antigen; CR, complement regulatory domain; EGF, epidermal growth factor; Me²⁺, divalent cation dependence; TM, transmembrane domain; WBC, white blood cell.

Inflammatory mediators regulate selectins in several different ways. Activation of endothelial cells with histamine or platelets with thrombin causes vesicles storing P-selectin to fuse with the plasma membrane, exposing the selectin on the cell surface. Various inflammatory agents stimulate endothelial cells to synthesize E- and P-selectin. Activation of white blood cells increases the affinity of L-selectin for mucins and later leads to its proteolytic release from the cell surface. Furthermore, selectin binding to mucins initiates intracellular signals that result in Ca^{2+} release inside the cell.

Other Adhesion Receptors

Table 32–6 lists a variety of adhesion receptors that fall outside the four main families. See Chapter 27 for CD45 and Chapter 33 for connexins.

Mucins

Selectins bind to cell surface glycoproteins called mucins. Their extracellular segments are rich in serine and threonine, which are heavily modified with acidic oligosaccharide chains (see Fig. 32–11). Because of their strong negative charge, these proteins extend like rods up to 50 nm from the cell surface. Mucins on endothelial cells or white blood cells interact with complementary selectins on the other cell type. Endothelial mucin CD34 interacts with white blood cell L-selectin, whereas endothelial P-selectin interacts with white blood cell PSGL-1 mucin.

Galactosyltransferase

At least one enzyme, galactosyltransferase, is also an important adhesion receptor. This enzyme is usually considered in another context, namely, protein glyco-

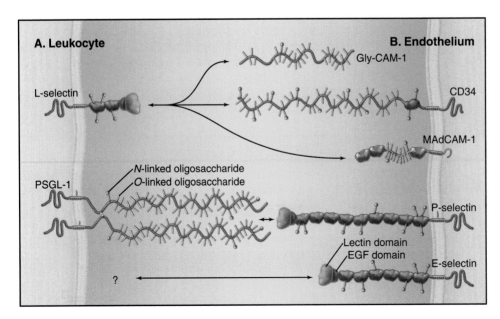

Figure 32–11 Structure of selectins and their mucin ligands. Domain architecture of selectins and mucins exposed on the surfaces of leukocytes (*A*) and endothelial cells (*B*). Complement regulatory domains of the selectins are shown in red. (Redrawn and modified from Rosen SD, Bertozzi CR: The selectins and their ligands. Curr Opin Cell Biol 6:663–673, 1994. Copyright 1994, with permission from Elsevier Science.)

table 32–6

OTHER CELL ADHESION MOLECULES

Examples	Structure	Extracellular Ligands	Me²⁺	Intracellular Ligands	Expression	Functions
CD44	Link protein-1 TM			?Ankyrin	Lymphocytes	Adhesion to endothelium
CD44E	Link protein-HS/CS-1 TM	Fibronectin, hyaluronan	No		Many epithelial cells	Adhesion to matrix
Connexin	Multispan, hexamer	Self	No		Epithelia, muscle, nerve	Gap junctions
Dystroglycans	Multi-subunit, TM	Laminin, agrin	Cal	Dystrophin	Muscle	Adhesion, synapse format
Galactosyl-transferase	Galactose transferase-1 TM	N-acetylglucosamine	No	?Actin filaments	Many cells, including sperm	Adhesion to cells & matrix
Glypican	4HS-GPI anchor	Fibronectin, collagen I	No	None	Endothelium, small muscle, epithelium	Adhesion to matrix
GPIB-IX	7 leucine-rich-1 TM	von Willebrand factor		Filamin	Platelets, endothelium	Adhesion
LCA (CD45)	50kD-1 TM-tyrosine phosphatase				WBCs	Tyrosine phosphatase
Mucins (CD34, CD43)	Sialylated oligosaccharide-1 TM	Selectins	No		Epithelia, leukocytes	Intercellular adhesion

CD, cellular differentiation antigen; CS, chondroitin sulfate; GPI, glycosylphosphatidylinositol; HS, heparan sulfate; LCA, leukocyte common antigen; Me²⁺, divalent cation dependence; TM, transmembrane domain; WBC, white blood cell.

sylation in the Golgi apparatus (see Chapter 20). However, the messenger RNA (mRNA) for galactosyltransferase has two alternative initiation sites, one of which adds 13 amino acids to the cytoplasmic, N-terminus of this transmembrane protein. The longer enzyme moves to the cell surface rather than being retained in the Golgi apparatus. On the cell surface, the enzyme can bind oligosaccharides that terminate in N-acetylglucosamine. These ligands are found on both cell surface and matrix proteins. The complex of transferase and ligand oligosaccharide is stable because the galactose-nucleotide substrate added to the oligosaccharide in the Golgi apparatus is not available outside the cell to complete the reaction. The short extension on the N-terminus is also required for the enzyme to interact with the actin cytoskeleton. The nature of the connection is not known, but overexpression of the cytoplasmic domain can saturate cytoskeletal binding sites and abrogate the ability of the enzyme to mediate adhesion. During fertilization, a surface galactosyltransferase mediates the initial contact of mouse sperm with the matrix surrounding the egg (called the zona pellucida). This association induces secretion of the contents of the sperm acrosomal vesicle, including an enzyme that destroys the transferase binding site on the matrix so that the sperm can proceed through the zona to fuse with the egg. Cell-to-cell interactions in very early embryos and development of the retina also require cell surface galactosyltransferase. The enzyme is present on the surface of most cells that migrate during embryogenesis and may contribute to their interactions with the matrix.

Adhesion Receptors with Leucine-Rich Repeats (GP IB-IX)

One platelet receptor for the adhesive glycoprotein called von Willebrand factor (see Fig. 32–14 and Example 2) is a disulfide-bonded trimer of transmembrane polypeptides, each with leucine-rich repeats in the extracellular domain. Such repeats form an α-β-β structure that binds protein ligands. Binding of von Willebrand factor to this receptor generates a signal that activates the platelet, enhancing affinity of integrin $\alpha_{IIb}\beta_3$ for fibrinogen and reorganizing the cytoskeleton.

Dystroglycan/Sarcoglycan Complex

In muscles, a complex of transmembrane glycoproteins links a network of dystrophin and actin filaments on the inside of the plasma membrane to two proteins of the extracellular basal lamina, $\alpha2$ laminin and agrin (Fig. 32–12). These protein associations stabilize the muscle plasma membrane from inside and outside. This muscle membrane skeleton resembles in concept and function the actin-spectrin network of red blood cells (see Fig. 6–10). Genetic defects or deficiencies in dystrophin, transmembrane linker proteins of the dys-

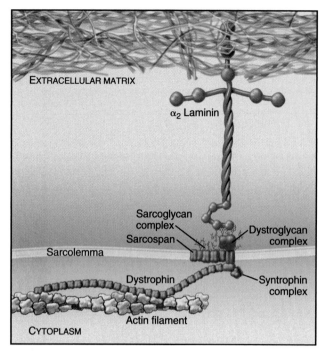

Figure 32-12 Drawing of the dystroglycan/sarcoglycan complex of the muscle plasma membrane. Dystroglycan is synthesized as a large precursor protein and then cut into the extracellular α subunit (which binds α₂ laminin) and the transmembrane β subunit (which binds dystrophin). The three transmembrane sarcoglycans and one sarcospan associate with β-dystroglycan. The C-terminus of dystrophin also binds a cytoplasmic complex of three syntrophins. (Based on a drawing by K. Amann and J. Ervasti, University of Wisconsin, Madison.)

troglycan/sarcoglycan complex or α2 laminin cause muscular dystrophy in humans, most likely due to the mechanical instability of the membrane, leading to cellular damage and eventual atrophy of the muscle. Chapter 42 provides additional details on their role in muscle function and disease. In other tissues, nonmuscle cells express many of these proteins (or their homologues), where they may contribute to adhesion to the extracellular matrix. Some pathogens use the dystroglycan complex to bind their cellular targets. Arenavirus, the cause of Lassa fever, binds directly to α-dystroglycan and the leprosy bacterium binds laminin-2.

example 1
Cellular Adhesion Between Leukocytes and Endothelial Cells in Response to Inflammation

Movement of white blood cells from blood to sites of inflammation in connective tissue illustrates how cells integrate the activities of selectins, mucins, integrins, Ig-CAMs, and chemoattractant receptors. Infection or inflammation in connective tissue attracts neutrophils and monocytes, the main phagocytes circulating in blood (see Chapter 30).

In the absence of inflammation, neutrophils flow rapidly over the surface of endothelial cells, but do not bind to them, because the appropriate pairs of adhesion molecules are not exposed or activated, or both. Infection or other inflammation in nearby tissues causes neutrophils to bind to the vascular endothelium and to move out of the blood into the tissue. Neutrophils adhere to the endothelium in three sequential, but overlapping steps (Fig. 32-13).

1. Locally generated inflammatory chemicals, including histamine (secreted by mast cells), bind to seven-helix receptors on endothelial cells and stimulate fusion of cytoplasmic vesicles (called Weibel-Palade bodies) with the plasma membrane. This exposes P-selectin, formerly stored in these vesicle membranes, on the cell surface facing the blood. These selectins bind mucins constitutively exposed on the surface of neutrophils, tethering them to the surface in < 1 msec. The association is weak, so the bonds are rapidly broken and remade, allowing the neutrophil to roll along the surface of the endothelium at rates greater than 10 μm per second as the blood flow pushes them along.

2. Chemotactic factors activate integrins on the neutrophil. These chemoattractants bind seven-helix receptors on the surface of the leukocyte and activate integrins. The signal transduction pathway is incompletely understood, but the consequence is that about 10% of the neutrophil integrins increase their affinity for their ligand by 200-fold. This makes the third step possible.

3. Activated neutrophil integrins bind tightly to Ig-CAMs on the surface of endothelial cells, immobi-

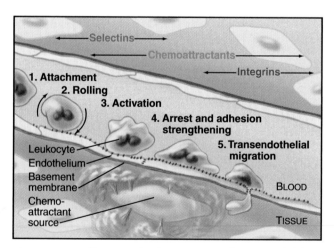

Figure 32-13 Five steps in the migration of a neutrophil from the blood to the connective tissue. *1,* Endothelial cells exposed to inflammatory agents like histamine expose selectins on their surface and snare mucins on neutrophils flowing in the bloodstream. As a neutrophil rolls along the surface (*2*) chemotactic factors activate their integrins (*3*) causing the neutrophil to bind tightly to Ig-CAMs on the endothelium (*4*). *5,* The neutrophil then migrates between the endothelial cells into the connective tissue. (Reference: Springer T: Traffic signals for lymphocyte and leukocyte emigration: The multi-step paradigm. Cell 76:301–314, 1994.)

lizing the neutrophil despite the force of the blood flow. Neutrophils stop rolling and initiate cellular motility, which eventually leads them to crawl between endothelial cells into connective tissue and toward the source of the chemoattractant.

These interactions are necessary to fight infections, so patients with defects in leukocyte adhesion suffer from acute and chronic infections. A genetic deficiency of β_2 integrins causes leukocyte adhesion deficiency. The affected individual's white blood cells bind weakly and roll on the endothelium through the selectin mechanism, but do not achieve the tight binding required to migrate out of the circulation. Consequently, these individuals are susceptible to bacterial infections. Similarly, a genetic defect in fucose metabolism causes a second type of leukocyte adhesion deficiency that involves interference with the synthesis of a carbohydrate ligand on leukocytes that binds endothelial selectins. Cells cannot roll, and so they fail to initiate the emigration process.

On the other hand, neutrophils are double-edged swords because they also generate reactive oxygen species that can damage tissues at sites of inflammation or at sites temporarily deprived of oxygen. Thus, movement of white blood cells into tissues contributes to damage that occurs when blood flow is restored to an ischemic tissue. Monoclonal antibodies to selectins can attenuate this injury. Drugs targeted to selectins

may be therapeutically useful in the future to mitigate damage after heart attacks or severe frostbite.

A similar mechanism and a partially overlapping set of receptors attract blood monocytes and eosinophils to sites of inflammation. Once in connective tissue, interactions of monocyte integrins with matrix molecules triggers the new gene expression causing them to differentiate into macrophages (see Chapter 30).

Lymphocytes patrol the body, circulating from the blood to lymphoid tissues and through the lymphatic circulation on their way back to the blood. This "recirculation" requires lymphocytes to recognize endothelial cells in specific lymphoid tissues where they exit from the blood. Lymphocytes use L-selectin, three different mucin-like proteins, and $\alpha_4\beta_2$ integrins to bind to these target endothelial cells. Lymphocytes from mice with an L-selectin null mutation do not roll on endothelial cells or accumulate normally in lymph nodes.

example 2
Platelet Activation and Adhesion

Platelets aggregate at sites where damage to vascular endothelial cells exposes the basal lamina (Fig. 32–14). This process requires the coordinated activity of a variety of receptors including integrins, leucine-rich repeat adhesion proteins, and seven-helix receptors. These reactions prevent bleeding and bruising, but inappropriate activation of platelets produces clots in

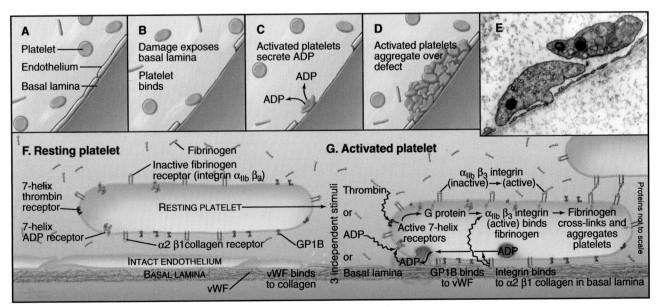

Figure 32-14 Platelet activation and aggregation at the site of a defect in the endothelium. *A* to *D*, Steps in platelet activation and aggregation. *E*, Electron micrograph of a thin section of a platelet adhering to the basal lamina through a tiny defect in the endothelium. *F*, Resting platelets circulate in the blood without interacting with the intact endothelium lining the vessel. *G*, Platelets are activated in three ways: (i) Where the basal lamina is exposed, von Willebrand factor (vWF) binds the collagen. Platelet GP1B-IX binds weakly to von Willebrand factor, allowing platelets to adhere to the exposed matrix. (ii) Binding of $\alpha_2\beta_1$ integrins to collagen results in firm adhesion. (iii) These interactions stimulate secretion of ADP, which binds seven-helix receptors and activates the $\alpha_{IIb}\beta_3$ integrins. Then $\alpha_{IIb}\beta_3$ integrins bind dimeric fibrinogen and aggregate platelets together. Platelet proteins are not to scale.

blood vessels, causing heart attacks and strokes. To understand the good effects and avert the bad, investigators have studied platelet activation and adhesion in great detail.

Resting platelets have a low tendency to aggregate, even though they circulate in a sea of integrin ligands, including fibrinogen. This lack of reactivity of resting platelets is explained by three factors. In resting platelets, the major platelet integrin, $\alpha_{IIb}\beta_3$, has a low affinity ($K_d \gg \mu M$) for its plasma ligand, fibrinogen. Similarly, the platelet receptor GP1b-IX, a platelet plasma membrane receptor with leucine-rich motifs, has a low affinity for circulating von Willebrand factor, an adhesive glycoprotein. The endothelium masks potential ligands, collagen, and von Willebrand factor in the basal lamina. The concentrations of soluble ligands, such as adenosine diphosphate (ADP) and thrombin are low under physiological conditions.

Damage to the endothelium usually initiates platelet activation by stripping back endothelial cells and exposing platelets to von Willebrand factor and collagen in the basal lamina. Initial rolling interactions with the basal lamina at high blood flow rates are mediated by interaction of GP1b-IX with von Willebrand factor bound to basal lamina collagen. $\alpha_2\beta_1$ Integrin mediates subsequent tight binding to collagen. Exposure to soluble agonists like ADP or thrombin also activates platelets and promotes their aggregation. Within seconds of activation, platelet $\alpha_{IIb}\beta_3$ integrins convert to a high affinity state ($K_d < \mu M$) and bind tightly to fibrinogen. Dimeric fibrinogen links platelets into aggregates.

Agonists activate platelet $\alpha_{IIb}\beta_3$ integrins through three different pathways:

1. Collagen binding to $\alpha_2\beta_1$ integrin directly stimulates platelets to secrete ADP, synthesize the lipid second messenger thromboxane A$_2$ (see Chapter 28), and activate $\alpha_{IIb}\beta_3$.
2. Damage to blood vessels activates the blood clotting proteolytic enzyme, thrombin, which binds two related seven-helix receptors and signals through trimeric guanosine triphosphate (GTP)–binding proteins, especially G$_q$ (see Chapter 27), to activate $\alpha_{IIb}\beta_3$. The pathway and mechanism are not yet clear.
3. von Willebrand factor binding to the platelet receptor GP1b-IX activates through a third, uncharacterized pathway.

   Two additional mechanisms augment all of these responses. Activated platelets secrete ADP, which activates a seven-helix receptor and amplifies the response to thrombin. Aggregation of platelets by binding dimeric fibrinogen further stimulates their response to ADP and thrombin.

Platelet aggregation is disadvantageous in the normal circulation, so several mechanisms actively inhibit platelet activation. Endothelial cells produce both nitric oxide and an eicosanoid, prostacyclin, which inhibit platelet activation. Nitric oxide acts through cyclic guanosine monophosphate (cGMP) and prostacyclin acts through cyclic adenosine monophosphate (cAMP) (see Chapter 28). Drugs that inhibit $\alpha_{IIb}\beta_3$ are being tested to treat heart attacks.

The most common bleeding disorder is von Willebrand disease, caused by defects in von Willebrand factor. In some cases, mutations reduce the activity or the circulating concentration of the factor. Other mutations make the factor overactive, so that it causes circulating platelets to aggregate and be removed from the blood. The resulting platelet deficiency causes bleeding. Genetic defects in the platelet receptor GP1b-IX cause the human bleeding disorder called Bernard-Soullier syndrome. Individuals with Glanzmann's thrombasthenia bleed abnormally because $\alpha_{IIb}\beta_3$ integrin is absent or defective and their platelets do not aggregate.

■ Selected Readings

Brown EJ, Fraizer WA: Integrin-associated protein (CD47) and its ligands. Trends Cell Biol 11:130–135, 2001.

Burridge K, Chrzanowska-Wodnicka M: Focal adhesions, contractility and signaling. Annu Rev Cell Dev Biol 12:463–519, 1996.

Critchley DR: Focal adhesions—The cytoskeletal connection. Curr Opin Cell Biol 12:133–139, 2000.

Gumbiner BM: Cell adhesion: The molecular basis of tissue architecture and morphogenesis. Cell 84:345–357, 1996.

Henry MD, Campbell KP: Dystroglycan: An extracellular matrix receptor linked to the cytoskeleton. Curr Opin Cell Biol 8:625–631, 1996.

Humphries MJ, Mould AP: An anthropomorphic integrin (a perspective on the integrin structure). Science 294:316–317, 2001.

Jones EY: Three-dimensional structure of cell adhesion molecules. Curr Opin Cell Biol 8:602–608, 1996.

Liotta LA, Clair T: Checkpoint for invasion. Nature 405:287–286, 2000.

Ruoslahti E: RGD and other recognition sequences for integrins. Annu Rev Cell Dev Biol 12:697–715, 1996.

Shapiro L, Colman DR: The diversity of cadherins and implications for a synaptic adhesive code in the CNS. Neuron 23:427–430, 1999.

Springer TA: Traffic signals for lymphocyte and leukocyte emigration: The multi-step paradigm. Cell 76:301–314, 1994.

Turner CE: Paxillin and focal adhesion signaling. Nature Cell Biol 2:E231–E236, 2000.

van der Merwe PA, Barclay AN: Transient intercellular adhesion: The importance of weak protein-protein interactions. Trends Cell Biol 19:354–358, 1994.

chapter 33

INTERCELLULAR JUNCTIONS

Animal cells require intracellular and extracellular support systems to form tissues such as epithelia, nerves, and muscles. Plasma membrane specializations, called cellular junctions, mediate these interactions between neighboring cells and between cells and the basal lamina (see Chapter 31). On the cytoplasmic side of the membrane, most types of junctions are anchored to filaments of the cytoskeleton. These physical connections—from cell to cell through junctions and across cells via the cytoskeleton—impart mechanical strength to the tissue.

Four types of intercellular junctions, each composed of a different transmembrane protein, connect the plasma membranes of adjacent cells (Table 33–1; Fig. 33–1). *Adherens junctions* and *desmosomes* use different cadherins (see Chapter 32) to link the plasma membranes of adjacent cells. The cytoplasmic tails of these cadherins are anchored to cytoskeletal filaments: actin filaments in the case of adherens junctions and intermediate filaments for desmosomes. *Tight junctions* not only link cells together, but they also create a seal that limits the diffusion of ions and small molecules between adjacent cells, allowing sheets of epithelial cells to form permeability barriers that are essential for many physiological functions at the organ level (see Chapter 10 for examples). Tight junctions also create a barrier to the movement of molecules in the plane of the plasma membrane. This helps epithelial cells maintain apical and basolateral domains of their plasma membrane with different biochemical compositions. This allows the surface of the cell facing the outside world to differ from that facing the interior of the organism. *Gap junctions* also link cells together, but their main function is to provide channels for small molecules to move from the cytoplasm of one cell into the cytoplasm of the neighboring cell.

Like fibroblasts (see Chapter 30), other tissue cells use integrins to adhere to the extracellular matrix. One type of integrin forms *hemidesmosomes* that link cytoplasmic intermediate filaments across the plasma membrane to the basal lamina. Other integrins spread out more diffusely, connecting cytoplasmic actin filaments to the basal lamina.

Each tissue uses a selection of junctions particularly suited to its physiological functions. All four types of intercellular junctions link columnar epithelial cells laterally to their neighbors, whereas hemidesmosomes attach epithelia to the underlying basal lamina (see Fig. 33–1). Stratified epithelial cells rely heavily on desmosomes and intermediate filaments to resist mechanical forces (see Chapter 38). Muscle cells (see Chapter 42) are surrounded by a basal lamina and linked together by desmosomal and adherens junctions. Hemidesmosomes and adherens junctions anchor muscle cells to tendons. Gap junctions connect heart and smooth muscle cells, but not skeletal muscle cells. Nerve cells in the peripheral nervous system (outside the brain and spinal cord) are enveloped by a basal lamina. Nerve cells in the central nervous system are not. Most nerve cells communicate chemically, but some use gap junctions for electrical communication.

Histologists and physiologists have long recognized that epithelial cells are specialized for adhering to each other and the underlying extracellular matrix. They have also learned that some epithelia form a tight barrier between the luminal surface and the underlying tissue spaces. Many of these interactions depend on extracellular calcium. The physical basis of these interactions became clear during the 1960s when electron micrographs of thin sections of intestinal epithelial cells revealed the variety of cellular junctions (see Fig. 33–1). Intestinal epithelial cells are particu-

table 33–1

MOLECULAR COMPONENTS OF CELL-CELL AND CELL-MATRIX JUNCTIONS

Junction	Target Molecule	Adhesive Protein	Cytoplasmic Proteins	Cytoskeletal Filaments
Sealing of the Extracellular Space				
Tight junction	Occludin	Occludin	ZO-1, ZO-2, cingulin,	Actin
	Claudin	Claudin	spectrin	
Communication Between Cells				
Gap junction	Connexin	Connexin		None
Adhesion to Other Cells				
Zonula adherens	Cadherin	Cadherin	Catenins, plakoglobin	Actin
Desmosome	Desmoglein	Desmoglein	Plakoglobin, desmoplakin	Intermediate
	Desmocollin	Desmocollin	Plakoglobin, desmoplakin	Intermediate
Adhesion to the Extracellular Matrix				
Hemidesmosome	Laminin	Integrin	Plectin, BP 180	Intermediate
Focal contact	Fibronectin	Integrin	Talin, vinculin, α-actinin	Actin

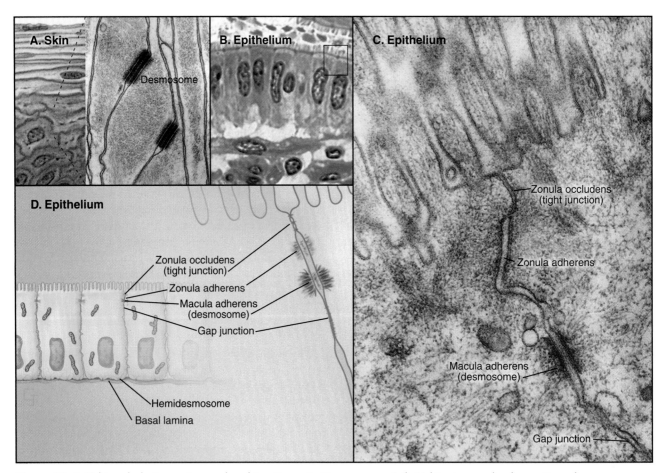

Figure 33–1 Light and electron micrographs of junctions. *A,* Desmosomes. *Left,* Light micrograph of a section of skin showing numerous desmosomes as pink dots between the cells. *Right,* Electron micrograph of a thin section of skin showing desmosomes. *B,* Light micrograph of a section of intestinal epithelium stained with hematoxylin-eosin showing the junctional complex (also called "terminal bars") as bright pink dots between the cells near their apex, just below the microvilli of the brush border. *C,* Electron micrograph of a thin section of intestinal epithelial cells showing the junctional complex consisting of a belt-like tight junction (also called the zonula occludens), a belt-like adherens junction (also called the zonula adherens), and desmosomes (also called the macula adherens), all in their characteristic relation to each other. The circumferential tight junction seals the extracellular space. The zonula adherens is anchored to the actin cytoskeleton. Desmosomes are attached to cytoplasmic intermediate filaments. *D,* Drawing showing the position of the junctional complex in the cell and the locations of gap junctions, basal lamina, and hemidesmosomes. (*A,* Courtesy of Don W. Fawcett, Harvard Medical School. *C,* Courtesy of Marilyn Farquhar, University of California, San Diego.)

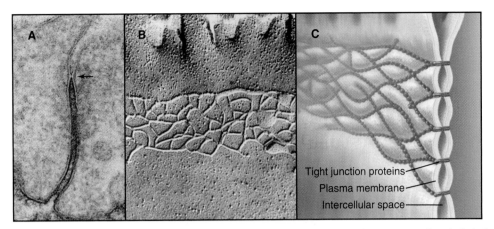

Figure 33–2 Epithelial tight junctions. *A,* Electron micrograph of a thin section of endothelial cells showing a point of contact between the plasma membranes at a tight junction *(arrow). B,* Electron micrograph of a replica of a freeze-fractured cell. This method exposes proteins within the lipid bilayer and reveals strands aligned along the points of contact between the plasma membranes. *C,* Interpretive drawing showing the strands at points of contact as rows of transmembrane proteins. (*A,* Courtesy of George Palade, University of California, San Diego. *B,* Courtesy of Don W. Fawcett, Harvard Medical School.)

larly favorable for this work, as they have all four types of intercellular junctions, as well as hemidesmosomes. Belt-like, tight junctions and adherens junctions encircle the apex of the cell. Desmosomes and gap junctions form patch-like lateral connections between the cells. Subsequent research has established the molecular architecture of all of these junctions.

Tight Junctions (Zonula Occludens)

Tight junctions, also called zonula occludens, get their name from the fact that they occlude the extracellular space between epithelial cells, forming a tight, belt-like gasket or seal that limits diffusion of water, ions, and larger solutes, as well as migration of cells (Fig. 33–2). This barrier accounts for the electrical resistance across sheets of epithelial cells. The quality of this seal, reflected in the electrical resistance, varies by several orders of magnitude depending upon the cell type and its activity. Extremely tight barriers are found where epithelia must maintain high ion gradients, such as in the distal tubules of the kidney where urine is concentrated. Leaky tight junctions are found where ion gradients across epithelia are small, but a barrier is required for large solutes, proteins, and leukocytes (e.g., in most blood vessels). Tight junctions are more permeable to cations than anions and generally restrict the diffusion of all solutes larger than about 1.8 nm in diameter. Sensitive methods have detected no water flow across tight junctions. Both cellular metabolic activity and intracellular signals generated by hormones and cytokines regulate the tight junction seal.

Epithelial tight junctions also define the boundary between biochemically distinct **apical** and **basolateral domains** of the plasma membrane. Plasma membranes on these two surfaces differ in lipid and protein compositions and functions. By locating different pumps and carriers in the two plasma membrane domains, cells can create a different extracellular environment in the basal compartment than the apical compartment, which commonly faces the external world. For example, the fluid in the lumen of the intestine is far different from that in the extracellular space between the cells and in the adjacent connective tissue only a few nanometers away. Chapter 10 covers several other examples where the permeability barrier created by tight junctions is important for physiology.

In electron micrographs of thin sections of tight junctions, the plasma membranes of adjacent cells appear to fuse together in a series of one or more contacts (see Fig. 33–2). Freeze-fracturing provides a different view. The contacts correspond to continuous strands of intramembranous particles that form a branching network in the plane of the lipid bilayer. Correlation of the architecture of these strands with the tightness of the seal has revealed that the number and continuity of these strands determines the tightness of the barrier to the diffusion of ions in the extracellular space.

Early models of tight junctions proposed a fusion between the lipid bilayers of the two membranes to account for the barrier to ion diffusion, but freeze-fracture images revealed that the strands consist of integral membrane proteins. These proteins were very difficult to identify until investigators found a monoclonal antibody that could bind to the cytoplasmic side of the plasma membrane at tight junction contacts. Using this antibody, they identified an integral

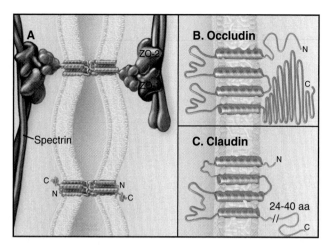

Figure 33-3 Tight junction proteins: occludin and claudin. *A,* Speculative model of tight junction structure with claudin linking the two membranes together and peripheral proteins ZO-1 and ZO-2 linking claudin to spectrin. *B* and *C,* The proposed topology of occludin and claudin.

membrane protein that they named **occludin**. It was so named because it was the first discovered to form the intramembrane particles that self-associate with related molecules in a neighboring plasma membrane to seal the extracellular space. The amino acid sequence of occludin suggested four transmembrane strands and two hydrophobic extracellular loops that were extremely rich in tyrosine and glycine residues (Fig. 33–3). The existence of other tight junction proteins was revealed when mice lacking the single occludin gene survived with normal tight junctions. It is now believed that a family of at least eight proteins, called **claudins,** constitutes the main structural proteins of tight junction strands. Claudins have four transmembrane sequences, but they are not related in sequence to occludin.

The structural basis of the permeability barrier remains to be established but presumably involves close association of the extracellular domains of claudins and occludin, both laterally and across the space between opposed membranes. The long C-terminal cytoplasmic segment of occludin binds a peripheral membrane protein called **ZO-1,** which in turn associates with a homologous protein **ZO-2** and spectrin. ZO-1 must have other anchors, perhaps claudins, as it associates with tight junctions in the absence of occludin. Additional cytoplasmic proteins, including cingulin and a small guanosine triphosphate (GTP)–binding protein, are associated with tight junctions. ZO-2 and cingulin appear to be specific for tight junctions, whereas ZO-1 also associates with cadherins in the adherens junctions of nonepithelial cells like fibroblasts and cardiac muscle cells.

Invertebrates seal the space between epithelial cells with so-called septate junctions, which differ in morphology from tight junctions but which associate

with a cytoplasmic protein with sequence homology to both ZO-1 and ZO-2. The similarities to tight junctions may be more extensive at the molecular level than revealed by the morphology. Fly embryos with mutations in the ZO-1 homologue (dlg) lose epithelial cell polarity and develop tumors.

The transepithelial barrier established by tight junctions is regulated by extracellular stimuli (e.g., hormones like vasopressin and cytokines like tumor necrosis factor; see Chapter 29), their downstream second messengers (e.g., Ca^{2+} and cyclic adenosine monophosphate [cAMP]; see Chapter 28), and effectors (e.g., protein kinases A and C; see Chapter 26). The mechanisms are not yet well understood, but posttranslational modifications of tight junctions may modify their assembly. Another possibility is that tension on the associated actin filaments may physically open passages through tight junctions. The metabolic state of the cell also influences tight junctions; depletion of adenosine triphosphate (ATP) causes tight junctions to leak without destroying the barrier between the apical and basolateral domains of the plasma membrane. Cells migrating across epithelia, such as white blood cells moving from the blood to the connective tissue (see Chapter 34), open tight junctions locally without disrupting the tight seal across the epithelium. Migratory cells induce a localized increase in cytoplasmic Ca^{2+} in the epithelial cells that is required for opening the tight junctions.

Several bacterial toxins affect the tight junction barrier. The ZO-toxin of *Vibrio cholerae* induces diarrhea by loosening tight junctions, independent of the classic cholera toxin, which induces secretion.

Gap Junctions

For many years, the dominance of the cell theory in biology, which suggested that isolation of cells was a general principle, discouraged curiosity about the possibility of direct intercellular communication. Early electrophysiological experiments on nerves and skeletal muscles reinforced the widespread belief that cells were autonomous. By chance, the cells used in these experiments *were* electrically isolated and communicated exclusively by secreting chemical messengers that bound to receptors on target cells (see Chapter 10). However, nerve and skeletal muscle cells were found to be exceptions to the general principle that cells in animal tissues communicate with each other by gap junctions. The generality of gap junctional communication means that sharing cytoplasmic components is common in animal cell biology.

In 1959, electrophysiological experiments on synapses between giant axons and the motor neurons that drive the flipper muscles of crayfish provided the first convincing evidence for direct electrical communication between cells. These **electrical synapses**

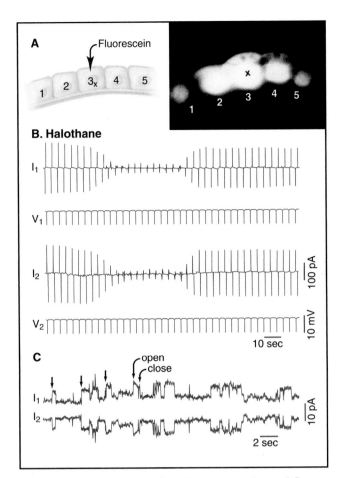

Figure 33-4 Gap junction physiology. *A,* Drawing and fluorescence micrograph showing the movement of a tracer dye between epithelial cells from the salivary gland of *Chironomus.* Cell 3 was injected with fluorescein (molecular weight-330), which spread to adjacent cells via gap junctions. *B* and *C,* Electrical recordings from pairs of cells coupled by gap junctions. *B,* Two cells (1 and 2) were voltage-clamped (see text describing Fig. 10–6) and subjected alternately to small depolarizing voltage changes (V_1, V_2). Being electrically coupled, they responded with opposite currents (I_1, I_2). The anesthetic halothane closes most of the channels, reducing the current in response to depolarization. *C,* When the cells are held at a constant depolarizing voltage in the presence of halothane, current records reveal the opening and closing of individual gap junction channels as opposite step changes in current. (*A,* From Lowenstein W: Physiol Rev 61:829, 1991. *B* and *C,* From Eghbali B, et al: Proc Natl Acad Sci 87:1328, 1990.)

transmit action potentials directly from one cell to the next without the delay required for secretion and reception of a chemical transmitter. This, in turn, allows exceptionally fast responses for escaping from predators. Heart muscle cells were found to be connected by similar electrical junctions. Over the next decade, two approaches revealed coupling between many non-excitable cells. Using microelectrodes, physiologists established that depolarization of one cell was transmitted with little resistance to adjacent epithelial cells (Fig. 33–4), although the amplitude of the change was found to decline with distance. Similarly, it was dis-

covered that fluorescent molecules, radioactive tracers, and essential nutrients could pass from the cytoplasm of one cell to the cytoplasm of neighboring cells.

Electron microscopists associated low-resistance communication between cells with the presence of plasma membrane specializations that they called gap junctions owing to the regular 2-nm separation of the adjacent cell membranes (Fig. 33–5). Light microscopy

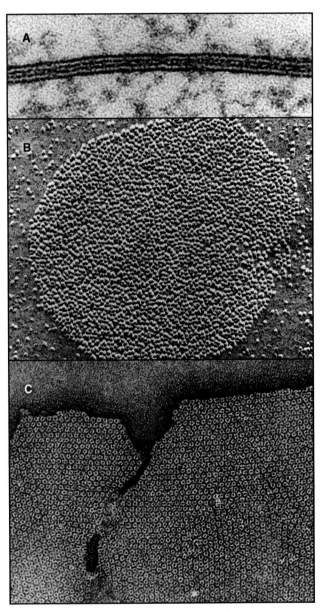

Figure 33-5 Electron micrographs of gap junctions. *A,* Thin section of embedded cells showing the closely apposed membranes of adjacent cells separated by a gap of 2 nm. *B,* Replica of a freeze-fractured cell showing an irregular array of particles exposed in the plane of the lipid bilayer. *C,* Negative staining of an isolated gap junction reveals the intercellular connexon channels packed together in a regular, two-dimensional array. Each connexon has a central channel filled with stain. (Micrographs courtesy of Don W. Fawcett, Harvard Medical School, from the work of N. B. Gilula, Scripps Research Institute, La Jolla, CA.)

PLASMADESMATA

Plants lack gap junctions, but many cells in plant tissues maintain cytoplasmic continuity with their neighbors through plasmadesmata, membrane-lined channels across the cell wall. A strand of modified endoplasmic reticulum fills most of the pore. Specialized proteins on the cytoplasmic surfaces of the surrounding plasma membrane and central endoplasmic reticulum are thought to line the pore, although not a single molecular component of plasmadesmata has yet been identified. Most plasmadesmata form by incomplete cytokinesis, but secondary plasmadesmata can form independently.

Molecules smaller than about 1 kD diffuse freely through plasmadesmata, but larger molecules, even whole viruses, can pass selectively through these channels. Constitutive diffusion of small molecules allows exchange of metabolites between cells. Regulated passage of larger molecules, including proteins such as transcription factors, allows developmental signals to move between cells and tissues. Permeability varies among tissues and with physiological states and developmental stages. For example, all cells in embryos are connected, whereas cells in some adult tissues are isolated. Actin filaments contribute to regulation of the pore size, but the signals controlling permeability are not known. Specialized viral proteins are required for viruses or their nucleic acids to move between cells.

bilayer. In the narrow intracellular gap, each connexon pairs with a connexon from the adjacent cell, forming a tight extracellular seal that precludes leakage of ions out of the cell. Vertebrates have a family of about 20 connexin genes that encode isoforms ranging in size from 26 kD to 60 kD. The transmem-

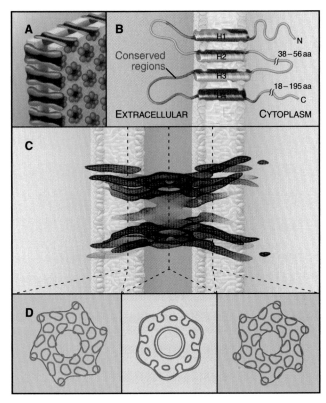

Figure 33-6 Molecular structure of the gap junction connexon. *A,* Drawing of gap junction connexons forming channels between the cytoplasms of adjacent cells. *B,* Transmembrane topology of connexins. Judging from the x-ray diffraction pattern and reconstructions from electron micrographs, the polypeptide chain crosses the lipid bilayer four times as α helices. A linear array of conserved polar residues on one face of helix 3 suggests that it lines the channel. Conserved residues *(maroon)* form the transmembrane and extracellular loops required for channel assembly. Cytoplasmic loops between helix 2 and 3 and the C-terminal tails vary in length among connexin isoforms. Removal of the C-terminal tail from connexin-43 alters its gating properties. *C,* Three-dimensional reconstruction of a gap junction channel at 7.5Å resolution by electron crystallography. The specimen was a two-dimensional crystal composed of a mutant connexin α1-Cx-263T lacking most of the C-terminal tail, which would project into the cytoplasm. This cut-away side view shows the interior of the channel and transmembrane densities formed by α helices. The yellow asterisk marks the narrowest part of the channel. *D,* Cross-sectional views at three levels, as indicated. The pink contours are cross sections of the 24 α helices. Secondary structures forming the tightly sealed channel across the extracellular gap are not resolved *(middle panel). (C* and *D,* Courtesy of Mark Yeager, Scripps Research Institute, La Jolla, CA; reference: Unger VM, et al: Three-dimensional structure of a recombinant gap junctional membrane channel. Science 283:1176–1180, 1999. Copyright 1999, American Association for the Advancement of Science.)

using antibody probes is now the optimal approach for surveying tissues for junctions.

Cells in most metazoans communicate by gap junctions. Coupled cells in vertebrates include the epithelial cells of the skin, endocrine glands, exocrine glands, the gastrointestinal tract, and renal-urinary tract, as well as smooth muscle, cardiac muscle, bone, some neurons, and glial cells. Even white blood cells may form transient gap junctions with endothelial cells. Cells in plant tissues also communicate with each other, but they use direct cytoplasmic connections, called **plasmadesmata,** rather than gap junctions (Box 33–1).

Gap junctions are plaques containing large *intercellular* channels that connect the cytoplasms of a pair of cells. These plaques exclude other transmembrane proteins and contain a few to thousands of channels. Half channels in each membrane are called **connexons.** They consist of six protein subunits, named **connexins,** which are proteins with four transmembrane α helices (Fig. 33–6). The lateral association of six **connexins** forms an aqueous channel across the lipid

brane helices and extracellular loops are more conserved than the variable N- and C-terminal cytoplasmic sequences. Connexins are named by molecular weight; for instance, connexin-43 (Cx-43) is the name for the 43-kD isoform. Remarkably, gap junctions were invented twice during animal evolution. Invertebrates form gap junctions from a completely different family of transmembrane proteins, call innexins, for invertebrate connexins.

Connexons are size filters, allowing hydrophilic molecules up to about 1 kD to diffuse between coupled cells (see Fig. 33–4). Various connexins differ somewhat in size and charge selectivity. The cylindrical transmembrane channel is 10 nm long with a diameter of 1.2 nm in mammals; in insects, the diameter is a little larger. The use of six subunits creates a larger channel than tetrameric voltage-gated ion channels or pentameric ligand-gated ion channels (see Chapter 9). These properties allow gap junction channels to pass ions (to establish electrochemical continuity between the cells), second messengers (to establish a common network of information), and metabolites (to allow sharing of resources).

Biophysicists have studied the properties of single connexon channels by patch-clamping (see Chapter 9) pairs of cells with few channels, a state that can be achieved conveniently by expressing connexins in cells lacking them, or by measuring electrical properties of purified connexons incorporated into lipid bilayers. Like other channels, connexons flip back and forth between two states: open and closed (see Fig. 33–4). The gating mechanism is not known, but analysis of electron micrographs of isolated gap junctions has suggested that the twisting of connexin subunits may open and close the channel. The conductance of the open state depends on the connexin isoform and varies from about 30 pS to 300 pS. Given the permeability of gap junctions to relatively large solutes, it is surprising that their conductance is in the same range as narrower ligand- and voltage-gated ion channels. Both the greater length and the arrangement of charged residues lining the channel may contribute to the unexpectedly low conductance of connexons.

Gap junctional communication is conditional, depending on both the number of channels and the fraction that is open or closed. The fraction of open channels is usually less than 1.0; it is about 0.2 in heart and as low as 0.01 in one nerve cell tested. Many factors regulate the reversible opening and closing of connexon channels, including the transjunctional voltage, cytoplasmic H^+ and Ca^{2+} concentrations, and protein kinases. Oleamide, a fatty acid amide produced by the brain, blocks gap junctional communication and induces sleep in animals. Organic alcohols (heptanol and octanol) and general anesthetics (halothane) can also close gap junction channels

reversibly, but these agents are not specific for gap junctions. The transjunctional potential (i.e., the potential difference between the coupled cells) gates most connexons, regardless of the plasma membrane potentials of these cells. Like other voltage-gated channels (see Chapter 9), individual transitions are fast, but the response to potential changes, on the scale of seconds, is very slow compared with other channels. High concentrations of cytoplasmic Ca^{2+} (100 to 500 μM) and cytoplasmic acidification also close connexons. These effects of membrane potential, H^+, and Ca^{2+} allow cells to terminate communication with neighboring cells that are damaged (depolarizing the plasma membrane and admitting high concentrations of Ca^{2+}) or metabolically compromised (allowing Ca^{2+} to leak out of intracellular stores and acidifying the cytoplasm).

Second messengers generated by signaling pathways control gap junction activity in two ways. For example, on a time scale of seconds, cAMP activates cAMP–protein kinase (PKA), which phosphorylates the C-terminal tail of some connexins, increasing or decreasing the fraction of open channels (depending on the connexin isoform and the cell type). In one well-studied example, the neurotransmitter dopamine regulates the size of a network of electrically coupled neurons in the retina of the eye. Dopamine activates a seven-helix receptor (see Chapter 26) on these "horizontal cells," stimulating the production of cAMP. This second messenger activates PKA to phosphorylate the connexons, reducing their open probability and the size of the neuronal network. On a time scale of hours, cAMP also promotes the assembly of gap junctions.

Most connexons pair with identical connexons on the partner cell to form homotypic gap junctional channels, but nonidentical pairs can form heterotypic channels with novel properties. Homotypic channels pass molecules equally well in both directions, but heterotypic channels can be asymmetrical. These hybrid channels may pass fluorescent tracers more readily in one direction than the other, or react more sensitively to the transjunctional potential of one polarity than the other. This may explain the asymmetrical coupling that is sometimes observed between both excitable and nonexcitable cells, such as neuronal gap junctions, which pass action potentials in one direction but not the other.

Intercellular communication through gap junctions allows cells to function as a syncytium in the plane of an epithelium, allows cardiac and smooth muscle cells to transmit the action potentials that set off waves of contraction (see Chapter 42), and allows osteocytes buried deep in bone to have a cellular supply line to acquire nutrients from distant blood vessels (see Chapter 34). Note that the concentrations of solutes need not be the same on the two sides of a gap junction, as

table 33–2

PHENOTYPES OF HUMANS AND MICE WITH MUTATIONS IN GAP JUNCTION SUBUNITS

Connexin	Species	Phenotype
Cx-26	Human	Dominant and recessive mutations with deafness
	Mouse	Embryonic lethal defect owing to defective glucose transport across the placenta
Cx-32	Human	X-linked point mutations, defective myelin, peripheral nerve degeneration
	Mouse	Defective liver glucose metabolism, increased incidence of liver tumors, mild nerve defect
Cx-37	Mouse	Female infertility, defect in communication of granulosa cells with oocyte
Cx-40	Mouse	Partial block of impulse conduction in heart
Cx-43	Mouse	Embryonic lethal heart defects (heterozygote mild heart conduction defect)
Cx-46	Mouse	Cataracts in lens of the eye
Cx-50	Mouse	Cataracts in lens of the eye, small eyes
	Human	Cataracts in lens of the eye

Note: Mutations are homozygous loss of function mutations unless noted otherwise.

the metabolic activity of the coupled cells may differ. Electrical synapses can transmit action potentials at very high frequencies (>1000 per second). In some parts of the brain, gap junctions also coordinate action potentials in groups of neurons.

Mutations in connexin genes cause human disease and pathology in mice (Table 33–2). The defects are remarkably specific, considering that most connexins are expressed in several tissues. This may reflect situations in which other connexins cannot compensate, or in which the absolute number of channels is crucial. Recessive mutations in the connexin-26 gene are the most common causes of inherited human **deafness.** As many as 1 in 30 people are carriers, and their mutations may contribute to hearing loss late in life. Connexin-26 participates in the transport of K^+ in the epithelia supporting the sensory hair cells in the ear. Patients with one of a variety of mutations in the connexin-32 gene can suffer from degeneration of the myelin sheath around axons, an X-linked variant of **Charcot-Marie-Tooth disease.** Many human tissues express connexin-32, but the pathologic processes are confined to myelin. The viability of myelin may depend upon intracellular gap junctions between layers of the myelin sheath that provide a pathway between the metabolically active cell body and the deep layers of the sheath near the axon. (Defects in myelin membrane proteins cause other forms of Charcot-Marie-Tooth disease.) In contrast to humans, mice lacking connexin-32 have mild myelin defects but more serious defects in liver function (metabolic defects and a high incidence of tumors). Mice with null mutations in connexin-43, the main connexin of gap junctions in

heart and other tissues, die shortly after birth. Their hearts beat, but a malformation of the heart is fatal. Other organs are only mildly abnormal.

Adherens Junctions and Desmosomes

Two types of adhesive junctions—adherens junctions and desmosomes—use homophilic interactions of cadherins (see Chapter 32) to bind epithelial cells to their neighbors. Cytoplasmic actin filaments reinforce adherens junctions (see Fig. 33–1), whereas cytoplasmic intermediate filaments anchor desmosomes (Fig. 33–7).

A belt-like adherens junction, called the **zonula adherens,** encircles epithelial cells near their apical surface. This continuous junction maintains the physical integrity of the epithelium. Homophilic interactions between densely clustered **E-cadherins** bind adjacent cells together. β-catenin and a related protein called plakoglobin bind the cytoplasmic domains of E-cadherin. α-Catenin links β-catenin and plakoglobin to the bundle of actin filaments in the zonula adherens (see Fig. 33–7).

Desmosomes provide strong adhesions between epithelial and muscle cells. In epithelia, these junctions are small, disk-shaped, "spot welds" between cells. Their architecture is relatively more complicated in the heart (see Chapter 42). Two types of cadherins, named **desmogleins** and **desmocollins,** participate in linkages between the plasma membranes of adja-

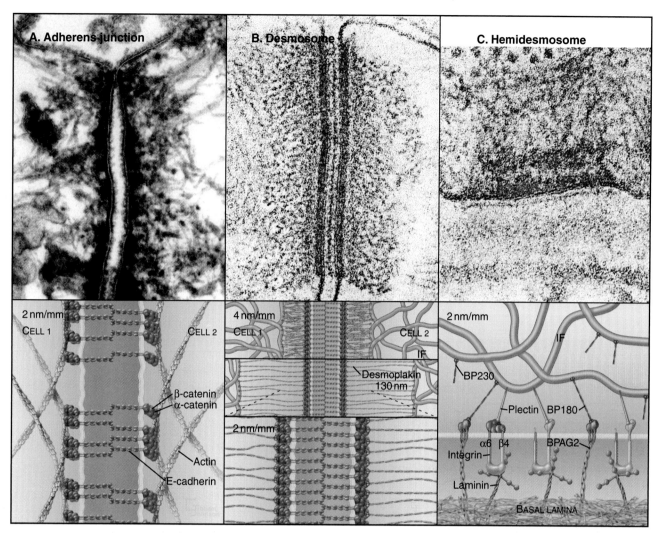

Figure 33-7 Comparison of adherens junction, desmosome, and hemidesmosome. *Top,* Electron micrographs of thin sections. *Bottom,* Molecular models. *A,* Adherens junction. Electron micrograph from the intestinal epithelium with partially dissociated cadherins. E-cadherins link two cells together. β- and α-catenin link the cytoplasmic domain of E-cadherin to actin filaments. *B,* Desmosome. Two types of cadherins—desmoglein and desmocollin—link adjacent cells together. The central dense stratum seen in the micrograph presumably corresponds to the interaction sites of the cadherins, although accessory proteins may participate. Desmoplakin and other accessory proteins link the cadherins and associated plakoglobin (related to catenin) to keratin intermediate filaments. Desmoplakin molecules are shown extended to their full length in the middle drawing, wheareas in desmosomes, they must be kinked or folded (as shown in the upper drawing), since the thickness of the desmoplakin layer is half that expected from extended molecules. *C,* Hemidesmosome. Integrin $\alpha_6\beta_4$ and type XVII collagen (also called BPAG2) attach to the basal lamina. Plectin and BPAG1 link the membrane proteins to keratin intermediate filaments. (*A,* Courtesy of Mark Mooseker, Yale University. *B,* Electron micrographs courtesy of Kathleen Green, Northwestern University. *C,* Electron micrograph courtesy of Jonathan Jones, Northwestern University.)

cent cells. Accessory proteins may be involved, as it has been difficult experimentally to constitute desmosomes with these cadherins alone. Desmosomal cadherins have similar extracellular domains, single transmembrane sequences, and cytoplasmic domains that interact with **plakoglobin** and **desmoplakin** but not β-catenin like other cadherins. Desmogleins have novel cytoplasmic domains that are not yet understood.

Desmoplakin and accessory proteins link desmosomal cadherins to intermediate filaments. Desmo-

plakin I and II, dimeric proteins related to plectin (see Chapter 38), consist of a coiled-coil rod with globular domains at each end. N-terminal globular domains bind desmosomal cadherins, whereas C-terminal domains bind directly to **epidermal keratins.** The binding site on keratin is the N-terminal, nonhelical domain. Mutations in this part of epidermal keratins can cause blistering skin diseases by compromising the integrity of desmosomes (see Chapter 38). Accessory proteins contribute to this connection between the cadherins and intermediate filaments. The best characterized is plakoglobin, which interacts with both the cytoplasmic domains of desmosomal cadherins and desmoplakin. Desmosomal cadherins somehow prevent plakoglobin from interacting with α-catenin and actin filaments. Plakoglobin gene knockouts in mice are lethal during embryogenesis owing to disruption of the heart.

Although all desmosomes share a common plan, their molecular composition varies in particular tissues. Mammals have three genes for desmogleins and three genes for desmocollins. Desmocollin messages are also alternatively spliced. Desmoglein-2 and desmocollin-2 are found in most desmosomes. Expression of the other isoforms is more restricted. For example, in epidermis, desmoglein-1 and desmocollin-1 are found only in the upper layers, whereas desmoglein-3 is in the basal layers. This explains the pathologic etiology in autoimmune blistering diseases. Patients with **pemphigus foliaceus** make antibodies that react with desmoglein-1 and disrupt desmosomes in the upper layers of the epidermis, whereas patients with **pemphigus vulgaris** produce autoantibodies to desmoglein-3 that have the same effect on the basal layers. The antibodies are directly responsible, as transfusion of human autoantibodies into a mouse reproduces the disease. Other organs are spared owing to the restricted expression of these two isoforms. Mutations in these desmoglein genes in mice result in skin blisters similar to pemphigus and attributable to compromised desmosomes.

Hemidesmosomes

Cells use hemidesmosomes to attach to the basal lamina. Adhesion to the extracellular matrix is fundamentally different than intercellular adhesion because integrins (see Chapter 32), rather than homophilic interactions of cadherins, provide the transmembrane link between the cytoskeleton and ligands in the extracellular matrix. Chapter 32 describes focal adhesions, which link cytoplasmic actin filaments through transmembrane integrins to the extracellular matrix. Hemidesmosomes are another type of integrin-based adhesive junction that links cytoplasmic intermediate filaments to the basal lamina. The morphologic resemblance of hemidesmosomes to half of a conventional desmosome (see Fig. 33–7) belies the fact that they are fundamentally different at the molecular level. Like desmosomes, hemidesmosomes have a dense plaque on the cytoplasmic surface of the plasma membrane

that anchors loops of intermediate filaments. The similarity ends there.

Two transmembrane proteins—$\alpha_6\beta_4$ **integrin** and **type XVII collagen**—concentrate in hemidesmosomes, and both are essential for assembly and stability. Outside the cell, $\alpha_6\beta_4$ integrin binds **laminin-5** in the basal lamina. Type XVII collagen is a trimeric transmembrane protein. The extracellular collagen triple helix is thought to form anchoring filaments between the membrane and the basal lamina. In a blistering skin disease called **bullous pemphigoid**, autoantibodies attack type XVII collagen, so the protein is also called bullous pemphigoid antigen-2, or BPAG2. This clinical observation and genetic deletions have established that both $\alpha_6\beta_4$ integrin and type XVII collagen are required for stable hemidesmosomes.

In the cytoplasm, plectin links the long tail of β_4 integrin to keratin intermediate filaments. The dense cytoplasmic plaque also contains BPAG1 (bullous pemphigoid antigen-1), another relative of plectin and desmoplakin, which may help bind intermediate filaments. Human mutations in plectin cause skin blisters associated with late-onset muscular dystrophy. A mouse null mutation of BPAG1 causes skin blisters, as well as defects in motor neurons.

Selected Readings

Burgeson RE, Christiano AM: The dermal-epidermal junction (basal lamina and hemidesmosomes). Curr Opin Cell Biol 9:651–658, 1997.

Crawford KM, Zambryski PC: Plasmadesmata signaling: Many roles, sophisticated statutes. Curr Opin Plant Biol 2:382–387, 1999.

Goodenough DA: Plugging the leak (a review of tight junction proteins). Proc Natl Acad Sci USA 96:319–321, 1999.

Jones JE, Hopkinson SB, Goldfinger LE: Structure and assembly of hemidesmosomes. BioEssays 20:488–494, 1998.

Kowalczyk AP, Bornslaeger EA, Norvell SM, et al: Desmosomes: Intercellular adhesive junctions specialized for attachment of intermediate filaments. Int Rev Cytol 185:237–302, 1999.

Kumar NM, Gilula NB: The gap junction communication channel. Cell 84:381–388, 1996.

Simon AM, Goodenough DA: Diverse functions of vertebrate gap junctions. Trends Cell Biol 8:477–483, 1998.

Stevenson BR, Keon BH: The tight junction: Morphology to molecules. Annu Rev Cell Dev Biol 14:89–109, 1998.

Yap AS, Brieher WM, Gumbiner BM: Molecular analysis of cadherin-based adherens junctions. Annu Rev Cell Dev Biol 13:119–146, 1998.

chapter 34

SPECIALIZED CONNECTIVE TISSUES

Animals use different proportions of matrix macromolecules to construct connective tissues with a range of mechanical properties to support their organs (see Figs. 30-1 and 34-1). Bone is a stiff, hard, solid; blood vessel walls are flexible and elastic; and the vitreous body of the eye is a watery gel. Plant cell walls are conceptually similar to the animal extracellular matrix but are composed of completely different molecules. This chapter begins with a discussion of simple connective tissues but concentrates on cartilage, bone, development of the skeleton, and the mechanisms that repair wounds, finishing with a discussion of the plant cell wall.

Loose Connective Tissue

Loose connective tissue consists of a sparse extracellular matrix of **hyaluronan** and **proteoglycans** supported by a few **collagen fibrils** and **elastic fibrils.** In addition to fibroblasts, the cell population is heterogeneous, including both indigenous and emigrant connective tissue cells (see Fig. 30-3). The loose connective tissue underlying the epithelium in the gastrointestinal tract is a good example of this heterogeneity (Fig. 34-1A), with lymphocytes, plasma cells, macrophages, eosinophils, neutrophils, and mast cells, as well as fibroblasts and occasional fat cells (see Chapter 30 for details on these cells). This variety of defensive cells is appropriate for a location near the lumen of the intestine, which contains microorganisms and potentially toxic materials from the outside world. Loose connective tissue is also found in and around other organs. The optically transparent vitreous body of the eye is an extremely simple loose connective tissue, where fibroblasts produce a highly hydrated gel

of hyaluronan and proteoglycans, supported by a loose network of type II collagen. Few defensive cells are required, as the interior of the eye is sterile.

Dense Connective Tissue

Collagen fibers, with or without elastic fibers, predominate over cells in dense connective tissue (see Fig. 34-1B). Fibroblasts are present to manufacture extracellular matrix but are relatively sparse. Other connective tissue cells are even rarer, as these tissues are not usually exposed to microorganisms. Collagen fibers can be arranged precisely, as in tendons or cornea (see Fig. 31-3), or less so, as in the wall of the intestine or the skin. Tendons consist nearly exclusively of type I collagen fibers, all aligned along the length of the tendon to provide the tensile strength required to transmit forces from muscle to bone. The cornea that forms the transparent front surface of the eye is also well organized into orthogonal layers of collagen fibrils.

Dense connective tissues can also be elastic. For example, the walls of arteries (see Fig. 31-8) and the dermal layer of skin (see Fig. 30-2C) consist of both collagen and elastic fibers. Energy from each heartbeat stretches the elastic fibers in the walls of arteries. Recoil of these elastic fibers propels blood between heartbeats.

About 1 of 5000 humans inherits a mutation in a gene for fibrillar collagens type III or type IV, which causes a range of connective tissue defects called **Ehlers-Danlos syndrome.** Most affected individuals have thin skin and lax joints. Severe mutations lead to rupture of arteries, bowel, or uterus, often with fatal consequences. The Ehlers-Danlos syndrome illustrates the

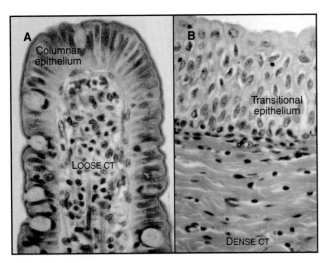

Figure 34-1 Connective tissues. *A,* Loose connective tissue (CT) underlying the columnar epithelium of the small intestine. Light micrograph of a section stained with Masson trichrome stain. *B,* Dense connective tissue (CT) underlying transitional epithelium in the wall of the ureter. Light micrograph of a section stained with hematoxylin-eosin. (Courtesy of D. W. Fawcett, Harvard Medical School.)

importance of these collagens with regard to the integrity of the affected tissues. Inheritance is dominant, as these collagens consist of trimers of three identical subunits. Given one mutant gene, only one in eight ($\frac{1}{2}$ × $\frac{1}{2}$ × $\frac{1}{2}$) procollagen molecules is normal.

Cartilage

Cartilage (Fig. 34−2) is tough, resilient connective tissue that is well suited for a variety of mechanical roles. It covers the articular surfaces of joints and supports large airways, such as the trachea, and skeletal appendages, such as the nose and ears. Cartilage also forms the entire skeleton of sharks and the embryonic precursors of many bones in higher vertebrates. The mechanical properties of cartilage are attributable to abundant extracellular matrix consisting of fine collagen fibrils and high concentrations of glycosaminoglycans and proteoglycans (Fig. 34−3).

Chondrocytes synthesize and secrete macromolecules for the cartilage matrix, which eventually surrounds them completely. Chondrocytes replenish the matrix as the macromolecules turn over slowly, but their ability to remodel and repair the matrix is limited. No blood vessels penetrate cartilage owing to several inhibitors of endothelial cell growth produced by chondrocytes. Thus, all nutrients must diffuse into cartilage from the nearest blood vessel in the **perichondrium,** a dense, fibrous, connective tissue capsule that covers the surface of cartilage. This capsule contains mesenchymal stem cells capable of differentiating into chondrocytes.

A meshwork of **type II collagen fibrils,** accounting for about 25% of the dry mass, fills the extracellu-

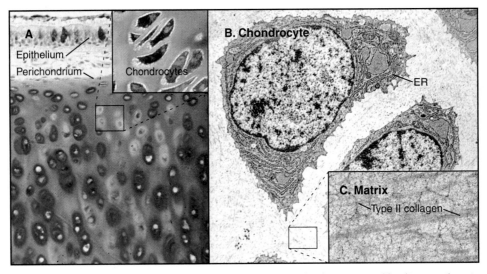

Figure 34-2 Cartilage and chondrocytes. *A,* Light micrograph of a section of hyaline cartilage in the wall of the respiratory tree stained with periodic acid–Schiff stain and alcian blue. The cartilage capsule of dense connective tissue (perichondrium) and the columnar epithelium lining the respiratory passage are at the top. *Inset,* Light micrograph of hyaline cartilage stained with toluidine blue. The proteoglycans in the matrix and the secretory pathway of the chondrocytes stain pink. The rough endoplasmic reticulum stains blue. Shrinkage during fixation and embedding creates the artifactual cavity or lacuna around each cell. *B,* Electron micrograph of a thin section of hyaline cartilage showing chondrocytes embedded in dense extracellular matrix. *C,* Electron micrograph of cartilage matrix at high magnification. This specimen was rapidly frozen and prepared by freeze-substitution to avoid collapse of the proteoglycans during dehydration and embedding. ER, endoplasmic reticulum. (*A,* Courtesy of D. W. Fawcett and E. D. Hay, Harvard Medical School. *B,* Courtesy of E. D. Hay, Harvard Medical School. *C,* Courtesy of E. B. Hunziker, M. Müller Institute, University of Bern.)

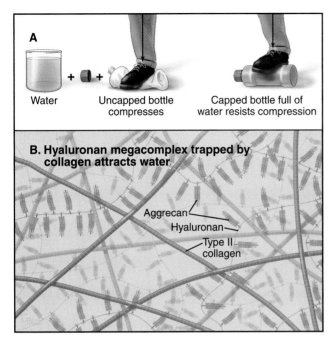

Figure 34–3 Macromolecular structure and mechanical properties of hyaline cartilage matrix. *A,* Hydrostatic model of the mechanical properties of cartilage. Water trapped in the extracellular matrix resists compression. Neither water alone *(in beaker)* nor a pliable container *(uncapped plastic bottle)* resist compression. However, if water fills a capped bottle, it resists compression. *B,* In the cartilage matrix, flexible strands of type II collagen trap proteoglycans, which attract large amounts of water. Trapped water resists compression because its "container," the network of collagen fibrils, does not stretch.

lar matrix. These slender collagen fibrils are hard to see even in electron micrographs but are extremely stable, with lifetimes estimated to be many years. Fibrils tend to line up parallel to surfaces, but otherwise are arranged randomly. Minor collagens type IX and type XI bind to the surface of type II fibrils. Type IX may be a cross-linker, and type XI may restrict fibril size. Expression of type X collagen is restricted to cartilage undergoing conversion to bone. The matrix contains several minor adhesive proteins, and other proteins inhibit invasion of blood vessels.

Glycosaminoglycans, including hyaluronic acid, constitute the second major class of matrix macromolecules. Molecules of the proteoglycan **aggrecan** attach to a hyaluronic acid backbone like the bristles of a test tube brush, forming so-called **megacomplexes** (see Fig. 31–14). Aggrecan also binds type II collagen. Highly charged glycosaminoglycans fill the extracellular space and attract water, the most abundant component of the matrix.

A hydrostatic mechanism allows cartilage to resist deformation (see Fig. 34–3). Collagen fibrils provide tensile strength (i.e., resistance to stretching) but do not resist compression or bending. Glycosaminoglycans strongly attract water, resulting in an internal swelling pressure that pushes outward against collagen

fibrils aligned parallel to the surface of the cartilage. The force of internal hydrostatic swelling pressure is balanced by the force produced by tension on the collagen fibrils. Remarkably, this internally stressed material can resist strong external forces like those on the articular surfaces of joints. A macroscopic analogue is a thin-walled plastic bottle filled with water. One can stand on the bottle provided that it is sealed, whereas neither the empty bottle nor the water could separately support any weight.

Specialized Forms of Cartilage

Hyaline cartilage, described earlier, is most common. It provides mechanical support for the respiratory tree, nose, articular surfaces, and developing bones. Elastic cartilage has abundant elastic fibers in addition to collagen, making the matrix much more elastic than hyaline cartilage. Elastic cartilage supports structures subjected to frequent deformation, including the larynx, epiglottis, and external ear. Fibrocartilage has features of both dense connective tissue (an abundance of thick collagen fibers) and cartilage (a prominent glycosaminoglycan matrix). It is tough and deformable, appropriate for its role in intervertebral disks, and insertions of tendons.

Differentiation and Growth of Cartilage

Cartilage grows by expansion of the extracellular matrix either from within or on the surface. For surface growth, mesenchymal cells in the perichondrium develop into chondrocytes that synthesize and secrete matrix materials. For internal growth, chondrocytes already trapped in the matrix divide and manufacture additional matrix, which is sufficiently deformable to allow for internal expansion.

Many growth factors, including transforming growth factor-β (TGF-β and its family members), fibroblast growth factors (FGFs), parathyroid hormone–related protein (PTHrP), and insulin-like growth factors (IGF-I and IGF-II), influence the growth of chondrocytes in culture. FGFs stimulate proliferation of mesenchymal precursors of chondrocytes, TGF-β promotes chondrocyte differentiation, and IGFs promote cartilage growth. Human diseases illustrate the physiological importance of these growth factors (Table 34–1). For example, without PTHrP, chondrocytes fail to proliferate in the growth plate of bones. Moreover, mutations in one of the receptors for FGF result in defective cartilage. It is expected that some combination of these and other growth factors, perhaps one or more of which is specific for cartilage, promotes the differentiation of the precursor cells into chondrocytes that secrete cartilage matrix molecules. Chondrocytes produce some of these growth factors (TGF-β, FGFs, and IGFs). During development, adjacent tissues can

table 34–1

EXAMPLES OF GENETIC DEFECTS OF CARTILAGE AND BONE

Gene/Protein	Species	Mutation	Phenotype
Transcription Factors			
Cbfa-1	Human	null for CBFA-1	+/− Human skeletal defects; −/− mouse no osteoblasts or bone
msx-1	Mouse	null for msx-1	Cleft palate
msx-2	Mouse	null for msx-2	Craniosynostosis (fusion of skull bones)
hoxa-2	Mouse	null for hoxa-2	Deletion of the second branchial arch; duplication of the first branchial arch
hoxd-13	Mouse	null for hoxd-13	Deletion of the fourth sacral derivatives; duplication of the third sacral derivatives
c-fos	Mouse	null for c-fos	Osteopetrosis; no osteoclasts
SOX9	Human	point mutations	Dominant defects in cartilage with severe skeletal deformities
Growth Factors			
BMP-4	Human	overexpression	Fibrodysplasia progressiva; ectopic bone formation
Shortear	Mouse	null for BMP-5 (TGF-β family)	Defective ears and sternum
Brachypodism	Mouse	null for GDF-5 (TGF-β family)	Reduced size of long bones; no joints
Growth hormone	Human	null for growth hormone	Reduced size of bones
PTHrP	Human	null for PTHrP	Reduced chondrocytic growth; epiphyseal plates fused at birth
op	Mouse	null for CSF-1	Osteopetrosis; reduced osteoclasts
opg1	Mouse	null for OPGL (TNF-like factor)	Osteopetrosis; no osteoclasts
Signal Transduction Components			
FGF receptor 1	Human	Point mutation FGFR-1	Pfeiffer's syndrome; cranial synostosis; long bone defects
FGF receptor 2	Human	Point mutation FGFR-2	Jackson-Weiss syndrome; cranial synostosis; long bone defects
FGF receptor 2	Human	Point mutation FGFR-2	Crouzon's disease; cranial synostosis
FGF receptor 3	Human	Activating point mutation	Achondroplasia; short, wide bones
c-Src	Mouse	null for c-src	Osteopetrosis; osteoclasts fail to attach to or degrade bone
Collagen and Other Structural Components of Cartilage and Bone			
COL1	Human	point mutations, deletions type I	Dominant osteogenesis imperfecta; fragile bones
COL2	Human	premature stop codon type II	Dominant Stickler's syndrome; chondrodysplasia, eye defects
	Human	point mutations type II	Dominant chondrodysplasia and osteoarthritis of variable severity
COL9A2	Human	splicing mutation type IX	Defective cartilage with degeneration of knee joint
COL10A1	Human	point mutations type X	Dominant Schmid's metaphyseal chondrodysplasia; abnormal growth plates, short bones
COL11A2	Human	exon skipping mutation type XI	Dominant Stickler's syndrome; chondrodysplasia, eye defects
	Human	point mutation type XI	Recessive severe chondrodysplasia; deafness; cleft palate
Cmd	Mouse	aggrecan missense mutation	Recessive cartilage deficiency; dwarfism; cleft palate
Perlecan	Mouse	deletion	Recessive defects in cartilage and bone formation
DTDST	Human	sulfate transporter	Recessive cartilage defects; short limbs; joint deformation
Cathepsin-K	Mouse	deletion	Osteopetrosis
Lysyl hydroxylase	Human	mutation, bone-specific enzyme	Bruck's disease; fragile bones

induce cartilage formation by secreting TGF-β and FGF. SOX9 is the key transcription factor mediating expression of cartilage-specific genes. Dominant mutations in this gene cause severe deformities of the skeleton.

Diseases Involving Cartilage

Cartilage fails in common human diseases, including arthritis and ruptured intervertebral disks. Mutations in the genes for cartilage proteins predispose individuals to disease (see Table 34–1). More than 25 different mutations of the gene for human type II collagen cause disorders of cartilage, ranging in severity from death in utero to dwarfism or osteoarthritis. Mutations in minor cartilage collagens cause a variety of symptoms, including degenerative joint disease (see Table 34–1). Type II collagen is a candidate for the antigen-inducing autoimmune inflammation in rheumatoid arthritis. A premature stop codon in chicken aggrecan causes lethal skeletal malformations.

▌ Bone

For most vertebrates, bones provide mechanical support and serve as the storage site for calcium. The great strength and light weight of bones are attributable to both the mechanical properties of the extracellular matrix and to efficient overall design, including tubular form and lamination (Fig. 34–4). A superficial layer of compact bone surrounds a medullary cavity that is filled with marrow or fat, or both, and is supported by struts of bone, arranged precisely along lines of mechanical stress. External surfaces of bones are covered by either dense connective tissue, called **periosteum,** or by cartilage at joint surfaces. A mono-layer of bone-forming cells called osteoblasts line the internal surfaces. Blood vessels supply the medullary cavity and penetrate compact bone through a network of channels. Although durable and strong, bone is remodeled continuously.

Extracellular Matrix of Bone

Bone is a composite material consisting of collagen fibrils (providing tensile strength) embedded in a matrix of calcium phosphate crystals (providing rigidity) (see Fig. 34–4E). Macroscopic analogues of the bone matrix are concrete reinforced by steel rods and fiberglass consisting of a brittle plastic reinforced by glass fibers. Each of these composites is stronger than its separate components. Simple extraction experiments illustrate the contributions of the two components. After removal of calcium phosphate with a calcium chelator, bone is so rubbery that it bends easily. After destruction of collagen by heating, bone is hard but brittle.

Fibrils of type I collagen, the dominant organic component of the matrix (Table 34–2), are arranged in sheets or a meshwork. Covalent crosslinks between the collagen molecules in fibrils make them inextensible. The matrix contains more than 100 minor proteins, including growth factors and adhesive glycoproteins, but few proteoglycans.

Calcium-phosphate crystals, similar to **hydroxyapatite** [$Ca_{10}(PO_4)_6(OH)_2$], comprise about two thirds of the dry weight of bone. These crystals begin growing within collagen fibrils and in holes between the ends of the staggered collagen molecules, eventually filling the spaces between the collagen molecules within the fibrils. The mechanisms that control nucleation of hydroxyapatite and the orientation of the crystals are still under investigation.

table 34–2

BONE PROTEINS

Name	Content	Functions
Bone morphogenic proteins	Minor	TGF-β homologues; cartilage stimulation and bone development and repair
Collagen type I	90%	Forms fibrils in the bone matrix
Osteocalcin	1%–2%	Binds to hydroxyapatite and weakly to Ca^{2+}; function unknown
Osteonectin	2%	Synthesized in developing and regenerating bone; binds collagen and hydroxyapatite; may nucleate hydroxyapatite crystallization in bone matrix
Osteopontin	Minor	RGD sequence; binds osteoclast integrins to bone surface
Proteoglycans	Minor	Decorin, biglycan, osteoadherin; may bind TGF-β
Sialoproteins	2%	RGD sequence; binds osteoclast integrins to bone surface

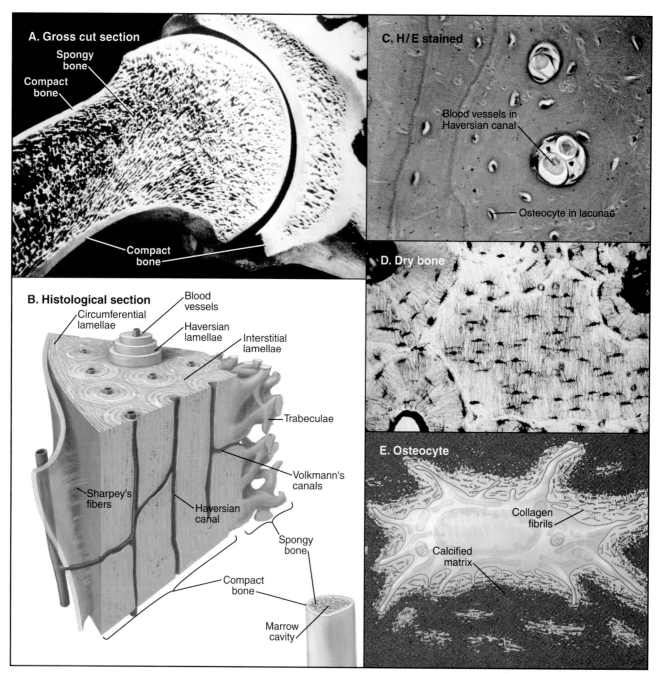

Figure 34–4 Organization of long bones. *A,* Longitudinal section of a shoulder joint of a dried bone specimen. Struts of trabecular spongy bone reinforce compact bone in the cortex. *B,* Drawing of a wedge of long bone. Circumferential lamellae form the outer layer just beneath the periosteum *(blue)* covering the surface. Osteons (Haversian systems) consist of concentric lamellae of calcified matrix and osteocytes arranged around a channel containing one or two capillaries or venules. Interstitial lamellae are fragments of osteons remaining after remodeling (see Fig. 34–10). Radial vascular channels connect longitudinal vascular channels to the medullary cavity or periosteum. *C,* Light micrograph of a cross section stained with hematoxylin-eosin showing circumferential lamellae on the left and two Haversian canals. *D,* Light micrograph of a cross section of dried bone showing a central interstitial lamella surrounded by three osteons. Narrow canaliculi connect the lacunae housing osteocytes. *E,* Drawing of an osteocyte surrounded by calcified matrix and extending filopodia into canaliculi. (Micrographs courtesy of D. W. Fawcett, Harvard Medical School.)

Bone Cells

Bone is an active tissue maintained by a balance of cellular activities. Osteoblasts and osteocytes produce extracellular matrix and establish conditions for its calcification. Osteoclasts resorb bone, as required for growth and remodeling. An imbalance of these opposing cellular activities causes human diseases. Osteoblasts arise from mesenchymal stem cells that also give rise to fibroblasts and chondrocytes (see Fig. 30–3). Osteoclasts form by fusion of blood monocytes.

A monolayer of **osteoblasts** on the surface of growing bone tissue uses a well-developed secretory pathway to synthesize and secrete organic components of the matrix (Fig. 34–5). Unmineralized bone matrix consists largely of type I collagen but includes factors that promote crystalization of calcium phosphate on the surface of these fibrils. Osteoblasts also control the differentiation, but not the activity, of osteoclasts (see later section).

Once an osteoblast has enclosed itself within bone matrix, it is called an **osteocyte.** Osteocytes are connected to each other by long, slender filopodia that run through narrow channels in the matrix. Gap junctions between the processes of osteocytes provide a continuous network of intercellular communication that stretches from cells adjacent to blood vessels to the most deeply embedded osteocyte. Osteocytes are less active than osteoblasts but lay down or resorb matrix in their immediate vicinity.

Many transcription factors and growth factors control differentiation and proliferation of osteoblasts. **Cbfa1** is the key transcription factor controlling the expression of multiple genes required to make bone matrix, including a few genes expressed exclusively by osteoblasts, enamel-making odontoblasts in teeth, and a subset of chondrocytes. Mouse embryos lacking Cbfa1 have no osteoblasts or osteoclasts. They make a cartilage skeleton that never transforms to bone. Humans and mice with just one active Cbfa-1 gene lack collarbones and experience a delay in the fusion of joints between skull bones. This syndrome is the most common human skeletal defect. Cbfa1 is part of a network of transcription factors with positive and negative influences on osteoblast differentiation and function. Homeobox transcription factors (Dlx5, Dlx6, Msx2, Bapx1) up-regulate Cbfa1, whereas Hoxa-2 inhibits Cbfa1. Indian Hedgehog (Ihh; see the discussion in Chapter 26 of Hedgehog receptors) triggers differentiation. Growth factors, including bone morphogenetic proteins (BMPs), stimulate Cbfa1 expression, whereas TGF-β inhibits its expression.

Circulating hormones influence osteoblasts and osteocytes. The parathyroid gland secretes its hormone to regulate the concentration of calcium in blood. Parathyroid hormone stimulates osteocytes to mobilize calcium from the surrounding matrix. The hormone leptin, secreted by fat cells, acts on cells of the hypothalamus in the brain to regulate appetite. In addition, these same neurons secrete an unidentified factor that inhibits bone production by osteoblasts. This explains why animals and people lacking leptin or leptin receptor are not only obese but also have dense bones.

Osteoclasts are multinucleated giant cells specialized for bone resorption (Fig. 34–6). They attach like a suction cup to the surface of bone. Interactions of a plasma membrane integrin ($\alpha_V\beta_3$) with bone matrix proteins (osteopontin and sialoprotein) help to create a leak-proof compartment on the bone surface. Osteoclasts amplify the plasma membrane that lines this closed space, forming a "ruffled border" composed of microvilli enriched with a **V-type H$^+$ transporting adenosine triphosphatase (ATPase)** (see Chapter 7) and chloride channels (see Chapter 9). The combined activities of the H$^+$ pump and these chloride channels allow the cell to secrete hydrochloric acid into the sealed extracellular compartment on the bone surface. This closed space acts like an extracellular lysosome: acid dissolves calcium phosphate crystals, and secreted proteolytic enzymes, including **cathepsin K,** digest collagen and other organic components. Degradation products are taken up by endocytosis and transported across the cell in vesicles for secretion on the free surface. Amino acids are reused, but collagen cross-linking groups are not, so they are excreted in

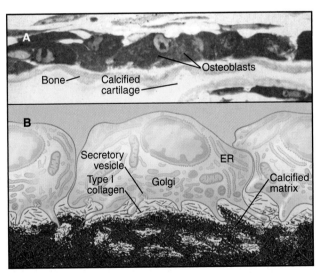

Figure 34–5 Osteoblasts. *A,* Light micrograph of a section of forming bone stained with toluidine blue. Osteoblasts with abundant, blue-stained, rough endoplasmic reticulum and a clear centrosomal region lay down bone matrix *(light green)* on the surface of calcified cartilage *(light pink). B,* Drawing of osteoblasts. ER, endoplasmic reticulum. (*A,* Courtesy of R. Dintzis and from the work of D. Walker, Johns Hopkins Medical School.)

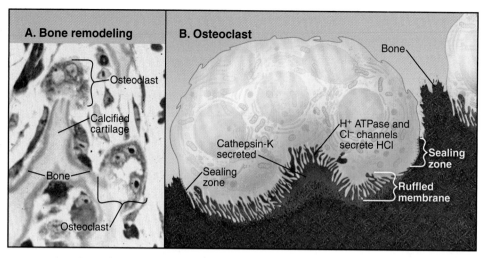

Figure 34–6 Osteoclasts. *A*, Light micrograph of a section of forming bone stained with toluidine blue showing two osteoclasts degrading bone and calcified cartilage. *B*, Drawing of an osteoclast attached to the bone matrix by a sealing zone, forming a resorption cavity *(pink)*. The cell pumps H⁺ and secretes lysosomal enzymes into this cavity to resorb the surface of the matrix. (*A*, Courtesy of R. Dintzis and from the work of D. Walker, Johns Hopkins Medical School.)

the urine where their concentration is a measure of bone turnover.

Just two external factors are required to stimulate blood monocytes to fuse and differentiate into multinucleated osteoclasts.

1. The circulating growth factor, macrophage-colony–stimulating factor **(M-CSF),** acts through a cytokine receptor (see Fig. 26–6) and the JAK-STAT pathway to regulate gene expression (see Fig. 29–12). Granulocyte-monocyte-colony-stimulating factor (GM-CSF) can substitute for M-CSF, but is only made late in development.
2. **RANKL** (RANK ligand, also called osteoprotegerin ligand [OPGL] or TRANCE) is a tumor necrosis factor (TNF) homologue that is displayed on the surface of bone marrow stromal cells, osteoblasts, and activated T lymphocytes. RANKL binds to a member of the TNF receptor family (see Fig. 26–11) on monocytes called RANK (receptor for activation of NF-κB). The combined activation of the cytokine receptor pathway and the NF-κB pathway triggers differentiation of osteoclasts. A soluble receptor for RANKL called OPG blocks activation of RANK. Mice lacking RANKL form no osteoclasts, and bone resorption fails. In addition, these mice lack lymph nodes, as RANKL also regulates lymph node development.

Many stimulators of osteoclast differentiation (parathyroid hormone, vitamin D) act indirectly by stimulating supporting cells to make RANKL. TNF stimulates osteoclasts directly. Estrogens inhibit osteoclast differentiation. The decline of estrogen levels after menopause enhances osteoclast differentiation and contributes to bone loss in older women. Osteoclast growth

factors merit more than academic interest because RANKL, TNF, and interleukin-1 (IL-1) mediate excess bone resorption at sites of chronic inflammation in rheumatoid arthritis and gum diseases.

Formation and Growth of the Skeleton

Both genetic and environmental information direct formation of the skeleton. Genetic information predominates in the master plan and initial development of skeletal tissues, as the size and shape of bones are characteristic for each species. Environmental information is important in remodeling of the skeleton in response to use. Mutations in genes for structural and informational molecules (see Table 34–2) have provided valuable clues about the genetic blueprint for the skeleton, but the understanding of these complex regulatory pathways is far from complete.

Genetic information is read out on at least two levels. First, master genetic regulators—including transcription factors encoded by **HOX** (homeobox) and **PAX** (paired box) genes—specify the developmental fate of each embryonic segment. Homeoboxes are DNA sequences encoding a family of 60-residue protein domains that bind DNA (see Chapter 14). The human genome contains 39 HOX genes arrayed in four linear arrays, similar to other animals, including flies and nematodes. HOX genes were discovered in flies as a result of mutations that cause "homeotic conversion," whereby the fate of one segment is converted into another, sometimes with bizarre results, such as the substitution of a leg for an antenna. The same thing happens in vertebrates: mouse embryos express Hoxd-4 in the second cervical (neck) vertebra and more posterior segments. Mutation of Hoxd-4 results in a failure of the second cervical vertebra to form normally. Instead, it takes on some of the features of the first cervical vertebra. Mutations in other HOX genes cause congenital malformations in humans. HOX transcription factors control the expression of downstream genes, including growth factors, but the pathway from HOX genes to determinants of three-dimensional architecture is incompletely understood.

Second, systematically circulating and locally secreted growth factors control the proliferation and differentiation of the cells of cartilage and bone. Mutations in these factors and their receptors also cause surprisingly specific human skeletal malformations. Circulating **growth hormone** produced by the pituitary gland is a major determinant of skeletal size. Individuals deficient in growth hormone are short in stature. Locally produced families of growth factors, including bone morphogenetic proteins (BMPs) and fibroblast growth factors (FGFs) and their receptors, control the development and growth of cartilage and bone during embryogenesis, in addition to stimulating repair after fractures. FGF receptors are tyrosine kinases. BMPs are related in structure and mechanism to transforming growth factor-β (TGF-β) (see Chapter 29) and are expressed in tissues other than bone and cartilage. BMPs are part of a system of positive and negative factors that regulate formation of cartilage, bone, and joints. For example, a BMP called GDF-5 specifies the position of joints, but joints form only if noggin protein, an inhibitor of other BMPs, is present.

Embryonic Bone Formation

Bone always forms by replacement of preexisting connective tissue. During embryonic development, flat bones, such as the skull and shoulder blades, form from **neural crest cell** precursors in loose connective tissue (Fig. 34–7). Somehow, one-dimensional information in the genome is read out as the three-dimensional pattern of a skull. Growth factors, vitamins (e.g., retinoic acid), and local matrix molecules, such as glycosaminoglycans, all influence the differentiation of these cells into osteoblasts at specific locations in connective tissue. Osteoblasts lay down struts of bone matrix in the loose connective tissue. As new bone is laid down on the surface of these bone spicules, some osteoblasts are trapped and become osteocytes. A similar process heals fractures.

During embryonic and postnatal development, genetic information precisely controls changes in the size and proportions of flat bones. For example, for the skull to increase in size both externally and internally, osteoclasts on the outer surface lay down new bone at the same rate at which osteoclasts resorb old bone inside (see Fig. 34–9). These cellular activities are carefully coordinated to change the proportions of the skull as the individual matures.

Long bones, such as the humerus, begin as cartilage models that are replaced by bone (Fig. 34–8). The initial steps are only vaguely understood at the cellular and molecular levels. Multiple, genetically programmed factors induce clusters of mesenchymal cells at specific locations to differentiate into chondrocytes that secrete type II collagen and glycosaminoglycans. This produces a miniature cartilaginous version of the adult bone. Bone then replaces this cartilage precursor in a series of steps. Over the course of about three days, chondrocytes grow in size, secrete type X collagen, and use matrix metalloproteinases to resorb some of their surrounding matrix. Matrix vesicles budded from chrondrocyte microvilli contribute to the calcification of the remaining cartilage matrix. These hyper-

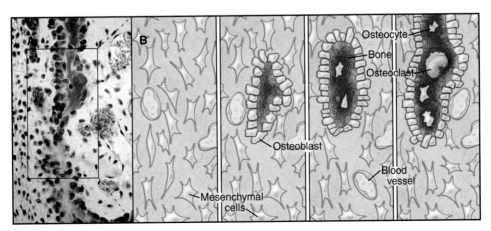

Figure 34–7 Bone formation by intramembranous ossification. *A*, Light micrograph of a section of forming bone stained with hematoxylin-eosin. Calcified bone matrix is maroon. *B*, Interpretive drawings. Connective tissue mesenchymal cells differentiate into osteoblasts, which lay down bone matrix *(blue)*. Osteoblasts become trapped as the matrix grows. (*A*, Courtesy of D. W. Fawcett, Harvard Medical School.)

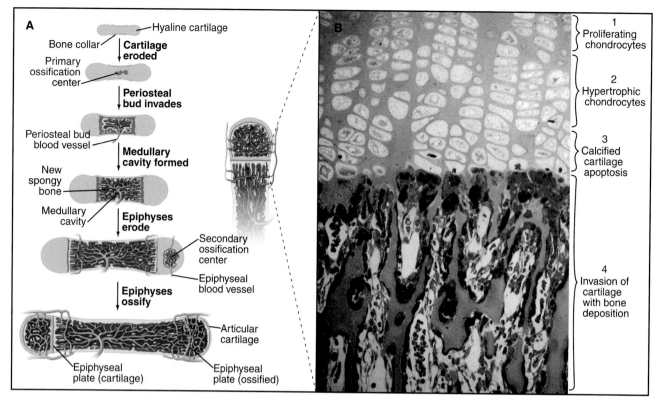

Figure 34-8 Formation of a long bone by replacement of a cartilage model *(light blue)*. A, The shaft grows in diameter as osteoblasts lay down bone *(tan)* on the outer surface of the primary collar of bone and osteoclasts remove bone from the inner surface to form and maintain the marrow cavity. The bone grows in length by interstitial expansion of the cartilage in the epiphyseal plate and its replacement by bone. B, Light micrograph of a section of an epiphyseal plate stained with toluidine blue. Cartilage growth, differentiation, and replacement by bone occurs in several zones. (1) Proliferation of chondrocytes and their production of matrix *(pink)* containing type II collagen is solely responsible for the longitudinal growth of the bone. (2) Hypertrophic chondrocytes enlarge and make type X collagen, as well as matrix metalloproteinases that resorb some of the surrounding matrix. (3) Chondrocytes die by apoptosis and the matrix calcifies. (4) Blood vessels and osteoblasts move into spaces vacated by chondrocytes and lay down bone *(blue)* on the surface of calcified cartilage. (Micrograph courtesy of R. Dintzis and from the work of D. Walker, Johns Hopkins Medical School.)

trophic chondrocytes generally die by apoptosis, but in tissue culture, they may differentiate into osteoblasts. Osteoblasts lay down bone matrix on the surface of the calcified cartilage. Cartilage is avascular owing to expression of inhibitors of blood vessel growth, but hypertrophic cartilage ceases to inhibit endothelial cell growth. This allows FGF-2, TGF-β, and vascular endothelium growth factor (VEGF) to attract capillaries as part of the transformation of cartilage to bone.

For a long bone to maintain its shape as it grows in size, deposition and removal of bone tissue must be highly selective. For the shaft to grow in diameter, new bone is laid down on the outer surface by osteoblasts at the same time as old bone is removed inside by osteoclasts (Fig. 34–9). Bones grow longer as a result of interstitial growth of cartilage in the **epiphyseal plate** and its continual replacement by bone. Growth of long bones stops at puberty when high

concentrations of estrogen and testosterone stop proliferation of epiphyseal chondrocytes so that bone replaces this cartilage. This closure of the epiphyses occurs over several years in a predictable order, so one can judge the maturity of a child by examining epiphyses by radiographic studies. Genetic variations in this process of maturation give rise to differences in stature. Metabolic and endocrine disorders can affect the timing of epiphyseal closure.

Bone Remodeling

Bone is amazingly dynamic and is remodeled continuously in response to stresses. Bone cells and matrix turn over every few years. Reorganization of bone requires two carefully coordinated steps: breakdown of preexisting bone by osteoclasts and replacement with new bone by osteoblasts. More than 100 years ago, Wolff realized that the strength of a bone depends on use. For example, bones of the racquet arm of tennis players are more robust than the bones of their other arm. Thus, mechanical forces on the bones must generate modulatory signals that control remodeling.

Elucidation of the mechanisms that transduce force into cellular responses has been challenging. A plausible mechanism is that bending and compression of bones stimulate osteocytes by forcing fluid to flow through the canalicular system. In fact, osteocytes are sensitive to pulsatile fluid flow over their surfaces, responding with production of prostaglandins (see Chapter 28). Possible participation of lipid second messengers is intriguing, as they can stimulate receptors on neighboring cells.

Formation of the cylindrical units of long bones called **osteons** is a good example of well-coordinated remodeling. The process involves two steps (Fig. 34–10). First, osteoclasts resorb preexisting bone to form long, cylindrical, resorption channels in the same way that a "Roto-rooter" clears debris from drain pipes. Second, osteoblasts fill in these channels by depositing concentric layers of lamellar bone against the walls. They lay down matrix at a rate of about 1 μm of thickness per day until bone completely surrounds the blood vessels trapped in the middle of the newly formed osteon. Because resorption channels cut randomly through the bone, fragments of older osteons are left behind during the remodeling of mature bone. These fragments are called **interstitial lamellae.** Resorption may release growth and differentiation factors from the mineralized matrix that provide a local stimu-

lus for the next round of bone formation by new osteoblasts.

Bone Diseases

Osteoporosis, a thinning of bones, is common in elderly people as a result of an imbalance of bone resorption over renewal. In the United States, osteoporosis results in 1.5 million painful fractures costing $14 billion annually. Almost 50% of women suffer from such a fracture at some time in their lives. Osteoporosis also occurs at reduced gravitational forces during space flight. The pathogenesis is not understood, but both behavioral (e.g., inactivity, poor nutrition, smoking) and multiple genetic factors have modest effects. One genetic factor may be naturally occurring variants of the nuclear receptor for vitamin D. This receptor is a transcription factor that is required for intestinal calcium uptake and calcification of bone. Minor variations in the gene for type I collagen may also contribute. Treatments (e.g., estrogen, calcium, fluoride, bisphosphonates) are empirical and only partially effective. Remarkably, statins (the inhibitors of HMG-CoA reductase (see Fig. 20–14) used to treat hypercholesterolemia) stimulate bone formation.

Osteopetrosis is failure of bone resorption, leading to an imbalance of renewal over resorption. This rare disease of osteoclasts is fatal in humans owing to bone marrow failure. The molecular defect in humans is not known, but the disease can be cured by transplantation of bone marrow stem cells to replace defective osteoclast precursors. Mutations in the genes for

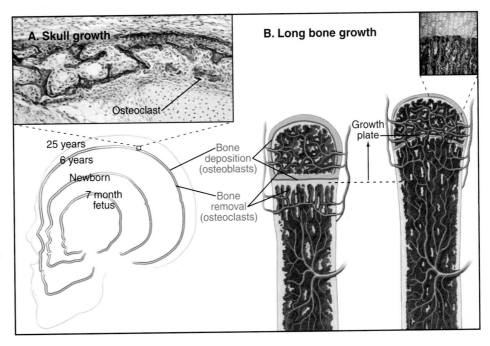

Figure 34-9 Bone growth. *A,* Light micrograph of a section of skull stained with Mallory's trichrome stain and an interpretive drawing. The skull expands during fetal development and growth to adulthood as osteoblasts lay down new bone on the outer surface *(blue)* and osteoclasts resorb bone *(pink)* on the inner surface. *B,* Long bones grow entirely by expansion of cartilage in the epiphyseal plate and its replacement by bone *(tan),* followed by resorption *(pink).* (*A,* Courtesy of D. W. Fawcett, Harvard Medical School.)

A. Skull growth

Osteoclast

25 years
6 years
Newborn
7 month fetus

B. Long bone growth

Bone deposition (osteoblasts)

Bone removal (osteoclasts)

Growth plate

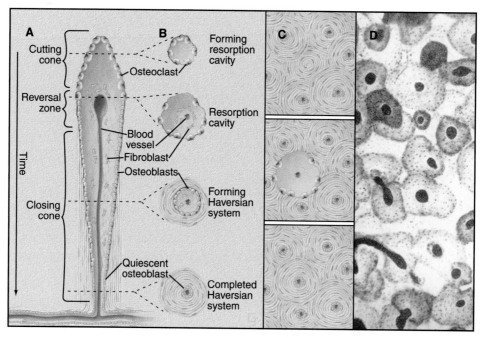

Figure 34–10 Bone remodeling. *A* and *B,* Longitudinal and cross sections of a time line illustrating the formation of an osteon. Osteoclasts cut a cylindrical channel through bone. Osteoblasts follow, laying down bone on the surface of the channel until the matrix surrounds the central blood vessel of the newly formed osteon. *C,* Steps in the formation of a new osteon. Parts of older osteons are left behind as interstitial lamellae. *D,* Microradiograph of a cross section of a long bone, illustrating the range of ages of the structures. A section of bone is placed on x-ray film, exposed to x-rays, developed, and examined by light microscopy. Older parts of the bone, such as the interstitial lamellae, are more heavily calcified and, therefore, absorb more of the x-rays, appearing lighter. Newly formed osteons appear the darkest, as they are the least calcified. Vascular spaces are empty and fully exposed by the x-rays. (*A,* Redrawn from Parfitt AM: The action of parathyroid hormone on bone. Metabolism 25:809–844, 1976. *D,* Courtesy of D. W. Fawcett, Harvard Medical School.)

three different types of proteins cause osteopetrosis in mice. A lack of the blood cell growth factor, colony-stimulating factor 1 (CSF-1 = M-CSF), precludes development of osteoclast precursors. Mice with a null mutation in the *c-Src* proto-oncogene (a cytoplasmic protein tyrosine kinase; see Chapter 27) are nearly normal except for severely impaired bone resorption. Osteoclasts are present but inactive. In the absence of the c-Fos transcription factor, no osteoclasts develop.

Osteogenesis imperfecta is the name of a variety of congenital fragile bone syndromes. Severely affected fetuses die in utero from multiple broken bones. Mildly affected individuals are born but suffer multiple fractures resulting in skeletal deformities. All affected individuals have mutations in the gene for type I collagen. Some are deletions or insertions, which may be mild. Most patients with severe disease have point mutations leading to replacement of a glycine by a large amino acid. This prevents the zipper-like folding of the collagen triple helix (see Chapter 31), even if only one chain is defective per molecule. This poisons assembly and accounts for the dominant phenotype. No one knows why these mutations in

type I collagen do not affect other tissues, such as skin, which are rich in type I collagen.

Wound Healing

Healing of minor skin wounds is a familiar occurrence that illustrates the mechanisms that control the assembly of connective tissue. Repair of the connective tissue in the dermis underlying the epithelium proceeds in three stages: formation of a blood clot, assembly of provisional connective tissue, and remodeling of the connective tissue (Fig. 34–11).

Tissue damage ruptures blood vessels, releasing blood that clots to stem the hemorrhage and fill the damaged area. The clot forms when injury activates the blood plasma proteolytic enzyme **thrombin,** which cleaves the plasma protein, **fibrinogen,** to form **fibrin.** Fibrin polymerizes and is cross-linked to itself and to **plasma fibronectin.** This provisional extracellular matrix of fibrin and fibronectin provides physical integrity for the clot and an environment for wound repair. Platelets activated during clotting secrete matrix molecules (thrombospondin, fibrinogen,

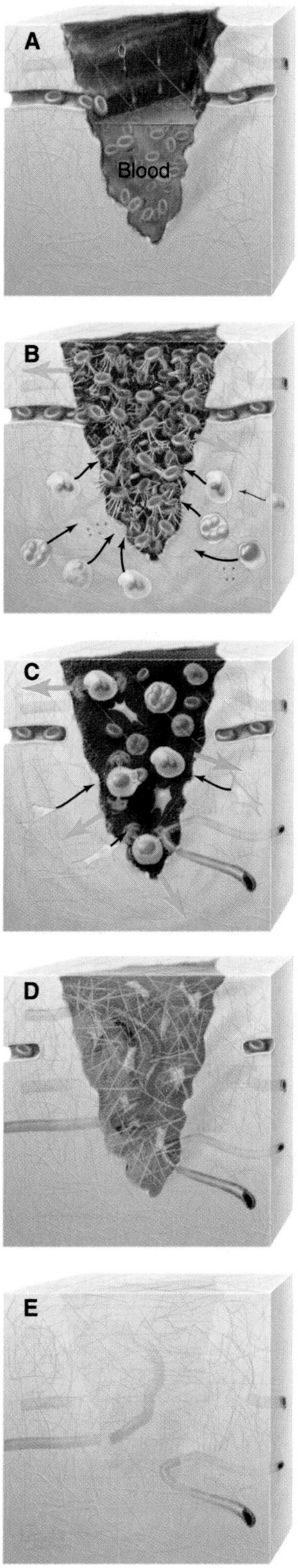

Figure 34-11 Repair of a wound in connective tissue. *A*, Wounding removes some tissue and damages blood vessels, releasing blood into the defect. *B*, Blood forms a clot of fibrin and fibronectin, releasing fibrin peptides, and platelets secrete PGDF and TGF-*β*, all of which attract neutrophils and monocytes. *C*, Neutrophils ingest any bacteria. Monocytes clean up debris and differentiate into macrophages, which secrete cytokines, attracting fibroblasts and blood vessels. *D*, Fibroblasts secrete type III collagen and hyaluronan, which, in turn, replace the fibrin clot. *E*, Fibroblasts remodel the provisional connective tissue with type I collagen, and blood vessels grow back into the new tissue.

fibronectin, and von Willebrand's factor) and growth factors (platelet-derived growth factor [PDGF], TGF-*β*, and TGF-*α*) that initiate the cellular events required to complete wound repair.

Chemotactic factors attract phagocytes from the blood into the wound. These factors include PDGF, chemokines, peptides cleaved from fibrinogen by thrombin, and peptides from any contaminating bacteria. Neutrophils arrive first, having attached to activated endothelial cells (see Fig. 32–15) and migrated into the connective tissue and clot. They ingest any bacteria. Second, monocytes (using a similar mechanism) migrate into the clot and clear foreign material and any dead neutrophils. The environment in a wound promotes transformation of monocytes into macrophages, which synthesize and secrete cytokines and growth factors that mediate the cellular processes that complete the repair process. In this way, platelets, monocytes, and fibroblasts form a relay, passing information from one cell to the next.

During the next phase of repair, macrophages, fibroblasts, and capillary endothelial cells migrate into the fibrin clot and reestablish the connective tissue. Endothelial cells form capillary loops that allow blood to flow and to provide oxygen. Initially, the endothelial cells are attracted by the growth factors released by platelets, but macrophages and dissolution of fibrin provide a more sustained supply of chemoattractants and growth factors. Integrin receptors for fibronectin allow fibroblasts to migrate into the clot. They secrete more fibronectin as they move. Within the clot, PDGF and TGF-β from microphages stimulate fibroblasts to secrete type III collagen, hyaluronan, SPARC (secreted protein acidic and rich in cysteine), and tenascin. Initially, this loose connective tissue is disorganized and weak. Hyaluronan predominates transiently, but after about five days, it is gradually replaced by proteoglycans and type I collagen.

Two events complete the repair of the matrix. First, fibroblasts differentiate into (smooth muscle–like) **myofibroblasts,** which contract the collagen matrix, closing the edges of the wound. This step is particularly important for large wounds. Second, fibroblasts remodel the provisional connective tissue to restore its original architecture with nearly normal physical strength. This requires resorption of provisional collagen fibrils by metalloproteinases (see Chapter 31) and assembly of more robust type I collagen fibrils.

While fibroblasts repair the connective tissue, the epithelium bordering the wound spreads by cell division and migration to cover the defect. This process of migration is initiated within hours of wounding. Both the loss of contacts with neighboring cells at the edge of the wound and the release of growth factors in the wound are thought to transform the static epithelial cells into rapidly migrating cells. Keratin filaments that predominate in the cytoskeleton of the skin epithelial cells are replaced with actin filaments. Hemidesmosomes that anchor the skin epithelial cells to the basal lamina are lost, and the cells migrate over the surface of the underlying matrix, which consists initially of fibrin and fibronectin and later of collagen. As they go, epithelial cells lay down a new basal lamina. Depending upon the size of the defect, proliferation of epithelial cells may be required to complete coverage of the surface. When it is covered, the cells begin to differentiate into stratified epithelium.

Many parallels exist between repair of a fractured bone and repair of a skin wound. Blood escapes from damaged blood vessels and clots at the fracture site. PDGF that has been released by platelets stimulates mesenchymal cells to proliferate in the surrounding tissue. These cells migrate into the clot along with blood vessels and macrophages. Stimulated by growth factors released initially by platelets and in a more sustained fashion by macrophages, mesenchymal cells differentiate into chondrocytes and osteoblasts that recapitulate the development of new bone to fill in the defect. Although the bone that is initially produced to join the fractured ends is poorly organized, fractures are mechanically stable within about six weeks. The fibrin clot is converted directly into bone if the broken bone is immobilized. A cartilage intermediate may form first if the fracture is allowed to move. Over a period of months, remodeling reestablishes the normal pattern of the bone. With time, remodeling can even straighten out bones mildly bent at fracture sites.

In all of these examples, wound healing is coordinated by a variety of growth factors and cytokines and supported by the environment provided by the extracellular matrix. For example, PDGF from platelets stimulates the proliferation of fibroblasts and attracts them to the fibrin clot at the site of a wound. TGF-β inhibits fibroblast proliferation but stimulates fibroblasts to make matrix molecules. The actions of cytokines and growth factors depend on the local environment in the matrix. In a fibrin clot, TGF-β binds to its receptor on cells rather than the matrix. In the normal connective tissue matrix, TGF-β binds to proteoglycans in preference to its cell surface receptors, and its effects are not felt. In a fibrin/fibronectin clot, cellular fibronectin receptors bind the matrix, stimulating production of matrix metalloproteinases that are appropriate for remodeling the matrix. In normal connective tissue with less fibronectin, cells produce less metalloproteinase.

The mechanisms that mediate physiological wound repair can also contribute to disease. For example, PDGF that is released from activated platelets in clots at the sites of wounds initiates the cellular events required for repair. On the other hand, when the endothelium lining of large arteries is damaged, platelets are activated by binding to the exposed basal lamina. This stimulates them to release PDGF, which promotes proliferation of fibroblasts and smooth muscle cells in the artery wall, an early step in the development of arteriosclerosis.

Plant Cell Wall

The cell walls of land plants are composite materials consisting of cellulose, other polysaccharides, and glycoproteins (Fig. 34–12). Wood and cotton are two familiar examples of cell wall material left behind after plant cells have died. Like the extracellular matrix of animals, plant cell walls not only provide mechanical support, but they also may influence development. Two types of forces act on cell walls. Internally, the vacuole of the plant cell applies turgor pressure. Cell walls also resist a variety of external mechanical forces that tend to deform the cell.

The main constituent of cell walls is **cellulose,** the most abundant biopolymer on earth. It is a long, unbranched polymer of glucose (Fig. 2–27A). Several dozen cellulose polymers associate laterally into 5- to 7-nm bundles called **microfibrils** (Fig. 34–12B). Two types of branched polysaccharides—**hemicellulose** and **pectin**—associate with cellulose in microfibrils.

Cellulose is synthesized by a complex of plasma membrane enzymes termed **cellulose synthases.** *Arabadopsis* has genes for about 30 different cellulose synthases. Genetic evidence suggests that active enzymes consist of two different synthase polypeptides. These transmembrane enzymes form a rosette of six particles that can easily be observed by electron microscopy. Each rosette extrudes 36 cellulose polymers across the plasma membrane to form a paracrystalline bundle outside the cell. These cellulose microfibrils in the cell wall and cytoplasmic microtubules tend to have the same orientation, usually perpendicular to the axis of cellular growth. Rosettes are believed to associate with cortical microtubules, perhaps moving along them as they lay down extracellular cellulose. However, cause-and-effect relationships are still being investigated.

Glycosyltransferases in the Golgi apparatus synthesize hemicellulose and pectin, which are transported in vesicles to the surface for secretion. Hemicellulose is a branched polysaccharide that coats microfibrils. Pectin is an acidic polysaccharide that forms a gel between microfibrils. Primary cell walls, laid down at the time of cellular growth and expansion, mature with the addition of glycoproteins and organic molecules, such as **lignins** (polymers of phenylpropanoid alcohols and acids), which contribute to the integrity of the "secondary" cell wall. Covalent and noncovalent bonds are thought to link cellulose and these other matrix molecules. The great strength and flexibility of tree branches illustrate the remarkable mechanical properties of mature cell walls.

Cellulose microfibrils are flexible and have a tensile strength greater than steel, so they do not stretch. For a plant tissue to expand, microfibrils must rearrange. Slippage and rearrangement of microfibrils are facilitated by **expansins,** a recently recognized class of matrix proteins unique to plants. Genetic defects in expansins inhibit the growth of plant tissues and the ripening of some fruits, such as tomatoes. Cell wall expansion apparently does not involve cleavage of

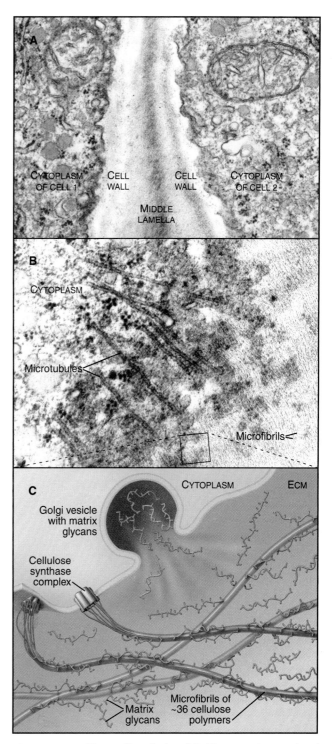

Figure 34-12 Plant cell wall. *A* and *B,* Electron micrographs of thin sections of cell walls in the root-like appendages of the parasitic weed dodder. *A,* Two cells are separated by an electron-translucent cell wall consisting of cellulose, xylogycan, and pectins. The darker area between the two cell walls is the middle lamella, which contains a high concentration of pectins. *B,* At high magnification, an oblique section through the plasma membrane and cell wall shows cellulose microfibrils aligned roughly parallel to cortical microtubules inside the plasma membrane. *C,* A drawing showing the biosynthesis of the cell wall. ECM, extracellular matrix. (*A,* Courtesy of K. C. Vaughn, U.S. Department of Agriculture, Stoneville, MD. *C,* Redrawn from Cosgrove DJ: Loosening of plant cell walls by expansins. Nature 407:321–326, 2000.)

any of the sugar polymers, so expansins are speculated to break noncovalent links between the polymers transiently, allowing turgor pressure to expand the volume of the cell. Expansins in grass pollen are one of the allergens responsible for hay fever.

Little is known about the molecular basis of plant cells adhering to their cell walls. By virtue of their physical connection with their product, cellulose synthases offer one means of attachment. Other plasma membrane proteins, including a family of serine/threonine kinases and some proteins with glycosylphosphatidylinositol (GPI) anchors, may contribute to adhesion by binding cell walls. Integrins are conspicuously missing from plant cells.

▌ Selected Readings

Cosgrove DJ: Assembly and enlargement of the primary cell wall in plants. Annu Rev Cell Dev Biol 13:171–201, 1997.

Cosgrove DJ: Loosening of plant cell walls by expansins. Nature 407:321–326, 2000.

Ducy P, Karsenty G: Genetic control of cell differentiation in the skeleton. Curr Opin Cell Biol 10:614–619, 1998.

Ducy P, Schinke T, Karsenty G: The osteoblast: A sophisticated fibroblast under central surveillance. Science 289:1501–1504, 2000.

Gorski JP, Olsen BR: Mutations in extacellular matrix molecules. Curr Opin Cell Biol 10:586–593, 1998.

Kohorn BD: Plasma membrane–cell wall contacts. Plant Physiol 124:31–38, 2000.

Marx SJ: Hyperparathyroid and hypoparathyroid disorders. N Engl J Med 343:1863–1875, 2000.

Olsen BR, Reginato AM, Wang W: Bone development. Annu Rev Cell Dev Biol 16:191–220, 2000.

Pyeritz RE: Ehlers-Danlos syndrome. N Engl J Med 342:730–732, 2000.

Teitelbaum SL: Bone resorption by osteoclasts. Science 289:1504–1508, 2000.

Watanabe H, Yamada Y, Kimata K: Roles of aggrecan, a large chondroitin sulfate proteoglycan, in cartilage structure and function. J Biochem 124:687–693, 1998.

Web site: ⟨http://cellwall.stanford.edu⟩.

CYTOSKELETON AND CELLULAR MOTILITY

chapter 35

OVERVIEW OF THE CYTOSKELETON AND CELLULAR MOTILITY

Most organisms depend on motility to sustain life itself (Fig. 35–1). Without a motile sperm, the egg would not be fertilized. Without cellular motility, a fertilized egg would not progress past the single-cell stage. Without active changes in cell shape and cellular migrations, complex embryos would not form. Without cellular motility, white blood cells would neither accumulate at sites of inflammation nor ingest invading microorganisms. Without active and rapid movements of organelles in axons and large plant cells, the peripheral parts of these cells would not be nourished. Without muscle contractions, we would be paralyzed and unable to implement any conscious decisions. Even a yeast, prevented from locomotion by its rigid cell wall, depends on internal movements for secretion and budding. Many prokaryotes use rotary flagella for locomotion. Thus, an understanding of the basis of cellular motility is central to our understanding of the functioning of all organisms.

Motor Proteins

A small handful of molecular machines is responsible for virtually all biological movements. The two most widespread mechanisms involve the physical movement of protein motors along protein polymers in cytoplasm. These motors use energy released from the hydrolysis of adenosine triphosphate (ATP) to take nanometer steps along their protein polymer tracks. These small steps apply force and move cargo attached to the motor. The cargo includes membrane-bound organelles and macromolecular complexes. Coordinated movements of thousands of motors power the locomotion of whole cells, including the contraction of muscles and the swimming of sperm.

Actin filaments and **microtubules** are the "tracks" for most biological movements. Different motors move along these two polymers: **myosins** along actin filaments and **dyneins** and **kinesins** along microtubules. The actin-myosin system is responsible for muscle contraction, cytokinesis, and organelle movements in plants. Microtubule motors power the beating of cilia and flagella, many organelle movements in animal cells, and chromosomal movements during mitosis. Although not usually considered to be molecular motors, nucleic acid polymerases and helicases (see Table 39–1 and Chapter 45) also use ATP hydrolysis to move along polymers of DNA or RNA.

At least four motility systems work without the aid of ATP-burning motor proteins (see Chapters 40 and 41). Actin polymerization drives extension of pseudopods. Hydrolysis of ATP bound to actin regulates recycling of subunits rather than being used directly to produce force. Assembly of an unrelated protein powers the amoeboid sperm of nematode worms. Calcium-sensitive contractile fibers cause rapid movements of some protozoa. ATP hydrolysis is used to create a store of Ca^{2+} used to trigger contraction. A proton or sodium ion gradient across the plasma membrane powers the rotary motor that turns bacterial flagella.

Cytoskeleton

Far from being a mere bag of water, cytoplasm is filled with protein polymers that resist deformation and transmit mechanical forces. This cytoskeleton is composed of actin filaments, microtubules, and **intermediate filaments.** Different protein subunits form each polymer (Fig. 35–2). Microtubules are rigid, hol-

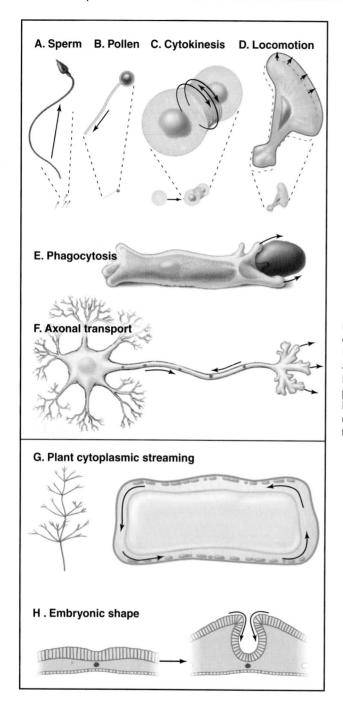

A. Sperm   B. Pollen   C. Cytokinesis   D. Locomotion

E. Phagocytosis

F. Axonal transport

G. Plant cytoplasmic streaming

H . Embryonic shape

Figure 35–1 These drawings provide examples of various biological movements: *A,* Sperm motility. *B,* Plant pollen tube growth. *C,* Cytokinesis of an animal cell. *D,* Locomotion of a fibroblast. *E,* Phagocytosis by a giant amoeba. *F,* Axonal transport and growth cone extension of a neuron. *G,* Plant cytoplasmic streaming around a central vacuole. *H,* Invagination of the neural tube in a vertebrate embryo.

low reinforcing rods that sustain both compression and tension. This makes them useful for supporting asymmetrical cellular processes and for bidirectional traffic generated by the motor proteins kinesin and dynein. Actin filaments are more flexible, so they must be cross-linked into bundles to bear compression forces or support asymmetrical processes. High tensile strength allows actin filaments to bear forces produced by myosins. Intermediate filaments are flexible cables having considerable tensile strength but little capacity to resist compression. Intermediate filaments prevent excessive stretching of cells by external forces. If intermediate filaments are defective, tissues are mechanically fragile.

The ability of actin filaments and microtubules to resist mechanical deformation and to transmit forces from motors allows the cytoskeletal-motility system to determine cell shape and, hence, the structure of both tissues and whole organisms. Furthermore, the dynamic nature of cytoskeletal polymers allows cells to

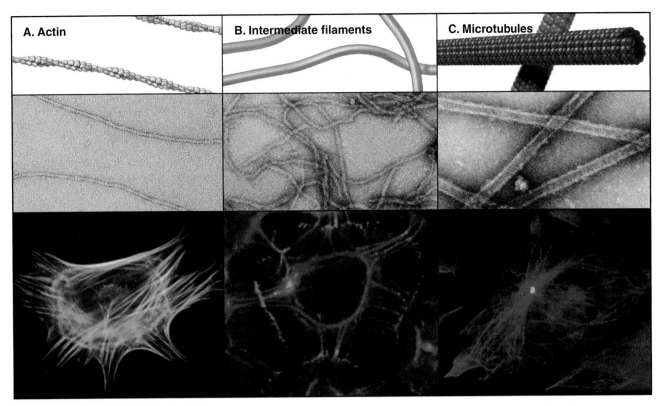

Figure 35-2 The three cytoskeletal polymers: *A,* Actin filaments. *B,* Intermediate filaments. *C,* Microtubules. The top panels illustrate the scale drawings used throughout this book. The middle panels show electron micrographs of negatively stained specimens of each polymer, all at the same magnification. The bottom panels show fluorescence light micrographs of cultured cells stained for each type of cytoskeletal polymer. (*A* [*bottom panel*], Courtesy of I. Herman, Tufts University. *B* [*bottom panel*], Courtesy of E. Smith and E. Fuchs, University of Chicago. *C* [*bottom panel*], Courtesy of G. Borisy, University of Wisconsin, Madison.)

change shape rapidly, in a timeframe of seconds. At each cell division, a band of actin filaments and myosin pinches the daughter cells apart. Active extension of cellular processes and active changes in shape produce asymmetrical cell shapes. Movements of chromosomes during mitosis and organelles in cytoplasm determine the cellular distribution of these components that are too large to move by diffusion. Together with the extracellular matrix, the shapes of individual cells define the shapes of tissues and organs.

Investigating Cell Motility and the Cytoskeleton

The physical properties of actin and microtubules have influenced what is known about these two cytoskeletal polymers. Microtubules are large and sparse enough to observe individually in living cells, so microscopists have collected a wealth of information about the distribution and dynamics of microtubules in cells. The small diameter and high concentration of actin filaments and intermediate filaments limit the observation of individual cytoplasmic filaments by light microscopy. Fluorescent labels permit the study of ensembles of actin filaments in live cells, but the research has emphasized the identification and characterization of proteins that regulate actin assembly and interactions.

The pioneering work on motor proteins focused on highly specialized systems: muscle contraction for actin and myosin and beating of cilia and flagella for microtubules and dynein. Now we recognize that these are extreme examples of general mechanisms, but it took years to appreciate the great diversity of variations on these general themes.

Organization of Chapters within this Section

Chapters 36 to 38 introduce the three cytoskeletal polymers and the proteins that regulate their assembly and dynamics. Chapter 39 covers the general principles by which motor proteins produce movements. The section concludes with three chapters showing how cells use cytoskeletal polymers and motors to produce a vast variety of movements: intracellular movements (Chapter 40); cell shape changes, cellular locomotion, and swimming (Chapter 41); and muscle contraction (Chapter 42). Mitosis and cytokinesis appear in the discussion of the cell cycle (Chapter 47).

▌ Selected Readings

Bray D: Cell Movements, 2nd ed. New York: Garland Publishing, 2000.

Kreis T, Vale R, eds.: Guidebook to the Cytoskeletal and Motor Proteins, 2nd ed. New York: Oxford University Press, 1999.

chapter 36

ACTIN AND ACTIN-BINDING PROTEINS

Actin filaments form a cytoskeletal and motility system in all eukaryotes (Fig. 36–1). As an essential part of the cytoskeleton, networks of cross-linked actin filaments resist deformation, transmit forces, and restrict diffusion of organelles. A network of cortical actin filaments excludes organelles (Fig. 36–2), reinforces the plasma membrane, and restricts the lateral motion of some integral membrane proteins. The **cortex** varies in thickness from a monolayer of actin filaments in red blood cells to more than 1 μm in amoeboid cells. Like fingers in a glove, bundles of actin filaments support slender protrusions of plasma membrane called **microvilli** or **filopodia.** Microvilli expand the cell surface for transport of nutrients and participate in sensory processes, including hearing. The actin cytoskeleton complements and interacts physically with cytoskeletal structures composed of microtubules (see Chapter 37) and intermediate filaments (see Chapter 38).

Actin contributes to cell movements in two ways. First, polymerization and depolymerization of the network of cortical actin filaments just inside the plasma membrane contribute to the extension of pseudopods, cell locomotion (see Chapter 41), and phagocytosis (see Chapter 23). Second, actin filaments are tracks for movements of the myosin family of motor proteins (see Chapter 39). Actin filaments and myosin filaments form the stable contractile apparatus of muscles (Fig. 36–3; see Chapter 42), as well as the transient **contractile ring** that pinches the two daughter cells apart at the end of mitosis (see Chapter 47). Myosins also power movement of some membranes along actin fila-

ments, complementing organelle movements by other motors along microtubules (see Chapter 40). Actin, myosin, and accessory proteins form bundles called **stress fibers** that apply tension between adhesive junctions on the plasma membrane (see Chapter 33), where cells attach to each other or to extracellular matrix (see Figs. 36–1 and 36–3). Stress fibers are prominent in tissue culture cells grown on glass or plastic and in endothelial cells lining major arteries.

Actin filaments are polarized, owing to the uniform orientation of the asymmetrical subunits along the polymer. One end is called the barbed end, the other the pointed end. This nomenclature comes from the appearance of actin filaments decorated with myosin (see Fig. 36–9). In many cell types, the barbed ends of the filaments are associated with the plasma membrane (see Fig. 36–2). Actin filaments in muscle are also anchored at their barbed ends (see Fig. 36–3A and Chapter 42). This makes mechanical sense, as actin filaments sustain tension better than compression, and because (with one interesting exception) all known actin-based motors are myosins that pull in a direction away from the barbed end. The plasma membrane is a prominent actin filament anchoring site, allowing force produced in the cytoplasmic actin network to change the shape of the membrane and to be transmitted to the substrate or adjacent cells.

More than 60 families of actin-binding proteins regulate the assembly and dynamics of actin-based structures in cytoplasm (see Table 36–1). Genetic defects in components of the actin cytoskeletal and motility system cause many human diseases, including muscular dystrophy, hereditary fragility of red blood cells (i.e., hemolytic anemias), and hereditary heart diseases called cardiomyopathies.

Chapter based, in part, on Pollard TD: Actin and actin binding proteins. In *Guidebook to the Cytoskeletal and Motor Proteins,* 1st ed. New York: Oxford University Press, 1993, pp 3–11.

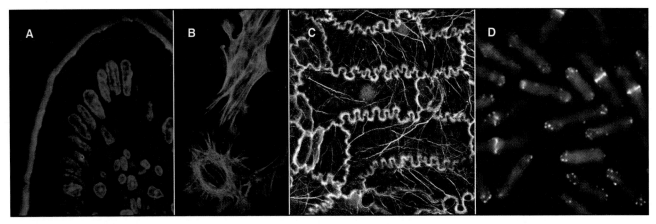

Figure 36–1 Fluorescence micrographs illustrating the distribution of actin filaments in cells. *A*, Intestinal epithelial cells stained with rhodamine-labeled phalloidin, a cyclic peptide that binds tightly to actin filaments. Actin filaments are concentrated in microvilli bordering the intestinal lumen. Nuclei are stained blue with DAPI. *B*, Cultured vascular smooth muscle cells. Actin filaments, stained red with a fluorescent antibody, are concentrated in stress fibers and in the cortex around the edges of these cells. *C*, Maize epidermis stained with rhodamine-labeled phalloidin. Actin filaments are concentrated in the cortex and in cytoplasmic bundles in these plant cells. *D*, Fission yeast *S. pombe*, stained with rhodamine-labeled phalloidin. Actin filaments are found in patches at the tips of growing cells and in the cleavage furrow of dividing cells. (*A*, Courtesy of C. Rahner, Yale University. *B*, Courtesy of I. Herman, Tufts Medical School. *C*, Courtesy of M. Frank, University of California, San Diego. *D*, Courtesy of W.-L. Lee, Salk Institute, La Jolla, CA.)

▌Molecular Inventory of the Actin System

The protein components of the actin system are ancient and abundant. Even rod-shaped bacteria have proteins very similar in structure to actin. These prokaryotic actins polymerize and, differently from eukaryotic actins, are required for rod-shaped bacteria to maintain their asymmetric shapes.

Actin, myosin, and a large variety of associated regulatory proteins are major constituents of all eukaryotic cells. In muscle, actin and myosin constitute more than 60% of the total protein. In nonmuscle cells, actin is often the most abundant protein, comprising up to 15% of protein, and actin-binding proteins may account for up to another 10% of cellular protein. Actin and myosin are thought to be among the five most abundant eukaryotic proteins on earth. Given this remarkable abundance, it is curious that actin was only discovered in muscle in the 1940s and in nonmuscle cells in the late 1960s. Since the mid-1970s, scientists have discovered two or more new classes of actin-binding proteins every year, but the inventory is probably still incomplete.

Most organisms have genes for several actin isoforms, and all known actin isoform diversity arises from multiple genes rather than from alternative splicing of mRNAs. Humans have 6 actin genes; *Dictyostelium* has more than 10, but budding yeast has only 1. These genes arose by duplication of a primordial actin gene and have diverged as the subtly different pro-

teins that they encode have acquired novel functions. Vertebrate muscle actin genes branched off from the main line of cytoplasmic actins at the level of primitive chordates (see Fig. 1–1*B*). Plant actin genes differ from animal actins and have diverged among themselves to a greater degree than animal actins.

The biochemical similarities of **actin isoforms** are more impressive than their differences. The sequences of pairs of actins are generally more than 90% identical, even between highly divergent species. Humans express β and γ isoforms in nonmuscle cells and four different α and β isoforms in various muscle cells (see Chapter 42). Many nonmuscle cells express both the β and γ isoforms, but red blood cells use only the β-actin.

In every case examined, actin isoforms copolymerize in the test tube, so it is remarkable that cells can sort actin isoforms into different structures. For example, β-actin is concentrated near the plasma membrane of cultured cells, whereas γ-actin is concentrated in stress fibers (Fig. 36–4). In muscle, α-actin forms the thin filaments of the contractile apparatus, whereas γ-actin localizes around mitochondria. Even the full array of known actin-binding proteins cannot yet explain how cells prevent copolymerization of the isoforms or concentrate isoforms in different locations.

▌Actin Molecule

Actin is folded into two domains that are stabilized by an adenine nucleotide lying in between (Fig. 36–5).

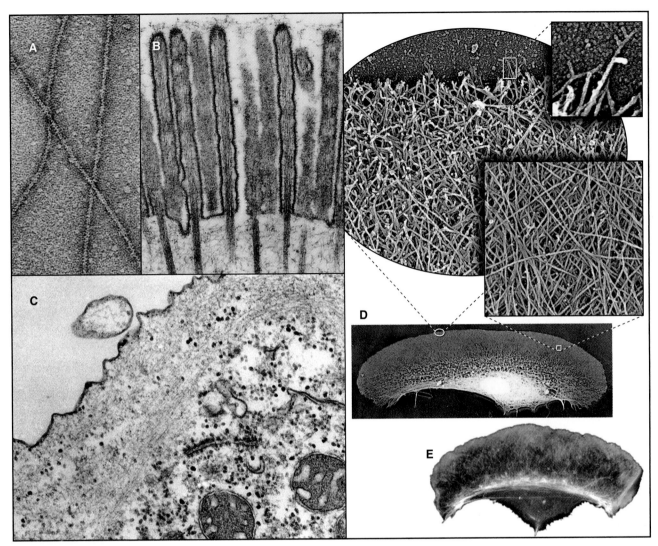

Figure 36-2 Micrographs of actin assemblies. *A,* Electron micrograph of filaments of purified actin prepared by negative staining. *B,* Electron micrograph of a thin section of an intestinal epithelial cell illustrating finger-like microvilli with tightly packed bundles of actin filaments linked to the surrounding plasma membrane by myosin-I. The barbed ends of these filaments are located at the tips of the microvilli. *C,* Electron micrograph of a thin section of *Acanthamoeba* showing the actin filament meshwork in the cortex beneath the plasma membrane. *D* and *E,* Cultured fish scale keratocytes, fixed while actively migrating toward the top of the figure. *D,* Electron micrograph of a whole mount of a cell illustrating the meshwork of branched filaments near the leading edge and longer, unbranched filaments deeper in the cytoplasm. Most filaments are oriented with their barbed ends forward. *E,* Staining for actin filaments with phalloidin (*blue*) and myosin II (*red*). (*A,* Courtesy of U. Aebi, University of Basel. *B,* Courtesy of L. Tilney, University of Pennsylvania, and M. Mooseker, Yale University. *D* and *E,* Courtesy of T. Svitkina and G. Borisy, University of Wisconsin, Madison.)

The polypeptide of 375 residues crosses twice between the two domains with the N- and C-termini near each other. The two domains are folded similarly, suggesting that actin arose by duplication of an ancestral gene. Remarkably, the adenine nucleotide binding site, fold, and overall shape of actin closely resemble two other proteins with very different functions: the glycolytic enzyme hexokinase (see Fig. 2–14) and the heat shock protein, Hsc70. All three proteins may have evolved originally in prokaryotes from the same primitive nucleotide-binding protein.

Actin binds adenosine triphosphate (ATP) or adenosine diphosphate (ADP) and a divalent cation, Mg^{2+} in cells, with nanomolar affinity. The affinity of actin for ATP is higher than for ADP, so given the higher concentration of ATP, unpolymerized actin in cells is saturated with ATP. The bound nucleotide exchanges relatively slowly with nucleotide in the

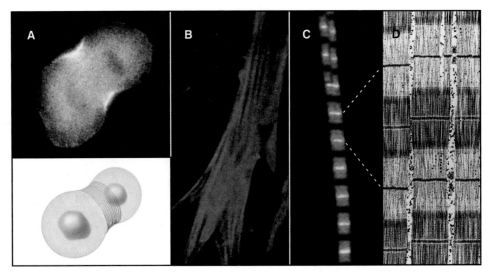

Figure 36–3 Micrographs of contractile bundles of actin filaments. *A,* Fluorescence micrograph of a dividing normal rat kidney cell stained with fluorescein-phalloidin. Actin filaments are concentrated in the contractile ring in the constricting cleavage furrow. The drawing illustrates the filaments in the contractile ring. *B,* Stress fibers in cultured endothelial cells stained with rhodamine-labeled antibodies. *C,* A fluorescence micrograph of a myofibril isolated from skeletal muscle and stained with fluorescein-phalloidin for actin filaments *(green)* and rhodamine-antibody to α-actinin, which stains Z disks yellow. *D,* An electron micrograph of a thin section of skeletal muscle. (*A,* Micrograph courtesy of Y.-L. Wang, University of Massachusetts, Worcester. *B,* Courtesy of I. Herman, Tufts Medical School. *C,* Courtesy of V. Fowler, Scripps Research Institute, La Jolla, CA. *D,* Courtesy of H. E. Huxley, Brandeis University.)

medium (Fig. 36–6). Actin monomer–binding proteins can inhibit or accelerate nucleotide exchange. Bound nucleotide stabilizes the actin molecule but is not required for polymerization in vitro. ATP-actin and ADP-actin polymerize at different rates.

Post-translational modifications of actins include acetylation of the N-terminus and (in most cases) methylation of histidine-68. In some insect flight muscles, the small protein ubiquitin (see Chapter 24) is attached covalently to about one in six actin molecules, yielding a 55-kD polypeptide that is stably incorporated into thin filaments. Some invertebrate

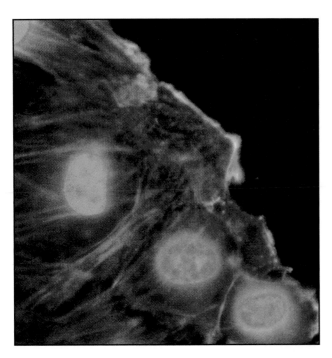

Figure 36–4 Sorting of actin isoforms. Fluorescence micrograph of cultured cells doubly stained with fluorescent antibodies specific for β-actin concentrated in the cortex *(orange)* and γ-actin concentrated in stress fibers *(green)*. Nuclei are stained blue with DAPI. (Courtesy of I. Herman, Tufts Medical School.)

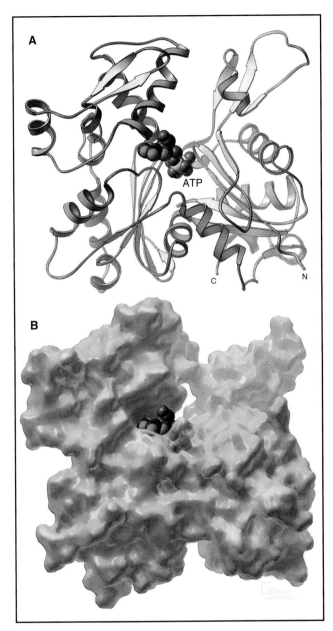

Figure 36-5 Atomic structure of actin. *A,* Ribbon model showing the polypeptide fold and the location of Mg-ATP, shown as space-filling. *B,* Surface rendering. ATP is almost completely buried in the cleft between the two lobes of the protein, where it makes extensive contacts with the protein. The barbed end of the molecule is at the bottom in this orientation. (PDB file: 1ATN. Reference: Kabsch W, et al: Atomic structure of the actin-DNase I complex. Nature 347:37–44, 1990.)

actins are phosphorylated on tyrosine-211. The functional significance of these modifications is still under investigation.

Actin-Related Proteins

After 20 years of believing that actins are one of the most evolutionarily conserved protein families, in the 1990s, scientists discovered several families of highly divergent **actin-related proteins (Arps)** (Fig. 36-7). Arps are found in a variety of eukaryotic organisms and species ranging from amoebas to humans and seem to be as ancient as actin itself. The residues forming the nucleotide-binding site are conserved, but the overall sequence identity is less than 60% compared with any conventional actin. Surface residues differ considerably, so Arps can participate in different molecular interactions from actin. Arp1 forms a short filament as part of the dynactin complex that links cargo to the microtubule motor dynein (see Fig. 40–4). Arp2 and Arp3 are two of seven subunits in a stable, abundant complex that controls actin polymerization in the cell cortex (see Fig. 36–18). These Arps are essential for the viability of budding yeast, which have genes for eight additional Arps.

Actin Polymerization

By the 1960s, electron microscopy and x-ray diffraction of whole muscle had revealed the helical geometry of actin filaments, but a detailed model required the atomic structure of the actin monomer (Fig. 36–8). The atomic model of the filament is still being refined; however, the present version accounts for most of the data on the structure of the filament, including x-ray fiber diffraction pattern, overall shape determined by electron microscopy, chemical cross-linking of amino acid side chains between subunits, and relative strength of lateral and longitudinal bonds between subunits. The polarity of the filament arising from the helical arrangement of symmetrical subunits was originally revealed by the asymmetrical arrowhead pattern

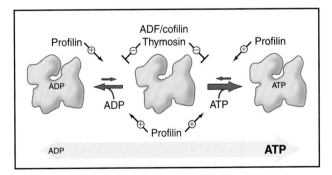

Figure 36-6 Regulation of actin nucleotide exchange by actin-binding proteins. Dissociation of the nucleotide requires opening of the nucleotide cleft by rotation of the two domains around a hinge at the base of the cleft. The rate-limiting step is dissociation of the bound nucleotide. ADF/cofilin proteins and β-thymosins inhibit nucleotide dissociation. Profilin promotes nucleotide dissociation by increasing the rates of both nucleotide dissociation and binding. The ability of profilin to promote nucleotide exchange, the higher affinity of actin for ATP than for ADP, and a higher concentration of ATP than ADP in cytoplasm account for why essentially all unpolymerized actin in cells has bound ATP.

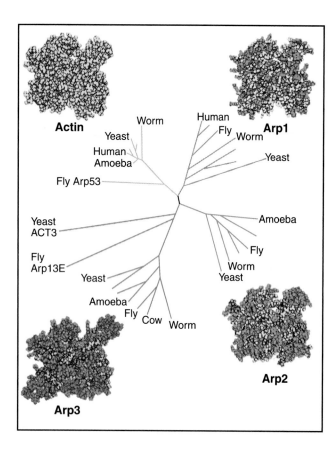

Figure 36-7 Comparison of actin and actin-related proteins (Arps). Space-filling models are based on the atomic structure of actin and the sequences of the Arps. Yellow residues are identical to actin, green residues are conservative substitutions, blue residues are nonconservative substitutions, and red residues are insertions. All of these proteins have similar internal architectures, including identical contacts with ATP, but their surfaces differ considerably. The phylogenetic tree, based on sequence comparisons, shows that the genes for actins and all of the Arps had a common ancestor. (From the work of J. Kelleher, Johns Hopkins Medical School; illustration redrawn from Mullins D, Kelleher J, Pollard TD: Actin' like actin. Trends Cell Biol 6:208–212, 1996. Copyright 1996, with permission from Elsevier Science.)

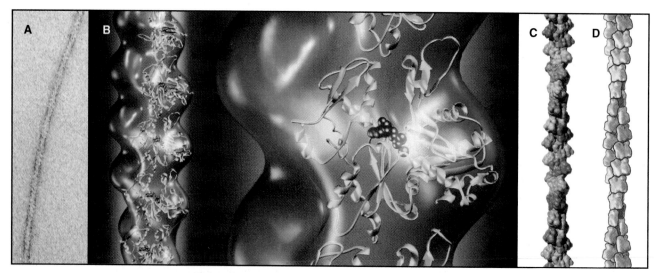

Figure 36-8 Structure of the actin filament. *A,* Electron micrograph of a negatively stained actin filament. *B,* Low-resolution reconstruction of an actin filament by image processing of electron micrographs (*blue*) with ribbon models of the subunits (*gold*) along one strand of the double helix. One subunit is enlarged to the right. The pointed end of the subunits with the nucleotide cleft is at the top and the barbed end is at the bottom. This orientation of the actin molecule in the filament uniquely accounts for the x-ray fiber diffraction pattern of oriented filaments and agrees with electron microscopy with probes on specific actin residues and chemical cross-linking between residues of adjacent subunits. *C,* Surface rendering of the atomic model. Subunits in the two long-pitch helices are shown as yellow-orange and blue-green. The short pitch helix, including every subunit, follows a yellow-green-orange-blue pattern. *D,* Scale drawing used throughout this text. (*A* and *B,* Courtesy of U. Aebi, University of Basel. *C,* Courtesy of R. Milligan, Scripps Research Institute, La Jolla, CA.)

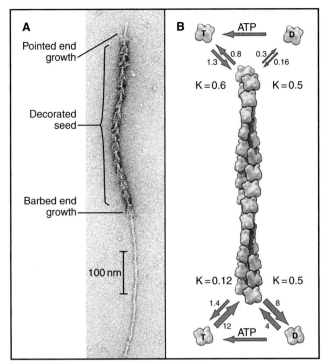

Figure 36-9 Kinetics of actin filament elongation. *A*, Electron micrograph of growth from an actin filament seed decorated with myosin heads to reveal the polarity. Growth is faster at the barbed end than at the pointed end. Rate constants for association and dissociation were determined by measuring the rate of elongation at the two ends as a function of monomer concentration. *B*, Rate constants for subunit association (units: $\mu M^{-1}s^{-1}$) and dissociation (units: s^{-1}) for Mg-ATP-actin and Mg-ADP-actin under physiological conditions. Ratios of the rate constants yield critical concentrations (K, units μM) for the various reactions. Note that the critical concentrations at the two ends are the same for ADP-actin (D) but differ for ATP-actin (T). (*A*, Courtesy of M. Runge, Johns Hopkins Medical School. *B*, Reference: Pollard TD: Rate constants for the reactions of ATP- and ADP-actin with the ends of actin filaments. J Cell Biol 103:2747–2754, 1986.)

reactions at the two ends have different rate constants (see Fig. 36–9). Association of subunits is rapid at both ends. Subunit association is a classic diffusion-limited reaction (see Chapter 3) at the rapidly growing barbed end and somewhat slower at the other end. Subunit dissociation is relatively slow at both ends, between 1 and 10 subunits per second. The rates of these reactions depend upon nucleotide bound to the associating or dissociating subunit.

In the presence of ATP, purified actin assembles almost completely, leaving as monomers the **critical concentration** of about 0.1 μM ATP-actin. Recall from Chapter 4 that the critical concentration is the monomer concentration giving equal rates of association

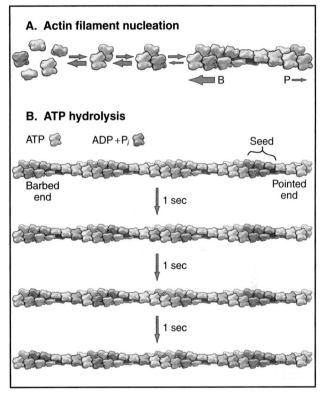

Figure 36-10 Actin filament nucleation, growth, and nucleotide hydrolysis. *A*, Nucleation: Formation of dimers and trimers is very unfavorable owing to rapid dissociation of subunits (see Chapter 4). Actin trimers are called nuclei because they initiate the highly favorable elongation reactions. This mechanism accounts for much experimental data, but is based largely on kinetic modeling and is limited to demonstrating that the model is consistent with the data. *B*, ATP hydrolysis by a polymer of ATP-actin (*yellow subunits*) is random and irreversible at a rate of 0.3 s^{-1}, yielding subunits with bound ADP and inorganic phosphate (*orange*). Phosphate dissociates slowly at a rate of 0.002 s^{-1} (not shown), converting half of the newly polymerized subunits to ADP-actin in 6 minutes. Bound ADP does not exchange with nucleotide in the medium. Phosphate binding is reversible, but the affinity is low, so most subunits bind only ADP. (Reference: Pollard TD, Blanchoin L, Mullin RD: Biophysics of actin filament dynamics in nonmuscle cells. Annu Rev Biophys Biomolec Struct 29:545–576, 2000.)

created when myosin binds to actin filaments (Fig. 36–9). These arrowheads define the barbed and pointed ends of the filaments.

Actin self-assembles by means of a series of bimolecular reactions (see Fig. 4–6; Fig. 36–10). Actin is isolated as a monomer at low salt concentrations. Physiological concentrations of monovalent and divalent cations bind to low-affinity sites on actin and promote polymerization. In vitro, actin trimers appear to be the nucleus that initiates polymer growth in the sense that the reactions required to form trimers are very unfavorable compared with reactions for elongation of polymers larger than trimers. To initiate new filaments, cells use regulatory proteins to overcome these unfavorable nucleation reactions.

Actin filaments grow and shrink by addition and loss of subunits at the two ends of the polymer. The

and dissociation. (At the barbed end, 0.1 μM actin gives an association rate (k_+A) of 1 s^{-1}, the same as the dissociation rate.) The critical concentration of ADP-actin is about 10 times higher than for ATP-actin. All actin above the critical concentration polymerizes into filaments.

Hydrolysis of the bound ATP during assembly modifies the behavior of actin filaments. During the seconds following incorporation of an ATP-actin subunit into a filament, bound ATP is hydrolyzed irreversibly to ADP and phosphate (see Fig. 36–10). Phosphate dissociates slowly over several minutes, yielding filaments with a core of subunits with tightly bound ADP. In contrast, nucleotide on subunits at the very ends of filaments exchanges with medium ATP. Phosphate is exchangeable along the length of filaments, and at the millimolar concentrations of phosphate in cytoplasm, this equilibrium results in phosphate being bound to some ADP-actin subunits and not others. ATP hydrolysis and phosphate dissociation determine the affinity of some regulatory proteins for actin filaments.

The critical concentrations for ATP-actin differ at the two ends of the filament as a result of nucleotide hydrolysis and phosphate release (see Fig. 36–9). At steady-state in the presence of ATP, the actin monomer concentration falls between the critical concentrations at the two ends. At this intermediate concentration of monomers, subunits add slowly to the barbed end at the expense of subunit loss from the pointed end. Polymer and monomer concentrations remain constant, whereas subunits migrate slowly through the polymer from the barbed end to the pointed end driven by ATP hydrolysis.

This flux of subunits may contribute to the turnover of actin filaments in cells, but the impression gained from in vitro experiments is that actin filaments are stable under physiological conditions. The flux of

subunits is slow, and neither end exhibits rapid fluctuations in length as microtubules do (see Chapter 37). In contrast to these expectations, several lines of evidence show that many actin filaments in live cells turn over much more rapidly than filaments of purified actin in a test tube. Accessory proteins likely regulate the short half-lives of actin filaments in live cells. The following section introduces some of these regulatory proteins and examines how they might participate in actin filament dynamics in cells.

Actin-Binding Proteins

A remarkable number of accessory proteins regulate the dynamics and organization of cellular actin filaments (Fig. 36–11; Table 36–1). Broadly, these proteins can be grouped into families that bind monomers, sever filaments, cap filament ends, cross-link filaments, stabilize filaments, or move along filaments. Many actin-binding proteins are modular, and some—including myosins (see Fig. 40–2) and cross-linking proteins (see later discussion)—share homologous actin-binding domains attached to divergent adapters. Like actin, actin-binding proteins are ancient. Many families of actin-binding proteins must have been present in primitive eukaryotes at the base of the phylogenetic tree because they are found in protozoa, myxomycetes, yeast, plants, and vertebrates.

Actin Monomer–Binding Proteins

Proteins that bind actin monomers work together to control the pool of unpolymerized actin in cells and the exchange of the nucleotide bound to actin.

- **β-Thymosins** are peptides of 43 residues that bind ATP-actin monomers with higher affinity than

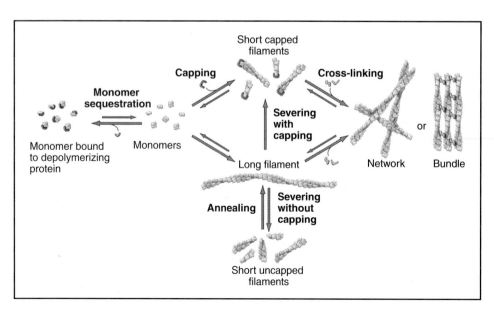

Figure 36–11 Families of actin-binding proteins. Monomer-binding proteins generally favor either ATP-actin (profilin and thymosin-β_4) or ADP-actin (ADF/cofilins). Capping proteins bind to either the barbed end (capping protein, gelsolin) or pointed end (tropomodulin, Arp2/3 complex) of filaments. Some severing proteins also cap (gelsolin, fragmin), whereas others do not (ADF/cofilins). Cross-linking proteins can form networks or bundles.

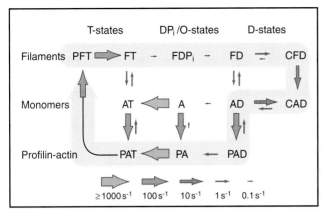

Figure 36-12 Actin polymerization cycle. Arrows indicate reaction rates adjusted for physiological concentrations. Shading indicates the main pathway followed by an actin molecule as it recycles between the monomer pool and filaments. A pool of ATP-actin bound to profilin elongates actin filaments with free barbed ends. Profilin rapidly dissociates, and filamentous actin hydrolyzes ATP and dissociates phosphate. ADF/cofilins promote disassembly of ADP-actin filaments. Profilin promotes the exchange of ADP for ATP. Thymosin-β_4, when present, sequesters a pool of unpolymerizable ATP-actin. Profilin transfers actin from this thymosin-actin pool to actin filaments. A, actin monomer; C, ADF/cofilin; D, ADP bound to actin; F, filamentous actin; P, profilin; Pi, phosphate bound to actin; T, ATP bound to actin.

The pool of unpolymerized actin exchanges rapidly among these proteins. The three proteins compete with each other and exchange on and off actin on a subsecond time scale, allowing an actin molecule to move from one protein to the next around a cycle (Fig. 36–12). ADF/cofilins bind ADP-actin subunits in filaments, as well as ADP-actin monomers, after they dissociate from filaments. During random dissociation and reassociation events, this ADP-actin binds profilin, which causes the rapid dissociation of ADP and its exchange for ATP. The profilin-actin-ATP complex is then stored until barbed filament ends are available for elongation. Soon after the profilin-actin complex adds to a barbed end, the profilin dissociates. In cells with a high concentration of thymosin, much of the ATP-actin is stored bound to thymosin. Profilin shuttles ATP-actin from thymosin to growing filaments.

Actin Filament–Capping Proteins

Capping proteins bind to either the barbed or pointed end of actin filaments, where they block subunit addition and dissociation. Many of these proteins also stimulate the formation of new filaments that grow only at their free end (Fig. 36–13). Some capping proteins also sever actin filaments (Fig. 36–14).

ADP-actin monomers. They inhibit both actin polymerization and nucleotide exchange. Thymosins have not been found in fungi, but they are the most abundant actin-binding proteins in some animal cells. For example, at a concentration of >200 μM in white blood cells, thymosin could sequester most of the unpolymerized actin.

- Members of the **ADF/cofilin** family are ubiquitous, essential eukaryotic proteins that bind ADP-actin monomers with higher affinity than ATP-actin. They inhibit nucleotide exchange but not polymerization. They bind and destabilize ADP-actin filaments (see later discussion).

- **Profilins** are also essential proteins found in all eukaryotes. Their affinity is highest for nucleotide-free actin monomers, followed by ATP-actin and ADP-actin. They stimulate nucleotide exchange and have a discriminating effect on polymerization; that is, they inhibit nucleation and elongation at the slow-growing (pointed) end but not growth at the fast-growing barbed end. This results from profilin binding to the barbed end of the actin subunit, where it sterically blocks most polymerization reactions but not association of the actin-profilin complex with the barbed end. Most unpolymerized actin in protozoa is bound to profilin. Profilin also binds certain membrane lipids (polyphosphoinositides) as well as polyproline repeats in a number of proteins. Both actin binding and polyproline binding are essential for profilin function.

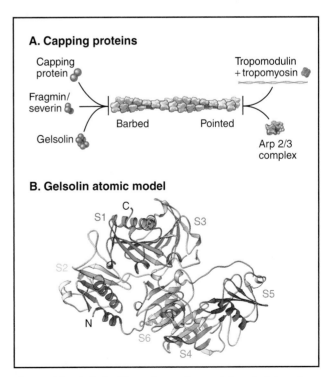

Figure 36-13 Actin filament–capping proteins. *A,* Interactions of capping proteins with the ends of actin filaments. Most of these proteins bind with high affinity to a filament end. Tropomodulin requires tropomyosin for high-affinity binding. *B,* Ribbon model of the atomic structure of gelsolin, showing the six homologous domains labeled S1 to S6. (PDB file: 1DON.)

table 36–1

CLASSIFICATION OF ACTIN-BINDING PROTEINS

Protein (Homologues and Synonyms)	Distribution	Subunits (N × kD)	K_d Actin Binding	Other Ligands	Diseases and Mutations
Monomer-binding					
Actobindin	Pr	1 × 9.8	3.3 μM dimers	—	—
β Thymosins	An	1 × 5	0.7 μM monomer	—	—
DNase I	An	1 × 29	0.1 nM monomer and pointed end	Calcium, DNA	—
Profilin	Eu	1 × 13–15	0.1 μM monomer	PIP$_2$, VASP, polyproline	Yst, Dros, mouse
Vitamin D–binding protein (Gc globulin)	An	1 × 58	1 nM monomer	Vitamin D, C5A complement	—
Small severing					
ADF/cofilin (acto-phorin, depac-tin, destrin)	Eu	1 × 15–19	0.1 μM ADP monomer, 0.5 μM ADP filament	PIP$_2$	Yst, Dros, *C. elegans*
Capping					
Arp2/3 complex	Eu	1 × 49, 1 × 44, 1 × 40, 1 × 35, 1 × 21, 1 × 20, 1 × 16	10 nM pointed end 0.5 μM filament side	Profilin Scar, WASp, cortac-tin	Yst
Capping protein (CapZ)	Eu	1 × 32–36(α) + 1 × 28–32(β)	1 nM barbed end	Dynactin com-plex, PIP$_2$	Yst, Dros, Dd
Fragmin (severin, gCAP39)	Pr, An	1 × 40	1 nM barbed end	—	Dd
Gelsolin (scin-derin)	Pr, An	1 × 80 or 83	50 nM barbed end, μM dimers, sides	Calcium, PIP$_2$	Dros, mouse, Hs Finnish amyloidosis
Tensin	An	1 × 96	Barbed end	P-tyrosine	
Tropomodulin	An	1 × 40	Pointed end, 1 nM with TM, 0.4 μM without TM	Tropomyosin (TM)	Dros
Villin (Cap 100)	Pr, An	1 × 93	7 μM filament, 0.3 μM filament for head domain	Calcium, PIP$_2$	—
Filament side binding					
Abp1p	Fu, An	1 × 67		—	Yst
Adducin	An	1 × 100 + 1 × 105	0.3 μM filament	Spectrin	—
Caldesmon	An	1 × 90 or 1 × 61	1 μM filament with tropomyosin	Calmodulin, tro-pomyosin, my-osin	—
Calponin	An	1 × 34	0.2 μM filament with tropomyosin	Calmodulin, tro-pomyosin	—
Coronin	Pr, Fu, An	1 × 51	5–40 nM filament	—	Dd, yst
Drebrin	An	1 × 95	0.1 μM filament	—	—
Nebulin		1 × 750	Filament		Hs Nemaline myopathy
Nuclear actin-binding protein	Pr	2 × 34	0.25 μM filament	DNA	—
Tropomyosin	Pr, Fu, An	2 × 28–32	Filament, coopera-tive	Self, troponin, caldesmon, calponin	Yst, Dros, Hs cardiomyop-athy
Troponin	An	1 × 18, TNC 1 × 21, TNI 1 × 31, TNT	Filament	Tropomyosin, calcium	TNT in Hs car-diomyopathy

table 36–1

CLASSIFICATION OF ACTIN-BINDING PROTEINS *Continued*

Protein (Homologues and Synonyms)	Distribution	Subunits (N × kD)	K$_d$ Actin Binding	Other Ligands	Diseases and Mutations
Cross-linking					
ABP-120	Pr	2 × 92	<1 μM filament	—	Dd
α-Actinin (actinogelin)	Pr, Fu, An	2 × 100	1–5 μM filament	Vinculin, zyxin, integrin, PIP$_2$, NMDA receptor, selectin	Dd, Dros, Hs muscular dystrophy
Anillin	An	1 × 132	Filament	—	Dros
Cortexillin	Pr	2 × 51	0.2 μM filament	—	Dd
Dematin (Band 4.9)	An	3 × 43–45	Filament	RBC membrane	—
eEF1A (ABP-50)	Eu	1 × 50	0.1–10 μM filament	GTP, ribosome, aminoacyl-tRNA, tubulin	Yst
Espin	An	1 × 95 or 29	0.1–0.2 μM filaments	—	Hs deafness
Fascin	An	1 × 56	Filament	β-catenin	Dros
Filamin (ABP-280)	An	2 × 240–280	0.5 μM filament	GP1B/1X	—
Fimbrin (plastin)	Eu	1 × 68	Filament	Ca^{2+}	Yst
Scruin	An	1 × 102	Filament	Calmodulin	—
Small cross-linking proteins (gelactins)	Pr	1 × 34	Filament	Ca^{2+}	Dd
Transgelin	Fu, An	1 × 23	Filament	—	—
Membrane-associated					
Actolinkin	An	1 × 20	Filament	Membranes	—
Annexin-II (calpactin I, lipocortin II)	An, Pl	2 × 38 + 2 × 10	0.2 μM filament	Calcium, acidic phospholipids	—
Dystrophin/utrophin	An	1 × 427/1 × 395	Filament, head 44 μM, tail 0.5 μM	β-dystroglycan	Hs muscular dystrophies
Ezrin/moesin/radixin	An	1 × 68 + oligomers	Filament	Self	—
Hisactophilin	Pr	1 × 13.5	Filament, 0.2 μM monomer	Membranes	Dd
Ponticulin	Pr, An	1 × 17	0.3 μM filament	Membranes	Dd
Protein 4.1	An	1 × 80	Filament	Spectrin, band 3, glycophorin	Hs hereditary elliptocytosis
Spectrin (fodrin, calspectin)	Pr, An	2 × 280 (α) + 2 × 246 (β)	1–25 μM filament	Ca^{2+}, self, ankyrin, calmodulin, band 4.1, adducin	Hs hereditary spherocytosis
Talin	Pr, An	1 × 272	Filament, 0.25 μM monomer	Vinculin, integrins, p125FAK	—
Microtubule-binding					
MAP-2	An	1 × 210	Filament sides	Microtubules, PKA, intermediate filaments	—
Tau	An	1 × 43–86	Filament sides	Microtubules	Alzheimer's disease
Intermediate filament–binding					
BPAG1	An	? × 280 or ? × 230	0.2 μM filaments	Intermediate filaments	Mouse dystonia musculorum
Motors					
Myosins I–XII	Eu	Various	1–100 μM with ATP, 4nM without ATP	Various (self, membranes)	Hs cardiomyopathy, deafness, retinitis

An, animals; Dd, Dictyostelium discoideum; Dros, Drosophila melanogaster; Eu, all eukaryotes; Fu, fungi; Hs, Homo sapiens; MAP-2, microtubule-associated protein 2; NMDA, N-methyl-D-aspartate; Pl, plants; Pr, protozoa; TM, tropomyosin; TNC, troponin C; TNI, troponin I; TNT, troponin T; tRNA, transfer RNA; Yst, yeast.

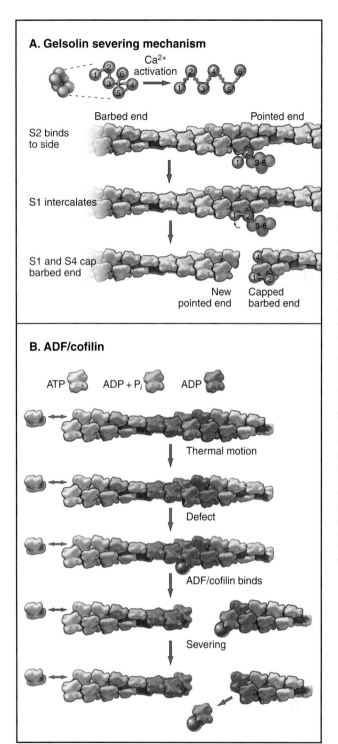

A. Gelsolin severing mechanism

Ca²⁺ activation

Barbed end   Pointed end

S2 binds to side

S1 intercalates

S1 and S4 cap barbed end

New pointed end   Capped barbed end

B. ADF/cofilin

ATP   ADP + Pᵢ   ADP

Thermal motion

Defect

ADF/cofilin binds

Severing

Figure 36–14 Actin filament–severing mechanisms. *A,* Gelsolin domains 2–6 bind to the side of an actin filament, increasing the likelihood that domain 1 will insert between actin subunits and disrupt the filament. The products are two filaments: one with a new pointed end and another with a new barbed end tightly capped by gelsolin. *B,* ADF/cofilin proteins bind to the side of ADP-actin filaments. ADF/cofilins are proposed to bind to ADP-actin subunits in a relatively rare conformation (indicated here by "defect"). Binding of several ADF/cofilins stabilizes the filament in a conformation with a tighter helical twist. ADF/cofilin binding to this conformation destabilizes and severs the filament. The products are two uncapped ends that are available for subunit dissociation. By creating uncapped ends and/or by promoting dissociation of ADP-actin from filament ends, ADF/cofilin enhances the turnover of actin filaments. (*A,* Reference: Robinson R, et al: Domain movement in gelsolin: A calcium-activated switch. Science 286:1939–1942, 1999. *B,* References: Maciver SK, et al: Characterization of actin filament severing by actophorin from *Acanthamoeba castellanii.* J Cell Biol 115:1611–1620, 1991; and McGough A, et al: Cofilin changes the twist of F-actin. J Cell Biol 138:771–781, 1997.)

• The **gelsolin** family of proteins all have six domains with similar folds but different sequences and functions. They bind tightly to the side and barbed end of actin filaments, trapping Ca²⁺ and blocking both the dissociation and association of actin subunits. Gelsolin also binds actin dimers, forming a nucleus that grows at the pointed end. Phosphatidyl 4,5-biphosphate (PIP₂) competes with actin for binding gelsolin.

• Three-domain capping proteins, such as **fragmin** and **severin,** are similar in structure and function to the first three domains of gelsolin. Genes for these capping proteins, found widely across the phylogenetic tree, are likely to have duplicated during evolution to give rise to gelsolin genes.

- **Heterodimeric capping proteins** consist of two subunits of approximately 30 kD. They cap barbed ends with high affinity, independent of Ca^{2+}, and promote nucleation of new pointed ends by stabilizing small actin oligomers. As with gelsolins, PIP_2 also inhibits capping by these proteins. Heterodimeric capping proteins are found in all eukaryotic cells. In striated muscle, they are thought to cap the barbed end of actin filaments in the Z disk (see Chapter 42).
- The **Arp2/3 complex** consists of two actin-related proteins (Arp2 and Arp3) tightly bound to five novel proteins (see Fig. 36–18). The complex caps the pointed end of actin filaments and is the only known cellular factor to nucleate actin polymerization in the barbed direction. It anchors a capped pointed end of the new filament to the side of another actin filament. This complex is ubiquitous and participates in the formation of many dynamic actin filaments in eukaryotes.
- **Tropomodulin** caps the pointed end of stable actin filaments in muscle, red blood cells, and other cells of higher organisms. High-affinity binding to these filaments requires tropomyosin, an α-helical protein that binds along the length of actin filaments (see Fig. 42–4).

Actin Filament–Severing Proteins

Three classes of proteins just introduced—gelsolin, fragmin/severin, and ADF/cofilin—also sever actin filaments into short fragments (see Fig. 36–14). Domain 2 of gelsolin binds to the side of an actin filament, positioning domain 1 to bind between subunits and disrupt the filament. This requires micromolar concentrations of Ca^{2+}. One gelsolin isoform is found inside cells; another is secreted into blood plasma, where it may sever actin filaments released from damaged cells. Fragmin and severin from slime molds (but not their vertebrate homologues) have similar Ca^{2+}-dependent severing activity. Independent of Ca^{2+}, ADF/cofilins bind ADP-actin subunits in filaments, change the helical twist of the filament, and promote severing and depolymerization.

Actin Filament Cross-Linking Proteins

Possession of two actin-binding sites enables cross-linking proteins (Fig. 36–15) to link filaments and to

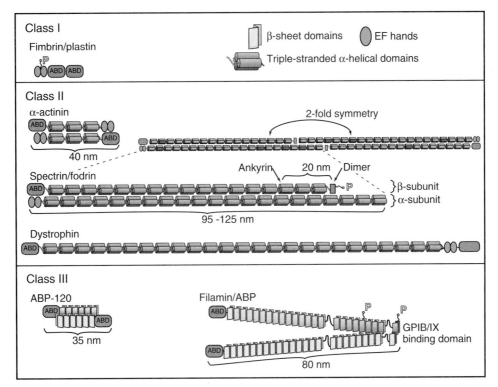

Figure 36–15 Actin filament cross-linking proteins sharing homologous actin-binding domains (ABD) (*red*). Cross-linking requires two actin-binding sites. This is achieved by incorporating two actin-binding domains into one polypeptide (fimbrin), forming dimers of subunits with one actin-binding domain (α-actinin, filamin), or having a second actin-binding site in the protein. The second actin-binding site of dystrophin is in the middle of the tail. (Redrawn from Matsudaira P.: Modular organization of actin crosslinking proteins. Trends Biochem Sci 16:87–92, 1991. Copyright 1991, with permission from Elsevier Science.)

stabilize higher-order assemblies of actin filaments. Some have a greater tendency to cross-link filaments in regular bundles, like those in microvilli (see Fig. 36–2), but depending on protein concentrations and filament lengths, most of these proteins seem to promote the formation of both random networks and regular bundles of filaments. α-Actinin is found in the cortical actin network, at intervals along stress fibers, and on the cytoplasmic side of cell adhesion plaques (see Chapter 32) as well as the Z-disk of striated muscles (see Chapter 42). Fimbrin and villin (a cousin of gelsolin with an extra actin-binding site) stabilize the regular actin filament bundles in microvilli. Filamin cross-links filaments in the cortex of many cells and also anchors these filaments to an integrin, a plasma membrane receptor for adhesive glycoproteins (see Chapter 32). The actin filament cross-linking proteins of the plasma membrane skeleton, such as spectrin (see Fig. 6–10) and dystrophin (see Fig. 32–12), have binding sites for integral membrane proteins in addition to actin filaments. Relatively little is known about how cells regulate cross-linking proteins, although Ca^{2+} can inhibit the binding of some α-actinins to actin.

Side-Binding Proteins: Stabilization of Actin Filaments and Regulation of Interaction with Myosin

Tropomyosin, nebulin, and **caldesmon** are extended proteins that bind along the sides of actin filaments. Tropomyosin increases the tensile strength of actin filaments; in striated muscles, it is also an essential component of the Ca^{2+}-sensitive regulatory machinery that controls the interaction of myosin and actin (see Fig. 42–4). Nebulin may determine the length of the actin filaments in skeletal muscle (see Chapter 42). Less is known about the function of caldesmon, but evidence is growing that caldesmon, together with tropomyosin, forms a Ca^{2+}-calmodulin–sensitive regulator of actin-myosin interaction in smooth muscle (see Chapter 42) and nonmuscle cells. Caldesmon is phosphorylated by cell cycle kinases and may play a role in the reorganization of actin filaments during mitosis.

Adapter Proteins

Animal and fungal cells use multidomain proteins as adapters between actin (or profilin-actin complexes) and other proteins, notably, small guanosine triphosphate (GTP)–binding proteins of the Rho family (see Chapter 27) and other signaling proteins (Table 36–2). Genetic experiments have implicated these proteins in actin-based functions. The multidomain protein **WASp** is defective in the inherited immunodeficiency and bleeding disorder called Wiskott-Aldrich syndrome.

The C-terminal domains of WASp (and related proteins N-WASp and Scar) activate the Arp2/3 complex to nucleate new actin filaments on the side of existing filaments (see Fig. 36–18). Other domains of WASp regulate this activity under the control of the small GTPase (guanosine triphosphatase) Cdc42, membrane polyphosphoinositides, and polyproline-binding proteins with SH3 domains. Another protein called **VASP** (vasodilator-stimulated phosphoprotein) and related proteins interact with membrane proteins, such as ActA of *Listeria* bacteria. They facilitate actin filament assembly by inhibiting barbed end capping, as in the actin filament comet tails that drive the intracellular motility of *Listeria* (see Fig. 40–13).

Functional Redundancy of Actin-Binding Proteins

The diversity and the apparent redundancy of actin-binding proteins is striking. Why should most organisms retain genes for 60 different actin-binding proteins if they have such a limited repertoire of functions: monomer binding, capping, severing, cross-linking, stabilizing, and motility? Why should a cell need more than one actin filament cross-linking protein? Null mutations show that some proteins are essential for normal physiology. These include Arp2/3 complex, profilin, cofilin, and capping protein in budding yeast and profilin in mice. On the other hand, organisms survive some null mutations, suggesting that some parts of the actin system are redundant. For example, in a laboratory environment, *Dictyostelium* was found to tolerate the loss of cross-linking proteins (α-actinin or ABP-120), severin, or one of two profilin genes with only minor defects in behavior and growth rate. Humans lacking dystrophin develop and grow normally for a few years but later succumb to muscle wasting. Mice without their single gelsolin gene reproduce normally, but have mildly defective platelets.

The data suggest that each actin-binding protein has a distinct function, conferring a small selective advantage. Multiple proteins sharing overlapping functions make the actin system relatively fail-safe so that it is difficult to detect the phenotypic consequences of particular proteins in mutant animals.

▌ Actin Dynamics in Live Cells

Actin filaments vary in stability depending upon the cell type. In muscle, essentially all of the actin is polymerized as thin filaments that turn over very slowly, on a time scale of weeks (see Chapter 42). Four proteins stabilize these filaments (see Fig. 42–6). Tropomyosin and nebulin run along the length of the filament, CapZ binds to the barbed end, and

table 36–2
MULTIDOMAIN ADAPTER PROTEINS

Protein family	Distribution	Domains	Ligands	Functions
FH-domain proteins *Formins, Diaphanous, Cykl, Bnil, Cdc12*	Animals, fungi	Formin-homology GBD Polyproline	? Rho, Cdc42 Profilin	Cytokinesis, yeast polarity
IQ-GAP	Animals, fungi	ABD WW IQ Ras-GAP Coiled-coil	Actin filaments Polyproline Calmodulin Rac, Cdc42 Self (homodimers)	Cytokinesis Actin filament cross-linking Localized in lamella, adherens junctions
VASP/ENA *Vasodilator-stimulated phosphoprotein*	Animals	EVH1 Polyproline EVH2	Listeria ActA, vinculin Profilin Actin	Bacterial motility Localized in lamella, stress fibers, focal contact
WASp, N-WASp *Wiskott-Aldrich syndrome protein*	Protozoa, animals, fungi	EVH1 GBD Polyproline WCA	Polyproline, WIP Cdc42>Rac>>Rho Grb2; other SH3 domains Actin, Arp2/3 complex	Stimulates nucleation of actin filaments by Arp2/3 complex

ABD, actin-binding domain; GAP, GTPase-activating protein; GBD, GTPase-binding domain; WIP, WASp-interacting protein

tropomodulin binds to the pointed end. These proteins inhibit breakage of the filaments and limit actin subunit exchange at either end.

In sharp contrast, the distribution of actin filaments changes dramatically as nonmuscle cells move, differentiate, and traverse the cell cycle (see Figs. 36–1 to 36–3). These changes were originally observed by light microscopy of live cells (Fig. 36–16) and light and electron microscopy of fixed cells. Later, actin was tagged with a fluorescent dye and loaded into live cells, so its dynamics could be followed directly (Fig. 36–17). Expression of actin tagged with green fluorescent protein (GFP) is even more convenient for following actin in live cells.

Actin dynamics are attributable, in part, to relocation of preexisting filaments; however, many, but not all, cytoplasmic actin filaments also turn over on a time scale of seconds to minutes. Only about half of the actin in resting cells is polymerized. The concentration of unpolymerized actin is 50–100 μM, which is 500 to 1000 times higher than the critical concentration for polymerization of purified actin. This large pool of unpolymerized actin allows cells to respond rapidly to growth factors or chemoattractants by assembling new filaments. Cells transduce incoming stimuli into signals that specify both the time and place within the cell where specialized actin-based structures assemble.

Continuous assembly and disassembly of actin filaments at the **leading edge** of cells is a dramatic example of rapid actin filament turnover (see Figs. 36–16 and 36–17). In stationary cells, polymerization near the plasma membrane pushes the underlying network of filaments in the cortex toward the center of the cell. In motile cells, the cortex is anchored to the substrate by integrins or other transmembrane adhesion proteins, so polymerization pushes the plasma membrane outward. By electron microscopy, this network consists of obliquely oriented actin filaments, with their fast-growing barbed ends generally facing the plasma membrane (see Fig. 36–2D).

Assembly of cortical actin filaments can be imaged directly by light microscopy in very flat cells (see Fig. 36–16). The effect of the drug **cytochalasin** (Box 36–1) illustrates the dynamics. In seconds, cytochalasin disrupts the cortical actin filament network. When cytochalasin is removed, the cortical actin network reforms rapidly from the leading edge.

Experiments with fluorescent probes on actin molecules (see Fig. 36–17) provide further insights. Purified actin can be labeled with a fluorescent dye and microinjected into live cells, where it incorporates into

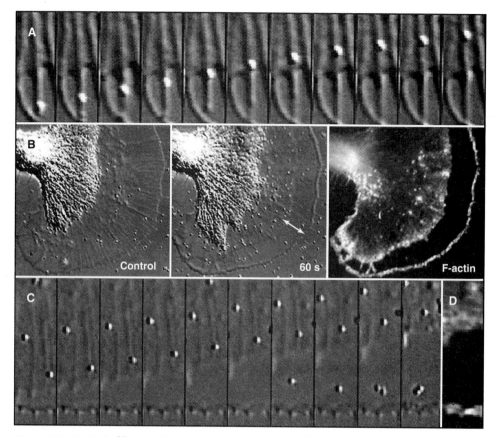

Figure 36-16 Actin filament dynamics at the leading edge of a growth cone of a neuron isolated from the mollusk *Aplysia*. Video-enhanced differential interference light microscopy shows the organization of the growth cone with a broad lamella of actin filaments that excludes organelles (*B, control*). This cortical network of actin filaments forms continuously at the edge of the cell, moves inward (upward in the orientation of the detailed time series shown in *A*) and then disassembles. Irregularities in the network or particles on the outer surface of the cell (bright white spot) allow this flux to be observed to move at a rate of about 3–6 μm/min (equivalent to filaments growing by 19–38 subunits/sec). *B* and *C,* Application of the drug cytochalasin D disrupts the cortical network over a period of 60 seconds, as illustrated in the middle panel of *B* (double-headed arrow marks the zone cleared of actin filaments) and the detailed time series in *C*. Staining with rhodamine-phalloidin (right panel in *B* and *D*) shows that a few filaments survive at the leading edge. Upon removal of cytochalasin, the network recovers, beginning near the leading edge, and resumes turnover of the filaments. (Courtesy of Paul Forscher, Yale University; based on Forscher P, Smith SJ: Actions of cytochalasins in a neuronal growth cone. J Cell Biol 107:1505–1516, 1988, by copyright permission of the Rockefeller University Press.)

the actin-containing structures, including the cortical network, pseudopods, stress fibers, and surface microspikes. The dye can be bleached locally inside a live cell to demonstrate the behavior of polymerized actin. Even in stationary cells, the bleached spot moves away from the edge of the cell and slowly recovers its fluorescence. Recovery after photobleaching is effected by replacement of bleached actin by diffusion of filaments, active movement of filaments, assembly of new filaments, subunit flux through filaments, or some combination of these processes. To assess the contribution of each process, a cell can be injected with actin carrying a "caged" dye. The caged dye is not fluorescent until a blocking group is removed locally by photolysis with a pulse from a

highly focused light. The fate of this small sample of polymeric actin can then be followed directly. Filaments in cortical cytoplasm lose their fluorescence over a period of minutes, an observation interpreted to mean that fluorescent subunits are released from filaments and diffuse away. In many cells, filaments also move as a group from the cell periphery toward the cell center, confirming that new filaments displace old filaments from the periphery.

Biochemical and genetic experiments have identified the same minimal set of proteins essential for maintaining the pool of unpolymerized actin, initiating and terminating new filaments, and controlling disassembly (Fig. 36–18). Biochemical reconstitution of the actin filament comet tail of the intracellular bacterium

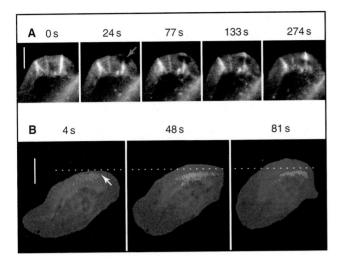

Figure 36–17 Documentation of actin filament dynamics at the leading edge with fluorescent actins. *A,* Fluorescence photobleaching experiment with a stationary cell. Fluorescent actin is injected into a cultured epithelial cell and allowed to incorporate into filaments. A laser pulse bleaches some of the fluorescent actin, leaving a dark spot (*arrow*) that reveals movement of the filaments toward the cell center. *B,* Caged fluorescent actin experiment with a motile cell. Fluorescent dye bound to actin is masked with a chemical group preventing fluorescence. After incorporation into actin filaments of a fish keratocyte (see Fig. 36–2*E*), dyes in one area of the cell are uncaged with a light pulse (*arrow*) and red fluorescence is followed with time. Fluorescent actin filaments are stationary with respect to the substrate as the cell moved forward (upward). The fluorescent spot of marked filaments fades with time owing to depolymerization and dispersal of the fluorescent subunits. (*A,* From Wang Y-L: Exchange of actin subunits at the leading edge of living fibroblasts: Possible role of treadmilling. J Cell Biol 101:597–602, 1985, by copyright permission of the Rockefeller University Press. *B,* Reprinted with permission from Nature. From Theriot JA, Mitchison TJ: Actin microfilament dynamics in locomoting cells. Nature 352:126–131, 1991. Copyright 1991, Macmillan Magazines Limited.)

Listeria (see Fig. 40–13) requires only actin heterodimeric Arp2/3 complex, ADF/cofilin, profilin, and capping protein.

The Pool of Unpolymerized Actin

Two complementary mechanisms appear to maintain the pool of unpolymerized actin: sequestration of actin monomers in complexes that do not nucleate or elongate filaments and capping of actin filament ends. Profilin (with help from thymosin in vertebrate cells) is the most attractive candidate for maintaining a pool of unpolymerized actin monomers under conditions in which they normally would polymerize. The concentrations of profilin and thymosin exceed the concentration of unpolymerized actin, and they bind tightly enough to reduce the free monomer concentration to the micromolar level. When bound to profilin or thymosin, actin monomers have limited capacity to nucleate new filaments. However, for profilin to be effec-

TOOLS TO STUDY ACTIN FILAMENTS: NATURAL PRODUCTS CAN STABILIZE OR DESTABILIZE ACTIN FILAMENTS

Destabilizers Cytochalasins, complex organic compounds synthesized by fungi, inhibit actin assembly in two ways. High-affinity binding to the barbed end of actin filaments inhibits subunit association and dissociation. Low-affinity binding to actin monomers promotes their dimerization and the hydrolysis of ATP bound to one subunit. In this way, cytochalasins catalyze the conversion of ATP-actin to ADP-actin. Cytochalasin (meaning "cell relaxing") is so named because it causes regression of the cleavage furrow during cytokinesis and disrupts many structures containing actin filaments in cells. Cytochalasins are used to test for the participation of actin filaments in cellular processes, but observations must be interpreted cautiously, given the complicated mechanism of action. Sponges synthesize toxins that destabilize actin filaments in cells by sequestering actin monomers (latrunculin A) or severing actin filaments (swinholide A).

Stabilizers Phallotoxins (such as phalloidin) are cyclic peptides synthesized by poisonous mushrooms. They bind and stabilize actin filaments by reducing the rate of subunit dissociation to near zero at both ends of the polymer. When introduced into cells by microinjection, phallotoxins inhibit processes that depend on actin filament turnover, including amoeboid movement. They are toxic to humans because they interfere with bile secretion. Fluorescent derivatives of phallotoxins are widely used to localize actin filaments in cells and tissues (see Fig. 36–1), as well as to quantify polymerized actin in cells and cell extracts. A sponge toxin, jasplakinolide, has effects similar to phallotoxins.

C2 toxin produced by *Clostridium botulinum* is an enzyme that catalyzes the ADP-ribosylation of cytoplasmic actins on arginine-177. *Clostridium perfringens* iota toxin does the same to muscle actin. ADP-ribosylated actin polymerizes poorly and caps the barbed end of actin filaments. The ability of these protein toxins to penetrate live cells, cap actin filaments, and alter actin polymerization accounts for their disruption of the actin cytoskeleton in cells and may contribute to their toxicity.

tive, the barbed ends of most filaments need to be capped, as rapid addition of actin-profilin complexes to free barbed ends would quickly deplete the pool of unpolymerized actin. Cells contain enough heterodimeric capping protein or gelsolin, or both, to cap the barbed ends of most filaments. Together, monomer binding and capping allow cells to maintain a large

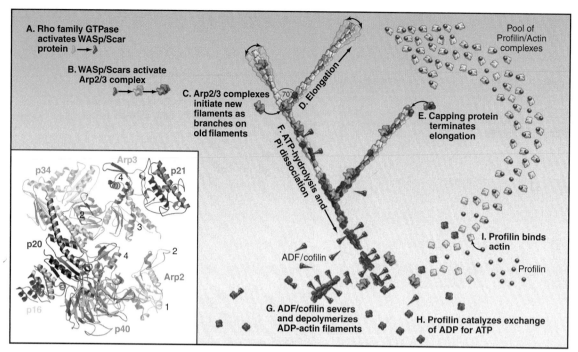

Figure 36-18 Branching nucleation of actin filaments by Arp2/3 complex and recycling of subunits to the unpolymerized pool by ADF/cofilins and profilin. *A to I* indicate the steps in this cycle. The inset shows a ribbon diagram of the crystal structure of Arp2/3 complex. The seven subunits are color coded and labeled. (Redrawn from Pollard TD, Blanchoin L, Mullins RD: Biophysics of actin filament dynamics in nonmuscle cells. Annu Rev Biophys Biomol Struct 29:545–576, 2000, with permission, from the *Annual Review of Biophysics and Biomolecular Structure,* Vol. 29, © 2000 by Annual Reviews www.AnnualReviews.org. *Inset,* PDB file: 1K88. Reference: Robinson R, Turbedsky K, et al: Crystal structure of Arp2/3 complex. Science 294:1679–1684, 2001.)

Figure 36-19 Cells polymerize actin and change shape in response to stimuli. The cellular slime mold *Dictyostelium* responds to cAMP by transiently polymerizing actin filaments, rounding, and then resuming motility in the direction of the source of cAMP. Two bursts of actin polymerization accompany this reorganization of the cell. *A,* Scanning electron micrograph and fluorescent actin filament staining of a resting cell. *B,* Similar micrographs of cells stimulated with cAMP. *C,* Time course of actin assembly with the times for cells shown in *A* and *B* indicated. (Courtesy of J. Condeelis and colleagues at the Albert Einstein College of Medicine, New York.)

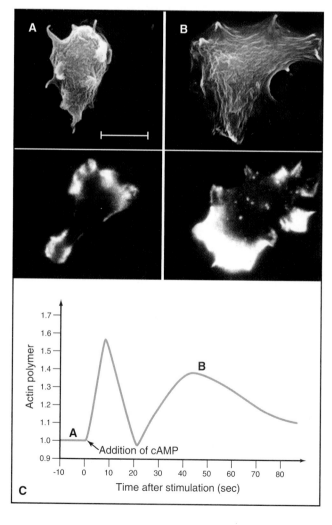

pool of actin subunits ready to elongate any barbed ends created by uncapping, severing, or nucleation.

Initiation and Termination of New Actin Filaments During Cell Motility

A variety of agonists stimulate the conversion of actin from the unpolymerized pool into actin filaments that contribute to the enlargement of pseudopodia and filopodia. Examples include the actions of cyclic adenosine monophosphate (cAMP) on *Dictyostelium* (Fig. 36–19), the bacterial chemotactic peptide formyl-methionine-leucine-phenylalanine on vertebrate white blood cells, and thrombin on vertebrate platelets. In each case, biochemical assays document an increase in the concentration of polymerized actin at the expense of the pool of unpolymerized actin. Polymerization depends on creation of uncapped barbed ends, which grow rapidly at rates estimated to be 50 to 500 subunits per second depending on the concentration of actin-profilin. Growth probably is brief, as the concentration of free capping protein is high enough to terminate growth in seconds by capping the growing barbed ends.

Three mechanisms are thought to create free barbed ends: uncapping, severing, and de novo formation of new barbed ends. In many cases, new barbed ends appear to form de novo. Arp2/3 complex is the prime candidate to initiate new barbed ends (see Fig. 36–18), as it is localized in sites where new filaments polymerize and it produces new actin filaments that grow as branches from the side of older filaments. Activated WASp stimulates this branching reaction, and Arp2/3 complex is found at these branches in cells (see Fig. 36–2D). Small Rho-family GTPases associated with the plasma membrane and polyphosphoinositides activate WASp. Because some filaments appear to form at sites lacking Arp2/3 complex, other initiating factors may exist. Plasma membrane polyphosphoinositides might uncap barbed ends by dissociating heterodimeric capping proteins or gelsolin. Ca^{2+} transients might induce gelsolin to sever actin filaments, creating capped barbed ends that would require uncapping before initiation of growth. Dephosphorylation activates ADF/cofilin proteins, which can sever filaments, creating free barbed ends.

Rapid Actin Filament Turnover and Subunit Recycling

Actin filaments at the leading edge of motile cells turn over much faster in the cellular environment than filaments of purified actin in vitro. A possible mechanism involves the hydrolysis of ATP and dissociation of the γ-phosphate, reactions that provide a timer to mark older filaments for depolymerization by regulatory proteins (see Fig. 36–18). Once phosphate dissociates, branches dissociate from Arp2/3 complex and ADF/cofilin proteins bind and sever these old filaments, in addition to promoting dissociation of ADP-actin subunits. Profilin stimulates exchange of ADP for ATP on dissociated subunits, recycling them back to the ATP-actin-profilin pool, ready to add to new barbed ends when they appear (see Fig. 36–12). Side-binding proteins such as tropomyosin appear to stabilize a subset of old filaments by protecting them against ADF/cofilins.

How Do Cells Organize Actin Assemblies?

Cells organize actin filaments in a variety of structures, including cortical networks, microvilli or filopodia, and contractile bundles (see Figs. 36–1 to 36–3). Although each cell in a population is unique, all cells of a particular type achieve a similar pattern of organization. How are these patterns specified? Although not yet understood in detail, the mechanisms appear to depend upon expression of an appropriate mixture of actin-binding proteins, a prerequisite for self-assembly of particular structures, as well as signals mediated by small **Rho-family GTPases (Rho, Rac, Cdc 42)** (Fig. 36–20).

Some specialized actin-containing structures assemble spontaneously from purified proteins. For example, actin forms bundles similar to microvilli when polymerized in the presence of fimbrin and villin, the two major cross-linking proteins found in microvilli. Overexpression of villin in cells induces extension of existing filopodia and formation of new **filopodia** (projections of the plasma membrane supported by an internal bundle of actin filaments, similar to microvilli). Thus, the pool of villin and fimbrin and other components limits the number of microvilli. In cells containing these building blocks, activation of the GTPase Cdc42 stimulates formation of filopodia (see Fig. 36–20) in a mechanism dependent upon N-WASp. The relation of branching nucleation to the assembly of the parallel bundle of filaments in filopodia is not yet understood.

Other actin filament structures assemble on membrane attachment sites. Plasma membrane proteins may provide sites to nucleate new filaments or bind preformed filaments, thus concentrating actin filaments in the cortex. The anion transporter in the red blood cell plasma membrane, called band 3, appears to be such a protein, as it anchors the membrane skeleton consisting of actin, spectrin, and associated proteins (see Fig. 6–12). A high concentration of actin filaments near the membrane attracts actin-binding proteins. Depending on the particular mixture of these proteins, cells assemble actin filaments into either a planar network (red blood cells), a random network (amoeboid cells), bundles for filopodia (epithelial cells), or bundles attached

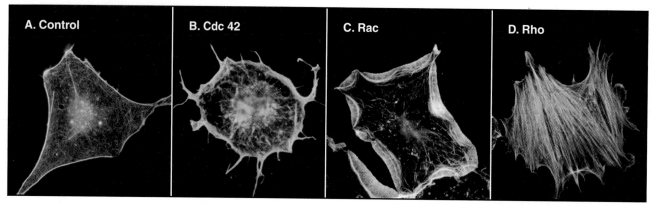

Figure 36–20 Rho-family GTPases trigger the assembly of actin-based structures. Fluorescence micrographs of Swiss 3T3 fibroblasts stained with rhodamine-phalloidin to reveal actin filaments. *A*, Resting cells. *B*, Cells microinjected with activated Cdc42 form many filopodia. *C*, Cells microinjected with activated Rac have a thick cortical network of actin filaments around the periphery. *D*, Stress fibers anchored at their ends by focal contacts are abundant in cells microinjected with an activated form of Rho. (Courtesy of Alan Hall, University of London.)

to membrane adhesion sites (epithelial cells and fibroblasts). An activated form of the GTPase Rac promotes the formation of cortical networks of actin filaments (see Fig. 36–20). Some intracellular pathogens, including the bacteria *Listeria* and *Shigella* and the vaccinia virus, usurp the host cellular machinery to assemble networks of actin filaments that propel them through the cytoplasm (see Fig. 40–13).

Physical forces also help to organize actin filaments. Bundles of actin filaments in stress fibers (see Fig. 36–1) and the contractile ring during cytokinesis (see Fig. 36–3 and Chapter 47) appear to be aligned, at least in part, by tension generated by myosin motors. Activated Rho is required for cytokinesis and also stimulates the formation of stress fibers (see Fig. 36–20) by activating **myosin II** through phosphorylation of its regulatory light chain (see Fig. 47–22). Rho stimulates two kinases that phosphorylate the regulatory light chain and inhibit the phosphatase that reverses the reaction. The success of forces in organizing actin filaments depends upon anchoring of the filaments to the plasma membrane—focal contacts in the case of stress

fibers (see Fig. 32–10) and the equatorial plasma membrane for the contractile ring (see Fig. 47–21). Cross-linking proteins are probably also essential for maintaining the integrity of these actin filament bundles under mechanical stress; accordingly, cross-linkers, such as α-actinin, are concentrated in these bundles.

Actin Filaments and the Mechanical Properties of Cytoplasm

Actin filaments are generally believed to provide the molecular basis for many of the mechanical properties of cytoplasm, a complicated, viscoelastic material. Viscoelastic means that the cytoplasm can both resist flow, like a viscous liquid (e.g., molasses), and store some mechanical energy when stretched or compressed, like a spring. Physiological concentrations of purified actin filaments are viscoelastic. At high concentrations, actin filaments also align spontaneously into large parallel arrays called liquid crystals.

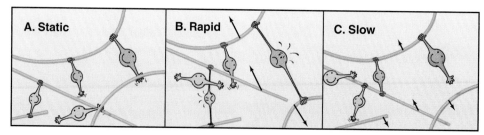

Figure 36–21 Dynamic cross-linking of actin filaments. Rapid binding and dissociation of cross-linking proteins allow networks of actin filaments to resist rapid deformations but to change shape passively when force is applied for a prolonged time. *A*, Cross-linked network in a static region. *B*, Cross-linking proteins resist deformation if force is applied rapidly. *C*, Cross-linking proteins provide little resistance to deformation if force is applied slowly since the crosslinks rearrange faster than the filaments are displaced. (Redrawn from Pollard TD, et al: Actin and myosin biochemistry in relation to cytokinesis. Ann NY Acad Sci 582:120–130, 1990.)

The physical properties of actin filaments depend on their length and their interactions. Cross-linking of actin filaments increases both their viscosity and elasticity. Severing actin filaments decreases their viscoelasticity. On the other hand, shorter filaments have an increased tendency to form bundles in the presence of cross-linking proteins, so severing can actually promote the formation of rigid actin filament bundles.

Many cross-linking proteins, including α-actinin, have a low affinity for actin filaments with a K_d in the micromolar range. At steady-state in vitro, bonds between these cross-linking proteins and actin break and re-form on a second or subsecond time scale. Consequently, gels of actin filaments and α-actinin are much more rigid when deformed rapidly than slowly (Fig. 36–21) because crosslinks can rearrange if given sufficient time. Dynamic crosslinks between filaments allow actin networks to remodel passively as cells move. Cells also remodel the actin cytoskeleton actively by turning over of filaments, as described previously.

▌ Selected Readings

Higgs HN, Pollard TD: Regulation of actin filament network formation through Arp2/3 complex: activation by a diverse array of proteins. Annu Rev Biochem 70:649–676, 2001.

Kaibuchi K, Kuroda S, Amano M: Regulation of the cytoskeleton and cell adhesion by the Rho family of GTPases in mammalian cells. Annu Rev Biochem 68:459–486, 1999.

Kreis T, Vale R, eds: Guidebook to the Cytoskeletal and Motor Proteins, 2nd ed. New York: Oxford University Press, 1999.

McLaughlin PJ, Weeds AG: Actin-binding protein complexes at atomic resolution. Annu Rev Biophys Biomolec Struct 24:643–675, 1995.

Pollard TD, Almo S, Quirk S, Vinson V, Lattman EE: Structure of actin binding proteins: Insights about function at atomic resolution. Annu Rev Cell Biol 10:207–249, 1994.

Pollard TD, Blanchoin L, Mullins RD: Biophysics of actin filament dynamics in nonmuscle cells. Annu Rev Biophys Biomolec Struct 29:545–576, 2000.

Schafer DA, Schroer TA: Actin-related proteins. Annu Rev Cell Dev Biol 15:341–365, 1999.

Schmidt A, Hall MN: Signaling to the actin cytoskeleton. Annu Rev Cell Dev Biol 14:305–339, 1998.

Stossel TP, Condeelis J, Cooley L, et al: Filamins as integrators of cell mechanics and signalling. Nature Rev Mol Cell Biol. 2:138–145, 2001.

Svitkina TM, Borisy GG: Progress in protrusion: The tell-tale scar. Trends Biochem Sci 24:432–436, 1999.

Van den Ent F, Amos LA, Löwe J: Prokaryotic origin of the actin cytoskeleton. Nature 413:39–44, 2001.

chapter 37

MICROTUBULES AND MICROTUBULE-ASSOCIATED PROTEINS

Microtubules are stiff, cylindrical polymers of α- and β-tubulin (Fig. 37–1) that provide support for a variety of cellular components and tracks for movements powered by a large number of motor proteins. Microtubules are 25 nm in diameter and grow longer than 20 μm in cells and 3 mm in vitro. The uniform orientation of dimers of α- and β-tubulin in the wall of microtubules give the polymer a molecular polarity. The **"plus" end** grows faster than the **"minus" end.**

A great simplifying principle that applies to organization of both the cytoskeleton and motility is that microtubules generally have a radial organization in many types of cells (Fig. 37–2A). Typically, the plus end is peripheral and the minus end is anchored in a **microtubule-organizing center:** the **centrosome** for cytoplasmic microtubules or **basal bodies** for axonemes (Fig. 37–3). In most animal cells, this microtubule organizing center is concentrated in a matrix surrounding the centrioles. The active component in microtubule nucleation is a minor tubulin isoform, γ-**tubulin** and associated proteins. Fungal microtubules grow from a **spindle pole body,** associated with the nuclear envelope and also containing γ-tubulin (see Fig. 37–2D). There are important exceptions to this radial organization of microtubules. About 40% of the microtubules in dendrites of nerve cells are oriented the other way around. The microtubule organizing center is more diffuse in columnar epithelial cells; microtubules originate from a broad zone near the apex of the cell (see Fig. 37–2B). In plant cells, γ-tubulin and microtubules are found throughout the cortex rather than in a discrete array, although they form a bipolar spindle during mitosis (see Fig. 37–2C).

Microtubules vary considerably in stability. Those forming the **axonemes** of the structural core of eukaryotic cilia and flagella are stable for days to weeks. Cytoplasmic microtubules turn over much more rapidly, within minutes in the case of the interphase array of microtubules and within seconds for mitotic spindle microtubules. These dynamic microtubules randomly undergo rapid depolymerization and then regrow over a period of seconds to minutes. This **"dynamic instability"** helps to remodel the network of microtubules in cytoplasm and contributes to some forms of motility, including the assembly of the mitotic spindle and movements of chromosomes during mitosis (see Chapter 47).

Because the same tubulin dimers can form dynamic single microtubules in cytoplasm and stable doublet microtubules in axonemes, it is believed that accessory proteins specify both the stability and diverse structures assembled from tubulin. More than a dozen **microtubule-associated proteins (MAPs)** bind tubulin dimers, stabilize polymers, associate with microtubule ends, or sever cytoplasmic microtubules. In the axonemes of cilia and flagella, more than 100 accessory proteins organize and stabilize the regular array of nine outer doublet microtubules and two central single microtubules (see Chapter 41).

The stiffness, length, and polarity of microtubules make them valuable for both cytoskeletal support and as tracks for microtubule-based motors. Because they resist compression, microtubules are called upon more frequently than actin filaments or intermediate filaments to support asymmetrical cellular structures, including axonemes, the mitotic spindle, and elaborate surface processes of some protozoa (Fig. 37–4). Interactions of microtubules with both actin filaments and intermediate filaments reinforce the cytoskeleton.

Microtubule motor proteins (see Chapter 39) power movements ranging from the slow movements of chromosomes on the mitotic spindle (see Chapter 47) to the rapid beating of cilia and flagella (see Chapter 41). Different motors move toward the plus and

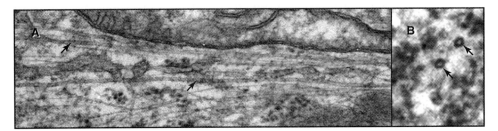

Figure 37-1 Microtubules *(arrows)* visualized in electron micrographs of thin sections of a cultured mammalian cell. *A*, Longitudinal section. *B*, Cross section. (Courtesy of R. Goldman, Northwestern University.)

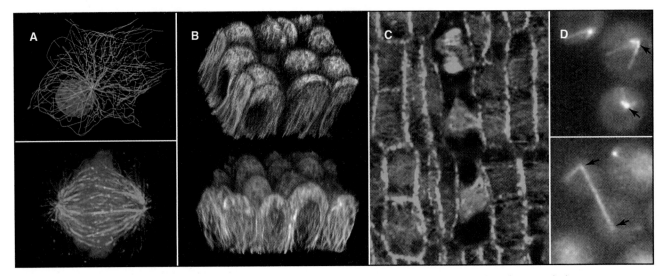

Figure 37-2 Arrangements of microtubules in various cells. *A* to *C*, Fluorescence micrographs of microtubules stained with antibodies to tubulin. *A*, Vertebrate tissue culture cells. *Upper panel*, Green microtubules radiate from the red centrosome near the blue nucleus of an interphase cell. *Lower panel*, A HeLa cell in mitosis with green microtubules radiating from the two poles toward the blue chromosomes and red centromeres (stained with anticentromere antibody). *B*, Columnar epithelial cells in tissue culture. Three-dimensional reconstructions show microtubules oriented along the long axis of the cell. *C*, Plant cells. Maize epidermal cells with green microtubules in the cortex and in the mitotic spindles of three dividing cells near the middle of the field. Nuclei are stained orange. *D*, Live budding yeast. The upper micrograph shows two interphase cells with microtubules radiating from the spindle pole bodies *(arrows)* associated with the nuclear envelope. These microtubules are marked with dynein fused to green fluorescent protein. The lower micrograph shows a cell late in mitosis with a bundle of microtubules extending from one spindle pole body to the other inside the nucleus. These microtubules are marked with tubulin fused to green fluorescent protein. (*A [upper panel]*, Courtesy of A. Khodjakov, Wadsworth Center, Albany, NY. *A [lower panel]*, Courtesy of D. W. Cleveland, University of California, San Diego. *B*, Courtesy of R. Bacallao, University of Indiana Medical School, Indianapolis. *C*, Courtesy of L. Smith, University of California, San Diego. *D*, Courtesy of P. Maddox, University of North Carolina, Chapel Hill.)

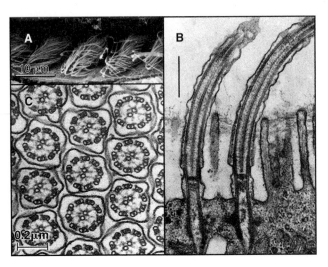

Figure 37-3 Cilia on mussel gill epithelial cells. *A*, A scanning electron micrograph reveals how the bending movements of the thread-like cilia are coordinated in waves. *B* and *C*, Transmission electron micrographs of cilia. *B*, Longitudinal section showing basal bodies and proximal parts of two cilia. *C*, Cross section of many cilia showing the nine outer doublets and the central pair of microtubules. (Courtesy of P. Satir, Albert Einstein College of Medicine, New York; Reference: Satir P: How cilia move. Sci Am 231:44–52, 1974.)

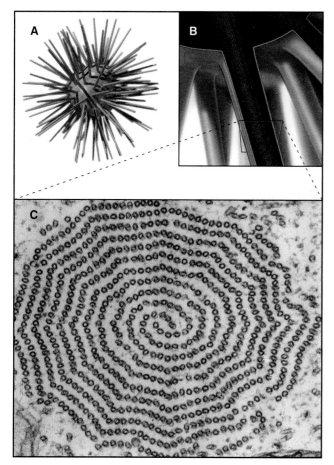

Figure 37-4 Cell surface projections supported by microtubules. *A* and *B*, Drawings of the radiolarian *Echinospherium* (a protozoan) showing projections called axopodia. *C*, Electron micrograph of a thin section across an axopodium showing the double spiral array of microtubules. (Courtesy of L. Tilney, University of Pennsylvania.)

minus ends of microtubules. The minus end–directed motor, dynein, drives the beating of cilia and flagella. Dynein and the kinesin family of plus end motors move membrane-bound organelles and other components, including RNA, along microtubules (see Chapter 40). Motors that move microtubules relative to one another play an important role in establishing the large-scale organization of microtubule arrays. These active movements determine, to a great extent, the distribution of cellular organelles and the shape of cells.

Tubulin Structure

The tubulin molecule is a heterodimer of α- and β-subunits that share a common fold and 40% identical residues (Fig. 37–5). Each subunit binds a guanine nucleotide, either guanosine triphosphate (GTP) or guanosine diphosphate (GDP). Tubulin dimers are stable and rarely dissociate at the 10- to 20-μM concen-

trations of tubulin found in cells. Neither the fold nor the GTP-binding site of tubulin resemble those of other GTP-binding proteins (see Chapter 27). Instead, loops between elements of secondary structure form a surface pocket that binds a guanine nucleotide like the enzyme glyceraldehyde-3-phosphate dehydrogenase binds nicotinamide-adenine dinucleotide (NAD). GTP on α-tubulin is buried in the dimer, so it does not exchange with solution GTP; hence, it is called the nonexchangeable N-site. GTP on β-tubulin is exposed in the dimer and exchanges slowly (K_d = 50 nM), so this is known as the exchangeable E-site. When incorporated into a microtubule, contacts with the adjacent subunit bury the β-subunit GTP and promote its hydrolysis. Neither bound guanine nucleotide can exchange when tubulin is buried in the wall of a microtubule. As explained later in this chapter, the nature of the nucleotide on the β-subunit profoundly affects microtubule assembly.

Although divergent in sequence, the bacterial protein **FtsZ** has the same fold as tubulin and likely had a common ancestor. FtsZ also forms polymers and is required for bacterial cell division (see Fig. 47–19).

Two modifications—acetylation of lysine-40 and removal of the C-terminal tyrosine of α-tubulin—have been correlated with increased microtubule stability, but no cause-and-effect relationship has been estab-

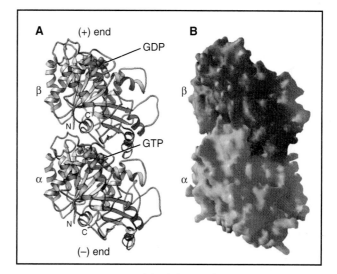

Figure 37-5 Atomic model of the α-tubulin–β-tubulin dimer. *A,* Ribbon diagrams with space-filling GTP on α-tubulin and GDP on β-tubulin. *B,* Surface rendering. This structure is historic, as it was the first atomic structure of a nonmembrane protein to be determined by electron crystallography, using sheets of tubulin protofilaments as the specimen. Each subunit consists of about 450 residues arranged in two domains. Each domain is a β sheet flanked by α helices. (PDB file: 1TUB. Reprinted with permission from Nature. From the work of Nogales E, Downing K: Structure of the alpha beta tubulin dimer by electron crystallography. Nature 391:199–203, 1998. Copyright 1998, Macmillan Magazines Limited.)

lished for either modification. The enzyme carboxypeptidase B removes the tyrosine, leaving a glutamic acid exposed. Another enzyme, tyrosine-tubulin ligase, can replace the tyrosine using ATP as the energy source to reform the peptide bond. Glutamic acid residues 445 of α-tubulin and 438 of β-tubulin are modified by the addition of a polymer of up to 6 glutamic acid residues to the γ-carboxyl. Other glutamic acids are modified by the addition of one or more glycines to the γ-carboxyl. Serine 344 of β-III tubulin can be phosphorylated, but its functional significance is not known.

Tubulin Diversity

Tubulins are remarkably conserved across the phylogenetic tree; more than 75% of the residues of animal α- or β-tubulins are identical to their plant homologues. On the other hand, species differ considerably in their variety of tubulin isoforms. Vertebrates have six to eight genes each for α- and β-tubulin, whereas budding yeast have but two α-tubulin genes and one β-tubulin gene. Unicellular ciliates like *Tetrahymena* assemble a greater variety of microtubule-based structures than humans have in their various tissues, using only one α- and one β-tubulin polypeptide. Most vertebrate cells express several tubulin isoforms, but exceptional cases, like bird red blood cells, express a single α-tubulin and β-tubulin. It is impressive that the sequences of homologous tubulins vary little, if at all, between different vertebrate species, whereas the various β-tubulin isoforms in one organism differ by about 10% in primary structure. γ-Tubulins are also conserved between species.

Two extreme views rationalize the significance of multiple α- and β-tubulin isoforms. On one hand, isoforms have different assembly properties and affinities for microtubule-associated proteins (MAPs) that may confer some advantage to the organism. This is illustrated by the failure of tubulin genes to substitute for each other in flies. Alternatively, the proteins themselves may be largely interchangeable (and all isoforms appear to copolymerize), but different genes may be required to ensure precise control of biosynthesis in particular cells at appropriate times during development. For example, the two α-tubulins of the filamentous fungus *Aspergillus* can substitute for each other, but two genes are required to control the expression of tubulin at specific times in the life cycle.

Four new tubulin isoforms called δ, ε, ζ, and η tubulin were discovered only recently. Their genes are found in protozoa, algae, and vertebrates but are conspicuously missing from fungi and plants. All of these new isoforms are localized to centrioles or basal bodies and seem to be required for their structure or function. The absence of these tubulins may account for the lack of centrioles in plants and fungi.

Structure of Microtubules

Microtubules are cylinders constructed of longitudinally oriented **protofilaments** with a 4-nm longitudinal repeat arising from the tubulin subunits (Fig. 37–6). Most cytoplasmic microtubules have 13 protofilaments, but microtubules in some cells have 11, 15, or 16 protofilaments. Microtubules assembled in vitro have 11 to 15 protofilaments, but 13 is the favored number. For years, microtubules were thought to be true helices, but most microtubules actually have a longitudinal seam or discontinuity between two of the

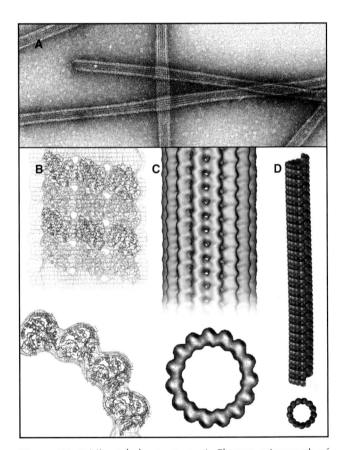

Figure 37–6 Microtubule structure. *A*, Electron micrograph of negatively stained microtubules. *B* and *C*, Longitudinal and cross sections of a reconstruction of a 13-protofilament microtubule made by image processing of electron micrographs. *B*, Atomic model made by fitting the tubulin dimer model into the reconstruction of the microtubule. *C*, Surface rendering of the reconstruction. *D*, Drawing of the microtubule used throughout this book. It shows the longitudinal seam between two protofilaments, which breaks the helical repeat of tubulin dimers. (*A*, Courtesy of D. B. Murphy, Johns Hopkins Medical School. *B* and *C*, Courtesy of R. Milligan, Scripps Research Institute, La Jolla, CA.)

protofilaments, breaking up perfect helical packing of the subunits (Fig. 37–6*D*). The other protofilaments are aligned identically with respect to their neighbors.

Microtubules are polar because all of the dimers have the same orientation. *β*-tubulin is oriented toward the plus end; *α*-tubulin toward the minus end. This polarity results in different rates of growth at the two ends. The plus end with exposed *β*-subunits grows faster than the minus end. For the purpose of marking polarity in electron micrographs of extracted cells, microtubules can be decorated with either exogenous dynein or with excess tubulin to form "hooks." These hooks form as curved sheets of tubulin along the length of microtubules exposed to tubulin in high concentrations of salt in the presence of the drug nocodazole. When the decorated microtubules are cut in cross section and examined by electron microscopy, the handedness of the hooks reveals the polarity of the microtubule. These hooks have no physiological significance but provided the primary evidence that the minus ends are usually associated with microtubule-organizing centers.

As might be expected from their cylindrical structure, microtubules are much stiffer than either actin filaments or intermediate filaments. If enlarged 1 million–fold to a diameter of 25 mm, microtubules would have mechanical properties similar to a steel pipe: quite stiff locally, but flexible over distances of several meters (micrometers in the cell). On the same scale, actin filaments would be like 8-mm steel wires and intermediate filaments would be akin to 10-mm braided steel cables. Thus, microtubules are resistant to compression and support asymmetrical structures much more effectively than the other cytoskeletal polymers.

Microtubule Assembly from GTP Tubulin

Microtubules assemble from GTP-tubulin subunits much like actin filaments (see Figs. 4–6 and 36–9). Superficially, the assembly of microtubules is a simple bimolecular reaction of tubulin dimers with the ends of the polymer. Association and dissociation of tubulin occurs only at the ends, not from the walls of microtubules. Growth is faster at the plus end than the minus end (Fig. 37–7), and assembly of GTP tubulin is much more favorable than that of GDP tubulin. The rate of elongation is proportional to the concentration of GTP-tubulin dimers above the **critical concentration** at each end. The rate constants (Table 37–1) are even similar to those for actin (see Fig. 37–9), although the analogy may be misleading, as the number of growing sites at the end of the polymer is unknown and is likely to be greater than one.

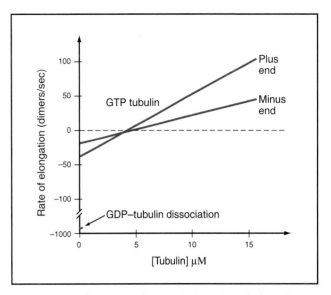

Figure 37–7 Elongation of pure tubulin microtubules. The rate of elongation at plus and minus ends is a function of GTP-tubulin dimer concentration. Slopes give association rate constants, x-intercepts give the critical concentrations, and the y-intercepts give the dissociation rate constants. The dissociation rate of GDP tubulin is shown as a single point at 733 s⁻¹ on the y-axis. (Data from Walker RA, et al: Dynamic instability of individual microtubules. J Cell Biol 107:1437–1448, 1988.)

Drugs (see Box 37–1) and environmental conditions can depolymerize microtubules. Pioneering light microscopic observations of live cells first established that mitotic spindle fibers (later shown to be microtubules) were sensitive to both cold and high hydrostatic pressure. This makes it possible to purify microtubules and tightly associated proteins by cycles of depolymerization in the cold and repolymerization at higher temperatures. Dissociated microtubule components in ice-cold cellular extracts polymerize when warmed to body temperature; pelleting in a centrifuge separates microtubules and any associated proteins from soluble components; resuspension in cold buffer depolymerizes the microtubules; and the cycle is repeated again until the desired degree of purity is achieved. Adaptations of tubulins or accessory proteins allow cold-water organisms to assemble microtubules in freezing temperatures.

Steady-State Dynamics of Microtubules In Vitro

If the GTP-tubulin reactions were all that contributed to assembly, microtubules would grow until the tubulin dimer concentration decreased to a critical concentration, after which polymers would be relatively stable. However, this is not what happens at steady-state in either test tubes or cells. In vitro the overall micro-

table 37–1

RATE CONSTANTS FOR THE ASSEMBLY OF MICROTUBULES IN VITRO AND IN CELLS

Reaction	Plus End	Minus End
In Vitro Elongation of Purified Tubulin		
Association of GTP tubulin	9 $\mu M^{-1}s^{-1}$	4 $\mu M^{-1}s^{-1}$
Dissociation of GTP tubulin	44 s^{-1}	23 s^{-1}
Association of GDP tubulin	Unknown	Unknown
Dissociation of GDP tubulin	733 s^{-1}	915 s^{-1}
Steady-State Dynamic Instability		
Frequency of catastrophe in vitro at 7 μM tubulin	0.0045 s^{-1}	0.003 s^{-1}
Frequency of rescue in vitro at 7 μM tubulin	0.02 s^{-1}	0.06 s^{-1}
Microtubule dynamic instability in live cells		
Frequency of catastrophe in vivo (interphase)	0.014 s^{-1}	
Frequency of catastrophe in vivo (mitosis)	0.017 s^{-1}	
Frequency of rescue in vivo (interphase)	0.046 s^{-1}	
Frequency of rescue in vivo (mitosis)	0	

Data from Walker RA, et al: Dynamic instability of individual microtubules. J Cell Biol 107:1437–1448, 1988.

tubule polymer and monomer concentrations are stable, but the microtubule number declines as some microtubules disappear and the survivors grow longer. Direct observation by light microscopy (Fig. 37–8*A*) shows that this behavior is attributable to random, rapid fluctuations in the length of microtubules. Amazingly, growing and shrinking microtubules coexist at steady-state; some shrinking microtubules disappear while others grow. This assembly behavior is called **dynamic instability.** Remarkably, microtubule assembly was studied in detail for more than a decade before dynamic instability was discovered.

At steady-state, individual microtubules grow slowly until they undergo a random transition to a phase of rapid shortening. This transition is called a **catastrophe.** As they shorten, tubulin is lost from the end at a rate of nearly 1000 dimers per second, so the polymer shrinks more than 0.5 μm per second. Electron micrographs of rapidly shortening microtubules show curved segments of protofilaments peeling out from the end (see Fig. 37–8). Dimers may dissociate rapidly from these curved protofilaments and sheets before or after they break free from an end. Rapid shortening is terminated by another random event called a **rescue,** after which the microtubule grows again at a steady rate. Rescue is more likely at the minus end than the plus end (see Table 37–1). Occasionally, a microtubule disappears completely during a shortening phase because its length reaches zero before a rescue event occurs.

Most investigators believe that hydrolysis of GTP bound to the (exchangeable) E-site on β-tubulin drives dynamic instability because GTP hydrolysis occurs during polymerization and because GDP-microtubules are so unstable. Dimeric tubulin hydrolyzes E-site GTP very slowly, but when incorporated into a microtubule, contacts with the adjacent α-subunit stimulate hydrolysis by 250-fold ($k \sim 0.3$ s^{-1}). The γ-phosphate then dissociates ($k = 0.02$ s^{-1}). In contrast,

box 37–1

PHARMACOLOGIC TOOLS FOR STUDYING TUBULIN AND MICROTUBULES

Tubulin dimers bind several therapeutically active plant alkaloids and synthetic chemicals. *Colchicine* (from the autumn crocus) and *nocodazole* (a synthetic chemical) inhibit microtubule assembly by binding dissociated tubulin dimers and reducing their affinity for microtubule ends. *Vinblastine* (from periwinkle) inhibits microtubule assembly by favoring alternate oligomeric assemblies. *Taxol* (from the bark of the western yew) binds β-tubulin and stabilizes microtubules. At substoichiometric concentrations, vinblastine and taxol are effective in cancer chemotherapy because they interfere with the dynamic instability of mitotic spindle microtubules and block cell division. Colchicine is used empirically to treat gout, a painful condition that results from the accumulation of uric acid crystals in joints and other tissues, but no one knows precisely how it works.

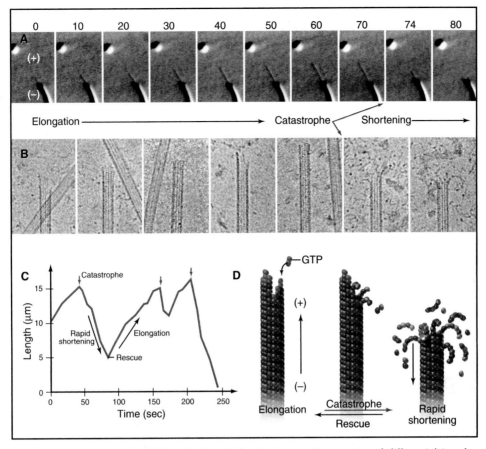

Figure 37-8 Dynamic instability of microtubules in vitro. *A*, Time series of differential interference contrast (DIC) light micrographs of a microtubule growing steadily from the broken end of an axoneme in the presence of 11-μM GTP tubulin. At 70 seconds, a catastrophe occurs and the microtubule shortens rapidly. *B*, Electron micrographs of frozen samples. Growing microtubules have flat or oblique ends interpreted as sheets of polymerized tubulin that have not yet closed up into a tube. Rapidly shortening microtubules have protofilaments and sheets peeling from the end. *C*, Time course of the fluctuations in the length of a microtubule from an experiment similar to *A*. *D*, Model for the transitions during steady-state dynamic instability of microtubules in vitro. GTP tubulin is blue-green; GDP tubulin is red-orange. (*A*, From Walker RA, et al: Dynamic instability of individual microtubules. J Cell Biol 107:1437–1448, 1988. *B*, From Mandelkow E-M, Mandelkow E, Milligan RA: Microtubule dynamics and microtubule caps: A time-resolved cryo-electron microscopy study. J Cell Biol 114:977–991, 1991. *A* and *B*, By copyright permission of the Rockefeller University Press. *C*, Reference: Erickson HP, O'Brien E: Microtubule dynamic instability and GTP hydrolysis. Annu Rev Biophys 21:145–166, 1992.)

the β-subunit does not provide analogous residues for the α-subunit, so its GTP is not hydrolyzed in the dimer or in microtubules. Thus, so-called GDP tubulin has GDP on the β-subunit and GTP on the α-subunit.

GTP hydrolysis creates microtubules with a core of potentially unstable GDP tubulin capped at both ends with GTP tubulin. GTP tubulin is thought to stabilize the ends of microtubules because microtubules assembled from dimers with slowly hydrolyzed GTP analogues bound to the β-subunit are unusually stable. GTP caps are maintained by exchange of tubulin dimer with bound GTP at the ends and by direct exchange of GTP onto the β-tubulin subunits exposed

at the plus end. The size of the GTP cap is expected to be small and has been difficult to measure, as few subunits are involved compared with the number of GDP subunits in the core of a microtubule (1600/μm).

Loss of the GTP cap is thought to cause a catastrophe. No one knows how many terminal subunits must have GDP before a catastrophe occurs, but computer models based on reasonable assumptions (including a single layer of GTP subunits in the cap) predict many features of dynamic instability. If the GTP cap is lost, the end shortens rapidly because the dissociation rate constant of GDP tubulin is very large compared with that of GTP tubulin. The energy derived from GTP hydrolysis is released during disintegration of the end of the microtubule, so hydrolysis can be viewed as a step that prepares the polymer for rapid depolymerization. "A catastrophe of an elongating microtubule is like removing the cork from a shaken bottle of champagne." (Michael Caplow, University of North Carolina) The tendency of GDP-tubulin protofilaments to curve into inside-out rings may contribute to their peeling rapidly off the ends of microtubules.

The GTP-cap hypothesis is an attractive explanation for catastrophes and is likely to be true in many respects. As expected, the frequency of catastrophes is inversely proportional to the concentration of GTP-tubulin dimers, declining to near zero at high concentrations. However, GDP ends do not inevitably shorten. If a microtubule is physically cut in the middle (presumably exposing two GDP ends), the plus end usually shortens as expected, but the newly exposed minus end continues to grow. If simply exposing GDP tubulin initiated a catastrophe, both ends would shorten. However, both ends do rapidly shorten within several seconds after dilution of the tubulin pool, indicating that long-term stability of both ends depends on GTP-tubulin association.

If rapid dissociation of GDP tubulin drives shortening, it is logical to assume that recapping with GTP tubulin would rescue a shortening microtubule. This hypothesis is also likely to be true in some ways, but the actual mechanism is complicated. For example, the frequency of rescue depends only weakly on the concentration of GTP tubulin.

It may seem odd that most microtubules grow at steady-state when the dimer concentration is close to the critical concentration. This is possible because catastrophes of other microtubules continuously liberate GDP-tubulin oligomers and dimers that slowly exchange GDP for GTP. This regenerates a pool of GTP-tubulin dimers at a concentration above the critical concentration to support elongation.

Initiation of Microtubules in Cells

Spontaneous nucleation of microtubules from tubulin dimers is so unfavorable that it may be irrelevant to living cells. In vitro, this slow nucleation accounts for a substantial lag of minutes during the formation of microtubules from purified tubulin. Presumably, tubulin dimers form oligomers that assemble into small sheets of protofilaments and eventually close to form a cylinder, but the details are still under investigation.

Instead of spontaneous nucleation, virtually all cellular microtubules arise from microtubule-organizing centers, including basal bodies (see Chapter 41)

and pericentrosomal material (Fig. 37–9). This organizing center surrounding centrioles contains 25-nm rings of about a dozen γ-tubulin molecules associated with multiple copies of 5 or 6 other proteins (Table 37–2). This **γ-tubulin ring complex** is shaped like a lock washer with a cap on one side. Loss of γ-tubulin interferes with microtubule nucleation in vivo. The γ-tubulin ring complex nucleates microtubules and caps their minus ends. One model is that the microtubule grows from the open face of the ring.

Microtubule-Associated Proteins

A growing number of proteins are known to regulate microtubule assembly and architecture (Table 37–3). Developmentally programmed gene expression establishes the mix of MAPs in each cell type. These mixtures influence the organization and dynamics of microtubules and, secondarily, the shape of the cell. Many additional accessory proteins are required to form axonemes of cilia and flagella (see Chapter 41).

The inventory of MAPs is biased toward proteins that stabilize microtubules. The original MAPs were discovered when they copurified from vertebrate brains along with microtubules during cycles of microtubule assembly and disassembly. The product is about 80% tubulin and 20% MAPs. Copurification se-

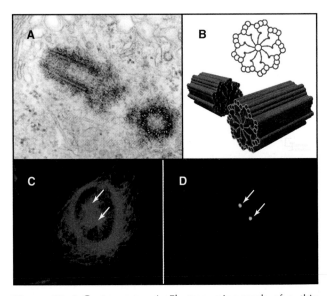

Figure 37–9 Centrosomes. *A,* Electron micrograph of a thin section of a centrosome showing the pair of centrioles surrounded by the pericentriolar microtubule-organizing material. *B,* Drawings of centrioles. *C* and *D,* A pair of fluorescence micrographs of HeLa cells stained simultaneously with antibodies to β-tubulin (*C*) and γ-tubulin (*D*). γ-Tubulin is concentrated in centrosomes (*arrows*). (*A,* Courtesy of D. W. Fawcett, Harvard Medical School. *C* and *D,* Courtesy of H. Joshi, Emory University Medical School.)

table 37–2
CENTROSOMAL PROTEINS

Name	Distribution	Composition	Properties	Functions
γ-Tubulin Ring Complex	Eukaryotes	12 × 50 kD (δ tubulin) Multiple 66 kD Multiple 97 kD Multiple 98 kD 1 × 118 kD Multiple 224 kD	Polymeric rings in pericentriolar material and yeast spindle pole bodies	Binds minus end of microtubules and nucleates their assembly
Centrosomin	*Drosophila*	115 kD	Coiled-coil protein in centrosomes	Required for spindle formation and recruitment of CP60 and CP190 to poles
CP60	*Drosophila*	48-kD oligomers	Nucleus in interphase; centrosome in mitosis	Binds microtubules; copurifies with CP190
CP190	*Drosophila*	120-kD ? dimer	Nucleus in interphase; centrosome in mitosis	Binds microtubules; copurifies with CP60
NuMA	Vertebrates	2 × 236 kD	Coiled-coil protein; nucleus in interphase; centrosome in mitosis	Interacts with dynein to focus microtubules at spindle poles
Pericentrin	Animals Plants	2 × 218 kD	Coiled-coil protein in pericentriolar matrix; insoluble	Required for spindle formation

lects a subset of MAPs that bind tightly to microtubules, but it misses important proteins that bind weakly, including the motor protein kinesin. New functional assays for proteins that bind transiently or weakly to microtubules are yielding additional MAPs. For example, a light microscopic assay for microtubule fragmentation has led to the severing protein katanin. Non-neuronal cells of animals, plants, fungi, and pro-

table 37–3
MICROTUBULE-ASSOCIATED PROTEINS

Name (Synonyms)	Distribution	Composition	Properties	Functions
Destabilizers				
Op18/stathmin (prosolin, metablastin)	Vertebrate cells	1 × 18 kD	Binds tubulin dimers	Enhances dynamic instability; null mice viable without defects
XKCM1 (MCAK)	Vertebrate	2 × 82 kD	Kinesin-related but not a motor	Promotes microtubule disassembly at kinetochores
Severing				
Katanin	Metazoans	1 × 84 kD 1 × 60 kD	MT-stimulated ATPase; ATP-dependent MT severing	
Stabilizers				
E-MAP 115	Vertebrate epithelial cells	? × 84 kD	Phosphorylation inhibits MT binding	May stabilize MTs
MAP1A	Axons of vertebrate neurons, glia, and other cells	1 × 277 kD 1 × 30 kD 1 × 28 kD 1 × 16 kD	150-nm rod	Promotes MT assembly

Table continued on following page

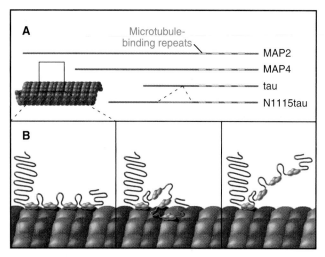

Figure 37-11 Tau, MAP2, and MAP4. *A,* Comparison of the primary structures, showing the homologous tubulin-binding motifs. *B,* The tubulin-binding motifs are thought to exchange rapidly among tubulin subunits on the surface of microtubules. (Redrawn from Butner KA, Kirschner M: Tau protein binds to microtubules through a flexible array of distributed weak sites. J Cell Biol 115:717–730, 1991, by copyright permission of the Rockefeller University Press.)

brains (Fig. 37–12*B*). It is also present in some neuronal cell bodies and glial cells. Alternate splicing produces seven tau isoforms from a single tau gene. Most of these isoforms have molecular weights of 40–50 kD, but high-molecular-weight tau, found mainly in peripheral nerves, is larger. Fetal brains express tau isoforms with three tubulin-binding motifs, whereas isoforms with four repeats predominate in adults. Multiple isoforms and partial phosphorylation of nearly 20 sites produce more than 30 tau species that can be resolved by electrophoresis. As expected from its ability to stabilize microtubules in vitro, reduction in the tau concentration in cultured nerve cells by antisense RNA expression reduces the numbers of microtubules and axon-like cellular processes. Nevertheless, mice survive the loss of their single tau gene with only minor alterations of their neurons. Compensation by other MAPs is postulated to account for the differences in the acute and chronic loss of tau.

In **Alzheimer's disease,** the most common dementia of older persons, and other degenerative diseases of the brain, tau forms **paired helical filaments** (Fig. 37–13) that aggregate in "neurofibrillary tangles" that are a hallmark of the disease and are used to judge its severity by light microscopy. Tau in these filaments is heavily phosphorylated on several sites, truncated by proteolysis, and cross-linked by a disulfide bond. These highly insoluble and proteolytically resistant paired helical filaments may result from, rather than cause, neuronal degeneration, although

mutations in the tau gene occur in some rare familial dementias.

MAP2 is concentrated in dendrites of neurons (see Fig. 37–12A). The mechanism giving preferential distribution of MAP2 in dendrites and tau in axons of the same cell is still largely a mystery. MAP4 shares many features with MAP2, but is expressed by glial cells in the nervous system and by many other cells and tissues.

High-molecular-weight **MAP1A** and **1B** form a distinct family that differs in many ways from the heat-stable tau family. These MAPs are heat-labile, lack the 18-residue tubulin-binding repeats, and are synthesized as polyproteins that are cleaved to form the heavy chain and one of the light chains. A region near the N-terminus is thought to bind light chains and microtubules. The C-terminus forms a rod-shaped projection on the surface of microtubules. Developing neurons express MAP1B earlier than any other known MAP. As in the case of tau, mice with null mutations of MAP1B are viable with minimal defects.

Other stabilizing proteins have novel properties: STOP binds microtubules, making them resistant to depolymerization by cold, dilution, or drugs. Calcium-calmodulin (see Chapter 28) inhibits STOP. Bird red blood cells express syncolin, which stabilizes the marginal band of microtubules. Tektins are fibrous proteins that stabilize microtubules in axonemes (see Chapter 41) and centrioles.

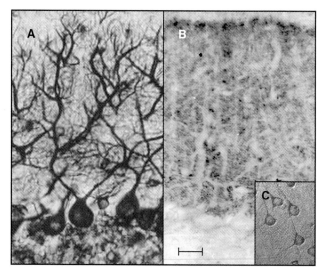

Figure 37-12 Distributions of tau and MAP2 in sections of the cerebellum from rat brain labeled with antibodies and subjected to a histochemical method producing a dark stain. *A,* MAP2 is concentrated in the cell bodies and dendrites of Purkinje cells. *B,* Tau is concentrated in the axons of granule cells, which appear here as small dark dots. *C,* Tau staining in the cell body and neurites of a pyramidal cell from another part of the brain. (Courtesy of L. Binder, Northwestern University Medical School.)

table 37–2

CENTROSOMAL PROTEINS

Name	Distribution	Composition	Properties	Functions
γ-Tubulin Ring Complex	Eukaryotes	12 × 50 kD (δ tubulin) Multiple 66 kD Multiple 97 kD Multiple 98 kD 1 X 118 kD Multiple 224 kD	Polymeric rings in pericentriolar material and yeast spindle pole bodies	Binds minus end of microtubules and nucleates their assembly
Centrosomin	*Drosophila*	115 kD	Coiled-coil protein in centrosomes	Required for spindle formation and recruitment of CP60 and CP190 to poles
CP60	*Drosophila*	48-kD oligomers	Nucleus in interphase; centrosome in mitosis	Binds microtubules; copurifies with CP190
CP190	*Drosophila*	120-kD ? dimer	Nucleus in interphase; centrosome in mitosis	Binds microtubules; copurifies with CP60
NuMA	Vertebrates	2 × 236 kD	Coiled-coil protein; nucleus in interphase; centrosome in mitosis	Interacts with dynein to focus microtubules at spindle poles
Pericentrin	Animals Plants	2 × 218 kD	Coiled-coil protein in pericentriolar matrix; insoluble	Required for spindle formation

lects a subset of MAPs that bind tightly to microtubules, but it misses important proteins that bind weakly, including the motor protein kinesin. New functional assays for proteins that bind transiently or weakly to microtubules are yielding additional MAPs. For example, a light microscopic assay for microtubule fragmentation has led to the severing protein katanin. Non-neuronal cells of animals, plants, fungi, and pro-

table 37–3

MICROTUBULE-ASSOCIATED PROTEINS

Name (Synonyms)	Distribution	Composition	Properties	Functions
Destabilizers				
Op18/stathmin (prosolin, metablastin)	Vertebrate cells	1 × 18 kD	Binds tubulin dimers	Enhances dynamic instability; null mice viable without defects
XKCM1 (MCAK)	Vertebrate	2 × 82 kD	Kinesin-related but not a motor	Promotes microtubule disassembly at kinetochores
Severing				
Katanin	Metazoans	1 × 84 kD 1 × 60 kD	MT-stimulated ATPase; ATP-dependent MT severing	
Stabilizers				
E-MAP 115	Vertebrate epithelial cells	? × 84 kD	Phosphorylation inhibits MT binding	May stabilize MTs
MAP1A	Axons of vertebrate neurons, glia, and other cells	1 × 277 kD 1 × 30 kD 1 × 28 kD 1 × 16 kD	150-nm rod	Promotes MT assembly

Table continued on following page

table 37–3

MICROTUBULE-ASSOCIATED PROTEINS *Continued*

Name (Synonyms)	Distribution	Composition	Properties	Functions
MAP1B (MAP5)	Vertebrate neurons and other cells	1 × 243 kD 1 × 30 kD 1 × 28 kD 1 × 16 kD	200-nm rod; expressed during brain development	Promotes MT assembly; null mutation well tolerated by mice
MAP2	Dendrites of vertebrate neurons	One gene, 4 isoforms: MAP2a 1 × 200 kD MAP2b 1 × 200 kD MAP 2c 1 × 42 kD	200-nm rod; 3 or 4 18-residue MT-binding repeats	Promotes MT assembly; binds regulatory subunit of PKA; binds actin
MAP 4 (MAP3, MAPU)	Vertebrate brain glia, many other cell types	1 × 135 kD	3 or 4 18-residue MT-binding repeats; phosphorylation inhibits MT binding	Promotes MT assembly and stability
STOP	Vertebrate cells	100 kD	Inhibited by either calcium/calmodulin or phosphorylation	Stabilizes MT against cold depolymerization
Syncolin	Chicken red blood cells	? × 280 kD	Relative of MAP2	Stabilizes marginal band MTs in red blood cells
Tau	Vertebrates; axon of neurons and other cells; big tau in peripheral nerves	One gene, 6 isoforms 1 × 40–50 kD; big tau 1 × 80 kD	3 or 4 18-residue MT-binding repeats; paired helical filaments in Alzheimer's disease	Promotes MT assembly and stability; mice tolerate null mutation
Tektin	Metazoan axonemes and cytoplasmic MTs	2 × 47–53 kD	Coiled-coil proteins	Stabilizes MTs in axonemes and centrioles
Dis1/TOG (XMAP215)	All eukaryotes	1 × 215 kD	60-nm long flexible molecule	Promotes plus-end MT assembly
XMAP230	Various *Xenopus* cell types	1 × 230 kD	Phosphorylated by mitotic kinases with lowered MT affinity	Stabilizes MTs against catastrophes
Linkers				
CLIP-170 (Restin)	Vertebrates, insects	170 kD	Phosphorylation inhibits MT binding	Binds endosomes to plus end of MTs
Gephyrin	Vertebrate neurons	? × 93 kD		Anchors glycine receptors to MTs
MAST (orbit)	Vertebrates, insects	? × 165 kD	Binds MT plus ends and CLIP-170	Binds kinetochores to plus ends
Other				
APC	Vertebrates, insects	1 × 300 kD	Binds and regulates β-catenin	Tumor suppressor; loss leads to colon polyps and cancer
Mapmodulin	Vertebrate cells	1 × 28 kD	Binds MT-binding repeats of tau, MAPs	Promotes dynein-driven organelle movements on MTs
Motors				
Kinesins	Eukaryotes	Multiple isoforms (see Chapter 40)	MT-stimulated ATPase plus-end motors	Organelle transport; mitotic spindle function
Cytoplasmic dynein (MAP1C)	Eukaryotes	2 × 410 kD 3 × 74 kD 4 × 55–59 kD ? × 8–21 kD	MT-stimulated ATPase; minus-end motor; binds dynactin complex	Organelle transport; mitotic spindle function

MT, microtubule; PKA, protein kinase A.

tozoa also have MAPs, but MAPS are generally more abundant in the brain. Genetic screens are also uncovering new proteins that regulate microtubules, such as the fission yeast protein Tea1p that associates the ends of microtubules and directs cellular elongation.

Most of what is understood about the functions of MAPs has been inferred from their distribution in particular parts of cells and from their effects on microtubules in biochemical assays. In a few cases, direct experimental evidence has shown that they modify the behavior of microtubules in living cells, but genetic experiments continue to produce surprises. For instance, mice with null mutations of tau, a major neuronal MAP, have no obvious defects (see Table 37–3).

Microtubule-Stabilizing MAPs

At least a dozen distinct MAPs stabilize microtubules (see Table 37–3). Most bind along the length of microtubules rather than capping an end. Several rod-shaped MAPs project from the microtubule surface, whereas tektins are long polymers that lie parallel to the protofilaments. Some are expressed widely, but others are restricted to specialized cells.

The **tau** family, including **MAP2** and **MAP4,** differ in size and pattern of expression but share many common features (Figs. 37–10 and 37–11).

- They share similar tubulin-binding motifs consisting of 18 residues arrayed in 3 or 4 imperfect tandem repeats separated by flexible linkers of 13 variable residues. Each repeat binds independently to a tubulin subunit.
- They are remarkably heat-stable, so purification may be accomplished simply by boiling to denature other proteins.
- All are rod-shaped, forming whisker-like projections on the surface of microtubules (see Fig. 37–10). The long side arm of MAP2 excludes structures, including other microtubules, from the immediate vicinity (see Fig. 38–9). This accounts for the wide spacing of microtubules in dendrites compared with axons, where the smaller tau predominates. Neither tau nor MAP2 cross-link to other microtubules, but they do bind actin filaments.
- Tau family MAPs can stabilize microtubules. For example, in the presence of tau, microtubules grow three times faster, shorten in half the time, and have catastrophes only 2% as frequently as pure tubulin microtubules. The rapid equilibrium of individual tubulin-binding repeats with the microtubule surface may allow tau to dampen microtubule dynamics without stopping tubulin association and dissociation altogether.
- Phosphorylation of the microtubule-binding motifs by MARKs (MAP affinity–regulating kinases) inhibits binding and destabilizes microtubules. The effects of phosphorylation by other kinases at other numerous potential sites are less well understood.
- An accessory protein, mapmodulin, regulates these MAPs by competing with microtubules for the microtubule-binding motifs. This competition may clear the way for motor proteins like dynein to move cargo along microtubules.

Tau, named for tubulin-associated protein, is the major MAP in the axons of neurons in vertebrate

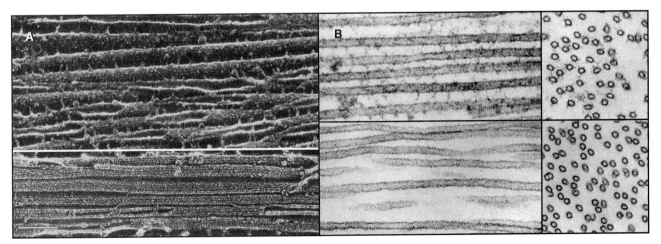

Figure 37–10 Electron micrographs of tau and MAP2 bound to microtubules. *A,* Frozen, deep-etched, and shadowed specimens of microtubules with tau *(upper panel)* and pure tubulin microtubules *(lower panel). B,* Thin sections of microtubules with MAP2 showing 40- to 100-nm projections *(upper panels)* and bare pure tubulin microtubules *(lower panels). (A,* Courtesy of N. Hirokawa, Toyko University. Reference: Hirokawa N, Shiomura Y, Okabe S: Tau proteins: The molecular structure and mode of binding on microtubules. J Cell Biol 107:1449–1459, 1988. *B,* Courtesy of D. B. Murphy, Johns Hopkins Medical School.)

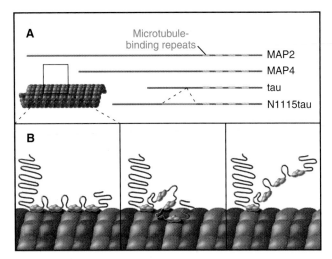

Figure 37-11 Tau, MAP2, and MAP4. *A*, Comparison of the primary structures, showing the homologous tubulin-binding motifs. *B*, The tubulin-binding motifs are thought to exchange rapidly among tubulin subunits on the surface of microtubules. (Redrawn from Butner KA, Kirschner M: Tau protein binds to microtubules through a flexible array of distributed weak sites. J Cell Biol 115:717–730, 1991, by copyright permission of the Rockefeller University Press.)

brains (Fig. 37–12*B*). It is also present in some neuronal cell bodies and glial cells. Alternate splicing produces seven tau isoforms from a single tau gene. Most of these isoforms have molecular weights of 40–50 kD, but high-molecular-weight tau, found mainly in peripheral nerves, is larger. Fetal brains express tau isoforms with three tubulin-binding motifs, whereas isoforms with four repeats predominate in adults. Multiple isoforms and partial phosphorylation of nearly 20 sites produce more than 30 tau species that can be resolved by electrophoresis. As expected from its ability to stabilize microtubules in vitro, reduction in the tau concentration in cultured nerve cells by antisense RNA expression reduces the numbers of microtubules and axon-like cellular processes. Nevertheless, mice survive the loss of their single tau gene with only minor alterations of their neurons. Compensation by other MAPs is postulated to account for the differences in the acute and chronic loss of tau.

In **Alzheimer's disease,** the most common dementia of older persons, and other degenerative diseases of the brain, tau forms **paired helical filaments** (Fig. 37–13) that aggregate in "neurofibrillary tangles" that are a hallmark of the disease and are used to judge its severity by light microscopy. Tau in these filaments is heavily phosphorylated on several sites, truncated by proteolysis, and cross-linked by a disulfide bond. These highly insoluble and proteolytically resistant paired helical filaments may result from, rather than cause, neuronal degeneration, although

mutations in the tau gene occur in some rare familial dementias.

MAP2 is concentrated in dendrites of neurons (see Fig. 37–12*A*). The mechanism giving preferential distribution of MAP2 in dendrites and tau in axons of the same cell is still largely a mystery. MAP4 shares many features with MAP2, but is expressed by glial cells in the nervous system and by many other cells and tissues.

High-molecular-weight **MAP1A** and **1B** form a distinct family that differs in many ways from the heat-stable tau family. These MAPs are heat-labile, lack the 18-residue tubulin-binding repeats, and are synthesized as polyproteins that are cleaved to form the heavy chain and one of the light chains. A region near the N-terminus is thought to bind light chains and microtubules. The C-terminus forms a rod-shaped projection on the surface of microtubules. Developing neurons express MAP1B earlier than any other known MAP. As in the case of tau, mice with null mutations of MAP1B are viable with minimal defects.

Other stabilizing proteins have novel properties: STOP binds microtubules, making them resistant to depolymerization by cold, dilution, or drugs. Calcium-calmodulin (see Chapter 28) inhibits STOP. Bird red blood cells express syncolin, which stabilizes the marginal band of microtubules. Tektins are fibrous proteins that stabilize microtubules in axonemes (see Chapter 41) and centrioles.

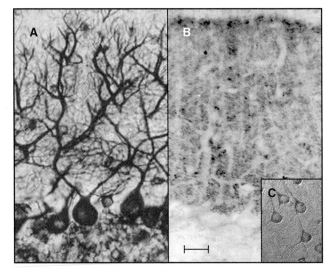

Figure 37-12 Distributions of tau and MAP2 in sections of the cerebellum from rat brain labeled with antibodies and subjected to a histochemical method producing a dark stain. *A*, MAP2 is concentrated in the cell bodies and dendrites of Purkinje cells. *B*, Tau is concentrated in the axons of granule cells, which appear here as small dark dots. *C*, Tau staining in the cell body and neurites of a pyramidal cell from another part of the brain. (Courtesy of L. Binder, Northwestern University Medical School.)

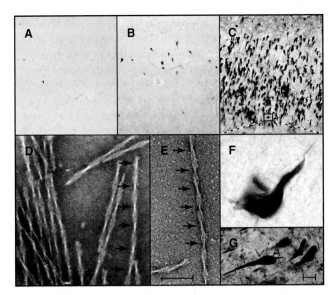

Figure 37–13 Neurofibrillary tangles of paired helical filaments in the brains of patients with Alzheimer's disease. *A to C,* Light micrographs of sections of the hippocampus of human brains stained with silver for neurofibrillary tangles. *A,* Stage I with few tangles. *B,* Stage III with moderate numbers of tangles. *C,* Stage V, advanced Alzheimer's disease, showing abundant tangles. *D,* Electron micrograph of paired helical filaments isolated from Alzheimer's neurofilbrillary tangles and prepared by negative staining. *E,* Electron micrograph of a negatively stained, paired, helical filament reassembled in vitro from recombinant tau protein. *F and G,* High-powered micrographs of neurofibrillary tangles from the brain of an Alzheimer's patient stained brown with an antibody to tau. (*A to C* and *G,* Courtesy of E. and H. Braak, University of Frankfurt. *D* and *E,* Courtesy of E.-M. Mandelkow, Max Planck Institute, Hamburg. *F,* Courtesy of L. Binder, Northwestern University Medical School.)

Microtulule-Destabilizing MAPs

In principle, cells might destabilize microtubules in three different ways. First, cellular factors might promote catastrophes, as proposed for Op18/stathmin. **Op18/stathmin** is a small protein that destabilizes microtubules in vitro by sequestering tubulin dimers and promoting catastrophes. The protein consists of a long α-helix that binds laterally to a pair of tubulin dimers, blocking their polymerization. Overexpression in cell lines reduces tubulin polymerization. Many malignant cells express unusually high levels of Op18 (hence its name, oncoprotein 18). Phosphorylation inhibits Op18 and may be required for tubulin to form a mitotic spindle.

Second, factors might actively remove subunits from the ends of microtubules. One family of kinesin-related proteins has such activity. These unusual kinesins were discovered independently in experiments searching for motor proteins active in mitosis (hence MCAK = mitotic centromere associated kinesin) and for factors that disassemble microtubules (XKCM1 =

Xenopus kinesin central motor 1). **XKCM1/MCAK** has a motor domain in the middle of the polypeptide chains but is not thought to be a motor that moves cargo. ATP hydrolysis by the motor domain is thought to stress the lattice of tubulin subunits at the plus end of microtubules and to promote disassembly. Depletion of MCAK results in the failure of chromosomes to move to the poles during anaphase of mitosis, presumably because microtubule shortening at centromere depends on these kinesins (see Chapter 47).

Third, actively severing microtubules creates additional ends for depolymerization. **Katanin** is a heterodimeric protein that can sever microtubules into short fragments, even when they are stabilized by taxol. These fragments depolymerize into tubulin dimers that are capable of reassembly. Severing requires ATP hydrolysis by katanin, which is a member of the AAA ATPase family that includes dynein and NSF. Activation of this severing function during mitosis may contribute to remodeling of the interphase microtubule network.

MAPs Associated with Growing Plus Ends

A growing number of proteins and protein complexes associate with microtubule plus ends. The founding example **CLIP-170** (Bik1p in budding yeast, Tip1p in fission yeast) links membranes (see Fig. 40–7) and the dynactin complex (see Fig. 40–4) to microtubule plus ends. In fission yeast-growing microtubules carry Tip1p with an associated protein Tea1p to the ends of the cell, where Tea1p directs the polar growth of the cell. A second family of plus end MAPs includes vertebrate EB1 (Bim1p in budding yeast, Ma13p in fission yeast). EB1 links the human tumor suppressor protein APC (see Fig. 32–8) to microtubule plus ends. Proteins in both of these families surf along microtubules near their growing plus ends. The mechanism is not known, but they appear to bind to newly incorporated tubulin subunits at the plus end. After a short time, they dissociate and recycle back to the growing tip. A third class of plus end MAPs is the **Dis1/TOG** family of proteins (called XMAP215 in frogs). This is the only family of MAPs found in animals, plants, and fungi. In a wide range of species, Dis1/TOG proteins appear to stabilize microtubule plus ends and to play an important role in assembly of mitotic spindles. Interestingly, a mixture of tubulin, XMAP-215, and the depolymerizing kinesin XKCM1 can recapitulate microtubule dynamic instability very similar to that seen in extracts from mitotic cells. Another MAP, the chromosomal passenger protein INCENP (see Chapter 47), targets the aurora-B kinase to the central spindle and may regulate its kinase activity toward spindle components. An emerging family of MAPs that includes *Drosophila*

MAST/Orbit appears to be required for kinetochores to hold on to the plus end of dynamic microtubules during mitosis.

Linker Proteins

Gephyrin was discovered in the spinal cord as a peripheral membrane protein associated with the cytoplasmic domain of neuronal plasma membrane receptors for the neurotransmitter glycine. Later experiments showed that gephyrin binds microtubules and is required for clustering of glycine receptors in the plane of the membrane. A physical link between the receptor and microtubules is hypothesized to account for clustering.

Microtubule Dynamics in Cells

Microtubule dynamics in cells (Fig. 37–14A) are remarkably similar to those simple buffers in vitro (see Table 37–1). Despite frequent catastrophes ($k = 0.01$ s^{-1}) during which they shorten rapidly (0.28 μm s^{-1}), interphase microtubules generally are long, both because the chance of rescue is high ($k = 0.05$ s^{-1}) and because growth during the elongation phase (at a rate of 0.11 μm s^{-1}) restores their length before the next catastrophe. As a result of this dynamic instability, the bulk of interphase microtubules have a half-life of about 10 minutes. A subset of microtubules is much more stable. These microtubules are enriched in detyrosinated and acetylated tubulin and are resistant to depolymerization by nocodazole. MAPs, such as members of the Dis1/TOG family, are postulated to stabi-

lize their plus ends. These proteins bind to microtubule plus ends and reduce the frequency of catastrophes. In addition, the minus ends of stable microtubules are anchored to and may be stabilized by γ-tubulin complexes in the centrosome. A few microtubules detach from the centrosome and undergo a treadmilling reaction whereby the plus end grows while the minus end shrinks (see Fig. 37–14B). Unknown cytoplasmic conditions favor treadmilling, which is slow for purified tubulin in vitro owing to the similar critical concentrations at the two ends (see Fig. 37–7).

Conditions in cells influence the dynamics and the resulting lengths of cytoplasmic microtubules. The most dramatic transition occurs as a cell enters mitosis (see Fig. 37–2). Mitotic microtubules are much shorter and more dynamic than interphase microtubules. A mitotic microtubule grows out from the centrosome at a pole of the mitotic spindle and depolymerizes completely after a brief lifetime unless a kinetochore on a chromosome captures and stabilizes its plus end. Conflicting evidence suggests that this behavior is caused either by an increased frequency of catastrophe or a decreased frequency of rescue. This modulation of microtubule stability undoubtedly involves mitotic kinases, but the mechanisms are still being investigated. Phosphorylation of some MAPs decreases their affinity for microtubules, and their dissociation destabilizes microtubules.

Both the tubulin isoform composition and associated proteins influence microtubule dynamics. Microtubules assembled from tubulin isoforms of intrinsically stable microtubules (marginal band of avian red blood cells) are more stable than brain microtubules. Associated proteins can either stabilize the polymer by reducing the frequency of catastrophes and the rate of shortening or destabilize microtubules as described above. In extreme cases, such as in ciliary axonemes, the microtubules remain stable for days, even under conditions that would depolymerize cytoplasmic microtubules. Tubulin purified from axonemes forms microtubules that are just as labile as cytoplasmic microtubules, so the difference must lie with the associated proteins.

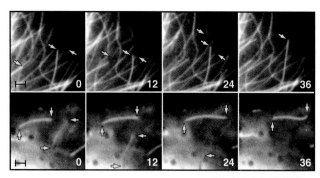

Figure 37–14 Dynamic instability of microtubules in vivo. Time series of fluorescence micrographs of a cultured vertebrate cell microinjected with rhodamine-labeled tubulin. *Upper row,* The plus ends of microtubules anchored at the centrosome grow and shrink randomly in the same cell *(arrows). Lower row,* Free microtubules treadmill, growing at their plus end at about the same rate as shortening proceeds at their minus end. Marking a spot on such microtubules shows that this is treadmilling rather than transport of a stable microtubule through cytoplasm. (Courtesy of G. Borisy, University of Wisconsin, Madison.)

Selected Readings

Cassimeris L: Accessory protein regulation of microtubule dynamics. Curr Opin Cell Biol 11:134–141, 1999.

Desai A, Mitchison TJ: Microtubule polymerization dynamics. Annu Rev Cell Dev Biol 13:83–118, 1998.

Drewes G, Ebneth A, Mandelkow E-M: MAPs, MARKS and microtubules dynamics. Trends Biochem Sci 23:307–311, 1998.

Dutcher SK: The tubulin family: Alpha to eta. Curr Opin Cell Biol 13:49–54, 2001.

Hardy J, Duff K, Hardy KG, Perez-Tur J, Hutton M: Genetic dissection of Alzheimer's disease and related dementias: Amyloid and its relationship to tau. Nature Neurosci 1:355–358, 1998.

Houseweart MK, Cleveland DW: Cytoskeletal linkers: New MAPs for old destinations. Curr Biol 18:R864–866, 1999.

Kreis T, Vale R, eds: Guidebook to the Cytoskeletal and Motor Proteins, 2nd ed. New York: Oxford University Press, 1999.

Moritz M, Agard DA: Gamma-tubulin complexes and micro-tubule nucleation. Curr Opin Struct Biol 11:174–181, 2001.

Nogales E, Whittaker M, Milligan RA, Downing KH: High resolution model of the microtubule. Cell 96:79–88, 1999.

Ohkura H, Garcia MA, Toda T: Dis1/TOG universal microtu-bule adaptors—one MAP for all? J Cell Sci 114:3805–3812, 2001.

Schroer TA: Microtubules don and doff their caps: Dynamic attachments at plus and minus ends. Curr Opin Cell Biol 13:92–96, 2001.

Walczak CE: Microtubule dynamics and tubulin interacting proteins. Curr Opin Cell Biol 12:52–56, 2000.

Waterman-Storer CM, Salmon ED: Microtubule dynamics: Treadmilling comes around again. Curr Biol 7:R369–372, 1997.

Wiese C, Zheng Y: γ-Tubulin complex and its interaction with microtubule organizing centers. Curr Opin Struct Biol 9:250–259, 1999.

chapter 38

INTERMEDIATE FILAMENTS

Intermediate filaments (Fig. 38–1) are flexible but strong polymers that provide mechanical support for cells, especially to prevent excessive stretching of cells in the tissues of higher organisms. Mutations in intermediate filament protein subunits in humans and experimental animals dramatically compromise the integrity of tissues, such as skin and muscle, that depend upon intermediate filaments. The most widespread class of intermediate filaments, the nuclear lamins, reinforce the inner nuclear envelope and may also have an important role in organizing the chromosome architecture in interphase (see Chapter 16). Lamin genes are thought to be evolutionary progenitors of the large family of genes for cytoplasmic intermediate filaments of higher animals. Special intermediate filaments are major constituents of nails and hair. Hair illustrates nicely the flexibility and high tensile strength of intermediate filaments.

A continuous network of intermediate filaments stretches from the nuclear envelope to attachments on the plasma membrane called desmosomes and hemidesmosomes (see Chapter 33). This network transmits mechanical forces from one cell to another cell through desmosomes and to the extracellular matrix through hemidesmosomes. This continuum of intermediate filaments gives skin its mechanical integrity. Molecular defects in intermediate filaments or junctions associated with intermediate filaments result in rupture of skin cells and blistering diseases.

In contrast to the highly conserved actins and tubulins, the protein subunits of intermediate filaments vary considerably in sequence and size. However, all possess an α-helical coiled-coil domain that forms the core of the filaments. The more variable N- and C-terminal domains of the subunits project from the surface of the filaments and give each class of filaments,

expressed in specialized cell types, distinctive features. This molecular heterogeneity made it difficult to appreciate the general features of intermediate filament structure and function until the sequences of the proteins were determined in the 1980s.

Structure of Intermediate Filament Subunits

Vertebrates have more than 50 genes encoding 6 classes of intermediate filament proteins (Table 38–1). Each isoform has a unique amino acid sequence, but all these proteins share a rod-like domain with variable head and tail domains at the two ends (Fig. 38–2).

The rod is a parallel coiled-coil of two α helices, usually about 47 nm long (Fig. 38–3A). Analysis of sequences, spectroscopic data, and x-ray fiber diffraction from materials composed of intermediate filaments, like wool, has firmly established this coiled-coil structure of the rod. Like other coiled-coils (see Fig. 2–12), **rod domains** of intermediate filament proteins have a heptad repeat, with the first and fourth residues providing a continuous row of nonionic interactions along the interface of the two helices. Zones of positive and negative charge alternate along the rod. When staggered appropriately, these zones provide complementary electrostatic bonds for assembly of filaments. About 20 highly conserved residues at each end of the rod are essential for filament elongation through head to tail interactions between dimeric molecules. Amino acid sequences suggest three interruptions in the coiled-coil (see Fig. 38–2). One of these interruptions is often the site of mutations in mild cases of skin blistering disorders. Assembly studies

595

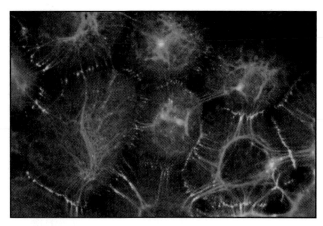

Figure 38-1 Fluorescence light micrograph of cultured epithelial cells stained with antibodies to keratin intermediate filaments (*orange*). Desmosomes are stained green. The network of keratin filaments stabilizes the cell against physical forces and reinforces desmosomal attachments between cells. (Courtesy of E. Smith and E. Fuchs, University of Chicago.)

with mutant proteins suggest that this part of the rod contributes to lateral associations within filaments.

Less is known about the structure and functions of the nonhelical N- and C-terminal domains, although nuclear magnetic resonance (NMR) studies provide evidence that these terminal domains are less tightly folded than the rod. The N- and C-terminal domains can influence assembly, and in some cases, project from the filament surface (see Fig. 38–3C) to interact with other cellular components.

Intermediate filament protein molecules are commonly referred to as "dimers," as they consist of two polypeptide chains. Some of the six classes of intermediate filament molecules are homodimers; others are heterodimers. **Lamins** and class III intermediate filament molecules are parallel dimers of identical polypeptides (see Fig. 38–3A), whereas **keratins** are obligate heterodimers of one acidic (class I) and one basic (class II) keratin polypeptide. Many intermediate filament molecules form relatively stable, partially overlapping, antiparallel molecular dimers (referred to as tetramers; see Fig. 38–3D) that are believed to be intermediates in polymer assembly.

Like other cytoskeletal proteins, sequence similarities are greater between species for each class of intermediate filament protein than for the different classes

table 38–1

CLASSIFICATION OF INTERMEDIATE FILAMENT (IF) PROTEINS BASED ON SEQUENCES OF THE ROD DOMAIN

Class	Type	Genes	Molecule	Distribution	Diseases
I	Acidic keratin	>15	40–65 kD, obligate heterodimer with class II	Epithelial cells	Blistering skin, corneal dystrophy, esophageal degeneration, brittle hair, liver cirrhosis, colon hyperplasia
II	Basic keratin	>15	51–68 kD, obligate heterodimer with class I	Epithelial cells	Similar to class I
III	Desmin	1	53 kD, homopolymers	Muscle cells	Generalized myopathy
	GFAP	1	50 kD, homopolymers	Glial cells	Mouse null viable
	Peripherin	1	57 kD	Peripheral > CNS neurons	
	Synemin	1	190 kD, interacts with other class III IFs	Muscle cells	
	Vimentin	1	54 kD, homopolymers and heteropolymers	Mesenchymal cells	Mouse null viable
IV	Neurofilaments				
	NFL	1	Obligate heteropolymers with NFM, NFH	Neurons	Mouse null viable
	NFM	1	Obligate heteropolymers with NFL, NFH	Neurons	
	NFH	1	Obligate heteropolymers with NFL, NFM	Neurons	Some mutations in amyotrophic lateral sclerosis
	α-Internexin	1	55 kD, homopolymers	Embryonic neurons	
V	Lamins	4	7 Isoforms, 62–72 kD, homodimers	Animal, plant nuclei	Cardiomyopathy, Emery-Dreifuss muscular dystrophy
VI	Nestin	1	230 kD, homopolymers	Embryonic neurons, muscle, other cells	

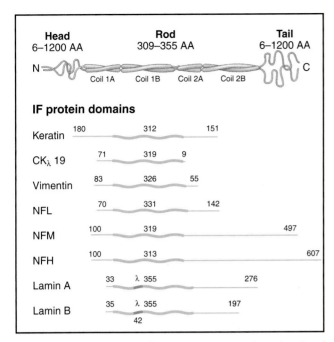

Figure 38-2 Intermediate filament (IF) proteins have head and tail domains of variable lengths flanking a central rod domain. Rod domains consist of a coiled-coil of about 310 residues that are 46.5 nm long. Lamins have an additional 42 residues in the rod (λ). Residues most important for assembly are at the beginning and end of the rod. End domains differ in sequence and size from 6 to 1200 residues.

of intermediate proteins within one species. For example, human **desmin** is much more similar to frog desmin than it is to human keratin. This strongly suggests that unique functional requirements of each class of intermediate filament protein arose early in animal evolution and have conferred strong selective pressure on the genes for each intermediate filament protein. Sequence comparisons and the detailed structure of the genes suggest that the ubiquitous nuclear lamins were the evolutionary progenitors of cytoplasmic intermediate filaments. According to this view, deletions in a primitive lamin gene removed 42 residues from the coiled-coil (also found in invertebrate intermediate filaments), the nuclear localization sequence, and the CAAX box (a C-terminal prenylation site). Further gene duplications and mutations in the rod and terminal domains led to genes for intermediate filament proteins with particular functional advantages for the differentiated cells of higher organisms in which they are selectively expressed.

▌ Polymer Structure

Intermediate filaments average about 10 nm in diameter and have up to 16 coiled-coils in a cross section (see Fig. 38–3). The internal structure may be less uniform than other cytoskeletal polymers. Subunits are

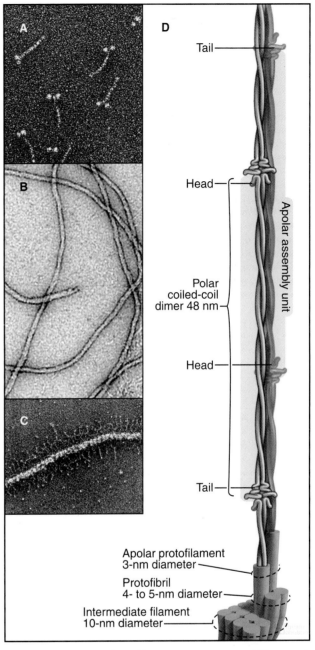

Figure 38-3 Intermediate filaments are constructed like a multistrand rope. *A,* Electron micrograph of metal-shadowed lamin molecules consisting of two polypeptides joined by a long coiled-coil with globular tail domains at the C-terminus. *B,* Electron micrograph of negatively stained keratin filaments. *C,* Electron micrograph of a rotary shadowed intermediate filament showing lateral projections. *D,* A model for intermediate filament structure. Antiparallel molecular dimers (referred to as tetramers because they have four polypeptides) are the building blocks. They polymerize in a staggered fashion to make apolar protofilaments. Two protofilaments associate laterally to make a protofibril. Four protofibrils associate to form the 10-nm intermediate filament. This model is consistent with x-ray fiber diffraction patterns, chemical cross-linking, and other data, but details of subunit packing remain to be determined. (*A* to *C,* Courtesy of U. Aebi, University of Basel. *D,* Based on Steinert P, et al: Conservation of the structure of keratin intermediate filaments. Biochemistry 32:10046–10056, 1993. Reprinted with permission from the American Chemical Society, copyright 1993.)

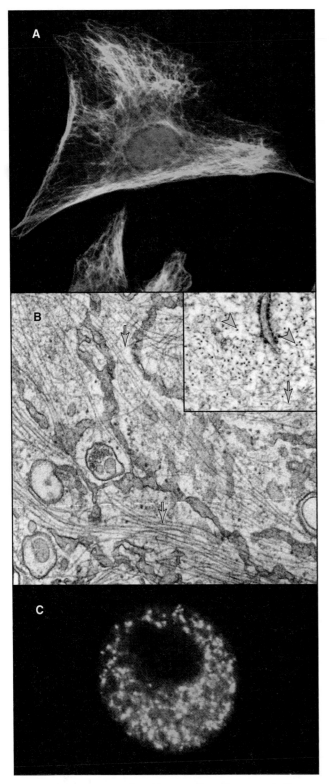

Figure 38–4 Micrographs of intermediate filaments. *A,* Fluorescence micrograph of a cultured fibroblast stained with antibodies to vimentin filaments *(green)* and microtubules *(red). B,* Electron micrograph of a thin section of a cultured baby hamster kidney cell showing longitudinal *(green arrows)* and cross sections *(green arrowheads)* of vimentin intermediate filaments. *C,* Fluorescence micrograph showing vimentin filaments dispersed in mitosis. (Courtesy of R. Goldman, Northwestern University.)

organized into thin polymers like the strands of a rope. Under dissociating conditions, they may unravel into several longitudinal strands. In electron micrographs of thin sections of cells (Fig. 38–4B) or after negative staining of isolated filaments (see Fig. 38–3B), intermediate filaments appear to have smooth surfaces and wavy profiles.

The most carefully studied intermediate filaments are built from four-chain, antiparallel molecular dimers that lack polarity, so intermediate filaments are generally thought to be apolar (i.e., both ends of the filament are equivalent; see Fig. 38–3D). This is a striking difference from actin filaments (see Chapter 36) and microtubules (see Chapter 37), which depend upon their polarity for many functions.

Assembly and Dynamics of Intermediate Filaments

Dissociated intermediate filament subunits spontaneously self-assemble into structures resembling intermediate filaments within a few minutes under physiological conditions in vitro. Assembly is highly favored judging from the low critical concentration. Subunits add to both the ends and the sides of the polymer, in contrast to actin filaments and microtubules, which grow only at their ends. The nucleation mechanism that initiates polymerization is still being investigated.

Rod domains form the backbone of intermediate filaments, so what is the role, if any, for the variable end domains? Some intermediate filaments appear to assemble normally in vitro and in vivo without one of the end domains, but whether these filaments can withstand the stresses found in tissues in vivo is untested. Other data suggest that end domains might modulate assembly.

Intermediate filaments are some of the most chemically stable cellular components, resisting solubilization by extremes of temperature as well as high concentrations of salt and detergents (Fig. 38–5). Nevertheless, intermediate filaments in some cells exchange their subunits within minutes to hours during interphase. One line of evidence has been derived from studies involving the microinjection of live cells with **vimentin** labeled with a fluorescent dye. Labeled vimentin incorporates into cytoplasmic filaments. After photobleaching a spot of fluorescent filaments with a laser, the fluorescence recovers over a period of several minutes, indicating that subunits in filaments exchange with a pool of unpolymerized molecules. (See Fig. 36–17 for a similar experiment with actin.) A second line of evidence comes from the effect of small peptides corresponding to parts of the rod domain that are crucial for assembly. When microinjected

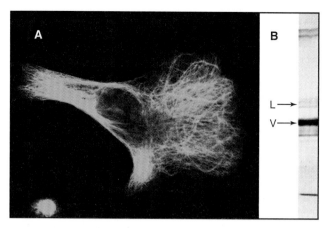

Figure 38-5 Intermediate filaments resist solubilization when cells are extracted. *A,* A fluorescence micrograph shows the network of vimentin filaments remaining after extraction of a CHO cell with the detergent Triton X-100, DNase, and a high concentration of salt to remove lipids, DNA, and soluble proteins. *B,* Gel electrophoresis reveals that lamins (L) and vimentin (V) are among the few proteins remaining in the detergent-resistant cytoskeletal fraction. (Courtesy of R. Goldman, Northwestern University.)

into cells, these peptides rapidly depolymerize vimentin filaments, presumably by binding to and depleting the pool of unpolymerized molecules. Vimentin and lamin filaments, but not all intermediate filaments, disassemble during mitosis in response to phosphorylation by mitotic kinases in some cells (Fig. 38–4*C*). Other intermediate filaments appear to be very stable, including keratin filaments in epithelial cells.

Post-Translational Modifications

Phosphorylation of intermediate filament subunits can dramatically affect polymer assembly and dynamics. The story is complex and incompletely understood, as each class of intermediate filament has multiple phosphorylation sites, and many protein kinases can phosphorylate these sites. The impact of phosphorylation depends critically on the particular residue modified.

In several cases, phosphorylation destabilizes the filaments and blocks assembly. The best examples are phosphorylation of lamins and vimentin by Cdkl:cyclin B kinase during mitosis. The enzyme phosphorylates serine residues near the ends of the rod domain. This destabilizes the filaments and contributes to the breakdown of the nuclear lamina (see Fig. 16–19 and Chapter 47) and depolymerization of cytoplasmic vimentin filaments (see Fig. 38–4*C*). Keratins are also phosphorylated during mitosis, but not directly by Cdkl:cyclin B kinase. During mitosis, the organization of keratins changes subtly without complete disassembly like other intermediate filaments.

The role of phosphorylation of intermediate filaments during interphase is less clear, but one attractive speculation is that these reversible reactions influence the structure of the cytoskeleton in response to various signals. Protein kinase C, protein kinase A, and calcium-calmodulin–dependent kinase phosphorylate all classes of intermediate filaments, so there is the potential for regulation by numerous inputs. Residues phosphorylated by each kinase and the effects of phosphorylation are still being characterized. Phosphorylation of intermediate filaments is dynamic, and phosphates turn over rapidly.

Neurofilaments, major structural components of nerve axons and dendrites, are an exception to the rule that phosphorylation destabilizes intermediate filaments. The most stable neurofilaments are heavily phosphorylated in the large C-terminal end domain (see Fig. 38–2), whereas the pool of unpolymerized molecules is not phosphorylated. The end domain containing the phosphorylation sites is not essential for assembly, so phosphorylation may influence other functions of these intermediate filaments.

Keratin intermediate filaments in hair are chemically cross-linked to each other by disulfide bonds and associated with matrix proteins, creating a tough composite material built on the same principles as fiberglass. Chemical reduction and oxidation of these disulfide bonds allows beauticians to modify the shape of hairs during "permanents." Permanents are considered permanent because they first reduce and then rebuild the disulfides once the hair is twisted into a new shape.

Expression of Intermediate Filaments in Specialized Cells

With rare known exceptions, animal and plant cells express nuclear lamins, whereas the repertoire of cytoplasmic intermediate filaments varies greatly in different cell types (see Table 38–1). It is assumed that each isoform has unique properties appropriate for cells that use them. Most cells express predominantly one class of cytoplasmic intermediate filament. For example, epithelial cells express keratin and muscles express desmin. A few cells, such as the basal myoepithelial cells of the mammary gland, express two types of intermediate filament subunits that sort into separate filaments with different distributions in the cytoplasm. Likewise, microinjection or expression of foreign intermediate filament subunits usually (but not invariably) results in correct sorting to the homologous class of filaments.

In tissues like skin and brain, cells express a succession of intermediate filament isoforms as they ma-

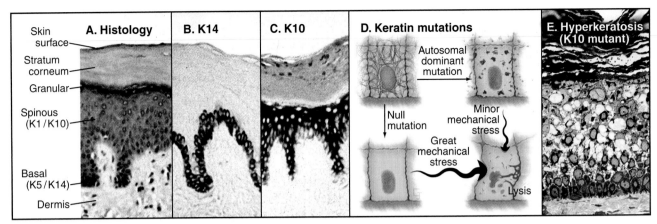

Figure 38-6 Expression of keratin (K) and effects of keratin mutations on the stratified squamous epithelium of skin. *A,* Light micrograph of a section of mouse skin stained with hematoxylin-eosin. *B,* Localization of keratin 14 in a section of skin using antibodies and a histochemical procedure that leaves a brown deposit. Proliferating cells in the basal layer express keratin 5 and keratin 14. *C,* Localization of keratin 10 to differentiating cells in intermediate layers of the epithelium. These cells eventually lose their nuclei and form the surface layers of cornified cells. *D,* Drawings illustrating the effects of keratin mutations on the structure of the epithelium. Dominant negative keratin mutations affect the assembly of keratin filaments wherever they are expressed. Human patients with epidermolysis bullosa have point mutations in keratin 5 or keratin 14 that disrupt the filaments in the basal cells, causing mechanical fragility and cellular rupture with mild trauma, resulting in blisters. Mutations in keratin 1 or keratin 10 cause cell rupture in the middle layers where they are expressed. Null mutations in keratin genes disrupt the epithelium to a lesser extent than dominant negative point mutations. *E,* Light micrograph of a histological section of skin illustrating how a mutation in keratin 10 disrupts cells in the spinous layer and causes hyperkeratosis (excess scaling of surface layers). (*A* to *C* and *E,* Courtesy of P. Coulombe, Johns Hopkins University. *D,* Reprinted with permission. Based on a drawing from Fuchs E., Cleveland DW: A structural scaffolding of intermediate filaments in health and disease. Science 279:514–519, 1998. Copyright 1998, American Association for the Advancement of Science.)

table 38-2

PROTEINS ASSOCIATED WITH INTERMEDIATE FILAMENTS

Name	Genes	Molecule	Distribution	Diseases
BPAG1	1	Alternate splicing forms BPAG1e and BPAG1n		Blistering skin and neuropathy in mice
BPAG1e		230 kD; membrane-anchored; binds keratin filaments to hemidesmosomes	Stratified epithelia	
BPAG1n		280 kD, including actin-binding domain; cross-links neurofilaments and actin filaments	Neurons	Axonal degeneration of sensory nerves
Filaggrin	1	37 kD; 10 filaggrins cut by proteolysis from profilaggrin precursor; aggregates keratin	Cornified epithelia	
Lamin-associated		Binds laminin to nuclear envelope	Nuclei of animals	
LAP1	1	57–70 kD isoforms, integral membrane protein		
LAP2	1	50 kD, integral membrane protein		
LBR	1	73 kD, 8 transmembrane spans		
Emerin	1	34 kD protein of the inner nuclear membrane	Animal cells	Emery-Dreifuss muscular dystrophy
Plectin	1	>500 kD homodimer; cytoplasm, focal contacts, hemidesmosomes; binds IF, actin filaments, microtubules, spectrin, MAPs	Animal cells	Blistering skin with muscular dystrophy in mice and humans

ture and differentiate. Human epidermis and its appendages (hair and glands) express 12 different keratin isoforms as they differentiate. Dividing cells at the base of the epidermis express mainly keratins 5 and 14, whereas terminally differentiating cells express keratins 1 and 10 (Fig. 38–6). The switch in keratin expression is associated with a marked increase in filament bundling, a feature that may contribute to the resistance of the surface layers of the skin to chemical dissociation. In the nervous system, supporting glial cells use a class III intermediate filament, whereas embryonic neurons first express α-internexin and later express the three different neurofilament isoforms (see Table 38–1). Although the smallest neurofilament isoform (NFL) can assemble on its own in vitro, NFL plus one of the larger isoforms (NFM or NFH) is required to form intermediate filaments in neurons.

Drosophila has a single nuclear lamin gene, but has no other gene for intermediate filament proteins. Perhaps the exoskeleton of this insect diminished the need for mechanical integrity provided by intermediate filaments. Yeasts lack even the gene for lamins and have no intermediate filaments.

Tumors often express the intermediate filament protein characteristic of the differentiated cells from which they arose. This is helpful to pathologists in diagnosing poorly differentiated cancers. For example, tumors of muscle cells express desmin rather than keratin, like epithelial cells, or vimentin, like mesenchymal cells.

Proteins Associated with Intermediate Filaments

A number of proteins bind intermediate filaments and link them to other cellular components, including membranes and other cytoskeletal components (Table 38–2). Three integral membrane proteins anchor nuclear lamins to the nuclear membrane. Plectin and BPAG1e link intermediate filaments to hemidesmosomes, and desmoplakin links keratin to desmosomes (see Fig. 33–7). Filaggrin helps to aggregate keratin filaments in the upper layers of skin. The splicing isoform of **BPAG1** in neurons, BPAG1n, includes an actin-binding domain homologous to those of α-actinin (see Fig. 36–15), so it cross-links neuronal intermediate filaments to actin filaments. Mice lacking BPAG1 have skin blisters secondary to compromised hemidesmosomes, as well as disorganized neuronal intermediate filaments that result in death of sensory neurons. **Plectin,** a giant protein consisting of a 170-nm coiled-coil with globular domains at each end (Fig. 38–7) binds an amazing number of cytoskeletal ligands. It cross-links intermediate filaments to each other and to the plasma membrane, microtubules, and

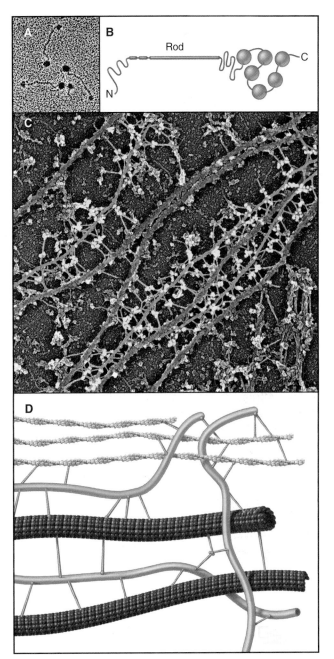

Figure 38-7 Plectin structure and activities. *A,* Electron micrograph of plectin molecules. *B,* Model of the domain structure of plectin. *C,* Electron micrograph of an extracted fibroblast cell reacted with gold-labeled antibodies to plectin. Gold particles (*yellow*) identify plectin molecules (*blue*) as linkers between intermediate filaments (*orange*) and microtubules (*red*). The specimen was prepared by rotary shadowing. The molecules are pseudocolored for clarity. *D,* Drawing of plectin (*blue*) connecting cytoskeletal polymers to each other. (*A,* From G. Wiche, University of Vienna. *C,* Courtesy of G. Borisy, University of Wisconsin, Madison.)

actin filaments. Recessive mutations in human plectin cause a rare form of muscular dystrophy associated with skin blisters. Motors associated with actin filaments and microtubules can use intermediate filaments as cargo and move them around in the cytoplasm.

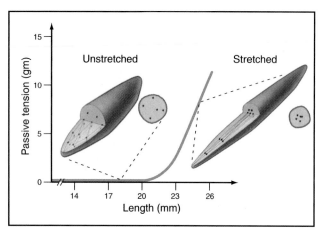

Figure 38-8 Smooth muscle cell intermediate filaments form an inextensible intracellular tendon that resists excessive stretching. The graph shows that a relaxed smooth muscle resists stretching very little up to a length of 21 mm. Resistance increases dramatically with further stretching. At short lengths, the three-dimensional network of intermediate filaments and dense bodies is open, offering little resistance to stretching. At the inflection point of the resistance curve, the filaments are extended linearly from one end of the cell to the other and so resist further stretching. (Based on Cooke P, Fay R: Correlation between fiber length, ultrastructure, and the length tension relationship of mammalian smooth muscle. J Cell Biol 52:105–116, 1972, by copyright permission of the Rockefeller University Press.)

▌ Distribution and Functions of Intermediate Filaments in Cells

Cytoplasmic intermediate filaments tend to cluster into wavy bundles that vary in compactness, forming a branching network between the plasma membrane and the nucleus (see Fig. 38–4). It is presumed that associations into bundles are mediated by the end domains of the intermediate filament subunits themselves or by associated proteins, or both. **Desmosomes** and **hemidesmosomes** anchor intermediate filaments to the plasma membrane (see Fig. 33–7). The connection to the nucleus is not well characterized.

Intermediate filaments function primarily as flexible but inextensible intracellular tendons that prevent excessive stretching of cells subjected to external or internal physical forces. This function is facilitated by interactions with microtubules, actin filaments, and membranes. For example, if a relaxed smooth muscle is stretched, the intracellular network of intermediate filaments connected by dense bodies (see Fig. 42–20) reorganizes from a polygonal three-dimensional network into a continuous strap that runs the length of the cell (Fig. 38–8). Up to the point where this network is taut, the cell offers little resistance to stretching. Once the network is taut, the cell strongly resists further stretching. The three-dimensional network of desmin filaments in smooth muscle is attached to the plasma membrane as well as to cytoplasmic dense

bodies. Actin filaments anchored to the dense bodies apply contractile force to the network of intermediate filaments.

Although the geometry is different in striated muscles, the concept is remarkably similar to smooth muscle. Desmin filaments surround the Z disks in addition to forming a looser, longitudinal basket around the myofibrils (see Fig. 42–8). The ends of both skeletal and cardiac muscle cells must be anchored to transmit their contractile forces. This is accomplished by intercellular junctions (see Chapters 33 and 42) that combine features of desmosomes or hemidesmosomes (anchoring intermediate filaments) and adherens junctions (anchoring actin filaments).

Keratin intermediate filaments are the major proteins in skin where they form a dense network connected to numerous desmosomes and hemidesmosomes (see Figs. 38–1 and 38–6). These junctions anchor a physically continuous network of intermediate filaments, imparting mechanical stability to the epithelium. If either the junctions or keratin filaments fail, cells pull apart or rupture and the skin blisters. Mutations that compromise intermediate filament assembly or their anchoring junctions illustrate the importance of this network. Point mutations near the ends of the keratin rod cause especially severe forms of inherited skin diseases (such as **epidermolysis bullosa** simplex) characterized by blistering and sensitivity to mechanical stress. Expressing keratins with similar mutations in transgenic mice reproduces the human disease. The specific epithelial tissue affected depends on the expression pattern of the defective keratin. For example, a mutation in the rod domain of keratin 14 or keratin 5 leads to disruption of the basal cells in the epidermis where these keratins are expressed. Likewise, mutations in keratin 10 or keratin 1 cause cellular rupture at higher levels in the epidermis where these keratins are found. Mutations in keratin 12 or keratin 3 cause sores in the cornea of the eye where they are expressed.

Expression of a mutant keratin can cause disease in heterozygotes with one normal keratin gene. This is called a **dominant negative mutation.** Defective subunits assemble imperfectly with normal keratin subunits and compromise the physical integrity and strength of the filaments. The affected cells can grow, divide, and even form desmosomes with neighboring cells, but they tear apart physically when subjected to the shearing forces that impact the skin during normal life activities. Young children are severely affected, but some affected individuals improve with age. They learn to avoid physical trauma to their skin and may also adapt biochemically in some way.

In contrast to these dominant negative keratin mutations, complete loss of intermediate filament proteins can be less severe (see Fig. 38–6*D*). Mice and humans

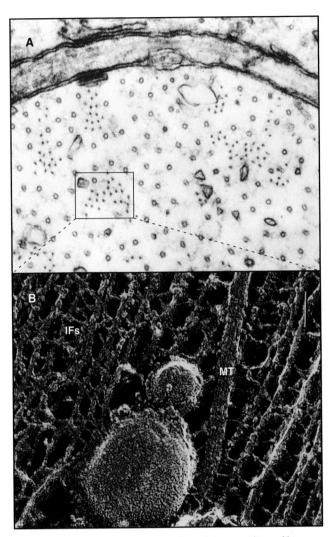

Figure 38-9 Electron micrographs of intermediate filaments (called neurofilaments) in axons of nerve cells. *A*, A thin cross section shows clusters of intermediate filaments and microtubules. *B*, A longitudinal freeze-fracture preparation shows a microtubule (MT; *red*) with associated vesicles and many intermediate filaments (IF; *orange*). (*A*, Courtesy of P. Eagle, Kings College, London. *B*, Courtesy of N. Hirokawa, University of Tokyo.)

lacking keratin 14 suffer from milder blistering than patients with dominant negative point mutations. Mice without functional keratin 8 or keratin 18 genes may die during embryonic development, but some survive with modest defects in their colon and liver. Remarkably, mice also survive deletion of both copies of the genes for class III intermediate filaments. Mice lacking desmin are viable, but with mildly disorganized muscle architecture that is aggravated by vigorous exercise. Humans who are heterozygous for desmin mutations can suffer severely from generalized muscle failure, including signs of heart disease.

Neurofilaments have a second function equal in importance to their mechanical properties. Once a nerve cell forms its synapses (see Chapter 10), it expresses large amounts of neurofilaments that fill the axon and expand its diameter (Fig. 38–9). Because the velocity of action potentials depends on the diameter of axons, this enhances electrical communication in the nervous system.

Lamins were originally thought to be merely a support network for the nuclear envelope but are now known to have other important functions as well. For example, perturbation of lamina assembly by expressing toxic fragments of lamins in cells can interfere with DNA replication. This may reflect a role for the lamina in organizing the chromosomal architecture in the interphase nucleus. Mutations in the lamin A gene also can give rise to Emery-Dreifuss muscular dystrophy, and this has been recapitulated in the lab by gene targeting in mice. Why lamina mutants should cause muscular dystrophy is not known, although a weakness in the nuclear envelope may be exacerbated by the contraction of muscle cells.

Selected Readings

Braun S, Panatel K, Muller P, Janni W, et al.: Cytokeratin-positive cells in the bone marrow and survival of patients with stage I, II or III breast cancer. N Engl J Med 342:525–533, 2000.

Evans RM: Vimentin: The conundrum of the intermediate filament gene family. Bioessays 20:79–86, 1998.

Fatkin D, MacRae C, Sasaki T, et al.: Missense mutations in the rod domain of the lamin A/C gene as causes of dilated cardiomyopathy and contraction system disease. N Engl J Med 341:1715–1724, 1999.

Fuchs E, Cleveland DW: A structural scaffolding of intermediate filaments in health and disease. Science 279:514–519, 1998.

Goebel HH: Desmin-related myopathies. Curr Opin Neurol 10:426–429, 1997.

Goldman RD, Chou YH, Prohlad V, Yoon M: Intermediate filaments: Dynamic processes regulating their assembly, motility and interactions with other cytoskeletal systems. FASEB J [Suppl] 2:S261–S265, 1999.

Herrmann H, Aebi U: Intermediate filaments and their associates: Multi-talented structural elements specifying cytoarchitecture and cytodynamics. Curr Opin Cell Biol 12:79–90, 2000.

Kreis T, Vale R, eds: Guidebook to the Cytoskeletal and Motor Proteins, 2nd ed. New York: Oxford University Press, 1999.

Martys JL, Ho CL, Liem RK, Gundersen GG: Intermediate filaments in motion: Observations of intermediate filaments in cells using green fluorescent protein-vimentin. Mol Biol Cell 10:1289–1295, 1999.

Wiche G: Role of plectin in cytoskeleton organization and dynamics. J Cell Sci 111:2477–2486, 1998.

chapter 39

MOTOR PROTEINS

Molecular motors power movements of subcellular components, such as organelles and chromosomes, along the two polarized cytoskeletal fibers: actin filaments and microtubules. No motors are known to move on the third component of the cytoskeleton, apolar intermediate filaments. Motor proteins also produce force locally within the network of cytoskeletal polymers, which transmit these forces to change the shape of cells and to power their locomotion. These movements determine the shape of each cell, and, ultimately, the architecture of tissues and whole organisms. Chapters 40 to 42 and 47 illustrate how motors move cells and their parts.

Remarkably, just three families of motor proteins—myosin, kinesin, and dynein—power most eukaryotic cellular movements (Fig. 39–1 and Table 39–1). This chapter focuses on general principles rather than on the heterogeneity of each family of motors. Most myosins move toward the barbed end of actin filaments, most dyneins move toward the minus end of microtubules, and most kinesins move toward the plus end of microtubules. A subset of kinesins moves toward the minus end of microtubules. Other chapters cover additional protein machines that produce molecular movements (see Table 39–1) during protein and nucleic acid synthesis, proton pumping, and bacterial motility.

Although specialized in terms of their polymer tracts and directions of movement, all of these motors are enzymes that convert chemical energy stored in adenosine triphosphate (ATP) into molecular motion that produces force upon the associated cytoskeletal polymer (Fig. 39–2). If the *motor* is anchored, the polymer may move. If the *polymer* is anchored, the motor and any attached cargo may move. If *both* are anchored, the force stretches elastic elements in the molecules transiently, but nothing moves and the en-

ergy is lost as heat. Cells use all of these options (see Chapters 40 to 42).

Biochemists originally discovered and purified these motors by means of enzyme activity or in vitro motility assays (see Figs. 39–4 and 39–9). With the prototype enzymes identified, investigators found further examples and variant isoforms of each motor by purification of the proteins, molecular cloning of DNAs, genome-wide DNA sequencing, or genetic screening. The three families of motor proteins are widespread in eukaryotes, but are not present in prokaryotic genomes. A bacterial gene distantly related to kinesin has been described, but characterization of the protein has not progressed to the point where its relation to eukaryotic motors is understood.

As detailed later in this chapter, myosin and kinesin appear to have shared a common origin with Ras family GTPases (see Chapter 27) during evolution, whereas dynein is a member of another family of ATPases. Over time, gene duplication and divergence gave rise to many variants of myosin, dynein, and kinesin with specialized functions (see Chapters 40 to 42). Typically, a relatively conserved motor domain is linked with a variety of adapter domains or accessory subunits specialized for self-assembly or interaction with particular cargos. For example, all myosins have similar motor domains that are linked to tails that allow self-assembly into filaments or, alternatively, binding to membranes or other cargo.

Myosins

The diverse family of myosins has a common structural unit called a **myosin "head"** that produces force on actin filaments (Fig. 39–3). The myosin head alone is sufficient to drive the movement of actin filaments,

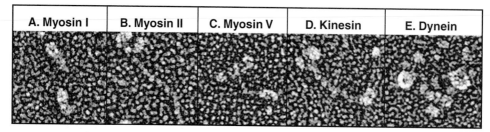

| A. Myosin I | B. Myosin II | C. Myosin V | D. Kinesin | E. Dynein |

Figure 39–1 Electron micrographs of ATPase motors prepared by rotary shadowing. *A,* Myosin I. *B,* Myosin II. *C,* Myosin V. *D,* Conventional kinesin. *E,* Cytoplasmic dynein. (Courtesy of J. Heuser, Washington University.)

at least in laboratory experiments. When supplied with ATP, the joint action of many myosin heads attached to a microscope coverslip causes actin filaments to glide across the surface at the same rate observed in contracting muscle (Fig. 39–4). Some myosins have one head; others have two. Myosins also have tails, which vary considerably (see Fig. 40–2). Tails anchor myosin molecules in polymers or on other cellular structures, including membranes. This chapter explains how heads work. Chapters 40 and 41 consider the functions of tails.

Myosin heads consist of at least two polypeptides: a heavy chain of about 850 residues and one or more light chains of less than 200 residues (see Fig. 39–3). The head of muscle myosin was originally isolated as a proteolytic fragment called subfragment-1. The N-

table 39–1

EXAMPLES OF MECHANOCHEMICAL ATPases AND OTHER SYSTEMS

Families	Track	Direction	Cargo	Energy
ATPases				
Myosins				
Muscle myosin	Actin	Barbed-end	Myosin filament	ATP
Myosin II	Actin	Barbed-end	Myosin, actin	ATP
Myosin I	Actin	Barbed-end	Membranes	ATP
Myosin V	Actin	Barbed-end	Organelles	ATP
Myosin VI	Actin	Pointed-End	? coated vesicles	ATP
Dyneins				
Axonemal	Microtubule	Minus end	Microtubules	ATP
Cytoplasmic	Microtubule	Minus end	Membranes, chromosomes	ATP
Kinesins				
Conventional	Microtubule	Plus end	Membranes, intermediate filaments	ATP
ncd	Microtubule	Minus end	?Microtubules	ATP
Other Mechanochemical Systems				
Polymerases				
Ribosome	mRNA	5′ to 3′	None	GTP
DNA polymerase	DNA	5′ to 3′	None	ATP
RNA polymerase	DNA	5′ to 3′	None	ATP
Conformational system				
Spasmin/centrin	None	None	Cell, basal body	Ca^{2+}
Polymerizing systems				
Actin filaments	None	Barbed end	Membranes	ATP
Microtubules	None	Plus end	Chromosomes	GTP
Worm sperm MSP	None	Not polar	Cytoskeleton	
?Associated proteins				
Rotary motors				
Bacterial flagella	None	Bidirectional	Cell	H^+ or Na^+ gradient
F-type ATPase	None	Bidirectional	None	H^+ or ATP
V-type ATPase pump	None		None	ATP

mRNA, messenger RNA; MSP, major sperm protein.

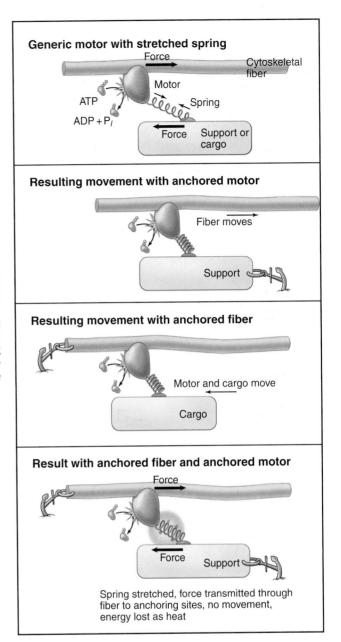

Figure 39-2 General features of ATPase motors. Motors bind stably to a support or cargo and transiently to a cytoskeletal fiber (actin filament or microtubule). Energy liberated by ATP hydrolysis produces force to stretch an elastic element somewhere in the physical connection between the cargo and the cytoskeletal fiber. The resulting motion depends on whether the force in the spring exceeds the resistance of the fiber or the cargo.

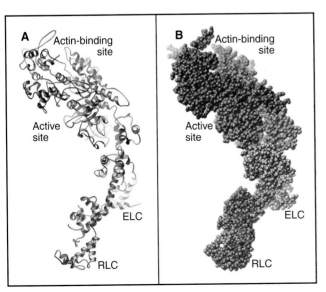

Figure 39-3 Atomic structure of the head of muscle myosin. *A,* Ribbon drawing of the polypeptide backbones. *B,* Space-filling model. *Green,* heavy chain residues 4–204; *red,* heavy chain residues 216–626; *purple,* heavy chain residues 647–843: *yellow,* essential light chain (ELC); *orange,* regulatory light chain (RLC). The myosin light chains consist of two globular domains connected by an α helix, like calmodulin and troponin C. (PDB file: 2MYS.)

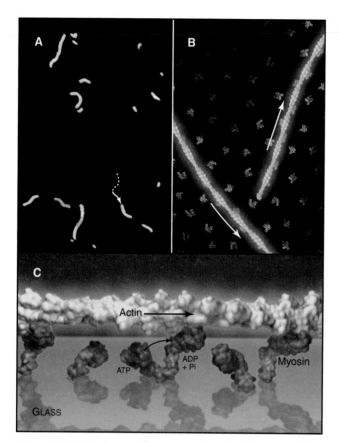

Figure 39-4 In vitro motility assay with actin filaments gliding over myosin attached to a microscope slide. *A,* Filaments are labeled with rhodamine-phalloidin to render them visible by light microscopy. ATP hydrolysis by myosin moves actin filaments over the surface. *B* and *C,* Drawings of actin filaments moving over myosin heads immobilized on a glass coverslip. (*A,* Courtesy of A. Bresnick, Albert Einstein College of Medicine, New York.)

terminal 710 residues of the heavy chain are folded into a globular **catalytic domain** that forms actin- and ATP-binding sites. At the core of the catalytic domain, a β sheet forms the floor of the nucleotide binding site. The walls of this site are flanked by α helices. The sheet and flanking helices have a topology similar to the Ras GTPases that participates in signaling (see Chapter 33) despite little sequence homology. The γ-phosphate of ATP inserts most deeply into the nucleotide binding site with the adenine exposed on the surface. Actin binds more than 4 nm away from the nucleotide on the other side of the molecule.

The second part of the head is the **light chain domain,** where one to six light chains wrap around and stabilize a long α helix formed by the heavy chain (see Fig. 39-3). Calmodulin serves as a light chain for some cytoplasmic myosins (see Fig. 40-2), but many light chains are specialized evolutionary relatives of calmodulin with novel functions. Light chains bind the heavy chain α helix in a manner similar to calmodulin

binding its target proteins (see Fig. 2-14 and Chapter 28). Some light chains, like calmodulin, bind divalent cations.

Myosin heads bind tightly and rigidly to actin filaments in the absence of ATP. This is called a **rigor** complex because it forms in muscle during rigor mortis when ATP is depleted after death. Myosin heads form a polarized structure, resembling a series of arrowheads when viewed from the side, along an actin filament (Fig. 39-5). The heads bind at an angle and wrap around the filament. Their orientation defines the barbed and pointed ends of the actin filament (see Chapter 37). All but one class of myosins move toward the barbed end of the filament. The exception is myosin VI, a cellular motor thought to move vesicles, which moves toward the pointed end.

The atomic structures of the myosin head and actin filament fit nicely into the three-dimensional structure of the decorated filament determined by electron microscopy, providing a reasonable model of the complex at near atomic resolution (see Fig. 39-5). The model shows each head in contact with two adjacent actins, but does not reveal important details, including atomic contacts, between the proteins. This model is the structural starting point for understanding the mechanics of force production. First, a look at the chemistry of the actomyosin adenosine triphosphatase (ATPase) is necessary, as the chemistry defines the pathway that produces force and movement.

Chemistry of the Myosin-Actin ATPase Cycle

Myosin uses energy from ATP hydrolysis to move actin filaments, so an appreciation of the mechanism requires an understanding of the steps in the biochemical reaction. Fig. 39-6*A* looks intimidating, but working through it one step at a time reveals its logic and simplicity. In this scheme, M is a myosin head, A is actin, T is ATP, D is ADP, and P is inorganic phosphate. Note that the mechanism consists of two parallel lines of chemical intermediates. On the bottom line, myosin is free of actin. On the top line, each myosin intermediate is bound to actin. First, consider the bottom line, which shows how myosin hydrolyzes ATP in the absence of actin. This series of reactions explains why myosin alone turns over ATP remarkably slowly, at a rate of only about 0.02 s^{-1}.

Step 1. At physiologic concentrations of ATP, myosin binds ATP in less than 1 msec, so this is not the rate-limiting step. Binding is accompanied by a conformational change in the myosin that can be detected by a change in the fluorescence of the protein itself.

Step 2. The enzyme catalyzes the hydrolysis of ATP. This reaction is moderately fast (>100 s^{-1}) and readily reversible. The equilibrium constant for hy-

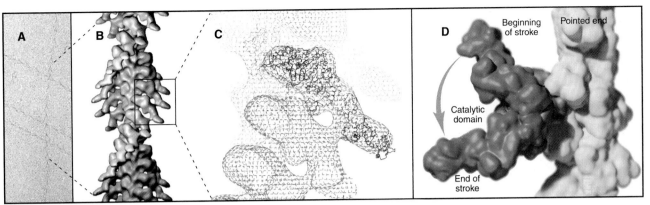

Figure 39–5 Actin filaments decorated with myosin heads. *A,* Electron micrograph of frozen-hydrated actin filaments saturated with myosin heads. *B,* Three-dimensional reconstruction from electron micrographs of an actin filament saturated with myosin heads. *C,* Superimposition of atomic models of the actin filament and one myosin head on the reconstruction of the decorated filament (blue cage-like surface). *D,* Space-filling atomic model of an actin filament with one attached muscle myosin head showing the light chain domain in two positions: (1) the end of the power stroke as observed in the absence of ATP *(blue)* and (2) the postulated beginning of the power stroke *(pink)* deduced from x-ray structures of isolated heads and spectroscopic studies. The catalytic domain *(red)* is fixed in one position on actin *(yellow).* (Courtesy of R. Milligan, Scripps Research Institute, La Jolla, CA.)

drolysis on the enzyme is near 1, so each ATP is hydrolyzed to adenosine diphosphate (ADP [*D* in the figure]) and inorganic phosphate (P) and re-synthesized several times before the products eventually dissociate from the enzyme. ATP splitting provides energy for a second conformational change, reflected in a further increase in the fluorescence of the myosin. It is presumed that this conformational change completes the "cocking" of the myosin in a structure prepared to undergo the molecular rearrangements that subsequently produce movement.

Step 3. Inorganic phosphate (P) slowly dissociates from the active site (at a rate of about 0.02 s^{-1}), perhaps by escaping through a narrow "back door" on the far side of the enzyme. This is the rate-limiting step of the reaction pathway. The loss of phosphate is coupled to conformational changes that return the myosin toward its "uncocked" basal state. The phosphate dissociation step has the largest negative free energy change, so it is presumed that energy derived from ATP binding and hydrolysis and stored in conformational changes in the myosin head is used to do work or dissipated as heat at this point in the reaction pathway.

Step 4. Once phosphate dissociates, ADP leaves rapidly from the "front door."

To summarize, in the absence of actin filaments, ATP binds rapidly to myosin, is rapidly but reversibly split, and the products slowly dissociate from the active site. The overall cycle of the enzyme is limited by a slow conformational change coupled to product dissociation, not binding or hydrolysis. Energy derived

from ATP binding and hydrolysis is used for a conformational change in the myosin head that is dissipated when phosphate dissociates.

Now focus on the upper line where myosin is associated with an actin filament. The chemical intermediates are the same, but some of the key rate constants differ for the actin-bound and free enzymes. Steps 1 and 2 are similar to those of free myosin, but step 3—the dissociation of phosphate—is much faster when a head is bound to an actin filament. As a result, myosin bound to actin traverses the ATPase cycle about 200 times faster than myosin free in solution, and ATP hydrolysis becomes the rate-limiting step. This effect of actin is referred to as "actin activation of the myosin ATPase." A practical advantage of this mechanism is that the ATPase cycle is essentially turned off unless a head interacts with an actin filament.

Finally, consider the vertical arrows representing transitions between bound and free states of each myosin chemical intermediate. All myosin intermediates bind rapidly to actin filaments, but the dissociation rate constants vary over a wide range depending upon the nucleotide bound to the active site of the myosin. Myosin with no nucleotide or with bound ADP alone dissociates very slowly and, therefore, binds tightly to actin filaments (see Fig. 39–5). Myosin with bound ATP or ADP + P$_i$ dissociates rapidly from actin, so it binds much less strongly.

These rapid binding and dissociation reactions allow myosin intermediates (MT and MDP) to hop on and off actin filaments on a millisecond time scale (indicated by the large vertical arrows in the box in Fig. 39–6*A*), a key feature of muscle contraction (see Chapter 42). As a result of this rapid equilibrium, a

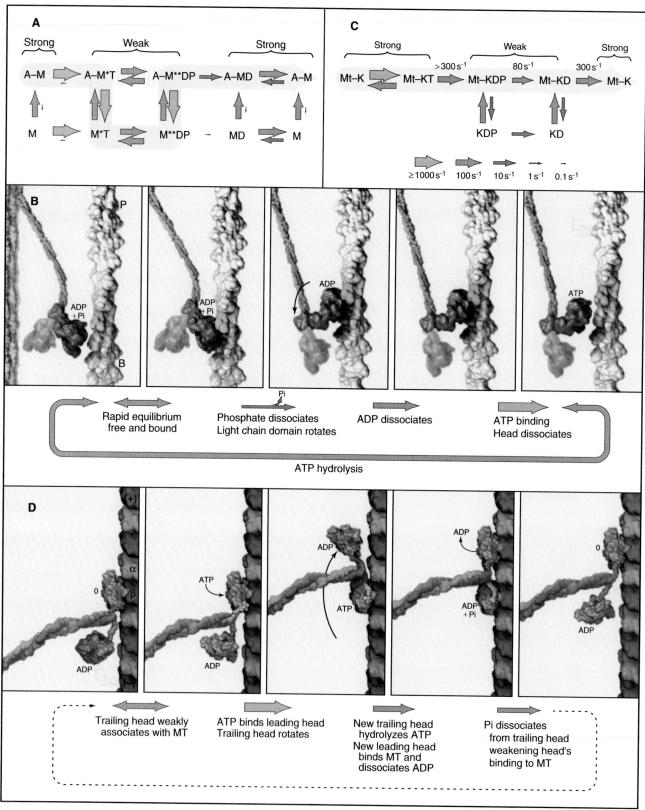

A

Strong   Weak   Strong

A–M ⟹ A–M*T ⇄ A–M**DP ⟹ A–MD ⇄ A–M

M ⟹ M*T ⇄ M**DP → MD ⇄ M

C

Strong   Weak   Strong

                >300 s⁻¹   80 s⁻¹   300 s⁻¹

Mt–K ⇄ Mt–KT ⟹ Mt–KDP ⟹ Mt–KD ⟹ Mt–K

KDP → KD

≥1000 s⁻¹   100 s⁻¹   10 s⁻¹   1 s⁻¹   0.1 s⁻¹

B

Rapid equilibrium free and bound   Phosphate dissociates Light chain domain rotates   ADP dissociates   ATP binding Head dissociates

ATP hydrolysis

D

Trailing head weakly associates with MT   ATP binds leading head Trailing head rotates   New trailing head hydrolyzes ATP New leading head binds MT and dissociates ADP   Pi dissociates from trailing head weakening head's binding to MT

See legend on opposite page

single pathway cannot be drawn through the reaction mechanism of ATP, myosin, and actin. One cycle of ATP hydrolysis takes about 50 msec. Starting with AM, ATP binds very rapidly and sets up a rapid, four-way equilibrium including AMT, MT, AMDP, and MDP—the major intermediates during steady-state ATP turnover. Because the products of ATP hydrolysis dissociate much more rapidly from AMDP than from MDP, the favored pathway out of this four-way equilibrium is through AMDP to AMD and back to AM. Because the fraction of myosin heads bound to actin in the AMDP state depends on the actin concentration, the overall ATPase rate depends on the actin concentration. At the high actin concentrations in cells, a significant fraction of myosin heads are associated with actin (about 10% to 20% in contracting muscle), but each molecule continues to exchange on and off actin filaments.

Myosin produces force when myosin in the AMDP state makes the transitions to the AMD and AM states. Production of force at this step makes sense for two reasons: first, the large free energy difference between AMDP and AMD provides energy to produce force; second, the force-producing AMD and AM intermediates bind tightly to actin, so that force between the motor and the actin track is not dissipated. However, for most myosins, these force-producing states occupy a small fraction of the whole ATPase cycle. ADP dissociates rapidly from AMD, and ATP binds rapidly to AM, dissociating myosin from the actin filament and initiating another ATPase cycle.

Transduction of Chemical Energy into Molecular Motion

Establishing the structural basis for the conversion of free energy into force has been the most challenging question in this field for 40 years. A combination of mechanical measurements, static atomic structures of myosin heads with various bound nucleotides, and spectroscopic observations of contracting muscle have revealed a likely mechanism: a dramatic conformational change in the myosin head associated with phosphate dissociation (see Fig. 39-6B).

The original approach was to measure the size of the mechanical step produced by myosin during one cycle of ATP hydrolysis. Elegant mechanical experiments on muscles have suggested that each cycle of ATP hydrolysis moves an actin filament about 5–10 nm relative to myosin. More recently, it has been possible to observe by light microscopy the movements of actin produced by single myosin molecules (Fig. 39-7). For each cycle of ATP hydrolysis, myosin moves an actin filament 5–15 nm and develops a force of about 3–7 pN. These single steps can be observed if the ATP concentration is low enough that the interval between the force-producing step and the binding of the next ATP is relatively long.

A second approach has been through biophysical studies of muscle and purified proteins using x-ray diffraction, electron microscopy, electron spin resonance spectroscopy, and fluorescence spectroscopy. These experiments consistently show little or no rotation of the catalytic domain of the heads relative to the actin filament, apparently ruling out tilting of the whole crossbridge as the major source of motion. The same types of experiments reveal pivoting of the light chain domain around a fulcrum just within the catalytic domain. For example, spectroscopic probes on light chains reveal a change in orientation when muscle is activated to contract, whereas the same probes on the catalytic domain do not rotate. Most graphically, three-dimensional reconstructions of electron micrographs and crystal structures of myosin heads with various bound nucleotides and nucleotide analogs show that the light chain domain of some myosins pivots by up to 90° (see Fig. 39-5D). These experi-

Figure 39-6 Comparison of the ATPase mechanisms of myosin and kinesin. *A,* A diagram of the actomyosin ATPase cycle showing the actin filament (A); myosin head (M); ATP (T); ADP (D); and inorganic phosphate (P). Transient-state kinetics revealed the major chemical intermediates and the rate constants for their transitions. Arrows are proportional to the rates of the reactions, with second-order reactions, adjusted for physiologic concentrations of reactants. One or two asterisks indicate conformational changes in the myosin head induced by ATP binding and hydrolysis. Myosin without nucleotide (M) and myosin with ADP (MD) bind much more tightly to actin filaments than do AMT and AMDP. The weakly bound AMT and AMDP intermediates are in a rapid equilibrium with free MT and MDP. The beige highlight shows the main pathway through the reaction. *B,* The postulated force-producing structural changes in the orientation of the light chain domain (*purple* and *blue*) coupled to the myosin ATPase cycle. *C,* A diagram of the kinesin-microtubule ATPase cycle for a single kinesin head showing the kinesin (K); microtubule (Mt); ATP (T); ADP (D); and inorganic phosphate (P). A single head remains associated with a microtubule for many rounds of ATP hydrolysis, as all ATPase steps are faster than the dissociation of any intermediate from the microtubule. The beige highlight shows the main pathway through the reaction. *D,* Postulated structural changes in double-headed kinesin coupled to the ATPase cycle resulting in hand-over-hand, processive stepping along of a microtubule. ATP binding to the empty head, associated with the microtubule, causes folding of its neck-linker (*green*), thereby thrusting the detached head forward. The new leading head binds the microtubule and dissociates its ADP, whereas the trailing head hydrolyzes ATP and dissociates phosphate, returning the heads to the original condition, but with the heads advanced 8 nm and in the opposite chemical states. (*B and D,* Based on sketches and data from R. Vale, University of California, San Francisco, and R. Milligan, Scripps Research Institute, La Jolla, CA.)

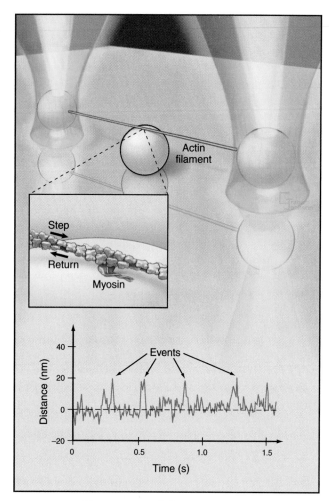

Figure 39-7 Measurement of the myosin step size. An actin filament is attached between two plastic beads, which are suspended by laser optical traps. The optical traps move the filament near a myosin molecule on the surface of another bead attached to the microscope slide, allowing a myosin head to attach to the actin filament. When supplied with ATP, a single myosin head can move the actin filament a short distance corresponding to the step size. The graph shows the time course of displacements of the actin filament and attached beads. Brownian motion limits the precision of the measurement of the size of these steps to a range of 5 to 15 nm. The duration of the step depends upon the ATP concentration because ATP dissociates the force-producing AM state, allowing the force of the optical traps to return the beads and the actin filament to their original position. (Reference: Finer JT, et al: Single myosin molecule mechanics: Piconewton forces and nanometre steps. Nature 368:113–119, 1994.)

count for the observed step size of 10 nm. This range of conformations depends on rearrangements in the polypeptide chain immediately around the γ-phosphate of ATP, similar to the changes in the Ras family of GTPases (see Fig. 27–7). However, some questions remain, as the nucleotides associated with the observed structures do not correspond to the expected steps in the force-producing cycle shown in the figure.

Regardless of the details, it is believed that the molecular motion produces movement indirectly in the sense that force-producing intermediates stretch elastic elements in the system, represented by a spring in Figure 39–2. The location of the spring in the myosin-actin complex is not known, but likely includes the light chain domain and, possibly, the proximal part of the tail. Movement of the motor relative to the track occurs as force shortens the spring. Elastic elements are stretched transiently, since dissociation of ADP and rebinding of ATP to the AM intermediate reverts the system to the rapid equilibrium of weakly bound intermediates, including dissociated heads. Any force left in the spring is lost as soon as the head dissociates from the actin filament.

The actual motion depends on the mechanical resistance in the system (see Fig. 39–2). If both myosin and actin are fixed, elastic elements are stretched for the life of the force-producing states (AMD and AM), and the energy is lost as heat when the head dissociates. This happens if one tries to lift an immovable object. If myosin is fixed and resistance on the actin is less than the force in the stretched elastic elements, the actin filament moves. This happens when muscles contract. The distance moved in each step depends on the resistance, as the spring stops shortening when the forces are balanced. Myosin and any cargo move for the same reason, provided actin is fixed and the resistance on the myosin and cargo is less than the force in the spring. This happens when certain types of myosin transport a cytoplasmic vesicle along an actin filament.

In most cases, multiple myosin heads must work together, as each one produces force less than 10% of the time during its ATPase cycle. Myosin V (see Chapter 40) is an exception. This two-headed myosin appears to move processively along an actin filament by virtue of the fact that each head spends about 70% of each ATPase cycle attached to the filament. This is accomplished by very slow ADP dissociation from the AMD intermediate, which hangs onto the filament for about 50 msec.

ments suggest that the light chain domain is bent more acutely in AMT and AMDP intermediates, and pivots to a more extended orientation, when phosphate dissociates. ADP dissociation produces an extension of this rotation in smooth muscle and some classes of cytoplasmic myosin. Experiments showing that the rate of actin filament gliding in an in vitro assay is proportional to the length of the light chain domain support the concept of rotation of the light chain domain. The observed range of orientations of the light chain domain relative to the catalytic domain can ac-

Microtubule Motors

The kinesin and dynein families of molecular motors are thought to be responsible for all movements along microtubules in cells. Dynein powers bending motions

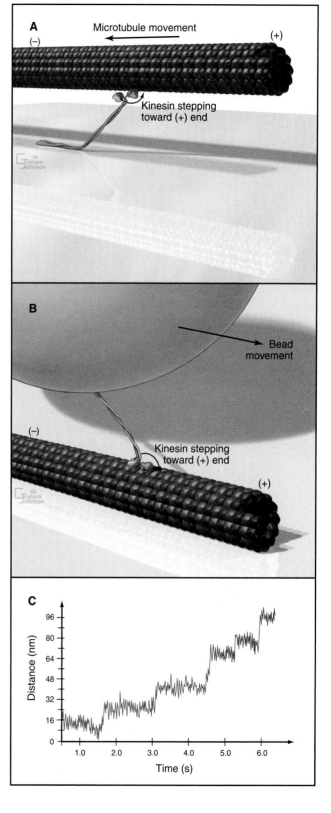

Figure 39-8 In vitro motility assays for microtubule motors. *A,* Gliding assay. Kinesin or dynein that is attached to a microscope slide uses ATP hydrolysis to move microtubules over the surface. A single kinesin can move a microtubule in this assay. Microtubules are imaged by video-enhanced differential interference contrast microscopy. *B,* Bead assay. Kinesin or dynein that is attached to a plastic bead uses ATP hydrolysis to move the bead along a microtubule attached to the microscopic slide. *C,* Experimental measurement of the kinesin step size using the bead assay. The bead is held in a laser optical trap to minimize Brownian motion, so that 8-nm steps can be recorded as a single, two-headed kinesin moves a bead processively along a microtubule, as in *B.* The position of the bead is recorded with nanometer precision by interferometry. (Reference: Svoboda K, et al: Direct observation of kinesin stepping by optical trapping interferometry. Nature 365:721–727, 1993.)

of eukaryotic flagella and cilia (see Chapter 41), as well as movements of various types of cargo in cytoplasm (see Chapter 40). Cargo includes membrane-bound organelles and vesicles, as well as chromosomes. Kinesins provide complementary movements of the same types of cargo.

In vitro motility assays (Fig. 39–8) established the ability of purified dynein and kinesin to move along microtubules. Dyneins move both themselves and any cargo toward the minus end of microtubules. Consequently, if dynein is immobilized in an in vitro assay, the plus end of a microtubule will lead as the dynein

TOOLS FOR STUDYING MOTOR PROTEINS

Few selective pharmacologic agents are available to inhibit motor proteins. A recently described kinesin inhibitor from marine sponges, *adocia*sulfate-2, may be an exception. It inhibits kinesins by blocking binding to microtubules. When injected into live cells, it disrupts kinesin-dependent processes. A small chemical named monasterol inhibits a mitotic kinesin, resulting in monopolar spindles. A small chemical—2,3-butanedione 2 monoxime (BDM)—inhibits actin-activated myosin ATPase and in vitro gliding movements of actin filaments over myosin, but must be used with caution because it lacks specificity. BDM is also reported to block L-type calcium channels and gap junctions, in addition to altering protein phosphorylation and depleting Ca^{2+} from smooth endoplasmic reticulum. Vanadate and ultraviolet light can inactivate dynein. Vanadate binds to the γ-phosphate site of dynein-ADP, but it binds similarly to other ATPases, so it is not specific. However, ultraviolet light has a novel effect on the dynein-ADP-vanadate complex: it cleaves and inactivates the dynein heavy chain.

"walks" toward the minus end of the microtubule. Most kinesins move in the opposite direction, toward the plus end, but some kinesin family members are minus-end-directed motors (see Chapter 40). Like myosins, microtubule motors have heads with ATPase activity and tails that serve as adapters for interacting with various cellular structures, including membranes, chromosomes, and other microtubules. Pharmacological agents (Box 39–1) can sometimes help to distinguish these various motors.

Kinesins

Members of the large kinesin family have a conserved motor domain (Fig. 39–9) attached to a variety of tails that are thought to interact with cargo (see Chapters 40 and 47). Like myosin, most kinesin motor domains are located at the N-terminus of the polypeptide chain, but a few are at the other end or even in the middle. Like myosins, kinesins use ATP hydrolysis to move along microtubule tracks, but the mechanics appear to be remarkably different from myosin. Single molecules of some kinesins can move a microtubule at full speed in an in vitro assay (see Fig. 39–8). In these cases, cooperation between two heads is required for the kinesin to maintain physical contact with the moving microtubule.

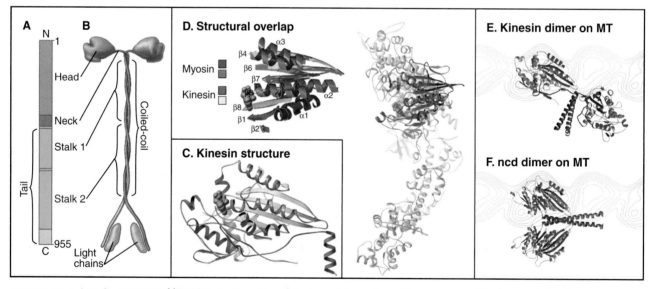

Figure 39–9 Atomic structure of kinesins. *A,* Domain architecture of the polypeptide sequence of the heavy chain of classic kinesin. *B,* Sketch of classic kinesin showing two heads and the coiled-coil tail with light chains bound at the distal end. *C,* Ribbon diagram of the polypeptide backbone of the kinesin head showing ATP as a space-filling model, the neck-linker residues *(red),* and the proximal part of the coiled-coil stalk. *D,* Superimposition of the core of the kinesin head on the catalytic domain of myosin showing the structural homology of the proteins. The detailed ribbon diagram shows only the homologous pieces of secondary structure. The overview *(right)* shows kinesin *(blue)* superimposed on the structure of the whole myosin head *(pink). E,* Atomic model of dimeric kinesin superimposed on a microtubule (MT) protofilament. *F,* Atomic model of dimeric ncd superimposed on a microtubule protofilament. Note that the N-terminus of ncd attaches to the tail in approximately the same position as the C-terminus of kinesin. (*C,* From Sack S, et al: X-ray structure of motor and neck domains from rat brain kinesin. Biochemistry 36:16155–16165, 1997. *C* and *E,* PDB file: 3KIN. *F,* PDB file: 2NCD. All structures courtesy of R. Vale, University of California, San Francisco.)

Classic kinesin has two heads at the N-terminus of an α-helical coiled-coil, much like myosin II, except both domains are much smaller (see Fig. 39–9). Each head, consisting of about 340 residues, is a motor unit that binds microtubules, catalyzes ATP hydrolysis, and moves microtubules. With some variation in amino acid sequence, this motor unit is common to the whole kinesin family. In classic kinesin, light chains are associated with the C-terminal bifurcation of the tail.

Because the **kinesin head** is less than half the size of a myosin head, and because the proteins lack appreciable sequence homology, determination of the atomic structure of kinesin (see Fig. 39–9) revealed a major surprise: the small kinesin molecule fits neatly inside the catalytic domain of myosin! In fact, this core of both motors is similar to the yet smaller Ras family GTPases (see Fig. 27–7), suggesting that all three families of nucleoside triphosphatases evolved from a common ancestor. The kinesin motor consists of a central, mixed, β sheet flanked by three helices on each side. ATP binds to a site homologous to the GTP-binding site of Ras, but the enzyme mechanisms differ in important ways. The microtubule-binding site was mapped at some distance from the ATP-binding site by making point mutations; it was confirmed by fitting the atomic model into three-dimensional reconstructions of kinesin bound to microtubules (Fig. 39–10).

Movement of kinesin along microtubules has two remarkable features. First, a two-headed kinesin can track faithfully along a single microtubule protofilament for long distances at 0.5 μm/sec. This processive movement, which may allow single kinesins to move organelles along microtubules in the cell, depends upon the ability of kinesin to remain associated with the microtubule as it moves toward the plus end. Second, kinesins move in discrete steps of 8 nm (see Fig. 39–9), the spacing of successive tubulin dimers in a microtubule. This large step is remarkable for the small (<10 nm) kinesin heads linked together at the neck region.

Single kinesin heads, produced experimentally by expression of truncated complementary DNAs (cDNAs), traverse a microtubule-stimulated ATPase cycle much like myosin, except that each head remains associated with the microtubule (presumably, the same tubulin subunit) through many cycles without dissociating (see Fig. 39–6). Like myosin, kinesin binds and hydrolyzes ATP rapidly. Phosphate dissociation is rate-limiting, followed by rapid ADP dissociation. KDP and KD bind microtubules less tightly than K or KT and may transiently dissociate from and rebind a microtubule, before returning to multiple cycles of ATP hydrolysis while bound to the microtubule.

Kinesin with two heads moves processively along a microtubule while remaining attached through doz-

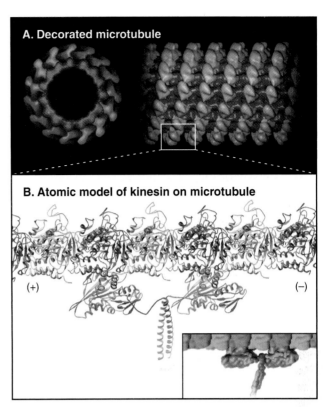

Figure 39–10 Interaction of kinesin with microtubules. *A*, Three-dimensional reconstruction from electron micrographs of kinesin heads *(blue)* bound to a microtubule *(brown)*. The primary interaction is with β-tubulin *(red)*. *B*, Atomic model of dimeric kinesin bound to the surface of a microtubule with the neck-linker peptide unfolded on the leading head *(brown, toward the plus end)* and the neck-linker peptide folded on the trailing head *(green)*. (*A*, Courtesy of R. Milligan, Scripps Research Institute, La Jolla, CA. *B*, Courtesy of R. Vale, University of California, San Francisco.)

ens of cycles of ATP hydrolysis (see Fig. 39–6D). The presence of a second head introduces a key feature: the two heads strongly influence each other, leading to reciprocal affinities of the heads for nucleotide (either ATP or ADP) and microtubules. One head binds nucleotide strongly and microtubules weakly; the other does the opposite. Hence, one head tends to bind the tubule and to dissociate its bound nucleotide rapidly. For example, if kinesin with ADP bound to both heads is mixed with microtubules, only one of the two heads binds the microtubule and dissociates its ADP.

Given an excess of ATP over ADP, ATP will bind to this open site on the head associated with the microtubule. This drives a switch that causes the weakly bound ADP head to bind the microtubule and the ATP head to dissociate. This interchange is consistent with the hypothesis (see Fig. 39–6D) that the heads step past each other such that the ADP head ends up on the tubulin dimer, 8 nm beyond the former binding site of the ATP head.

The key to this complicated head-over-head stepping of the two heads is postulated to be the folding and unfolding of a segment of the heavy chain linking the motor domain to the tail. When ATP is bound to the motor domain, this "neck-linker" peptide associates tightly with the motor domain, as shown in the x-ray structure of dimeric kinesin (see Figs. 39–6 and 39–9). When no nucleotide or ADP is bound to the motor domain, the neck-linker peptide is flexible and only loosely bound to the motor domain.

These structural changes allow the ATPase cycle to drive hand-over-hand stepping, as illustrated in Figure 39–6D. Many details of this mechanism remain to be elucidated. Note how much the deliberate stepping of kinesin differs from myosin. Myosin heads act independently, dancing rapidly and reversibly on and off an actin filament, whereas kinesin heads cooperate so that at least one head is bound to the microtubule at every point in the ATPase cycle.

Some kinesins, such as *Drosophila* ncd, move backward, toward the minus rather than the plus end of microtubules. This difference is not explained by the architecture of the motor domain, as ncd is nearly identical to kinesin (see Fig. 39–10). The ncd ATPase mechanism is similar to kinesin, although there is less cooperation between the heads and lower processivity. Why should ncd move backward? The most obvious difference is that the ncd motor domain is attached to the tail by its N-terminus, rather than C-terminus, as in kinesin. However, this cannot be the explanation because transplantation of kinesin heads to the C-terminus of a tail or of ncd heads to the N-terminus of a tail does not necessarily reverse their motor activity. Experiments with more complicated chimeric proteins suggest that the neck-linker peptide and the proximal part of the ncd tail determine the direction of movement. The ncd tail may simply orient the two heads in a way that favors binding of the detached head to the tubulin dimer in the minus, rather than the plus, direction as kinesin does.

Dyneins

Dyneins are microtubule-based motor proteins with completely different evolutionary origins than myosins and kinesins. Dyneins are members of the AAA family of ATPases that also includes hsp100 chaperones, the microtubule severing protein katanin, the clamp loader proteins for DNA polymerase processivity factors and NSF (the N-ethylmaleimide-sensitive membrane fusion protein). The sequences of these proteins have diverged so greatly during evolution that it took years to realize that they are related. These proteins consist of multiple ATP-binding domains that work together in diverse cellular processes.

Dyneins consist of gigantic heavy chains of 380 kD and a variety of smaller polypeptides (Fig. 39–11). The N-terminal 1800 residues form the tail that interacts with these accessory chains and cargo molecules. The C-terminal 2350 residues form six AAA modules, predicted to be folded much like those known from the atomic structures of homologous modules from related proteins. Modules 1 to 4 bind ATP, but only module 1 hydrolyzes ATP during the interactions with microtubules that generate movements. A ring consisting of the six AAA modules forms the globular head of dynein. Between the fourth and fifth AAA modules, the dynein heavy chain forms a rod-like loop with an ATP-sensitive microtubule-binding site at the end. The rod is formed by an anti-parallel coil of the folded back heavy chain.

Isoforms of the dynein heavy, intermediate, and light chains allow construction of a wide variety of different dyneins with many common features but with specialization for different functions. Dyneins have two or three heavy chains and the corresponding number of heads. Each type of heavy chain associates with certain light chains and intermediate chains. Subunits in the base of the molecule target dynein isoforms to particular locations. For example, axonemes of cilia and flagella incorporate at least 7 different dyneins (see Fig. 41–11), and cytoplasmic dyneins bind specific cargo, such as organelles or chromosomes (see Chapters 40 and 47).

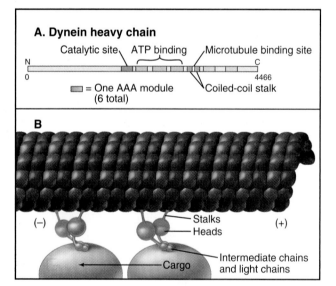

Figure 39–11 Dynein structure. *A,* Linear drawing of a dynein heavy chain showing the location of six AAA modules and two sequences predicted to form an antiparallel coiled-coil with an ATP-sensitive microtubule binding site in the connecting loop. The first AAA module forms the catalytic site. Modules 2, 3 and 4 bind but do not hydrolyze ATP. Modules 5 and 6 do not bind ATP. *B,* Model of a cytoplasmic dynein with two heads. Light and intermediate chains bind cargo and 10-nm stalks link the globular heads to the microtubule. Reconstructions of electron micrographs resolve subdomains in the 16 nm globular head corresponding to the six AAA modules and one or two other domains.

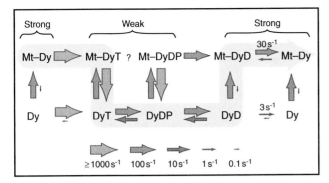

Figure 39-12 Dynein-microtubule ATPase mechanism. Arrows are proportional to the rates of the reactions, with second-order reactions adjusted for physiologic concentrations of reactants. The beige highlight shows the main pathway through the reaction. Dy, dynein; Mt, microtubule; T, ATP; D, ADP; P, inorganic phosphate.

The dynein ATPase cycle resembles the actomyosin ATPase mechanism in broad outline but differs in important details, particularly the rate-limiting reactions (Fig. 39–12). Dynein largely dissociates from the microtubule when it binds ATP. The dynein-ADP + P_i intermediate also binds weakly to microtubules. After the rapid dissociation of inorganic phosphate, the dynein-ADP complex rebinds to the microtubule. Binding to a microtubule stimulates the rate of ADP dissociation from dynein about 10-fold, from about 3 s^{-1} to about 33 s^{-1}, by accelerating a rate-limiting conformational change. Consequently, microtubules stimulate the dynein ATPase to levels required for the rapid beating of cilia at up to 100 cycles per second. Free dynein turns over ATP relatively rapidly (3 s^{-1}). However, in cilia and flagella, control mechanisms keep dynein turned off except during beating, as ATP hydrolysis is tightly coupled to the production of motion (see Chapter 41).

Further work is required to learn how the ATPase cycle drives the motion of dynein toward the minus end of microtubules. An attractive hypothesis is that the microtubule-binding stalk is used as a fulcrum to amplify conformational changes in the globular domain during the ATPase cycle. It is not understood how ATP binding to the active site might dissociate such a distant binding site from the microtubule. In vitro motility assays have not yet resolved the size of the step associated with each ATP hydrolysis, but they suggest that a small number of axonemal dyneins can generate rapid oscillatory movements of microtubules.

▌ **Selected Readings**

Geeves MA, Holmes KC: Structural mechanism of muscle contraction. Annu Rev Biochem 68:687–728, 1999.

Hackney DD: The kinetic cycles of myosin, kinesin and dynein. Annu Rev Physiol 58:731–750, 1996.

Kreis T, Vale R, eds: Guidebook to the Cytoskeletal and Motor Proteins, 2nd ed. New York: Oxford University Press, 1999.

Mandelkow E, Johnson KA: The structural and mechanochemical cycle of kinesin. Trends Biochem Sci 23:429–433, 1998.

Mocz G, Gibbons IR: Model for the motor component of dynein heavy chain based on homology to the AAA family of oligomeric ATPases. Structure 9:93–103, 2001.

Rayment I: The structural basis of the myosin ATPase activity. J Biol Chem 271:15850–15853, 1996.

Ruppel KM, Spudich JA: Structure-function analysis of the motor domain of myosin. Annu Rev Cell Dev Biol 12:543–574, 1996.

Vale RD, Fletterick RJ: The design plan of kinesin motors. Annu Rev Cell Dev Biol 13:745–778, 1997.

Vale RD, Milligan RA: The way things move: Looking under the hood of molecular motor proteins. Science 288:88–95, 2000.

Vallee RB, Gee MA: Make room for dynein. Trends Cell Biol 8:490–494, 1998.

Weiss A, Leinwand LA: The mammalian myosin heavy chain gene family. Annu Rev Cell Dev Biol 12:417–440, 1996.

chapter 40

INTRACELLULAR MOTILITY

Virtually every component inside living cells moves to some extent, but the magnitude and velocity of these movements varies by orders of magnitude depending on the cell (Table 40–1 and Fig. 40–1). At one extreme, the bulk cytoplasm of algae and giant amoebae streams tens of micrometers per second. At the other extreme, small molecules and macromolecules diffuse through cytoplasm essentially unnoticed. The cytoskeletal network of polymers has a pore size of less than 50 nm, so particles larger than the pores must be transported actively. For example, messenger RNA (mRNA) moves from its site of synthesis in the nucleus through nuclear pores into the cytoplasm and then may be carried actively to specific parts of the cell. The nucleus rotates back and forth in most cells. Lysosomes, mitochondria, secretory vesicles, and endosomes all move about actively in cytoplasm, frequently between the centrosome and the cell periphery. Intracellular pathogenic bacteria and viruses subvert the host cell's actin system to propel themselves randomly through the cytoplasm. Virus particles move along microtubules.

Just four ancient mechanisms (see Fig. 40–1) appear to account for the great variety of intracellular movements in eukaryotes: (1) transport of cargo along microtubules by kinesin or dynein; (2) polymerization and depolymerization of microtubules; (3) transport of cargo along actin filaments by myosin (which produces contraction when other actin filaments are the cargo); and (4) polymerization and depolymerization of actin filaments. Motor-driven movements on microtubules in animal cells generally receive the most attention, but taking a broad view across biology, the other mechanisms are also very important. This chapter covers a variety of intracellular movements to highlight each of these mechanisms; many more examples are found in chapters on membrane traffic (see Chapters 17 to 23 and mitosis, Chapter 47). These examples illustrate how hard it is to predict the underlying mechanism without careful inspection at the molecular level. For orientation, the first section covers the variety of specialized motor proteins in the myosin, kinesin, and dynein families.

Specialized Motor Proteins

All eukaryotes have multiple genes for myosins, kinesins, and dyneins (Figs. 40–2 and 40–3). Even the slimmed down genome of budding yeast includes genes for five myosins, six kinesins, and one dynein. Single cells can express more than a dozen different motors, and more complex organisms express diverse members of each of these families in different tissues. Sequence analysis of myosins and kinesins suggests that the major classes of these motors are universal, beginning with primitive cells at the bottom of the eukaryote radiation (see Fig. 1–1). The genes for many isoforms have been preserved over hundreds of millions of years, suggesting that each motor has a special function, such as serving as a binding site for particular cargo. Note that the genes for a particular class of motor, whether from protozoa or vertebrates, are more closely related to each other than to other classes of motors in the same organism.

Motor proteins have two parts: a **motor domain** that utilizes adenosine triphosphate (ATP) hydrolysis to produce movements (covered in Chapter 39), and a **tail** that allows the motors to self-associate or to bind particular cargo. Within each family, the motor domains are more conserved than the tails. Thus, it seems likely that the tails determine the specialized functions of each motor isoform.

table 40–1

VELOCITIES OF INTRACELLULAR MOVEMENTS

System	Velocity (μm s^{-1})	Mechanism
Microtubule motors		
Anterograde fast axonal transport, squid	1	Individual kinesin motors
Retrograde fast axonal transport, squid	2	Individual dynein motors
Chromosome movement in anaphase of mitosis, animal cells	0.003–0.2	Motors plus depolymerization
Endoplasmic reticulum sliding, Newt cell	0.1	Individual kinesin motors
Slow axonal transport, rat nerves	0.002–0.1 net 1 (intermittent)	Motors on microtubules
Microtubule polymerization		
Endoplasmic reticulum tip elongation, Newt cell	0.1	Microtubule polymerization
Actin-myosin motors		
Cytoplasmic streaming, *Nitella*	60	Myosin motors on tracks
Cytoplasmic streaming, *Physarum*	500	Actin-myosin contraction
Actin polymerization		
Actin-propelled comet, *Listeria*	0.5	Actin polymerization

The Myosin Superfamily

Myosins are the only known motors that use actin filaments for tracks. Biochemical and molecular genetic explorations have identified 18 families of myosin, classified on the basis of the amino acid sequences of their motor domains (see Fig. 40–2). Myosin tails are more variable, but generally all of the tails within a class are also related to each other. All 18 classes of myosin have deep phylogenetic roots tracing back to a common eukaryotic ancestor. The genes for the various classes separated more than a billion years ago. Some myosin families are restricted to limited parts of the phylogenetic tree. For example, myosin VIII and myosin XI are found only in plants, which lack other myosin families. In many cases, later gene duplications gave rise to multiple isoforms within each class of myosin, presumably accommodating specialized functions that confer selective advantage. For example, smooth muscle myosin genes appeared relatively recently, arising from the duplication of a gene for a cytoplasmic myosin II. Many myosin genes have been lost during evolution. This is particularly striking in the case of budding yeast, which has only two myosin Is, two myosin Vs, and one myosin II. A warning for those who delve into the myosin literature: nomenclature can be confusing. For example, myosin V from budding yeast is commonly known as Myo2p from its gene name.

Few cytoplasmic myosins have been characterized in depth, but in all but one case tested, myosins have been found to move toward the barbed end of actin filaments using ATP hydrolysis and an energy-transducing mechanism similar to muscle myosin (see Fig. 39–6). The exception is **myosin VI**, which moves toward the pointed end of actin filaments. Some class-

es of myosin use modifications of the ATPase cycle for specialized functions. For example, ADP release from myosin V is rate limiting. This slow step allows myosin V to walk slowly for long distances along an actin filament rather than dancing lightly on and off actin like muscle myosin II.

The number of **light chains** varies from one to seven per heavy chain. Calmodulin (see Fig. 2–14) serves as a light chain in some cases, specialized light chains in others.

Myosin tails are striking in their diversity of structure and ligand-binding activities. Many tails form coiled-coils, so those myosins have two heads like muscle myosin. A few have single heads. The tail of myosin II is best understood. This α-helical coiled-coil forms the bipolar filaments (see Fig. 4–7 and Fig. 5–4.) that are essential for the antiparallel sliding of actin filaments during muscle contraction (see Chapter 42) and cytokinesis (see Fig. 47–21). The single-headed myosin Is have short tails, including a basic domain with affinity for acidic phospholipids. Some myosin I tails also have an SH-3 domain (see Fig. 27–11) that binds proline-rich sequences in other proteins. Some myosin I tails bind actin filaments independent of the motor domain, enabling them to cross-link actin filaments. A domain in the tail of myosin X stimulates guanosine triphosphate (GTP) hydrolysis by the small G protein, Rho.

Establishing the biological functions of the various myosins has been a challenge. Biochemical characterization of ligands and localization in cells provide some clues, but genetic or biochemical knockouts often have mild effects, probably owing to overlapping functions of the myosins and the capacity of some cells to adapt to their loss, at least under laboratory conditions. The first example was also the clearest,

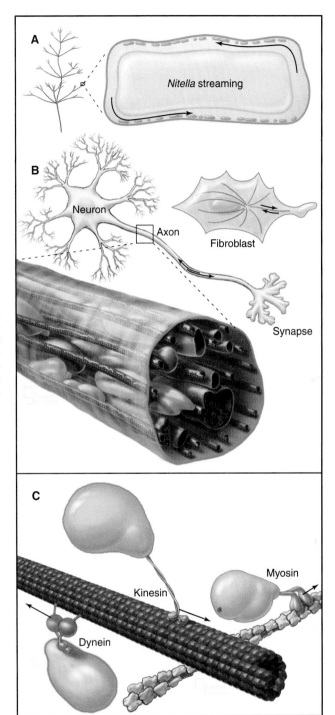

Figure 40-1 Mechanisms of intracellular movement. *A*, The green alga *Nitella* moves cytoplasmic organelles along bundles of actin filaments located in the cell cortex. *B*, Fibroblasts and neurons move organelles bidirectionally along microtubules. *C*, Microtubule-based and actin filament–based motors. The microtubules are depicted as red; actin filaments are yellow.

namely that immunologic inhibition of or genetic deletion of **myosin II** inhibits cytokinesis (see Chapter 47). Mouse and yeast mutations show that **myosin V** participates in the movement of pigment granules and other cellular components. Mutations show that **myosin I** is required for endocytosis, as expected from its concentration at sites of phagocytosis and macropinocytosis. In microvilli of intestinal epithelial cells, myosin I links actin filaments laterally to the plasma membrane (see Fig. 36–2). Myosins VI and VII are es-

sential in auditory and vestibular cells in the ear, as loss-of-function mutations cause deafness in mice and humans. Similarly, fly photoreceptor cells degenerate without myosin III.

Many different mechanisms have evolved to regulate cytoplasmic myosins. As in smooth muscle (see Fig. 42–21), phosphorylation of the regulatory light chain activates myosin II in animal nonmuscle cells. In addition, phosphorylation of the heavy chain regulates the polymerization of some myosin IIs. Lower eukary-

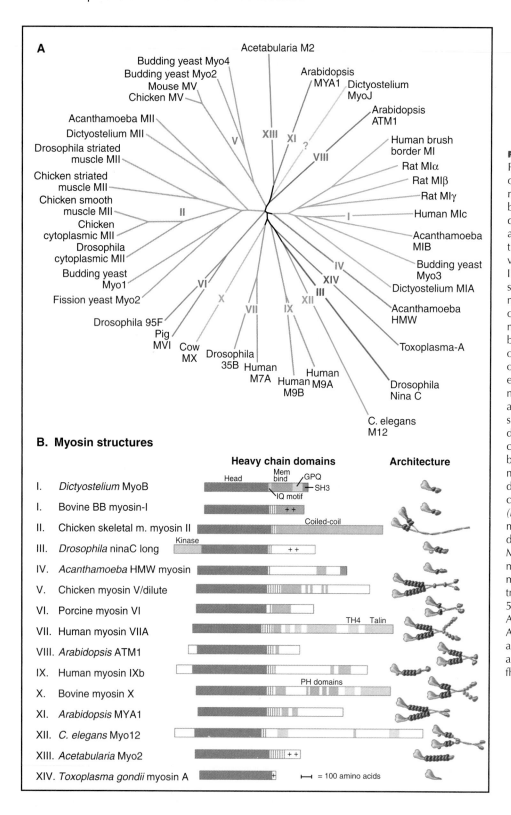

A

Acetabularia M2

Budding yeast Myo4
Budding yeast Myo2
Mouse MV
Chicken MV

Arabidopsis
MYA1   Dictyostelium
MyoJ

Acanthamoeba MII

Dictyostelium MII

Drosophila striated
muscle MII

Chicken striated
muscle MII

Chicken smooth
muscle MII

Chicken
cytoplasmic MII

Drosophila
cytoplasmic MII

Budding yeast
Myo1

Fission yeast Myo2

Drosophila 95F
Pig
MVI
Cow
MX   Drosophila
35B   Human
M7A   Human
M9B   Human
M9A

V   XIII   XI
?
VIII

II

VI

X
VII   IX   XII

IV
XIV
III

I

Arabidopsis
ATM1

Human brush
border MI

Rat MIα
Rat MIβ
Rat MIγ
Human MIc

Acanthamoeba
MIB

Budding yeast
Myo3

Dictyostelium MIA

Acanthamoeba
HMW

Toxoplasma-A

Drosophila
Nina C

C. elegans
M12

B. Myosin structures

Heavy chain domains   **Architecture**

Mem
bind   GPQ
Head   SH3
I.   *Dictyostelium* MyoB   IQ motif

I.   Bovine BB myosin-I   + +

II.   Chicken skeletal m. myosin II   Coiled-coil

Kinase
III.   *Drosophila* ninaC long   + +

IV.   *Acanthamoeba* HMW myosin

V.   Chicken myosin V/dilute

VI.   Porcine myosin VI

TH4   Talin
VII.   Human myosin VIIA

VIII.   *Arabidopsis* ATM1

IX.   Human myosin IXb

PH domains
X.   Bovine myosin X

XI.   *Arabidopsis* MYA1

XII.   *C. elegans* Myo12

XIII.   *Acetabularia* Myo2   + +

XIV.   *Toxoplasma gondii* myosin A   ⊢—⊣ = 100 amino acids

Figure 40-2 Myosin family. *A*, Phylogenetic relationships based on sequences of motor domains. Note the very early branching of 15 myosin classes denoted by Roman numerals and of many isoforms within these classes (e.g., cytoplasmic versus striated muscle myosin II). Thus, much of myosin diversity is very ancient. Genes for myosins in related species (for clarity, illustrated here only by mouse and chicken myosin V) branched only recently. Many of the specific names are based on gene names and are not enumerated here. *B*, Drawing of myosin heavy chain domains and molecular models of myosin isoforms showing catalytic domains *(rose)*; IQ motifs, light chain binding sites *(rose bars)*; basic domains with affinity for membrane lipids *(violet)*; SH3 domains *(dark green)*; coiled-coil *(orange)*; kinase domain *(light blue)*; and pleckstrin homology domain *(blue)*. (Redrawn from Mermall V, Post P, Mooseker MS: Unconventional myosins in cell movement, membrane traffic and signal transduction. Science 279:527–533, 1998. Copyright 1998, American Association for the Advancement of Science. See also Myosin Home Page, available at ⟨www.http://blocks.fhcrc.org/~myosin⟩.)

otes use both light chain phosphorylation to activate and heavy chain phosphorylation to inhibit myosin II. Heavy chain phosphorylation activates myosin I from lower eukaryotes, whereas calcium binding to the calmodulin light chains regulates myosin I from the intestinal brush border. Less is known about the regulation of other classes of myosin.

The Kinesin Superfamily

Early in evolution, gene duplication and recombination produced at least nine families of kinesins having motor domains associated with a variety of tails (see Fig. 40–3; Table 40–2). Classification systems based on the sequences of motor domains group kinesins

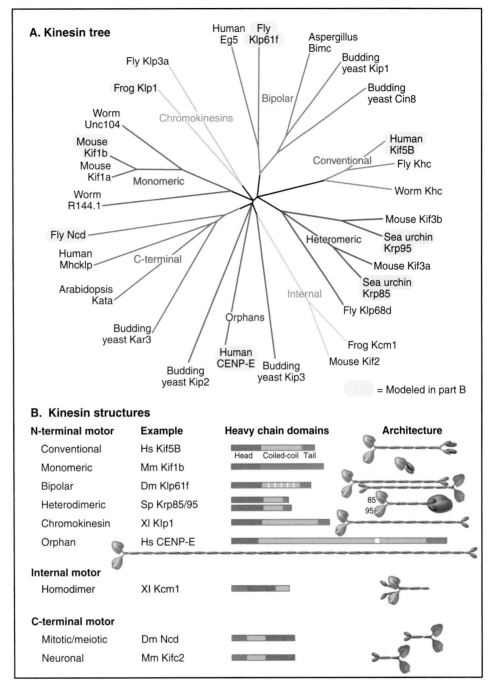

Figure 40–3 Kinesin family. *A,* Phylogenetic relationships of a selection of kinesins based on the sequences of the motor domains. *B,* Drawing of kinesin heavy chain domains and molecular models of kinesin isoforms showing the catalytic domain *(red);* coiled-coil *(orange);* and tails *(blue).* (*A* and *B,* Based on data of R. Case and R. Vale, University of California, San Francisco; see also the Kinesin Home Page available at ⟨www.http://blocks.fhcrc.org/~kinesin⟩.)

that also have similar tails and functions. The motor domain is most often located at the N-terminus, but some classes have motor domains in the middle or at the C-terminus of the polypeptide. Most kinesins are dimeric, with two polypeptides joined in a coiled-coil. Most are homodimers, but one class consists of two different polypeptides with motor domains plus another large subunit. Most kinesins move along microtubules toward their plus ends, but C-terminal kinesins, such as ncd, move toward the minus end and internal motor kinesins may not move at all. Whether located at the N- or C-terminus, the motor domains

are similar in structure; peptide sequences that link the head to the tail determine the direction of movement on microtubules (see Chapter 39).

Kinesins transport a variety of cargo, including chromosomes and organelles, along microtubules. **Chromokinesins** have DNA binding sites that allow them to bind to the surface of mitotic chromosomes and carry them toward the metaphase plate (see Chapter 47). **CENP-E** is concentrated at kinetochores. **Bipolar kinesins** form an antiparallel dimer of two-headed kinesins that can interact with a pair of oppositely polarized microtubules and push apart the poles of the

table 40-2

KINESIN SUPERFAMILY: CLASSIFICATION AND EXAMPLES OF KINESIN-FAMILY MOTOR PROTEINS

Class	Examples	Subunits (kD)	Velocity	Functions
N-terminal motor				
Conventional	Human KHC	2×110, 2×70	+0.9	Organelle movement
Monomeric	Mouse KIF1B	1×130	+0.7	Mitochondria movement
Bipolar	Fly KLP61F	4×121	+0.04	Pole separation, mitosis
Heterodimeric	Urchin KRP85/95	1×79, 1×84, 1×115	+0.4	Organelle movement
Chromokinesin	*Xenopus* Kp11	2×139	+0.2	Chromosome movement
Orphan	Human CENP-E	2×340	+0.1	Kinetochore-microtubule binding
Internal motor				
Homodimeric	Mouse KIF2	2×81	+0.5	Axonal transport
	MCAK/XKCM1	2×83	?	Microtubule disassembly
C-terminal motor				
Mitotic	Fly ncd	2×78	−0.2	Mitotic/meiotic spindle
Neuronal	Mouse KIFC2	2×86	?	Organelle movement

Velocities in μm s^{-1}. Adapted from Vale RD, Fletterick RJ: Annu Rev Cell Dev Biol 13:745–777, 1997. More data on kinesins are available at the Kinesin Home Page ⟨www.http://blocks.fhcrc.org/~kinesin⟩.

mitotic spindle. A variety of evidence implicates kinesin in organelle movements, but the interactions of kinesins with membranes are not yet well understood. Most kinesins appear to be constitutively active, so much may remain to be learned about their regulation.

The Dynein Superfamily

Dyneins are giant ATPases that move along microtubules toward their minus ends (see Chapter 39). The

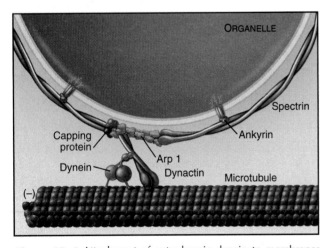

Figure 40-4 Attachment of cytoplasmic dynein to membranes by the dynactin complex. Dynein moves toward the minus end of a microtubule. It is linked to a vesicle by the dynactin complex associated with spectrin on the membrane surface. Dynactin complex consists of a short filament of Arp1 capped on its barbed end by capping protein, p50 dynamitin, and p150^{glued}, which binds both Arp1 and microtubules. (Redrawn from Holleran E, et al: The role of the dynactin complex in intracellular motility. Int Rev Cytol 182:69–109, 1998.)

minus ends of microtubules are associated with the microtubule-organizing center near the centrosome of many cells, or near the terminal web at the apical surface of epithelial cells (see Chapter 37). Animals have multiple genes for dynein heavy chains, multiple splice isoforms of intermediate chains, and multiple isoforms of light chains. However, owing to the technical challenge of working with such large genes and proteins, the full extent of dynein diversity is not yet known. Tissues express these dynein isoforms differentially, and the heavy chain isoforms target to specific cellular organelles, such as the Golgi apparatus. A null mutation in the gene for a mouse cytoplasmic dynein heavy chain leaves the Golgi apparatus dispersed throughout the cytoplasm and is lethal during embryogenesis. Calcium and a cyclic adenosine monophosphate (cAMP)–dependent protein kinase (see Chapter 41) regulate dynein in cilia and flagella, but little is known about the regulation of cytoplasmic dynein.

Specific dynein isoforms associate with microtubules in axonemes (see Chapter 41), kinetochores of chromosomes during mitosis (see Chapter 47), and membranes of organelles that move along cytoplasmic microtubules. A 20S protein assembly called the **dynactin complex** links dynein to membranes and is required for their transport along microtubules (Fig. 40-4). This complex consists of a short filament of the actin-related protein, Arp1, and seven other subunits, including heterodimeric capping protein. A 150-kD subunit (p150^{glued}) binds to an intermediate chain of dynein. The Arp-1 filament interacts with spectrin associated with the membrane. Mutations in *Drosophila* p150^{glued} cause developmental defects in the eye and brain.

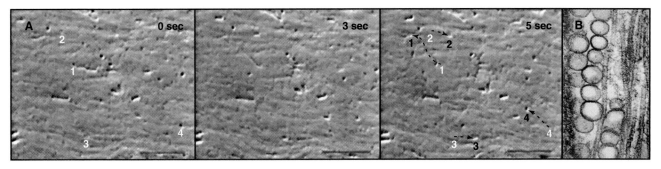

Figure 40-5 Fast transport in cytoplasm isolated from squid giant axons. *A*, Three frames from a series of video-enhanced differential interference contrast (DIC) micrographs show movement of organelles in both the anterograde *(right)* and retrograde *(left)* directions. Four large organelles are marked with numbers. Movement, as indicated with an arrow, is from the white to the black number. These organelles are colored green at zero time, blue at 3 seconds, and red at 5 seconds. The original video record shows hundreds of smaller organelles moving steadily in either an anterograde or a retrograde direction at 1–2 μm/second. *B*, Electron micrograph of a thin section showing vesicles associated with microtubules in axoplasm. (*A*, Courtesy of S. Brady, University of Texas Southwestern Medical School, Dallas. *B*, Courtesy of R. H. Miller, Case Western Reserve Medical School.)

Rapid Movements Along Microtubules

Organelles in most cells move at relatively high velocities, on the order of one micrometer per second (see Table 40–1) along linear microtubule tracks. Thus, the organization of microtubules determines the patterns of these movements (see Fig. 38–2 and 40–1). These movements of organelles share many features with intraflagellar transport of proteins in cilia and flagella (see Chapter 41). Analysis of microtubule-based movements is particularly favorable in axons of nerve cells because axons are long (up to 1 m) but narrow, the microtubules have a uniform polarity, and organelles move at constant rates in both directions. Furthermore, nerve cells contain high concentrations of microtubules and microtubule motors; indeed, cytoplasmic tubulin, cytoplasmic dynein, and kinesin were all originally isolated from brain.

High-contrast light microscopy of living axons reveals that most membrane-bound organelles move steadily either toward (anterograde) or away from (retrograde) the end of the axon (Fig. 40–5). **Retrograde movements** (2.5 μm s^{-1}) are faster than **anterograde movements** (0.5 μm s^{-1}). At these rates, a round trip from a cell body in the spinal cord of a human to the foot and back takes only 3 weeks. This may seem slow, but if a 0.1-μm vesicle were the size of a small car, it would be moving anterograde at 50 miles per hour and retrograde at 250 miles per hour. In the axons of vertebrate neurons, mitochondria and autophagic vesicles move back and forth in both directions. Their net movement toward the nerve terminal or cell body depends on physiological conditions.

Rapid axonal transport provides the periphery of a nerve cell with fresh membrane components and re-trieves endosomes from the end of the axon. Small, round, and tubular vesicles, including components of synaptic vesicles (see Chapter 10), move toward the end of the axon, where they enter the cycle of synaptic vesicle turnover. Multivesicular bodies derived from lysosomes form at the nerve terminus and travel in a reterograde direction back to the cell body. This can be illustrated by constricting a nerve mechanically to block transport, which causes different organelles to pile up on either side (Fig. 40–6).

Microtubule-based motor proteins bound to moving organelles power fast axonal transport (see Fig. 40–1). The plus-end motors of the kinesin family are responsible for anterograde movements toward the nerve terminal, and the minus-end motor dynein is responsible for movement in the retrograde direction. Herpesvirus and rabies virus also use dynein for long-distance transport on microtubules from the terminals of sensory nerves to the cell body, where viral DNA enters the nucleus for replication. In vitro kinesin and dynein can move plastic beads in the appropriate directions at the same velocities as they move organelles. Movements of organelles along microtubules have been reconstituted with purified dynein and kinesin. Final proof of the responsible motors depends on genetic tests. A null mutation of mouse KIF1A, a monomeric kinesin, reduces the anterograde transport of synaptic vesicles. However, kinesin mutations in flies do not give a clear-cut, fast transport phenotype, most likely because of the presence of multiple plus-end motors. Because dynein piles up on both sides of constrictions in axons, the dynein used for retrograde transport is probably carried to the nerve terminal as cargo on vesicles that are moved in an anterograde direction by kinesin. Vesicles that move on microtubules can transfer to and move along actin filaments, so

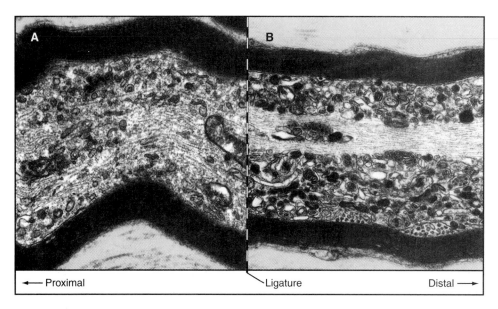

Figure 40-6 Electron micrographs showing the result of nerve ligation. *A,* The cytoplasm proximal to the ligation demonstrates the accumulation of vesicles and mitochondria, which were being transported toward the nerve terminal to the right. *B,* The cytoplasm distal to the ligation shows the accumulation of lysosomes, multivesicular bodies, and mitochondria, which were being transported toward the cell body to the left. (From Hirokawa N et al: J Cell Biol 111: 1027–1037, 1990, by copyright permission of the Rockefeller University Press.)

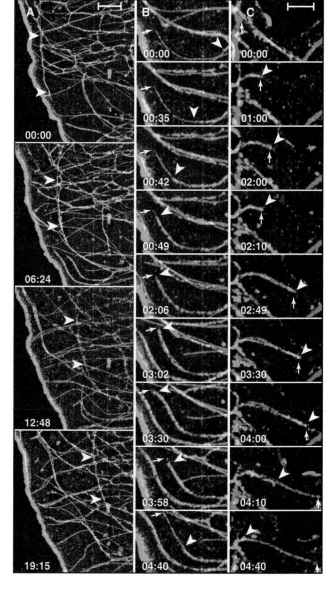

Figure 40-7 Two modes of microtubule-dependent movement of the endoplasmic reticulum in a Newt epithelial cell. The cell was microinjected with rhodamine-labeled tubulin *(red),* which incorporates into microtubules, and a lipophilic green fluorescent dye (DiOC₆), which labels endoplasmic reticulum. Time series are indicated in minutes and seconds. *A,* Fluorescence micrographs illustrate the dynamics of microtubules *(red)* and endoplasmic reticulum *(green),* over a period of 19 minutes. Arrowheads mark a strand of endoplasmic reticulum moving away from the leading edge. Scale bar is 5 μM. *B,* Time course of the movement of a strand of endoplasmic reticulum toward the end of a microtubule, followed by retraction. This type of movement is thought to be driven by a kinesin motor attached to the tip of the elongating membrane *(arrowhead).* *C,* Time course of the movement of a strand of endoplasmic reticulum attached to the tip of a growing microtubule *(arrowhead),* followed by retraction of the membrane along the microtubule. Scale bar for *B* and *C* is 5 μM. (Courtesy of C. Waterman-Storer and E. D. Salmon, University of North Carolina, Chapel Hill. Reference: Waterman-Storer C, Salmon ED: Endoplasmic reticulum membrane tubules. Curr Biol 8:798–806, 1998. Copyright 1998, with permission from Elsevier Science.)

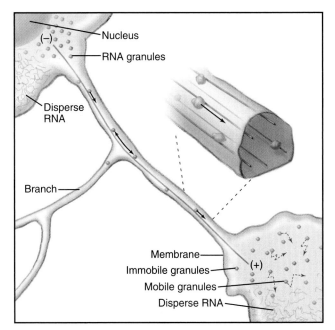

Figure 40-8 Transport of mRNA for myelin basic protein in a cultured oligodendrocyte, a glial cell isolated from brain. mRNA synthesized in the cell body (or, in this case, labeled with a fluorescent dye and microinjected into the cell body) is packaged with proteins in a ribonucleoprotein particle, transported from the cell center along microtubules at a steady rate of 0.2 μm/second, and released at the periphery where it moves randomly at 1 μm/second. (Redrawn from Ainger K, et al: Transport and localization of exogenous myelin basic protein mRNA microinjected into oligodendrocytes. J Cell Biol 123: 431–441, 1993, by copyright permission of the Rockefeller University Press.)

myosin may be used for local movements of vesicles at the nerve terminus and in the cortex of the axon.

Many questions remain open regarding the control of microtubule motors during fast transport, including: how the bidirectional movements of mitochondria are biased by the physiological state of the cell to achieve net transport; how kinesins remain active and dynein inactive during the long trip to the nerve terminal; and how cytoplasmic dynein on retrograde cargo is activated locally at the nerve terminal and kept active during movement to the cell body.

Other cells use the same molecular mechanisms to move organelles in the cytoplasm. Secretory vesicles use plus-end motors to move from the Golgi apparatus to the plasma membrane. Endosomes use dynein to move from the plasma membrane toward the cell center. The distribution of the endoplasmic reticulum depends on intact microtubules. Strands of the endoplasmic reticulum align with microtubules in cultured cells (Fig. 40–7). This codistribution is achieved in two ways: (1) motors can transport tubules of endoplasmic reticulum bidirectionally on microtubules, and (2) other tubules of the endoplasmic reticulum can attach to the plus end of microtubules and ride the microtubule tip as it grows and shrinks during dynamic instability (see later discussion). The latter is the

best example of movement of an organelle driven by microtubule assembly. The condensation of the Golgi near the centrosome depends on intact microtubules and dynein motors that transport Golgi vesicles toward the minus ends of the microtubules. Mitochondria are a complicated example, as they move bidirectionally on microtubules in animal cells but depend on actin filaments in yeast. These examples illustrate how not only the dynamics of the organelles, but also the overall organization of a cell, depend on the activity of microtubule motors. Thus, cellular structure is determined actively, not passively.

The distribution of nucleoprotein complexes in the cell also depends on active movements. Microtubule assembly and microtubule motors participate in the assembly of the mitotic spindle and chromosome movement during mitosis (see Chapter 47). RNAs use microtubules for movements through the cytoplasm (Fig. 40–8). Specific RNA sequences promote the assembly of protein-containing particles that move at steady rates on microtubules over long distances in the cell. The movements are in the plus direction, so a kinesin family member may be responsible. Microtubules and motors also transport specific mRNAs to help establish the polarity of fly embryos. Because mutations in the actin-binding protein tropomyosin can also affect RNA distribution, actin may participate as well. Investigators are still compiling the complete inventory of macromolecular cargos that move actively along microtubules or actin filaments.

Intracellular Movements Driven by Microtubule Polymerization

Microtubule polymerization and depolymerization has long been known to play a central role in the assembly of the mitotic apparatus and the movement of chromosomes (see Chapter 47), as well as the establishment of cellular asymmetry (see Chapter 41), but only recently have cell biologists begun to appreciate its potential for moving organelles. An in vitro proof-of-principle experiment (Fig. 40–9) revealed that chro-

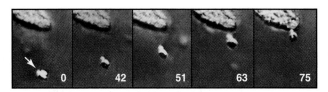

Figure 40-9 Transport of an isolated chromosome on a shortening microtubule in vitro. A microtubule was grown from brain tubulin on the extracted carcass of a ciliate, *Tetrahymena*. A chromosome *(arrow)* was added as a test cargo and captured by the end of the microtubule. When the concentration of tubulin was reduced, the microtubule shortened, carrying along the chromosome attached to its tip. This transport occurs in the absence of ATP or GTP. (Courtesy of J. R. McIntosh, University of Colorado, Boulder.)

mosomes can attach to the end of a microtubule and ride along the end as it depolymerizes, even in the absence of ATP or GTP. One explanation is that multiple weak bonds between the chromosome and the side of the microtubule near its end can rearrange rapidly enough to maintain attachment, even as tubulin subunits dissociate from the end.

Endoplasmic reticulum provides the best example of an intracellular organelle that harnesses microtubule growth for movement as an alternative to motor-driven movements along microtubules (see Fig. 40–7). A "tip attachment complex" yet to be characterized maintains a connection between the endoplasmic reticulum and the end of a microtubule as its length

varies secondary to cycles of polymerization and depolymerization.

Bulk Movement of Cytoplasm Driven by Actin and Myosin

Bulk streaming of cytoplasm is most spectacular in plant cells (see Fig. 40–1A). Although confined within rigid walls, plant cell cytoplasm streams vigorously at very high velocities (up to 60 μm s^{-1}). At this rate, cytoplasm moves 5 m per day. Such **cytoplasmic streaming** is best understood in the giant cells of the green alga, *Nitella* (Fig. 40–10). Streaming occurs con-

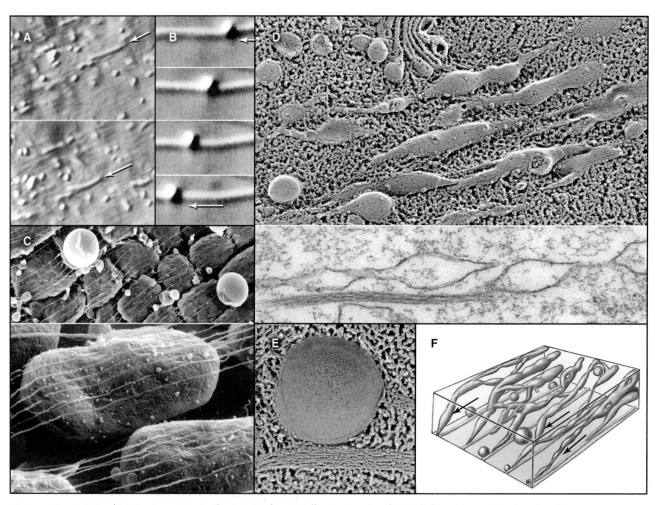

Figure 40–10 Cytoplasmic streaming in the green alga *Nitella*. *A,* A pair of DIC light micrographs showing the movement of organelles in cytoplasm. The arrow marks a strand of endoplasmic reticulum. *B,* Time series of DIC light micrographs showing movement of a vesicle isolated from *Nitella* along a bundle of actin filaments isolated from *Nitella*. *C,* Scanning electron micrographs of the cortex isolated from *Nitella* showing the bundles of actin filaments associated with chloroplasts. *D,* Transmission electron micrographs of a freeze-fracture preparation *(upper)* and thin section *(lower)* showing endoplasmic reticulum associated with actin filament bundles. *E,* Freeze-fracture preparation of a vesicle associated with an actin filament bundle. *F,* Drawing depicting the movement of endoplasmic reticulum along actin filament bundles dragging along bulk cytoplasm. (Courtesy of B. Kachar, National Institutes of Health. Reference: Kachar B, Reese T: The mechanism of cytoplasmic streaming in characean algal cells. J Cell Biol 106:1545–1552, 1988, by copyright permission of the Rockefeller University Press.)

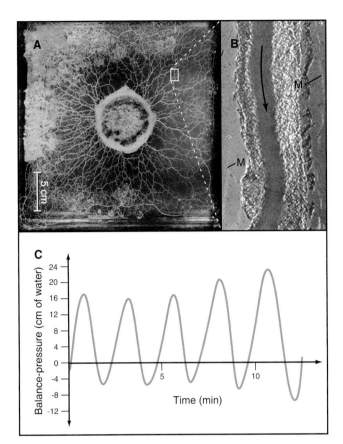

Figure 40–11 Cytoplasmic streaming in the acellular slime mold *Physarum polycephalum. A,* Photograph of *Physarum,* a giant multinucleated single cell growing in a baking dish. *B,* Blur photomicrograph made with polarization optics by taking a time exposure showing the bulk streaming of the endoplasm in a cytoplasmic strand *(long arrow).* M is mucus. *C,* Time course of pressure changes produced by shuttle streaming of cytoplasm through a strand. (*B,* From Nakajima H: The mechanochemical system behind streaming in *Physarum.* In Allen RD, Kamiya N, eds. Primitive Motile Systems in Cell Biology. New York: Academic Press, 1964, pp. 111–123. *C,* Reference: Kamiya N. The mechanism of cytoplasmic movement in a myxomycete plasmodium. Symp Soc Exp Biol 22:199–214, 1968.)

dragging along other cytoplasmic components, including organelles and soluble molecules. The biochemical properties of this myosin must be fascinating because the velocity of streaming is nearly 10 times faster than the fastest muscle contraction.

An actomyosin mechanism different from that in plants produces equally spectacular cytoplasmic streaming in the acellular slime mold *Physarum.* In these giant, multinucleated cells, cytoplasm flows back and forth rhythmically at high velocities through tubular channels (Fig. 40–11). Cycles of contraction and relaxation of cortical actin filament networks push the relatively fluid endoplasm back and forth in a manner akin to squeezing a toothpaste tube. Myosin II is thought to generate the cortical contraction, as it is present in high concentration in this cell and can contract actin filament gels in vitro. (This, incidentally, was the first nonmuscle myosin to be purified in the late 1960s.) The cortical contractions that are so prominent in *Physarum* are also used by giant amoebae for cell locomotion (see Fig. 41–1), for cytokinesis (see Fig. 47–21), and for folding of epithelial sheets (see Fig. 41–3).

Actin-Based Movements of Organelles in Other Cells

Like *Nitella,* budding yeasts transport vesicles along bundles of actin filaments from the mother to the bud (Fig. 40–12), although this vesicle movement does not appear to produce cytoplasmic streaming. Myosin V is the motor, given the fact that vesicles fail to move

tinuously in a thin layer of cytoplasm between the large central vacuole and chloroplasts immobilized in the cortex. On each side of the cell, a zone of stationary cytoplasm separates streams moving in opposite directions. The physiological function of this streaming is not clearly understood.

Bulk streaming in *Nitella* is brought about by movement of endoplasmic reticulum along tracks consisting of bundles of polarized actin filaments associated with chloroplasts (see Fig. 40–10). Actin filaments in these bundles have the same polarity, and cytoplasm streams toward their barbed ends. In *Nitella* extracts, membrane vesicles move along actin filament bundles at the same high velocities characteristic of the cytoplasmic streaming. An extraordinary myosin pulls endoplasmic reticulum along cortical actin tracks,

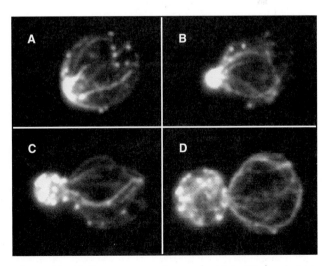

Figure 40–12 Fluorescence micrographs (*A* to *D*) showing actin filament bundles and patches at various stages in the cell cycle of the budding yeast *Saccharomyces cerevisiae.* Myosin V uses these actin filament bundles to deliver vesicles (including the vacuole), certain mRNAs, and at least one enzyme (chitin synthase) from the mother to the bud. (Courtesy of J. A. Cooper, Washington University.)

from mother to bud in null mutants of myosin V genes. Yeasts also depend on actin filaments and a myosin V to transport certain mRNAs from the mother to the bud, where they determine cell fate.

Given the ability of myosins to move organelles in plant and fungal cells, it seems likely that animal cells use the same mechanisms. In fact, vesicles isolated from nerve cells can move along both actin filaments and microtubules. Owing to the short actin filaments in animal cells, the amplitude of movements on actin is expected to be relatively small, making them more difficult to detect than the long-distance movements of organelles along highly extended microtubules. Nevertheless, in many cells, actin filaments are strategically positioned to transport secretory vesicles the last micrometer or so to the plasma membrane.

Cytoplasmic Movements Driven by Actin Polymerization

Some intracellular pathogenic bacteria, including *Listeria* and *Shigella,* move through the cytoplasm at about 0.5 μm s^{-1} on actin filament rockets (Fig. 40–13B). Polymerization of actin filaments at one pole of the bacterium produces an asymmetrical force that drives it forward. The rocket tail of cross-linked actin filaments is stationary and depolymerizes distally at the same rate that it grows next to the bacterium, so it remains a constant length. Proteins localized asymmetrically on the surface of the bacterium mobilize from

the host cell some of the same proteins that organize the assembly of actin filaments at the leading edge of motile cells (see Fig. 36–18 and Fig. 41–5). These include Arp2/3 complex and VASP (vasodilator-stimulated phosphoprotein) so the mechanisms may be similar. One exception is that the small GTPases implicated in cellular actin assembly are not required for the constitutive assembly of actin by bacteria. Under some conditions, cellular endosomes can induce actin filament rockets and undergo movements similar to *Listeria*, rather than using microtubules. It is not yet known how widely this phenomenon is used for intracellular motility. Vaccinia virus also usurps the actin assembly system to drive movement over the surface of the host animal cell at one stage in its life cycle (see Fig. 40–13A). Similar propulsive, cytoplasmic rocket tails can be induced in some cells by a plastic bead placed on the plasma membrane.

Slow Transport of Cytoskeletal Polymers and Associated Proteins in Axons

Many neuronal proteins move slowly from their site of synthesis in the cell body toward the ends of axons and dendrites. This transport is essential, as protein synthesis is restricted to the cell body, whereas more than 99% of cell volume can be in axons and dendrites. If nerve cells were smaller or less asymmetrical, one might not even notice such slow movements.

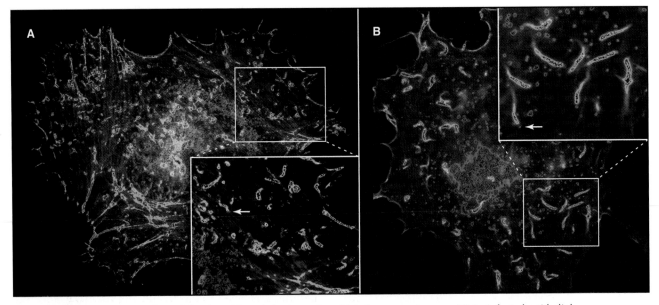

Figure 40–13 Movements of vaccinia virus (A) and the bacterium *Listeria monocytogenes* (B) in infected epithelial cells. Fluorescence micrographs with actin filaments stained green with fluorescein-phalloidin and pathogens stained orange. Both pathogens usurped the actin assembly machinery of the cell to assemble a cross-linked network, shaped like a comet tail, which pushes the organism (*arrows*). *Listeria* moves through the cytoplasm. Vaccinia moves on the cell surface. (Courtesy of F. Frischknecht and M. Way, European Molecular Biology Laboratory, Heidelberg.)

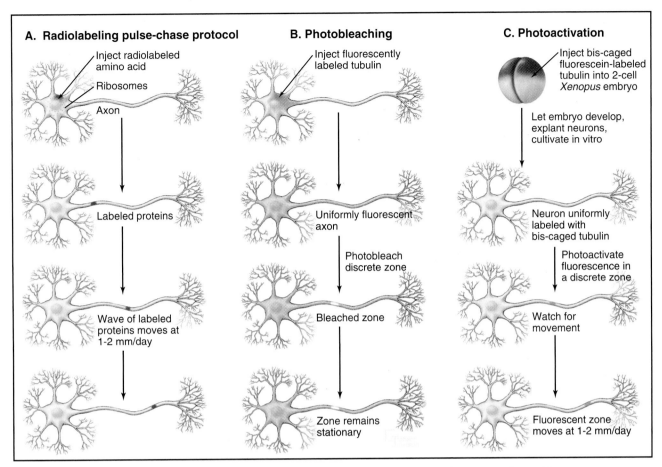

A. Radiolabeling pulse-chase protocol

Inject radiolabeled amino acid

Ribosomes

Axon

Labeled proteins

Wave of labeled proteins moves at 1-2 mm/day

B. Photobleaching

Inject fluorescently labeled tubulin

Uniformly fluorescent axon

Photobleach discrete zone

Bleached zone

Zone remains stationary

C. Photoactivation

Inject bis-caged fluorescein-labeled tubulin into 2-cell *Xenopus* embryo

Let embryo develop, explant neurons, cultivate in vitro

Neuron uniformly labeled with bis-caged tubulin

Photoactivate fluorescence in a discrete zone

Watch for movement

Fluorescent zone moves at 1-2 mm/day

Figure 40–14 Experiments on slow axonal transport. *A,* Pulse-chase experiment. Radioactive amino acids are injected into the spinal cord or eye of an experimental animal. In the nerve cell body, radioactive tracer is incorporated into proteins, which are transported out the axon. Some proteins are incorporated into stationary structures and left along the way. *B,* Photobleaching experiment. A cultured nerve cell is injected with tubulin labeled with a fluorescent dye. Tubulin fills the cytoplasm and axon as it grows out. A section of the axon is then bleached with a strong pulse of light. This bleached zone is stationary over a period of minutes. *C,* Photoactivation experiment. Tubulin labeled with a caged fluorescent dye is injected into a *Xenopus* embryo. Later, nerve cells are isolated from the embryo and grown in culture where they extend axons rapidly. When the cage is removed from the fluorescent dye with a pulse of light, fluorescent tubulin can be followed by fluorescence microscopy. Fluorescence moves slowly as a block. (Redrawn from D. W. Cleveland and P. N. Hoffman: Slow axonal transport models come full circle. Cell 67:453–456, 1991. Copyright 1991, with permission from Elsevier Science.)

These movements along axons can be followed by labeling the proteins with radioactive amino acids during their synthesis in the cell body (Fig. 40–14A). Proteins moved by slow axonal transport are classified into two groups based on their velocities. Tubulin, intermediate filament proteins, and spectrin, which comprise the "slow component-a" move exceedingly slowly, about 0.1 to 1.0 mm per day (or 1–10 nm/ sec). In a human, these molecules take more than 3 months to travel from their site of synthesis in the spinal cord to the foot. "Slow component-b" moves about 10 times faster and includes 10 times more protein than slow component-a. It is a heterogeneous mixture of proteins, including clathrin, glycolytic enzymes, and actin.

Defining the mechanism of slow transport has

been challenging and contentious because various experimental approaches have yielded apparently conflicting results (see Fig. 40–14). Radioactive labeling has established the existence of movements and has shown that the moving proteins decline in concentration as they move away from the cell body (see Fig. 40–14A). Photobleaching of fluorescent tubulin and actin in axons of cultured neurons has demonstrated that the bulk of these cytoskeletal polymers are stationary (Fig. 40–14B), whereas fluorescent tubulin, photoactivated inside an axon of a cultured *Xenopus* neuron, has been found to move as a block at a rate characteristic of slow transport (see Fig. 40–14C).

This puzzle was resolved when it became possible to image single fluorescent intermediate filaments in axons of live nerve cells. It turns out that these filaments are stationary most of the time (up to 99%), but occasionally, they move rapidly (0.2 to 2 μm s^{-1}) for up to 20 μm. Most of their movements are away from the cell body, accounting for the net movement. These rapid but intermittent movements depend on microtubules and are presumably driven by motor proteins. Similar experiments with other slowly transported proteins are needed to establish whether or not they use the same mechanism.

▌ Selected Readings

Brady ST: Neurofilaments run sprints not marathons. (Slow axonal transport.) Nature Cell Biol 2:E43–45, 2000.

Brown SS: Cooperation between microtubule- and actin-based motor proteins. Annu Rev Cell Dev Biol 15:63–80, 1999.

Chou YH, Helfand BT, Goldman RD: New horizons in cytoskeletal dynamics: Transport of intermediate filaments along microtubule tracks. Curr Opin Cell Biol 13:106–109, 2001.

Dramsi S, Cossart P: Intracellular pathogens and the actin cytoskeleton. Annu Rev Cell Dev Biol 14:137–166, 1998.

Goldstein LSB, Phip AV: The road less traveled: Emerging principles of kinesin motor utilization. Annu Rev Cell Dev Biol 15:141–183, 1999.

Hasson T, Mooseker MS: Vertebrate unconventional myosins. J Biol Chem 271:16431–16434, 1996.

Hermann GJ, Shaw JM: Mitochondrial dynamics in yeast. Annu Rev Cell Dev Biol 14:265–304, 1998.

Hirokawa N: Kinesin and dynein superfamily proteins and the mechanism of organelle transport. Science 279:519–526, 1998.

Holleran EA, Karki S, Holzbaur ELF: The role of the dynactin complex in intracellular motility. Int Rev Cytol 182:69–109, 1998.

Mermall V, Post PL, Mooseker MS: Unconventional myosins in cell movement, membrane traffic and signal transduction. Science 279:527–533, 1998.

Milisav I: Dynein and dynein-related genes. Cell Motil Cytoskel 39:261–272, 1998.

Nixon RA: The slow axonal transport of cytoskeletal proteins. Curr Opin Cell Biol 10:87–92, 1998.

Rosenbaum JL, Cole DG, Diener DR: Intraflagellar transport: The eyes have it (review). J Cell Biol 144:385–388, 1999.

Vale RD, Fletterick RJ: The design plan of kinesin motors. Annu Rev Cell Dev Biol 13:745–777, 1997.

chapter 41

CELLULAR MOTILITY

Cells move at rates that range over four orders of magnitude (Fig. 41–1; Table 41–1). At one extreme, ciliates and sperm swim rapidly through water and giant amoebas crawl rapidly over solid substrates. At the other extreme, rigid cell walls prevent many fungal, algal, and plant cells from moving. However, even some plant cells move rapidly, such as pollen, which extends tubular pseudopods (see Fig. 35–1). Most cells, including human white blood cells, nerve growth cones, and fibroblasts move at intermediate rates. The examples presented in this chapter illustrate general principles of cellular motility.

Cells produce forces for motility in many different ways, most commonly using the same four mechanisms that produce intracellular movements (see Chapter 40): contraction of actin-myosin networks; movement of motors on microtubules; reversible assembly of actin filaments; or reversible assembly of microtubules. However, the repertoire of molecular mechanisms is larger. Some cells use contraction of calcium-sensitive fibers, reversible assembly of novel cytoskeletal polymers, or the rotary motion of bacterial flagellar motors. As in intracellular motility, the mechanisms complement each other, even in cases in which movements depend mainly on one system. For example, microtubules contribute to actin-based pseudopod extension by helping to specify the polarity of the cell.

Most cells possess the basic machinery for cellular motility, so the striking variability in their rates of movement arises from differences in the organization of this machinery and the emphasis placed on various types of movements. For example, both nonmotile yeast and contractile muscle cells contain actin, myosin, heterodimeric capping protein, α-actinin and tropomyosin. These are minor proteins in yeast but constitute the bulk of the protein found in muscle (see Chapter 42). The contractile apparatus in muscle is highly organized for rapid, one-directional contractions, whereas yeasts use similar proteins for cytokinesis and intracellular transport.

Cell Shape Changes Produced by Extension of Surface Processes

Simple alteration of cellular shape is the most primitive type of cellular motility. This can be brought about by assembly of new cytoskeletal polymers or by rearrangement of preexisting cytoskeletal assemblies. Actin filaments, microtubules, or other cytoskeletal fibers can support these changes. A few highly exaggerated examples illustrate the principles involved.

During fertilization, echinoderm sperm use actin polymerization to extend a long filopodium to penetrate the protective jelly surrounding the egg (Fig. 41–2A). Actin subunits for this **acrosomal process** are stored with profilin (see Chapter 36) in a concentrated packet near the nucleus. Contact with an egg stimulates actin filaments to polymerize, starting from a dense structure near the nucleus. Subunits add to the distal (barbed) end of growing filaments, driving the elongation of the process and the surrounding membrane at a rate of 5–10 μm s^{-1}. Actin subunits diffuse rapidly enough from their storage site to drive this rapid elongation, which pushes the plasma membrane forward.

A similar mechanism may explain the growth of the actin filament bundles that support filopodia and microvilli (see Chapter 36) on most other cells, including nerve growth cones, fibroblasts, and epithelial cells. Actin filaments of brush border microvilli are organized and stabilized by proteins that cross-link the filaments to each other (fibrin and villin) and to the plasma membrane (myosin I). During embryonic development, the pool of cellular actin does not form

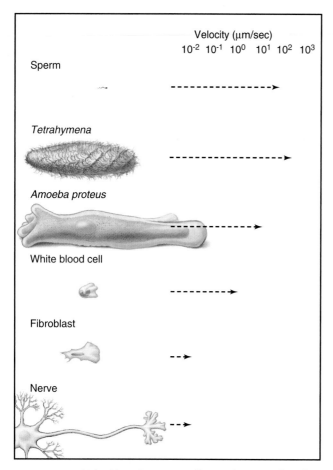

Figure 41–1 Velocities of moving cells vary by more than four orders of magnitude. Scale drawings of cells with a range of velocities.

microvilli until the epithelial cells synthesize these accessory proteins. Similarly, cells with few microvilli can be induced to make more simply by increasing the level of villin.

Sperm of the horseshoe crab, *Limulus*, use a novel acrosomal process to penetrate an egg (see Fig. 41–2*B*). They preassemble a coiled bundle of actin filaments cross-linked by a protein called scruin. This bundle is like a tightly coiled spring. When a sperm encounters an egg, an unknown signal triggers a rearrangement of the crosslinks, causing the actin bundle to unwind. It threads its way through a channel in the nucleus and emerges at the anterior end of the sperm head. The uncoiling bundle drives the extension of a process surrounded by plasma membrane that literally screws its way through the egg jelly to fertilize the egg.

A group of ciliates called heliozoans, named for their similarity to a cartoon of the sun, use microtubules instead of actin filaments to extend, support, and retract long, thin processes bounded by the plasma membrane (see Fig. 38–4). Microtubules in these **axopodia** are cross-linked into a precise geometrical array that accounts for the rigidity of these long processes. Axopodia are dynamic, collapsing in a few seconds after mechanical stimulation by prey organisms, which are dragged toward the cell body for phagocytosis. The collapse is caused by rapid depolymerization of the microtubules. Ca^{2+} influx appears to trigger depolymerization of the microtubules, but the details of the mechanism are not known. This ability to use reversible microtubule assembly to support transient cell surface projections is unusual.

Cell Shape Changes Produced by Contraction

Cells can change shape by localized or oriented cytoplasmic contractions. Muscle contraction (see Chapter 42) and cytokinesis (see Chapter 47) are the best examples, but similar contractions remodel many embryonic tissues. Localized contractions at the base or apex of cells in a planar epithelium cause evaginations or invaginations that form the neural tube (see Fig. 32–7) and that bud glands off from the gastrointestinal tract and respiratory tract (Fig. 41–3). As in cytokinesis

table 41–1

VELOCITIES OF CELLULAR MOVEMENTS

System	Unitary Velocity ($\mu m\ s^{-1}$)	Summed Velocity ($\mu m\ s^{-1}$)	Motile Mechanism
Striated muscle contraction (biceps)	5–10	4–8×10^5	Actin-myosin ATPase
Filopodium extension, *Thyone* sperm	10	10	Actin polymerization
Pseudopod extension, fibroblast	0.02	0.02	Actin polymerization
Pseudopod extension, human neutrophil	0.1	0.1	Actin polymerization
Pseudopod extension, *Amoeba proteus*	?	10	?Actin-myosin ATPase
Pseudopod extension, nematode sperm	1	1	Assembly of major sperm protein
Retraction of axopodium, heliozoan	>100	>100	Disassembly of microtubules
Spasmoneme contraction, *Vorticella*	?	23,000	Calcium-induced conformational change
Swimming, *E. coli*		25	Flagellum powered by rotary motor
Swimming, sea urchin sperm		15	Microtubule-dynein ATPase

Ext

B.

Figur
in spa
zed a
tripho
nucle<
the b<
Cappi
inorga
cofilin
of AD
initiate
depoly
PAK,
dynan
Revie\
Inset,

41–4
then
tion (
T
of th
many
come
Arp2
of otl
serve
Rho-f
actin<
36), i
erodi
filam<
the r
the h
bias

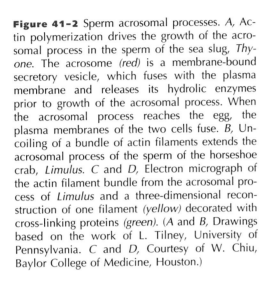

Figure 41-2 Sperm acrosomal processes. *A*, Actin polymerization drives the growth of the acrosomal process in the sperm of the sea slug, *Thyone*. The acrosome *(red)* is a membrane-bound secretory vesicle, which fuses with the plasma membrane and releases its hydrolic enzymes prior to growth of the acrosomal process. When the acrosomal process reaches the egg, the plasma membranes of the two cells fuse. *B*, Uncoiling of a bundle of actin filaments extends the acrosomal process of the sperm of the horseshoe crab, *Limulus*. *C* and *D*, Electron micrograph of the actin filament bundle from the acrosomal process of *Limulus* and a three-dimensional reconstruction of one filament *(yellow)* decorated with cross-linking proteins *(green)*. (*A* and *B*, Drawings based on the work of L. Tilney, University of Pennsylvania. *C* and *D*, Courtesy of W. Chiu, Baylor College of Medicine, Houston.)

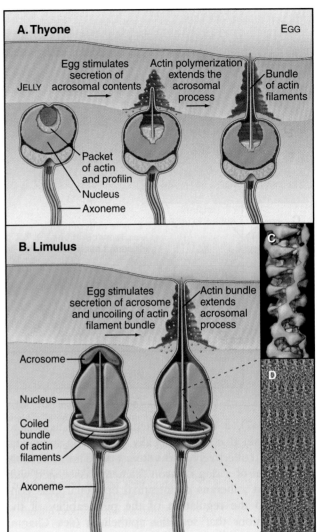

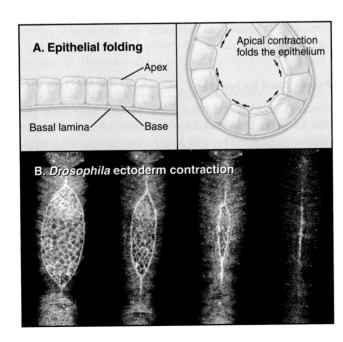

Figure 41-3 Actomyosin contractions mold the shape of epithelia during embryonic development. *A*, Contraction of the apical pole of columnar epithelial cells changes their shape and invaginates an epithelium, as in the formation of the neural tube. *B*, Contraction around the margin of the ectoderm pulls this epithelium over the surface of a *Drosophila* embryo. Time series of fluorescence micrographs of live embryos expressing an actin-binding fragment of the protein moesin, which has been fused to green fluorescent protein. (*B*, Courtesy of D. Kiehart, Duke University. Reference: Kiehart DP, et al: Multiple forces contribute to cell sheet morphogenesis for dorsal closure in *Drosophila*. J Cell Biol 149:471–490, 2000.)

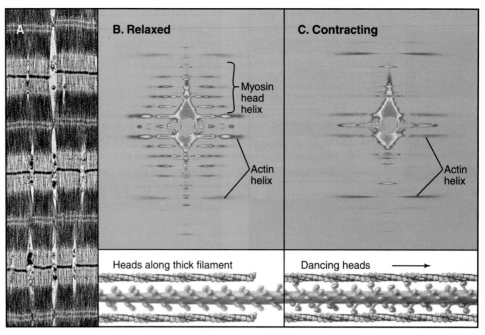

Figure 42–13 Cross-bridge dynamics revealed by x-ray diffraction patterns of whole muscle. *A,* Electron micrograph showing the orientation of the muscle in the x-ray beam. *B* and *C,* Fiber diffraction patterns from relaxed and contracting skeletal muscles with interpretive drawings of cross-bridges in each state. Reflections from myosin heads arranged on the thick-filament helix are strong in relaxed muscle. Reflections from the actin helix are stronger than the thick-filament helix in contraction. The myosin and actin reflections are each labeled in only one of four equivalent quadrants. During contraction, a few myosin heads attach transiently to actin, increasing the strength of the actin helix reflections, but most are disordered. (Micrograph and x-ray patterns courtesy of H. E. Huxley, Brandeis University.)

actin-myosin complex, dissociating the cross-bridge and starting a new ATPase cycle.

Relationship of Cross-bridge Behavior to the Mechanical Properties of Muscle

Under normal conditions, each sarcomere shortens less than 1 μm. However, the whole muscle shortens macroscopically because it has thousands of sarcomeres in series. For example, a human biceps muscle 20 cm long has about 80,000 sarcomeres in series from end to end. When each contracts 0.25 μm, the muscle shortens 2 cm. Because the system maintains a constant volume, each sarcomere and the whole muscle increase in diameter as they shorten. Although the individual filaments slide past each other relatively slowly (about 5 μm/second), muscles contract rapidly because the motion of each sarcomere in the series is added together. In our example, without resistance, the biceps contracts 2 cm in 100–200 msecs.

The behavior of cross-bridges explains why the velocity of muscle contractions of an active muscle depends on the external load (see Fig. 42–12). Contraction velocity is maximal when opposed by no load. Without a load, the molecular motion stored in elastic elements of each cross-bridge is largely converted into movement of actin filaments relative to

myosin filaments. Under these conditions, the filaments in muscle slide past each other at a rate of about 5 μm per second, the same speed observed for free actin filaments moving over myosin heads in vitro (see Fig. 39–4). For this rapid sliding to occur, myosin heads not producing force must not impede movement. If bound tightly to actin, they would interfere mechanically with rapid sliding. This is avoided by the rapid equilibrium of the myosin intermediates between being bound to actin and being free (see Fig. 39–6). Myosin heads with bound ATP or ADP-P$_i$ do not produce force when they bind transiently to a given actin subunit. These brief encounters do not retard sliding driven by force producing cross-bridges.

Muscle produces maximum force when the contraction rate is zero (see Fig. 42–12). The conformational change in the myosin head stretches elastic elements in the cross-bridge, but the force cannot overcome the resistance from the load on the muscle. Consequently, the filaments do not slide, and energy stored in each stretched elastic element is lost as heat when the cross-bridge dissociates at the end of the ATPase cycle. The maximum force depends on the numbers of sarcomeres in parallel, that is, the cross-sectional area of the muscle. Thus, muscles respond to strengthening exercises by growing in diameter.

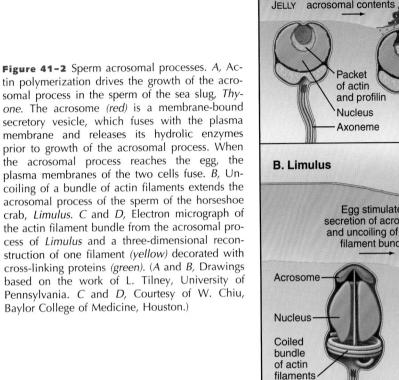

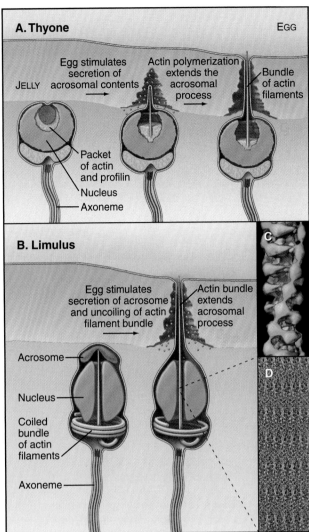

Figure 41-2 Sperm acrosomal processes. *A,* Actin polymerization drives the growth of the acrosomal process in the sperm of the sea slug, *Thyone.* The acrosome *(red)* is a membrane-bound secretory vesicle, which fuses with the plasma membrane and releases its hydrolic enzymes prior to growth of the acrosomal process. When the acrosomal process reaches the egg, the plasma membranes of the two cells fuse. *B,* Uncoiling of a bundle of actin filaments extends the acrosomal process of the sperm of the horseshoe crab, *Limulus. C* and *D,* Electron micrograph of the actin filament bundle from the acrosomal process of *Limulus* and a three-dimensional reconstruction of one filament *(yellow)* decorated with cross-linking proteins *(green).* (*A* and *B,* Drawings based on the work of L. Tilney, University of Pennsylvania. *C* and *D,* Courtesy of W. Chiu, Baylor College of Medicine, Houston.)

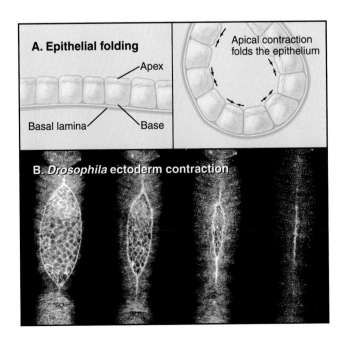

Figure 41-3 Actomyosin contractions mold the shape of epithelia during embryonic development. *A,* Contraction of the apical pole of columnar epithelial cells changes their shape and invaginates an epithelium, as in the formation of the neural tube. *B,* Contraction around the margin of the ectoderm pulls this epithelium over the surface of a *Drosophila* embryo. Time series of fluorescence micrographs of live embryos expressing an actin-binding fragment of the protein moesin, which has been fused to green fluorescent protein. (*B,* Courtesy of D. Kiehart, Duke University. Reference: Kiehart DP, et al: Multiple forces contribute to cell sheet morphogenesis for dorsal closure in *Drosophila.* J Cell Biol 149:471–490, 2000.)

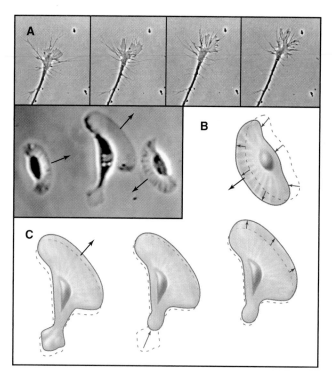

Figure 41-4 Motility by pseudopod extension. *A,* Time series at 1-minute intervals of phase-contrast light micrographs of a growth cone of a cultured nerve cell. The growth cone extends filopodia and then fills in the space between with an actin-filled lamella. *B* and *C,* Movements of cultured fish epidermal keratocytes. Phase-contrast light micrograph of live cells and drawings of cells. *B,* The dotted profile of the cell at an earlier point in time shows how these cells glide forward at a steady rate using actin polymerization to expand a broad anterior lamella and myosin-based contraction to retract the posterior. *C,* This time series shows a cell with an adhesive rear that is retracted intermittently as the leading edge moves forward. (*A,* Courtesy of D. Bray, University of Cambridge. *B* and *C,* Courtesy of J. Lee, University of Connecticut, Storrs, and K. Jacobson, University of North Carolina, Chapel Hill.)

(Chapter 47), a bundle of actin filaments associated with myosin II contracts locally, deforming individual cells and, collectively, the whole epithelium. Similarly contraction of a ring of actin filaments associated with the zonula adherans of intestinal epithelial cells contributes to the regulation of the permeability of the tight junctions that seal the epithelium (see Chapter 33). These localized cellular contractions are presumably controlled by the phosphorylation of the myosin II light chain, but the signal transduction mechanisms are still being investigated. Closure of the epidermis over a *Drosophila* embryo also requires a circumferential ring of actin filaments and myosin II (see Fig. 41–3).

Locomotion by Pseudopod Extension

The ability to crawl over solid substrates or through extracellular matrix is essential for many cells (Fig. 41–4). Perhaps the most spectacular example is the slowly moving **growth cone** of a nerve axon. Although moving a mere 0.1 μm per second or less, these structures navigate precisely over distances ranging from micrometers to meters to establish all of the connections in a human nervous system consisting of billions of neurons and about 1 million miles of cellular processes! During vertebrate embryogenesis, neural crest cells also migrate long distances before differentiating into pigment cells and sympathetic neurons. Fibroblasts depend on locomotion to lay down collagen fibrils (see Chapter 31). White blood cells require motility to move from the blood circulation to sites of inflammation (see Chapter 34) and to engulf microorganisms by phagocytosis (see Chapter 23).

This type of locomotion requires coordination of three different events. The cell must extend its leading edge, adhere to the substrate, and (if the whole cell is to move) retract its tail along with any attachments. Cells vary considerably in how they meet these requirements (see Fig. 41–4). Actin and associated proteins provide the molecular basis for locomotion in most cells, but a completely different system produces remarkably similar movements in nematode sperm (see a later section).

Pseudopod Extension

Pseudopods that lead the way in cell migration are rich in actin filaments (see Fig. 36–2*D* and *E*), and extension of pseudopods is sensitive to the drug cytochalasin, which disrupts actin filaments (see Fig. 36–16). In the best understood examples, growth of actin filaments at the **leading edge** pushes the plasma membrane forward. Filaments grow at their barbed ends near the plasma membrane and disassemble deeper in the cytoplasm (see Fig. 36–17). Details vary from cell to cell. Epithelial cells from fish scales (see Fig. 41–4*B*) advance forward on a broad front with the filaments remaining stationary relative to the substrate (see Fig. 36–17). These cells literally polymerize their way forward. Nerve growth cones (see Fig.

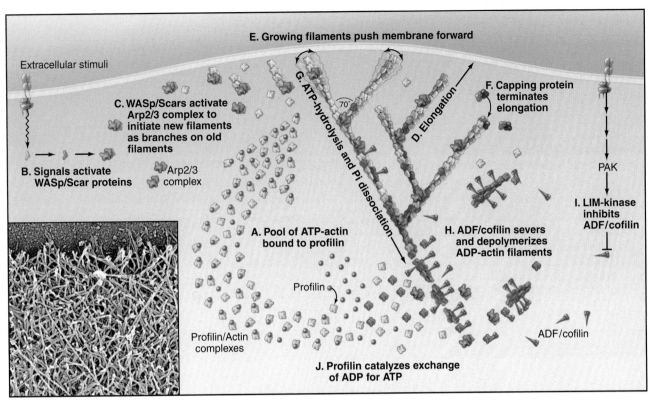

Figure 41-5 A model for actin filament assembly and disassembly at the leading edge. The reactions are separated in space for clarity, but actually occur together along the leading edge. *A,* Cells contain a large pool of unpolymerized actin bound to profilin. *B,* Stimulation of cell surface receptors produces activated Rho-family guanosine triphosphatases (GTPases) and other signals that activate WASp/Scar proteins. *C,* These proteins, in turn, activate nucleation of new actin filaments by Arp2/3 complex on the side of existing filaments. *D,* The new filaments grow in the barbed direction until they are capped (see *F*). *E,* Growing filaments push the plasma membrane forward. *F,* Capping protein terminates elongation. *G,* Polymerized ATP-actin *(yellow)* hydrolyzes the bound ATP to ADP and inorganic phosphate (Pi) *(orange),* followed by slow dissociation of phosphate yielding ADP-actin *(red). H,* ADF/cofilins bind and sever ADP-actin filaments and promote disassembly of ADP-actin. *J,* Profilin promotes the exchange of ADP for ATP, refilling the pool of unpolymerized ATP-actin bound to profilin. *I,* Some of the same stimuli that initiate polymerization can also stabilize filaments when LIM-kinase phosphorylates ADF/cofilins, inhibiting their depolymerizing activity. *Inset,* Electron micrograph of the branched network of actin filaments at the leading edge. PAK, p21-activated kinase. (Redrawn from Pollard TD, Blanchoin L, Mullins RD: Biophysics of actin filament dynamics in nonmuscle cells. Annu Rev Biophys Biomol Struct 29:545–576, 2000, with permission from the *Annual Review of Biophysics and Biomolecular Structure,* Vol. 29, © 2000 by Annual Reviews, www.AnnualReviews.org. *Inset,* Courtesy of T. Svitkina and G. Borisy, University of Wisconsin, Madison.)

41–4*A*) and other cells extend short filopodia and then fill in the spaces between them with a combination of new cortical actin filaments.

The molecular mechanism orchestrating assembly of the leading edge (Fig. 41–5) is thought to share many features with the formation of actin filament comets by intracellular bacteria (see Fig. 40–13). **Arp2/3 complex** nucleates new filaments on the side of other filaments, forming the branching network observed in cells. Motile cells activate this process with Rho-family GTPases (see Chapter 27) and other signals acting through **WASp/Scar proteins,** (see Chapter 36), rather than by a bacterial membrane protein. Heterodimeric **capping protein** limits the growth of the filaments, but phosphatidyl 4,5-bisphosphate (PIP$_2$) in the membrane may dissociate capping protein from the barbed end of filaments near the membrane and bias their growth forward. Actin filament cross-linking

proteins stabilize pseudopods. Human melanoma cells lacking **filamin** form unstable pseudopods all around their peripheries and locomote abnormally (Fig. 41–6). These tumor cells revert to normal behavior if they express filamin. Similarly, *Dictyostelium* lacking ABP120 (a smaller homologue of filamin) forms fewer pseudopods. Severing proteins such as ADF/cofilins are thought to disassemble the actin filaments deep in the cytoplasm, recycling actin and accessory proteins for multiple rounds of assembly as the cell moves forward.

Chemotaxis

Extracellular chemical clues can define the direction of locomotion by influencing the formation and persistence of pseudopods. The response to a positive signal is called chemotaxis. For example, *Dictyostelium* re-

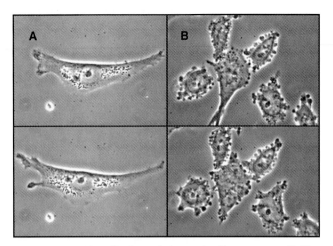

Figure 41–6 Contribution of the actin filament cross-linking protein filamin to the stability of the leading edge of human melanoma cells. Pairs of phase-contrast light micrographs, taken at different times, of living cells grown in serum containing medium on a plastic surface. *A,* Melanoma cells expressing filamin have normal leading lamella. *B,* Melanoma cells lacking filamin form spherical blebs around their margins and migrate very little. (Courtesy of C. Cunningham and T. P. Stossel, Harvard Medical School. Reference: Cunningham C, et al: Actin-binding protein requirement for cortical stability and efficient locomotion. Science 255:325–327, 1992. Copyright 1992, American Association for the Advancement of Science.)

sponds positively to a source of cyclic adenosine monophosphate (cAMP), the chemotactic chemical that these cells use to form colonies prior to making spores. Within seconds, a cell forms a new pseudopod and moves toward the cAMP (Fig. 41–7). cAMP binds a seven-helix receptor in the plasma membrane (see Chapter 26) that activates trimeric G proteins (see Chapter 27). Downstream events require Rho-family GTPases, especially Cdc42, and induce the formation of new actin filament barbed ends. Local polymerization and cross-linking of these actin filaments (see Fig. 37–19) expands the cortex facing the source of cAMP into a new pseudopod. By a similar mechanism, chemokines and bacterial metabolites—especially small peptides from the N-termini of bacterial proteins, such as **N-formyl-methionine-leucine-phenylalanine** (referred to as FMLP in the literature)—are chemotac-

tic for white blood cells. They attract leukocytes from the circulation to sites of infection (see Fig. 32–15).

Negative signals also influence pseudopod persistence and the direction of motility. A classic example is the negative effect of contact with another cell. Loss of **contact inhibition** of motility by tumor cells contributes to their tendency to migrate among other cells and spread throughout the body. The mechanism of this "contact inhibition" of motility is still being investigated. Repulsive chemical signals are important for axon guidance (see later section).

Influence of the Substrate

Pseudopods must establish contacts with the substrate for the cell to move forward. Both the chemical and physical nature of the substrate influence these adhesions and cellular movement. Cells tend to move up gradients of adhesiveness but stop if adhesion is too strong. Rapidly moving white blood cells attach weakly and transiently, whereas slowly moving fibroblasts and epithelial cells form longer lasting, integrin-mediated focal contacts (see Chapter 32). Weak binding of integrins to the extracellular matrix molecules, such as fibronectin, allows adherence without immobilization, so cultured cells move up gradients of fibronectin coated on glass. Similarly, neural crest cells migrate preferentially through specific regions of embryonic connective tissue thought to be marked by adhesive proteins in the extracellular matrix.

Role of Myosin in Motility

Although actin polymerization drives many pseudopods, the very rapid growth of pseudopods by giant amoebae is best explained by actin-myosin contractions in the cortex or front of the pseudopod, or both (see Fig. 41–1). These contractions cause cytoplasm to stream forward into the advancing pseudopod where actin filaments form a cortical gel through which cytoplasm continues to flow. The participation of myosin in other pseudopods is less clear. Local inactivation of myosin V in growth cones compromises extension of filopodia, but its role is not yet clear. *Dictyostelium* mutants lacking myosin II or individual isoforms of

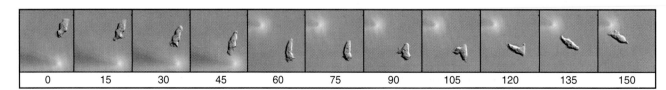

Figure 41–7 Chemotaxis of a *Dictyostelium* amoeba toward cAMP *(gold)* released from a micropipette. A time series of differential interference micrographs shows the rapid formation of a new pseudopod and reorientation of the direction of movement when the position of the micropipette is moved at the 60-second time point. (Courtesy of Susan Lee and Richard Firtel, University of California, San Diego.)

myosin I can still extend pseudopods, although mutants lacking three different myosin I isoforms are impaired in their ability to move toward attractive chemical signals. If myosins participate, they may pull forward actin filaments, the plasma membrane, or other components along preexisting actin filaments into an advancing pseudopod.

Myosin does appear to contribute to retraction of the cell body behind advancing pseudopods. Growth cones draw out a long cellular process from a stationary cell body, but most motile cells must retract their tails to move forward. Adherent, slowly moving cells like fibroblasts exert significant tension on the underlying substrate. When this tension overcomes the attachments at the rear of the cell, the rear shortens elastically; this is then followed by further active shortening (see Fig. 41–4C). Concentration of myosin II in the rear of cells suggests that it generates the tension. *Dictyostelium* cells lacking myosin II have a defect in polarity; mutant cells extend pseudopods around the whole periphery rather than favoring the front of the cell.

Microtubules help cells maintain the polarized shape required for persistent directional locomotion, but they are not required for pseudopod extension. On the other hand, small cells can move directionally and respond to chemotactic stimuli after their microtubules are depolymerized or even when the nucleus and centrosome are removed surgically.

Growth Cone Guidance: A Model for Regulation of Motility

Growth cones of embryonic nerve cells use a combination of positive and negative cues to navigate with high reliability to precisely the right location to create a synapse (Fig. 41–8). This combinatorial strategy is much more complex than the simple chemoattraction of white blood cells to soluble bacterial peptides, as is appropriate for the more complicated task of connecting billions of neurons to each other and to targets, such as specific muscle cells. Cues for growth cone guidance come from soluble factors and cell surface molecules, each requiring a specific receptor on the growth cone. As in other systems, extracellular matrix molecules provide a substrate for growth cone movements. Precisely positioned expression of cue molecules and their receptors guides growth cones along a staggering number of different pathways. The following are some well-characterized examples:

- *Positive chemoattractants.* Localized cells in the nervous system, such as those in the floor plate of the developing spinal cord, secrete soluble chemoattractant proteins like **netrin.** Gradients of netrin provide long-range guidance for growth cones of

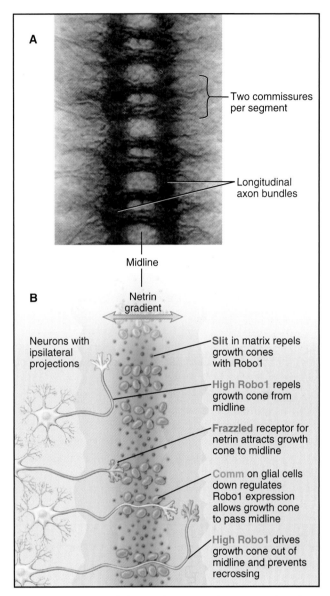

Figure 41–8 *Drosophila* growth cone guidance. *A,* Light micrograph of a filleted embryo showing the nerve cord stained brown with an axon marker. The axons of about 90% of neurons cross the midline a single time before running longitudinally in fascicles on each side of the midline. *B,* Drawing showing the ligands and receptors that guide growth cones across the midline and prevent their return to the ipsilateral (original) side. Frazzled receptors for netrin attract the growth cone to the midline where Comm down-regulates the activity of Robo1, a repulsive receptor for Slit, allowing axons to cross the midline. (*A,* Courtesy of John Thomas, Salk Institute, La Jolla, CA.)

cells possessing netrin receptors (DCC-like, Frazzled) to migrate toward a netrin source. Growth cones without these receptors ignore this cue.

- *Negative chemorepellents.* A variety of cells express **semaphorins,** a family of transmembrane and secreted proteins that repel growth cones expressing appropriate receptors. Neuropilins are receptors for soluble semaphorins (SemaIII). Plexins are transmembrane receptors for cell surface semaphorins (SemaI). Semaphorin binding to these receptors causes growth cones to collapse or turn away.

- *Matrix repellents.* **Slit,** a large extracellular matrix protein, repels growth cones with slit receptors, immunoglobulin cell adhesion molecules ([Ig-CAMs] called Robo1 and Robo2). Mutations in these receptors cause growth cones to ignore slit.
- *Cell adhesion proteins.* Ig-CAM cell surface adhesion proteins (see Chapter 32), such as **fasciculin II,** prompt growing axons to bundle together in bundles called fascicles by homophilic interactions. Growth cones can be attracted out of these bundles to particular targets, such as muscle cells, that secrete chemoattractants or proteins that antagonize fascicuclin II adhesion.

Navigation of growth cones in *Drosophila* embryos illustrates the participation of multiple cues (see Fig. 41–8). These insights came largely from the effects of mutations in genes for the various receptors and their ligands. Growth cones of neurons on one side of the nerve cord cross the midline to the opposite side and migrate to their targets with great fidelity. Netrins secreted by cells at the midline attract growth cones expressing the netrin receptor. However, midline cells also secrete high levels of a matrix protein, Slit, which repels growth cones. Growth cones manage to cross the midline by overcoming this repulsion. Near the midline, growth cones encounter cells with a

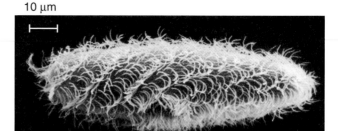

10 μm

Figure 41–10 Scanning electron micrographs of coordinated beating of cilia of *Paramecium*. Waves of effective strokes pass regularly over the cell surface from one end to the other to keep the cell moving steadily forward. (Courtesy of T. Hamasaki, Albert Einstein College of Medicine, New York. Reference: Lieberman SJ, Hamasaki T, Satir P: Ultrastructure and motion analysis of permeabilized Paramecium. Cell Motil Cytoskel 9:73–84, 1988.)

novel transmembrane protein called Comm. Acting through an unidentified receptor, Comm down-regulates the activity of the slit receptor on the growth cone. This allows the growth cone to ignore Slit and cross the midline. Once across the midline, growth cones up-regulate the slit receptor so that once they complete the journey across the midline, they never cross back to the side of origin. Local cues alert particular growth cones of motor neurons to branch off of fascicles to innervate individual muscle cells. The molecular connections of these growth cone guidance receptors to the cytoskeleton are under investigation.

Locomotion by Cilia and Flagella

Microtubule-based axonemes that produce the beating of cilia and flagella are not only exceedingly complex but also remarkably ancient. Diplomonads and trichomonads at the very bottom of the eukaryotic radiation (see Fig. 1–1) have flagella that share the essential features of human cilia and flagella. This highly efficient organelle for rapid swimming developed 1 to 2 billion years ago and is retained essentially unchanged in most parts of the eukaryotic phylogenetic tree. Most protists, algae, and animals have axonemes. So do some fungi, ferns, and plants.

Cilia and flagella are distinguished from each other by their beating patterns (Fig. 41–9), but are nearly identical in structure. In fact, the flagella of the alga *Chlamydomonas* can alternate between propagating waves typical of flagella and the oar-like rowing motion of cilia. Subtle differences in the mechanism that converts the dynein-powered sliding of the axonemal microtubules into movements determines which beating pattern is produced.

Both cilia and flagella can propel cells. They cycle rapidly, beating up to 100 times per second. Propagation of bends along the length of individual flagella

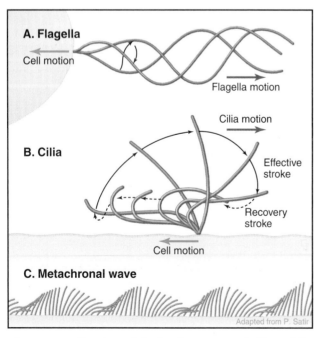

A. Flagella
Cell motion
Flagella motion

B. Cilia
Cilia motion
Effective stroke
Recovery stroke
Cell motion

C. Metachronal wave

Adapted from P. Satir

Figure 41–9 Drawings of the beating patterns of cilia and flagella. *A,* Sinusoidal waves of a sperm flagellum. *B,* Ciliary power and recovery strokes. *C,* Coordinated beating of cilia on the surface of an epithelium. (Adapted from P. Satir, Albert Einstein College of Medicine, New York.)

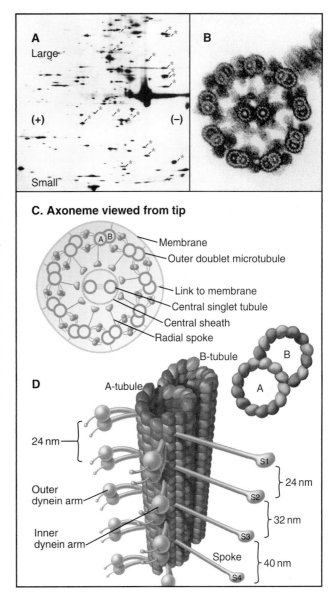

Figure 41-11 Composition and structure of the axoneme. *A,* Two-dimensional gel electrophoresis separating more than 100 polypeptides of the axoneme of *Chlamydomonas.* Marked polypeptides *(blue asterisk)* are components of radial spokes. *B,* Electron micrograph of a thin cross section of a ciliary axoneme stained with tannic acid. *C,* Drawing of a cross section of an axoneme. *D,* Perspective drawing of a short section of an outer doublet showing inner and outer dynein arms and radial spokes. In this example, the outer arm dyneins have two heads. In some species, they have three heads. (*A,* Courtesy of B. Huang, Scripps Research Institute, La Jolla, CA. *B,* Courtesy of R. Linck, University of Minnesota, Minneapolis. *D,* Redrawn from Amos LA, Amos WB: Molecules of the Cytoskeleton. New York: Guilford Press, 1991.)

pushes the cell ahead. Coordinated beating of many cilia can move large cells (Fig. 41–10). Reversal of the direction of the power stroke allows a cell to swim forward or backward. Alternatively, if the cell is immobilized, like epithelial cells lining an animal respiratory tract, coordinated beating of cilia propels fluid and particles over their apical surface. Ctenophores fuse the membranes of many cilia together to make macrocilia that propel the organism like oars.

Although nature has produced some fascinating variations, most cilia and flagella consist of **axonemes** composed of a 9 + 2 arrangement of microtubules surrounded by the plasma membrane (Figs. 41–11 and 41–12). The 9 **outer doublets** consist of 1 complete A-microtubule of the usual 13 protofilaments, with an incomplete B-microtubule composed of 10 protofilaments appended to its side. Tektin, a filamen-

tous protein in the wall of the A-microtubule, may help attach the B-microtubule. Like many other microtubular structures, the distal end of axonemal microtubules is the plus end. The **central pair** are typical 13-protofilament microtubules.

More than 200 accessory proteins reinforce the 9 + 2 microtubules (see Fig. 41–11), making axonemes stiff but elastic. Circumferential links join outer doublets to each other. Central pair microtubules are connected by a bridge and decorated by elaborate projections. Radial links extend from the central sheath toward the outer doublets. Genetic analysis has established that radial links consist of 17 different polypeptides, but little is known about most of the other minor accessory proteins.

A family of axonemal **dyneins** bound to outer doublets generates force for movement but are not

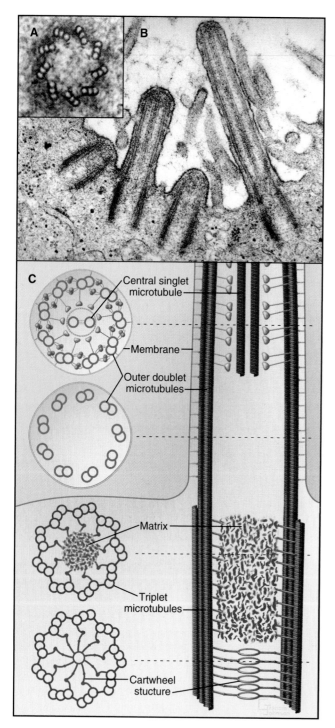

Figure 41-12 Basal bodies. *A,* Electron micrograph of a thin cross section of a basal body. *B,* Electron micrograph of thin longitudinal section of basal bodies and proximal axonemes of cilia. *C,* Drawings of a longitudinal section and cross sections of the flagella of *Chlamydomonas.* (*A* and *B,* Courtesy of D. W. Fawcett, Harvard Medical School. *C,* Redrawn from Amos LA, Amos WB: Molecules of the Cytoskeleton. New York: Guilford Press, 1991; originally from Cavalier-Smith TJ: Basal body and flagellar development. J Cell Sci 16:529, 1974, Company of Biologists Ltd.)

essential for assembly of axonemes. *Chlamydomonas* outer-arm dyneins are all the same, consisting of three different heavy chains, each forming a flexible stem, a globular head, and a thin stalk with an adenosine triphosphate (ATP)–sensitive binding site for the adjacent B-tubule (see Fig. 41–11). Inner arms are more heterogeneous. Six have one dynein heavy chain and one head, but one type has two heads. These seven different inner-arm dyneins are arranged in an orderly

pattern that repeats every 96 nm along the A-tubule of each outer doublet. Intermediate chains and light chains are present in a basal structure that anchors dynein stems and heads to A-tubules.

Dynein-powered sliding of outer doublets relative to each other bends axonemes. Sliding was first inferred from electron micrographs of the distal tips of microtubules in bent cilia. Later, sliding was observed directly by loosening connections between outer dou-

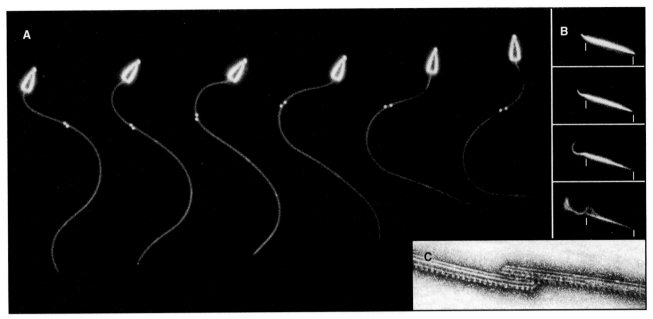

Figure 41-13 Sliding movements of outer doublets of axonemes. *A,* Time series of dark-field light micrographs of a sea urchin sperm extracted with the detergent Triton X-100 and reactivated with ATP. Gold microbeads attached to two different outer doublets document their displacement as the tail bends. *B,* Time series of dark-field light micrographs of a fragment of a sea urchin flagellar axoneme treated with trypsin. The addition of ATP results in outer doublets sliding past each other out of the ends of the axonemal fragment. *C,* Electron micrograph of two outer doublets that have slid past each other in an experiment similar to that in *B.* (*A,* Courtesy of Charles Brokow, California Institute of Technology. Reference: Brokaw CJ: Microtubule sliding in swimming sperm flagella. J Cell Biol 114:1201–1215, 1991, by copyright permission of the Rockefeller University Press. *B,* Courtesy of Ian Gibbons, University of California, Berkeley. Reference: Summers KE, Gibbons I: ATP-induced sliding of tubules in trypsin-treated flagella of sea-urchin sperm. Proc Natl Acad Sci USA 68:3092–3096, 1971. *C,* Courtesy of P. Satir, Albert Einstein College of Medicine, New York. Reference: Sale WS, Satir P: Direction of actin sliding of microtubules in Tetrahymena cilia. Proc Natl Acad Sci USA 74:2045–2049, 1977.)

blets with proteolytic enzymes and then adding ATP to allow dynein to push the microtubules past each other (Fig. 41–13*B*). Sliding can now be followed precisely in axonemes stripped of their membrane by marking outer doublets with small gold beads (see Fig. 41–13*A*). As outer doublets slide past each other, the positions of the beads change. Dynein attached to one doublet "walks" toward the base of the adjacent microtubule, pushing its neighbor toward the tip of the axoneme.

Biochemical extraction or genetic deletion of specific dynein isoforms alter the frequency and wave form of axonemal bending. Inner arms are required for flagellar beating, and deletion of even a single type of inner-arm dynein can alter the wave form. Outer arms are not essential, but influence the beat frequency and add power to the inner arms. Humans with **Kartagener's syndrome** lack visible dynein arms and have immotile sperm and cilia. As a result, affected males are infertile and both men and women have serious respiratory infections owing to poor clearance of bacteria and other foreign matter from the lungs. Axonemal dynein also has a major influence on the body plan. Individuals with Kartagener's syndrome and mice missing a single dynein heavy chain have an

equal chance of having their internal organs, such as heart and liver, either on the normal side or the opposite side, a condition called **situs inversus.** Cilia are thought to direct key growth factors to one side of the body. In the absence of this motion, the placement of the organs is left to chance.

The mechanism of beating is intrinsic to the axoneme, as demembranated sperm swim normally when provided with ATP, even without the plasma membrane or soluble cytoplasmic components (see Fig. 41–13*A*). Experiments with these demembranated sperm models revealed that the dynein adenosine triphosphatase (ATPase) activity is tightly coupled to movement. The beat frequency is proportional to ATPase activity, regardless of whether the frequency is limited by varying the viscosity of the medium or enzyme activity is limited by varying the ATP concentration.

Local variation in the rate of sliding of microtubules along the length of an axoneme produces bending, but no one understands how this differential sliding is converted into sinusoidal waves of flagella or the power and recovery strokes of cilia. Two factors are likely to be involved. First, mechanical constraints must contribute to the conversion of microtubule slid-

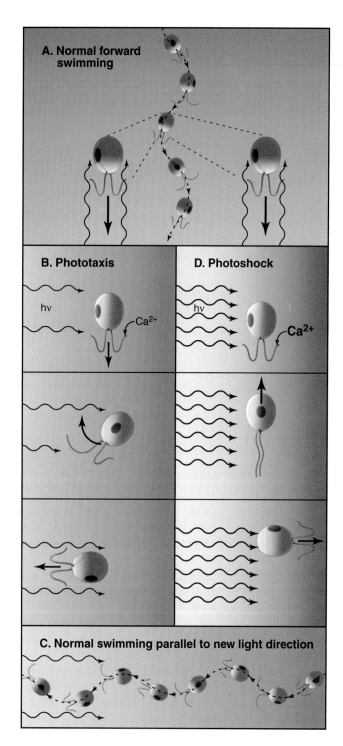

Figure 41-14 *Chlamydomonas* phototaxis. *A,* Normal swimming toward the light using a cilia-like rowing motion of the flagella. Absorption of light by the eyespot keeps the cell oriented. *B,* Moderate-intensity light from the side causes the release of Ca²⁺ from outside the cell into the cytoplasm. The two flagella react differently, causing the cell to turn toward the light. Once the cell is reoriented, the flagella beat equally, and the cell swims toward the light (*C*). *D,* High-intensity light releases a high concentration of Ca²⁺ and causes transient flagella-like motion of the flagella. This backward swimming allows the cell to reorient and to swim away from the light.

ing into coordinated bending. Destruction of the links between outer doublets frees them to slide past each other, rather than bending the axoneme. Second, the activity of the dyneins must be activated and inactivated in a coordinated fashion around the circumference of the axoneme as a bend passes along its length. Arms on opposite sides of an axoneme must alternate their activity or axonemes would twist rather than bend. One idea is that the central pair and radial spokes might act as a distributor (like that in older automobile engines) to coordinate the activity of the motors. This is an attractive theory because the central pair rotates during flagellar bending, at least in some species. Furthermore, mutations leading to the loss of all or part of the radial spokes can paralyze the flagella. On the other hand, the situation is complicated, as compensatory mutations in dynein or other genes (or even low ATP concentrations) can restore motility without changing the spoke deficiency.

Although beating of an axoneme is autonomous, it

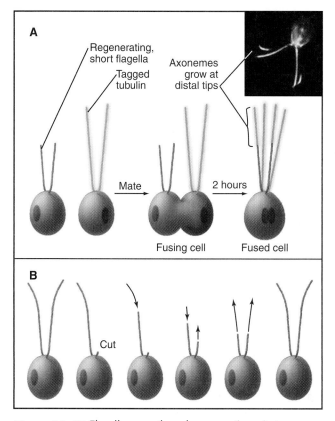

Figure 41–15 Flagellar growth and regeneration. *A,* Incorporation of protein subunits at the tip of growing *Chlamydomonas* flagella is revealed by an experiment involving the fusion of two cells, one expressing tubulin with an epitope tag that reacts with a specific antibody, and the other regenerating its flagella. As shown in the fluorescence micrograph, tagged tubulin is incorporated only at the distal tips of the growing flagella. Cells with paralyzed flagella made this experiment more convenient. *B,* Time course of regeneration of *Chlamydomonas* flagella following amputation of one flagellum. The surviving flagellum shortens transiently before both grow out together. (*A,* From K. Johnson, Haverford College. Reference: Johnson KA, Rosenbaum JL: Polarity of flagellar assembly in Chlamydomonas. J Cell Biol 119:1605–1611, 1992, by copyright permission of the Rockefeller University Press. *B,* Based on the work of J. Rosenbaum, Yale University.)

is regulated by signal transduction pathways. Phototaxis of *Chlamydomonas* is a particularly clear example of how fluctuations in intracellular Ca^{2+} can modify flagellar activity. The release of Ca^{2+} affects the two flagella differentially and allows a cell to steer toward or away from light (Fig. 41–14). Ciliates also have mechanosensitive channels that depolarize the plasma membrane when the organism collides with something. This opens voltage-sensitive plasma membrane Ca^{2+} channels, admitting Ca^{2+}, which reverses the direction of ciliary beat. Both calcium and cAMP-dependent phosphorylation of outer-arm dynein can change the beat frequency (all the way to zero) or alter the wave form.

A **basal body,** a modified centriole similar to those in the centrosome of animal cells, anchors each axoneme in the cortex of the cell (see Figs. 41–12 and 37–3*B*). Note that the nine outer doublets of the axoneme grow directly from an extension of the nine outer triplet microtubules of the basal body, rather than from amorphous pericentriolar material that initiates interphase microtubules (see Fig. 37–9). In sperm, one centriole serves as the basal body. In some protozoa, basal bodies are used as centrioles during mitosis. In ciliated cells, basal bodies replicate en mass from amorphous filamentous material to provide a basal body for each of the numerous axonemes.

Axonemes grow at their tips by incorporation of subunits synthesized in the cytoplasm (Fig. 41–15). These subunits travel actively in packets to the growing tip, a process called **intraflagellar transport.** Kinesin-family motors move these packets of proteins toward the tip of the axoneme along the outer doublets just beneath the plasma membrane. A specialized dynein transports particles back toward the cell body. Similarly, transmembrane proteins of the plasma membrane also move bidirectionally along microtubules of the underlying axoneme, presumably powered by motor proteins. This process is remarkably similar to fast axonal transport but on a smaller scale.

In some species, including *Chlamydomonas*, flagella regenerate if they are severed from the cell (see Fig. 41–15). Absence of the flagellum activates expression of genes required to supply subunits for regrowth of the axoneme. In about 1 hour, the cell regrows replacement flagella and the genes are turned off. Even more remarkable, if only one of the two flagella is lost, the remaining flagellum shortens rapidly to provide components required to make two half-length flagella. Then protein synthesis slowly provides additional subunits to restore both flagella to full length.

Cells in many tissues produce a single **primary cilium** by growth of an immotile axoneme from one of their centrioles. In a growing number of examples, primary cilia have been implicated in sensory processes. Nematode olfactory neurons have their odorant receptors concentrated in the membranes of modified cilia. Rod and cone photoreceptors in the eye are modified cilia with a basal body and a vestigial axoneme (see Chapter 29).

Specialized Microtubular Organelles

Some protozoa use dynein to generate beating movements of large arrays of cytoplasmic microtubules called **axostyles** (Fig. 41–16). The mechanism seems to be similar to an axoneme, although the organization is clearly different. Singlet microtubules are held together in sheets by cross-linking structures, and the sheets slide past each other as a result of the action of

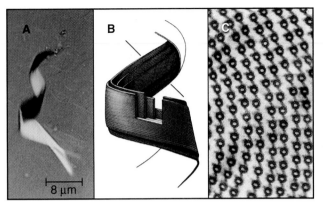

Figure 41–16 Motile axostyle of *Saccinobaculus,* a protozoan parasite of termites. The twisting motions of this intracellular assembly of microtubules cause the whole parasite to twist and turn in the gut of termites. *A,* Polarization light micrograph of an isolated axostyle. *B,* Drawing of part of the axostyle showing the arrangement of sheets of cross-linked microtubules. *C,* Transmission electron micrograph of a cross section of the axostyle showing microtubules cross-linked into sheets with dynein arms between the sheets. (Courtesy of R. Linck, University of Minnesota, Minneapolis; from Woodrum D, Linck R: Structural basis of motility in the microtubular axostyle. J Cell Biol 87: 404–414, 1980, by copyright permission of the Rockefeller University Press.)

dynein motors on adjacent sheets. The process is coordinated so that the axostyle beats regularly. This distorts the whole organism, allowing it to wiggle about.

Other Motile Systems

Although actin and microtubules account for most eukaryotic cell motility, at least three completely different motile systems evolved and remain in use today. Of these, at least calcium-sensitive contractile fibrils are present in human cells, so more research may reveal additional novel mechanisms relevant to animal cell motility.

Calcium-Sensitive Contractile Fibers

Ciliates like *Vorticella* contract faster than any muscle owing to the shortening of a **spasmoneme,** a fibril of a calcium-sensitive protein called spasmin (Fig. 41–17*A*). Other ciliates like *Stentor* have similar contractile fibrils called myonemes in their cortex. These fibrils consist of 3-nm filaments that shorten when they bind calcium. The mechanism is not understood, but it seems likely to involve a conformational change in each subunit. Rapid shortening is achieved by coupling many of these subunits in series. The fibers relax when calcium dissociates. This allows an active mechanism driven by sliding microtubules to reextend the cell. The calcium source in *Vorticella* is thought to be

a tubular system of membranes associated with the contractile fibers. These membranes may be similar to endoplasmic reticulum in muscle, concentrating free calcium from the cytoplasm and releasing it when stimulated. Energy for contraction is ultimately supplied by ATP-driven pumps that create a calcium gradient between the lumen of the membrane system and cytoplasm.

Proteins similar to those in contractile fibers of *Vorticella* are found in the rootlets that anchor axonemal basal bodies in the cortex of cells, as well as centrosomes of vertebrate cells. These proteins, called **centrin** or **caltractin,** are related to other calmodulin-like, calcium-binding proteins. Algal caltractin has four conserved calcium-binding sites, but some sites may be inactive in the yeast and human homologues. Algae and yeasts with mutations in the genes for caltractin cannot duplicate or separate the microtubule organizers (centrosomes or spindle pole bodies; see Chapter 47) used for mitosis. The role, if any, of calcium-sensitive contractions in these activities is under investigation.

An Actin Substitute in Nematode Sperm

Nematode sperm use amoeboid movements to find an egg rather than swimming with flagella like other sperm (Fig. 41–18). The behavior of these sperm is so similar to a small amoeba or a white blood cell that anyone would have guessed that it is based on the

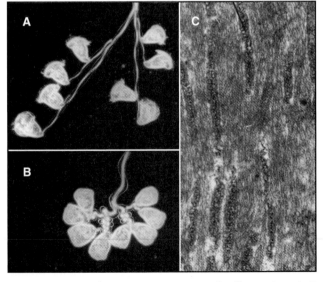

Figure 41–17 Calcium-sensitive contractile fibers. *A* and *B,* Light micrographs of a group of vorticellid protozoa suspended from the bottom of a leaf, taken before (*A*) and after (*B*) contraction of their spasmonemes. *C,* Electron micrograph of a thin section of contractile fibers and tubular membranes that store and release calcium. (Courtesy of W. B. Amos, MRC Laboratory of Molecular Biology, Cambridge, England.)

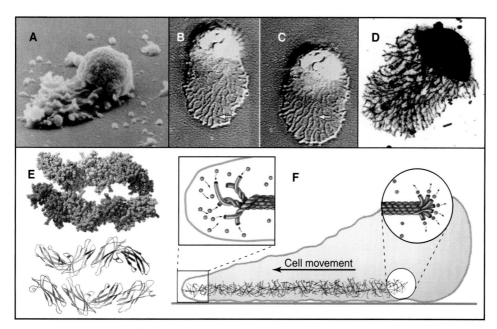

Figure 41-18 Motility of nematode sperm. *A,* Scanning electron micrograph of an amoeboid sperm showing the anterior pseudopod and trailing cell body. *B* and *C,* Time series of differential interference contrast light micrographs showing movement of a live sperm by assembly of a network of fibers at the leading edge. Arrows mark the same point in the network, which is stationary with respect to the substrate. *D,* Transmission electron micrograph of an extracted sperm showing the fibers. *E,* Atomic model of a short segment of the sperm filaments consisting of a polymer of major sperm protein (MSP). *F,* Schematic diagram of the cycle of MSP assembly at the leading edge and disassembly at the cell body. (Courtesy of T. Roberts, Florida State University, Tallahassee, and M. Stewart, MRC Laboratory of Molecular Biology, Cambridge, England.)

assembly of actin filaments. Although actin is a major protein in adult worms, it is only a minor protein in sperm. Instead, sperm pseudopods are filled with 10-nm filaments assembled from a 14-kD protein called **major sperm protein.** These filaments function remarkably like actin, despite the fact that they have no bound nucleotide and no known associated motor protein. High-resolution light microscopy of migrating cells has shown that 10-nm filaments assemble at the leading edge of the pseudopod and remain stationary with respect to the substrate as the expanding pseudopod advances. Isolated membrane vesicles can initiate the assembly of a comet tail of major sperm protein, just like *Listeria* does with actin (see Fig. 40–13). Filament bundles disappear at the interface between the pseudopod and the spherical cell body, presumably by depolymerization. The control mechanism and energy source for turning over these filaments are still under investigation. Remarkably, this highly efficient motility system is still unknown in other parts of the phylogenetic tree.

Bacterial Flagella

Bacteria use a reversible, high-speed, rotary motor driven by H^+ or Na^+ gradients to power their flagella (Figs. 41–19 and 41–20). Bacterial flagella differ in every respect from eukaryotic cilia and flagella. The bacterial flagellum itself is an extracellular protein wire, not a cytoskeletal structure like an axoneme inside its plasma membrane. Flagella act like the propellers of a motor boat when turned by its motor, embedded in the plasma membrane. Motion of the bacterium is produced by one or more flagella, all rotating in the same direction. When multiple flagella rotate counterclockwise, they form a bundle that propels *Escherichia coli* 30 μm/second. If the bacterium were the size of an automobile, this would be equivalent to a speed exceeding 400 miles per hour. When flagella reverse their direction and rotate clockwise, the bundle of flagella flies apart and the cell tumbles in one place (see Fig. 29–12). Chemotactic stimuli control the probability of the change in the direction of rotation, ensuring that the cell swims away from harm and toward nutrients. (See Chapter 4 for a discussion of the structure and assembly of the flagellar filament and Chapter 29 for an explanation of the signal transduction mechanism.)

Assays for rotation of individual flagella have been informative about the mechanism of flagellar motion. When a flagellum is attached to a glass slide by means of antibodies to the flagellar filament, the bacterium rotates, providing decisive evidence for rotation of flagella (see Fig. 41–19). Similarly, beads attached to

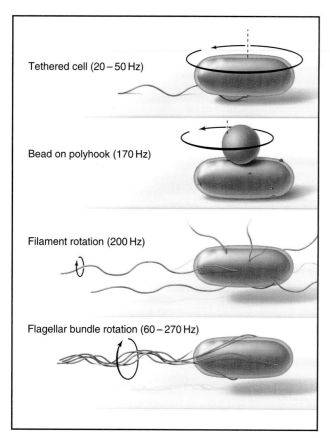

Figure 41-19 Rotation of bacterial flagella. Drawings show different manifestations of the rotation of flagella. If a flagellum is attached to a surface, the bacterium rotates. If a short flagellum is attached to a bead, the bead rotates. Individual flagella and bundles of flagella rotate on free bacteria. (Redrawn from Schuster SD, Khan S: The bacterial flagellar motor. Annu Rev Biophys Biomol Struct 23:509–539, 1994, with permission from the *Annual Review of Biophysics and Biomolecular Structure*, Vol. 23, © 1994 by Annual Reviews, www.AnnualReviews.org.)

short flagella are observed to rotate. The rotational speed depends on the resistance. The motor of a single immobilized flagellum can rotate a whole *E. coli* 10 to 50 times per second, whereas an unloaded motor can rotate up to 1600 times per second in some species.

The rotary engine driving the flagellar filament is constructed from two parts: a cylindrical **basal body** on the end of the filament; and a surrounding ring of proteins embedded in the plasma membrane (see Fig. 41–20). Genetic screens for motility mutants have identified all of the protein components of the motor, and their presumed functions were defined by analysis of the behavior of these mutants. Most of these proteins are present in isolated basal bodies. Two proteins essential for rotation—MotA and MotB—are found in the cell membrane surrounding the basal body. Flagella are immotile in cells lacking either one of these proteins. Expression of the missing membrane protein in cells with preformed but immotile flagella reactivates flagellar rotation, with the speed increasing in a stepwise fashion. An attractive interpretation is

that the speed increases as a result of the addition of individual, independent, torque-producing units, one after another, to the engine. At the same time, a ring of 10 to 12 integral membrane proteins reappears in the plasma membrane, so they are generally believed to be part of the motors. MotA protein has four hydro-

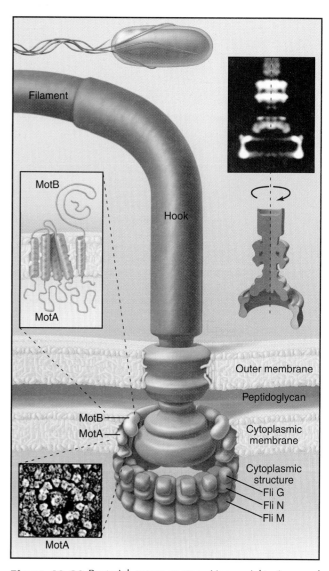

Figure 41-20 Bacterial rotary motor. *Upper right,* Averaged electron micrographs of isolated flagellar basal bodies and a three-dimensional reconstruction of this large structure, estimated to have a molecular mass of 4400 kD. *Middle,* Molecular model of the rotary motor in place in the bacterial membrane. *Lower left,* Electron micrograph of a freeze-fractured bacterium illustrating the ring of intramembranous particles thought to correspond to MotA and MotB. (*Upper right,* Courtesy of D. DeRosier, Brandeis University. Reference: Thomas DR, Morgan DG, DeRosier DJ: Rotational symmetry of the C ring. Proc Natl Acad Sci USA 96:10134–10139, 1999. Copyright 1999, National Academy of Sciences, U.S.A. *Middle:* Redrawn from Schuster SD, Khan S: The bacterial flagellar motor. Annu Rev Biophys Biomol Struct 23:509–539, 1994, with permission from the *Annual Review of Biophysics and Biomolecular Structure*, Vol. 23, © 1994 by Annual Reviews www.AnnualReviews.org. *Lower left,* Courtesy of S. Khan, Albert Einstein College of Medicine, New York.)

phobic sequences and the MotB protein has one, leading to the model shown in Figure 41–20.

Movement of protons (or, in some bacteria, Na^+) down a concentration gradient from outside the bacterium through the motor to the cytoplasm drives rotation. Transfer of one proton across the membrane provides approximately the same energy as the hydrolysis of an ATP. Pumps driven by light, oxidation, or ATP hydrolysis (see Chapter 7) generate the **proton gradient.** Flagellar rotation stops when bacteria are starved, and it resumes when nutrients are supplied to allow reestablishment of the membrane proton gradient. MotA is the strongest candidate for the proton channel because mutations in its gene inhibit both flagellar rotation and proton permeability. The big question is how does the transfer of protons generate the torque that turns the basal body? Several explicit models can account for the observed behavior of the motor, but differences among the models are unlikely to be resolved without atomic structures of the proteins.

▌ Selected Readings

Branda CS, Stern MJ: Cell migration and axon growth cone guidance in *Caenorhabditis elegans.* Curr Opin Genet Dev 9:479–484, 1999.

Bray D: Cell Movements, 2nd ed. New York: Garland Publishing, 2000.

Culotti JG, Merz DC: DCC and netrins. Curr Opin Cell Biol 10:609–613, 1998.

DeRosier DJ: The turn of the screw: The bacterial flagellar motor. Cell 93:17–20, 1998.

Dutcher SK: Flagellar assembly in two hundred and fifty easy-to-follow steps. Trends Genet 11:398–404, 1995.

Eisenbach M, Caplan SR: Bacterial chemotaxis: Unsolved mystery of the flagellar switch. Curr Biol 8:R444–446, 1998.

Holwill ME, Foster GF, Hamasaki T, Satir P: Biophysical aspects and modeling of ciliary motility. Cell Motil Cytoskel 32:114–120, 1995.

Katoh K, Kikuyama M: An all-or-nothing rise in cytoplasmic $[Ca^{2+}]$ in Vorticella sp. J Exp Biol 200:35–40, 1997.

Mueller BK: Growth cone guidance: First steps towards a deeper understanding. Annu Rev Neurosci 22:351–388, 1999.

Porter ME: Axonemal dyneins: Assembly, organization and regulation. Curr Opin Cell Biol 8:10–17, 1996.

Roberts TM, Stewart M: Actin' like actin. The dynamics of the nematode major sperm protein (msp) cytoskeleton indicate a push-pull mechanism for amoeboid cell motility. J Cell Biol 149:7–12, 2000.

Rosenbaum JL, Cole DG, Diener DR: Intraflagellar transport: The eyes have it. J Cell Biol 144:385–388, 1999.

Schuster SD, Khan S: The bacterial flagellar motor. Annu Rev Biophys Biomol Struct 23:509–539, 1994.

Song HJ, Poo MM: Signal transduction underlying growth cone guidance by diffusible factors. Curr Opin Neurobiol 9:355–365, 1999.

Supp DM, Potter SS, Brueckner M: Molecular motors: The driving force behind mammalian left-right development. Trends Cell Biol 10:41–45, 2000.

Suter DM, Forscher P: An emerging link between cytoskeletal dynamics and cell adhesion molecules in growth cone guidance. Curr Opin Neurobiol 8:106–116, 1998.

Svitkina TM, Borisy GG: Progress in protrusion: The tell-tale scar. Trends Biochem Sci 24:432–436, 1999.

Van Vactor D, Flanagan JG: The middle and the end: Slit brings guidance and branching together in axon pathway selection. Neuron 22:649–652, 1999.

Welch MD: The world according to Arp: Regulation of actin nucleation by the Arp2/3 complex. Trends Cell Biol 9:423–427, 1999.

Witman G: Chlamydomonas phototaxis. Trends Cell Biol 3:403–408, 1993.

chapter 42

MUSCLES

Vertebrates have three types of specialized contractile cells—smooth muscle, skeletal muscle, and cardiac muscle—that use actin and myosin to generate powerful, unidirectional movements (Fig. 42–1). These muscles have much in common but differ in their activation mechanisms, arrangement of contractile filaments, and energy supplies. This provides three options for physiological responses. The nervous system controls the timing, force, and speed of skeletal muscle contraction over a wide range. Cardiac muscle generates its own rhythmic, fatigue-free contractions that spread through the heart in a highly reproducible fashion. Neurotransmitters, acting like hormones, regulate the force and frequency of heartbeats over a narrow range. Nerves, hormones, and intrinsic signals control the activity of smooth muscles, which contract slowly but maintain tension very efficiently.

This chapter explains the molecular and cellular basis for the distinctive physiological properties of the three types of muscle. These specialized muscle cells adapt and exaggerate the same molecular strategies used by other cells to produce contractions, to adhere to each other and the extracellular matrix, and to control their activity.

Skeletal Muscle

Skeletal muscle cells are designed for rapid, forceful contractions. Accordingly, they have a massive concentration of highly ordered contractile units composed of actin, myosin, and associated proteins (Fig. 42–2). Actin and myosin filaments are organized into **sarcomeres,** semi-crystalline arrays that give the cells a striped appearance in the microscope. For this reason, they are called striated muscles. Contraction is generated by adenosine triphosphate (ATP)–fueled, myosin-

powered sliding of actin-based thin filaments past myosin-containing thick filaments. Speed is achieved by linking many sarcomeres in series. Force is determined by the number of sarcomeres contracting in parallel.

Although skeletal muscle *cells* have only two states—inactive (relaxed) or active (contracting)—skeletal *muscles* produce a wide range of contractions, varying from slow and delicate to rapid and forceful. These **graded contractions** are achieved by varying the *number* of muscle cells activated by voluntary or reflex signals from the nervous system (see Fig. 42–14). Nerve impulses stimulate a transient rise in cytoplasmic calcium that activates the contractile proteins.

Organization of the Skeletal Muscle Contractile Apparatus

Skeletal muscle cells (also called muscle fibers in the physiological literature) are among the largest cells in vertebrates. During development, muscle cells that reach up to several centimeters long form by the fusion of mononucleate progenitor cells called myoblasts. Mature cells have many nuclei distributed along their length. A basal lamina (see Fig. 31–18C) surrounds and supports each muscle cell. At the ends of each cell, actin thin filaments are anchored to the plasma membrane at myotendinous junctions, which are similar to focal contacts (see Fig. 32–10). Integrins provide the physical connection across the membrane to the basal lamina and to collagen fibrils of tendons that is required to transmit contractile force to the skeleton.

Organization of the Actomyosin Apparatus

Interdigitation of thick, bipolar, myosin filaments and thin actin filaments in sarcomeres is so precise (Fig. 42–3) that it yields an x-ray diffraction pattern

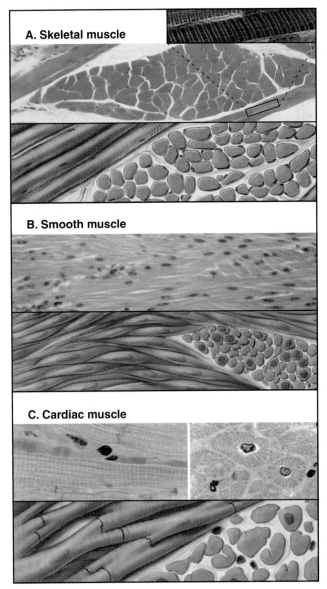

Figure 42-1 Light micrographs and interpretive drawings of histological sections of skeletal, cardiac, and smooth muscles. *A,* Skeletal muscle cells are shaped like cylinders and may be up to 50 cm long. Multiple nuclei are located near the plasma membrane. Striations are seen in the inset, a longitudinal section at high magnification. *B,* Smooth muscle cells are spindle-shaped with homogeneous cytoplasm and single nuclei. *C,* Cardiac muscle cells are striated and have one or two nuclei. Adhesive junctions called intercalated disks (bright pink vertical bars in the longitudinal section, left) bind these short cells together end to end.

(see Fig. 42–13) revealing the spacing of the filaments and the helical repeats of their subunits to a resolution of about 3 nm. **Z disks** at both ends of the sarcomere anchor the barbed ends of the actin filaments, so their pointed ends are near the center of the sarcomere. Myosin heads project from the surface of **thick filaments,** whereas their tails are anchored in the filament backbone. Thick and **thin filaments** overlap, with the myosin heads only a few nanometers away

from adjacent actin filaments. The alignment and interdigitation of the filaments facilitate the sliding interactions required to produce contraction.

An important, simplifying architectural feature is that sarcomeres are symmetrical about their middle (see Fig. 42–3). Consequently, the polarity of myosin relative to the actin filaments is the same in both halves of the sarcomere, allowing the same force-generating mechanism to work at both ends of the bipolar myosin filaments. Sarcomeres are organized end to end into long, cylindrical assemblies called **myofibrils** (see Fig. 42–2) that retain their contractility even after isolation from muscle.

Thin Filaments

Thin filaments consist of actin and the tightly bound regulatory proteins, **troponin,** and **tropomyosin** (Fig. 42–4). At low Ca^{2+} levels, troponin and tropomyosin inhibit the actin-activated adenosine triphosphatase (ATPase) of myosin. Tropomyosin, a 40-nm-

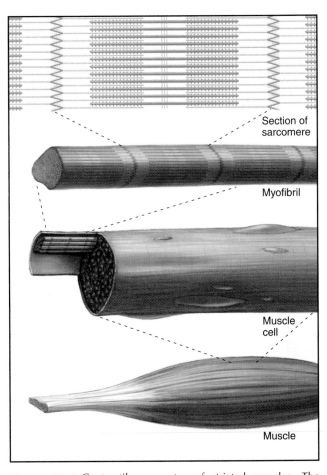

Figure 42-2 Contractile apparatus of striated muscles. The contractile unit is the sarcomere, an interdigitating array of thick and thin filaments. Sarcomeres are arranged end to end into long, rod-shaped myofibrils that run the length of the cell. Mitochondria and smooth endoplasmic reticulum separate myofibrils, facilitating their isolation by homogenization and differential centrifugation.

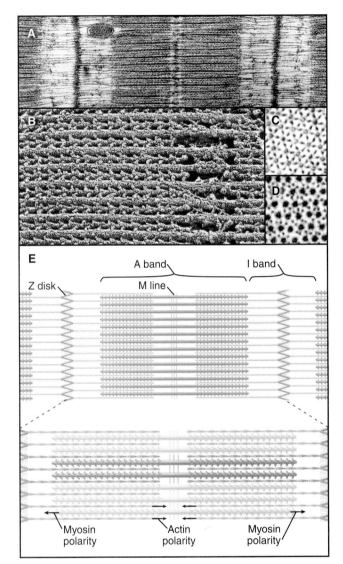

Figure 42-3 Electron micrographs and drawings of sarcomeres. *A,* Longitudinal thin section showing the array of thin filaments anchored to Z disks and overlapping bipolar thick filaments cross-linked in the middle at the M line. *B,* Longitudinal freeze-fractured, etched, and shadowed sarcomere showing myosin cross-bridges attached to thin filaments near the bare zone in the center *(right)* of a sarcomere. *C* and *D,* Cross sections of insect flight muscle and vertebrate skeletal muscle showing the double hexagonal arrays of thick and thin filaments. *E,* Drawings indicating the polarity of the thick and thin filaments. (*A* and *C,* Courtesy of H. E. Huxley, Brandeis University. *B* and *D,* Courtesy of J. Heuser, Washington University.)

long coiled-coil of two α-helical polypeptides (see Fig. 2–12), binds laterally to seven contiguous actin subunits and head to tail to neighboring tropomyosins, forming a continuous strand along the whole thin filament. Troponin (TN) consists of three different subunits called TNC, TNI, and TNT (Table 42–1). TNT anchors troponin to tropomyosin. Like calmodulin (see Fig. 2–14 and Chapter 28), TNC is a dumbbell-shaped protein with four EF-hand motifs to bind divalent ca-

tions. Two high-affinity sites at the C-terminus bind Mg^{2+}. Two low-affinity sites at the N-terminus are empty in resting muscle but bind Ca^{2+} when muscle is activated. In the troponin complex, TNC wraps around an N-terminal α-helix of TNI, but the structure of the rest of troponin is not yet known.

A protein meshwork in the Z disk anchors the barbed end of each thin filament (Fig. 42–5). Some crosslinks between actin filaments consist of α-actinin, a short rod with actin-binding sites on each end (see Fig. 36–15). **Cap-Z,** the muscle isoform of capping protein, binds the barbed ends of the thin filaments with high affinity, limiting actin subunit addition or loss. Other Z-disk proteins are less well characterized, in part because they are insoluble and difficult to isolate.

Tropomodulin associates with both tropomyosin and actin to cap and stabilize the pointed end of thin filaments (see Fig. 42–4B). In skeletal muscle, a gigan-

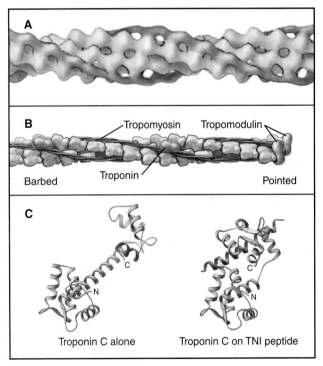

Figure 42-4 Thin filament structure. *A,* Three-dimensional reconstruction from electron micrographs of a thin filament from vertebrate skeletal muscle showing actin and the position of tropomyosin in relaxed muscle. *B,* Drawing of a model of a thin filament from active muscle. Each tropomyosin is associated with seven actin subunits. The structure and binding sites of troponin and tropomodulin have been inferred from biochemical experiments. *C,* Ribbon diagrams of the atomic structures of troponin C, free and bound to a troponin I peptide. Two divalent cation-binding EF-hands are found at each end, separated by a long α helix. In cells, two high-affinity sites at the C-terminal end are permanently occupied with Mg^{2+}. Two low-affinity sites at the other end are unoccupied in relaxed muscle but bind Ca^{2+} when muscle is activated. (*A,* Courtesy of W. Lehman, Boston University. *C,* PDB files: 1AX2 and 1TROP.)

table 42–1

SARCOMERE PROTEINS

Name	Size (kD)	Domains	Functions
Thick filament			
Myosin	2 × 200	Heavy chain	Motor, backbone of thick filament
	2 × 20	Light chain	
	2 × 18 or 25	Light chain	
C protein	1 × 128	Ig, FNIII	Stabilizes, thick filament
Paramyosin	2 × 100	Coiled-coil	Core of invertebrate thick filaments
M Line			
MM-creatine phosphokinase	2 × 43		Glycolytic enzyme
M protein	1 × 165	IgC2, FNIII	M-line structure
Myomesin (skelemin)	1 × 185	IgC2, FN III	Link M-disk to desmin
Thin Filament			
Actin	1 × 43		Backbone of the thin filament
Tropomyosin	2 × 35	Coiled-coil	Blocks myosin binding
Troponin C	1 × 18	4 × EF-hand	Calcium-binding component of troponin
Troponin I	1 × 21		Inhibitory component of troponin
Troponin T	1 × 31		Tropomyosin-binding component of troponin
Tropomodulin	1 × 43		Binds tropomyosin at the pointed end of the actin filament
Nebulin		>200 × 35 residues	May bind thin filament; absent from heart
Z disk			
α-Actinin	2 × 100	Actin binding	Cross-links thin filaments in the Z disk
CapZ	1 × 31 + 1 × 32		Blocks the barbed end of thin filaments
Elastic filaments			
Titin	1 × 2500	FNIII, IgC2, MLCK	Elastic connection from Z disk to M line
Minititin	1 × 650	FN III, IgC2	Connects thick filament to Z disk in insects

FN, fibronectin; Ig, immunoglobulin; MLCK, myosin light chain kinase.

tic filamentous protein, nebulin, runs from one end of the thin filaments to the other. Tropomyosin and nebulin are thought to reinforce the tensile strength of thin filaments. Together with tropomodulin, they may also set the length of thin filaments.

Thick Filaments

The self-assembly of myosin II (see Chapter 4, Example 2) establishes the bipolar architecture of striated muscle thick filaments (Fig. 42–6). Some features of thick filaments are invariant, such as a backbone consisting of myosin tails, a surface array of myosin heads, the 14.3-nm stagger between rows of heads, and a central bare zone formed by antiparallel packing of tails. Filaments may vary in length, diameter, and organization of the helical array of heads in various species. Invertebrate thick filaments have a core of paramyosin, a second coiled-coil protein, not found in vertebrates.

Several accessory proteins stabilize thick filaments (see Table 42–1). Thick filaments in most striated muscles are girdled at intervals by semi-circular bands of a protein that is, coincidentally, called "C protein." C protein consists of fibronectin III and immunoglobulin domains. The **"M line"** in the center of the sarcomere is a three-dimensional array of protein crosslinks that maintains the precise registration of thick filaments. At least three structural proteins and the enzyme MM-creatine phosphokinase (which transfers phosphate from creatine-phosphate to adenosine diphosphate [ADP]) are located in the M line.

Titin Filaments

A third array of protein filaments lies parallel to the thin and thick filaments, connecting the Z disk to the thick filaments and the M line (Fig. 42–7). Hard to preserve for electron microscopy, these diaphanous filaments were neglected for years. Each filament is a

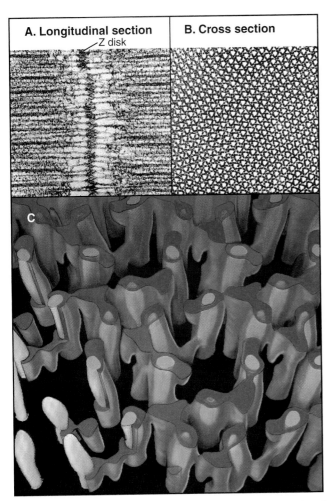

Figure 42-5 Z-disk structure. *A* and *B,* Electron micrographs of thin sections perpendicular to and in the plane of the Z disk. *C,* Three-dimensional reconstruction, based on electron micrographs of the Z disk, showing the network of protein crosslinks that anchor the barbed ends of the yellow actin filaments. (Courtesy of J. Deatherage, National Institutes of Health; modified from Cheng NQ, Deatherage JF: Three dimensional reconstruction of the Z disk of sectioned bee flight muscle. J Cell Biol 108:1761–1774, 1989, by copyright permission of the Rockefeller University Press.)

and lysine (the PEVK domain). Extreme stretching unfolds and extends the polypeptide as the repeated domains lose their compact structure one by one.

Intermediate Filaments

Desmin intermediate filaments (see Chapter 38) help align the sarcomeres laterally. They surround each Z disk (Fig. 42–8), linking it to its neighbors and to specialized attachment sites on the plasma membrane. Desmin mutations in humans cause disorganization of myofibrils, resulting in generalized muscle failure. Myofibrils near the cell surface are attached to

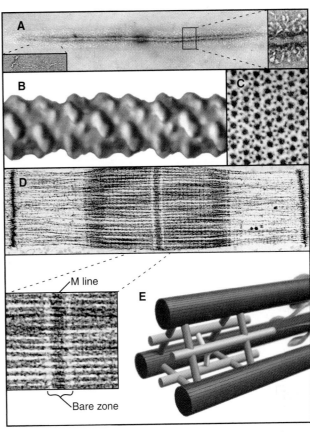

Figure 42-6 Structure of bipolar thick filaments. *A,* Electron micrograph of a thick filament isolated directly from skeletal muscle and prepared by negative staining. A myosin molecule is shown at the same magnification at the lower left. The myosin tails form the backbone of the thick filament and allow the two myosin heads to swing out from the side (see the enlarged *inset* on the right). *B,* Reconstruction from electron micrographs of part of a rabbit skeletal muscle thick filament. The surface bumps are myosin heads. *C,* Cross section of vertebrate skeletal muscle showing the double hexagonal arrays of thick and thin filaments. *D,* Electron micrograph of a highly stretched sarcomere with the M line in the middle. *E,* Drawing of protein links between thick filaments in the M line. (*A,* Courtesy of John Trinick, Bristol University. Reference: Knight P, Trinick J: Structure of the myosin projections on native thick filaments from vertebrate skeletal muscle. J Mol Biol 177:461–482, 1984. *B,* Courtesy of M. Stewart, MRC Laboratory of Molecular Biology, Cambridge, England. *C,* Courtesy of J. Heuser, Washington University. *D,* Courtesy of H. E. Huxley, Brandeis University.)

single polypeptide named **titin** (after mythological giants), so named because of its remarkable size: more than 30,000 amino acids folded into a linear array of 300 immunoglobulin and fibronectin II domains measuring more than 1.2 μm long. Titin is thought to be the largest protein encoded by the human genome. Titin filaments are elastic and account for the passive resistance to stretching of relaxed muscle. Their connection to the Z disk keeps the thick filaments centered in the sarcomere during contraction. If titin molecules are broken experimentally, thick filaments slide out of register toward one Z disk during contraction. The elasticity during short, physiological stretches is provided by the reversible unraveling of a segment of the polypeptide rich in proline, glutamic acid, valine,

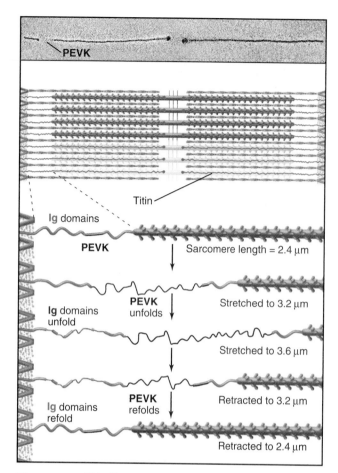

Figure 42-7 Titin filaments. *Upper panel,* Electron micrographs of single, isolated titin molecules prepared by heavy metal shadowing. Titin molecules are long enough to extend from the Z disk to the M line. *Middle panel,* Drawing of a sarcomere, to the same scale as the electron micrograph, with the thick filaments removed from the bottom half to illustrate how titin molecules anchor thick filaments to the Z disk and extend to the M line. *Lower panel,* Drawing illustrating a model for the elasticity of titin. Modest stretches extend the PEVK domain reversibly. Extreme extension unfolds immunoglobulin or fibronectin III domains. (Redrawn from Reif M, Gautel M, Oesterhelt F, et al: Reversible unfolding of individual titin immunoglobulin domains by AFM. Science 276:1090–1092, 1997.)

the plasma membrane at specializations called costameres. In addition to desmin, costameres contain several cytoskeletal proteins (vinculin, talin, spectrin, and ankyrin) found in focal contacts and adherens junctions of nonmuscle cells (see Chapters 32 and 33).

Organization of the Muscle Membrane System

Structural Proteins of the Plasma Membrane: Defects in Muscular Dystrophies

A transmembrane complex of proteins stabilizes the muscle plasma membrane and links it to the basal lamina (Fig. 42–9 and Table 42–2). These proteins escaped detection until the late 1980s when mutations in the **dystrophin** gene were discovered to cause the most common type of human **muscular dystrophy,** Duchenne's muscular dystrophy. Patients with this disease lack dystrophin and suffer from muscle degeneration in their youth. Dystrophin is a very large member of the α-actinin superfamily of actin-binding proteins (see Fig. 36–15). The **dystroglycan/sarcoglycan complex** copurifies with dystrophin after solubilization of the membrane with detergents. The extracellular α subunit of dystroglycan binds to α2 laminin in the basal lamina (see Chapter 31).

Genetic defects or deficiencies involving dystrophin, its associated membrane proteins, or α2 laminin cause various forms of human muscular dystrophy (see Table 42–2). The age of onset and clinical features depend on which protein is defective, but in all cases, the accelerated death of muscle cells exceeds the capacity of the tissue to repair itself. Progressive weakness and the failure of respiratory muscles is ultimately fatal. Although single proteins are defective, the plasma membrane often lacks the whole complex. For example, individuals lacking dystrophin have diminished dystroglycans and sarcoglycans. On the other hand, patients with severe muscular dystrophy secondary to defects in sarcoglycans can have normal levels of dystrophin and dystroglycans.

Dystrophin and its associated membrane proteins are believed to support the muscle plasma membrane mechanically, similar to the spectrin-actin network of red blood cells (see Fig. 6–10). Red blood cells deficient in spectrin are easily lysed by mechanical stress during circulation. Similarly, stress produced by con-

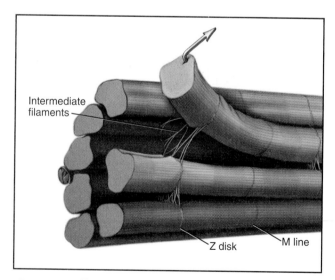

Figure 42-8 Desmin intermediate filaments in skeletal muscle. Desmin filaments *(orange)* connect Z disks laterally to each other and to the plasma membrane at specializations called costameres. (Redrawn from Lazarides E: Intermediate filaments as mechanical integrators of cellular space. Nature 283:249–256, 1980.)

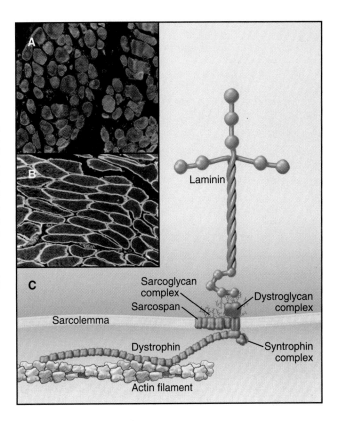

Figure 42-9 Dystrophin and associated proteins stabilize the plasma membrane of skeletal muscle. *A* and *B,* Fluorescent antibody staining of cross sections of human skeletal muscle showing the localization of dystrophin at the plasma membrane of a normal individual (*B*) and its absence in an individual with Duchenne's muscular dystrophy (*A*). *C,* Model of the transmembrane complex of proteins that links dystrophin and actin filaments in cytoplasm to laminin in the basal lamina outside the cell. (*A* and *B,* Courtesy of L. Kunkel, Harvard Medical School. *C,* Based on a drawing of K. Amann and J. Ervasti, University of Wisconsin, Madison.)

traction is more likely to rupture a muscle plasma membrane lacking dystrophin, dystroglycan/sarcoglycan complex, or laminin. Even a minor compromise of the mechanical integrity of the muscle plasma membrane caused by a defect in one of these proteins may rupture and kill muscle cells during years of contraction. Other factors may also contribute to the disease. For example, the cytoplasmic Ca^{2+} concentration is abnormally high in dystrophic muscle cells as a result of abnormal Ca^{2+} leakage.

Dystroglycans and a dystrophin homologue, utrophin, participate in clustering acetylcholine receptors

table 42–2

DYSTROPHIN COMPLEX

Protein	Synonyms	Size (kD)*	Partners	Expression	Diseases
Dystrophin		427	β-Dystroglycan, actin	Muscle, brain	DMD, mdx mouse
Utrophin		395	β-Dystroglycan, actin	Muscle, other cells	
α-Dystroglycan	DAG156	56 *156	Laminin, agrin	Many tissues	
β-Dystroglycan	DAG43	43	Dystrophin, utrophin	Many tissues	
α-Sarcoglycan	Adhalin	50 *52		Muscle	ARMD, LGMD, cardiomyopathy
β-Sarcoglycan	DAG43	43		Muscle	ARMD, LGMD
γ-Sarcoglycan	DAG35	35		Muscle	SCARMD, LGMD
α2-Laminin	Merosin	350	α-Dystroglycan	Muscle, other cells	CMD, dy/dy mouse
Agrin		55	α-Dystroglycan, AChR	Muscle	
α-Syntrophins		55			
β-Syntrophins		48	Dystrophin, utrophin	Muscle more than other cells	

*The first entry is the polypeptide molecular weight; if there is a second entry with an asterisk (*), that is the apparent molecular weight after post-translational modifications.

Abbreviation key for human diseases: *DMD,* Duchenne's muscular dystrophy (X-linked recessive); BMD, Becker's muscular dystrophy (X-linked recessive); ARMD, autosomal recessive muscular dystrophy; LGMD, limb-girdle muscular dystrophy (autosomal recessive); SCARMD, severe childhood autosomal recessive muscular dystrophy; CMD, childhood muscular dystrophy (autosomal recessive).

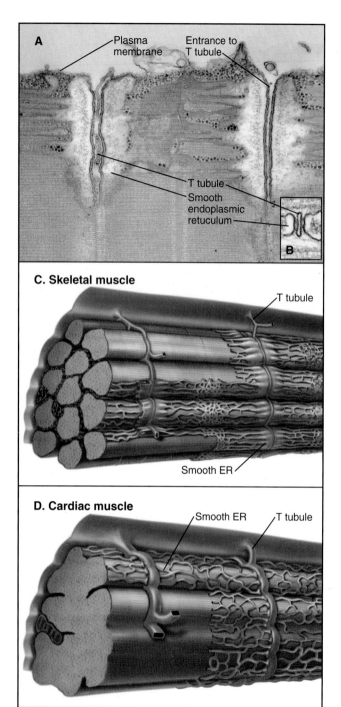

Figure 42–10 Plasma membrane specializations of striated muscles. *A* and *B*, Electron micrographs of thin sections of fish skeletal muscle showing invaginations, called T tubules, which cross the whole muscle cell and associate closely with smooth endoplasmic reticulum (ER). The complex of a T tubule with smooth endoplasmic reticulum on both sides is called a triad. Foot processes, consisting of voltage-sensitive calcium channels in a T tubule paired with calcium release channels in the endoplasmic reticulum, connect the T tubule to the smooth endoplasmic reticulum. (Figure 42–15 provides molecular details.) *C* and *D*, Drawings of the three-dimensional arrangement of T tubules and smooth endoplasmic reticulum relative to the sarcomeres in skeletal and cardiac muscle. (*A* and *B*, Courtesy of C. Franzini-Armstrong and K. Porter, University of Pennsylvania.)

at the neuromuscular junction, the chemical synapse between motor neurons and skeletal muscle (see Fig. 10–8). When, during development, a motor neuron arrives at the surface of its target muscle cell, the neuron secretes an adhesive protein called agrin, which is incorporated into the basal lamina, immediately adjacent to the nerve terminal. Dystroglycan binds agrin and positions associated acetylcholine receptors at the site where they receive acetylcholine secreted by the nerve in response to an action potential.

Interaction of Plasma Membrane Invaginations with the Smooth Endoplasmic Reticulum

The plasma membrane of skeletal muscle cells, like the plasma membrane of nerve cells (see Chapter 9), is excitable and invaginates deeply to form so-called **T tubules** that run across the entire cell (Fig. 42–10). Depending on the species and type of striated muscle (skeletal versus cardiac), T tubules may be located either at the level of the Z disks or thick filament ends. Inside the muscle cell, T tubules interact extensively with the smooth endoplasmic reticulum that surrounds each myofibril. Historically, this smooth endoplasmic reticulum has been called **sarcoplasmic reticulum.** Terminal cisternae of smooth endoplasmic reticulum are closely associated with the passing T tubules by foot processes that can be visualized by electron microscopy. Together, T tubules and smooth endoplasmic reticulum constitute a signal-transducing apparatus that converts depolarizations of the plasma membrane into a spike of cytoplasmic Ca^{2+} that triggers contraction (see later discussion).

Molecular Basis of Skeletal Muscle Contraction

The Sliding Filament Mechanism

The key to understanding muscle contraction was the discovery that thick and thin filaments maintain constant lengths and slide past each other as sarcomeres (and the muscle) shorten (Fig. 42–11). About the same time, it was appreciated that cross-bridges (now recognized to be myosin heads) can connect actin and myosin filaments (see Fig. 42–11) and that tension produced during contraction is proportional to the overlap of actin and myosin filaments (Fig. 42–12). Supported by biochemical and ultrastructural evidence for actin-myosin interaction, these pioneering observations led to the theory that cross-bridges between the thick and thin filaments produce force for contraction. Forty years of research on cross-bridges have yielded a detailed picture of the chemistry and molecular mechanics underlying the force-producing reactions. A review of the steps of the actomyosin-ATPase cycle (Fig. 40–6) may be helpful in under-

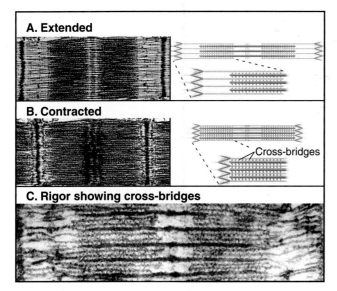

Figure 42-11 Sliding filaments. Electron micrographs and interpretive drawings of longitudinal sections of a sarcomere from a relaxed muscle (A) and a contracted skeletal muscle (B). The lengths of the thin and thick filaments are constant as the sarcomere shortens, demonstrating that the filaments slide past each other during contraction. C, Cross-bridges between thick and thin filaments from a muscle in rigor. (Micrographs courtesy of H. E. Huxley, Brandeis University.)

standing the contraction mechanism. Three different physiological states reveal information about cross-bridge mechanisms.

- *Relaxed.* One extreme is relaxed muscle. When the concentration of cytoplasmic Ca²⁺ is low, tropomyosin and troponin inhibit the interaction of myosin heads with actin filaments, so few myosin heads are bound. Without long-lived physical connections between the filaments, muscle offers little resistance to passive stretching. X-ray diffraction (Fig. 42–13) shows that the myosin heads (in the myosin-ATP and myosin-ADP-P$_i$ (myosin with bound ADP and phosphate) states; see Fig. 39–6) are closely associated with the backbone of thick filaments and arranged in a helical array determined by the thick filament structure (see Fig. 42–6B).
- *Rigor.* The other extreme occurs after death. Depletion of ATP allows all myosin heads to bind tightly to actin filaments (see Figs. 42–3B, 42–11C, and 39–5). By x-ray diffraction, the myosin heads bound to actin filaments contribute to the strength of the reflections from the actin filament helix. The strong physical connections between the filaments prevent stretching, making the muscle stiff, hence the term rigor mortis. This extreme condition is informative because it illustrates what happens structurally and mechanically when all of the cross-bridges engage actin filaments.

- *Contracting.* The most interesting, but most complicated, state is *actively contracting* muscle. Myosin heads "walk" along actin filaments toward their barbed ends, pulling Z disks toward the center of the sarcomere. Thousands of sarcomeres shorten in series, causing the whole muscle to shorten. ATP is consumed and force is produced. The thick filament helical pattern is very weak by x-ray diffraction (see Fig. 42–13). Actin reflections are stronger than relaxed muscle, but not as strong as rigor. Disordered myosin heads must lie between the thick and thin filaments as each one dances asynchronously on and off of actin filaments.

Most myosin heads in contracting muscle have bound ATP or ADP-P$_i$ and oscillate rapidly among the four "weakly bound" states illustrated in Figure 39–6. During some of the transient interactions of myosin-ADP-P$_i$ with actin, phosphate dissociates from myosin, and the light chain domain rapidly reorients (Figs. 39–5 and 39–6), stretching elastic elements in the cross-bridge. Energy in this stretched spring can be used over a period of milliseconds to displace the actin filament relative to the cross-bridge and contracting the muscle. When ADP dissociates from the actin-myosin-ADP intermediate, ATP rapidly binds to the

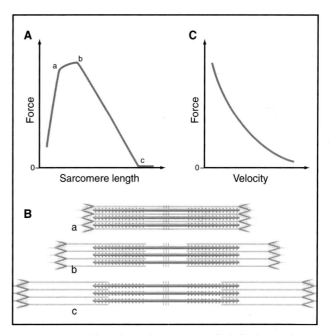

Figure 42-12 Physiological properties of skeletal muscle. *A,* Dependence of maximum tension on the length of the sarcomeres. *B,* Interpretive drawings. *C,* Relationship of force and velocity during muscle contraction. (*A,* Reference: Gordon AM, Huxely AF, Julian F: The variation in isometric tension with sarcomere length in vertebrate muscle fibres. J Physiol 171:28P–30P, 1964. *C,* Ruch TC, Patton HD (eds): Physiology and Biophysics. 19th ed. Philadelphia: WB Saunders, 1965, ch. 5, Fig. 14.)

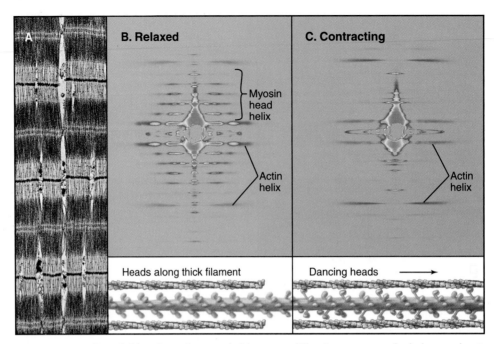

Figure 42-13 Cross-bridge dynamics revealed by x-ray diffraction patterns of whole muscle. *A,* Electron micrograph showing the orientation of the muscle in the x-ray beam. *B* and *C,* Fiber diffraction patterns from relaxed and contracting skeletal muscles with interpretive drawings of cross-bridges in each state. Reflections from myosin heads arranged on the thick-filament helix are strong in relaxed muscle. Reflections from the actin helix are stronger than the thick-filament helix in contraction. The myosin and actin reflections are each labeled in only one of four equivalent quadrants. During contraction, a few myosin heads attach transiently to actin, increasing the strength of the actin helix reflections, but most are disordered. (Micrograph and x-ray patterns courtesy of H. E. Huxley, Brandeis University.)

actin-myosin complex, dissociating the cross-bridge and starting a new ATPase cycle.

Relationship of Cross-bridge Behavior to the Mechanical Properties of Muscle

Under normal conditions, each sarcomere shortens less than 1 μm. However, the whole muscle shortens macroscopically because it has thousands of sarcomeres in series. For example, a human biceps muscle 20 cm long has about 80,000 sarcomeres in series from end to end. When each contracts 0.25 μm, the muscle shortens 2 cm. Because the system maintains a constant volume, each sarcomere and the whole muscle increase in diameter as they shorten. Although the individual filaments slide past each other relatively slowly (about 5 μm/second), muscles contract rapidly because the motion of each sarcomere in the series is added together. In our example, without resistance, the biceps contracts 2 cm in 100–200 msecs.

The behavior of cross-bridges explains why the velocity of muscle contractions of an active muscle depends on the external load (see Fig. 42–12). Contraction velocity is maximal when opposed by no load. Without a load, the molecular motion stored in elastic elements of each cross-bridge is largely converted into movement of actin filaments relative to

myosin filaments. Under these conditions, the filaments in muscle slide past each other at a rate of about 5 μm per second, the same speed observed for free actin filaments moving over myosin heads in vitro (see Fig. 39–4). For this rapid sliding to occur, myosin heads not producing force must not impede movement. If bound tightly to actin, they would interfere mechanically with rapid sliding. This is avoided by the rapid equilibrium of the myosin intermediates between being bound to actin and being free (see Fig. 39–6). Myosin heads with bound ATP or ADP-P$_i$ do not produce force when they bind transiently to a given actin subunit. These brief encounters do not retard sliding driven by force producing cross-bridges.

Muscle produces maximum force when the contraction rate is zero (see Fig. 42–12). The conformational change in the myosin head stretches elastic elements in the cross-bridge, but the force cannot overcome the resistance from the load on the muscle. Consequently, the filaments do not slide, and energy stored in each stretched elastic element is lost as heat when the cross-bridge dissociates at the end of the ATPase cycle. The maximum force depends on the numbers of sarcomeres in parallel, that is, the cross-sectional area of the muscle. Thus, muscles respond to strengthening exercises by growing in diameter.

Regulation of Skeletal Muscle Contraction

Control of Skeletal Muscle by Motor Neurons

Neural stimuli that activate skeletal muscles arise in two ways (Fig. 42–14). In organisms with well-developed central nervous systems, most neural signals that activate skeletal muscles result from conscious decisions, providing voluntary control over skeletal muscles. Other signals result from reflex responses to stimulation of sensory nerves. Specialized muscle cells innervated with both motor and sensory nerves function as stretch receptors, relaying information about length and tension back to the spinal cord where reflexes coordinate the motor neuron output. Neural inputs from both sources converge on **motor neurons** located in the brainstem and spinal cord of vertebrates. Axons of these motor neurons branch in the muscle to contact one or more muscle cells. A motor neuron together with its target muscle cells form a **motor unit.** In the most precisely controlled muscles, such as the extraocular muscles, some motor neurons innervate single muscle cells.

The contractile activity of a muscle is graded in terms of the speed and force of the contraction, so that individual muscles can produce both delicate and powerful movements. Nerve stimulation determines the contractile force in two ways: (1) the number of active motor units determines how many muscle cells produce force, and (2) the rate of stimulation adjusts the force produced by active cells. Every time a muscle cell is stimulated, all of the sarcomeres are activated, but the force that they produce increases as the rate of stimulation increases, up to a maximum of about 200 times per second. The shortening velocity of an active muscle depends simply on force produced and the resistance (see Fig. 42–12C). If a large force or high velocity of contraction is required, many motor units are called into action and stimulated repetitively. To sustain contraction, motor nerves fire repeatedly. By varying the number of active cells in a muscle and rate of stimulation, the nervous system sets the force required for a particular movement.

Synaptic Transmission at Neuromuscular Junctions

The terminal branch of each motor neuron axon forms a synapse called the **motor end plate** or **neuromuscular junction** on the muscle surface (see Fig. 10–8). These nerve endings are filled with synaptic vesicles containing the neurotransmitter **acetylcholine.** Arrival of an action potential at the nerve terminal stimulates fusion of synaptic vesicles with the nerve plasma membrane, releasing acetylcholine into the cleft between nerve and muscle. In less than a millisecond, acetylcholine diffuses across the extracellular space and binds to acetylcholine receptors con-

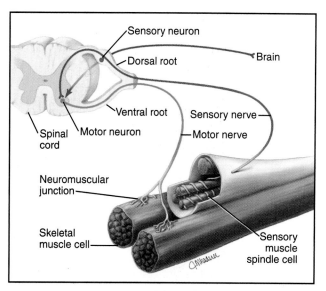

Figure 42–14 Innervation of skeletal muscle. Motor neurons in the spinal cord stimulate one or (usually) more skeletal muscle cells. Two neural pathways control motor neurons. Some stimuli come from neurons in higher centers of the brain. This pathway provides voluntary control over muscle contraction. Other stimuli come through local reflex circuits from sensory detectors, including muscle spindle cells. These signals help coordinate muscle contraction in response to changing forces on the muscle.

centrated in the adjacent muscle plasma membrane. Acetylcholine binding opens the receptor cation channel, initiating a new action potential that spreads over the muscle cell plasma membrane and down into the T tubules.

Coupling Action Potentials to Contraction

An action potential in a T tubule triggers the release of Ca^{2+} from smooth endoplasmic reticulum into the cytoplasm (Fig. 42–15). Ca^{2+} binding to troponin allows myosin to interact with the thin filament, initiating contraction. This signal transduction process is called excitation-contraction coupling. Ca^{2+} release in skeletal muscle is the best characterized example of a general regulatory mechanism used by many cells (see Chapter 28).

Three transmembrane proteins located in the T tubule and the terminal cisternae of the smooth endoplasmic reticulum cooperate to generate the transient Ca^{2+} signal (Fig. 42–16). The operation of this system is described after introducing its components.

1. A voltage-sensitive calcium channel (see Chapter 9) senses action potentials in the T tubule. These channels are called **dihydropyridine (DHP) receptors** owing to their affinity for this class of drugs. The actual Ca^{2+} channel of dihydropyridine receptors is not essential for skeletal muscle, as shown by the fact that external Ca^{2+} is not required for contraction in the short term.

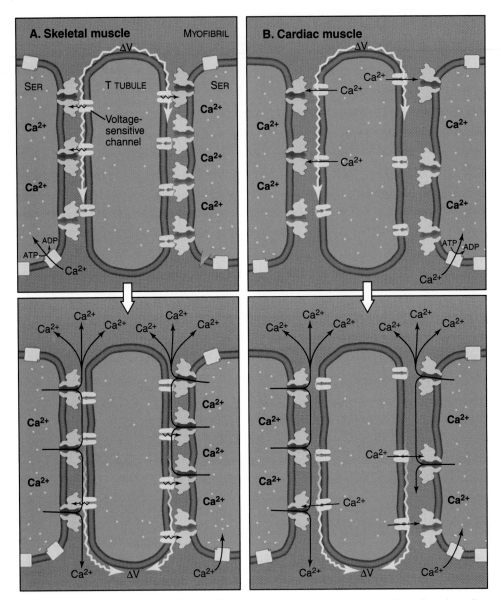

Figure 42–15 A molecular model for the calcium release mechanism in skeletal and cardiac muscles. Both muscles use voltage-sensitive calcium channels in the T tubule membrane and calcium release channels in the smooth endoplasmic reticulum (SER). *A*, Direct coupling in skeletal muscle. An action potential in the T tubule (Δv) activates the voltage sensor (turning from grey to blue). This then, through a direct contact, opens the calcium release channel (turning from grey to pink). Cytoplasmic Ca^{2+} levels rise only briefly because calcium-ATPase pumps Ca^{2+} back into the lumen of the SER. *B*, Calcium-induced Ca^{2+} release in cardiac muscle. An action potential opens the voltage-sensitive Ca^{2+} channel in the T tubule, releasing Ca^{2+} into the cytoplasm. This Ca^{2+} opens the calcium release channel in the SER.

2. Ca^{2+} release channels (see Fig. 28–13), concentrated in the terminal cisternae of smooth endoplasmic reticulum, release Ca^{2+} into the cytoplasm. A drug called ryanodine binds these channels and inhibits Ca^{2+} release. Every second **ryanodine receptor** is connected to a cytoplasmic loop of a DHP receptor, forming bridges called feet between the T tubule to the endoplasmic reticulum (see Fig. 42–10*B*).

3. The E1E2 **calcium-ATPase** (see Fig. 7–7) actively pumps Ca^{2+} from cytoplasm into the endoplasmic reticulum against a concentration gradient of greater than 10^4. Several low-affinity, high-capacity Ca^{2+}-binding proteins buffer the millimolar concentration of Ca^{2+} inside the smooth endoplasmic reticulum. For example, numerous carboxyl groups on the surface of calsequestrin bind Ca^{2+} with a millimolar K_d. This rapidly reversible reac-

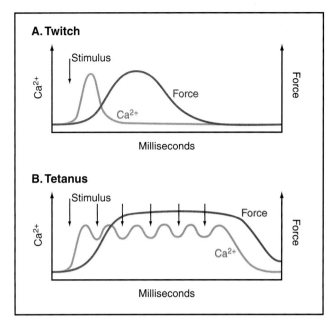

A. Twitch

B. Tetanus

Figure 42-16 Ca^{2+} triggers contraction of skeletal muscle. In these experiments, the Ca^{2+}-sensitive protein aequorin was injected into live muscle cells to provide a signal for the cytoplasmic Ca^{2+} concentration. *A*, Single stimulus. Cytoplasmic Ca^{2+} concentration increases transiently, followed by a short contraction. This brief contraction persists after cytoplasmic Ca^{2+} decreases to the resting level. *B*, Multiple stimuli. Each stimulus releases a new pulse of Ca^{2+}, prolonging the contraction in so-called tetanus. (Reference: Ridgway EB, Ashley CC: Calcium transients in single muscle fibers. Biochem Biophys Res Commun 29:229–234, 1967.)

tion increases the Ca^{2+} storage capacity of endoplasmic reticulum without sacrificing the speed of Ca^{2+} release. Accessory subunits anchor calsequestrin to the Ca^{2+} release channel, ensuring a local supply of Ca^{2+} for release into cytoplasm when muscle is activated.

An action potential in a T tubule results in a transient rise in cytoplasmic Ca^{2+}—from 0.1 μM to about 2 μM (see Fig. 42–16)—in the following way. The action potential causes a short-lived conformational change in the DHP receptors that is transmitted directly to associated ryanodine receptor Ca^{2+} release channels. Many Ca^{2+} channels open transiently, allowing Ca^{2+} to diffuse down the steep concentration gradient from lumen to cytoplasm. Physical connections between ryanodine receptors may spread their activation laterally, ensuring synchronous activation of a patch of channels. The structural changes in these channels that release Ca^{2+} are not yet understood.

After a single action potential, the rise in the cytoplasmic Ca^{2+} level lasts but a few milliseconds for three reasons. First, Ca^{2+} release channels close quickly. Second, cytoplasmic Ca^{2+} binds to troponin C and other proteins. Third, Ca^{2+} pumps efficiently transport cytoplasmic Ca^{2+} back into the lumen of the

smooth endoplasmic reticulum, even before the muscle develops maximum force. Ca^{2+} pumps are continuously active, keeping cytoplasmic Ca^{2+} concentration low. Repeated action potentials are required to prolong the rise in cytoplasmic Ca^{2+} (see Fig. 42–16*B*).

Transduction of the Calcium Spike into Contraction

Troponin-tropomyosin on thin filaments cooperates with myosin to turn on contraction in response to a Ca^{2+} spike. At rest, two Ca^{2+}-binding sites of troponin C are largely unoccupied (owing to their low affinity for Ca^{2+} and the low Ca^{2+} concentration), and the troponin-tropomyosin complex partially blocks the binding site for myosin heads on actin (Fig. 42–17). This prevents most of the weak-binding myosin intermediates with ATP or ADP-P_i in the active site from

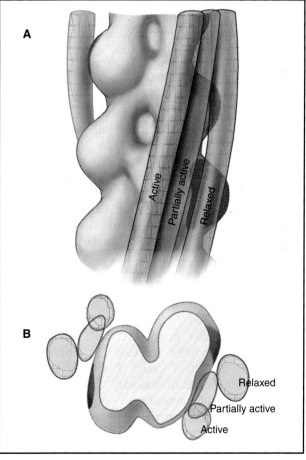

Figure 42-17 Thin filament activation mechanism. Reconstructions from electron micrographs showing a short segment of thin filament (*A*) and a cross section of a thin filament (*B*). Ca^{2+} binding to troponin C partially activates the filament by moving tropomyosin away from its lateral position in relaxed muscle where it overlaps the myosin-binding site on actin *(red)*. Myosin binding to the partially activated filament moves tropomyosin further out of the way into the active position. (Redrawn from data of W. Lehman, Boston University.)

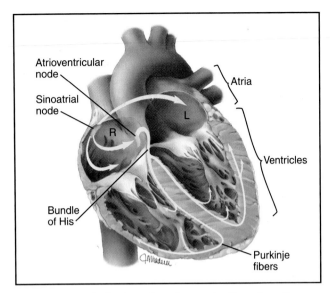

Figure 42–19 Activation of cardiac contraction. An action potential starts at the sinoatrial node and travels through atrial muscle cells to the atrioventricular node. After a short delay, the action potential spreads through the interventricular septum in modified cardiac muscle cells, called Purkinje's fibers, and then through muscle cells to the whole ventricle. The action potential follows the same path each time, giving rise to electrical signals that can be detected on the body surface by electrocardiogram (EKG). Damage during myocardial infarctions changes the EKG pattern and may cause arrhythmias.

the **atrioventricular node,** the action potential and contraction spread through the ventricle.

Like skeletal muscle, plasma membrane action potentials stimulate cardiac muscle cells to contract by releasing Ca^{2+} to activate troponin-tropomyosin. However, the Ca^{2+} release mechanism differs in important details from skeletal muscle. In particular, extracellular Ca^{2+} is required for heart but not skeletal muscle. Action potentials open voltage-sensitive calcium channels (dihydropyridine receptors) in T tubules, releasing Ca^{2+} locally. This small burst of Ca^{2+} opens nearby ryanodine receptors in the smooth endoplasmic reticulum, releasing a flood of Ca^{2+} to trigger contraction. This excitation-contraction coupling can be defective when heart muscle cells grow larger in response to abnormal demands, as in high blood pressure. The defect may be explained by growth separating T tubules from smooth endoplasmic reticulum, either physically or functionally, thereby decreasing the probability that Ca^{2+} entering through dihydropyridine receptors will trigger Ca^{2+} release from the endoplasmic reticulum.

Motor nerves do not stimulate cardiac muscle directly, but the heart is rich in autonomic nerves from the sympathetic and parasympathetic nervous systems. These nerves secrete acetylcholine and norepinephrine, which act as hormones to modulate the rate and force of contraction (see Fig. 10–12).

Molecular Basis of Inherited Heart Diseases

Because the heart is so vital to survival, relatively minor molecular defects, which might escape detection in an experimental animal, command attention in humans. About 1 of 500 persons carries a mutation in a gene that compromises cardiac function (Table 42–4). For example, many different point mutations in the myosin heavy chain can compromise its function. Affected individuals are typically heterozygous for these mutations, and the mutant myosin interferes with the function of the normal myosin. Over a period of

table 42–4

GENETIC DEFECTS IN CARDIAC DISEASE

Gene/Protein	Normal Function	Disease Manifestations
Actin	Thin filament	Dilated cardiomyopathy, heart failure
Titin	Passive elasticity	Dilated cardiomyopathy, heart failure
Dystrophin	Membrane stabilization	Dilated cardiomyopathy, heart failure
β-Myosin heavy chain	Thick-filament motor	Hypertrophic cardiomyopathy, arrhythmias
Myosin essential light chain	Myosin motor	Hypertrophic cardiomyopathy, arrhythmias
Myosin regulatory light chain	Myosin motor	Hypertrophic cardiomyopathy, arrhythmias
Myosin C protein	Thick-filament structure	Hypertrophic cardiomyopathy, arrhythmias
Troponin T	Calcium regulation	Hypertrophic cardiomyopathy, arrhythmias
Troponin I	Calcium regulation	Hypertrophic cardiomyopathy, arrhythmias
Tropomyosin	Calcium regulation	Hypertrophic cardiomyopathy, arrhythmias
NKX2–5	Transcription factor	Congenital atrioseptal defects
TBX5	Transcription factor	Multiple congenital defects between heart chambers
HERG	Potassium channel	Long QT syndrome, arrhythmias
KVLQT1	Potassium channel	Long QT syndrome, arrhythmias
minK	Potassium channel	Long QT syndrome, arrhythmias
SCN5A	Sodium channel	Long QT syndrome, arrhythmias

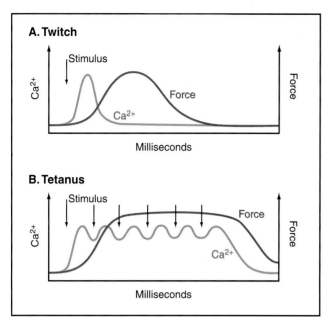

A. Twitch

Stimulus

Ca²⁺

Force

Ca²⁺

Force

Milliseconds

B. Tetanus

Stimulus

Ca²⁺

Force

Force

Ca²⁺

Milliseconds

Figure 42-16 Ca²⁺ triggers contraction of skeletal muscle. In these experiments, the Ca²⁺-sensitive protein aequorin was injected into live muscle cells to provide a signal for the cytoplasmic Ca²⁺ concentration. *A*, Single stimulus. Cytoplasmic Ca²⁺ concentration increases transiently, followed by a short contraction. This brief contraction persists after cytoplasmic Ca²⁺ decreases to the resting level. *B*, Multiple stimuli. Each stimulus releases a new pulse of Ca²⁺, prolonging the contraction in so-called tetanus. (Reference: Ridgway EB, Ashley CC: Calcium transients in single muscle fibers. Biochem Biophys Res Commun 29:229–234, 1967.)

tion increases the Ca²⁺ storage capacity of endoplasmic reticulum without sacrificing the speed of Ca²⁺ release. Accessory subunits anchor calsequestrin to the Ca²⁺ release channel, ensuring a local supply of Ca²⁺ for release into cytoplasm when muscle is activated.

An action potential in a T tubule results in a transient rise in cytoplasmic Ca²⁺—from 0.1 μM to about 2 μM (see Fig. 42–16)—in the following way. The action potential causes a short-lived conformational change in the DHP receptors that is transmitted directly to associated ryanodine receptor Ca²⁺ release channels. Many Ca²⁺ channels open transiently, allowing Ca²⁺ to diffuse down the steep concentration gradient from lumen to cytoplasm. Physical connections between ryanodine receptors may spread their activation laterally, ensuring synchronous activation of a patch of channels. The structural changes in these channels that release Ca²⁺ are not yet understood.

After a single action potential, the rise in the cytoplasmic Ca²⁺ level lasts but a few milliseconds for three reasons. First, Ca²⁺ release channels close quickly. Second, cytoplasmic Ca²⁺ binds to troponin C and other proteins. Third, Ca²⁺ pumps efficiently transport cytoplasmic Ca²⁺ back into the lumen of the

smooth endoplasmic reticulum, even before the muscle develops maximum force. Ca²⁺ pumps are continuously active, keeping cytoplasmic Ca²⁺ concentration low. Repeated action potentials are required to prolong the rise in cytoplasmic Ca²⁺ (see Fig. 42–16B).

Transduction of the Calcium Spike into Contraction

Troponin-tropomyosin on thin filaments cooperates with myosin to turn on contraction in response to a Ca²⁺ spike. At rest, two Ca²⁺-binding sites of troponin C are largely unoccupied (owing to their low affinity for Ca²⁺ and the low Ca²⁺ concentration), and the troponin-tropomyosin complex partially blocks the binding site for myosin heads on actin (Fig. 42–17). This prevents most of the weak-binding myosin intermediates with ATP or ADP-P$_i$ in the active site from

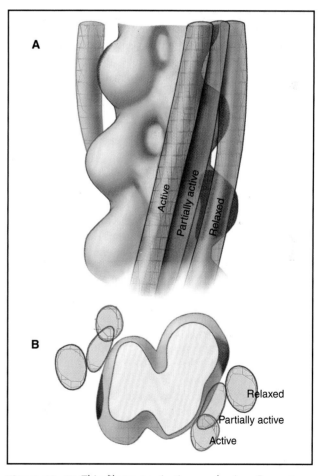

A

Active

Partially active

Relaxed

B

Relaxed

Partially active

Active

Figure 42-17 Thin filament activation mechanism. Reconstructions from electron micrographs showing a short segment of thin filament (*A*) and a cross section of a thin filament (*B*). Ca²⁺ binding to troponin C partially activates the filament by moving tropomyosin away from its lateral position in relaxed muscle where it overlaps the myosin-binding site on actin *(red)*. Myosin binding to the partially activated filament moves tropomyosin further out of the way into the active position. (Redrawn from data of W. Lehman, Boston University.)

binding the thin filament. When released into cytoplasm, Ca^{2+} binds troponin C, releasing TNI and resulting in a small shift in the position of tropomyosin on the thin filament. This shift increases the probability that myosin-ADP-P_i heads will bind to the thin filament, dissociating their bound P_i and producing force. The initial binding of the first force-producing heads shifts the long tropomyosin molecule a bit further away from the myosin binding sites, allowing adjacent actins to interact freely with other myosin heads. The end-to-end association of tropomyosins facilitates this cooperative switch by exposing more distant actin subunits in the thin filament to myosin. The response of troponin to Ca^{2+} involves a shift in a segment of TNI from a binding site on actin to a site on Ca^{2+}-activated TNC, allowing tropomyosin to move.

Thus, the combined effects of Ca^{2+} and myosin make the thin filament receptive to myosin binding. Activation is cooperative because both Ca^{2+}-binding sites on troponin C must be occupied; because the effects of Ca^{2+} binding and myosin binding are transmitted to neighboring tropomyosins through their end-to-end attachments; and because every myosin that binds accentuates the response. This cooperativity makes the on-off switch respond very sharply to a relatively small, 10- to 20-fold change in the cytoplasmic Ca^{2+} concentration. The efficiency of this switch is underscored by the fact that the energy consumption of a muscle cell increases more than 1000-fold when it is activated. Activation of slow skeletal muscle and cardiac muscle is less cooperative, as their troponin C has only one Ca^{2+}-binding site.

Note the delay between the Ca^{2+} spike and the onset of tension (see Fig. 42–16). The Ca^{2+}-sensitive switch is sharp but slow owing to the slow response of thin filaments to Ca^{2+} binding. Note also that muscle continues to produce force well after the cytoplasmic Ca^{2+} concentration returns to resting levels. Ca^{2+} binds troponin C rapidly (within milliseconds) but dissociates slowly (within tens of milliseconds). Thus, Ca^{2+} spike saturates troponin C, and the muscle remains active even after free Ca^{2+} has returned to the endoplasmic reticulum lumen. Force declines slowly as Ca^{2+} dissociates from troponin C and returns to the smooth endoplasmic reticulum.

A single action potential produces a short contractile "twitch" (see Fig. 42–16). Maximum contractile force is produced by a series of closely spaced action potentials, leading to a sustained rise in cytoplasmic Ca^{2+} and prolonged activation of actomyosin. The extended contraction is called tetanus.

Regulation by Myosin Light Chains

The participation of skeletal muscle myosin light chains in the regulation of contraction varies among species. The skeletal muscles of mollusks are one extreme; myosin light chains bind Ca^{2+} and provide the main on/off switch for contraction. When the Ca^{2+} concentration is low in resting muscle, no Ca^{2+} binds to light chains and the actin-myosin ATPase is off. Ca^{2+} that is released during activation binds to the light chains, turning on the ATPase and contraction. At the other extreme, the light chains of vertebrate skeletal muscle myosin do not bind Ca^{2+} and do not participate in activation. However, *phosphorylation* of vertebrate skeletal muscle light chains modulates contractile activity by increasing force production at suboptimal Ca^{2+} concentrations. Horseshoe crab skeletal muscle uses a dual system: Ca^{2+} binding to troponin-tropomyosin on thin filaments and Ca^{2+}-regulated phosphorylation of myosin light chains both stimulate contraction.

Specialized Skeletal Muscle Cells

All skeletal muscle cells are built on the same principles, but vertebrates actually have several different types of skeletal muscle cells, each with distinct contractile protein isoforms. The myosin and actin isoforms are coded by different genes, whereas alternative splicing of one primary transcript (see Fig. 15–9) creates more than 50 isoforms of troponin T!

Physiological properties, such as the speed of contraction and the rate of fatigue, provide criteria for classifying muscle cells (Table 42–3). The isoforms of myosin (and probably the other contractile proteins) determine the speed of contraction, whereas the content of mitochondria and myoglobin determines the endurance and overall color of the muscle. White muscle cells depend largely on glycolysis to supply ATP, accounting for their rapid fatigue compared with red muscle cells, which are specialized for oxidative metabolism with abundant mitochondria and myoglobin.

Some muscles consist of only fast-twitch white muscle cells or slow-twitch red muscle cells, but most muscles are a mixture of two or more cell types. For example, in chickens, the leg muscles responsible for supporting the body, walking, and maintaining balance over long periods of time are rich in red muscle cells. On the other hand, the chicken breast muscles,

table 42–3
MUSCLE CELL TYPES

Physiological Type	Myosin Type	Mitochondria	Fatigue
Fast, white	Fast	Few	Rapid
Intermediate	Fast	Medium	Medium
Fast, red	Fast	Many	Slow
Slow, red	Slow	Many	Slow

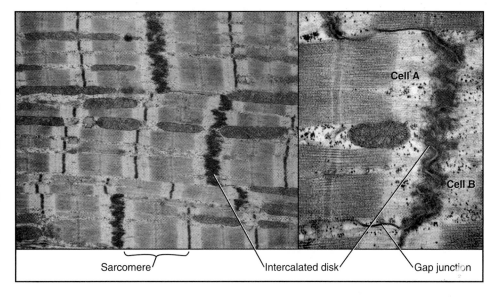

Figure 42–18 Electron micrographs of a longitudinal section of two cardiac muscle cells. Sarcomeres are similar to skeletal muscle. Intercalated disks anchor neighboring cells together, and gap junctions couple the cells electrically. (Courtesy of D. W. Fawcett, Harvard Medical School.)

Sarcomere   Intercalated disk   Gap junction

used for energetic flapping of the wings for short periods, are mainly white muscle cells.

The pattern of *nerve stimulation* determines the muscle cell type by controlling which genes are expressed (and presumably, how the troponin T messenger RNA [mRNA] is processed). This has been demonstrated by transplanting motor nerves between fast and slow muscles. Over a period of weeks, slow isoforms replace fast isoforms and vice versa. Even more surprising, the same result is achieved by stimulating muscles electrically with fast or slow patterns of impulses. No one knows how this happens.

The proportion of each cell type in a muscle is determined genetically, so world-class sprinters (with a high proportion of fast, white fibers) and marathoners (with a high proportion of slow red fibers) are born with advantages for their specialties. Training can lead to hypertrophy of specific cell types and improved performance. Endurance training also leads to an increased proportion of slow cells.

Cardiac Muscle

To maintain the circulation of blood, heart muscle is specialized for repetitive, fatigue-free contractions driven at regular intervals by action potentials from specialized pace-making cells. Gap junctions allow these action potentials to spread from one muscle cell to the next. The arrangement of the contractile apparatus into sarcomeres is similar to skeletal muscle.

The Contractile Apparatus of Cardiac Muscle

Cardiac muscle cells have sarcomeres with thick and thin filaments like skeletal muscle (Fig. 42–18), but they have more mitochondria, larger T tubules, less smooth endoplasmic reticulum, and a smaller version of nebulin called nebulette. The atrium has one major myosin isoform. Two ventricular myosin isoforms differ in ATPase activity and speed of contraction. Humans almost exclusively express only one of these isoforms. In rats, thyroid hormone regulates expression of these isoforms. Both are expressed normally, but one predominates in hypothyroidism and the other in hyperthyroidism. Heart expresses different isoforms of TNI and TNT than skeletal muscle. If damaged in a heart attack, cardiac cells release TNI and TNT into the blood. Measurement of cardiac TNI and TNT in blood is now the most sensitive chemical test for heart attacks.

Short, modestly branched, cardiac muscle cells have centrally located nuclei and squared-off ends (see Fig. 42–1) where neighboring cells attach to each other at specialized adhesive junctions called **intercalated disks** (see Fig. 42–18). These junctions have properties of both adherens junctions (binding actin filaments) and desmosomes (binding intermediate filaments). Membranes of adjacent cells are bound together by Ca^{2+}-dependent cadherins (see Chapter 32).

Pacemaker Cells

Modified cardiac muscle cells in the right atrium (**sinoatrial node**) spontaneously depolarize their plasma membrane at regular intervals to initiate each heartbeat (see Figs. 10–11 and 42–19). Special nonselective cation channels allow Na^+ to leak into these cells and K^+ to leak out, depolarizing the plasma membrane and triggering an action potential. The action potential spreads from cell to cell through gap junctions (see Chapter 33), activating all cells in the atrium within a few hundred milliseconds. After a delay in

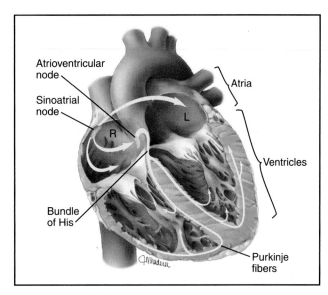

Figure 42-19 Activation of cardiac contraction. An action potential starts at the sinoatrial node and travels through atrial muscle cells to the atrioventricular node. After a short delay, the action potential spreads through the interventricular septum in modified cardiac muscle cells, called Purkinje's fibers, and then through muscle cells to the whole ventricle. The action potential follows the same path each time, giving rise to electrical signals that can be detected on the body surface by electrocardiogram (EKG). Damage during myocardial infarctions changes the EKG pattern and may cause arrhythmias.

the **atrioventricular node,** the action potential and contraction spread through the ventricle.

Like skeletal muscle, plasma membrane action potentials stimulate cardiac muscle cells to contract by releasing Ca^{2+} to activate troponin-tropomyosin. However, the Ca^{2+} release mechanism differs in important details from skeletal muscle. In particular, extracellular Ca^{2+} is required for heart but not skeletal muscle. Action potentials open voltage-sensitive calcium channels (dihydropyridine receptors) in T tubules, releasing Ca^{2+} locally. This small burst of Ca^{2+} opens nearby ryanodine receptors in the smooth endoplasmic reticulum, releasing a flood of Ca^{2+} to trigger contraction. This excitation-contraction coupling can be defective when heart muscle cells grow larger in response to abnormal demands, as in high blood pressure. The defect may be explained by growth separating T tubules from smooth endoplasmic reticulum, either physically or functionally, thereby decreasing the probability that Ca^{2+} entering through dihydropyridine receptors will trigger Ca^{2+} release from the endoplasmic reticulum.

Motor nerves do not stimulate cardiac muscle directly, but the heart is rich in autonomic nerves from the sympathetic and parasympathetic nervous systems. These nerves secrete acetylcholine and norepinephrine, which act as hormones to modulate the rate and force of contraction (see Fig. 10–12).

Molecular Basis of Inherited Heart Diseases

Because the heart is so vital to survival, relatively minor molecular defects, which might escape detection in an experimental animal, command attention in humans. About 1 of 500 persons carries a mutation in a gene that compromises cardiac function (Table 42–4). For example, many different point mutations in the myosin heavy chain can compromise its function. Affected individuals are typically heterozygous for these mutations, and the mutant myosin interferes with the function of the normal myosin. Over a period of

table 42-4

GENETIC DEFECTS IN CARDIAC DISEASE

Gene/Protein	Normal Function	Disease Manifestations
Actin	Thin filament	Dilated cardiomyopathy, heart failure
Titin	Passive elasticity	Dilated cardiomyopathy, heart failure
Dystrophin	Membrane stabilization	Dilated cardiomyopathy, heart failure
β-Myosin heavy chain	Thick-filament motor	Hypertrophic cardiomyopathy, arrhythmias
Myosin essential light chain	Myosin motor	Hypertrophic cardiomyopathy, arrhythmias
Myosin regulatory light chain	Myosin motor	Hypertrophic cardiomyopathy, arrhythmias
Myosin C protein	Thick-filament structure	Hypertrophic cardiomyopathy, arrhythmias
Troponin T	Calcium regulation	Hypertrophic cardiomyopathy, arrhythmias
Troponin I	Calcium regulation	Hypertrophic cardiomyopathy, arrhythmias
Tropomyosin	Calcium regulation	Hypertrophic cardiomyopathy, arrhythmias
NKX2–5	Transcription factor	Congenital atrioseptal defects
TBX5	Transcription factor	Multiple congenital defects between heart chambers
HERG	Potassium channel	Long QT syndrome, arrhythmias
KVLQT1	Potassium channel	Long QT syndrome, arrhythmias
minK	Potassium channel	Long QT syndrome, arrhythmias
SCN5A	Sodium channel	Long QT syndrome, arrhythmias

years, the heart attempts to compensate for the contractility defect through hypertrophy, but the thickened heart wall compromises cardiac relaxation and filling of the chambers with blood. More serious, heart hypertrophy eventually causes defects in activation and abnormal rhythms that can be fatal. The rate of progress of these so-called **hypertrophic cardiomyopathies** depends on the particular mutation. Individuals with defects in C protein develop hypertrophy in their 50s and can live normal life spans. By contrast, those with defects in troponin T can be affected as teenagers and die of arrhythmias in their 20s. These severe mutations of cardiac contractile proteins account for about half of the deaths of apparently healthy young athletes. Myosin mutations are intermediate in severity. Mutations in actin and dystrophin cause a disease of an opposite sort. Individual cells hypertrophy, but many die and are replaced by connective tissue, leading to thinning of the wall of the heart and defective contractility.

Smooth Muscle

The Contractile Apparatus

Smooth muscle cells are specialized for slow, powerful, efficient contractions controlled by a variety of involuntary mechanisms. Smooth muscle cells are generally confined to internal organs, such as blood vessels (where they regulate blood pressure), the gastrointestinal tract (where they move food through the intestines), and the respiratory system (where their excessive contraction contributes to asthma and other allergic reactions). The cytoplasm of spindle-shaped smooth muscle cells (see Fig. 42–1) appears homogeneous by light microscopy because the contractile proteins are not organized in regular arrays like sarcomeres of skeletal and cardiac muscle. A basal lamina and variable amounts of collagen and elastic fibers surround each cell.

In terms of organization and biochemistry, smooth muscle cells (Fig. 42–20) resemble nonmuscle cells more than they do skeletal or cardiac muscle. For example, the gene for smooth muscle myosin arose relatively recently from a cytoplasmic myosin II gene (see Fig. 40–2). These myosins also share the same regulatory light chain. Long myosin thick filaments are interspersed among the thin filaments, but not in a regular way like striated muscles. Thin filaments are composed of actin and tropomyosin, along with two regulatory proteins, caldesmon and calponin, rather than troponin. Thin filaments are arranged obliquely in the cell, some with their barbed ends attached to dense plaques on the plasma membrane, others to **dense bodies** in the cytoplasm. Like Z disks in striated muscles, dense bodies also anchor desmin inter-

mediate filaments, forming a continuous, inextensible, internal "tendon" running from end to end into the cell, preventing excess stretching (see Fig. 38–8).

Smooth muscle cells contract like a concertina (Fig. 42–21) because tension generated by myosin and actin is applied to discrete spots on the plasma membrane. This compression can be seen in light micrographs as irregular cells with "corkscrew" nuclei. Given that smooth muscle cells have less myosin than striated muscle, it is remarkable that they develop the same force. This is explained by two factors. First, the force-generating unit, the myosin filament, is larger in smooth muscle than skeletal muscle. Deploying a given amount of myosin in large thick filaments in a long sarcomere produces more force than the same myosin in small filaments arranged in a series of short sarcomeres. Second, individual smooth muscle myosin molecules produce a larger force than skeletal muscle myosin, at least in in vitro assays.

Regulation of Smooth Muscle Contraction

Stimuli that trigger smooth muscle contraction vary widely, but they all seem to act through seven-helix receptors coupled to trimeric G proteins. Hormones stimulate contraction of the uterus, whereas motor nerves stimulate instrinsic eye muscles that close the pupil. Gap junctions couple some groups of smooth muscle cells, so their activation is propagated and coordinated within the tissue.

Depending on the muscle, Ca^{2+} for contraction enters the cytoplasm through either voltage-dependent calcium channels in the plasma membrane or IP_3 (inositol, 1,4,5-triphosphate)–induced Ca^{2+} release from smooth endoplasmic reticulum (see Fig. 42–21). Drugs that block plasma membrane calcium channels can distinguish these two pathways experimentally. In intestines, parasympathetic nerves release acetylcholine to stimulate seven-helix muscarinic receptors (see Chapters 10 and 26). Associated trimeric G proteins activate cation channels that depolarize the plasma membrane and allow Ca^{2+} to enter through voltage-sensitive calcium channels. Gap junctions couple gut smooth muscle cells, allowing excitation to spread from cell to cell. Calcium channel blockers strongly inhibit activation of gut smooth muscle. At the other end of the spectrum, vascular smooth muscle depends on IP_3 to release Ca^{2+} from intracellular stores rather than from outside the cell.

Following stimulation, intracellular Ca^{2+} increases rapidly but transiently, declining to a value above resting level as the receptors desensitize (see Chapter 28). Ca^{2+} pumps in both smooth endoplasmic reticulum and plasma membrane clear the cytoplasm of Ca^{2+} so that Ca^{2+} levels decrease to resting levels and the muscle relaxes when the activating stimulus is removed.

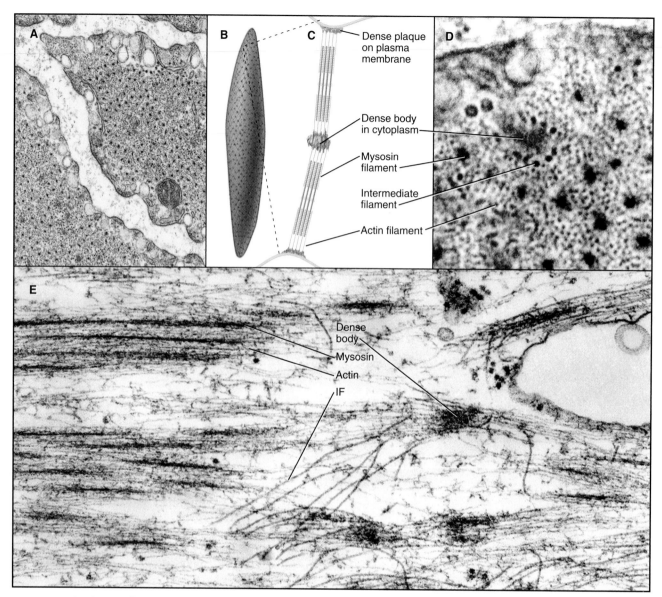

Figure 42-20 Contractile apparatus of smooth muscle. *A,* Electron micrograph of a thin cross section. *B* and *C,* Simplified schematic drawings of the organization of the contractile units, which stretch across the cell between plasma membrane attachment plaques. Contractile units consist of myosin filaments connecting thin filaments attached to a dense body or plasma membrane plaque. *D,* High-power electron micrograph showing a dense body and cross sections of three types of filaments. *E,* Electron micrograph of a longitudinal section of an extracted vascular smooth muscle cell illustrating associations of actin filaments and intermediate filaments (IF) with dense bodies, and myosin filaments interacting with actin filaments. (*A, D,* and *E,* Courtesy of A. V. Somlyo and A. P. Somlyo, University of Virginia, Charlottesville. References: Somlyo AP, et al: Filament organization in vertebrate smooth muscle. Philos Trans R Soc Lond [Biol] 265:223–229, 1973; Bond M, Somylo AV: Dense bodies and actin polarity in vertebrate smooth muscle. J Cell Biol 95:403–413, 1982, by copyright permission of the Rockefeller University Press.)

Relaxing agents, acting through cyclic guanosine monophosphate (cGMP) or cAMP (see Chapter 28), promote clearance of cytoplasmic Ca^{2+}. Epinephrine relaxes smooth muscles of the respiratory system by another method. Stimulation of β-adrenergic receptors activates potassium channels that hyperpolarize the plasma membrane and reduce Ca^{2+} entry. This approach is used to treat asthma.

After a considerable delay (> 200 msec) following the Ca^{2+} spike, contractile force develops slowly. The delay is attributable to the time required for a sequence of three biochemical reactions: Ca^{2+} binding to calmodulin (see Chapter 28); calcium-calmodulin activation of **myosin light chain kinase;** and phosphorylation of myosin regulatory light chains, turning on the myosin-actin ATPase cycle (see Fig. 42–21). Un-

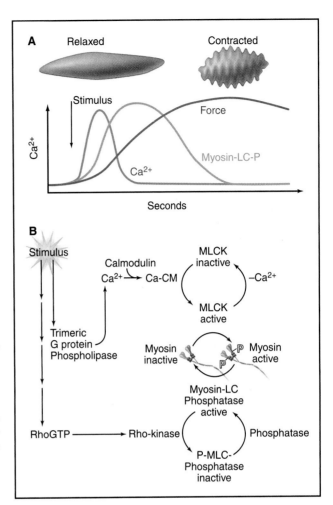

Figure 42-21 Activation of smooth muscle contraction. *A,* Drawings show how the spindle-shaped smooth muscle cell becomes pleated as it contracts owing to the attachment of the actin filaments at intervals along the plasma membrane. The graph shows the time course of activation, consisting of release of Ca^{2+} into the cytoplasm, phosphorylation of myosin regulatory light chains, and then the slow development of force. Myosin light chain phosphorylation (LC-P) is required to initiate, but not to prolong, the contraction of smooth muscle. *B,* Biochemical pathways controlling phosphorylation of myosin regulatory light chains. Receptor stimulation leads to production of IP_3 by phospholipase C and release of Ca^{2+} into cytoplasm. Ca^{2+} binds calmodulin (CM), which activates myosin light chain kinase (MLCK) by binding the kinase's autoinhibitory peptide and displacing it from the active site. Active MLCK phosphorylates activating sites on the regulatory light chain. Light chain phosphatase reverses phosphorylation of myosin. Activation of the small GTPase Rho with GTP stimulates Rho-kinase, which phosphorylates and inactivates light chain phosphatase. This makes the system more sensitive to any level of Ca^{2+}, as light chain phosphorylation is prolonged. P-MLC-, phosphorylated myosin light chain. (*A,* Redrawn from the work of K. Kamm and J. Stull, University of Texas Southwestern Medical School, Dallas.)

phosphorylated myosin II from smooth muscle and vertebrate nonmuscle cells is inactive.

Phosphorylation of myosin light chains is required to initiate but not maintain contraction, so slowly cycling, unphosphorylated myosins maintain peak force with little expenditure of energy. Regulation of unphosphorylated cross-bridges is not well understood, but they appear to be activated cooperatively by a small population of phosphorylated myosin heads. Caldesmon, a calcium-calmodulin binding protein associated with tropomyosin on actin filaments, may allow myosin heads to cycle very slowly or remain bound even in the presence of ATP.

The sensitivity of light chain phosphorylation to Ca^{2+} depends on a parallel signaling pathway that partially inhibits myosin phosphatase, thus increasing the number of phosphorylated myosin cross-bridges and force at any given Ca^{2+} concentration (see Fig. 42-21). Receptors coupled to trimeric G proteins activate the small GTPase RhoA, which stimulates a protein kinase that inhibits myosin light chain phosphatase. Malfunction of this Ca^{2+}-sensitizing mechanism may contribute to some forms of high blood pressure, since in hypertensive animals, drugs that inhibit Rho-activated kinase relax smooth muscle and lower blood pressure.

▌ Selected Readings

Bolton TB, Prestwich SA, Zholos AV, Gordienko DV: Excitation-contraction coupling in gastrointestinal and other smooth muscles. Annu Rev Physiol 61:85–115, 1999.

Franzini-Armstrong C, Protasi F, Ramesh V: Comparative ultrastructure of Ca^{2+} release units in skeletal and cardiac muscle. Ann NY Acad Sci 853:20–30, 1998.

Geeves MA, Holmes KC: Structural mechanism of muscle contraction. Annu Rev Biochem 68:687–728, 1999.

Gordon AM, Homsher E, Regnier M: Regulation of contraction in striated muscle. Physiol Rev 80:853–924, 2000.

Kiriazis H, Kranias EG: Genetically engineered models with alterations in cardiac membrane calcium-handling proteins. Annu Rev Physiol 62:321–351, 2000.

Littlefield R, Fowler VM: Defining actin filament length in striated muscle: Rulers and caps or dynamic instability? Annu Rev Cell Biol 14:487–525, 1998.

Severs NJ: The cardiac muscle cell. Bioessays 22:188–199, 2000.

Somlyo AP, Somlyo AV: Signal transduction by G-proteins, rho-kinase and protein phosphatase to smooth muscle and non-muscle myosin-II. J Physiol [London] 522:177–185, 2000.

Squire JM, Morris EP: A new look at thin filament regulation in vertebrate striated muscle. FASEB J 12:761–771, 1998.

Tobacman LS: Thin filament-mediated regulation of cardiac contraction. Annu Rev Physiol 58:447–481, 1996.

Towbin JA: The role of cytoskeletal proteins in cardiomyopathies. Curr Opin Cell Biol 10:131–139, 1998.

Wagenknecht T, Rademacher M: Ryanodine receptors: Structure and macromolecular interactions. Curr Opin Struct Biol 7:258–265, 1997.

CELL CYCLE

chapter 43

INTRODUCTION TO THE CELL CYCLE

Three patterns of growth regulation used by most cells in multicellular organisms can all be observed in a typical stratified epithelium (Fig. 43–1). The basal layer of the epithelium is composed of stem cells that divide only occasionally. They can activate the cell cycle on demand and then return to a nondividing state. When specific signals induce stem cells to proliferate, one daughter cell usually remains a stem cell and the other enters a pool of rapidly dividing cells. These dividing cells supply the upper layers of the epithelium with cells that stop dividing and gradually differentiate into the specialized cells that cover the surface.

These growth behaviors are not unique to epithelial cells. The nervous system contains a few stem cells and a few dividing cells, but most neurons, once differentiated, can live for more than 100 years without dividing again. Like stem cells, fibroblasts of the connective tissue are typically nondividing, but they can be stimulated to enter the cell cycle following wounding or other stimuli (see Fig. 34–11).

These patterns of cell behavior are all manifestations of the **cell cycle**, a term originally used to describe the behavior of cells as they grow and divide. An improved understanding of the molecular events of cell cycle control has revealed that the same components that regulate cell growth and division also play a key role in the cessation of cell division that accompanies cell differentiation. Control of the cell cycle is of major importance in human disease, as cancer is a perturbation of normal cell cycle regulation.

Principles of Cell Cycle Regulation

The goal of the cell cycle in most cases is to produce two daughter cells that are accurate copies of the par-

ent. The cell cycle integrates a continuous **growth cycle** (the increase in cell mass) with a discontinuous **division** or **chromosome cycle** (the replication and partitioning of the genome into two daughter cells). It has been said that "successful cellular reproduction requires a cell to integrate the discontinuous (or stage specific) events that occur once or a few times per cell cycle with the continuous processes of metabolism, maintenance, and growth that occur throughout the cell cycle and, indeed, even when the cell is not cycling."* The chromosome cycle is driven by a sequence of enzymatic cascades that produce a linear sequence of discrete biochemical "states" of the cytoplasm. Each state arises by destruction or inactivation of key enzymatic activities characteristic of the preceding state and expression or activation of a new cohort of activities. This is explained in detail later in this chapter. An example is mitosis, when an important class of protein kinases called cyclin-dependent kinases (see later section) is highly active. Proteolytic destruction of key components of these kinases renders them inactive and triggers the exit from mitosis and entry into the G_1 phase (Fig. 43–2).

Biochemical pathways termed **checkpoints** control transitions between cell cycle stages. (Box 43–1 defines key terms used in this chapter.) Checkpoints modulate progression of cells through the cycle in response to external or internal signals. Four checkpoints are particularly well characterized. The **restriction point** in the G_1 phase is sensitive to the size and physiological state of the cell and to its interactions with the surrounding extracellular matrix. Cells that do

---

* Pringle JR, Hartwell LH: The *Saccharomyces cerevisiae* cell cycle. In The Molecular Biology of the Yeast *Saccharomyces,* Life Cycle and Inheritance. Ed. Strathern JN, Jones EW, and Broach JR. Cold Spring Harbor, NY: Cold Spring Harbor Press, 1981, p. 98.

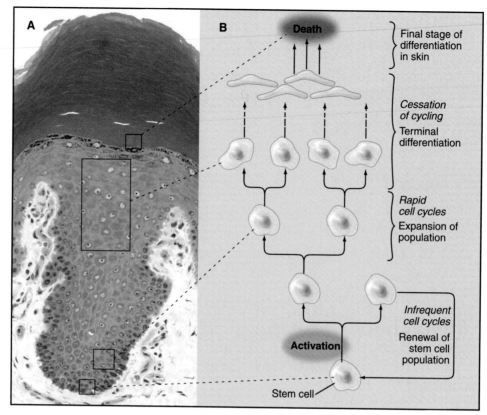

Figure 43-1 *A*, Light micrograph of a section of skin, a stratified squamous epithelium. *B*, Diagram showing the different types of cell cycles at the various levels of this epithelium.

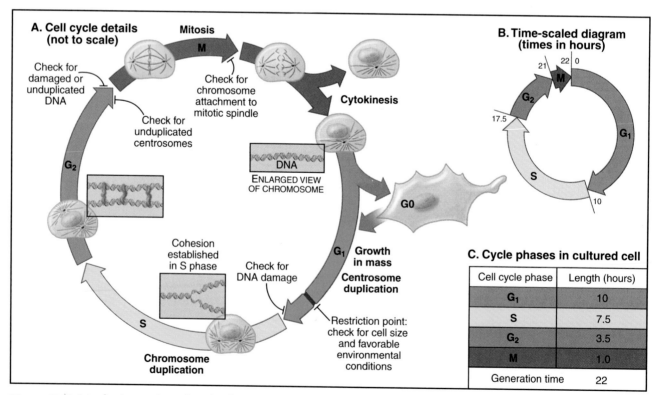

Figure 43-2 Introduction to the cell cycle phases. *A*, Diagrams of cellular morphology and chromosome structure across the cell cycle. *B*, Time scale of cell cycle phases. *C*, Length of cell cycle phases in cultured cells.

box 43–1

SELECTED KEY TERMS

Mitosis: The part of the cell cycle when a fully grown cell segregates the replicated chromosomes to opposite ends of a molecular scaffold, termed the spindle, and then cleaves between them in a process known as *cytokinesis* to produce two daughter cells. In general, each daughter cell receives a complement of genetic material and organelles identical to that of the parent cell.

Interphase: The portion of the cell cycle when cells grow and replicate their DNA. Interphase has three sections. The G_1 (first gap) *phase* is the interval between mitosis and the onset of DNA replication. The S (synthetic) *phase* is the time during which DNA is replicated. The G_2 (second gap) *phase* is the interval between the termination of DNA replication and the onset of mitosis. In multicellular organisms, many differentiated cells no longer actively divide. These nondividing cells (which may physiologically be extremely active) are in the G_0 *phase,* a branch of the G_1 phase.

Checkpoints: Biochemical pathways that regulate cell cycle transitions in response to the physiological condition of the cell and the state of its environment. The *restriction point* is a checkpoint early in the cell cycle at which cells decide whether to commit themselves to DNA replication and division, to delay before proceeding, or to enter a nondividing state. Other checkpoints regulate the entry into and exit from the S phase mitosis.

not receive appropriate growth stimuli from their environment arrest at this point in the G_1 phase and may commit suicide by apoptosis (Chapter 49). The **DNA damage checkpoints** monitor the integrity of DNA. Cells with damaged or partly replicated DNA arrest their progression through the cycle in late G_1 or G_2 phase, so that this damage can either be repaired or the cell can undergo programmed cell death by apoptosis. The **metaphase checkpoint** (also called the **spindle assembly checkpoint**) delays the onset of chromosome segregation in mitosis until all chromosomes have attached properly to mitotic spindle. One way in which checkpoints work is by modulating the activity of the cyclin-dependent kinases by a variety of mechanisms, including post-translational modification, targeted proteolysis of essential cofactors, binding of inhibitors, and changes in intracellular location.

Phases of the Cell Cycle

In 1882, Flemming described a process of nuclear division that he termed **mitosis** (from the Greek *mito,* or thread) after the appearance of the condensed chromosomes. Because cells only appeared to be active during mitosis, the rest of the cell cycle was referred to as **interphase** (or "resting stage").

Once DNA was recognized as the agent of heredity, it was deduced that DNA must be duplicated at some time during interphase so that daughter cells each receive a full complement of the genetic material. A single key experiment identified the relationship between the timing of DNA synthesis and the

mitotic cycle and defined the four cell cycle phases as they are known today (Fig. 43–3). Each cell is born at the completion of **mitosis.** The chromosomal DNA is replicated during **S phase** (synthetic phase). The remaining two phases are gaps between mitosis and the S phase. The **G_1 phase** (first gap phase) is the interval between mitosis and DNA replication. The **G_2 phase** (second gap phase) is the interval between the completion of DNA replication and mitosis.

G_1 Phase

The G_1 phase is typically the longest and most variable cell cycle phase. If the supply of nutrients is poor, or if cells receive an antiproliferative stimulus, such as a signal to embark on terminal differentiation, they may delay their progress through the cell cycle in G_1 or exit the cycle and enter G_0 (see the section that follows). Progress through G_1 is regulated by two cell cycle control checkpoints, the **restriction point** and the **G_1 DNA damage checkpoint.** Both control points are lost in many cancer cells; these cells continue to attempt to divide even in the absence of appropriate environmental signals and in the presence of DNA damage.

G_0 and Growth Control

Most cells in the bodies of multicellular organisms are differentiated to carry out specialized functions and no longer divide. Such cells are considered to be in a special compartment of the G_1 phase called the **G_0**

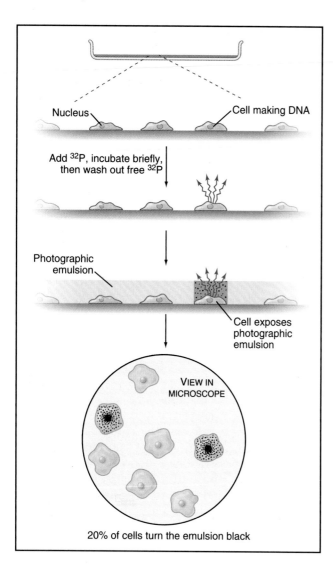

Figure 43-3 To determine whether cells synthesized DNA during a defined portion of the cell cycle or constantly throughout the entire cycle (as is the case in bacteria, for example), Howard and Pelc fed a radioactive precursor to DNA (^{32}P) to onion root tip cells, spread the cells in a thin layer on a microscope slide, and overlayered the slide with photographic emulsion. After incubation in the dark, the emulsion was developed like film and examined with a light microscope. The nuclei of cells that were engaged in active DNA replication during the period of exposure to ^{32}P incorporated the radioactive label into DNA and exposed the photographic emulsion above them. Two possible outcomes were predicted. If cells synthesized DNA constantly during interphase, then all cells would incorporate the radioactive label. Conversely, if each cell only synthesized DNA during a discrete portion of the cell cycle, then only those cells engaged in active replication during the period of exposure to ^{32}P would expose the photographic emulsion. When the slides were examined, 20% of the interphase cell nuclei were labeled, proving that cells synthesize DNA only during a discrete portion of interphase. Mitotic cells were unlabeled. Assuming that the cells traverse the cycle at a more or less constant rate, it was possible to calculate the length of the synthetic phase. Overall, the time between successive divisions—the generation time—was about 30 hours in the root tip cells. If about 20% of the cells were labeled, then about 20% of the 30-hour generation time must be spent in DNA synthesis. Thus, 0.2 × 30, or 6 hours, was spent in replication. (Drawing based on the work of Pelc HA, Sr: Synthesis of DNA in normal and irradiated cells and its relation to chromosome breakage. Heredity Suppl 6:261–273, 1953.)

phase. G_0 cells are not dormant; indeed, they are often actively engaged in protein synthesis and secretion, and they may be highly motile. The G_0 phase is not necessarily permanent. In some cases, G_0 cells may be recruited to reenter the growth cycle in response to a variety of stimuli. This return to growth is highly regulated, as the uncontrolled growth of cells in a multicellular organism can lead to cancer.

S Phase

Chromosomes of higher eukaryotes are very large. For example, an average human chromosome contains about 150×10^6 base pairs of DNA. Replication of such a chromosome is initiated at many different sites, termed **origins of replication**, along the chromosomal DNA. In budding yeast, the approximately 400 origins are spaced an average of 30,000 base pairs apart. Each region of the chromosome that is repli-

cated from a single origin is referred to as a **replicon**. In higher eukaryotes, the unit of chromosomal replication is a cluster of replicons. Each replicon cluster replicates at a characteristic time during the S phase. In general, actively transcribed regions of the genome replicate early in S phase, whereas regions of inactive heterochromatin (see Chapter 13) replicate late.

During the G_1 phase, chromosomes become modified, or "licensed," to replicate as a consequence of the binding of particular proteins to the origins of replication to form a **prereplication complex**. As replication is initiated at each origin, essential components of the prereplication complex are inactivated, thereby preventing any regions of the chromosome from replicating twice in any given cell cycle. Passage through mitosis and subsequent reentry into the G_1 phase is required for reformation of the prereplication complex. This "licensing" cycle is driven at least in part by fluctuations in the activity of cyclin-dependent kinases.

G₂ Phase

During the G₂ phase, cells "proofread" the DNA structure and make preparations for mitosis. If unreplicated or damaged DNA is detected, a protein kinase cascade, known as the **G₂ DNA damage checkpoint**, is triggered. This cascade ultimately leads to the inactivation of cyclin-dependent kinases required for entry into mitosis. The resultant increase in the length of the G₂ phase is called **G₂ delay**. Defects in enzymes in this checkpoint pathway can lead to cancer.

M Phase

During M phase (or **mitosis**) and subsequent **cytokinesis,** chromosomes and cytoplasm are partitioned into two daughter cells. Chromosome segregation is controlled by the **metaphase checkpoint,** which delays the onset of sister chromatid separation until all chromosomes are properly aligned on the mitotic spindle. This checkpoint is also called the spindle assembly checkpoint, but this book uses *metaphase checkpoint* for two reasons. First, the checkpoint blocks the metaphase-anaphase transition in response to a wide variety of signals. Second, the checkpoint does not actually monitor assembly of a bipolar spindle. Abnormal multipolar spindles often do not activate the checkpoint and give rise to highly aberrant anaphase chromosome segregation.

Mitosis is normally divided into five discrete phases. **Prophase** is defined by the onset of chromosome condensation. In the cytoplasm, a dramatic change in the dynamic properties of the microtubules (the half-life of which decreases from ~10 minutes to ~30 seconds) is accompanied by the separation of the duplicated centrosomes (centrioles and associated pericentriolar material in animal cells), each of which nucleates the formation of one pole of the **mitotic spindle. Prometaphase** begins when the nuclear envelope breaks down (in higher eukaryotes) and chromosomes begin to attach randomly to microtubules emanating from the two poles of the forming mitotic spindle. Once both kinetochores on a chromosome are attached to opposite spindle poles, the chromosome slowly moves to a point midway between the poles. When all chromosomes are properly attached, the cell is said to be in **metaphase. Anaphase** is heralded by the abrupt separation of the two **sister chromatids** from one another. The metaphase-anaphase transition requires the proteolytic degradation of molecules that regulate sister chromatid pairing. During anaphase, the separated sister chromatids move to the two spindle poles **(anaphase A),** which themselves move apart **(anaphase B).** As the chromatids approach the spindle poles, the nuclear envelope re-

forms on the surface of the chromatin. At this point, the cell is said to be in **telophase.** Finally, during telophase, a **contractile ring** of actin and myosin assembles as a circumferential belt in the cortex midway between spindle poles and constricts the equator of the cell. This process, called **cytokinesis,** separates the two daughter cells from one another.

▪ The Biochemical Basis of Cell Cycle Transitions

Transitions between cell cycle phases are triggered by a network of protein kinases and phosphatases that is tied to the discontinuous events of the chromosome cycle by the cyclic accumulation, modification, and destruction of several key components. This section provides a general introduction to the most important components of this network.

Cyclin-Dependent Kinases

Genetic analysis of the cell cycle in the fission yeast, *Schizosaccharomyces pombe,* identified a gene called *cdc2⁺* (*cell division cycle* [Box 43–2]) that was essential for cell cycle progression during both the G₁ ⇒ S and G₂ ⇒ M transitions. The product of this gene, a protein kinase of 34,000 D originally called p34^{cdc2}, is the prototype for a family of protein kinases that is crucial for cell cycle progression in all eukaryotes. This mechanism of cell cycle control is so well conserved that a human homologue of p34^{cdc2} can functionally replace the yeast protein, restoring a normal cell cycle to a *cdc2* mutant yeast!

Humans have more than 10 distinct protein kinases related to p34^{cdc2}. To be active, these enzymes must each associate with a regulatory subunit called a cyclin (see section that follows). Thus, they have been termed *cyclin-dependent kinases* **(CDKs).** p34^{cdc2}, now termed Cdk1, seems to function primarily in the regulation of the G₂ ⇒ M transition in animal cells. A second family member, Cdk2, is involved in regulation of the G₁ ⇒ S and G₂ ⇒ M transitions, whereas two other family members—Cdk4 and Cdk6—are involved in passage of the restriction point (Table 43–1). Cdk7 is important for activation of other CDKs, and also appears to participate in RNA transcription and repair of damaged DNA. Other CDKs participate in diverse processes ranging from transcriptional regulation to neuronal differentiation, and may play as-yet-undiscovered roles in cell cycle regulation.

Cyclins

The defining feature of CDKs is that they require binding of **cyclins** for catalytic activity. Cyclins are a di-

box 43–2

USE OF GENETICS TO STUDY THE CELL CYCLE

Studies of the distantly related budding and fission yeasts *Saccharomyces cerevisiae* and *Schizosaccharomyces pombe* (see Fig. 1–1) have been extremely important for understanding the cell cycle for several reasons. First, the proteins that control the cell cycle are remarkably conserved between yeasts and mammals. Second, both yeast genomes are sequenced, simplifying characterization of novel gene products. Third, genetic analysis is facilitated, as both yeasts grow as haploids and both efficiently incorporate cloned DNA into their chromosomes by homologous recombination.

These two yeasts have evolved very different strategies for cell division. Budding yeasts divide by assembling a single bud on the surface of the cell every cell cycle. Fission yeasts divide by fission of an elongated cell by a mechanism similar to cytokinesis in animal

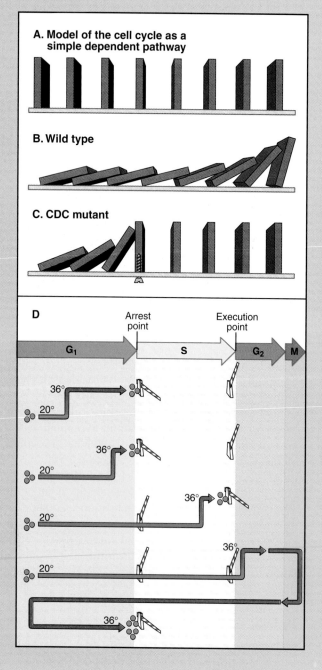

Figure 43–4 *A* to *C,* The cell cycle may be modeled as a simple dependent pathway. A CDC mutation can block further progression along the pathway, typically at a characteristic point in the cell cycle. *D,* Diagram explaining the arrest and execution points for a CDC mutant. This figure assumes that the cells enter the cycle from the left side in synchrony. Periods of growth at 23°C (permissive temperature) are shown in blue. Periods of growth at 36°C (restrictive temperature) are shown in red. The execution point is the point in the cell cycle where the gene has fully executed its function (i.e., where it is no longer needed to finish that cell cycle). The arrest point is the first point in the cell cycle where the gene's function is essential. If a cell enters the cycle lacking this function, this is where the cycle will stop. The arrest and execution points shown are what would be predicted for genes encoding components essential for DNA replication.

box 43–2

USE OF GENETICS TO STUDY THE CELL CYCLE *Continued*

cells. During mitosis, the nuclear envelope of both yeasts remains intact, so the chromosomes segregate on a spindle inside the nucleus. The stage of the cell cycle is revealed by the cellular morphology in the light microscope. For budding yeast, unbudded cells are in G_1, cells with buds smaller than the mother cell are in S phase, and cells whose buds are similar in size to the mother cell are in G_2. For fission yeast, cell length provides a yardstick for estimating cell cycle position.

The cell cycles of both yeasts differ from those of animal cells. In budding yeast, much of the 90-minute cell cycle is spent in G_1. Thus, the system controlling the $G_1 \Rightarrow S$ transition is particularly amenable to study. In contrast, a fission yeast spends most of its 2-hour cell cycle in G_2. S phase follows separation of sister chromatids prior to cytokinesis. Thus, the control of the $G_2 \Rightarrow M$ transition is readily studied in fission yeast.

Genetic studies have revealed that the yeast cell cycle is a *dependent pathway* whereby events in the cycle occur normally only after earlier processes are completed. The cell cycle can be modeled as a line of dominoes, with each domino corresponding to the action of a gene product that is essential for cell cycle progression (Fig. 43–4), and with the nth domino only falling when knocked down by the $(n-1)^{th}$ domino. According to the model, mutations in genes essential for cell cycle progression cause an entire culture of yeast to accumulate at a single point in the cell cycle (the point at which the defective gene product *first becomes essential*). This is referred to as the **arrest point**. Figure 43–4 shows this by including a "mutant" domino that does not fall over when struck by the upstream domino. Mutants that meet this criterion are called **cell division cycle mutants** or **CDC mutants**. Genetic screens for CDC mutants have identified many important genes involved in cell cycle control.

Because CDC genes are essential for cell cycle progression, it would be impossible to propagate strains of

yeast carrying CDC mutants unless the mutants have a **conditional lethal** phenotype. The most commonly used conditional lethal mutations are **temperature sensitive (ts)**. Many yeast temperature-sensitive mutants are viable at 23°C (the **permissive temperature**) but cease dividing at 36°C (the **restrictive temperature**). Temperature-sensitive proteins often have an altered amino acid sequence, but occasionally, the lack of a gene product altogether can cause a *ts* phenotype.

Fission yeasts with CDC mutants affecting the entry into mitosis have distinctive morphologies. Cells that are unable to carry out mitosis continue their growth cycle and become greatly elongated (Fig. 43–5*C*). In contrast, mutant cells that enter mitosis prematurely in the cell cycle are shorter than normal. Mutations that produce tiny cells are called *wee* mutants (see Fig. 43–5*B*). This simple morphologic assay allowed straightforward classification of yeast CDC genes into those that stimulate progression through mitosis and those that retard entry into mitosis.

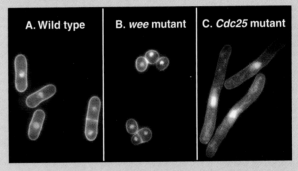

Figure 43–5 The phenotype of wild-type fission yeast cells (*A*) together with phenotypes of a CDC mutant (*B*) that accelerates the entry into mitosis (*wee1*) and a CDC mutant (*C*) that delays entry into mitosis (*cdc25*). Cell walls and nuclei are stained. (Courtesy of H. Ohkura, Wellcome Trust Institute for Cell Biology, University of Edinburgh.)

---

verse group of proteins ranging in size between 35 kD and 90 kD, all with a similar core structure based upon two symmetrical domains of five α helices. One of these domains, called the cyclin box, is highly conserved and is the defining structural feature of these proteins. Cyclins were discovered in rapidly dividing invertebrate embryos as proteins that accumulate gradually during interphase and are abruptly destroyed during mitosis. This cyclic accumulation and destruction is the derivation of their name. Subsequently, at least 16 different cyclins have been identified in humans. Some cyclins function during G_1 phase, others during G_2 phase, and still others during M phase; some may function independent of the cell cycle.

Positive Regulation of CDK Structure and Function

The activity of CDKs is regulated with extraordinary care. Like other eukaryotic protein kinases (see Chapter 27), CDKs have a bilobed structure with the active site in a deep cleft between a small N-terminal and larger C-terminal domain. However, newly synthesized monomeric CDKs differ from other kinases in that they appear to have only partially completed the folding process. The mouth of the catalytic pocket is blocked by a flexible loop, called the T loop. In addition, a short α helix containing a glutamic acid needed for coordination of the adenosine triphosphate (ATP)

table 43-1

INVENTORY OF THE ENZYMES OF THE CELL CYCLE ENGINE

Cyclin-Dependent Kinases and Their Cyclin Partners

Kinase	Cyclin (+ Other) Partner	Function
Cdk1 (p34^{cdc2})	A B$_1$, B$_2$ (*Xenopus* has 5 B-type cyclins) Cdk1-cyclin B also binds p9	*Mammals:* triggers G$_2$ → M transition. *Yeasts:* triggers G$_1$ → S and G$_2$ → M transitions. Cyclin A is synthesized in S and destroyed starting at prometaphase. Cyclins B are synthesized in S/G$_2$ and destroyed following the completion of chromosome attachment to the spindle.
Cdk2	A, E	Triggers G$_1$ → S transition
Cdk3	?	Poorly understood; may trigger G$_1$ → S transition
Cdk4, Cdk6	D$_1$–D$_3$	Phosphorylation of the retinoblastoma susceptibility protein (pRb) in G$_1$; triggers passage of the restriction point and cyclin E synthesis. Synthesis of D cyclins is controlled by extracellular growth factors.
Cdk5	p35 (G)	Neuronal differentiation
Cdk7 (CAK)	H Also binds assembly factor MAT1	Cdk activation by phosphorylation of the T loop. Also in the TFIIH complex, it is important for regulation of RNA polymerase II transcription and DNA repair (see Chapter 14).
Cdk8	C	Regulation of RNA polymerase II transcription
Cdk9	T	Regulation of RNA polymerase II transcription

Inhibitors of Cyclin-Dependent Kinases

Inhibitor	Cdk Substrates	Function
CKI: p21$^{Cip1/Waf1}$	Most CDK-cyclin complexes	Induced by p53 tumor suppressor; cell cycle arrest after DNA damage; binds PCNA (see Chapter 45) and inhibits DNA synthesis; cell cycle arrest in senescence and terminal differentiation. At low levels, it may help to assemble active Cdk-cyclin complexes.
CKI: p27^{Kip1}	Most CDK-cyclin complexes	Cell cycle arrest in response to growth suppressors, like TGF-β, and in contact inhibition and differentiation
CKI: p57^{Kip2}	Most CDK-cyclin complexes	Important in development of the palate
Ink4b: p15^{Ink4b}	Cdk4, Cdk6	Cell cycle arrest in response to TGF-β; also altered in many cancers
Ink4a: p16^{Ink4a}	Cdk4, Cdk6	Cooperates with the retinoblastoma susceptibility protein (pRb) in growth regulation; cell cycle arrest in senescence; altered in a high percentage of human cancers. This gene overlaps the gene for p19^{ARF}, an important regulator of the p53 tumor suppressor protein.
Ink4c: p18^{Ink4c}	Cdk4, Cdk6	Cell cycle arrest in response to growth suppressors
Ink4d: p19^{Ink4d}	Cdk4, Cdk6	Cell cycle arrest in response to growth suppressors

Other Components

Enzyme	Substrates	Function
Wee1 kinase	Cdk1 Y^{15}	Nuclear kinase; inhibits Cdk1–cyclin B in G$_2$ phase
Myt1 kinase	Cdk1 T^{14} + Y^{15}	Cytoplasmic kinase; inhibits Cdk1–cyclin B in G$_2$ phase
Cdc25A phosphatase	?	Promotes G$_1$ → S transition
Cdc25C phosphatase	Cdk1 Y^{14}, T^{15}	Promotes G$_2$ → M transition. Dephosphorylates Cdk1 complexed to cyclins A, B at T^{14} and Y^{15}.
APC/C^{Cdc20}	Securin, others	E3 ubiquitin ligase active during M; requires high CDK activity to function; destruction of securin, cyclins and other substrates essential for the onset of anaphase; contains 10–12 subunits + the Cdc20 activator/specificity factor

table 43-1

INVENTORY OF THE ENZYMES OF THE CELL CYCLE ENGINE *Continued*

Other Components

Enzyme	Substrates	Functions
APC/C^Cdh1	Cyclins A, B, many others	E3 ubiquitin ligase active in the exit from mitosis and during G_1; requires low CDK activity to function; keeps CDK activity low in G_1 through cyclin proteolysis; contains 10–12 subunits + the Cdh1 activator/specificity factor
SCF	Cyclin E, CDK inhibitors, many others	Class of E3 ubiquitin ligases containing Skp1 + Cullin + Rbx1 + an F-box protein. *Caenorhabditis elegans* has >60 F-box proteins, acting as specificity factors recognizing substrates phosphorylated as specific sites. There are many SCF complexes.

SCF, Skp1, Cullin, F-box–containing E3 ubiquitin ligase; TFIIH, basal transcription factor for RNA polymerase II (see Chapter 14); TGF, transforming growth factor.

is misoriented so that this residue faces away from the catalytic cleft. As a result, ATP bound by the monomeric kinase is distorted and cannot transfer its γ phosphate to protein substrates (Fig. 43–6A).

At least four different mechanisms regulate CDK activity (Fig. 43–7). On the one hand, enzyme activity is stimulated by cyclin binding and by phosphorylation of the T loop. On the other, CDKs can be inhibited by phosphorylation of residues adjacent to the ATP-binding site and by binding of inhibitory proteins.

Binding of the cyclin subunit causes a profound change in CDK structure, starting with the retraction of the T loop back from the mouth of the catalytic pocket (see Fig. 43–6B). In addition, the secondary structure of the N-terminal domain is altered, causing the short helix mentioned earlier to reorient by 90 degrees so that its critical glutamate now faces into the catalytic pocket and interacts with the ATP phosphates. This causes the bound ATP to assume a con-

formation suitable for reaction with substrates. In the roof of the ATP-binding pocket, cyclin binding also causes two residues—threonine[14] and tyrosine[15]—to reorient so that they become accessible to protein kinases involved in regulation of CDK activity (see later section).

Despite these changes, the CDK-cyclin complex has only partial catalytic activity. Complete activation requires the action of a kinase, called CAK (*C*DK-*a*ctivating *k*inase), which phosphorylates threonine[160] in the T loop (this is the residue that gives the loop its name). In vertebrates, CAK is composed of Cdk7–cyclin H. Phosphorylated threonine[160] fits into a charged pocket on the surface of the enzyme, flattening the T loop back even further from the mouth of the catalytic pocket (see Fig. 43–6C and 43–7A). This has a profound effect, stimulating the catalytic activity by up to 300-fold. This occurs, in part, because the T loop now forms part of the substrate-binding surface. In addition, threonine[160] phosphorylation stabilizes the

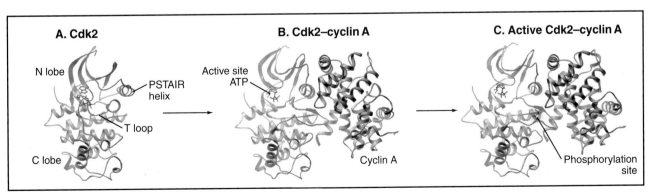

Figure 43-6 Atomic structures of cyclin-dependent kinases. *A,* Cdk2. The PSTAIR helix, found in most CDKs, is named after a sequence of six amino acids (one letter code). (PDB file: 1DM2.) *B,* Cdk2–cyclin A (kinase at basal activity level). (PDB file: 1FIN.) *C,* Cdk2–cyclin (kinase fully active following phosphorylation of threonine[160]). (PDB file: 1JST.)

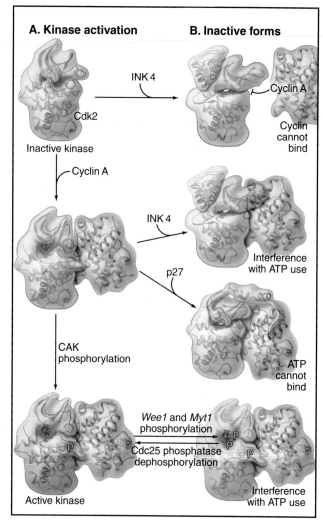

A. Kinase activation

B. Inactive forms

Figure 43-7 Positive and negative regulation of cyclin-dependent kinases. *A,* Pathway of activation by cyclin binding and phosphorylation. *B,* Pathways of inactivation by inhibitor binding and phosphorylation. (PDB files: Cdk2-INK4, 1BI7; Cdk2-INK4-cyclin A, composite of 1FIN and 1BI7; Cdk2-p27-cyclin A, 1JSU.)

association of Cdk2 with cyclin A, as well as Cdk7, and cyclin H in CAK itself, apparently because the phosphorylated T loop contributes to cyclin binding.

One further activation step involves binding of a small subunit called p9 (a 9000-D protein) to the C-terminal domain of the CDK, away from the active site. Although p9 does not alter CDK structure significantly, it is an essential component of the dominant mitotic CDK (Cdk1–cyclin B–p9). Moreover, p9 may influence substrate or cofactor binding.

Negative Regulation of CDK Structure and Function

At least two mechanisms inactivate CDKs and slow or stop the cell cycle (see Fig. 43–7). During the G_2

phase, CDK activity is held in check by the phosphorylation of two amino acid residues (threonine[14] and tyrosine[15]) in the roof of the ATP-binding site by the protein kinases Myt1 and Wee1. This phosphorylation interferes with ATP binding and hydrolysis by the enzyme. Because threonine[14] and tyrosine[15] are only accessible to the regulatory kinases following cyclin binding, this phosphorylation of CDKs depends, at least in part, on the availability of cyclins.

Three Cdc25 phosphatases (see Fig. 27–5) reverse these inhibitory phosphorylations. Cdc25A appears to be involved in the regulation of the $G_1 \Rightarrow S$ transition, whereas Cdc25B and Cdc25C appear to function at $G_2 \Rightarrow M$. Cdc25C is an important target of the G_2 DNA damage checkpoint that operates during G_2 to prevent cells from undergoing mitosis with damaged DNA (see Chapter 46).

A second strategy for inactivating CDKs involves the binding of small inhibitory subunits of the CKI (cyclin-dependent kinase inhibitor) and INK4 (inhibitor of Cdk4) families. CKI molecules, usually known by their molecular weights as p21[Cip1/Waf1], p27[Kip1], or p57[Kip2], inactivate all of the CDKs involved in cell cycle progression. The p27[Kip1] molecule inactivates the Cdk2–cyclin B complex in two ways (see Fig. 43–8B). A portion of the N-terminal segment of p27[Kip1] associates with the cyclin subunit, while another portion invades the N-terminal domain of CDK, profoundly disrupting its structure. In addition, a region of the inhibitory peptide is a molecular mimic of ATP, binding in the ATP-binding pocket through interactions with residues that normally coordinate ATP. This effectively prevents binding of ATP to the enzyme.

Members of the INK4 family (p15[Ink4b], p16[Ink4a], p18[Ink4c], and p19[Ink4d]) preferentially inactivate Cdk4 and Cdk6. They do this in two ways (Fig. 43–8A). First, they bind to N- and C-terminal lobes of mono-

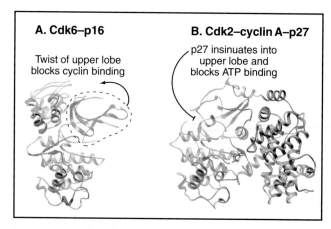

A. Cdk6–p16

Twist of upper lobe blocks cyclin binding

B. Cdk2–cyclin A–p27

p27 insinuates into upper lobe and blocks ATP binding

Figure 43-8 Atomic structures of cyclin-dependent kinases with bound inhibitors. *A,* Crystal structures of Cdk4 with bound inhibitor p16[Ink4a]. *B,* Cdk2–cyclin A with bound p27[Kip1].

box 43–3

STUDIES OF THE CELL CYCLE IN VITRO

Amphibian oocytes and eggs are storehouses of most of the components needed for cell cycle progression. Oocytes are arrested in G_2 until a surge of the hormone progesterone causes them to "mature" into eggs, which are then naturally arrested in metaphase of the second meiotic division (see Chapter 48). After fertilization, the embryo of the South African clawed frog *(Xenopus laevis)* undergoes a rapid burst of cell divisions. An initial cell cycle 90 minutes in length is followed by a rapid succession of 10 cleavages spaced only 30 minutes apart to produce an embryo of 2000 cells (Fig. 43–9). Thirty minutes per cycle is insufficient to transcribe and translate all of the genes needed to make the daughter cells produced at each division. The frog solves this problem by making oocytes extremely large (~500,000 times the volume of a typical somatic cell) and storing within them vast stockpiles of the structural components needed to make cells. As a result, only DNA and a very few proteins need be synthesized during the early embryonic divisions. In addition to structural components, many factors that regulate normal cell cycle progression are also stockpiled in the oocyte. The net result is that the *Xenopus* oocyte is an excellent source of material for cell cycle analyses.

Remarkably, it is possible to make cell-free extracts from *Xenopus* eggs that progress through the cell cycle in vitro (Fig. 43–10). Nuclei from G_1 cells, when added to these extracts, efficiently replicate their DNA and proceed through the cell cycle into mitosis, complete with chromosome condensation, nuclear envelope

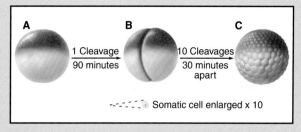

Figure 43–9 Summary diagram of *Xenopus'* early development showing how cleavages subdivide the egg. *A,* Fertilized egg. *B,* Two-cell stage. *C,* Multicellular embryo. Compare size of somatic cell and egg.

breakdown, chromosome alignment on a spindle, and anaphase segregation of sister chromatids! Because these events occur in a cell-free milieu, they are readily accessible to biochemical manipulation. For example, antibodies and other proteins can be added to the extracts, and their effect on the cell cycle can readily be determined. Thus, the *Xenopus* extract system offers one of the best tools for testing the role of various proteins in the cell cycle in higher eukaryotes.

A crucial experiment using frog eggs involved the extraction, with a microneedle, of a small portion of cytoplasm from a mature metaphase-arrested egg and its subsequent injection into a fully grown oocyte. The oocyte rapidly entered M phase, with concomitant chromosome condensation and nuclear envelope disas-

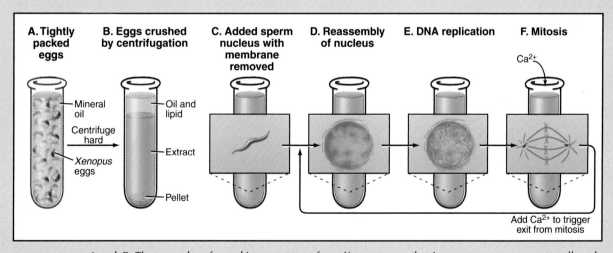

Figure 43–10 *A* and *B,* The procedure for making an extract from *Xenopus* eggs that is competent to carry out cell cycle oscillations in vitro. *C* to *F,* The sequence of cell cycle events that occur in a cycling *Xenopus* extract. These cycles consist of alternating S and M phases. G_1 and G_2 phases are minimal (as they are during early development of the frog).

Box continued on next page

STUDIES OF THE CELL CYCLE IN VITRO *Continued*

sembly (Fig. 43–11). This stimulation to enter M phase is called *maturation*, and the unknown factor present in the egg cytoplasm that induced oocyte maturation was termed **MPF**, or **maturation-promoting factor** (now often referred to as **M phase–promoting factor**). The

identification of MPF involved many biochemists, geneticists, and developmental biologists, and took 17 years. Gratifyingly, MPF turned out to be a complex of the product of the second cell cycle gene identified in the fission yeast, Cdc2 (Cdk1) with a cyclin and p9.

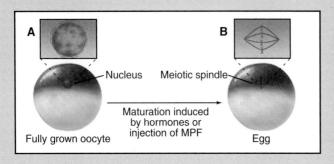

Figure 43-11 The $G_2 \Rightarrow M$ transition in frog oocytes, a process called maturation. *A,* Oocyte. *B,* Mature egg. Maturation may be induced naturally by hormones or experimentally by injecting cytoplasm from an egg arrested in metaphase of meiosis division II. This cytoplasm contains MPF (M phase–promoting factor), which promotes the $G_2 \Rightarrow M$ transition.

A — Nucleus — Fully grown oocyte — Maturation induced by hormones or injection of MPF — Meiotic spindle — Egg — *B*

meric CDK on the side opposite the catalytic cleft. In doing so, they twist the orientation of these lobes relative to one another, thus distorting the molecule so that cyclin D does not bind. INK4 family inhibitors also inhibit preformed Cdk4/6–cyclin D complexes by binding to the CDK and distorting the ATP-binding site so that the kinase uses ATP much less efficiently.

Binding of CDK inhibitors is an important part of growth regulation during the G_1 and G_0 phases of the cell cycle (see Chapter 44). These inhibitors play a critical role in the cell cycle arrest that occurs in response to DNA damage and to antiproliferative signals. The p16^{Ink4a} gene is disrupted in up to 30% of human cancers.

Role of Protein Destruction in Cell Cycle Control

Mitosis is a state of the cytoplasm dominated by high levels of active Cdk1–cyclin B–p9. Phosphorylation of key components by this kinase leads to dramatic reorganization of the cell and, ultimately, to separation of sister chromatids on the mitotic spindle. Once chromatids are separated, the cell must progress to a state with low levels of CDK activity so that nuclear envelope reassembly, spindle disassembly, and cytokinesis can occur. Thus, exit from mitosis requires CDK inactivation. This occurs through the action of the ubiquitin-mediated proteolytic machinery that targets, among

other key proteins, A- and B-type cyclins and a protein called securin, which is a key regulator of the onset of sister chromatid separation at anaphase. Destruction of cyclins inactivates the Cdk1 and Cdk2 kinases, allowing various phosphatases to reverse the action of CDKs to bring mitosis to a close.

Ubiquitin-mediated destruction of cyclins is a complex and interesting process that involves the action of a series of enzymes (see Chapter 24). First, an E1 enzyme (**ubiquitin-activating enzyme**) activates the small protein **ubiquitin** by forming a thioester bond between the C-terminus of ubiquitin and a cysteine on the enzyme. Activated ubiquitin is then transferred to another thioester bond on an E2 enzyme (**ubiquitin-conjugating enzyme**). The E2 may either transfer ubiquitin directly to a target protein, or it may combine with a third component (an E3 or ubiquitin-protein ligase) to do so. E3s either facilitate transfer of ubiquitin from E2 to the substrate or they act as thioester intermediates. They are thought to be important for imparting substrate specificity.

The product of this pathway is a target protein carrying a chain of ubiquitin molecules conjugated via the ϵ amino group of a lysine. Such polyubiquitinated proteins are targets for the cylindrical 26S **proteasome.** This large multienzyme complex functions like a cytoplasmic garbage disposal, grinding target proteins down to short peptides and spitting out intact ubiquitin monomers for reuse in further rounds of protein degradation. Originally, it was thought that the

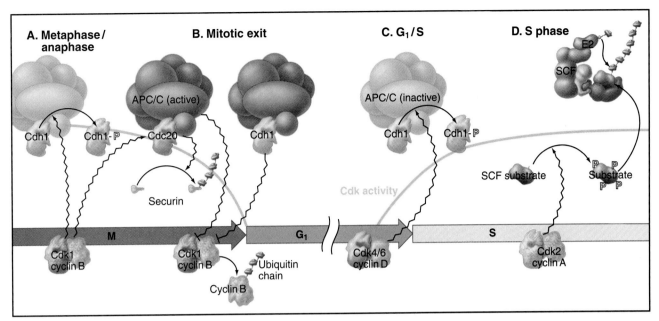

Figure 43–12 Ubiquitin E3 activities and their role in cell cycle control. *A,* At the metaphase-anaphase transition, the APC/C with associated Cdc20 triggers anaphase onset by signaling the degradation of securin. The Cdh1 form of the APC/C is inactive as Cdh1 phosphorylated by Cdk1–cyclin B is unable to bind. *B,* At the end of mitosis, the APC/C first with associated Cdc20 and then with associated Cdh1 degrades cyclin B and triggers the exit from mitosis into G$_1$. *C,* APC/C^{Cdh1} remains active throughout G$_1$ until activation of Cdk4/6–cyclin D again causes Cdh1 to fall off. *D,* After the onset of S phase, the degradation of cell cycle substrates is driven by SCF, which targets substrates of kinases, such as Cdk2–cyclin A, for destruction.

role of the proteasome was solely to remove damaged proteins from the cytoplasm; however, this enzyme is now appreciated as a central factor in cell cycle control.

The key specificity factor in the regulated proteolysis of the cyclins is a large (20S) complex of 10 to 12 subunits called the ***a*naphase-*p*romoting complex/ cyclosome (APC/C)** (Fig. 43–12). Although the APC/ C possesses E3 activity, little is known about how it targets ubiquitin to its substrates. The APC/C is inactive during the S and G$_2$ phases of the cell cycle but becomes active during mitosis, at least in part as a result of phosphorylation by Cdk1–cyclin B–p9. There are at least two forms of APC/C, depending upon which of two specificity factors is bound to the complex. One of these—Cdc20—is involved in targeting the APC/C to substrates in mitosis. This form of APC, called APC/C^{Cdc20}, is **activated** by CDK activity and seems to have primary responsibility for triggering the termination of mitosis. A second form of the APC/ C binds a different specificity factor, Cdh1. APC/C^{Cdh1} is **inactivated** by CDK activity because phosphorylation of Cdh1 by CDKs stops it from associating with the APC/C. APC/C^{Cdh1} is thought to function during the final exit from mitosis and throughout the G$_1$ phase to ensure that mitotic CDK-cyclin activities are repressed. This repression of CDK activity plays a critical role in preparing chromatin for the initiation of DNA replication (see Chapter 45).

A different E3 activity plays a critical role in the G$_1 \Rightarrow$ S transition, as well as in the transition from early to late S phase. This activity, called SCF (for Skp1, Cullin, F-box, three key subunits of this enzyme), is described in Chapter 44. Table 43–1 lists some properties of the enzymes involved in driving the cell cycle.

▌ Changing States of the Cytoplasm During the Cell Cycle

The biochemical activities that drive the cell cycle subdivide the cell cycle into five discrete states (Fig. 43–13). Mitosis itself can be subdivided into two states. **Early mitosis,** extending from prophase through metaphase, is a state in which mitotic CDKs (Cdk1 and Cdk2, in combination with cyclins A and B) are highly active. At prometaphase, the APC/C degrades cyclin A, but other substrates are resistant. During **late mitosis,** the onset of anaphase is triggered by a change to a state dominated by active APC/C^{Cdc20}. Securins and cyclins are destroyed and CDKs are inacti-

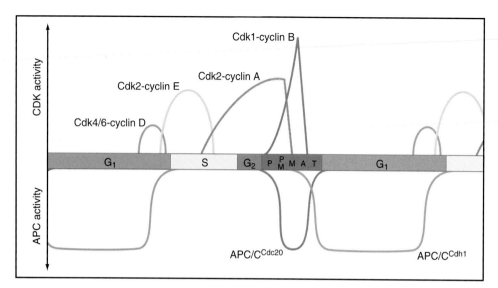

Figure 43-13 Diagram showing the changing patterns of CDK and APC activation in the various cell cycle states. Between G_2 and G_1 are shown the various stages of mitosis: P, prophase; PM, prometaphase; M, metaphase; A, anaphase; T, telophase.

vated. This state continues through telophase into the next G_1 phase. In the **early G_1 phase,** APC/C^{Cdh1} dominates from telophase through the restriction point in late G_1. Cyclins are destroyed and CDK inhibitors of the CKI and Ink4 family ensure that CDK activity is low. This period of low CDK activity is required for cytokinesis, spindle disassembly, chromosome decondensation, nuclear envelope reassembly, reactivation of transcription, reassembly of the Golgi, and assembly of prereplication complexes. During the **G_1/S phase,** appropriate growth signals from the environment stimulate the cell to synthesize D-type cyclins, producing a pulse of Cdk4/6 activity. This triggers passage of the restriction point, leading to synthesis of cyclin E and stimulating a sharp rise in CDK activity. CDKs then dominate, inactivating APC/C^{Cdh1}, targeting the CDK inhibitory peptides for destruction by SCF, and triggering the onset of DNA replication. During **mid-S–early mitosis,** CDK activity remains high throughout the remainder of the cell cycle, and the APC/C is switched off. Proteolysis of cyclin E by SCF leads to a transition from G_1 to mitotic cyclins, ultimately triggering entry into mitosis.

Although this sounds complicated, the underlying principles are actually quite straightforward. The following chapters discuss the cell cycle transitions in greater detail and show how checkpoints modulate the process in response to a changing environment.

■ Selected Readings

Ekholm SV, Reed SI: Regulation of G(1) cyclin-dependent kinases in the mammalian cell cycle. Curr Opin Cell Biol 12:676–684, 2000.

Evan GI, Vousden KH: Proliferation, cell cycle and apoptosis in cancer. Nature 411:342–348, 2001.

Hartwell LH, Weinert TA: Checkpoints: Controls that ensure the order of cell cycle events. Science 246:629–634, 1989.

Kirschner M: Intracellular proteolysis. Trends Cell Biol 9: M42–M45, 1999.

Morgan DO: Cyclin-dependent kinases: Engines, clocks and microprocessors. Annu Rev Cell Biol 13:261–291, 1997.

Nigg EA: Cell division: Mitotic kinases as regulators of cell division and its checkpoints. Natl Rev Mol Cell Biol 2: 21–32, 2001.

Nurse P: A long twentieth century of the cell cycle and beyond. Cell 100:71–78, 2000.

Peters J-M: SCF and APC: The Yin and Yang of cell cycle regulated proteolysis. Curr Opin Cell Biol 10:759–768, 1998.

Pines J: Four-dimensional control of the cell cycle. Natl Cell Biol 1:E73–E79, 1999.

Russell P: Checkpoints on the road to mitosis. Trends Biochem Sci 23:399–402, 1998.

Sherr CJ: Cancer cell cycles. Science 274:1672–1677, 1996.

Zachariae W, Nasmyth K: Whose end is destruction: Cell division and the anaphase-promoting complex. Genes Dev 13:2039–2058, 1999.

chapter 44

THE G₁ PHASE AND THE REGULATION OF CELL PROLIFERATION

During the G_1 phase of the cell cycle, each cell makes a key decision: whether to continue through another cycle and divide, or to remain in a nondividing state either temporarily or permanently. During development of metazoans, this is the time when cells exit the cell cycle as the first step toward forming differentiated tissues. In adults, strict regulation of the timing and location of cell proliferation is critical to avoid cancer.

Cells enter the G_1 phase after completing mitosis, at the end of a proliferation cycle. To clear the way for the decision to proliferate or differentiate, the cell must erase the bias toward proliferation carried over from the preceding cell cycle. This is accomplished by inactivating cyclin-dependent kinases (CDKs; see Chapter 43) through proteolytic destruction of cyclin subunits and synthesis of inhibitory proteins. The absence of CDK activity turns on a regulatory network that represses the transcription of many genes that promote cell cycle progression. While this repressive network is active, the cell cannot proceed through the cell cycle unless it is continuously stimulated by growth-promoting signals from the extracellular matrix or growth factors (see Chapters 26 and 29). These stimuli have the potential to drive another round of DNA replication and mitosis, but first, the cell must pass a major decision point late in G_1 called the **restriction point** (Fig. 44–1).

In metazoans, many cells cease cycling in the G_1 phase, either temporarily or permanently, entering instead a state known as G_0 (Fig. 44–1). This frequently accompanies their acquisition of specialized, differentiated characteristics. Occasionally, it is desirable in tissues for cells in G_0 to reenter the cell cycle in order to replace cells lost through death or tissue injury. These cells reenter the G_1 phase after being prepared by an orderly progression in which successive waves of genes are activated.

This chapter describes how cells regulate their progress through the G_1 phase, exit into the G_0 phase, and return to the cycle. It also considers some of the points at which defects in growth control lead to cancer. Because the activities involved in the restriction point are key to regulation of cell cycle progression, the chapter begins by discussing this control point in detail, despite the fact that it occurs relatively late in the G_1 phase.

The Restriction Point: A Critical G₁ Decision Point

All eukaryotes have a major cell cycle decision point late in the G_1 phase that monitors cell size, the condition of the chromosomes, and the cell's external environment. Healthy cells do not embark on a round of DNA replication and division until they reach an appropriate minimum size. This is important, because after cell division, one daughter cell is often smaller than the other. The smaller daughter cell needs more time to grow before it divides if a constant size of the cells in the population is to be maintained.

The influence of cell size on the division cycle was first demonstrated in an elegant microsurgery experiment (Fig. 44–2). Two *Amoeba proteus* cells were grown under identical conditions in parallel cultures. Each day, a portion of the cytoplasm was amputated from one of the amoebas, leaving the other untouched as a control. Under those circumstances, the cell that suffered the amputations did not divide for 20 days. During this time, the control amoeba divided 11 times. When the amputations were stopped, the amoeba that

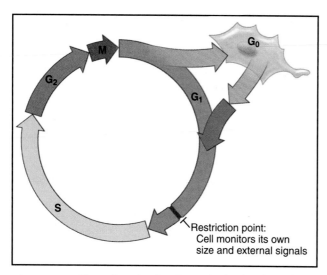

Figure 44–1 The cell cycle, showing major landmarks in the G_1 phase.

ing in G_1. Furthermore, all three populations of treated cells resumed the cell cycle and entered S phase at about the same time following restoration of the missing nutrient. This was surprising because amino acids are needed to make protein, serum provides growth factors, phosphate is needed for synthesis of DNA, and phospholipids are needed to make membranes. This experiment was interpreted as evidence that all three types of starvation caused cells to arrest at an equivalent point in the G_1 phase, termed the **restriction point.** The restriction point is defined as the point after which the cell cycle will proceed even if mitogenic factors are withdrawn (Fig. 44–3). This supremely important aspect of cell cycle control prevents cells from dividing at inappropriate times and in inappropriate places. Defects in restriction point control are among the most common causes of cancer.

Genetic analysis of budding yeast has also revealed a point in the G_1 phase after which cells appear to be committed to completion of the cycle. Cells starved for nutrients arrest at, or just prior to, this point, termed **START.** The mammalian restriction point resembles yeast START in a number of aspects, but they are not exactly equivalent owing to differences between animal and yeast cell cycles.

had been operated upon divided within 38 hours. The interpretation of this experiment was that the repeated amputations prevented the experimental amoeba from ever attaining a size sufficient to undergo division.

During the G_1 phase, cells also monitor their DNA for damage left over from the previous cell cycle. If damage is detected, the cell will either stop cycling or undergo apoptosis (see later section). This monitoring system is similar to that used for the G_2 checkpoint, covered in Chapter 46.

An essential aspect of growth control during the G_1 phase involves monitoring the external environment for nutrient availability and for signals to proliferate (**mitogenic** signals) coming from other cells and from the extracellular matrix. In a classic experiment, when cells growing in culture were starved by deprivation of amino acids, serum, or phosphate, they stopped grow-

■ Regulation of Cell Proliferation by the Restriction Point

The restriction point is a **checkpoint,** or molecular "gate" to cell cycle progression that regulates the expression of genes required for cell cycle progression. The gate is based upon the retinoblastoma susceptibility protein (**pRb**) and a family of essential transcription factors known as **E2F.** Interaction of these two proteins with target promoters turns off many genes and blocks

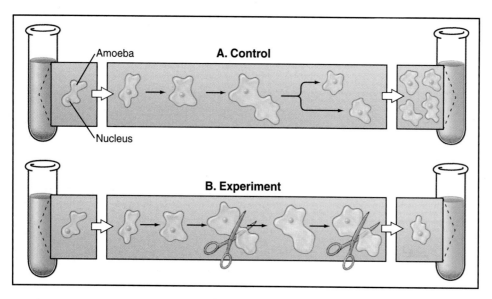

Figure 44–2 A microsurgery experiment demonstrates that amoebae will not divide if they are kept from attaining a sufficient size. *A,* Control cell continues to divide. *B,* Experimental cell does not divide. (Reference: Prescott DM: Relation between cell growth and cell division, II: The effect of cell size on cell growth rate and generation time in Amoeba proteus. Exp Cell Res 11:86–98, 1956.)

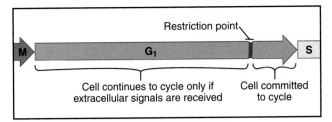

Figure 44–3 At the restriction point, cells assess external and internal stimuli and decide whether to commit to a further round of DNA replication and division.

cell cycle progression. To pass the restriction point, the cell must phosphorylate pRb, which then dissociates from E2F. This allows E2F to activate, rather than repress, transcription of the target genes. Cells that can phosphorylate pRb pass the restriction point and complete a cell cycle, whereas cells that cannot phosphorylate pRb remain arrested in the G₁ phase.

E2F binds DNA as a heterodimer with a subunit called DP1. Unphosphorylated pRb binds tightly to the E2F/DP1 heterodimer, and the E2F/DP1/pRb complex associates with the promoter region of genes regulated by E2F (Fig. 44–4A). pRb recruits histone deacetylases, enzymes that remove acetyl groups from the amino-terminal tails of histones (see Chapter 13). Histone deacetylation causes compaction of chromatin structure, thereby interfering with RNA polymerase II transcription. Thus, by locally promoting histone deacetylation, the E2F/DP1/pRb complex represses specific genes required for cell cycle progression.

Passage of the restriction point occurs when CDKs (see Chapter 43 and Table 43–1) phosphorylate pRb and release it from the E2F/DP1 complex (see Fig. 44–4B). CDK activity in early G₁ is regulated by adjusting the relative levels of D-type cyclins and the small inhibitory proteins p27^{Kip1} and p21^{Cip1}. Regulation of cyclin D transcription and stability provide the crucial links between extracellular growth stimuli and the cell cycle.

The E2F/DP1 heterodimer remains bound to its target promoter regions after phosphorylated pRb dissociates from E2F. Free E2F/DP1 is a potent transcription factor, promoting expression of genes that stimulate both reentry of G₀ cells back into the cycle and their subsequent passage through the cell cycle. These genes encode proteins required for DNA synthesis (DNA polymerase α_1, accessory factors and enzymes that synthesize nucleotide precursors; see Chapter 45), proteins that promote cell cycle progression (cyclins E and A, Cdk1), and proteins that regulate cell cycle progression (pRb). This molecular switch from the presence of E2F/DP1/pRb trimers to E2F/DP1 dimers at the promoters of essential cell cycle genes is the molecular key to the restriction point gate.

How is phosphorylation of pRb held in check in

nonproliferating cells? Any of the Cdk-cyclin pairs involved in cell cycle progression can phosphorylate pRb, but in practice, the enzymes available in the G₁ phase are Cdk4–cyclin D, Cdk6–cyclin D (referred hereafter as Cdk4/6–cyclin D), Cdk2–cyclin E, and Cdk2–cyclin A. Unless cells receive signals from mitogens (growth factors promoting cell proliferation), cyclin D is highly unstable (with a half-life of 10 minutes), so it never accumulates to levels sufficient to make a significant amount of Cdk4/6–cyclin D kinase. E2F controls the expression of the genes for cyclins E and A, so these cyclins are present at only low levels while pRb acts as an inhibitor with E2F. Furthermore, levels of p27^{Kip1} are high in pre-restriction point G₁ cells. This means that any Cdk2–cyclin E or Cdk2–

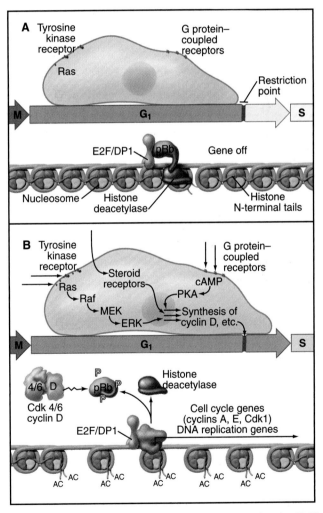

Figure 44–4 Regulation of cell cycle progression by the E2F/DP1/pRb complex. *A,* The E2F/DP1/pRb complex recruits histone deacetylases (see Chapter 13) and represses specific genes required for cell cycle progression. This blocks cell cycle progression at the restriction point. *B,* Phosphorylation of pRb by CDKs alleviates this block and permits passage of the restriction point. cAMP, cyclic adenosine monophosphate; MEK, mitogen-activated protein kinase kinase; PKA, protein kinase A.

cyclin A that is present will be inactive owing to binding of the p27^Kip1 inhibitor (see Figs. 43–7 and 43–8).

How do cells convert signals from growth factors and the extracellular matrix into a decision to open the restriction point gate? Stimulation of either receptor tyrosine kinases (see Chapters 26 and 29) or integrins (Chapter 32) initiates a signal transduction pathway starting with Ras activation of Raf and leading to activation of the mitogen-activated protein (MAP) kinase/extracellular signal–regulated kinase (ERK) cascade (see Fig. 29–6). Activation of this cascade stimulates transcription of D-type cyclins (see Fig. 44–4). D-type cyclins break through the barrier to cell cycle progression imposed by pRb, but they cannot do this alone.

In pre-restriction point G₁ cells, cyclin D is made, but the protein is continually exported from the nucleus back to the cytoplasm, where it is unstable (Fig. 44–5). In addition to stimulating synthesis of cyclin D, mitogens also stimulate transcription of p21^Cip1. This protein and p27^Kip1 are *positive* cofactors for Cdk4/6–cyclin D complexes that promote enzyme activity in two ways. First, they enhance assembly of complexes of cyclin D with Cdk4 and Cdk6. Second, they promote the nuclear import of Cdk4/6–cyclin D, thereby leading to activation of CDKs by CDK-activating kinase (a nuclear enzyme; see Chapter 43), as well as an increase in the stability of cyclin D. All of this depends on the continuous presence of mitogenic signals; if these cease, then cyclin D stability rapidly declines again.

This response to mitogens breaks the blockade on cell cycle progression imposed by pRb as follows. Cdk4/6–cyclin D–p21^Cip1/p27^Kip1 complexes begin to phosphorylate pRb. This permits the initial expression of certain E2F-responsive genes, including those encoding cyclin E and cyclin A. In addition, Cdk4/6–cyclin D can act as a sponge, soaking up p21^Cip1 and p27^Kip1. This liberates active Cdk2–cyclin E enzyme. Cdk2–cyclin E is responsible for a second wave of pRb phosphorylation on as many as 16 possible sites, leading to the wholesale liberation of E2F and a surge in transcription of genes that promote cell cycle progression. These factors needed for DNA replication trigger the onset of S phase and progression through the cell cycle. As the cell cycle proceeds, pRb phosphorylation is maintained first by Cdk2–cyclin A, and then later by Cdk1–cyclin B until the exit from mitosis. pRb is dephosphorylated at the mitosis-G₁ transition, thereby enabling it once again to bind E2F and close the restriction point gate to progression through G₁.

The Restriction Point and Cancer

Cancer is a complex class of diseases in which genetic changes within clones of cells lead to production of cell populations whose uncontrolled growth can disrupt tissue function and can ultimately kill the organism. About one in three humans is affected by cancer during their lifetime. This may sound very high, but considering that a human is composed of about 10^{14} cells, any one of which could in theory become transformed into a cancer cell over a lifetime of many decades, the disease is actually remarkably rare on a per cell basis. Why is this so? Cancer is rare, at least in part, because multiple genetic alterations are required to transform a normal cell into a cancer cell. In addition, the cell cycle is highly regulated, and activities that tend to drive cellular proliferation are held in check by a web of feedback pathways. Also, some cancer-causing mutations are actually deleterious in normal cells. As a result of these controls, most cells with disturbed growth control pathways are eliminated by backup mechanisms that cause them to commit suicide by apoptosis (see Chapter 49).

Many, though not all, types of cancer are caused by a disregulation of cell growth in the G₁ and G₂ phases. This is readily seen in the laboratory when cells are grown on plastic tissue culture dishes. Most normal cells grow until they cover the surface completely, forming a monolayer. When the monolayer is confluent (i.e., when cells are touched by other cells on all sides), cells stop dividing, arresting their cell cycle progression in G₁. This is called **contact inhibition** of growth. Cancer cells lack this control, so they keep growing and piling up on top of one another as long as the nutrient supply lasts (Fig. 44–6). Cells that lose this aspect of growth regulation are said to be **transformed**.

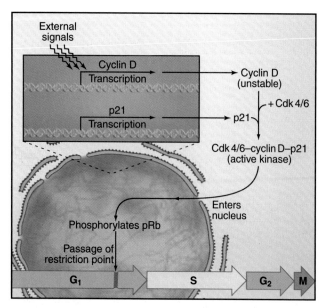

Figure 44–5 How growth factors regulate Cdk4/6 activity: the role of D-type cyclins and p21.

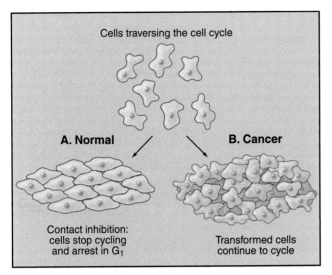

Figure 44-6 Loss of growth control in transformed cells. *A,* Normal cells. *B,* Cancer cells.

Malfunction of the restriction point is a common contributor to transformation. In fact, one or more components of the p16/cyclin D/Cdk-4/Rb system is mutated in most human cancers. In addition, several cancer-causing viruses, such as simian virus 40 (SV40) and adenovirus, make proteins that facilitate the G₁ → S transition by binding pRb and liberating E2F.

Cancer cells have abnormalities in the activities of two classes of genes. **Oncogenes** are genes whose inappropriate *activation* can cause oncogenic (cancerous) transformation of cells. The protein products of most oncogenes are regulators of cellular growth and proliferation, typically, components of signal transduction pathways that are controlled by feedback mechanisms. **Tumor suppressors** are genes whose *inactivation* can lead to cancerous transformation. Their protein products typically inhibit products of oncogenes or negatively regulate cell proliferation. Several genes involved in restriction point control can act as oncogenes, and at least two can act as tumor suppressors.

More than 100 oncogenes have been identified thus far. Most normally function in signal transduction pathways that lie downstream of signals that stimulate cell cycle progression. Their inappropriate activation can mimic the effects of persistent mitogenic stimulation, thereby uncoupling cells from normal environmental controls and leading to uncontrolled proliferation and cancer. For example, Ras proteins are involved in signaling pathways that lead to activation of the MAP/ERK kinase cascade and expression of cyclin D (see Fig. 44–4). Inappropriate activation of Ras tricks the cell into thinking that it is receiving mitogenic signals, leading it to express cyclin D, phosphorylate pRb, and proliferate. Ras proteins are among the most commonly mutated genes in human cancers. Other proteins involved in restriction point control can

also act as oncogenes if hyperactivated. These include E2F1, cyclin D, and Cdk4. In each case, activation of the protein causes inappropriate transcription of genes promoting cell cycle progression, bypassing the restriction point, and leading to uncontrolled cell cycles and cancerous transformation (Fig. 44–7).

pRb is one of the best characterized tumor suppressor genes. As discussed earlier, the primary function of pRb is to block cell cycle progression until

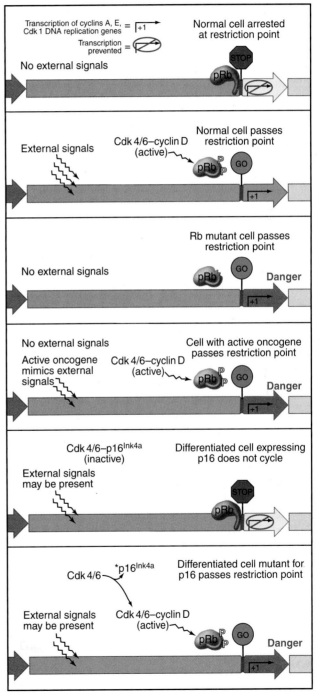

Figure 44-7 How activated oncogenes or mutations in the pRb or p16 tumor suppressor proteins can lead to abnormal passage of the restriction point and cancer.

inactivated in response to mitogenic stimulation. It is, therefore, not surprising that loss of pRb can lead to inappropriate cell cycle progression and cancer (see Fig. 44–7). Rare individuals who inherit one inactivated Rb gene are predisposed to develop retinoblastomas as children and osteosarcomas as adults. Localized loss of the other Rb gene through a somatic mutation in a single cell during later life can trigger cancer development. Retinoblastoma is less frequent and occurs later in life in individuals who inherit two good Rb genes, as two rare somatic mutations (two "hits") are required. Homozygous loss of pRb is lethal during embryogenesis, as the protein is essential for promoting differentiation of a number of organs and tissues. E2F is a tumor suppressor because it opposes cell cycle progression prior to the restriction point when partnered with pRb; however, it can also act as an oncogene, as it promotes the cell cycle when pRb is inactivated.

P16^{Ink4a} is another important tumor suppressor involved in G₁ growth control. Normally, it suppresses CDK4/6 activity in nondividing cells (see Chapter 43 and the section that follows). By helping to keep CDK4/6 inactive, p16^{Ink4a} reinforces the ability of pRb to maintain the growth arrest of G₁ cells. Mutations in p16^{Ink4a} are found in 25% to 70% of human cancers (see Fig. 44–7).

The G₀ Phase and Growth Control

Most cells in multicellular organisms are differentiated (adapted to carry out specialized functions) and no longer divide. They typically form specialized tissues, each of which has a distinctive structural organization that is important for function. Unscheduled cell division severely disrupts the organization of such tissues (Fig. 44–8). Accordingly, tissues strictly regulate both the location and the frequency of cell division. These divisions normally occur at a low rate, producing new cells in numbers just sufficient to replace those that die. Under special circumstances, however, such as in response to wounding (see Fig. 34–11), the rate of cell division increases dramatically. This highlights an important constraint on cell cycle control in multicellular organisms. *To make organized tissues, cells must exit from the cell cycle, but some cells must also retain the ability to reenter the active cell cycle when needed to repair injuries.*

Cells that stop cycling in order to differentiate normally do so in the G₁ phase. Such cells are said to be in a special compartment of G₁ called **G₀** (see Fig. 44–1). G₀ may last hours or days, or even for the life of the organism, as it does for most neurons. It is important to note that *nondividing cells are not dormant*: G₀ cells continue to expend energy for many

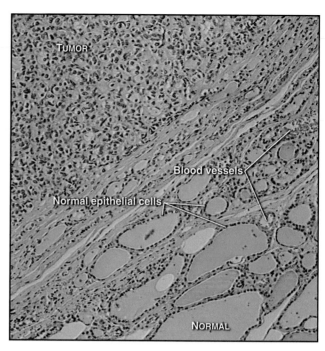

Figure 44–8 Disruption of normal tissue architecture by cancer cells growing without proper cell cycle regulation. *Lower right,* Normal thyroid tissue. *Upper left,* A thyroid tumor with loss of the normal gland structure. (Courtesy of Clara Sambade, IPATIMUP, Porto, Portugal.)

ongoing processes. Because of turnover, all cells must continuously synthesize proteins; many specialized G₀ cells consume large amounts of energy to synthesize and secrete proteins. All cells expend energy to maintain intracellular pH and ionic composition; action potentials consume additional energy in excitable cells. All cells use energy for intracellular motility; energy metabolism is particularly dramatic in muscle cells that are responsible for all body movements. Thus, G₀ cells should be regarded as active cells that just happen no longer to be engaged in cell division.

Why do cells stop cycling and enter the G₀ phase? First, cells may receive external signals that stimulate withdrawal from the cell cycle. This often initiates differentiation of tissues. Second, cells may find themselves in an environment with insufficient growth factors to drive proliferation. Such conditions trigger many cell types to undergo suicide by apoptosis (see Chapter 49), but other cells enter a nondividing state. Third, at least in cell culture, cells that have divided more than a critical number of times undergo **senescence**, entering a viable but nondividing state. Senescence is a terminal G₀ state from which cells normally cannot exit.

One external signal that arrests progress through the cycle is transforming growth factor β (TGF-β), one of a family of growth-regulating proteins with a major role in differentiation and tissue morphogenesis (Fig. 44–9). TGF-β, acting through a receptor serine/threonine kinase (see Chapter 26), increases the expression of the small CDK-inhibiting protein p15^{Ink4b} by up to 30-fold (see Table 43–1). Like other Ink4 family members, p15^{Ink4B} specifically inactivates Cdk4–cyclin D complexes. p15^{Ink4B} binding also releases p27^{Kip1} from the Cdk4–cyclin D complexes, permitting it to transfer to Cdk2–cyclin E complexes in the nucleus and further inhibit cell cycle progression. The Ink4 proteins also displace p21^{Cip1} and p57^{Kip2} from Cdk4/6–cyclin D complexes. They, too, then inhibit Cdk2–cyclin A and E complexes.

In addition to its role in stopping cell cycle progression in response to TGF-β, p27^{Kip1} also helps to arrest the cell cycle when normal cells become crowded by neighboring cells (contact inhibition) or when the environment lacks growth factors. Genetic analysis in mice indicates that p27^{Kip1} regulates cell cycle progression during development. Indeed, mice lacking p27^{Kip1} are 30% larger than their normal litter mates by several weeks of age. This increase in size occurs at least partly because cells in many organs undergo extra rounds of division.

An analogous mechanism appears to arrest the cell cycle during the differentiation of muscle cells. The transcription factor MyoD is a master regulator of muscle differentiation. MyoD activates transcription of p21^{Cip1}, and it is believed that this may help arrest proliferation and start muscle differentiation (see Fig. 44–9). p21^{Cip1} stops cell cycle progression in at least two ways. First, by binding CDK-cyclin complexes, it blocks them from promoting cell cycle progression. Second, p21^{Cip1} binds to the DNA replication factor PCNA (proliferating cell nuclear antigen) (see Chapter 45) in a way that blocks chromosomal replication, but

not repair of DNA damage. p57^{Kip2} is also involved in myogenesis, although its regulation and role are less well understood.

Growth arrest of aged cells (senescence) appears to involve several of the mechanisms just discussed. Increased expression of both p16^{Ink4a} and p21^{Cip1} may contribute to the establishment of senescence. In this case, at least part of the signal to proliferate appears to come from the chromosomal telomeres, as overexpression of telomerase (see Chapter 12) can prevent cells from undergoing senescence in tissue culture.

Once cells exit the cycle, reentry is inhibited by multiple redundant pathways in addition to the CDK inhibitors. Current evidence indicates that many of these factors ultimately work by promoting interaction of pRb with E2F to keep the E2F-responsive cell cycle genes inactive. In addition to this selective repression of cell cycle-promoting genes by E2F, transcription may generally be more suppressed in G₀ cells. Often, the chromatin is more condensed in G₀ cells than in cycling cells, in part as a result of the replacement of histone H1 with a specialized variant (H1°). H1° represses transcription and replication, in general, by promoting a more condensed chromatin packing. However, not all gene expression is suppressed in differentiated cells, many of which synthesize large amounts of specific proteins (e.g., secreted digestive enzymes by the pancreas).

▌ Exit from the G₀ Phase

Cells in the G₀ phase may reenter the growth cycle in response to specific stimulation, often induced by injury or normal cell turnover. Cultured fibroblasts are favored for studies of this process, as they readily enter the G₀ phase when serum (and, thus, growth factors) is removed from the medium for several days, and they reenter the active cell cycle upon restoration of serum. The pattern of gene expression induced in this culture system mimics that found in tissues in response to wounding. This reflects the lifestyle of fibroblasts in connective tissue. When a tissue is wounded in vivo (see Fig. 34–11), fibroblasts divide so that they can colonize the wound and lay down new extracellular matrix to repair the damage.

Cultured fibroblasts complete the transition from quiescence to growth in three stages, referred to as **competence, entry,** and **progression** (Fig. 44–10). During the competence and entry stages, the cell takes roughly 6 hours to restore its machinery to synthesize mRNA and protein. The competence stage in fibroblasts requires platelet-derived growth factor (PDGF) (see Chapter 29). The subsequent entry stage requires (epidermal growth factor) (EGF) and insulin rather than PDGF. In the presence of appropriate nutrients,

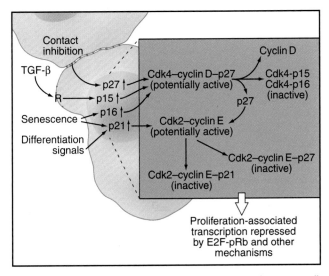

Figure 44–9 Mechanisms by which external stimuli act on Cdk inhibitors to cause cells to enter the nondividing G₀ state from the G₁ phase of the cell cycle.

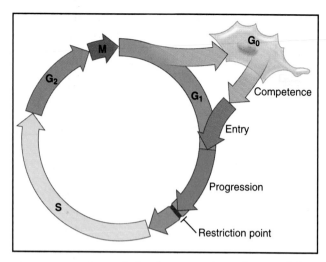

Figure 44–10 Stages during the return of growth-arrested fibroblasts from G_0 to active proliferation and the cell cycle.

G_0 fibroblasts continue into about a 4-hour progression stage, when normal transcription and translation prepare the cell for DNA synthesis. Insulin-like growth factor-I (IGF-I) is the only growth factor required during this stage. Progression advances the cell to the G_1 restriction point, about 2 hours prior to the $G_1 \rightarrow S$ transition in a typical cell cycle.

Cultured fibroblasts produce three waves of gene expression following stimulation by serum. More than 100 **"immediate early"** genes are transcribed in the first wave (Fig. 44–11). Members of the Jun, fos, myc, and zinc finger families of transcription factors (see Chapter 14) activate numerous downstream genes required for cell growth and division. Other immediate early genes encode tissue remodeling factors, cytokines (growth factors), extracellular matrix components (fibronectin), plasma membrane receptors (integrins), and cytoskeletal proteins (actin, tropomyosin, vimentin), as well as activities involved in angiogenesis (blood vessel formation), inflammation, and coagulation. These proteins facilitate the movement of fibroblasts into wounds and initiate the repair of tissue damage.

Expression of a second wave of **"delayed early"** genes precedes the onset of S phase. Genes activated after the onset of S phase are referred to as **"late"** genes. Both delayed early and late gene transcription requires synthesis of proteins, including the transcription factors encoded by immediate early genes. Delayed early genes encode a variety of proteins required for cell growth, including cyclin D and several other proteins that regulate cellular proliferation.

In addition to these patterns of increased gene transcription, cell cycle progression during the return from G_0 is also promoted by a decrease in the transcription of several of the CDK-inhibiting proteins (see Fig. 44–11).

Proteolysis and G₁ Cell Cycle Progression

Just as controlled destruction of proteins is key to the transition of cells from mitosis to the G_1 phase (see Chapter 43), proteolysis also fulfills a number of key roles during cell cycle progression. For example, when Cdk2-cyclin E is activated following synthesis of cyclin D, it phosphorylates its $p27^{Kip1}$ inhibitor. This allows $p27^{Kip1}$ to be recognized by a specific class of ubiquitin ligase (E3) called **SCF** (see Chapter 24 and the explanation that follows). The resulting destruction of $p27^{Kip1}$ leads to a burst of Cdk2-cyclin E activity that contributes to initiation of S phase. Later in the S phase, phosphorylation of the DP subunit of E2F causes dissociation of the transcription factor from DNA, recognition by SCF, and degradation. This is essential to complete S phase. SCF also targets cyclins D1 and E for destruction, the former when growth factors are limiting and the latter during progression through S phase.

SCF is a versatile class of E3, deriving its name from three of its subunits: *S*kp1, *C*dc53/*C*ullin and *F*-box proteins (Fig. 44–12). A fourth subunit, Rbx1, was discovered only later. SKP1 provides the structural core for SCF, bridging the F-box protein and Cdc53/cullin. Cdc53/cullin provides a docking site for Rbx1 and a ubiquitin-conjugating enzyme (E2) called Cdc34. Rbx1 activates Cdc34. The F-box protein recognizes the specific substrate to be destroyed. There are many different forms of SCF, recognizing a wide range of substrates and defined by the differing F-box proteins they contain. *Saccharomyces cerevisiae* has 15 F-box proteins, whereas *Caenorhabditis elegans* has at least 100. Often, F-box recognition depends on phosphorylation of the target protein. This provides a convenient

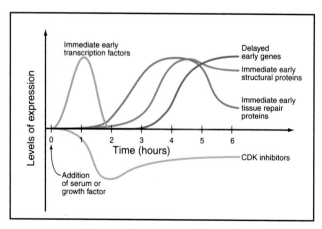

Figure 44–11 Patterns of expression of immediate and delayed early genes during the return of growth-arrested fibroblasts from G_0 to active proliferation and the cell cycle.

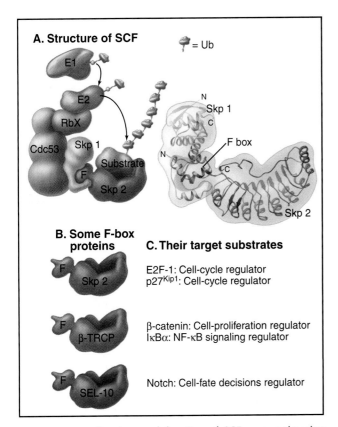

A. Structure of SCF

B. Some F-box proteins

C. Their target substrates

E2F-1: Cell-cycle regulator
p27^{Kip1}: Cell-cycle regulator

β-catenin: Cell-proliferation regulator
IκBα: NF-κB signaling regulator

Notch: Cell-fate decisions regulator

Figure 44–12 Structure and function of SCF, a complex that targets proteins for cell cycle–regulated destruction. *A,* Structure of SCF. SCF recognizes target proteins through its F-box subunit (Skp2 in this case), which often binds to specific phosphorylated forms of the target. *B,* Examples of several F-box proteins with their known target proteins.

mechanism for cell cycle regulation, as many SCF target proteins are phosphorylated by kinases, like Cdks, that are active only during specific windows of the cell cycle. Thus, the target proteins are destroyed only during those cell cycle windows.

Integrity of Cellular DNA Monitored by a Late G₁ Checkpoint

S phase is a point of no return in the history of any dividing cell. Because of the semi-conservative mechanism of DNA replication, whereby existing DNA strands serve as templates for the newly synthesized strands, any DNA defect that passes unnoticed through S phase becomes perpetuated as a mutation that is transmitted to all future progeny of the cell. Furthermore, any single-stranded nick in DNA becomes a full-fledged chromosome break if present during replication. To avoid these problems, cells have a quality control mechanism to ensure that chromosomal DNA is undamaged prior to replication in S phase.

This quality control mechanism involves a **checkpoint** late in the G₁ phase. Checkpoints are modular

subroutines superimposed on the normal cell cycle. When activated, checkpoints block progression through the cycle, either temporarily or, in some cases, permanently. In certain cases, checkpoint activation leads to cell death by apoptosis. Checkpoints are activated by sensor proteins that detect problems—typically, DNA damage in the case of the G₁ checkpoint. Sensor proteins activate protein kinases that modify target proteins, which then block cell cycle progression. This discussion of checkpoints is continued and expanded in Chapter 46.

The **p53** tumor suppressor protein is essential for the G₁ DNA damage checkpoint; the checkpoint is lost in p53 knockout mice. p53 is a transcription factor whose role in the G₁ DNA damage checkpoint appears to involve activation of a set of target genes, including the CDK inhibitor p21^{Cip1}. Fibroblasts from mice lacking the p21 gene are impaired in their ability to arrest in G₁ after DNA damage. However, p53 is also thought to be able to induce G₁ arrest by mechanisms not requiring p21^{Cip1}. p53 also participates in other checkpoints during G₂ and mitosis (see Chapter 46).

P53 is widely studied, in part because it is mutated or deleted in about half of all human cancers. Families carrying a mutated p53 allele have Li-Fraumeni syndrome, a condition associated with an elevated risk of cancers. Mice lacking p53 are viable, but develop cancers while young. This reveals an important fact about checkpoints. In many cases, checkpoint components are not essential as long as nothing untoward occurs. Checkpoints exist primarily as backup mechanisms to deal with problems that arise during cell cycle progression. However, the elevated cancer rates in Li-Fraumeni syndrome indicate that although p53 is not essential for the passage of every cell cycle, it is essential for genetic stability and for maintaining a proper balance among cell proliferation, differentiation, and death during the lifetime of a mammal.

P53 is very powerful medicine for the cell cycle. If present in excessive amounts, it is extremely toxic. For this reason, p53 is regulated by a partner protein called **Mdm2**, a ubiquitin ligase (E3) whose job it is to keep p53 levels low under circumstances in which the cell cycle is running normally (Fig. 44–13). Loss of the Mdm2 gene in mice is lethal unless the p53 gene is also lost. Mdm2 protein shuttles in and out of the nucleus (see Chapter 16). p53 also has a nuclear export signal, and when these two proteins associate in the cytoplasm, Mdm2 promotes the rapid degradation of p53 by the ubiquitin/proteasome system (see Chapter 24). Because p53 directly stimulates expression of Mdm2, a negative feedback mechanism keeps levels of p53 low.

Following DNA damage, p53 is phosphorylated by several protein kinases, including ataxia-telangiecta-

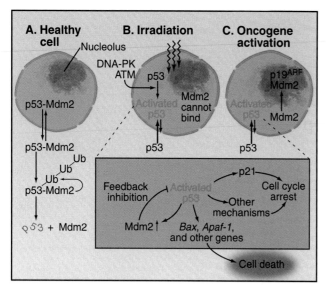

Figure 44-13 P53 regulation and the DNA damage checkpoint in G₁. *A,* Healthy cell. *B,* After irradiation, Mdm2 can no longer bind p53, which accumulates in active form in the nucleus. *C,* After oncogene activation, Mdm2 is sequestered in the nucleolus, and active p53 accumulates in the nucleus. Activated p53 can induce either cell cycle arrest or cell death.

sia–mutated (ATM) kinase and DNA-dependent protein kinase (DNA-PK). DNA-PK also phosphorylates Mdm2. Exactly which kinase does what is still a matter of some debate, but the net result is that these phosphorylations prevent Mdm2 from binding p53. As a result, p53 is stabilized, and its concentration in the nucleus increases dramatically. This results in a burst of transcription of p53-regulated genes.

ATM and DNA-PK are related to the lipid kinase, phosphatidylinositol 3-kinase (see Chapters 27 and 28), but their only known substrates are proteins (see also Chapter 46). Humans with mutations of ATM have a disease, called ataxia-telangiectasia, with defects in induction of the DNA repair cell cycle checkpoint, and they are predisposed to cancer. Mice lacking DNA-PK suffer from severe combined immunodeficiency (SCID) owing to defects in gene rearrangements during immunoglobulin maturation.

P53 uses a different mechanism to defend the cell against cancer caused by inappropriate activation of oncogenes that disrupt normal cell cycle controls. Dysregulated cell cycle progression stimulates expression of the tumor suppressor protein p19^ARF, which binds and sequesters Mdm2 (but not p53) in the nucleolus. This allows p53 to accumulate in the nucleus, where it activates a pathway promoting cell death by apoptosis. Thus, aberrantly growing cells are removed and the body is protected. P53 induces cell death by stimulating transcription of a number of genes involved in cell killing by apoptosis. Of the known p53 target genes, *Bax*, CD95 (*Fas/Apo1*), and *Apaf-1* are discussed in Chapter 49.

The p19^ARF gene (in humans, the protein is smaller and so is called p14^ARF) is quite unusual as it is located within the p16^Ink4a gene. In fact, the genes not only overlap, but they share a common exon. Nevertheless, the two proteins have no common amino acid sequences because the shared exons are read in different frames in the mature messenger RNAs (mRNAs) for the two proteins. Thus, the p16^Ink4a/p19^ARF locus encodes two vital protective factors with different jobs. It is not surprising that this key locus is a very frequent target for mutations in human cancers.

■ Is G₁ Regulation Equivalent to pRb Regulation?

The restriction point is essentially a regulatory gate controlled by pRb. When pRb is dephosphorylated, it binds to E2F and the restriction point is closed, blocking cell cycle progression. Phosphorylation of pRb by CDKs liberates the E2F transcription factor, the restriction point gate is then opened, and cell cycle progression proceeds. In reality, the situation is more complex, but it is a useful approximation to say that the regulation of cell cycle progression through G₁, in many cases, hinges upon the regulation of the phosphorylation of the pRb tumor suppressor protein.

■ Selected Readings

Bartek J, Bartkova J, Lukas J: The retinoblastoma protein pathway in cell cycle control and cancer. Exp Cell Res 237:1–6, 1997.

Chin L, Pomerantz J, DePinho RA: The INK4a/ARF tumor suppressor: One gene—two products—two pathways. Trends Biochem Sci 23:291–296, 1998.

Ekholm SV, Reed SI: Regulation of G(1) cyclin-dependent kinases in the mammalian cell cycle. Curr Opin Cell Biol 12:676–684, 2000.

Elledge SJ: Cell cycle checkpoints: Preventing an identity crisis. Science 274:1664–1672, 1996.

Johnson DG, Walker CL: Cyclins and cell cycle checkpoints. Annu Rev Pharmacol Toxicol 39:295–312, 1999.

Kitazono A, Matsumoto T: "Isogaba Maware": Quality control of genome DNA by checkpoints. BioEssays 20:391–399, 1998.

Lavia P, Jansen-Durr P: E2F target genes and cell-cycle checkpoint control. Bioessays 21:221–230, 1999.

Planas-Silva MD, Weinberg RA: The restriction point and control of cell proliferation. Curr Opin Cell Biol 9:768–772, 1997.

Polymenis M, Schmidt EV: Coordination of cell growth with cell division. Curr Opin Genet Dev 9:76–80, 1999.

Prives C: Signaling to p53: Breaking the MDM2-p53 circuit. Cell 95:5–8, 1998.

Sherr CJ: Cancer cell cycles. Science 274:1672–1677, 1996.

chapter 45

THE S PHASE AND DNA REPLICATION

Accurate replication of DNA, which is crucial for cellular propagation and survival, occurs during the S phase (DNA *s*ynthesis phase) of the cell cycle. This chapter begins with a brief primer on the events of replication, and then discusses its regulation. Next, it covers the proteins that bind origins of replication and ensure that each region of DNA is replicated once and only once per cell cycle. It closes by discussing how the structure of the nucleus influences replication.

▮ DNA Replication: A Primer

One of the most exciting predictions of the Watson: Crick model for the structure of DNA was a mechanism for DNA replication. Because DNA strand pairing is determined by complementary base pairing, it was logical to propose the existence of enzymes called DNA polymerases that would move along a single strand of DNA, recognize each base in turn, and insert the proper complementary base at the end of the growing chain. Thus, one *might* have surmised that only a single enzyme was required for DNA synthesis. In fact, DNA replication in eukaryotic cells involves a complex macromolecular machine.

Before discussing DNA replication and its regulation, an introduction to some terminology describing the geometry of replicating DNA is required. The exact site on the chromosomal DNA where replication begins is termed the **origin of bidirectional replication.** As the term bidirectional implies, two sets of DNA replication machinery head off in opposite directions from the origin. Each set of replication machinery, together with the DNA that it is replicating, is called a **replication fork** because at the site of replication, one parental DNA molecule splits into two (Fig. 45–1). It is not known whether replication forks move along the DNA like a train along a track, or whether the fork sits at a stationary site (referred to as a replication factory) through which the DNA is "reeled in" as it is replicated.

The bidirectional nature of DNA replication causes a fundamental problem, as synthesis of all known DNA polynucleotides proceeds in a 5′ to 3′ direction (Fig. 45–2). In the fundamental reaction, an activated triphosphate group at the 5′ position of the incoming nucleoside triphosphate precursor forms a phosphodiester bond with an OH group at the 3′ position of the deoxyribose sugar at the terminus of the nascent DNA chain. Replication of the so-called **leading strand** poses no problems, with newly synthesized DNA laid down in a 5′ to 3′ direction. However, the other strand faces in the opposite direction, apparently requiring DNA polymerase to synthesize DNA in the wrong direction (i.e., adding nucleotides in a 3′ to 5′ direction) for the replication fork to move away from the origin. No DNA polymerase with this polarity has been found. Instead, this **lagging strand** replicates in a series of short segments. Every time the DNA strands have been peeled apart (unwound) by 250 nucleotides or so, a polymerase/primase complex (see later section) initiates DNA synthesis on the lagging strand, with the polymerase running back toward the replication origin in a 5′ to 3′ direction. Thus, synthesis on the lagging strand proceeds in a direction *opposite to the overall direction of fork movement.* Synthesis of each lagging strand fragment stops when DNA polymerase runs into the 5′ end of the previous fragment. Thus, the lagging strand is copied in a highly *discontinuous* fashion into short fragments known as **Okazaki fragments** (named after their discoverer; see Fig. 45–1). The enzymes and events at the replication fork are considered in greater detail in a later section.

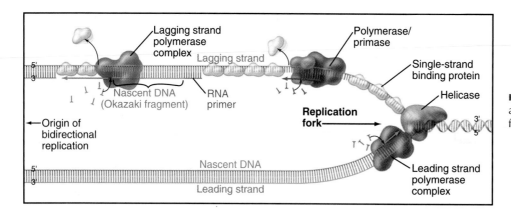

Figure 45–1 Key components and events at the replication fork.

Origins of Replication

Replication of the large genomes of eukaryotes during a relatively short S phase, which can be limited to as little as a few minutes in some early embryos, presents

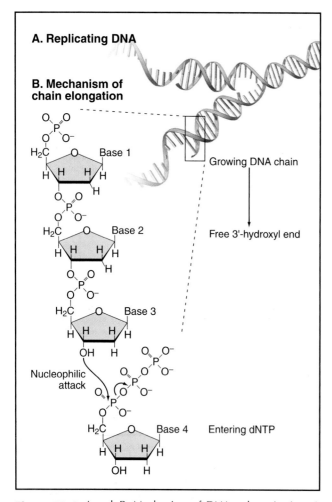

Figure 45–2 *A* and *B*, Mechanism of DNA polymerization. A 3′ OH group at the end of a growing DNA chain makes a nucleophilic attack on the α-phosphate of a triphosphate precursor in the active site of polymerase (enzyme not shown here). dNTP, nucleoside triphosphate.

a challenge. How do cells guarantee that all of the DNA is replicated? The replication apparatus simply does not move quickly enough to copy all of the DNA in a eukaryotic chromosome during the time available if it starts at a single **origin of replication** (a specific sequence on the DNA; see later section), as it does in the bacterium *Escherichia coli*. Instead, eukaryotes initiate replication at many origins distributed along the chromosome: 400 in budding yeast and about 60,000 in human cells. These origins are positioned so that all of the DNA can be replicated in the available time.

How is the "firing" of all of these origins orchestrated so that each is used once and only once per S phase? If any origin were to fire more or less than once, the consequences would be dire, with either duplication or loss of genes. This problem is controlled by a mechanism termed "licensing." Each origin is licensed to replicate once per cell cycle. Replication of the origin removes the license, which cannot normally be renewed until the cell has completely traversed the cycle and has passed through mitosis.

A unit of chromosomal DNA whose replication is initiated at a single origin is termed a **replicon.** The origin is defined genetically as a **replicator** element. The classic replicon is the *E. coli* chromosome (which is 4×10^6 bp in size); this has a single replicator site called *oriC* (Fig. 45–3). A protein termed the **initiator** (in the case of *E. coli*, the product of the DnaA gene) binds to this origin and either directly or indirectly promotes melting of the DNA duplex, giving the replication machinery access to two single strands of DNA. Other factors bind to the initiator, and their concerted action produces a wave of DNA replication proceeding outward in both directions along the DNA (a replication "bubble") at about 750 to 1250 bases per second.

An average human chromosome contains about 150×10^6 bp of DNA. Because the replication machinery in mammals moves only about 20 to 100 bases per second (probably reflecting the fact that the DNA is packaged into chromatin; see Chapter 13), it would take up to 2000 hours to replicate this length of

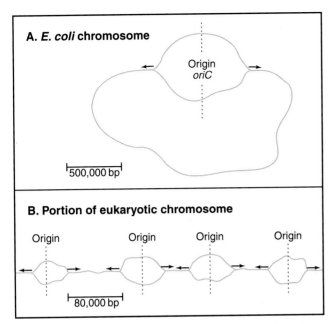

Figure 45-3 *A,* The *E. coli* chromosome is a simple replicon with a single origin of replication. In cells, this chromosome has a complex, highly supercoiled structure. *B,* Eukaryotic chromosomes have multiple origins of replication.

DNA from a single origin! In most human cells, the duration of S phase is about 8 hours. This means that at least 25 to 125 origins of replication would be required to replicate an average chromosome in the allotted time. In fact, origins of replication are much more closely spaced than this. It has been estimated that mammalian origins of replication are spaced about 100,000–150,000 bp apart. Thus, approximately 60,000 origins of replication participate in replication of the entire human genome.

To explain the events at origins of replication, the budding yeast *Saccharomyces cerevisiae* serves as a good example. Its DNA replication is better understood than that of any other eukaryote.

Replication Origins in *S. cerevisiae*

More than 400 origins of replication participate in replicating the entire budding yeast genome. A major breakthrough in understanding DNA replication in *S. cerevisiae* was the identification of short (100–150 bp) segments of DNA that act as replication origins in vivo when cloned into a yeast plasmid (circular DNA molecule). These **autonomously replicating sequences** (or **ARS elements**) allow yeast plasmids to replicate in parallel with the cellular chromosomes (Fig. 45–4). It has since been confirmed that ARS elements are often, although not always, bona fide replication origins in their native chromosomal context. Replication always initiates within ARS elements, but

not all ARS elements act as origins of DNA replication in every cell cycle.

The average spacing between yeast replication origins is about 30,000 bp, with the maximum spacing between adjacent origins being about 130,000 bp. Even this longest spacing should readily be replicated within the 30 minutes available during S phase. Because the number of origins exceeds the number required to replicate the genome within the allotted time, some origins need not "fire" every cell cycle. The probability that a specific origin is used in a given cell cycle ranges from less than 0.2 to more than 0.9.

The ARS element does two things to establish an origin of replication. First, it has conserved sequences that act as binding sites for a protein complex that marks it as a potential origin. Second, it has nearby sequences that can readily be induced to unwind (or to become un–base-paired).

Budding yeast ARS elements share a common DNA sequence motif called the **ARS core consensus**

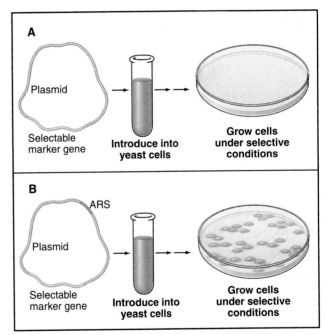

Figure 45-4 The plasmid assay for identification of an autonomously replicating sequence (ARS) element (origin of DNA replication) in budding yeast. The plasmid at left has a selectable marker gene (e.g., a gene required for the synthesis of an essential amino acid) plus (in panel *B*) an ARS element. This plasmid is transferred into growing yeast cells that are defective in the marker gene carried by the plasmid, and these cells are then plated out on agar medium lacking the essential amino acid. Only cells containing a form of the plasmid that can be replicated will grow to make colonies. *A,* A plasmid lacking an ARS fails to replicate and is lost from the cells. These cells cannot grow into colonies on plates lacking the essential amino acid. *B,* If the plasmid contains an ARS element, it replicates along with the chromosomal DNA and is maintained in the population. These cells grow into colonies in the absence of the essential amino acid.

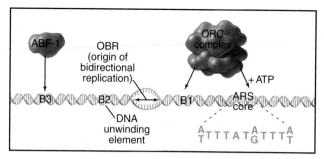

Figure 45-5 The structure of the ARS1 element. ORC binds to the ARS core sequence plus element B1. B2 is a sequence that can readily be induced to unwind. The OBR (origin of bidirectional replication) is the site where DNA synthesis actually begins. B3 is a binding site for an auxiliary factor called ABF-1 that is both a transcriptional activator and an activator of the ARS element.

sequence: 5′-(A/T)TTTAT(A/G)TTT(A/T)-3′ (Fig. 45–5). Single base mutations at several locations within this sequence completely inactivate ARS activity. Other, less well-conserved DNA sequences also contribute to the activity of the ARS as a replication origin. One of these, termed B1, together with the ARS core, forms the binding site for a complex of six proteins termed the *origin recognition complex* or **ORC** (see later section). The DNA unwinding element referred to earlier is thought to be another short sequence (B2) located a bit further along the DNA. When the origin actually initiates DNA replication, synthesis starts at an origin of bidirectional replication midway between the ORC binding site and the DNA unwinding element.

ORC was first identified by its ability to bind the 11-bp ARS core sequence (see Fig. 45–5). This binding has two noteworthy features. First, it requires adenosine triphosphate (ATP), which remains associated with the ORC complex. ORC with bound ATP may be poised for further assembly processes or some later function in the initiation of DNA replication. Second, in yeast, the ORC complex remains bound to origins of replication across the entire cell cycle. Thus, something other than the presence of ORC must be responsible for regulating the periodic activation of origins in S phase (see later section). In metazoans, ORC behavior is more complex and is not fully understood.

ARS elements typically contain binding sites for other sequence-specific DNA binding proteins, such as transcription factors. For example, the ARS1 element contains a sequence (B3 in Fig. 45–5) that is bound by a transcription factor called ABF-1 (*ARS-binding factor* 1). Deletion of the ABF-1 binding site only slightly reduces the ability of ARS1 to act as a replication origin in vivo. Furthermore, ABF-1 can be replaced by several other transcription factors (by switching their DNA binding sequences for the B3

sequence), and these artificial ARS elements replicate with an efficiency essentially identical to that of the wild type element.

There are important functional links between origins of replication and promoter elements that stimulate the transcription of genes (see Chapter 14). In addition to their role in DNA replication, several ORC components also seem to regulate transcription. Crosstalk between the machinery used for transcription and DNA replication may explain why regions of chromosomes with actively transcribed genes typically replicate early in S phase (see discussion that follows).

Replication Origins in Mammalian Cells

Far less is known about the structure and function of mammalian origins of DNA replication than about ARS elements in budding yeast. Many attempts have been made to develop an assay equivalent to the ARS assay for mammalian DNA, but with few successes. In fact, for years, a controversy has raged over whether vertebrate chromosomes have discrete origins of DNA replication. This question arose, in part, from studies of DNA replication in *Xenopus* eggs. Once activated by fertilization or by various experimental tricks, *Xenopus* eggs divide about an hour later and then undergo a rapid sequence of cell cycles, each of which lasts about 30 minutes. Any DNA injected into these eggs is rapidly and efficiently replicated. Both prokaryotic and eukaryotic DNA is replicated with similar efficiency, and careful studies have demonstrated that this replication initiates at random (i.e., does not use defined origins). This promiscuous initiation of DNA replication is now thought to be a specialized adaptation by early embryos to permit replication of the chromosomes in the very brief temporal window available.

Following a great deal of study, the existence of preferred origins of DNA replication in mammalian cells is beginning to be accepted. These origins are much more complex than their budding yeast counterparts. Mammalian origin activity is affected by a number of factors, including DNA sequence, DNA modifications, chromatin structure, and nuclear organization. Interestingly, DNA methylation, which is typically associated with transcriptional inactivation (see Chapter 13), can stimulate activity at certain replication origins.

At present, two types of mammalian replication origins are known. The first is exemplified by the origin of replication adjacent to the lamin B2 gene (Fig. 45–6*B*). This origin "fires" within the first several minutes of S phase, and a variety of methods have succeeded in mapping it to a stretch of less than 500 bp. Within this region, a single origin of bidirectional replication appears to be used. Thus, the current assumption is that the lamin B2 origin of replication

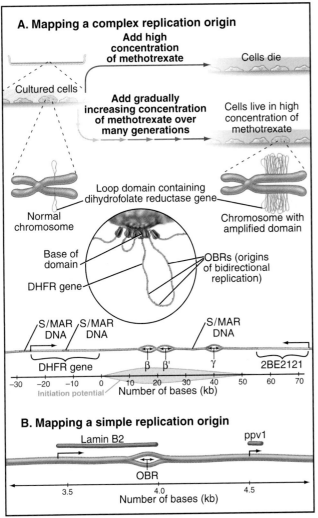

A. Mapping a complex replication origin

Add high concentration of methotrexate → Cells die

Cultured cells

Add gradually increasing concentration of methotrexate over many generations → Cells live in high concentration of methotrexate

Normal chromosome

Loop domain containing dihydrofolate reductase gene

Chromosome with amplified domain

Base of domain

DHFR gene

OBRs (origins of bidirectional replication)

S/MAR DNA   S/MAR DNA   S/MAR DNA

DHFR gene   β β'   γ   2BE2121

−30 −20 −10 0 10 20 30 40 50 60 70
Initiation potential   Number of bases (kb)

B. Mapping a simple replication origin

Lamin B2   ppv1

OBR

3.5   4.0   4.5
Number of bases (kb)

Figure 45-6 DNA replication origins in mammals. *A,* A complex DNA replication origin near the dihydrofolate reductase (DHFR) gene. Normal cells are killed by exposure to methotrexate, but it is possible to select resistant cell lines by growing them in progressively increasing concentrations of the drug, selecting at each stage for cells that survive. Use of this procedure on hamster cells has resulted in a cell line that contains about 1000 copies of a 230,000-bp domain containing the dihydrofolate reductase gene. This region of DNA is replicated using origins found within a 55,000-bp region adjacent to the dihydrofolate reductase gene. Low levels of initiation of replication occur throughout the entire 55,000-bp region, but most initiation occurs at three specific origins called β, β', and γ. *B,* A simple DNA replication origin. Replication of the DNA adjacent to the lamin B2 gene appears to initiate entirely from a single origin, as shown. S/MAR, scaffold/matrix attachment regions (see Chapter 13); ppv1, a gene next to the lamin B2 gene.

resembles the well-characterized budding yeast origins.

The replication origin lying just downstream of the gene for dihydrofolate reductase (DHFR) appears to be significantly more complex. The enzyme DHFR is essential for biosynthesis of thymidine. This origin is accessible to experimental study because it is possible

to select for cells with this chromosomal region amplified into hundreds or even thousands of copies (see Fig. 45–6). By looking for the first regions of the amplified DNA to replicate, the origin of replication was initially located within a region of about 55,000 bp.

However, controversy resulted when attempts were made to map the origin more precisely. Certain methods indicate that initiation occurs at random across the entire region. However, other methods have localized a probable origin of replication to a single 500-bp stretch of the DNA. It now appears that both answers are correct. Although initiation can occur randomly throughout the entire region, most initiation events occur at three preferred sites, termed Ori-β, Ori-β', and Ori-γ (see Fig. 45–6). Each origin encompasses about 0.5–2 kb of DNA.

There is still much to be learned about mammalian origins of DNA replication. In particular, it will be important to determine which aspects of origin function are conserved between yeasts and mammals, and which differences have arisen to deal with the more complex metazoan chromosomes.

■ Assembly of the Prereplication Complex

To preserve the integrity of the genome, each origin of replication must "fire" only once per cell cycle. Although the mechanism underlying this important cell cycle control is incompletely understood, budding yeasts provide an insight into how it works.

As stated earlier, yeast ORC is stably bound to replication origins throughout the yeast cell cycle. However, ORC is not the trigger for DNA replication. Rather, it can be thought of as a "landing pad" upon which the protein complex responsible for the initiation of DNA replication assembles. During late anaphase or very early G_1 phase, two proteins, called **Cdc6p** and **Cdt1,** bind to the ORC complex at origins of replication. ORC-Cdc6p-Cdt1 then recruits a complex of Mcm proteins (see next paragraph) to the origin and loads it onto the DNA. This complex of ORC, Cdc6p, CDT1, and Mcm proteins is known as the **prereplication complex** (Fig. 45–7). A prereplication complex assembles at every replication origin before the onset of S phase.

Mcm (*m*inichromosome *m*aintenance) **proteins** were identified in a screen for genes of budding yeast that are required for the stability of small artificial chromosomes. A number of *Mcm* genes were identified by this assay, with a structurally related group of proteins, termed Mcm 2–7, being required for DNA replication. Mcm 2–7 proteins form a hexameric complex that is thought to be shaped like a doughnut. Somehow, Cdc6p-Cdt1 uses ATP hydrolysis to thread

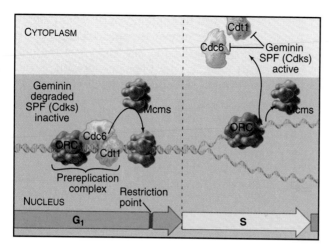

Figure 45–7 Components of the prereplication complex and their fate after the initiation of DNA replication.

DNA through the central hole of the Mcm doughnut. Although the function of the Mcm proteins is not known for certain, it has been suggested that the Mcm hexamer is a DNA helicase, an enzyme that uses ATP hydrolysis to separate DNA strands (see later section).

It is currently thought that assembly of the prereplication complex is the key point of regulation at which origins are "licensed" so that they replicate only once per cell cycle. Licensing is accomplished by at least three mechanisms. The first involves regulation of Cdc6p activity by Cdks. Cdc6p-Cdt1 loads Mcm proteins onto DNA only in the *absence* of a protein kinase activity called "SPF" (S phase–promoting factor). SPF is thought to be composed of particular Cdk-cyclin pairs. In mammalian cells, these include Cdk1 or Cdk2 complexed with cyclins E, A, and B; in yeasts, the single Cdk is complexed with B-type cyclins. As discussed in Chapter 43, Cdks, including SPF, are inactivated at the exit from mitosis by destruction of their cyclin cofactors, and by synthesis of specific inhibitory proteins. Their activity remains low until cells pass the restriction point, when levels of Cdk2–cyclin E, and subsequently, Cdk2–cyclin A, rise again (see Chapter 43). Therefore, licensing of replication origins can only occur between the onset of anaphase and passage of the restriction point. Once the restriction point is passed, SPF-Cdk activity prevents the reformation of prereplication complexes until after mitosis. The importance of this mechanism was demonstrated particularly clearly in the fission yeast *Schizosaccharomyces pombe*, in which inactivation of Cdk1 during the G_2 phase was found to lead to assembly of prereplication complexes on already replicated DNA. These cells then undergo further rounds of "illegal" DNA replication without division.

Vertebrates use a protein called **geminin** to regulate origin "licensing." Geminin prevents Cdc6-Cdt1

from loading Mcm proteins onto DNA. The anaphase-promoting complex/cyclosome (APC/C) (see Chapter 43) degrades geminin, keeping its concentration very low from anaphase through late G_1 when prereplication complexes assemble. Accumulation of geminin starting in S phase prevents the assembly of new prereplication complexes until after the next mitosis. Yeasts lack geminin.

A third way to regulate origin "licensing" involves sequestering molecules required to assemble the replication complex in the cytoplasm following the onset of S phase. If nuclei from G_1 cells are added to a cell-free system of DNA replication based on the use of *Xenopus* egg extracts (see Chapter 43), these nuclei will replicate their nuclei once and only once. Nuclei from G_2 cells will not replicate. However, in both cases, if holes are punched in the nuclear membranes and then subsequently repaired, then the replicated nuclei will re-replicate their DNA in the extracts. This suggests that factors in the cytoplasm that cannot normally get through the nuclear envelope can permit replicated nuclei to assemble prereplication complexes and re-replicate their DNA. In yeast, factors excluded

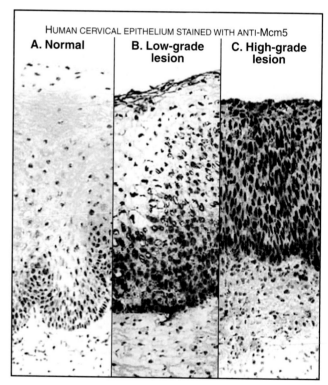

Figure 45–8 *A* to *C*, Sections of human cervix stained with antibodies to Mcm5. Normal G_0 cells in this stratified epithelium lack Mcm5 and other replication proteins. Cancer cells express Mcm5 at higher levels as they become more malignant. (Adapted from Williams GH, Romanowski P, Morris L, et al: Improved cervical smear assessment using antibodies against proteins that regulate DNA replication. Proc Natl Acad Sci USA 95:14932–14937, 1998. Copyright 1998, National Academy of Sciences, U.S.A.)

from the nucleus after replication include Mcm proteins. In vertebrates, one excluded factor is Cdt1.

Components of the prereplication complex are absent from differentiated (G_0) cells. In fact, immunodetection of these proteins in cervical smears is currently being explored as a sensitive method for the early detection of cancer cells (Fig. 45–8).

Signals That Start Replication

A classic experiment (Fig. 45–9) demonstrated that (1) a cytoplasmic inducer triggers the transition into S phase, and (2) this inducer triggers DNA replication in a G_1 nucleus, but not a G_2 nucleus. The inducer is very likely a combination of protein kinases, including the SPF Cdk-cyclin pairs, as well as a specialized kinase, Cdc7p-Dbf4p. In mammals, the first Cdk-cyclin pair that is important for S-phase entry is Cdk2–cyclin E, whose activity is maximal at the G_1/S transition (Fig. 45–10). This kinase phosphorylates pRb, thereby further opening the restriction point "gate" and allowing E2F to function as a transcription factor and stimulate the transcription of genes involved in DNA replication (see Chapter 44). In addition to cyclin E itself, E2F target genes include cyclin A, Cdc25A, enzymes required for synthesis of DNA precursors (DHFR, thymidine kinase, and thymidylate synthase), origin-binding proteins Cdc6p and ORC1, and two components of the replication machinery (DNA polymerase α and proliferating cell nuclear antigen [PCNA]; see later section).

Cdk2–cyclin E is also thought to phosphorylate the Cdk inhibitor p27^{Kip1}, rendering it a target for the SCF complex, which marks it for destruction by the proteasome (see Chapter 43). SCF gets its name from three of its components: Skp1, cullin, and F-box proteins. Skp1, in turn, got its name (*S*-phase *k*inase-associated *p*rotein) because it was first identified in a

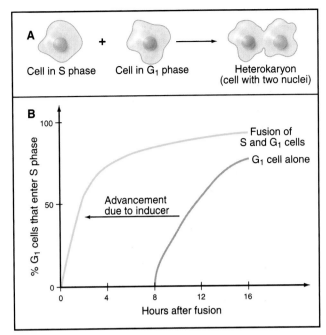

Figure 45–9 Cell fusion experiment showing the existence of a positive inducer of S phase. *A*, Synchronized cells in different stages of the cycle were fused to yield two nuclei in a single cytoplasm. *B*, If the fusion involved nuclei from G_1 and S cells, the G_1 nucleus was induced to enter S phase sooner than expected. If the fusion involved nuclei from S and G_2 cells, the G_2 nucleus failed to re-replicate its DNA (not shown). (Redrawn from Rao PN, Johnson RT: Mammalian cell fusion: Studies on the regulation of DNA synthesis and mitosis. Nature 225:159–164, 1970.)

complex with Cdk2–cyclin A. In fact, this kinase may be important for targeting various proteins for destruction by SCF, which recognizes its substrates only after they have been phosphorylated at certain key positions (see also Fig. 44–12). One example of this is provided by E2F$_1$. Once cells have entered S phase, Cdk2–cyclin A phosphorylates the DP1 subunit of

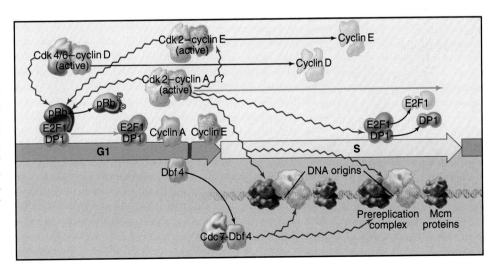

Figure 45–10 Cdk4/6–cyclin D first opens the restriction point gate, and this is reinforced by a positive feedback loop involving Cdk2–cyclin E and Cdk2–cyclin A. Cdk2–cyclin A phosphorylation then marks cyclin E and E2F$_1$ for degradation. In addition, phosphorylation by Cdk2–cyclin A and Cdc7-Dbf4 activates replication origins for synthesis.

E2F$_1$. This causes the DP1-E2F$_1$ complex to be released from the DNA and leads to the degradation of E2F$_1$ (see Fig. 45–10). Cyclin E is degraded when cells enter S phase, and this may also be triggered by Cdk2–cyclin A. (D-type cyclins are also degraded at this time by SCF.)

In addition to acting as a molecular "hit man," Cdk2–cyclin A is also essential for cells to enter S phase. In live cells, selective destruction of either cyclin A or its messenger RNA (mRNA) prevents entry into S phase. Furthermore, transforming growth factor-β causes cell cycle arrest, in part by repressing cyclin A transcription (see Chapter 44). Cdk2–cyclin A has two targets that are essential for entry into S phase: Cdc6p and a protein known as Cdc45p (see later section).

The second kinase involved with initiation of DNA replication is Cdc7p with its associated subunit Dbf4p. This kinase seems to act at the level of individual DNA replication origins. Careful analysis has revealed that Cdc7p-Dbf4p is required for firing of origins in both early and late S phase. Cdc7p is capable of phosphorylating several Mcm proteins. Thus, one possible function of this kinase is to modify the Mcm complex somehow starting the replication process. Dbf4p, which is responsible for targeting Cdc7p to origins, is very unstable from anaphase through G$_1$ phase. This period of Dbf4 instability coincides with the time of the cell cycle during which prereplication complexes are being assembled, and it may provide a mechanism to ensure that origins do not fire prematurely until the cell is ready to enter S phase.

---

table 45–1

BIOCHEMICAL ACTIVITIES REQUIRED FOR REPLICATION OF DNA IN EXTRACTS FROM EUKARYOTIC CELLS

Activity	Protein* (Size†)
Origin recognition	
SV40 virus and original cell-free extracts	SV40 large T antigen (82 kD)
Eukaryotes	ORC (*origin recognition complex* (120, 72, 62, 56, 53, 50 kD)
Origin activation	Protein phosphatase 2A (34, 32 kD)
DNA unwinding (helicase)	SV40 large T antigen
	Mcm proteins? (cellular counterpart)
Stabilization of single-stranded DNA	RPA (subunits: 70 [ssDNA binding], p32, p11)
polymerase/primase	DNA polymerase α (subunits: p180 [polymerase], p70 [stimulates primasome assembly], p58 [stability and activation of p48], p48 [primase]); no editing function
Replicative polymerases	DNA polymerase δ (p125 [polymerase], p48, + plus others?)
	DNA polymerase ε (205, 70 kD); both have 3′–5′exonuclease editing capability
Processivity factor	PCNA (36 kD); ring-shaped clamp that slides along the DNA; keeps polymerases δ and ε attached to the template strand so that they make longer chains; involved in coordination of cell cycle control and replication and repair
PCNA loader	RFC (145, 40, 38, 37, 36.5 kD); binds primer: template junction; loading factor for PCNA; important for polymerase switch
Closing factors:	
Removal of RNA primer	Fen1 5′ ⇒ 3′ exonuclease (46 kD) + RNaseH (49, 39 kD)
Ligation of discontinuous DNA fragments	DNA ligase I (102 kD)
Release of superhelical tension	DNA topoisomerase I (100 kD)
Disentanglement of daughter strands	DNA topoisomerase II (175 kD)

*The identities of several of the components involved in the reactions listed were first worked out using a model system for DNA replication in vitro. These systems were based on the replication of DNA isolated from a simian virus (SV40) in cellular extracts. This virus has a small circular genome with a defined origin of replication. The reason why SV40 virus is so suitable for model studies is that it uses only one viral protein, the *large T antigen,* for its DNA replication. All the rest of the replication functions come from the host human cell.

†Unless otherwise specified, size of subunits in humans is given.

Mechanism of DNA Synthesis

At the onset of DNA replication, each origin of replication has bound to it the ORC complex, Cdc6p-Cdt1, and multiple hexameric Mcm complexes. (For a description of the major activities involved in DNA replication, see Table 45–1.) For replication to start, paired DNA strands must be separated. This permits the DNA polymerase to bind and begin synthesizing the daughter strand.

Locally, DNA replication appears to begin with phosphorylation of Cdc6p and Mcm proteins (Fig. 45–11A). The role of Mcm phosphorylation (by the Cdc7p-Dbf4p kinase) is not yet known. Cdc6p phosphorylation by Cdk2–cyclin A may cause the protein to let go of the Mcm proteins, possibly helping to start replication. Phosphorylated Cdc6p and Cdt1 then leave the DNA and move to the cytoplasm, where their fate varies in different organisms. In cycling mammalian cells, cytoplasmic Cdc6p is stable and waits for the next cell cycle to rebind replication origins. In yeast, cytoplasmic Cdc6p is destroyed.

Studies of viral and bacterial DNA replication have established that the next step is activation of a DNA helicase, an enzyme that uses ATP hydrolysis to peel apart the paired strands of the DNA double helix. Despite exhaustive efforts, the helicase has not yet been firmly identified in eukaryotes, but it is striking that helicases in both viruses and bacteria are hexameric protein complexes. This, in addition to other experimental evidence, has led to the belief that the hexameric Mcm complex is the eukaryotic DNA helicase. For an introduction to DNA replication in *E. coli,* see Box 45–1.

Cdc6p release is accompanied by binding of **Cdc45p** and a single-strand DNA-binding protein, **RPA,** to the origin (see Fig. 45–11B). Cdc45p appears to associate with the Mcm proteins, and this promotes the binding of RPA. It now appears likely that this complex somehow activates the Mcm helicase. Cdc45p and RPA then recruit DNA polymerase to the origin (see Fig. 45–11C). As the helicase starts to separate the DNA strands, moving outward in both directions from the origin of bidirectional replication, RPA stabilizes the separated strands, ensuring that they do not simply base-pair with one another again.

The separated DNA strands are ready for replication, but DNA synthesis always involves the addition of an incoming nucleoside triphosphate to a free 3′ OH group at the terminus of a preexisting nascent polynucleotide (see Fig. 45–2). In the absence of a nascent DNA chain, how does DNA polymerase get started? This problem is solved by a DNA-dependent RNA polymerase called a primase, which, like other RNA polymerases, can initiate synthesis de novo without the need for a 3′ OH group. In eukaryotes, all DNA chains are started by a complex of DNA poly-

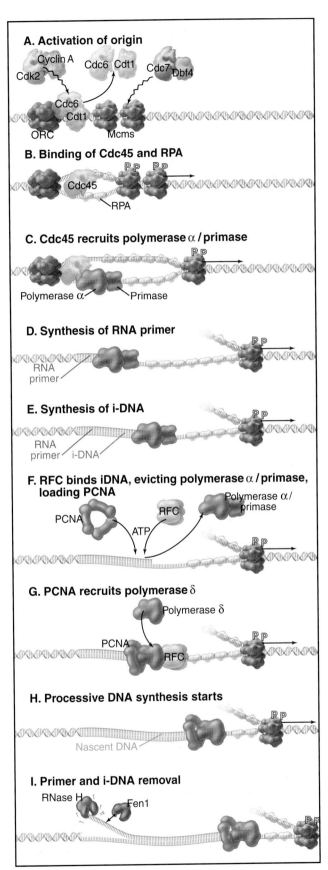

Figure 45-11 *A* to *I,* The main events of DNA replication. (For a more detailed description, see text.)

box 45–1

DNA REPLICATION IN *ESCHERICHIA COLI*

The DNA replication system of *Escherichia coli* has been reconstituted entirely from purified components. Analysis of this system reveals many similarities with eukaryotic replication, indicating that this process is highly conserved. *E. coli* DNA replication can be subdivided into three phases: initiation, elongation, and termination. Thus far, at least 28 polypeptides are known to be involved.

Initiation *E. coli* chromosomal DNA replication initiates within a 245-bp region, termed *oriC*. This region contains four 9-bp binding sites for the *E. coli* initiator protein, DnaA. Nearby are three repeats of a 13-bp A:T-rich sequence. *oriC* also contains specific binding sites for two small histone-like proteins called HU and IHF. Replication is initiated with the cooperative binding of 10 to 20 DnaA monomers to their specific binding sites (Fig. 45–12). In order to be active, these monomers must each have bound ATP. Binding of DnaA permits unwinding of the DNA at the 13-bp repeats, in a reaction that requires the histone-like proteins. Next, DnaC binds to DnaB and escorts it to the unwound DNA. DnaB is the key helicase that will drive DNA replication by unwinding the double helix, but it binds DNA poorly on its own in the absence of its DnaC escort. Once DnaB has docked onto the DNA, DnaC is released and the helicase can then start to unwind the DNA, provided that ATP, SSB, and DNA gyrase are present. SSB is a single-stranded DNA binding protein that stabilizes the unwound DNA, and DNA gyrase is a topoisomerase (see Chapter 13) that removes the twist that is generated when the two strands of the double helix are separated.

Elongation As in eukaryotes, *E. coli* DNA replication involves a leading strand, with the daughter DNA synthesized as a single continuous molecule, as well as a lagging strand, with the DNA synthesized as discontinuous Okazaki fragments. All daughter strands are started by an RNA primase that deposits primers of 11 ±1 nucleotides. The enzyme that actually synthesizes the DNA is the polymerase III holoenzyme, which has at least 10 subunits. This contains polymerase and proofreading subunits and is held to the DNA by a doughnut-like "sliding clamp" (β). β is loaded onto the DNA by a pentameric complex in a process that requires ATP. The parallel with PCNA and RFC in eukaryotes is striking. Activities specific for the lagging strand include RNase H, which removes the RNA primers;

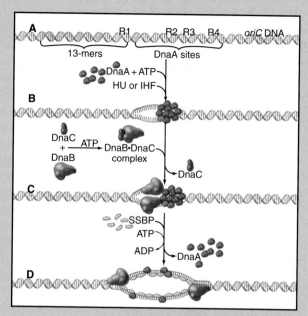

Figure 45–12 Diagram showing factors involved in the initiation of DNA replication in *E. coli*. *A,* DNA sequences at OriC. *B,* Unwinding of the origin. *C,* Binding of helicase. *D,* The template now ready for binding of DNA polymerase. (Adapted from Baker TA, Wickner SH: Genetics and enzymology of DNA replication in *Escherichia coli*. Annu Rev Genet 26:447–477, 1992.)

DNA polymerase I, which fills in the gaps left behind by primer removal; and DNA ligase, which links the Okazaki fragments together. DNA replication in *E. coli* is significantly faster than it is in eukaryotes, with the fork moving at a rate of about 1000 bp per second. This increased speed is presumed to be at least partially attributable to the absence of nucleosomes on the bacterial chromosome.

Termination A specialized termination zone is found on the circular *E. coli* chromosome opposite *oriC*. This zone contains binding sites called *ter* sites, to which the *ter* binding protein binds. This protein appears to block the movement of DNA helicases, such as DnaB, thereby stalling the DNA replication fork. Following termination of replication, a specialized topoisomerase, the product of the *parC* and *parE* genes, is required to separate the daughter chromosomes from one another.

---

merase α and a primase subunit, collectively known as **Pol α/Primase.** Primase synthesizes a complementary RNA chain of about 10 nucleotides to which DNA polymerase α adds another 20 to 30 nucleotides of so-called "initiator DNA" (iDNA) (see Fig. 45–11*D* and *E*). These initiating reactions are potentially hazardous, because DNA polymerase α lacks any proofreading

ability. Any errors in matching up an incoming base would create a mutation. Given the huge number of initiation events required to replicate an entire genome, this potential for errors is not acceptable. Thus, the RNA primer and most or all of the initiator DNA laid down by Pol α/Primase are subsequently replaced (see the discussion that follows).

Once Pol α/Primase has done its job, two further essential factors act. A pentameric protein complex called *r*eplication *f*actor *C* (**RFC**) binds the 3' end of the initiator DNA. RFC uses energy from ATP hydrolysis to load the trimeric protein **PCNA** onto the DNA (see Fig. 45–11*F* and *G*). The PCNA trimer is doughnut-shaped, and when the DNA is inserted into its central hole, it is topologically locked onto the DNA. RFC binding and PCNA loading displace Pol α/Primase from the DNA, and PCNA then recruits **DNA polymerase** δ (and probably also polymerase ϵ) to the DNA. Moving along with the sliding platform of PCNA, these polymerases then process along the DNA, synthesizing DNA continuously on the leading strand (see Fig. 45–11*H*). On the lagging strand, they synthesize about 250 bp of DNA until they run into the next Okazaki fragment. Cdc45p has been suggested to be a scaffolding factor that holds the Mcm hexamer and the replicative DNA polymerases together as the fork moves.

Both polymerases δ and ϵ have associated exonuclease activities. This enables them to proofread the newly synthesized DNA and correct any mistakes that they have made. This may explain the amazing fidelity of DNA replication (with a typical frequency of 1 error per 10^9 base pairs polymerized).

The final steps of DNA replication are removal of the RNA primer (and probably initiator DNA) and ligation of adjacent stretches of newly synthesized DNA. Removal of the primer can be accomplished in two ways (see Fig. 45–11*I*). On the one hand, an RNA exonuclease called **RNase H** can chew in from the 5' end of the primer. However, this enzyme cannot remove the last ribonucleotide that is joined to initiator DNA. That requires a second nuclease, called **Fen1.** Alternatively, Fen1 can do the whole job itself if it gets help from a helicase. In this case, the helicase peels the RNA (and possibly the initiator DNA) away from the template, creating a sort of flap. Fen1 then cleaves at the junction where the flap is peeled away, removing the unwanted nucleotides in one step. In yeast, the participating helicase is called Dna2.

Following removal of initiator RNA, the Pol δ/PCNA complex extends the upstream nascent chain until it runs into the 5' end created by Fen1. DNA ligase I then joins the two stretches of DNA together.

Higher-Order Organization of DNA Replication in the Nucleus

A wide variety of experimental evidence has revealed that the unit of replication in eukaryotic chromosomes is not the individual replicon, but rather a replicon cluster. Evidence for this higher-order organization of

DNA replication within the nucleus was first obtained by fiber autoradiography. Cells were fed radioactive precursors for DNA synthesis and then examined by electron microscopy. (For an explanation of this technique, see Fig. 43–2.) Now it is easier to observe the spatial distribution of DNA replication during the S phase using BrdU, a nucleotide base analogue that is readily incorporated into DNA by the replication machinery in place of thymidine (this is called by its more correct name of Br-dUTP in Fig. 45–13). Incorporation of BrdU into DNA makes the newly synthesized daughter DNA strand heavier, allowing its separation from the parental DNA by centrifugation on a cesium chloride density gradient (see Chapter 5). In addition, specific antibodies recognizing DNA containing either BrdU or the related reagents IdU and CldU can be used to localize the changing patterns of DNA synthesis as cells traverse S phase. More recently, analogs have been developed where the Br in Fig. 45–13*A* has been replaced by a fluorescent group. This allows the newly replicated DNA to be observed directly.

These methods reveal up to 1000 sites of active replication, called **replication foci,** at any one time during S phase in a mammalian cell nucleus (see Fig. 45–13*B, C, E,* and *F*). Given that each of these replication foci is active for only about 1 hour out of the 8- to 10-hour S phase, a cell will replicate DNA at about 10,000 of these foci. Given roughly 60,000 origins in a mammalian cell, each replication focus represents five or six replication origins that are activated coordinately. These replication foci, which have been termed replication factories, may be associated with the nuclear matrix or nucleoskeleton (see Chapter 13).

Temporal Control of Replication During the S Phase

The term "S phase" may give the impression that all DNA replicates more or less synchronously, but this is far from true. At any given time during S phase, only 10% to 15% of the replicons actively synthesize DNA. Some replicate earlier, others later. Importantly, this pattern of replication is not random: some origins consistently replicate early in S phase, whereas others consistently replicate late in S phase. Overall, the human genome can be subdivided into at least 1000 "zones," each of which replicates at a characteristic time during S phase. The organization of replication zones corresponds roughly to the organization of chromosomes into banding patterns: early-replicating regions typically correspond to gene-rich R bands, whereas late-replicating regions typically correspond to gene-poor G-bands (see Fig. 45–13*D;* compare with Fig. 13–9). A similar division of chromosomes

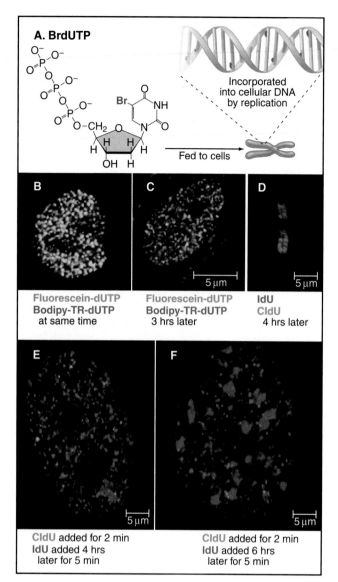

Figure 45–13 Visualization of DNA replication within the nucleus. *A,* The protocol for fluorescent labeling of newly replicated DNA. BrdUTP is introduced into DNA in place of dTTP. The incorporated BrdU molecules are detected by fluorescence labeling with labeled antibodies. *B,* In a related technology, green-dUTP and red-dUTP, when added together, show the many sites of DNA replication in a cell nucleus. Because both UTP analogues are incorporated simultaneously into the DNA, the sites of replication appear yellow. *C,* Green-dUTP is followed by red-dUTP added 3 hours later. The later sites of DNA replication show very little overlap with the earlier sites. *D,* Mitotic chromosome from a cell that was labeled early in S phase with IdU *(green),* and then 4 hours later with CldU *(red).* The late- and early-replicating regions of the chromosome are segregated into discrete bands. *E,* CldU *(green)* added early in S phase and IdU *(red)* added 4 hours later show little overlap. *F,* CldU *(green)* added early in S phase and IdU *(red)* added 6 hours later show no overlap. The large red blocks of labeling seen with the IdU are characteristic of the pattern of replicating heterochromatin seen late in S phase. Bodipy-TR-dUTP, a red fluorescent form of dUTP; BrdUTP, Bromo-deoxyuridine triphosphate; CldU, Chlorine-dUTP; Fluorescein-dUTP, a green fluorescent form of dUTP; IdU, Iodine-dUTP. All are used in place of dTTP (thymidine triphosphate) in DNA synthesis. (*B* and *C,* Courtesy of P. R. Cook, University of Oxford; from Manders EMM, Kimura H, Cook PR: Direct imaging of DNA in living cells reveals the dynamics of chromosome formation. J Cell Biol 144:813–821, 1999. *D,* Courtesy of A. I. Lamond, University of Dundee, Scotland; from Ferreira J, Paolella G, Ramos C, et al: Spatial organization of large-scale chromatin domains in the nucleus: A magnified view of single chromosome territories. J Cell Biol 139:1597–1610. *E* and *F,* From Ma H, Samarabandu J, Devdhar RS, et al: Spatial and temporal dynamics of DNA replication sites in mammalian cells. J Cell Biol 143:1415–1425, 1998. *Journal of Cell Biology* illustrations used by copyright permission of the Rockefeller University Press.)

into early- and late-replicating regions also holds true for budding yeast, although many fewer replication origins are involved.

As described earlier, BrdU labeling experiments show that the basic unit of chromosomal DNA replication is a cluster of about five replication origins that "fire" coordinately. What must now be superimposed on this view of the replicating chromosome is a second level of regulation: the time at which each replicon cluster "fires" during S phase. This can be seen clearly by synchronizing cells at the beginning of S phase, releasing them from cell cycle arrest, and then exposing them to BrdU at various times thereafter. This experiment reveals very distinctive patterns of DNA synthesis occurring at different times during S phase (see Fig. 45–13*B, C, E,* and *F*). Early on, euchromatin replicates throughout the nucleus. Later,

replicating regions appear concentrated around nucleoli and other areas of more condensed chromatin. Then, toward the end of S phase, replication is largely concentrated in blocks of heterochromatin. These observations show that DNA replication occurs throughout the nucleus, wherever DNA is located; DNA does not move to a small number of discrete sites to be replicated (as had been thought).

The most striking aspect of these patterns of DNA synthesis is their reproducibility from one cell cycle to the next. For example, regions of DNA labeled early in S phase overlap little or not at all with DNA labeled 3 hours later (see Fig. 45–13*C* and *E*). However, DNA labeled at corresponding points of S phase in two successive cell cycles superimposes almost entirely. Thus, the chromosomal substructure that gives rise to replication foci is stable from one cell cycle to the next. This strongly suggests that particular regions of chromosomes are organized into reproducible structural domains, and that each domain has a particular "window" during S phase during which it replicates.

The timing of replication of particular replication origins has been studied most carefully in budding yeast. First, a procedure was developed whereby all cells in a population could be induced to enter S phase synchronously. Next, the shift in the density of the DNA following BrdU incorporation was used to distinguish between DNA that had replicated and DNA that had not (Fig. 45–14). It then became relatively simple to take DNA probes from different regions of the chromosome and determine when each replicated

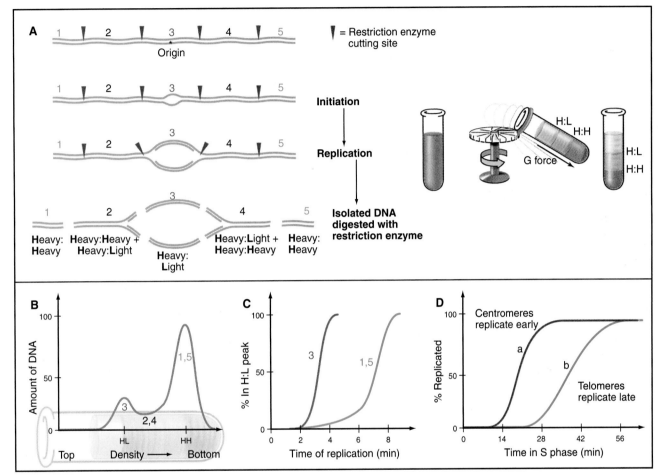

Figure 45-14 *A* to *C,* An experimental protocol that permits measurement of the time of replication of particular chromosomal regions in *Saccharomyces cerevisiae.* This protocol is based on a classical density shift experiment of Messelson and Stahl that proved that DNA replication is semi-conservative. *S. cerevisiae* are grown for several generations in medium containing ^{13}C and ^{15}N heavy isotopes. As a result, their DNA is fully substituted with heavy isotopes. At the beginning of the experiment, the cells are synchronized so that they enter S phase in a single wave. At the same time, the heavy (H) isotope medium is removed and replaced with "light medium" (L) containing ^{12}C and ^{14}N. At various times after the initiation of S phase, aliquots of cells are removed and the DNA is isolated. The DNA is then cleaved with restriction enzymes so that the chromosomes are cut into many fragments. DNA from each time point is then subjected to CsCl density gradient centrifugation. When any local region of DNA is replicated, its density alters from heavy/heavy to heavy/light. After very short incubations with light isotopes, only DNA near the origin of replication will be heavy/light; all other DNA will be heavy/heavy. These two populations of molecules are separated from one another by the density gradient centrifugation. To examine the timing of replication of a specific gene, a cloned segment of DNA corresponding to the region of interest is used to probe (by DNA hybridization) the heavy/heavy and heavy/light peaks from each gradient. The time of replication of each locus is the time at which the restriction fragment being detected by DNA hybridization moves from the heavy/heavy peak to the heavy/light peak. The numbers in panels *B* and *C* refer to the numbered regions of the chromosomes shown in *A. D,* Data from such a replication timing experiment show that, in budding yeast, centromeres replicate early in the S phase and telomeres replicate late. To generate *curve a,* fractions from a gradient like that shown in *B* were hybridized to a cloned centromere region. To generate *curve b,* fractions from the same gradient were hybridized to a cloned telomere region probe. Note that in mammalian cells centromeres replicate late and telomeres replicate earlier.

(changed its density) during S phase. This protocol demonstrated that each ARS element replicates at a characteristic time during S phase.

Two possible explanations for the sequence of replication patterns seen for different chromosomal regions are as follows

1. As mentioned earlier, the involvement of transcription factors in the initiation of DNA replication might give transcriptionally active loci (where these factors are already bound) a head start over other regions of the chromosomes, permitting them to initiate DNA replication first. Thus, local chromatin structures, established as a result of gene expression, might somehow influence the time of replication. This model can explain certain examples in which the timing of replication of a particular locus varies in different cell types. For example, a greater than 200-kb of mammalian DNA domain containing the β-globin gene (encoding the protein component of hemoglobin) is replicated from a single origin lying just upstream of the gene. This domain replicates early in erythroid cells in which the β-globin gene is expressed, but later in nonerythroid cells, in which the gene is inactive.

2. Specific factors may activate particular origins of replication at the correct times during S phase. In yeast, the Cdc7p-Dbf4p kinase must act on later origins of replication for them to "fire." This kinase may permit the binding of Cdc45p and RPA, both of which bind to origins only as they are about to "fire" throughout S phase. In addition, the Rad53p protein kinase regulates firing of late origins of replication in budding yeast. Rad53p (known as Chk2 in higher eukaryotes) is an important component of the DNA damage checkpoint (see Chapter 46). If DNA is damaged during S phase, Rad53 can repress the firing of the late origins, thus preventing completion of the replication of damaged DNA. The G_2 DNA damage checkpoint detects this block to replication and blocks cell cycle progression (see Chapter 46).

Thus, Rad53 appears to be required for the dependence of late origin firing on completion of early replication.

Synthesis of the Histone Proteins

Chromatin contains approximately equal weights of DNA and core histones. Human cells have about 66×10^6 copies of each core histone, assuming a genome size of 6.56×10^9 bp and 200 bp per nucleosome (see Chapter 7). Because about 90% of histone transcription occurs during S phase, enormous amounts of these proteins are made during a relatively brief period. Histone synthesis apparently keeps pace, in part, because there are about 40 sets of histone genes.

Synthesis of histones during the S phase is tightly coupled to ongoing DNA replication. If replication is blocked by either addition of drugs or by temperature-sensitive mutants, histone synthesis declines abruptly shortly thereafter. This link between histone synthesis and DNA replication appears to involve at least three components (Fig. 45–15).

First, *transcription of the histone genes rises* three- to five-fold as cells enter S phase. Each histone gene has a cell cycle–responsive element in its promoter to which a transcription factor binds specifically during S phase.

Second, the *processing of histone mRNAs increases* 6- to 10-fold as cells enter S phase. Histone mRNAs are not polyadenylated, and the primary transcripts are considerably longer than the mature forms. Processing of the 3′ end of histone pre-mRNAs involves the U7 snRNP (see Chapter 15), a portion of which recognizes histone mRNA and base-pairs with it during processing. Cell cycle–dependent regulation of processing appears to involve changes in the accessibility of the necessary portion of U7 snRNA. This region is inaccessible in G_0 cells but becomes accessible when cells that have reentered the cycle begin S phase. The mechanism for this change in RNA conformation is not known. It could involve binding or release of a regu-

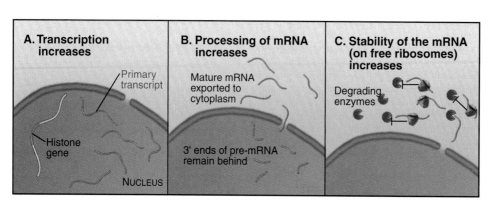

A. Transcription increases

Primary transcript

Histone gene

NUCLEUS

B. Processing of mRNA increases

Mature mRNA exported to cytoplasm

3′ ends of pre-mRNA remain behind

C. Stability of the mRNA (on free ribosomes) increases

Degrading enzymes

Figure 45–15 *A* to *C,* Three ways in which histone expression is elevated during the S phase.

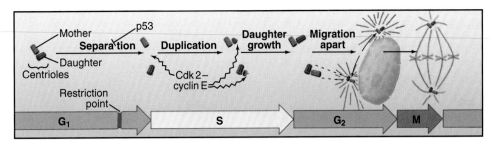

Figure 45–16 The centrosome duplication cycle.

latory factor, or both, or a conformational change in U7 snRNP.

Third, *changes in the stability of the mRNA* also regulate histone synthesis. Normally, the level of histone mRNA on free polysomes drops rapidly by about 35-fold as cells enter G_2 phase. If DNA synthesis is interrupted during the S phase, a region at the 3′ end of the mature message somehow targets the mRNA for degradation. If this region is removed from the 3′ terminus of the histone mRNA, the normal link between ongoing replication and mRNA stability is lost. Furthermore, this sequence, transposed onto the 3′ terminus of a globin mRNA, renders that mRNA sensitive to degradation if DNA synthesis is blocked. Degradation of histone mRNA requires ongoing protein synthesis, and it has been speculated that histones themselves participate in the control.

Duplication of the Centrosomes

Although the bulk of attention on S phase focuses on the duplication of the chromosomes, at least one other essential function required for stability of the genome also occurs at this time. This is duplication of the centrosomes, which will go on at the next mitosis to set up the poles of the mitotic spindle responsible for accurate partitioning of the replicated chromosomes. The "heart" of the centrosome (see Chapter 37) is a pair of centrioles oriented at right angles to one another (Fig. 45–16). These centrioles separate from one another at the beginning of S phase; during the course of S phase, a daughter centriole is assembled at right angles to each mother. Centriole duplication appears to be under the same cell cycle controls as entry into S phase: phosphorylation by the Cdk2–cyclin E or Cdk2–cyclin A kinases is required. It is not yet known which of the more than 100 protein components of centrosomes must be phosphorylated in order to per-

mit centrosomal duplication. Interestingly, it was proposed more than 100 years ago that defects in centrosomal duplication might lead to genomic instability and cancer. Recent results suggest that this is the case, and at least one centrosome-associated protein kinase appears to have undergone abnormal regulation in some cancer cells.

With the completion of DNA replication and duplication of the centrosomes, the cell is ready to divide. First, however, it must conduct one last series of checks to ensure that the genome has been replicated correctly and that no harmful DNA damage has occurred in the interim. These checks, together with other ongoing preparations for mitosis, are the principal events of the G_2 phase (see Chapter 46).

Selected Readings

Baker TA, Wickner SH: Genetics and enzymology of DNA replication in *Escherichia coli*. Annu Rev Genet 26:447–477, 1992.

Donaldson AD, Blow JJ: The regulation of replication origin activation. Curr Opin Genet Dev 9:62–68, 1999.

Doxsey S: Re-evaluating centrosome function. Nature Rev Mol Cell Biol 2:688–698, 2001.

Gilbert DM: Making sense of Eukaryotic DNA replication origins. Science 294:96–100, 2001.

Jónsson ZO, Hübscher U: Proliferating cell nuclear antigen: More than a clamp for DNA polymerases. BioEssays 19:967–975, 1997.

Kearsey SE, Maiorano D, Holmes EC, Todorov IT: The role of MCM proteins in the cell cycle control of genome duplication. BioEssays 18:183–190, 1996.

Leatherwood J: Emerging mechanisms of eukaryotic DNA replication initiation. Curr Opin Cell Biol 10:742–748, 1998.

Stillman B. Cell cycle control of DNA replication. Science 274:1659–1664, 1996.

Waga S, Stillman B: The DNA replication fork in eukaryotic cells. Annu Rev Biochem 67:721–751, 1998.

chapter 46

THE G₂ PHASE AND CONTROL OF ENTRY INTO MITOSIS

The G$_2$ phase was originally defined simply as a gap between the completion of DNA replication and the onset of mitosis. In fact, definition of this phase is not entirely straightforward, as progression from interphase into mitosis is gradual, with early mitotic prophase sharing characteristics of both interphase and mitosis. This chapter defines the G$_2$ phase as the period from the end of S phase until mid-prophase, that is, until activation of the main mitotic kinase, Cdk1–cyclin B1.

The G$_2$ phase has attracted considerable attention owing to recent advances in our understanding of biochemical changes that trigger the transition into mitosis, and because a major G$_2$ checkpoint is often disrupted in cancers. This chapter begins with the biochemical basis for the G$_2$/mitosis (M) transition and concludes with regulation of this transition by the G$_2$ checkpoint.

Enzymology of the G₂/Mitosis Transition

The transition between G$_2$ and mitosis is the most dramatic morphologic and physiological change that occurs during the life of a growing cell, matched only by the dramatic changes that occur during death by apoptosis (see Chapter 49). Entry into mitosis is controlled by a network of stimulatory and inhibitory protein kinases and phosphatases, presided over by Cdk1–cyclin B1. Chapter 43 introduced the components involved in the G$_2$/M transition.

Cdk1, the driving force for entry into mitosis, is present at a constant level throughout the cell cycle and appears to be distributed diffusely throughout the cell. Cdk1 regulation is multifaceted (see Fig. 43–7),

including binding of cyclin cofactors, inhibition and activation by phosphorylation, binding of inhibitory molecules, and changes in subcellular localization.

Mammalian cells have at least three **B-type cyclins:** B1, B2, and B3. Cyclin B1 is essential for triggering the G$_2$/M transition, and disruption of its gene has lethal consequences. Cyclin B1, newly synthesized during the latter part of the cell cycle, accumulates in the cytoplasm, where it appears to be associated with microtubules. This appearance is deceiving, however, as cyclin B1 actively shuttles in and out of the nucleus, being imported by importin β and then rapidly exported to the cytoplasm by Crm1 (see Chapter 16). Cyclin B1 associates with Cdk1 and carries it along on its journeys in and out of the nucleus.

As cells progress through G$_2$ phase to mitosis, Cdk1 first binds its essential cyclin cofactors and then, in quick succession, is activated by a protein kinase called **CAK** (*C*DK-*a*ctivating *k*inase, actually Cdk7–cyclin H) and inactivated by another kinase, **Wee1.** This combination of stimulatory and inhibitory modifications means that Cdk1 is poised for a burst of activation. Ultimately, Cdk1–cyclin B1 is activated during prophase by the **Cdc25** protein phosphatase (see Chapter 27), which removes the inhibitory phosphates and triggers the G$_2$/M transition (Fig. 46–1).

Why did such an elaborate system evolve to regulate the G$_2$/M transition? The answer appears to lie in the exquisite sensitivity provided by such an interlocking network of stimulatory and inhibitory activities. On the one hand, this network ensures a rapid, almost explosive, final transition into mitosis. On the other, it provides a number of ways to delay the G$_2$/M transition if the cell detects damage to chromosomes. Mitosis with chromosomal damage can lead to cell death or cancer.

Kinases acting on Cdk1 are found both in the

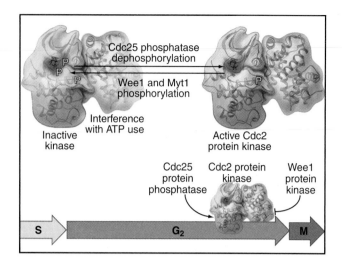

Figure 46-1 Diagram summarizing the role of protein phosphorylation in Cdk regulation during the G₂ phase.

nucleus and cytoplasm. Wee1 and CAK are both located in the nucleus. CAK phosphorylates Cdk1 on T^{161}, triggering a refolding of the active site cleft and rendering the enzyme able to bind to its substrates (see Chapter 43). Activation of Cdk1 by CAK is subsequently counteracted by Wee1 kinase, which phosphorylates Y^{15} adjacent to the adenosine triphosphate (ATP)–binding site, thereby preventing ATP binding and inactivating the enzyme. The Wee1 gene was discovered in *S. pombe*. Wee1-defective yeasts enter mitosis prematurely, dividing when smaller than normal (hence the name *wee*) (Fig. 46–2). A second *S. pombe* kinase, Mik1, also phosphorylates Cdk1. Human Wee1 is actually more similar to Mik1 than Wee1.

At least two cell cycle regulators are localized to the Golgi apparatus: the inhibitory kinase Myt1 and cyclin B2. Myt1 is a Wee1-like enzyme that phosphorylates Cdk1 on both T^{14} and Y^{15}. Golgi-associated Cdk1–cyclin B2 appears to have a single specialized task: disassembly of the Golgi apparatus during mitosis (see Chapter 47). Myt1 probably keeps Cdk1–cyclin B2 inactive during interphase.

Cdc25 phosphatase (see Fig. 27–5), the trigger for the G₂/M transition, is actually a family of three related proteins: Cdc25A, Cdc25B, and Cdc25C. These proteins are regulated both by stimulatory and inhibitory phosphorylation and by alterations in their subcellular localization. Cdc25A has a still mysterious function at the G₁/S transition. Cdc25B and Cdc25C have independent roles in the G₂/M transition.

The dual-specificity protein phosphatase Cdc25C removes phosphates from serine (S), threonine (T), and tyrosine (Y) residues, including the inhibitory phosphates from T^{14} and Y^{15} of Cdk1. Cdc25C is relatively inactive during interphase for two reasons. First, phosphorylation on two residues (S216 and S287) creates binding sites for a protein called 14-3-3 (see Fig. 27–11). This seems to inhibit nuclear import of Cdc25C, in some cases causing the protein to accumulate in the cytoplasm. Second, to be fully activated, Cdc25 requires phosphorylation of its amino-terminal region. This is triggered by a protein kinase called Polo (see next paragraph), and then completed by its substrate, Cdk1–cyclin B1, creating a powerful positive feedback amplification loop that provides the burst of CDK activity that triggers entry into mitosis.

Since Cdk1–cyclin B1 is inactive unless activated by a Cdc25 phosphatase, a molecular trigger is required to start the amplification cycle. **Polo** family kinases are one candidate to activate Cdc25C. Polo family kinases are involved in a variety of mitotic events, including formation of a bipolar spindle, cytokinesis, and passage through certain cell cycle checkpoints. These kinases, which reside at the centrosome during interphase, are still poorly understood, and little is known about their relevant substrates other than

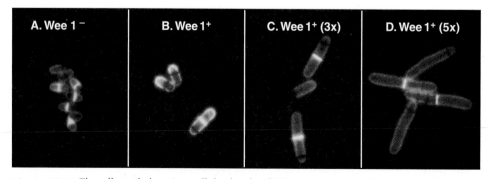

Figure 46-2 The effect of changing cellular levels of Wee1 protein on cell cycle progression in fission yeast. *A*, cells lacking functional Wee1 protein enter mitosis too soon in the cell cycle and are smaller than wild-type cells *(B)*. *C* and *D*, cells expressing excess Wee1 protein are too effective at inactivating Cdk1 and are severely delayed in their ability to enter mitosis (hence, their larger size). (From Russell P, Nurse P: Negative regulation of mitosis by Wee1+, a gene encoding a protein kinase homolog. Cell 49:559–567, 1987. Copyright 1987, with permission from Elsevier Science.)

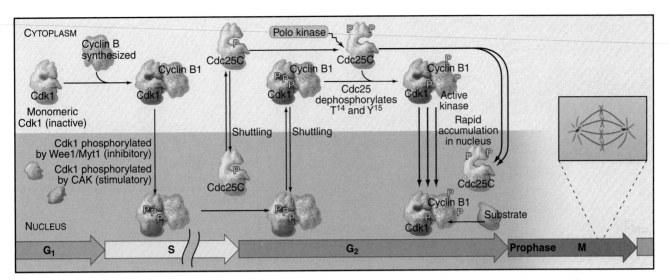

Figure 46–3 Summary of the roles of protein phosphorylation and subcellular localization in regulating the onset of mitosis.

Cdc25. Cdc25B participates in a second mechanism to trigger the Cdk1–cyclin B1/Cdc25C amplification cycle. Cdc25B is activated much earlier in the cell cycle than Cdc25C, with activity first detected in late S phase, and peaking during G₂ phase. Thus, this phosphatase is well positioned to initiate the G₂/M transition. Cdc25B activity is limited in S and G₂ phases when its concentration is kept low, in part owing to its short half-life of less than 30 minutes. Overexpression of Cdc25B during S or G₂ phase is sufficient to push cells prematurely into mitosis. Fig. 46–3 summarizes the network regulating Cdk1–cyclin B activation. The experimental systems used in the discovery of many of these factors are introduced in Box 46–1.

Changes in Subcellular Localization at the G₂/M Transition

The mechanism by which cells achieve the burst of Cdk1–cyclin B1 activity that pushes them over the brink from G₂ into M phase is not known. It was originally thought that this worked by keeping the critical components segregated during interphase, and then rapidly bringing them together in the cell nucleus to initiate the G₂/M transition. However, this model is inconsistent with the observation that cell-free extracts prepared from *Xenopus* eggs can undergo periodic cycles of Cdk1 activation and inactivation in the absence of any nuclei.

Three key factors involved in the G₂/M transition move continually throughout interphase (see Fig. 46–3). Cyclin B1 (with associated Cdk1), Cdc25C, and Cdc25B have both nuclear import and nuclear export signals, so they shuttle in and out of the nucleus.

During interphase, all three spend most of their time in the cytoplasm. Inhibitory phosphorylations of Cdk1 and Cdc25C keep Cdk1 activity low.

Early in prophase, phosphorylation of cyclin B1 inactivates its nuclear export signal (see Chapter 16), allowing Cdk1–cyclin B1 to accumulate rapidly in the nucleus within 5 minutes (Fig. 46–8). Cdc25C also stops shuttling at the G₂/M transition, probably as a result of phosphorylation, apparently by Polo kinase. The best evidence seems to indicate that the Cdk1–cyclin B that accumulates in the nucleus is already active, but it may be that restriction of Cdk–cyclin B complex to the nucleus together with Cdc25C significantly increases their local concentration (the volume of the nucleus is much less than the volume of the cytoplasm) and may contribute to the final burst of Cdk1–cyclin B1 activation.

Cdk2–Cyclin A and the Initiation of Prophase

As noted in Chapter 45, Cdk2–cyclin A plays a critical role during S phase. Several lines of evidence have revealed that this enzyme also helps to trigger the G₂/M transition. First, inactivation of cyclin A, either by mutation in *Drosophila* or by injection of anti–cyclin A antibodies into cultured cells, arrests the cell cycle in G₂. Second, Cdk2–cyclin A activity peaks at G₂/M, before the peak of Cdk1–cyclin B1 activity. Finally, if activated Cdk2–cyclin A complexes are injected into cells just after completion of S phase, cells enter mitosis prematurely.

Cdk2–cyclin A is likely to regulate several events

box 46–1

DISCOVERY OF FACTORS ESSENTIAL FOR THE G₂/MITOSIS TRANSITION

The best early evidence for the existence of an inducer of the G_2/M transition was obtained when mitotic cells were physically fused with interphase cells in culture. This caused the interphase cells to enter into mitosis abruptly (as judged by nuclear envelope breakdown and chromosome condensation). The phenomenon was termed **premature chromosome condensation (PCC)**. The mitotic inducer could work in any cell cycle phase (Fig. 46–4). If mitotic cells were fused with cells in G_1 phase, interphase chromosomes condensed into long, single filaments. If the interphase cell was in G_2 phase, double filaments were seen. If the interphase cell was in the S phase, a complex pattern of single and double condensed regions was seen. These were separated by regions of decondensed chromatin corresponding to sites of active DNA replication at the time of fusion.

Working independently, developmental biologists interested in the control of cell division during early development in frogs also discovered an activity that could cause interphase cells (in this case, oocytes) to enter the M phase. They found that oocyte maturation (nuclear envelope breakdown and chromosome condensation) could be induced experimentally by microinjection of the cytoplasm of mature eggs (which are arrested in the metaphase of meiosis II) into oocytes (which are in G_2 phase). The active factor in egg cytoplasm was called **MPF (maturation-promoting factor)** (Fig. 46–5). It was realized early on that MPF might be related to the inducer of mitosis detected in the PCC experiments. In fact, extracts from mitotic tissue culture cells could induce meiotic maturation when injected into oocytes. Similar extracts from cells in other phases

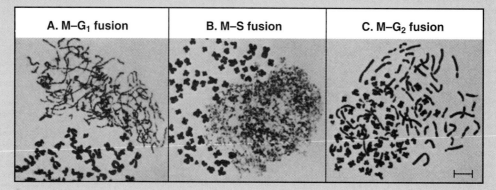

Figure 46–4 Fusion of mitotic and interphase cells causes the interphase cells to enter mitosis prematurely, no matter where they are in the cell cycle. The resulting prematurely condensed chromosomes are single threads if the interphase cell was in G_1 phase *(A)*, or double threads if the cell was in G_2 phase *(C)*, and a complex mixture of both interspersed with uncondensed regions if the cell was in S phase *(B)*. (From Hanks SK, Gollin SM, Rao PN, et al.: Cell cycle-specific changes in the ultrastructural organization of prematurely condensed chromosomes. Chromosoma 88:333–342, 1983.)

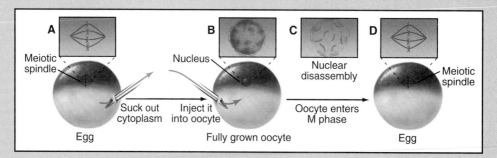

Figure 46–5 Diagram of the experimental protocol that identified MPF. *A*, The box shows the meiotic spindle in a *Xenopus* egg arrested in metaphase II of meiosis. *B*, The box shows the interphase nucleus in a mature oocyte. Following injection of MPF, the nucleus disassembles (*C*, and the cell assembles a meiotic spindle (*D*). Disassembly of the oocyte nucleus and entry into M phase is called maturation, and the factor triggering this event was named maturation promoting factor, or MPF.

box 46-1

DISCOVERY OF FACTORS ESSENTIAL FOR THE G₂/MITOSIS TRANSITION *Continued*

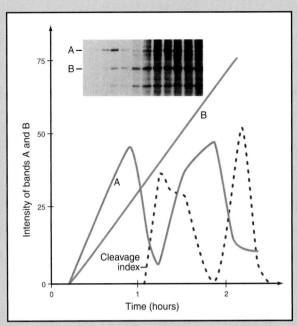

Figure 46-6 The original identification of a cyclin. Newly synthesized proteins (labeled with ³⁵S-methionine) in fertilized sea urchin eggs were separated by SDS polyacrylamide gel electrophoresis. It was noted that the protein-labeled A (which was named cyclin) accumulated, was greatly reduced at the metaphase/anaphase transition, and then began to accumulate again. Protein B, which is not involved in cell cycle regulation, accumulated progressively over this time. (From Evans T, Rosenthal ET, Youngblom J, et al: Cyclin: A protein specified by maternal mRNA in sea urchin eggs that is destroyed at each cleavage division. Cell 33:389–396, 1983. Copyright 1983, with permission from Elsevier Science.)

of the cell cycle did not cause the G₂/mitosis transition in oocytes.

Other developmental biologists studying protein synthesis in starfish and sea urchin embryos noticed a curious protein that seemed to accumulate across the cell cycle, but was then destroyed during mitosis. They were well aware of the work on MPF, and immediately suspected that their protein, which they called cyclin, might be somehow involved in MPF activity (Fig. 46-6).

In a third line of investigation, geneticists working on yeasts realized that the cell cycle could be dissected through the isolation of specific mutants, called CDC (*cell division cycle*) mutants. These studies were carried out in parallel in *Saccharomyces cerevisiae,* which has a very short G₂ phase and is ideal for the analysis of G₁ events, and *Schizosaccharomyces pombe,* which has a very short G₁ phase and is ideal for the analysis of G₂

events. The analysis of the cell cycle with these mutants dominated cell cycle research to the extent that many human genes important in cell cycle control bear the CDC name if they are related to well-characterized yeast genes. The best known genes to come out of this analysis were *Cdc2* and *Cdc25,* both of which were determined genetically to encode proteins that actively promote the G₂/M transition. Other genes, such as *Wee1,* were found to encode activities that act as antagonists that inhibit the G₂/M transition.

When active MPF was eventually purified from *Xenopus* eggs (Fig. 46-7), the purified fractions turned out to consist primarily of two polypeptide chains of 45,000 D and 32,000 D. The 32,000-D component of MPF is the *Xenopus* equivalent of the fission yeast Cdc2 (now known as Cdk1) gene product. The 45,000-D component of MPF is a *Xenopus* B-type cyclin.

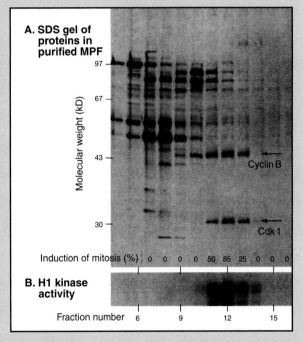

Figure 46-7 Purification of MPF *(A).* This shows an SDS polyacrylamide gel of the column fractions from the final column used in purification. The numbers at the bottom show the percentage of oocytes that entered M phase when a portion of each column fraction was injected (the classical MPF assay). The roughly 32-kD band is Cdk1 (p34^cdc2^). The roughly 45-kD band is cyclin B. *B,* This shows the ability of the various column fractions to phosphorylate histone Hl. This is the standard assay for active Cdk enzymes. (Redrawn from Lohka M, Hayes MK, Maller JL: Purification of maturation-promoting factor, an intracellular regulator of early mitotic events. Proc Natl Acad Sci (USA) 85:3009–3013, 1988.)

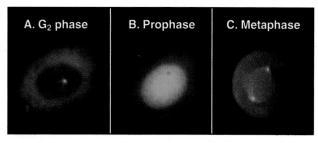

Figure 46-8 *A to C,* Rapid movement of cyclin B1 from the cytoplasm into the nucleus at the onset of prophase, and subsequent association with the spindle during mitosis. (Courtesy of Christina Karlsson and Jonathon Pines, Wellcome/CRC Institute, Cambridge, England.)

at the transition from the G_2 phase to prophase, including changes in microtubule behavior and chromosome condensation. Late in G_2, the half-life of microtubules drops dramatically from about 10 minutes to about 30 seconds (see Chapter 47). This, coupled with enhanced ability of centrosomes to initiate microtubule polymerization, completely transforms the organization of the microtubule cytoskeleton. Centrosomes take on the appearance of spindle poles and migrate apart over the surface of the nucleus. At the same time, chromatin begins to condense in the nucleus. The mechanism of chromosome condensation is not known, but a protein complex called condensin is likely to be involved (see Chapter 13). Condensin does not associate tightly with chromosomes during interphase; association with chromosomes requires phosphorylation of two of its subunits by a CDK. This occurs at G_2/M. As chromosomes condense, several mitosis-specific kinetochore proteins move into the nucleus and associate with kinetochores (see Chapter 12).

These events occur while most Cdk1–cyclin B1 is in the cytoplasm. It is, therefore, likely that Cdk2–cyclin A triggers at least the nuclear events of prophase (Fig. 46–9). In fact, microinjection of a specific inhibitor of Cdk2–cyclin A causes prophase cells to return rapidly to interphase: chromosomes decondense, rounded prophase cells flatten, and the interphase microtubule network returns. Commitment to mitosis appears to be irreversible only after Cdk1–cyclin B1 enters the nucleus.

∎ Summary of the Main Events of the G₂/M Transition

Synthesis of cyclin B1 in the latter portion of the S and G_2 phases leads to assembly of Cdk1–cyclin B dimers. This enzyme shuttles in and out of the nucleus, spending most of its time in the cytoplasm associated with microtubules (Fig. 46–10). In late S and G_2 phases, activation of Cdc25B activates Cdk1–cyclin A, which initiates mitotic prophase, beginning with changes in microtubule dynamics and chromosome condensation. Two events trigger entry into the active phase of mitosis. First, a kinase (possibly more than one) phosphorylates Cdc25C. This both activates it and prevents it from shuttling, causing it to accumulate in the nucleus. Second, another kinase (or kinases) phosphorylates cyclin B1, blocking its export from the nucleus and causing Cdk1–cyclin B1 to accumulate rapidly in the nucleus. Cdc25C activates Cdk1–cyclin B1 by removing inhibitory phosphates on T^{14} and Y^{15}. This starts in the cytoplasm and then may be stimulated as the two proteins concentrate in the nucleus. There, the action of Cdk1–cyclin B1 on the

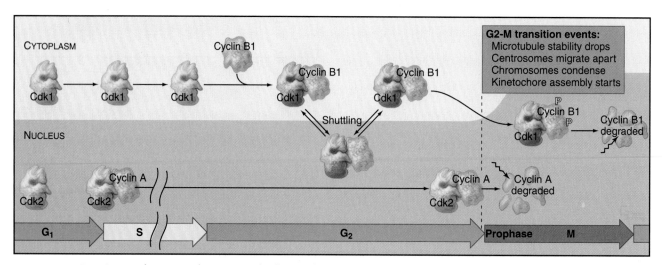

Figure 46-9 Locations and patterns of activation of Cdk2–cyclin A versus Cdk1–cyclin B.

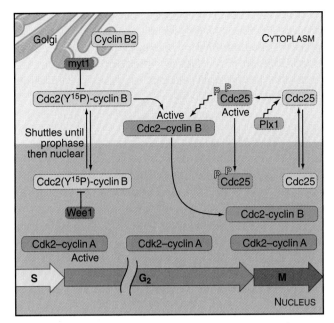

Figure 46-10 Summary of the Cdk regulation mechanism. Plx1, Polo kinase.

nuclear lamina triggers nuclear envelope breakdown and drives the cell into mitosis.

The G₂ Checkpoint

Chapter 44 explained the critical decision each cell makes in G₁ phase: whether to initiate a new cycle of proliferation or to stop cycling and differentiate. A second major decision is required in the G₂ phase: whether it is safe to enter mitosis and separate sister chromatids. Separation of sister chromatids is a potential danger point for a cell. If DNA is damaged after it is replicated, the cell can use information present in sister chromatids (which would have one good copy and one bad copy) to guide the repair process. However, once sisters are separated, such a corrective mechanism is impossible. In addition, if a cell enters mitosis before completing replication of its chromosomes, the attempt to separate sister chromatids results in extensive chromosomal damage. To minimize these hazards, cells use a major checkpoint late in the G₂ phase to stop the cycle if DNA is damaged or DNA replication is incomplete.

Exposure of cells to agents that damage DNA, including certain chemicals or ionizing radiation, halts the cell cycle temporarily in the G₂ phase. This **G₂ delay** gives cells an opportunity to repair damaged DNA before entering mitosis. Studies of radiation-induced G₂ delay in budding yeast have identified a major cell cycle checkpoint in G₂ with which the cell

monitors the status of its DNA. Cells defective in this checkpoint are much more sensitive to radiation injury than wild-type cells because they continue to divide, despite the presence of broken or otherwise damaged chromosomes (Fig. 46–11). This continued division leads to cell death, presumably due to accumulated chromosomal defects, as well as chromosome loss.

The G₂ checkpoint is also responsible for monitoring the completion of DNA replication. Remarkably, this aspect of the checkpoint even works in vitro in cell-free extracts. As described in Chapter 43, highly concentrated extracts made from *Xenopus* eggs can be induced to undergo a cyclic alteration in cell cycle phases, even in the absence of added nuclei. Passage through the different phases can be followed by

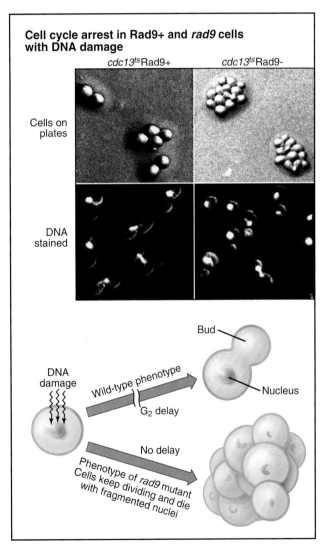

Figure 46-11 Cells defective in the G₂ checkpoint (*Rad9* mutants of budding yeast) cannot delay their entry into mitosis in the presence of damaged DNA, and thus divide themselves to death. (Courtesy of Ted Weinert, University of Arizona, Tucson.)

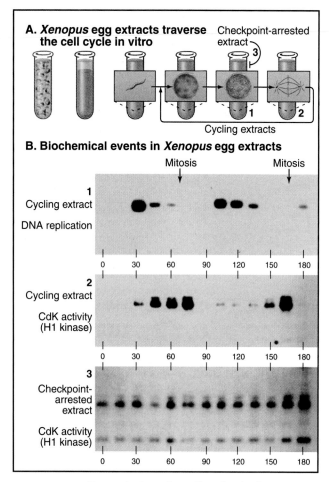

A. *Xenopus* egg extracts traverse the cell cycle in vitro   Checkpoint-arrested extract

Cycling extracts

B. Biochemical events in *Xenopus* egg extracts

Figure 46–12 Reconstitution of a cell cycle checkpoint in vitro. *A,* Cell cycle transitions in a cell-free extract. *B (panel 1),* DNA replication was measured by adding ³²P-labeled dCTP to the extract and subsequently isolating the DNA, running it in a gel, and detecting incorporation of the radioactive label by autoradiography. *Panel 2,* Cdk1–cyclin B activity was assayed based on the ability of active enzyme to phosphorylate added histone H1 (which was likewise subjected to gel electrophoresis and autoradiography). These panels show that DNA replication and Cdk activity alternate in these in vitro cell cycles. Cdk activity declines precipitously at the end of mitosis. *Panel 3,* If the concentration of nuclei is increased beyond a threshold level and an inhibitor of DNA replication is added, the G₂ checkpoint detects the partly replicated DNA and stops the extract from entering mitosis. Cdk activity now remains at about 10% of the level needed to trigger mitosis. (*B,* Redrawn from Dasso M, Newport JW: Completion of DNA replication is monitored by a feedback system that controls the initiation of mitosis in vitro: Studies in *Xenopus*. Cell 61:811–823, 1990. Copyright 1990, with permission from Elsevier Science.)

monitoring the activity of Cdk1–cyclin B kinase, which is high in mitosis and low in interphase. In the absence of nuclei, an inhibitor of DNA polymerases (such as the fungal toxin aphidicolin) has no effect on such extracts, which continue to cycle unabated between S and M phases. On the other hand, if the extract contains more than 400 nuclei/μL undergoing

synchronous cycles of DNA replication and mitosis, aphidicolin brings the cycling to a halt before M phase. This experiment appears to reconstitute the G₂ checkpoint in vitro (Fig. 46–12). Furthermore, it suggests that partly replicated nuclei release an inhibitory signal that stops the cycle.

▌G₂ Checkpoint and Cancer

Defects in the G₂ checkpoint are associated with cancer. This may seem strange, as cells do not reach the G₂ phase unless they are already committed to a cycle of proliferation. In fact, mistakes that occur during mitosis most likely lead to cancer when they disrupt the function of the G₁ checkpoint in the next cell cycle. This is probably best understood in terms of one or two specific examples.

Suppose a cell receives a dose of radiation that damages a nucleotide base in the gene for the retinoblastoma susceptibility protein (pRb; see Chapter 44). If this damage happens in the S or G₂ phases, information in the undamaged copy of the gene may be used to repair the damage. Delaying the cell cycle increases the chance of successful repair. On the other hand, if the checkpoint fails, the cell enters mitosis, sister chromatids are separated from one another, and this damage is never repaired. As a consequence, one daughter cell from that division has a defective pRb gene, impairing its ability to regulate its growth at the restriction point in the next G₁ phase. Loss of tumor suppressor genes like pRb and p53 is a major cause of cancer (see Chapter 43).

In a second scenario, suppose that a cell enters mitosis after receiving a dose of ionizing radiation that has broken several chromosomes. Broken chromosome ends are unstable in cells, and there is a strong possibility that they will either join up with other broken chromosomes or be inserted into regions of intact chromosomes. One consequence might be the fusion of a region of one chromosome that contains sequences that specify the high-level production of a gene product with a region of another chromosome that encodes a gene product that is normally expressed only at very low levels. This sounds unlikely, but actually is not rare. A famous case is **Burkitt's lymphoma,** in which the gene encoding c-myc (a potent promoter of cell proliferation) from chromosome 8 is inserted into the immunoglobulin heavy chain gene cluster on chromosome 14. Immunoglobulins are expressed at high levels in B lymphocytes, and this chromosome translocation results in lymphoma, a cancer of lymphocytes.

The G₂ checkpoint avoids these problems by detecting DNA damage and either delaying entry into mitosis until the damage is fixed or triggering cell suicide by apoptosis. The checkpoint works by modulating the activities of the components that control the G_2/M transition.

How the G₂ Checkpoint Works

The G_2 checkpoint involves three sorts of components: sensors, kinases, and effectors. When sensors detect damage to DNA, they become activated. In turn, they activate specialized protein kinases that transmit this information to a series of effector molecules. Effectors then either directly or indirectly block cell cycle progression.

Most of the components involved in the G_2 checkpoint have been identified in genetic studies of yeasts. *Rad* (radiation-sensitive) genes are so named because mutants are ultrasensitive to ionizing radiation. Many, but not all, Rad mutants are defective in the DNA damage checkpoint. *Hus* (hydroxyurea-sensitive, hydroxyurea being an inhibitor of DNA replication) mutants are unable to detect unreplicated DNA and are defective in the DNA replication checkpoint. Rad and Hus checkpoints operate in parallel, and are usually lumped together under the terms **"G₂ checkpoint"** or **"DNA structure checkpoint."** Many, but not all, components are shared by these two checkpoint pathways.

Little is known about how sensors for the G_2 checkpoint work (Fig. 46–13). At least five genes are involved in sensing DNA damage. Three of these—hRad9, hRad1, and hHus1—form a complex in humans. Detailed analysis of the sequences of these proteins has revealed similarities to PCNA, an essential cofactor of DNA polymerase δ/ϵ (see Chapter 45) that also has a key role in DNA damage repair. PCNA (proliferating cell nuclear antigen) is a toroidal (doughnut-shaped) trimeric molecule that surrounds the DNA and slides along it. The hRad9, hRad1, and hHus1 trimer may form a similar structure that somehow detects DNA damage as it slides along DNA.

Rad17 protein shares some similarities with a component of replication factor C (RFC), an essential pentameric DNA replication factor, which loads PCNA onto DNA. Perhaps Rad17 combines with bona fide RFC components to load the hRad9, hRad1, and hHus1 trimer onto DNA. This speculation is supported by the observation that mutants in four of the RFC subunits are defective in G_2 checkpoint control in yeasts and *Drosophila*.

Having detected damage, the various sensors transmit this information to a family of very large proteins kinases (>2000 amino acids) that resemble the lipid kinase phosphatidylinositol 3-kinase (see Chapters 28 and 29). Rather than phosphorylating phospha-

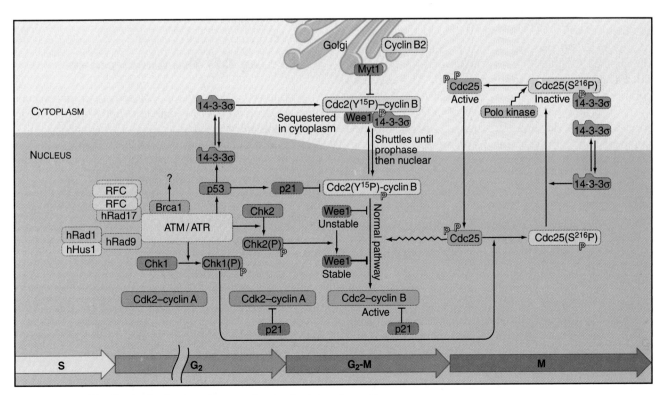

Figure 46-13 The G_2 checkpoint is an integrated network of signaling pathways.

tidylinositol, these G$_2$ checkpoint kinases phosphorylate proteins that stop the G$_2$/M transition. The best known of these G$_2$ checkpoint kinases is **ATM**, encoded by the gene defective in the human inherited disorder **ataxia-telangiectasia.** Ataxia-telangiectasia is complex, characterized by (among other things) premature aging, sensitivity to ionizing radiation, and an elevated risk of cancer. Evidence that ATM is important for checkpoint controls comes from the observation that caffeine, a molecule that can override cell cycle checkpoints in cultured cells, is a relatively specific inhibitor of ATM. Another member of the inositol 1,4,5-triphosphate (IP-3) kinase family, ATR (ataxia-telangiectasia and Rad3–related), is also involved in G$_2$ checkpoint control but may also have other roles, as it is essential for cellular life.

When ATM and ATR are informed of DNA damage, they phosphorylate at least two important substrates: the famous tumor suppressor protein **p53,** and a protein kinase called **Chk1** (*ch*eckpoint *k*inase 1). Chk1 is activated by phosphorylation and then it, in turn, phosphorylates the essential mitotic inducer Cdc25C on S^{216}. This has two consequences. First, it inhibits the activity of Cdc25C. This is thought to be the major mechanism of Cdc25C inactivation by the G$_2$ checkpoint. Second it produces a binding site for a member of the 14-3-3 group of adapter proteins (see Fig. 27–11). These proteins bind sites on target proteins containing serines flanked by several other characteristic amino acids, but only when the critical serine is phosphorylated. This is an example of the general mechanism whereby phosphorylation regulates interactions between proteins in response to physiological signals (see Chapter 27). As a result of 14-3-3-binding, Cdc25C is sequestered in the cytoplasm. This may also contribute to blocking the G$_2$/M transition.

p53 is another major target of ATM/ATR in response to DNA damage. Although p53 is not required to arrest the cell cycle in G$_2$ phase in response to DNA damage, it is absolutely required to prolong this cell cycle arrest. p53 regulates expression of proteins important for the G$_2$ checkpoint. One is **p21,** which inhibits Cdk1–cyclin A 100-fold better than it inhibits Cdk1–cyclin B1. p21 expression provides an effective way of blocking the initiation of prophase by Cdk1–cyclin A. p21 also participates in the G$_1$ DNA damage checkpoint. A second target of p53 in the G$_2$ checkpoint is another 14-3-3 protein, 14-3-3σ. 14-3-3σ binds Cdk1–cyclin B1 and interferes with its ability to shuttle between the nucleus and cytoplasm. As a result, Cdk1–cyclin B1 remains in the cytoplasm. The 14-3-3σ/Cdk1–cyclin B1 complex also contains the Wee1 inhibitory kinase, apparently providing a further level of assurance that cyclin B1–associated Cdk1 kinase remains inactive. Disruption of the gene for 14-3-3σ is fatal for cells if they sustain DNA damage. Instead of

activating their G$_2$ checkpoint, they enter an aberrant state with characteristics of both mitosis and apoptosis, and then die.

In yeasts, Chk1 is required only for the DNA damage checkpoint. If its gene is inactivated, the checkpoint that blocks G$_2$/M in response to incomplete DNA replication remains fully functional. A genetic screen for components of the replication checkpoint pathway has revealed a kinase known in humans as Chk2. Like Chk1, Chk2 is activated by the ATM/ATR kinases. Activated Chk2 phosphorylates Wee1 kinase, which normally inhibits Cdk1–cyclin B1, causing a significant stimulation in its activity. This is likely to result, at least in part, from stabilizing the Wee1 kinase, a target of the SCF/proteasome protein degradation pathway (see Chapters 24 and 44). This stimulation of Wee 1 activity promotes inactivation of Cdk1, thereby inhibiting the G$_2$/M transition. Mutations in the Chk2 gene are associated with Li-Fraumeni syndrome (a cancer-related syndrome originally shown to be associated with mutations in the p53 gene), suggesting that this kinase may function in both the replication and DNA damage checkpoints.

Rapid progress is being made in understanding checkpoint control in response to DNA damage, and it is likely that many new targets of the ATM/ATR kinase signaling pathway will be identified. However, our present body of knowledge has afforded an appreciation for the strategies that cells use to block the G$_2$/M transition in response to problems with the structure or replication of DNA.

▮ Turning Off the Checkpoint

The ability to block the G$_2$/M transition gives cells time to deal with DNA damage, but equally importantly, cells must be able to turn off this checkpoint if and when the damage is repaired. How this is done is still a mystery. The mechanism may be passive. The signaling pathways that activate ATM/ATR and turn on the G$_2$ checkpoint pathway appear to depend upon phosphorylation of sensor molecules. If these activating phosphate groups are continuously being removed by competing phosphatases, then the signal blocking cell cycle progression will decay automatically following repair of the damage.

Limited evidence suggests that more active factors may also contribute to termination of G$_2$ checkpoint arrest. The Polo protein kinase phosphorylates Ccd25C, which has been previously phosphorylated on S^{216} by Chk1 and is held in the cytoplasm in a complex with 14-3-3 protein. Phosphorylation of Cdc25C by the polo-like kinase disrupts the binding of 14-3-3 protein. This appears to directly promote activation of the Cdc25C, and also enables it to again shuttle into the nucleus. Overcoming checkpoint arrests may be a major job of polo-like kinases.

Transition to Mitosis

The complex web of stimulatory and inhibitory activities that regulate CDK activity in the G_2 phase enables an exquisite control of the G_2/M transition. On the one hand, it poises Cdk1–cyclin B in a state ready for the explosive burst of activation that triggers the G_2/M transition. At the same time, the complex pathway affords many points at which the process may be regulated. These are the basis of the G_2 checkpoint control that prevents cells from segregating their chromosomes until genomic DNA has passed stringent quality control standards. Eventually, however, if all goes well, Cdk1–cyclin B1 is activated, and the cell embarks on mitosis, probably the most dramatic event of its life.

Selected Readings

Johnson DG, Walker CL: Cyclins and cell cycle checkpoints. Annu Rev Pharmacol Toxicol 39:295–312, 1999.

Kitazono A, Matsumoto T: "Isogaba Maware": Quality control of genome DNA by checkpoints. BioEssays 20:391–399, 1998.

Morgan DO: Cyclin-dependent kinases: Engines, clocks and microprocessors. Annu Rev Cell Biol 13:261–291, 1997.

Nigg EA: Cell division: Mitotic kinases as regulators of cell division and its checkpoints. Nat Rev Mol Cell Biol 2: 21–32, 2001.

O'Connell MJ, Walworth NC, Carr AM: The G2-phase DNA-damage checkpoint. Trends Cell Biol 10:296–303, 2000.

Ohi R, Gould KL: Regulating the onset of mitosis. Curr Opin Cell Biol 11:267–273, 1999.

Pines J: Four-dimensional control of the cell cycle. Nat Cell Biol 1:E73–E79, 1999.

Smits VA, Medema RH: Checking out the G(2)/M transition. Biochim Biophys Acta 1519:1–12, 2001.

Wahl GM, Carr AM: The evolution of diverse biological responses to DNA damage: Insights from yeast and p53. Nat Cell Biol 3:E277–E286, 2001.

Weinert T: DNA damage and checkpoint pathways: Molecular anatomy and interactions with repair. Cell 94:555–558, 1998.

chapter 47

MITOSIS

The division of a somatic cell into two daughter cells is called mitosis. The daughters are usually identical copies of the parent cell, but the process can be asymmetrical. For example, division of stem cells gives rise to one stem cell and another daughter cell that goes on to mature into a differentiated cell, such as those in blood (see Fig. 30–7).

Mitosis involves a dramatic reorganization of both the nucleus and cytoplasm brought about by activation of a number of protein kinases, including Cdk1–cyclin B–p9 (see Chapter 43). After activation in the cytoplasm by Cdc25 phosphatase, Cdk1–cyclin B–p9 migrates into the nucleus where it joins Cdk1–cyclin A, which was activated somewhat earlier (see Chapter 46). These two Cdk1 kinase complexes operate both at an executive level as master controllers, and as workhorses that directly phosphorylate many proteins whose functional and structural status is altered during mitosis.

Mitosis is an ancient eukaryotic process, and a number of variations emerged during evolution. Many single-celled eukaryotes, including yeast and slime molds, undergo a **closed mitosis**, in which spindle formation and chromosome segregation occur within an intact nuclear envelope (to which the spindle poles are anchored). This chapter focuses on **open mitosis**, as used by most plants and animals, in which the nuclear envelope disassembles before the chromosomes segregate. For convenience of discussion, mitotic events are subdivided into six phases: **prophase**, **prometaphase**, **metaphase**, **anaphase**, **telophase** and **cytokinesis** (Fig. 47–1). This chapter describes each of these phases in turn.

Prophase

Prophase, the transition from G_2 into mitosis, begins with the first visible condensation of the chromosomes and disassembly of the nucleolus (Fig. 47–2). In the cytoplasm, the interphase network of long microtubules centered around a single centrosome is converted into two radial arrays of short microtubules surrounding the duplicated centrioles and their associated centrosomal material (see Chapter 37). These two **asters** separate by migrating over the surface of the nucleus. Most types of intermediate filaments disassemble, the Golgi and endoplasmic reticulum fragment, and both endocytosis and exocytosis are curtailed.

Nuclear Changes in Prophase

Chromosome condensation, the landmark event at the onset of prophase, often begins in isolated patches of chromatin at the nuclear periphery. Later, chromosomes condense into distinct paired threads, termed **sister chromatids**, which are closely paired along their entire length. Although chromosome condensation was first observed more than a century ago, the biochemical mechanism is just beginning to be understood.

Condensin, a complex of five proteins, is a major constituent of mitotic chromosomes, and it appears to have a key role in mitotic chromosome condensation (see Chapter 13; Fig. 47–3). Phosphorylation of two condensin subunits by Cdk1–cyclin B–p9 stimulates their entry into the nucleus and association with chromatin as cells enter prophase. Condensin was discovered in a study of proteins that associated with mitotic

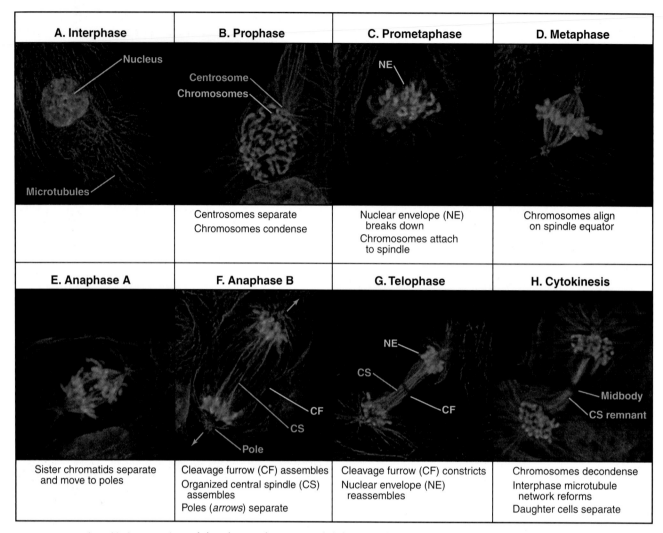

A. Interphase	**B. Prophase**	**C. Prometaphase**	**D. Metaphase**
	Centrosomes separate Chromosomes condense	Nuclear envelope (NE) breaks down Chromosomes attach to spindle	Chromosomes align on spindle equator
E. Anaphase A	**F. Anaphase B**	**G. Telophase**	**H. Cytokinesis**
Sister chromatids separate and move to poles	Cleavage furrow (CF) assembles Organized central spindle (CS) assembles Poles (*arrows*) separate	Cleavage furrow (CF) constricts Nuclear envelope (NE) reassembles	Chromosomes decondense Interphase microtubule network reforms Daughter cells separate

Figure 47-1 *A to H,* An overview of the phases of mitosis and definition of the most important terms. *Prophase—prometaphase,* The Cdk1 kinases trigger condensation of replicated sister chromatids, disassembly of the nuclear envelope and Golgi, and a dramatic reorganization of the cytoskeleton. These changes abolish the barrier between the chromosomes and cytoplasm. As cytoplasmic microtubules contact the condensed chromosomes, they attach at the kinetochores (see Chapter 12). Interaction of motor proteins on the chromosomes with microtubules produces jostling movements that culminate with the chromosomes aligned at the mid-plane of a bipolar scaffolding of microtubules (the spindle). *Metaphase–anaphase,* Once all of the chromosomes achieve a bipolar attachment to the spindle, an inhibitory signal is switched off. This leads to activation of a proteolytic network that destroys proteins responsible for holding sister chromatids together, and also inactivates Cdk1 by destroying its cyclin B cofactor (see Chapter 43). These changes trigger separation of the sister chromatids, which then move toward opposite spindle poles. *Telophase—cytokinesis,* Targeting of nuclear envelope components back to the surface of the chromatids subsequently leads to the reformation of two daughter nuclei. In most cells, the two daughter nuclei and the surrounding cytoplasm are partitioned by cytokinesis following the contraction of an actin-myosin ring.

chromosomes in *Xenopus* egg extracts. If condensin is depleted from *Xenopus* extracts, mitotic chromosome condensation is defective, pointing to a key role of the complex. Exactly how the complex acts is not known; however, it appears to introduce a superhelical twist into DNA molecules. The onset of condensation correlates with phosphorylation of histones H1 by Cdk1–cyclin B-p9 and H3 by **Aurora-B protein kinase.** It is now thought that local chromatin unfolding, triggered by histone phosphorylation, permits binding of other

factors, such as the condensin complex, that subsequently condense the chromosome.

DNA **topoisomerase II** also appears to be required for chromosome condensation. Topoisomerase II may contribute to the process as an element of the chromosome scaffold (see Chapter 13). More likely, its enzymatic activity may permit the untangling and separation of entwined sister chromatid DNA molecules, allowing condensin to form discrete condensed chromosomes.

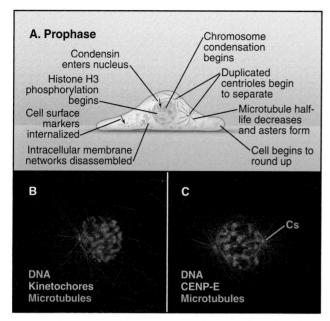

A. Prophase

Condensin
enters nucleus

Histone H3
phosphorylation
begins

Cell surface
markers
internalized

Intracellular membrane
networks disassembled

Chromosome
condensation
begins

Duplicated
centrioles begin
to separate

Microtubule half-
life decreases
and asters form

Cell begins to
round up

B
DNA
Kinetochores
Microtubules

C
Cs
DNA
CENP-E
Microtubules

Figure 47-2 Introduction to prophase. *A,* Summary of the major events of prophase. *B,* Distribution of DNA *(blue),* microtubules *(red),* and kinetochores *(green)* in a prophase PtK2 (rat kangaroo) cell. Kinetochores have duplicated and appear as pairs of dots. *C,* Distribution of DNA *(blue),* microtubules *(red),* and CENP-E *(green)* in a prophase human cell. CENP-E is a large kinesin motor that is involved in monitoring the attachment of kinetochores to the spindle.

Cytoplasmic Changes in Prophase

Most of the cytoskeleton reorganizes during prophase. Particularly dramatic are the changes in the microtubule array, which changes from an extensive network throughout the cytoplasm into two dense, radial arrays of short, dynamic microtubules around each centrosome. These are called **asters.** Each aster eventually becomes one **pole** of the mitotic spindle. During prophase, the two asters usually migrate apart across the surface of the nuclear envelope, signaling the start of spindle assembly. Spindle assembly is discussed in detail in a later section.

Mitotic microtubules behave like interphase microtubules in many ways (see Chapter 37). They are nucleated at their minus ends at centrosomes, they grow by addition of tubulin subunits at their free plus ends, and they undergo random catastrophes during which they rapidly shorten. To a large extent, the prophase changes in microtubule organization can be explained by two simple biochemical changes: (1) increased microtubule-nucleating activity of centrosomes and (2) altered dynamic instability properties of the microtubules (see Chapter 37; Table 47–1). Interphase microtubules have a high probability of recovering from catastrophes so they grow quite long. Mitotic microtubules grow more rapidly from the centrosomes but exist only transiently. This is because when they un-

dergo a catastrophe, they shorten all of the way back to the centrosome, with little chance of rescue. These differences in dynamic instability can be reproduced in vitro in mitotic and interphase cellular extracts. They appear to arise, at least in part, from counterbalancing interactions between microtubule-associated

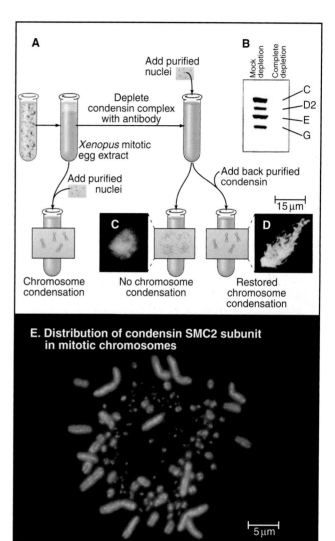

A
Add purified
nuclei

Deplete
condensin complex
with antibody

Xenopus mitotic
egg extract

Add purified
nuclei

Add back purified
condensin

15 µm

B
Mock depletion
Complete depletion
C
D2
E
G

Chromosome
condensation

C
No chromosome
condensation

D
Restored
chromosome
condensation

**E. Distribution of condensin SMC2 subunit
in mitotic chromosomes**

5 µm

Figure 47-3 The condensin complex is important for mitotic chromosome condensation. *A,* The biochemical protocol that led to the purification of the condensin complex. *B,* SDS, polyacrylamide gel (see Chapter 5) reveals the members of the condensin complex and demonstrates that they can be removed using a specific antibody. *C,* If condensins are removed, chromosome condensation fails. *D,* If purified condensin complex is added back to the depleted extract, chromosome condensation is recovered. *E,* An immunofluorescence micrograph shows the distribution of the condensin subunit SMC2 on mitotic chromosomes of the chicken. The tiny chromosomes, called microchromosomes, are commonly seen in birds. (*B* to *D,* Half-tones from Hirano T, Kobayashi R, Hirano M: Condensins, chromosome condensation protein complexes containing XCAP-C, XCAP-E and a *Xenopus* homolog of the *Drosophila* Barren protein. Cell 89:511–521, 1997. Copyright 1997, with permission from Elsevier Science).

table 47–1

COMPARISON OF MICROTUBULE DYNAMICS IN INTERPHASE AND MITOTIC NEWT LUNG CELLS

Parameter	Interphase	Mitosis
Elongation rate	7 μm/min	14 μm/min
Elongation time before catastrophe	71 seconds	60 seconds
Shortening rate	17 μm/min	17 μm/min
Probability of rescue from catastrophe*	0.046/sec	0
Length	100 μm	14 μm

*Most cellular microtubules grow constantly by addition of subunits to their free ends but occasionally stop growing and begin shrinking rapidly (a "catastrophe"). Unless shrinking is reversed (a "rescue"), the microtubule completely disappears. (Data from Gliksman NR, Skibbens RV, Salmon ED: How the transition frequencies of microtubule dynamic instability regulate microtubule dynamics in interphase and mitosis. Mol Biol Cell 4:1035–1050, 1993.)

proteins of the Dis1 family, which promote microtubule stability, and internal motor kinesins (see Fig. 40–3), which promote microtubule instability.

Other cytoskeletal elements that disassemble during prophase include most, but not all, classes of intermediate filaments (including the nuclear lamins) and specialized actin filament structures, such as stress fibers. However, the junctional complexes between adjoining cells are maintained in epithelial cells. This is presumably essential to retain the organization of the tissues. As a result of the cytoskeletal reorganization, most cells round up during prophase. This is particularly evident for cells cultured on a flat substrate, but cells in tissues also change their shape dramatically during mitosis.

Protein synthesis stops during mitosis as a result of the action of Cdk1–cyclin B-p9 kinase. Phosphorylation of ribosomal elongation factor EF2a stops ongoing protein synthesis and assembly of new ribosomes. Phosphorylation of several nucleolar proteins disassembles the nucleolus.

The Golgi apparatus and endoplasmic reticulum fragment or vesiculate during prophase (Fig. 47–4). In addition, other membrane-mediated events, including fluid-phase pinocytosis, endocytosis, exocytosis, and intracellular sorting of membrane components (see Chapters 22 and 23), may greatly decrease. Golgi fragmentation is driven by Cdk1–cyclin B-p9, which phosphorylates the membrane protein GM130. This phosphorylation blocks interaction of GM130 with protein p115 on Golgi transport vesicles. Interaction of GM130 and p115 is essential for fusion of the transport vesicles back into Golgi stacks (see Chapter 22). At the same time, COPI-mediated budding of transport vesicles from the Golgi continues unabated. The net result is that the Golgi buds apart into small vesicles. Golgi reassembly begins again during anaphase, following the inactivation of Cdk1–cyclin B-p9.

Prometaphase

In cells that undergo an open mitosis, **prometaphase** begins abruptly with disassembly of the nuclear envelope (Fig. 47–5). Microtubules growing outward from the spindle poles penetrate holes in the nuclear envelope, make contact with the chromosomes, and attach to them at specialized structures called **kinetochores** (see Chapter 12). Interactions of the two opposing kinetochores of paired sister chromatids with microtubules from opposite poles of the spindle ultimately result in alignment of the chromosomes in a group midway between the poles. This sets the stage for segregation of sister chromatids to daughter cells later in mitosis.

Nuclear Changes in Prometaphase

During prophase, kinetochores transform from nondescript balls of condensed chromatin into organized

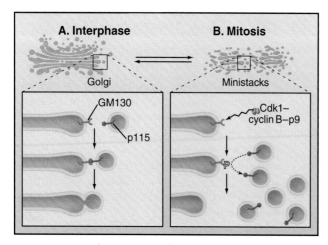

Figure 47–4 Golgi apparatus dynamics in interphase (A) and mitosis (B). Disassembly in mitosis is driven by phosphorylation of components blocking fusion of Golgi membranes.

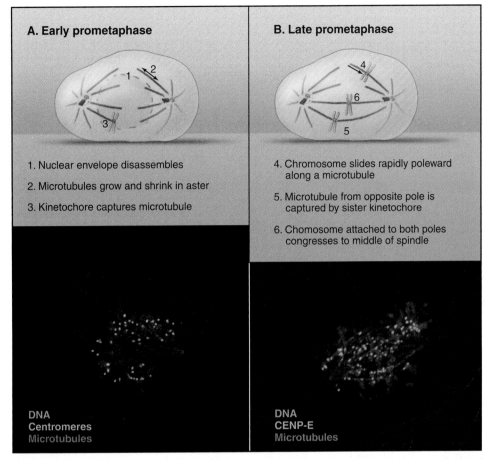

Figure 47-5 Introduction to prometaphase. *A,* Summary of the major events of early prometaphase *(upper).* Distribution of DNA *(blue),* microtubules *(red),* and kinetochores *(green)* in a prometaphase PtK2 cell *(lower). B,* Summary of the major events of late prometaphase *(upper).* Distribution of DNA *(blue),* microtubules *(red),* and CENP-E *(green)* in a prometaphase human cell *(lower).*

plaques on the surface of the chromosomes. By early prometaphase, the characteristic trilaminar disk structure (see Chapter 12) can be seen. Each sister chromatid has a kinetochore (called **sister kinetochores**). These structures are located 180 degrees apart on opposite faces of the mitotic chromosome. Thus, only one of the two sister kinetochores faces a given spindle pole at any one time.

Nuclear envelope disassembly involves the removal of two membrane bilayers, the nuclear pores, and a fibrous meshwork, called the **nuclear lamina**, that underlies the inner bilayer. Nuclear envelope breakdown is not understood in detail, but it is widely believed to be triggered by the phosphorylation of the nuclear lamins at two sites flanking the central coiled-coil. This causes the lamina network to disassemble into subunits (see Chapter 16; Fig. 16-19). Cdk1-cyclin B-p9 kinase can phosphorylate these residues in vitro; however, other kinases may also phosphorylate the lamins in vivo. Expression of mutated lamins lacking mitotic phosphorylation sites in cultured cells prevents breakdown of the nuclear lamina during mitosis.

In cells expressing mutant lamins, chromosomes still attach to spindle microtubules, indicating that, despite the persistence of a portion of the lamina, some degree of nuclear envelope breakdown still occurs.

Nuclear envelope components are dispersed in the cytoplasm from prometaphase until telophase (Fig. 47-6). The mechanism is a matter of recent controversy. For many years, it had been thought that the nuclear membrane broke up into small vesicles that were then dispersed in the cytoplasm. This is still the most likely fate of the nuclear envelope in fertilized amphibian eggs, a common experimental system for these studies. However, recent experiments have provided compelling evidence that, at the onset of prometaphase in somatic cells, the nuclear envelope is absorbed into the endoplasmic reticulum, which fragments but remains as an extensive tubular network throughout mitosis. Whatever the fate of the membrane, it is clear that lamin B remains associated with it, whereas lamins A and C and many proteins of the nuclear pore complexes are dispersed as soluble subunits.

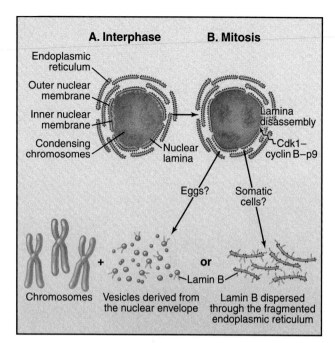

Figure 47–6 Two contrasting models explaining the fate of the nuclear envelope during the transition from interphase (*A*) to mitosis (*B*) in a higher eukaryote.

Organization of the Spindle

In order to discuss the assembly of the mitotic spindle, it is first necessary to describe its organization. The mature metaphase spindle is a bilaterally symmetrical structure with centrally located chromosomes flanked by arrays of microtubules radiating from the poles (Fig. 47–7). Spindle structure is largely determined by the action of at least seven different types of kinesins plus cytoplasmic dynein (see Chapter 39). These motors often work in opposition to one another. As a result, the spindle is a highly dynamic structure whose morphology changes as the balance of forces shifts as a result of differential regulation of the various motors. An important consequence of this is that chromosome movements and changes in spindle morphology typically are complex events reflecting the net vectorial output of the multiple antagonistic and synergistic motors involved. This can be seen clearly in experiments in which one or more kinesins are inactivated either by drugs or by switching a temperature-sensitive mutant to the nonpermissive temperature. This often results in the rapid collapse of the spindle upon itself.

Three predominant classes of microtubules are present in the metaphase spindle. **Kinetochore microtubules** have their plus ends embedded in the kinetochore and their minus ends at or near the spindle pole. They characteristically form bundles, called kinetochore fibers, which contain anywhere from 1 microtubule in the budding yeast to more than 200 microtubules in higher plants. Each human kineto-

chore captures about 20 microtubules. Because each half-spindle has about 1100 microtubules, up to about 80% of the spindle microtubules may be present in kinetochore fibers. **Interpolar microtubules** are distributed throughout the body of the spindle and do not attach to kinetochores. It was originally thought that the minus ends of these microtubules are attached to the pole, with the plus end free. However, only a

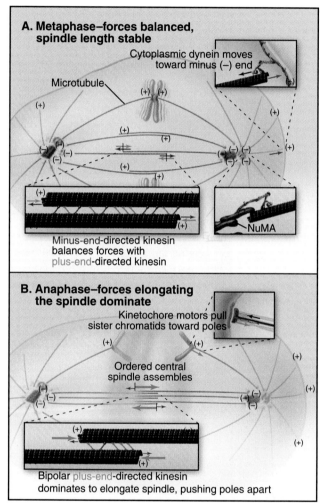

Figure 47–7 Role of motors in spindle structure. The mitotic spindle is a dynamic entity whose structure at any given moment depends on the balance of forces that act to slide microtubules relative to one another and to pull the poles together or apart. *A*, In metaphase the structure is at steady state. The forces that tend to elongate the spindle, including cytoplasmic dynein (which moves toward microtubule minus ends, pulling the poles out toward the cell cortex) and bipolar kinesins (which move toward microtubule plus ends, pushing the poles apart), are counterbalanced by other kinesins that move toward microtubule minus ends (and pull the poles together). Dynein and its associated protein, NuMA, also have an important role in organization of the spindle pole. *B*, In anaphase the influence of the minus-end–directed kinesins declines sharply and the spindle undergoes a dramatic elongation. During anaphase, bipolar kinesins also have an important role in organizing the central spindle, which is essential for subsequent assembly of the cleavage furrow.

minority of the interpolar microtubules reach the pole. Most minus ends terminate near the pole but are not physically linked to it. Thus, many interpolar microtubules appear to be free at both ends. Many of these microtubules penetrate between and through the chromosomes and extend for some distance beyond them, so that the central spindle contains a large number of interdigitated antiparallel microtubules. Tracking these spindle microtubules by electron microscopy has revealed a tendency for the interdigitated microtubules of opposite polarity to pack next to one another. **Astral microtubules** project out from the poles and have a role in orienting the spindle in the cell through interactions with the cell cortex.

Each unit of a spindle pole, with its kinetochore and interpolar and astral microtubules, is referred to as a **half-spindle**. All of the microtubules within the half-spindle have the same polarity, with their minus ends at the pole.

Spindle Assembly and Chromosome Attachment

In metazoans, spindle assembly starts in prophase with the separation of the asters. In most cells, each aster is organized around a centrosome, consisting of a centriole pair and associated pericentriolar material. γ-**Tubulin** ring complexes in the pericentriolar material efficiently nucleate microtubules, so that each aster acts as a **microtubule organizing center** (MTOC). By the end of prophase, the spindle consists of two asters linked by a few interpolar microtubules. Cytoplasmic dynein at the cell cortex exerts an outward force separating the asters, whereas C-terminal motor kinesins on the interpolar microtubules exert a counterbalancing force holding the asters together.

This balance of forces changes at nuclear envelope breakdown, when bipolar kinesins are released from the nucleus. When phosphorylated by Cdk1–cyclin B–p9, bipolar kinesins target to the central spindle, where they cross-link adjacent antiparallel interpolar microtubules. Bipolar kinesins tend to move toward the plus ends of microtubules. If such a motor attaches to two adjacent antiparallel microtubules and begins to move, it will cause them to slide apart. Thus, bipolar kinesins on the spindle tend to exert a force that pushes the spindle poles apart. This overcomes the action of C-terminal motor kinesins, and the combined force of the bipolar kinesins and cytoplasmic dynein causes the spindle to lengthen. Also at this time, the asters mature into focused spindle poles as cytoplasmic dynein transports a microtubule cross-linking protein called **NuMA** (nuclear mitotic apparatus protein, also newly released from the nucleus) to the minus ends of microtubules at the poles.

In large cells lacking centrosomes, such as eggs, spindles form despite the absence of centrosomes, as microtubules are also stabilized when they come in close proximity with chromosomes. Surprisingly, this involves components of the machinery that traffics macromolecules through nuclear pores (see Fig. 16–17). Import factors importin α and β can act as inhibitors of mitotic aster formation by sequestering several proteins essential for the process. These include NuMA. The effect of chromosomes is likely attributable to the presence of chromosome-associated RCC1, the Ran–guanosine triphosphate (GTP) exchange factor, which creates an environment rich in Ran-GTP around the chromosomes. This Ran-GTP apparently releases the astral assembly factors from importin α and β, allowing spindle assembly to occur. This dual role of the nuclear trafficking factors is surprising, although perhaps not as surprising as the dual role of cytochrome c in energy metabolism (see Chapter 10) and cell death (see Chapter 49).

Prometaphase asters are pulsating arrays of microtubules that probe the cytoplasm looking for binding sites that will capture and stabilize their distal plus ends. As the nuclear envelope breaks down, the nuclear interior, with its condensed chromosomes, becomes accessible to the microtubules for the first time. When the plus ends of microtubules encounter kinetochores, they are **captured** (bound) by them. Capture reduces by about five-fold the chance of catastrophic depolymerization for that microtubule. Microtubules that are not captured and stabilized soon have a catastrophe and rapidly depolymerize back to the centrosome, thus providing subunits for other growing microtubules.

In most cells where the two spindle poles and chromosomes are all within 10–15 μm of one another at the time of nuclear envelope breakdown, chromosomes attach to the spindle rapidly, and the initial events of microtubule capture cannot be observed clearly. However, these events are readily visualized in newt lung epithelial cells, where the spindle poles may be more than 50 μm apart at nuclear envelope breakdown. In these cells, attachment of chromosomes most distant from the poles can be greatly delayed and thus much more readily observed in the microscope. Initial attachment of a newt lung cell chromosome to a microtubule often involves a lateral interaction between the corona region of the kinetochore (see Fig. 12–5) and the side of a microtubule (Fig. 47–8). Following lateral attachment, the chromosome moves rapidly along the microtubule toward the pole. It is thought that cytoplasmic dynein mediates this initial chromosome attachment and movement. In smaller cells, kinetochores are typically impaled directly by the plus end of a microtubule.

Capture of the first microtubule by a kinetochore causes its chromosome to move initially toward the spindle pole from which that microtubule originated. Subsequent capture of a microtubule emanating from

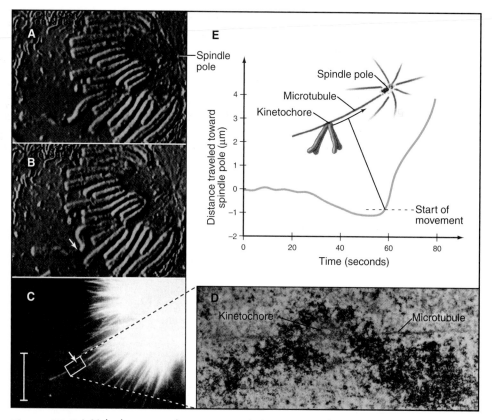

Figure 47-8 Initial chromosomal movements during prometaphase. *A* and *B*, Chromosomal movements initiate with the capture of a microtubule by the kinetochore. This results first in movement toward the pole from which that microtubule originated. These images come from a study in which living cells, observed by differential interference microscopy, were subjected to rapid chemical fixation just after a chromosome had attached to the spindle (*arrow*). *C*, Attachment of the chromosome to the spindle was confirmed by indirect immunofluorescence staining for tubulin and, ultimately, by thin-section electron microscopy (*D*). *E*, The graph shows the movements of the chromosomes before and after attachment. (From Rieder CL, Alexander SP, Rupp G: Kinetochores are transported poleward along a single astral microtubule during chromosome attachment to the spindle in newt lung cells. J Cell Biol 110:81–95, 1990, by copyright permission of the Rockefeller University Press.)

the opposite spindle pole by the sister kinetochore provides a counterforce that tugs the chromosome in the opposite direction. This **bipolar orientation** produces a balance of opposing forces that, together with the action of kinesin family motor proteins distributed along the chromosome arms, results in the slow movement of the chromosome toward a point midway between the spindle poles. These movements are accompanied by coordinated growth and shrinkage of microtubules: shrinkage of the microtubules at the leading kinetochore and growth at the trailing kinetochore.

The attachment of microtubules to kinetochores can be reproduced and studied in vitro by mixing together chromosomes, isolated centrosomes, and tubulin subunits. Under these circumstances, the plus ends of microtubules growing out from the centrosomes attach to the chromosomes. Surprisingly, chromosome-bound microtubules can either lengthen or shorten *at the attached end* without detaching from the chromosome. This is thought to be important to

the mechanism of chromosome movements during mitosis.

One potential error that can occur at this stage of mitosis is for both sister kinetochores to become attached to a single spindle pole. This is rare, owing to positioning of sister kinetochores on opposite faces of the chromosome. However, if it does occur, one or both kinetochores must detach for the chromosome to achieve a bipolar orientation subsequently. Reorientation is favored because attachment to opposite spindle poles is more stable than attachment to a single pole. This is the case because the tension generated by bipolar orientation (where the chromosome is simultaneously pulled toward opposite spindle poles) preferentially stabilizes microtubule connections to both kinetochores. Thus, *tension* between opposite spindle poles has a significant effect on the stability of the chromosome-microtubule connection. The kinetochore tension-sensing mechanism appears to involve a large kinesin, CENP-E (*cen*tromere *p*rotein-E; see later section).

Metaphase

When all of the chromosomes have attained bipolar orientations and moved to positions midway between the two spindle poles, the cell is said to be in **meta- phase** (Fig. 47–9). The compact grouping of chromo- somes at the middle of the spindle is referred to as the **metaphase plate**. A **metaphase checkpoint** (also called a spindle-assembly checkpoint; see Chap- ter 43) delays progress through mitosis at this point until all chromosomes have achieved a bipolar orien- tation (or until it is overridden by an intrinsic cell cycle clock). In yeast cells, chromosomes do not line up at the middle of the spindle, but the checkpoint still can detect whether all chromosomes have achieved a bipolar orientation.

Microtubule Flux Within the Metaphase Spindle

Although the average length of the kinetochore micro- tubules is approximately constant during metaphase, the microtubules change continuously in three ways. First, there is constant net addition of new tubulin subunits (about 10 subunits per second) to the plus end of the microtubules where they are attached to the kinetochore. Second, an equivalent number of tu- bulin subunits is continuously lost slowly from the minus end of the kinetochore tubules at the spindle

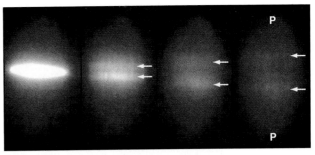

Figure 47–10 Tubulin flux in metaphase. Cells entering mitosis are injected with tubulin subunits modified chemically by at- tachment of a caged fluorescent dye. Such a dye becomes fluo- rescent after being irradiated with ultraviolet light. When cells enter metaphase and labeled tubulin is incorporated into the spindle, the central spindle is illuminated with a narrow stripe of ultraviolet light. This activates a narrow band of fluores- cent tubulin subunits. With time, these subunits approach the spindle poles (P). Because the length of kinetochore microtu- bules is constant during this time, the labeled tubulin molecules must migrate along the microtubule toward the pole (arrows). This can occur if new subunits are added to the microtubule at the kinetochore and old subunits are removed at the pole. (Courtesy of Arshad Desai and the MBL Cell Division Group, Marine Biology Laboratory, Woods Hole, MA; from Mitchison TJ, Salmon ED: Mitosis: A history of division. Reprinted by permission from Nature Cell Biol 3:E17–E21, 2001; copyright 2001, Macmillan Magazines Ltd.)

poles. Therefore, tubulin subunits slowly migrate through kinetochore microtubules from the kineto- chore to the pole (Fig. 47–10). This is referred to as **subunit flux** or treadmilling. Third, all microtubules attached to each kinetochore change coordinately in length during chromosomal oscillations (see next sec- tion).

Chromosome Oscillations During Metaphase

Contrary to popular belief, chromosomes are highly mobile during metaphase. Even though they remain, on the whole, balanced at the middle of the spindle, the chromosomes jostle one another and undergo nu- merous small excursions toward one pole or the other (Fig. 47–11). These oscillations are slow, about 1.5 μm/minute (gain or loss of about 40 tubulin sub- units per microtubule per second), perhaps because they involve simultaneous shortening or lengthening of the approximately 20 microtubules in each kineto- chore fiber. The oscillatory movements reverse every few seconds. Although the movements of paired sister chromatids are usually coordinated, uncoordinated movements can stretch or compress centromeric chro- matin. Thus, although each kinetochore can act inde- pendently, some mechanism (perhaps tension sensors in the kinetochore) usually coordinates their actions.

Both active movements by motor proteins and fluctuations in the length of kinetochore microtubules may contribute to chromosome oscillations during metaphase. Debate continues over which of the two is

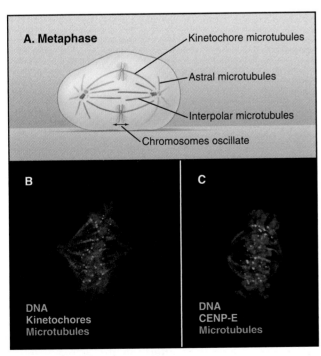

Figure 47–9 Introduction to metaphase. A, Summary of the major events of metaphase. B, Distribution of DNA (blue), mi- crotubules (red), and kinetochores (green) in a metaphase PtK2 cell. C, Distribution of DNA (blue), microtubules (red) and CENP-E (green) in a metaphase human cell.

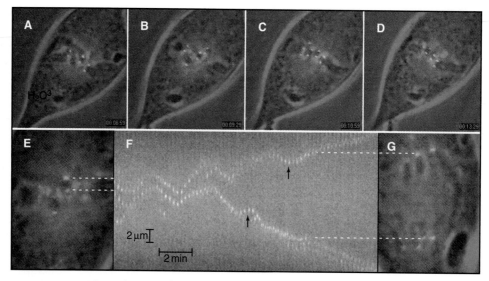

Figure 47-11 Kinetochore oscillations between P (poleward) and AP (away from the pole) movement during late prometaphase and anaphase in PtK1 (rat kangaroo) cells. *A to D,* Images showing the movements of several pairs of sister kinetochores. *E and G,* Higher-magnification views of sister kinetochores (marked with lines) in prometaphase and anaphase, respectively. *F,* Kymograph (collage of images of a vertical strip showing the same two kinetochores at various time points during the movie) showing the movements of these two kinetochores. Arrows mark transient AP movements during anaphase. Kinetochores, labeled with GFP-Cdc20 *(green),* are combined with phase-contrast images of the cell *(red).* Spindle poles are near the top and bottom of the figure. (Micrographs courtesy of E. D. Salmon, University of North Carolina, Chapel Hill.)

more important in driving chromosomal movements in mitosis. Motors, such as cytoplasmic dynein located in the kinetochore corona and along spindle microtubules, have the potential to move chromosomes toward microtubule minus ends (i.e., toward the spindle poles), but during anaphase, these may function more as clamps that attach the chromosomes to the microtubules than as engines for chromosome movement. Other kinesin motors influence the dynamic instability of the kinetochore microtubules. Members of the internal motor class of kinesins, found near kinetochores, use adenosine triphosphate (ATP) hydrolysis to promote microtubule disassembly rather than movement. Other kinesins located on chromosomes include CENP-E, an exceptionally large kinesin found in the kinetochore corona, where it may be involved in sensing chromosomal attachments to the spindle (see later section). In addition, **chromokinesins** associated with the chromosome arms appear to be important for stable alignment of chromosomes on the central spindle at metaphase.

Biochemical Signals for the Transition Out of Metaphase: The Metaphase Checkpoint

Segregation of replicated chromosomes into daughter cells is extremely accurate. For example, budding yeasts lose a chromosome only once in 100,000 cell divisions. Perhaps surprisingly, the frequency of chro-

mosome loss is 20- to 400-fold higher for human cells grown in culture. To achieve this level of accuracy, most cells delay entry into anaphase until all chromosomes achieve a bipolar orientation. This delay is caused by a cellular quality control pathway or checkpoint—the **metaphase checkpoint**—that senses the completion of chromosome alignment and spindle assembly at metaphase. This checkpoint is often called the spindle assembly checkpoint, but as it actually monitors kinetochore activity rather than spindle structure, we prefer the present nomenclature.

Genetic analysis of budding yeast and studies of vertebrate cells have revealed that this checkpoint involves several protein kinases plus other factors. Checkpoint proteins are mostly cytoplasmic during interphase and associate with the kinetochores at prophase or prometaphase. They then dissociate from kinetochores that have made stable attachments to the spindle. The components of the system are conserved from yeast to man.

Two of the kinases are known as Bub1p (budding uninhibited by benzimidazole) and BubR1 (Bub-*re*-lated kinase-1). When *bub* genes are mutated, yeast cells continue to divide even when the spindle is destroyed by drugs like benzimidazole. BubR1 is located in the outer plate of the kinetochore, where it interacts with the giant kinesin motor protein, **CENP-E.** Cytoplasmic CENP-E associates with chromosomes when the nuclear envelope breaks down at prometa-

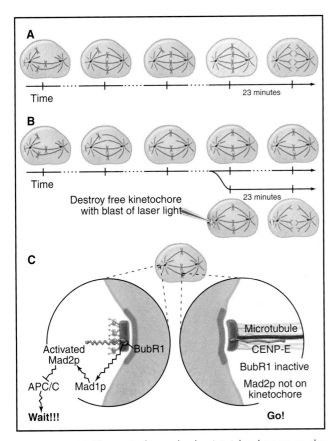

Figure 47-12 The metaphase checkpoint (also known as the spindle assembly checkpoint). Signaling by unattached kinetochores stops the cell from entering anaphase until all chromosomes have made a proper bipolar spindle attachment. *A,* As long as there is a chromosome that is not properly attached to the spindle *(reddish cells),* the cell does not enter anaphase. The cell enters mitosis about 20 minutes after chromosome attachment is complete *(green cells). B,* In a cell with a persistently maloriented chromosome, anaphase entry is delayed *(reddish cells).* If the unattached kinetochore is destroyed with a high-powered laser, the cell enters anaphase about 20 minutes later. This proves that the unattached kinetochore sends an inhibitory signal. *C,* Distribution of signaling molecules in the kinetochore. The microtubule motor protein CENP-E in the fibrous corona appears to act as a tension sensor, communicating the status of microtubule binding to the BubR1 kinase, with which it interacts. BubR1 and related kinases may send the inhibitory signal from unattached kinetochores that prevents cells from entering anaphase until all chromosomes are properly attached (see text for discussion of the other signaling components).

phase (see Figs. 47–2, 47–5, and 47–9). During metaphase, it is found in the kinetochore corona and along the kinetochore microtubules. At anaphase, most CENP-E disassociates from the chromosomes, although some remains at the kinetochores. The NH_2-terminal end of CENP-E, the kinesin motor domain, binds to microtubules, whereas the COOH-terminal end associates with BubR1 in the kinetochores. These two domains are linked by a long coiled-coil. Given this ar-

rangement, CENP-E is well suited to be the "tension detector" within the kinetochore.

BUB kinases regulate a protein called Mad1p (mitotic arrest–defective protein), which, in turn, activates a protein called **Mad2p.** The MAD genes were originally identified in yeast in a genetic screen for cells that tried to divide when the spindle was disassembled by drugs. Activated Mad2p inhibits the onset of anaphase by interacting with Cdc20, a key substrate-recognition factor for the APC/C (anaphase-promoting complex/cyclosome; see Chapters 43 and 46). APC/C is a ubiquitin-protein ligase (E3 enzyme; see Chapters 24 and 43) that marks target proteins for destruction by proteasomes by decorating them with ubiquitin. Its key substrates include a protein called securin (see section that follows) and cyclin B.

The current model for the operation of the metaphase checkpoint is that, as cells enter mitosis, the BUB and MAD proteins bind to all kinetochores and produce activated Mad2p, which associates with the APC/C^{Cdc20} and keeps it inactive. One by one, as chromosomes achieve a bipolar attachment to the spindle, the inhibitory signals are removed. It is only when the last chromosome has achieved a proper attachment that the last source of inhibitory Mad2p complexes is extinguished. Because the Mad2p complexes are short-lived, inhibition of the APC/C^{Cdc20} ceases shortly thereafter, triggering the onset of anaphase.

As predicted by this model, perturbing the function of Mad2p causes a catastrophic, premature entry into anaphase, regardless of the status of chromosome alignment. This leads to an unequal distribution of sister chromatids to daughter cells, causing a genetic imbalance of the daughter cells known as **aneuploidy.** Experiments have shown that microinjection of antibodies to Mad2p into cells causes this effect. Certain types of human colon cancers lack BubR1 function, and this may contribute to genetic instability and progression of a tumor from benign to malignant.

Anaphase

The onset of **anaphase,** with the physical separation of sister chromatids, is one of the most dramatic events of the entire cell cycle (Fig. 47–13). Sister chromatids move to opposite spindle poles (**anaphase A**) and the poles move apart (**anaphase B**). Anaphase is also the time when the mitotic spindle activates the cell cortex in preparation for cytokinesis.

Biochemical Mechanism of Anaphase Onset

The transition from metaphase to anaphase is triggered by a sudden drop in Cdk1 activity. This begins gradually with cyclin A destruction at the onset of

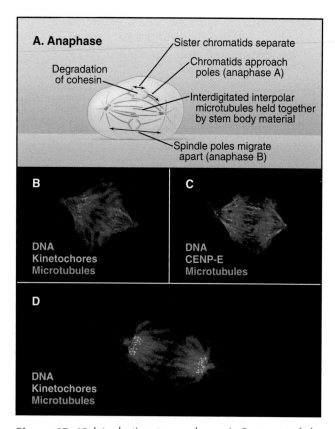

Figure 47-13 Introduction to anaphase. *A,* Summary of the major events of anaphase. *B,* Distribution of DNA *(blue),* microtubules *(red),* and kinetochores *(green)* in an early anaphase PtK2 cell. *C,* Distribution of DNA *(blue),* microtubules *(red),* and CENP-E *(green)* in a mid-anaphase human cell. Some CENP-E has moved from kinetochores to microtubules. *D,* Distribution of DNA *(blue),* microtubules *(red),* and kinetochores *(green)* in a late-anaphase PtK2 cell.

prometaphase, which is completed by mid-metaphase. The transition is completed by APC/C-directed cleavage of several key protein targets, including securin (see below) and cyclin B, by proteasomes.

Although important, the proteolytic degradation of cyclin and the transition to low levels of Cdk1 activity are not required for anaphase onset. Expression of a nondegradable cyclin mutant results in cells blocked in late mitosis with high levels of Cdk1 kinase activity, separated condensed sister chromatids, a disassembled nuclear envelope, and a persistent mitotic spindle. However, sister chromatid separation can be prevented by complete inhibition of the ubiquitin-mediated protein degradation pathway, indicating that degradation of proteins other than the cyclins is important for sister chromatid separation. Thus, inactivation of Cdk1−cyclin B-p9 kinase activity is required for the eventual exit from mitosis, but not the metaphase-anaphase transition per se.

Sister chromatid separation is regulated by the chromosomes themselves, not the mitotic spindle. Sis-

ter chromatids can separate in some cell types even when all of the microtubules are depolymerized. This appears to rule out any need for pulling by the spindle in this process. It follows that sister chromatid separation at anaphase does not reflect a sudden activation of motors that move chromosomes. In fact, these motors are already active during metaphase. If a laser microbeam is used to destroy one sister kinetochore of a chromosome aligned at the metaphase plate, severing the connection of that chromatid to the spindle pole, the chromosome immediately moves away from the metaphase plate toward the spindle pole to which it remains attached.

Studies of the budding yeast have prompted a major breakthrough by revealing three factors that reg-

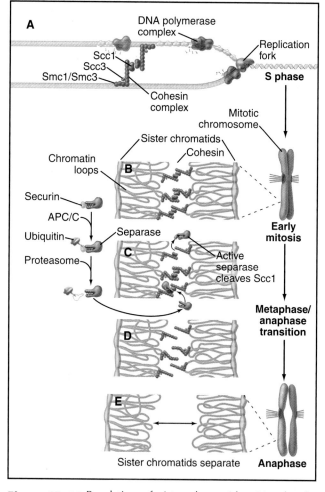

Figure 47-14 Regulation of sister chromatid pairing by the cohesin complex. *A,* The cohesin complex is loaded onto the chromosomes during DNA replication. *B,* The mechanism by which cohesins promote sister chromatid pairing is not known; this is one speculative model. *C,* At the onset of anaphase, degradation of the securin inhibitor liberates active separase enzyme, which then cleaves cohesin subunit Scc1. *D* and *E,* Following Scc1 cleavage, the two sister chromatids are able to separate from one another and move toward the spindle poles.

ulate sister chromatid separation: a protein complex known as **cohesin,** a protease known as **separase,** and an inhibitor of the protease known as **securin** (Fig. 47–14). This system is conserved from yeast to man.

Cohesin is a complex of four proteins that resembles the condensin complex described earlier and in Chapter 13 (see Figs. 13–15 and 47–3). Like condensin, cohesin has two large subunits that are members of the SMC (structural maintenance of chromosomes) family. These proteins, SMC1 and SMC3, are complexed with proteins called Scc1 (which has other names omitted here for simplicity) and Scc3. Two other associated proteins are required for the stable loading of this complex onto DNA during replication. Yeast or *Drosophila* cells with mutations in components of this complex separate sister chromatids prematurely in mitosis, resulting in chaotic chromosome mis-segregation. Interestingly, these mutants are also defective in repair of DNA damage. This system is very ancient; an SMC-related protein is required for orderly chromosome segregation in bacteria.

Exactly how cohesin holds sister chromatids together is unknown, but the complex may function as a kind of molecular zipper. Experiments with yeast have shown that the complex functions only if it binds chromosomes during DNA replication. In yeast, the complex stays associated with chromosomes at a number of preferred sites until the onset of anaphase. In vertebrates, most cohesin dissociates from the chromosome arms during prophase, but some remains associated with centromeres until the onset of anaphase.

Two separate protease activities trigger sister chromatid separation at anaphase. First, the newly activated APC/C tags securin with ubiquitin, leading to its destruction by proteasomes. Securin normally binds and inhibits a protease called separase, which is distantly related to caspases, key proteases in apoptosis (see Chapter 49). Degradation of securin releases separase to cleave the Scc1 subunit of cohesin. Cleavage of Scc1 triggers separation of sister chromatids and, therefore, the onset of anaphase. An additional level of control is provided by the fact that phosphorylation of the separase cleavage site on Scc1 by the Polo kinase substantially increases the cleavage of Scc1 by separase. This provides a mechanism whereby the activity of the protease system directed by the APC/C can be integrated and coordinated with the activities of the mitotic kinases, of which Polo is a key regulator (Chapter 46).

Human securin is overexpressed in some pituitary tumors, and the protein can act as an oncogene in cultured cells (see Chapter 44). The link with cancer may be that the misexpressed securin disrupts the normal timing of chromosome segregation, thereby leading to chromosome loss and ultimately contributing to cancer progression.

Chromosomal Passenger Proteins Regulate Numerous Mitotic Events

Chromosomal passenger proteins, including *in*ner *cen*tromere *p*rotein (**INCENP**) and its binding partners, **Aurora-B kinase** and **survivin**, are closely associated with chromosomes during prometaphase and metaphase. However, this association is not permanent. At the metaphase-anaphase transition, they associate with the overlapping interpolar microtubules of the central spindle, ultimately winding up in the intercellular bridge during cytokinesis (see later section). Some INCENP and Aurora-B proteins also associate with the cell membrane at the site of cytokinesis. Essential functions of chromosomal passengers in mitosis include phosphorylation of histone H3, promotion of condensin binding and chromosome assembly, chromosome segregation at anaphase, and the completion of cytokinesis. Current evidence suggests that INCENP targets Aurora-B kinase to its points of action. The role of survivin is not yet known.

Mitotic Spindle Dynamics During Anaphase

Anaphase is dominated by the orderly movement of the sister chromatids to opposite spindle poles brought about by the combined action of motor proteins and changes in the length of microtubules. Anaphase chromosome movements have two major components. **Anaphase A**, the movement of the sister chromatids to the spindle poles, requires a shortening of the kinetochore fibers. **Anaphase B** is the elongation of the spindle and separation of the spindle poles. The poles separate partially because of interactions between the antiparallel interpolar microtubules of the central spindle and partially because of intrinsic motility of the asters. Most cells use both components of anaphase, but in extreme cases, one component is strongly exaggerated relative to the other.

Evidence that anaphase A chromosome movement does not require movement of microtubules has come from observations of live cells injected with fluorescently labeled tubulin subunits (Fig. 47–15). These subunits assemble into the spindle so that it becomes fluorescent. Early in anaphase, when a laser is used to bleach a narrow zone in the fluorescent tubulin across the spindle between the chromosomes and the pole, the chromosomes approach the bleached zone much faster than the bleached zone approaches the spindle pole. This shows that the chromosomes "eat" their way along the kinetochore microtubules toward the pole.

Current evidence suggests that both motor molecules on the chromosomes and shortening of the kinetochore microtubules contribute to chromosome

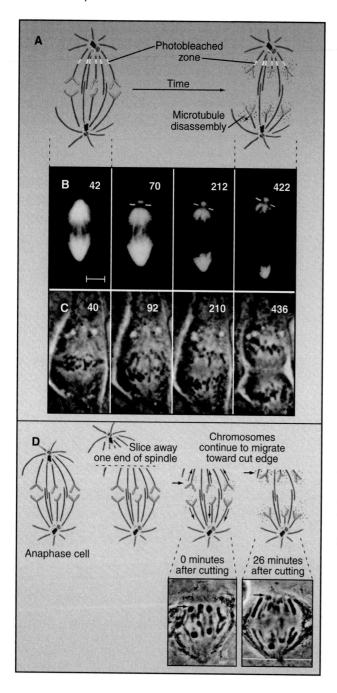

Figure 47–15 Two classic experiments that demonstrate that chromosomes move under their own power along microtubules during anaphase. *A* to *C,* Demonstration that kinetochore microtubules do not move during anaphase A. *Diagram:* Mitotic cells are injected with a fluorescently labeled tubulin that rapidly becomes incorporated into the spindle. Just after anaphase onset, a laser is used to photobleach a stripe (marked with two lines) across the spindle near the upper pole. The live cell was monitored over time by fluorescence (*B*) and phase contrast (*C*) microscopy. The chromosomes approach the bleached stripe much faster than the stripe approaches the spindle pole. The numbers are time in seconds. *D,* Microsurgery experiment in which the end of a spindle of an insect spermatocyte is cut off with a microneedle. Chromosomes continue to move toward the spindle pole, even after the pole has been amputated, confirming that the motor for movement must be on or near the chromosomes. (*A* to *C,* From Gorbsky GJ, Sammak PJ, Borisy GG: Microtubule dynamics and chromosome motion visualized in living anaphase cells. J Cell Biol 106:1185–1192, 1988. *D,* From Nicklas RB: The motor for poleward chromosome movement in anaphase is in or near the kinetochore. J Cell Biol 109:2245–2255, 1989. *A* to *D,* By copyright permission of the Rockefeller Univeristy Press.)

movement in anaphase A. Both theory and experiment (see Fig. 40–9) show that microtubule disassembly can move chromosomes. Energy for this movement comes from hydrolysis of GTP bound to assembled tubulin, which is stored in the conformation of the tubulin subunits. Chromosomes appear to use motor molecules like CENP-E to hold onto disassembling microtubules. These motors must "run" toward the poles without losing their grip as the microtubules disassemble behind them.

A second factor contributing to the separation of sister chromatids during anaphase is separation of the

spindle poles themselves, a process referred to as anaphase B. This overall lengthening of the spindle is produced partially by sliding apart of the interdigitated half-spindles and partially by intrinsic motility of the poles themselves. Anaphase B appears to be triggered by the inactivation of the C-terminal motor kinesins, so that all of the major motor forces now favor spindle elongation. This is accompanied by reorganization of the interpolar microtubules into a highly organized **central spindle** between the separating chromatids. Within the central spindle, an amorphous dense material called **stem body matrix** stabilizes bundles of antiparallel microtubules and holds together the two interdigitated half-spindles. The central spindle contains a variety of kinesins, including bipolar kinesins and orphan kinesins of the unrelated CHO1/Mklpl and CENP-E families (see Fig. 40–3). CHO1 kinesins, which are most closely related to budding yeast Kip3, are required for cytokinesis. In animal cells, cytokinesis is regulated, at least in part, by the organized central spindle (see later discussion).

Spindle elongation during anaphase B may also be partly attributable to active movements by the spindle poles themselves. In fact, during the latter stages of anaphase B, the spindle pole, with its attached kinetochore microtubules, appears to move away from the interpolar microtubules as the spindle lengthens. This astral movement involves interaction of the astral microtubules with cytoplasmic dynein molecules anchored in the cortical cytoplasm.

Telophase

During **telophase**, the nuclear envelope re-forms on the surface of the separated sister chromatids, which typically cluster in a dense mass near the spindle poles (Fig. 47–16). Some further anaphase B movement may still occur, but the most dramatic change in cellular structure at this time is the constriction of the cleavage furrow and subsequent cytokinesis.

Reassembly of the Nuclear Envelope

Nuclear envelope reassembly begins during anaphase and is completed during telophase (Fig. 47–17). The mechanism of nuclear envelope reassembly is debated, in part because the fate of the nuclear membrane during mitosis is unclear (see earlier discussion). If, as long thought, the nuclear envelope disassembles to discrete vesicles, then envelope reassembly can be regarded as a classical membrane-sorting problem (see Chapter 17), reflecting the fact that mitotic cells contain multiple populations of membrane vesicles derived from a number of organelles. In eggs, there are at least two or three discrete populations of membrane vesicles derived from the nuclear envelope alone. On the other hand, if the nuclear membrane is absorbed into the endoplasmic reticulum during mitosis in somatic cells, as recently proposed, then reassembly must involve diffusion of membrane components within the membrane network and their stabilization at preferred binding sites at the periphery of the chromosomes.

Lamin subunits disassembled in prophase are recycled to reform the nuclear envelope at the end of mitosis. Reassembly of the nuclear lamina is triggered by removal of mitosis-specific phosphate groups and methyl-esterification of several COOH side chains on

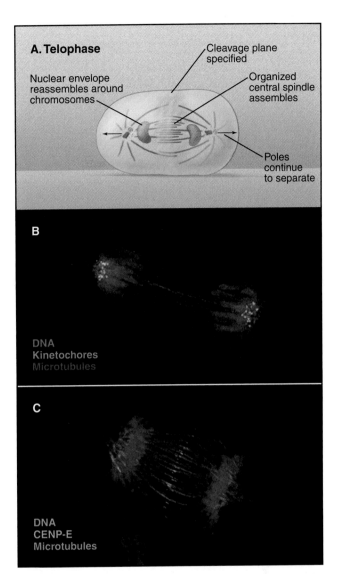

Figure 47–16 Introduction to telophase. *A,* Summary of the major events of telophase. *B,* Distribution of DNA *(blue),* microtubules *(red),* and kinetochores *(green)* in a telophase PtK2 cell. *C,* Distribution of DNA *(blue),* microtubules *(red),* and CENP-E *(green)* in a telophase human cell. Note that CENP-E, which acts like a chromosomal passenger protein, has now largely transferred to the overlapping microtubules of the central spindle. Low levels of CENP-E also remain at the kinetochores, however.

lamin B (see Chapter 16). B-type lamins are among the earliest components of the nuclear envelope to target to the surface of the chromosomes, which they do during mid-anaphase. Either at this time, or shortly thereafter, other integral membrane components of the inner nuclear membrane, including the lamin B receptor and certain nuclear pore components, also target to the forming envelope. Lamin A enters the reforming nucleus later during telophase, after the reassembly of nuclear pore complexes and reestablishment of nuclear import pathways. Its assembly into the peripheral lamina occurs slowly over a period of several hours in

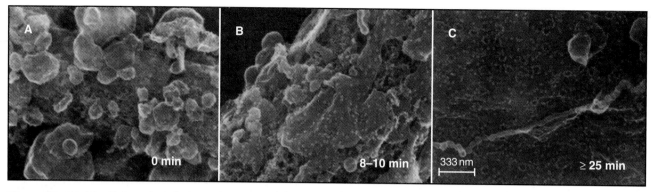

Figure 47-17 *A* to *C*, Scanning electron microscopy of the stages of assembly of membrane vesicles on the surface of chromosomes in a *Xenopus* extract. A solution containing membrane vesicles was added to isolated chromatin from *Xenopus* sperm, fixed, and then imaged by field emission scanning electron microscopy. Each panel shows the time of incubation prior to fixation. *(A and C,* From Wiese C, Goldberg MW, Allen TD, et al: Nuclear envelope assembly in *Xenopus* extracts visualized by scanning EM reveals a transport-dependent "envelope smoothing" event. J Cell Sci 110:1489–1502, 1997, Company of Biologists Ltd. Micrographs courtesy of K. L. Wilson, Johns Hopkins Medical School.)

the G_1 phase. Transport of lamins through the nuclear pores appears to be an essential step in nuclear reassembly. If lamin transport is prevented, chromosomes remain highly condensed following cytokinesis, and the cells fail to reenter the next S phase.

Cytokinesis

Cytokinesis is the process that divides the mitotic cell into two daughter cells (Fig. 47–18). In animals, daughter cells are normally separated from one another by a **contractile ring**, a transient array of actin filaments attached to the plasma membrane at sites around the equator of the dividing cell. The interac-

tion of these actin filaments with bipolar myosin II filaments applies tension to the membrane, much like the contraction of smooth muscle. Because the contractile ring is confined to a narrow band of cortex, it forms a **cleavage furrow**, constricting the plasma membrane locally and pinching the cell in two. A control mechanism ensures that this ring forms around the cell equator so that constriction occurs between the two separated sets of sister chromatids. Other controls ensure that activation of the contractile ring is delayed until after the sister chromatids are segregated to opposite poles of the mitotic spindle. For a description of other strategies of cytokinesis in bacteria, yeasts, and plants, see Box 47–1.

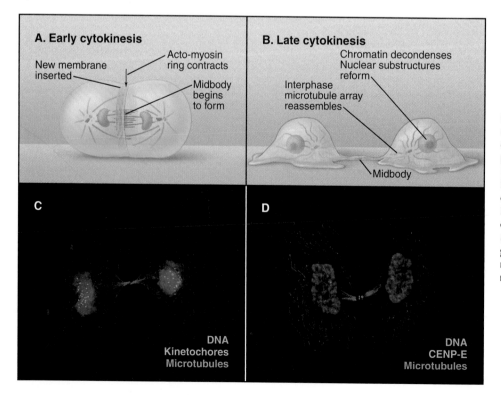

Figure 47–18 Introduction to cytokinesis. *A* and *B,* Summary of the major events of telophase. *C,* Distribution of DNA *(blue),* microtubules *(red),* and kinetochores *(green)* in a PtK2 cell undergoing cytokinesis. *D,* Distribution of DNA *(blue),* microtubules *(red),* and CENP-E *(green)* in a human cell undergoing cytokinesis. CENP-E has now largely transferred to the midbody structure.

Although cytokinesis has been studied for more than 100 years, it continues to pose a number of challenges. In part, this is because of a limited understanding of the components involved. In addition, a biochemical assay for cleavage furrow assembly and function has yet to be developed, thus severely limiting understanding of the mechanism of cytokinesis. Nevertheless, real progress has been made in recent years through genetic analysis in the fission yeast and fruit fly.

Signals Regulating the Position of the Cleavage Furrow

A wealth of experimental data from many classic studies on fertilized eggs suggest that a **cleavage stimulus,** emitted by the mitotic spindle, specifies the position of the cleavage furrow midway between the spindle poles and perpendicular to the long axis of the spindle, thereby ensuring that daughter nuclei are separated by the cleavage process (Fig. 47–19). In fertilized eggs, the poles, with their large astral arrays of microtubules, are regarded as the source of the cleavage stimulus, as furrows can be induced to form midway between two poles even when no chromosomes are present. Even in cells, such as fission yeast, with closed mitosis, the mitotic apparatus determines the position of the cleavage, perhaps utilizing the spindle pole bodies in the nuclear envelope as the source of the signals.

The molecular nature of the cleavage stimulus itself remains a mystery, although several of its features are known.

1. The signal moves from the spindle of echinoderm eggs to the cortex in a straight line at about 7 μm/minute. Because microtubules are required, the signal may migrate or be carried toward the cortex along the microtubules.
2. The cortex becomes committed to respond to the cleavage stimulus after being exposed to it for only about 1 minute. In fertilized eggs, furrowing commences after a brief lag and propagates around the equator, even if the spindle is now removed. Cortical commitment results in production of a self-propagating furrow that can spread hundreds of micrometers across the surface of very large cells, such as fertilized eggs.
3. The cleavage stimulus appears to be emitted throughout anaphase. Spindles can induce multiple furrows if they are experimentally repositioned within the cell.

In animal somatic cells, there is now compelling evidence that the organized central spindle plays a critical role, both early and late in cytokinesis. This has been studied best in *Drosophila*, in which mutants that cannot form a central spindle fail to initiate cyto-

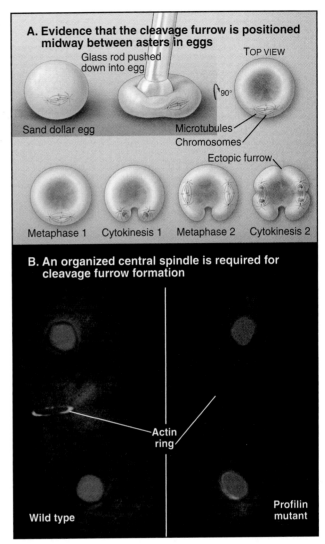

A. Evidence that the cleavage furrow is positioned midway between asters in eggs

Glass rod pushed down into egg

TOP VIEW

Sand dollar egg

Microtubules
Chromosomes

Ectopic furrow

Metaphase 1   Cytokinesis 1   Metaphase 2   Cytokinesis 2

B. An organized central spindle is required for cleavage furrow formation

Actin ring

Wild type

Profilin mutant

Figure 47–19 In eggs, the cleavage furrow forms midway between spindle asters. In animal cells, the central spindle is important. *A,* A classical experiment in which a sand dollar egg is caused to adopt a toroid shape. At cytokinesis 2, the egg cleaves into four cells with a furrow forming between the back sides of the two spindles. For a description of this and other classical experiments in cytokinesis, see the book by Rappaport in the Selected Readings list. *B, Left,* A wild-type *Drosophila* spermatocyte undergoing cytokinesis, with the contractile ring stained in yellow. *Right,* In a profilin mutant, no central spindle forms, and the cell fails to form a contractile ring. (Courtesy of Professor Maurizio Gatti, University of Rome; from Giansanti MG, Bonaccorsi S, Williams B, et al: Cooperative interactions between the central spindle and the contractile ring during *Drosophila* cytokinesis. Genes Dev 12:396–410, 1998.)

kinesis. Components of the central spindle that are required for cytokinesis include kinesins and the chromosomal passenger proteins INCENP, Aurora-B kinase, and survivin. The *Drosophila* CHO1 bipolar kinesin is absolutely essential for cytokinesis. In its absence, there is no central spindle, and no cleavage furrow forms. The chromosomal passengers, on the other hand, appear to act later in the process. If their

box 47–1

VARIATIONS ON A THEME: CYTOKINESIS IN BACTERIA, FUNGI, AND PLANTS

Bacteria Cytokinesis in bacteria shares several similarities with the process in animal cells (Fig. 47–20). Most bacterial cells cleave as a result of constriction of a ring of the FtsZ protein (*filamentous temperature-sensitive;* mutants in *fts* genes cannot divide and make long filaments). This is called the Z ring. FtsZ has been crystal-lized, and the structure is remarkably similar to eukaryotic tubulins. Furthermore, as for tubulins, FtsZ function requires GTP hydrolysis. The Z ring is positioned at the cell equator by the action of three genes: MinC, MinD, and MinE (*minicell* mutants divide at inappropriate locations and give birth to tiny cells). MinD is an enzyme

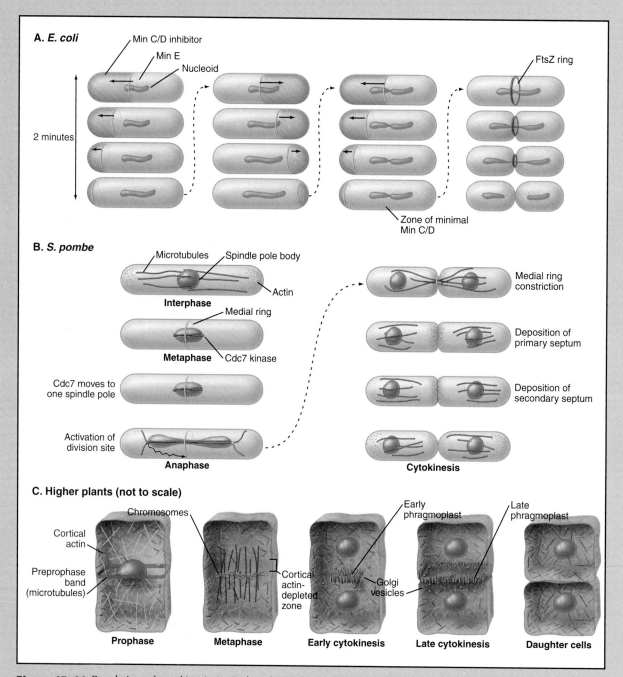

Figure 47-20 Regulation of cytokinesis in *Escherichia coli* (*A*), *Schizosaccharomyces pombe* (*B*), and higher plants (*C*). See text for details.

box 47–1

VARIATIONS ON A THEME: CYTOKINESIS IN BACTERIA, FUNGI, AND PLANTS
Continued

that recruits MinC to the cell cortex, where it inhibits Z-ring formation. MinE is an antagonist of MinC/MinD action. This system works in a truly remarkable way. MinE forms a ring at the cell equator that migrates along the inner surface of the cell membrane until it reaches the end of the cell, at which point it disassembles. The ring then re-forms in the center of the cell and sweeps off in the other direction, toward the other end of the cell. As it moves, MinE inactivates the MinC/MinD inhibitory complex on the cell cortex. The inhibitory complex rapidly reestablishes itself on the cell cortex behind the moving MinE ring. It takes about 2 minutes for each sweep of the MinE ring along half of the cell, and this cycle is repeated continuously until the FtsZ ring assembles at the cell center. No one knows how MinE and FtsZ locate the center of the cell. Interestingly, chloroplasts use a similar system for their division, and FtsZ has been detected in mitochondria of certain primitive eukaryotes. Mitochondria of higher eukaryotes appear to use another GTPase, dynamin, for a similar cleavage mechanism.

Fission Yeast Like plants, fission yeasts have a rigid cell wall. Nonetheless, they adopt a mechanism of cytokinesis that shares a number of aspects with cytokinesis in animal cells. During interphase, the fission yeast nucleus occupies a central position in a basket of microtubules that extend along the long axis of the cell. Actin is concentrated in small patches in the cortex at the two growing ends of the cell. As the cells enter mitosis, actin relocalizes from these patches to form a ring around the cell equator above the nucleus. This so-called medial ring contains, in addition, myosin II, tropomyosin, and a number of other components. The mechanism of medial ring positioning is not known, but it may be determined by the location of the spindle pole bodies, disk-like structures in the nuclear envelope that nucleate microtubules and act as the poles of the mitotic spindle. The spindle is inside the nucleus in these cells, as the nuclear membrane does not break down during mitosis. As the nucleus is partitioned into two parts during anaphase, the primary septum begins to form at the medial ring. Septum formation begins at the cell cortex, and a contractile ring of actin and myosin appears to draw the leading edge of this structure inward as it contracts. Actin is also found in patches along the sides of the forming septum at sites of assembly. The septum is a three-layered structure, with the primary septum flanked by two secondary septae. Cell separation is achieved by digestion of the primary septum. Septum formation is regulated by a network of protein kinases and other factors encoded by the Sid (septation initiation–defective) genes. These gene products function at the spindle pole bodies. One Sid protein, Sid4p, is found at the spindle pole body throughout the cell cycle and may be the "landing pad" for other members of this system. Several other Sid proteins bind to both spindle pole bodies at the onset of mitosis but then concentrate at a single pole as mitosis progresses. These include at least one protein kinase, a small GTPase, and its regulatory factors. The mechanisms and reason for this movement to a single pole are unknown, although several of the components only move after Cdk1–cyclin B are inactivated. This provides a link between cytokinesis and the exit from mitosis. It appears that the last participants in this system are a protein kinase and its binding partner. These normally are found in the spindle pole bodies, but they move to the site of cell division at the time of septation, after the other Sid genes have completed their functions. This movement is probably the signal for septum assembly.

Plants Chromosome segregation in plant cells is very similar to that in animals, and many of the components are conserved. However, significant differences occur between plant and animal cell mitosis. Some of these arise from the fact that plant cells have a rigid cell wall and cannot divide by a contractile ring mechanism. Centrosomes are absent in plants, and during interphase, microtubules radiate out from the surface of the cell nucleus in all directions. In mitosis, the spindle does not focus to sharp poles at metaphase; instead, it assumes a barrel shape with flat poles. Early in mitosis, a band of microtubules and actin filaments forms around the equator of the cell above the cell nucleus. This so-called preprophase band disassembles as cells enter prometaphase. Because the entire cell cortex is covered by a meshwork of actin filaments, disassembly of the preprophase band actually leaves an actin-poor zone in a ring where cytokinesis will ultimately occur. This is called the cortical division site. In late anaphase, two nonoverlapping, antiparallel arrays of microtubules form over the central spindle. This structure, the phragmoplast, gradually expands laterally until it makes a double disk of short microtubules with their plus ends adjacent at the plane of cell cleavage. In addition to microtubules, the phragmoplast contains actin filaments and vesicles derived from the Golgi and endoplasmic reticulum. The Golgi vesicles, which contain various cell wall materials, move along the phragmoplast to the equator, where they fuse and form the new cell wall. Cell wall formation begins at the cell cortex and gradually spreads inward until the two cells are partitioned from one another. It is the cortical division site, and not the spindle, that determines the site of cleavage. This has been shown in experiments in which mitotic cells were centrifuged to displace the spindle from the central location where it initially formed. Late in mitosis, the phragmoplast formed at the mid-zone of the displaced spindle, but this phragmoplast then migrated until it found the plane of the preprophase band, and that was where cytokinesis occurred.

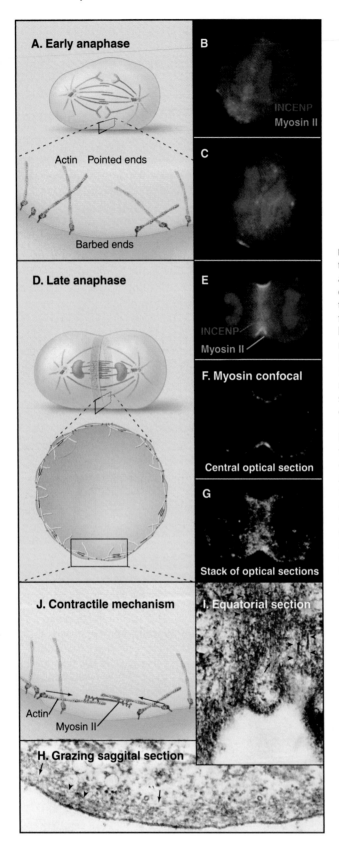

Figure 47-21 INCENP and myosin in the contractile ring. *A, D,* and *J,* Organization of actin and myosin in the contractile ring just before and during mid-cytokinesis. *B,* INCENP *(red)* concentrates at the site where the cleavage furrow will form just before myosin *(green)*. *C,* A cell with both INCENP and myosin at the site of ring formation prior to the initiation of contraction. *E,* INCENP and myosin concentrate in the contractile ring during contraction. *F* and *G,* Confocal micrographs clearly show the distribution of myosin in the contractile ring. *H* and *I,* Electron micrographs showing actin filaments in the contractile ring. *Arrowheads:* thick filaments thought to be myosin-II filaments. *Arrows:* actin filaments. (*F* to *I,* Courtesy of P. Maupin, Johns Hopkins Medical School. References: Maupin P., Pollard TD: Arrangement of actin filaments and myosin-like filaments in the contractile ring and actin-like filaments in the mitotic spindle of dividing HeLa cells. J. Ultrastr Res 94:92–103, 1986; Maupin P, et al: Differential localization of myosin-II isozymes in human cultured cells and blood cells. J Cell Sci 107:3077–3090, 1994; Eckley DM, et al: Chromosomal proteins and cytokinesis. J Cell Biol 136:1169–1183, 1997.)

function is perturbed, cytokinesis initiates but then fails, and the cleavage furrow regresses. This likely reflects essential action of the Aurora-B kinase and its targeting factor INCENP in the completion of cytokinesis. In the nematode worm *C. elegans*, another central spindle component required for cytokinesis is a Rho-GAP (guanosine triphosphatase [GTPase]–activating) protein (see Chapter 27) that appears to act on the small GTPase RhoA to allow the completion of cytokinesis. Rho and related GTPases Rac and Cdc42 have all been implicated in cytokinesis. They all participate in complex signaling pathways, including activation of actin polymerization (see Fig. 41–5) and motor activities of myosin II (see Fig. 42–21).

Structure and Function of the Contractile Ring

Exposure of the cell cortex to the cleavage stimulus culminates in the assembly of a **contractile ring.** This consists of a very thin (0.1–0.2 μm) array of actin filaments attached to the plasma membrane at many sites around the equator. Within the ring, myosin II is assembled into small, bipolar filaments that are interdigitated with actin filaments. Constriction of the ring probably involves a sliding filament mechanism, as in muscle (see Chapter 42). During the early stages of furrowing, the contractile ring maintains a constant volume, but the structure disassembles completely by the end of cleavage. Thus, during the later stages of cytokinesis, contraction is accompanied by disassembly of the ring.

The exact order of addition of components during the formation of the contractile ring is unknown. The process begins in mid-anaphase with targeting of the chromosomal passenger protein INCENP and anillin to the cortex at the cell equator (Fig. 47–21). Like INCENP, anillin is nuclear during interphase. Genetic evidence suggests that anillin is a very early component of the contractile ring. Anillin can bind and bundle actin filaments, but also has a phospholipid-binding domain, suggesting that it may interact directly with the membrane. The actin filament–binding protein radixin localizes to the contractile ring after INCENP, presumably via interactions with its binding partner, the integral membrane protein, and contractile ring component Cdc43. Radixin is a substrate for Rho-kinase, providing a possible explanation for the requirement for small GTPases in cytokinesis.

The contractile apparatus itself forms by the recruitment of actin and myosin II from preexisting structures (Fig. 47–22). The actin filaments in the ring apparently get there by a number of routes. Some were presumably located in the proper area of the cell cortex prior to arrival of the cleavage stimulus, as the entire cortex has a meshwork of actin filaments prior to entry into mitosis. Others are apparently recruited intact into the contractile ring from adjacent areas of the cortex, whereas still others may form de novo in the developing ring by assembly from monomers. Genetic analysis shows that profilin, an actin-binding protein that promotes actin filament assembly, and a profilin-binding protein are required early in contractile ring assembly.

The myosin II of the contractile ring is derived from various interphase structures. In cultured vertebrate cells, most of the myosin II comes from stress fibers (see Fig. 36–3) that break down during prophase. Myosin II is dispersed throughout the cytoplasm until anaphase, when it concentrates in the cor-

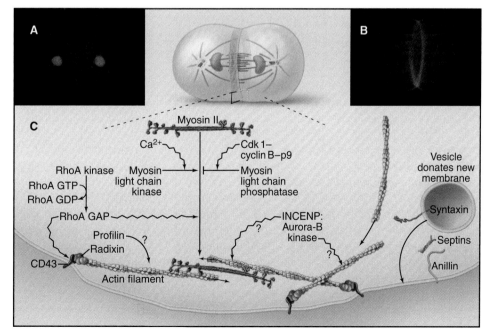

Figure 47–22 Components involved in cytokinesis. *A* and *B*, Invertebrate egg undergoing cytokinesis. *A*, The DNA is stained blue. *B*, The contractile ring is stained yellow. *C*, Diagram showing possible distributions of some of the components known to be involved in contractile ring assembly and function. (*A* and *B*, Micrographs courtesy of Professor Issei Mabuchi, University of Tokyo.)

tex, especially around the equator where the furrow forms.

The role of myosin II as the motor for cytokinesis was established by antibody microinjection and confirmed by genetic inactivation of both the myosin II heavy chain and its regulatory light chain. Amoeboid cells of the slime mold *Dictyostelium* that lack the myosin II heavy chain growing in solution can still extend pseudopodia, round up during mitosis, and complete nuclear division, but they cannot form a cleavage furrow. Paradoxically, these same cells can make relatively normal cleavage furrows if they are tightly adherent to a substratum during mitosis. How this alternative mechanism of furrowing works is not known, but it raises the possibility that another pathway may cooperate with the contractile ring in forming the cleavage furrow.

It now appears that the initiation of ring contraction is induced by a local release of calcium, called a **calcium transient**. This may activate the enzyme **myosin light chain kinase**, which, in turn, activates myosin II concentrated in the contractile ring. Much of the evidence for the involvement of a calcium transient in the regulation of cytokinesis has been indirect. For example, exposure of dividing cells to agents that stimulate the release of calcium accelerates the appearance and rate of propagation of the cleavage furrow. Direct injection of calcium can also stimulate cytokinesis locally, whereas injection of compounds that bind calcium can inhibit cytokinesis. A cytoplasmic calcium transient occurs around the equator prior to assembly and contraction of the cleavage furrow.

As the contractile ring pulls the cell membrane inward, the single cell that entered mitosis is gradually cleaved into two daughter cells. This process requires a significant net increase in the surface area of the cell. The new membrane is inserted adjacent to the leading edge of the furrow, and although its source is not yet known, a number of the proteins involved have now been identified. The best studied of these are the **septins**, which are required for cytokinesis in yeast and animals. Septins are GTP-binding proteins that can bind syntaxins, proteins of the t-SNARE class (see Chapter 21) that are required on target membranes to promote fusion of target vesicles during exocytosis. Specific syntaxins are required for cytokinesis in both plants and animals. In addition to being found in the cleavage furrow, septins are also found in the **exocyst** complex, a protein complex of seven or more subunits involved in secretion, that is thought to target vesicles to particular sites on the membrane. Together, these observations suggest that septins might target membrane vesicles to the cleavage furrow, where they might act as linkers between cytoskeleton and membrane (see Fig. 47–22).

In most cells, contraction of the cleavage furrow

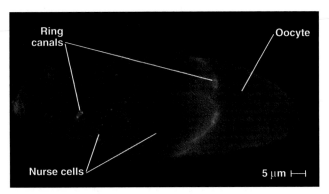

Figure 47–23 Indirect immunofluorescence of a *Drosophila* egg chamber shows actin in red and the ring canal protein *kelch* in green. The co-localization of the two colors in the ring canals makes them appear yellow. Ring canals are sites where cytokinesis arrests at a late stage, leaving channels of communication between daughter cells. In the *Drosophila* oocyte, ring canals connect nurse cells to each other and to the oocyte. Late in oocyte development, a contraction of the nurse cells forces much of their cytoplasmic contents through the ring canals and into the oocyte. This is one way in which the oocyte gains the stockpile of components that are needed for early development of the fly embryo. (Courtesy of Reed Kelso and Lynn Cooley, Yale University.)

ultimately reduces the cytoplasm to a thin intercellular bridge between the two daughter cells. The intercellular bridge contains a highly ordered, anti-parallel array of microtubules derived from the spindle, and it has a dense knob derived from the stem body matrix at its center. This is referred to as the **midbody**. The intercellular bridge eventually breaks by an as-yet-unknown mechanism that appears to require the CHO1 orphan-class kinesin, at least in *C. elegans* embryos. The remaining fragment with the midbody is then frequently shed into the medium. Thus, many of the components of the central spindle and stem body are apparently used for one series of mitotic events and then discarded.

In some tissues, intercellular bridges remain open as ring canals. After a number of successive rounds of "division," what remains is a complex network of interconnected and intercommunicating cells. In mammals, this is particularly notable in spermatogenesis, where groups of several hundred cells may remain connected to one another by ring canals. Figure 47–23 shows a similar situation during *Drosophila* oogenesis, whereby persistent ring canals provide a route for so-called nurse cells to transfer their cytoplasmic contents to the developing egg, thus greatly increasing its stockpile of proteins and mRNAs available for use in early development.

Regulation of the Timing of Cytokinesis

Although there is ample evidence that the level of Cdk1–cyclin B-p9 activity regulates the timing of cytokinesis, the mechanism is unclear. One possibility is that, following the onset of cyclin B destruction at the beginning of anaphase, declining levels of the kinase may promote the assembly of the central spindle, thereby providing the stimulus to activate the onset of cleavage.

Alternatively, it is possible that Cdk1−cyclin B-p9 indirectly regulates the activity of myosin light chain kinase, which activates myosin II by phosphorylating serine-19 and threonine-18 on the regulatory light chain. Phosphorylation of these residues initiates contraction of smooth muscle (see Fig. 42−21). It now appears that Cdk1−cyclin B-p9 or a downstream kinase phosphorylates myosin light chain phosphatase, stimulating its activity and preventing activation of myosin II until anaphase. Inactivation of Cdk1−cyclin B-p9 at the onset of anaphase may lead to dephosphorylation of light chain phosphatase, thereby lowering its activity. The net effect would be to allow the Ca^{2+} that is transient around the equator to activate myosin light chain kinase and trigger contraction of the furrow.

▌ Selected Readings

Adams RR, Carmena M, Earnshaw WC: Chromosomal passengers and the (Aurora) ABCs of mitosis. Trends Cell Biol 11:49−54, 2001.

Collas P, Courvalin J-C: Sorting nuclear membrane proteins at mitosis. Trends Cell Biol 10:5−8, 2000.

Hirano T: Chromosome cohesion, condensation, and separation. Annu Rev Biochem 69:115−144, 2000.

Mitchison TJ, Salmon ED: Mitosis: A history of division. Nat Cell Biol 3:E17−E21, 2001.

Nasmyth K, Peters JM, Uhlmann F: Splitting the chromosome: Cutting the ties that bind sister chromatids. Science 288: 1379−1385, 2000.

Rappaport, R: Cytokinesis in Animal Cells. Developmental and Cell Biology Series. Cambridge: Cambridge University Press, 1996.

Robinson DN, Spudich JA: Towards a molecular understanding of cytokinesis. Trends Cell Biol 10:228−237, 2000.

Sawin KE: Cytokinesis: Sid signals septation. Curr Biol 10: R547−R550, 2000.

Sharp DJ, Rogers GC, Scholey JM: Microtubule motors in mitosis. Nature 407:41−47, 2000.

Straight AF, Field CM: Microtubules, membranes and cytokinesis. Curr Biol 10:R760−R770, 2000.

Sullivan SM, Maddock JR: Bacterial division: Finding the dividing line. Curr Biol 10:R249−R252, 2000.

Wittmann T, Hyman A, Desai A: The spindle: A dynamic assembly of microtubules and motors. Nat Cell Biol 3: E28−E34, 2001.

chapter 48

MEIOSIS

Meiosis is a specialized program of two coupled cell divisions used by eukaryotes as the basis for sexual reproduction. The unique events of meiosis occur in the first division, termed **meiosis I**. The second division, **meiosis II**, is very similar in many respects to mitosis (see Chapter 47 and Box 48–1). Meiosis is an ancient process that occurs in virtually all higher eukaryotes including the animal, fungal, and plant kingdoms.

Each human somatic cell has 23 pairs of chromosomes (46 in all) known as **homologues.** One of each pair is donated by each parent in the egg and sperm, respectively. The number of homologues, 23, is known as the **haploid** chromosome number. In animals, the only haploid cells are gametes (sperm and eggs). At fertilization, haploid gametes fuse to form a zygote, restoring the **diploid** chromosome number of 46. In plants, the haploid phase is represented by gametophytes, which produce ovules and pollen. In most fungi, such as yeasts, haploid and diploid forms are alternate phases of the life cycle.

Meiosis I involves the pairing and orderly segregation of homologous chromosomes from one another. Sister chromatids, replicated in the premeiotic S phase, remain paired with one another throughout. As a result, the haploid daughter cells produced by meiosis I have half the number of chromosomes. Therefore, meiosis I is also known as the **reductional division.** In meiosis II, as in mitosis, sister chromatids segregate from each other, and the number of chromosomes remains the same. Meiosis II is called the **equational division.**

The pairing and orderly segregation of homologues in meiosis I are achieved by a unique process that typically requires genetic recombination between the homologous chromosomes. This recombination occurs during the lengthy and highly specialized prophase of meiosis I.

Meiosis: An Essential Process for Sexual Reproduction

Without meiosis, there would be no sex because every fusion of gametes would result in an increase in the number of chromosomes in the progeny. Sexual reproduction is an important survival strategy that offers organisms a mechanism for altering the genetic makeup of offspring. This strategy has been conserved throughout higher eukaryotes and is inextricably linked with the mechanism of meiosis.

Homologous (maternal and paternal) chromosomes separate from each other in meiosis I. For each pair of homologues, the choice of spindle orientation in meiosis I is random (i.e., each homologue has two equivalent choices of direction in which to migrate). Thus, for humans (with 23 pairs of homologous chromosomes), each gamete has 2^{23} (more than 8 million) possible chromosome configurations as a result of the independent assortment of chromosomes alone. This process does not create new versions of genes, but it guarantees the production of offspring with novel *combinations* of chromosomes.

Meiosis I also brings about the production of novel *versions* of chromosomes. This is because each chromosome must typically undergo at least one genetic recombination (crossover) event to segregate properly at anaphase of meiosis I. If the chromosomes of all the individuals of a species were identical, meiosis and sexual reproduction would only provide different combinations of the same chromosomes. Instead,

---

Chapter by WCE and Maria del Mar Carmena.

---

box 48–1

IMPORTANT DIFFERENCES BETWEEN MEIOSIS AND MITOSIS

- **Meiosis involves two cell divisions.** The two meiotic divisions are preceded by a round of DNA replication. There is no DNA replication between meiosis I and meiosis II.
- **The products of meiosis are haploid.** The products of mitosis are diploid.
- **The products of meiosis are genetically different.** After recombination and random assortment of homologues in meiosis I, the sister chromatids that segregate in meiosis II are different from each other. In normal mitosis, sister chromatids are identical.
- **Prophase is longer in meiosis I.** Proper orientation and segregation of homologous chromosomes is achieved thanks to the pairing, synapsis (synaptonemal complex formation), and recombination that occur in a lengthened prophase during the first meiotic division. In humans mitotic prophase lasts well under an hour, while meiotic prophase lasts many days in males and many years in females.
- **Recombination is increased in meiosis.** Recombination occurs in prophase I of meiosis at a rate 100- to 1000-fold higher than in mitosis. The process has two main consequences: the formation of chiasmata and

the introduction of genetic variation. Chiasmata are structures that physically link the homologous chromosomes after crossover and play an important role in meiotic chromosome segregation.
- **Kinetochore behavior is different in meiosis.** During meiosis I, kinetochores of sister chromatids attach to spindle microtubules emanating from the same pole. Homologous kinetochore pairs connect to opposite poles. In mitosis, sister kinetochores attach to spindle microtubules coming from opposite poles.
- **Chromatid cohesion is different in meiosis.** Sister chromatid cohesion is essential for orientation of bivalents (paired homologous chromosomes) on the metaphase I spindle. During anaphase of meiosis I, cohesion is destroyed between sister chromatid arms and chiasmata are released in order to allow segregation of homologues. Cohesion at the sister centromeres persists until the onset of anaphase II, when it is lost to permit segregation of sisters. In prometaphase of meiosis II, sister chromatids are only joined by the centromeres, whereas at the beginning of mitotic prometaphase, sisters are joined all along the arms.

---

mutation and recombination provide the genetic variation that is the basis for evolution. Recombination involves exchange of chromosomal segments and production of new chromosomes that are a patchwork of segments from the maternal and paternal homologues. The combined effects of recombination and random assortment of homologues in meiosis I yields a vast number of possibilities of different gametes. Genetic recombination, in concert with the random reassortment of chromosomes, provides an important source of genetic diversity that permits eukaryotic populations to adapt to changing environmental conditions.

▌ The Language of Meiosis

Meiosis is sometimes thought to be confusing because it has a language of its own, characterized by a number of new and unusual terms. In fact, the best way to understand meiosis is in terms of the essential biological processes that are involved. This reduces the process to only four essential key terms: pairing, synapsis, recombination, and segregation. Each of these is the subject of a section of this chapter, and so they are defined only briefly here.

Pairing is the alignment of homologous chromosomes within the cell nucleus. This can be seen by

fluorescence in situ hybridization (Fig. 13–10) as the two chromosomes lying near to one another in side-by-side register. Pairing is important because this process is intimately coupled with the scanning process through which DNA sequences on one chromosome find the corresponding DNA sequences on the homologous chromosome in the presence of the billions of base pairs of DNA in the cell nucleus.

Synapsis refers to a process in which the paired homologous chromosomes become intimately associated with one another. A specialized scaffolding structure called the synaptonemal complex mediates this process.

Recombination is a key event of meiotic prophase. It involves physical exchange of DNA between the homologous chromosomes. The first stages of recombination start during pairing; the process is completed following synapsis. In fact, recombination can occur without synapsis under specialized circumstances. Recombination is key to meiosis because specialized chromatin structures called chiasmata form at sites where recombination has been completed and are responsible for keeping the homologous chromosomes paired with one another until anaphase of meiosis I.

Meiosis is all about the *segregation* of the paired homologous chromosomes, and this process shows some key differences from mitosis (see Box 48–1).

When the homologues are balanced at the metaphase plate of the meiosis I spindle, it is the chiasmata that hold them together and counteract the pulling force of the spindle on the kinetochores. Chiasmata are held in place by cohesion between the chromatid arms, which is released at anaphase of meiosis I. Centromeres of the sister chromatids remain associated with one another throughout the whole of meiosis I. This means that, at anaphase, when the chiasmata are released, the paired sister chromatids migrate to the poles of the spindle. As a result, the progeny of meiosis I has the haploid number of chromosomes.

Stages of Meiosis

Pairing, synapsis, and recombination all take place during **prophase** of meiosis I (Fig. 48–1). In the discussion of these processes, it will, therefore, be necessary to refer to the five stages of meiotic prophase: leptotene, zygotene, pachytene, diplotene, and diakinesis. The following brief description of these stages is provided as an aid to understanding the more comprehensive discussion that follows.

The start of **leptotene** is marked by the appearance of individualized chromosomes whose telomeres

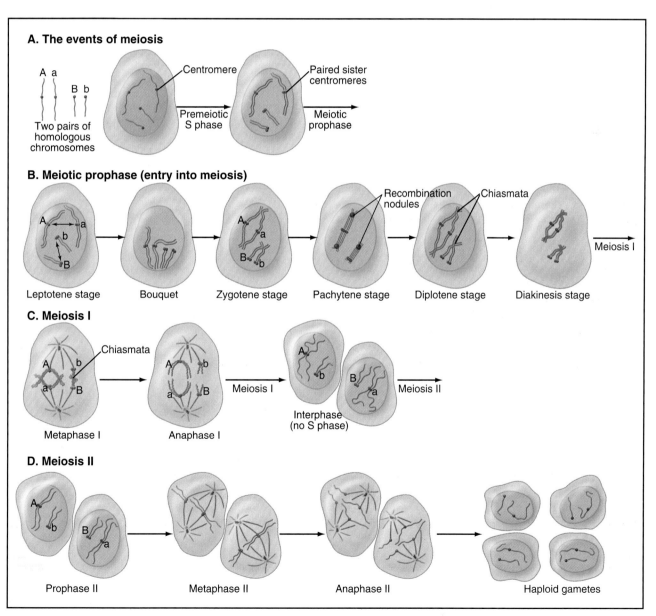

Figure 48-1 A to D, Overview of the phases of meiosis, showing important structures and regulatory molecules (see text for a more detailed explanation).

soon begin to attach to the inside of the nuclear membrane. Paired sister chromatids begin to condense as arrays of loops flanking a dense, proteinaceous axial element. **Zygotene** describes the portion of prophase during which homologues come together in a process known as **synapsis** (Fig. 48–2). This is intimately linked with the assembly of the **synaptonemal complex.** In early zygotene, the telomeres are clustered together at a spot on the nuclear envelope, giving rise to the "bouquet" arrangement of chromosomes. In **pachytene,** synapsis is complete, with the homologues joined together by the synaptonemal complex.

Early in **diplotene,** the synaptonemal complex disintegrates and chromosomes decondense. Later on, they start condensing again. Sister chromatids remain closely associated, whereas homologous chromosomes tend to separate from each other, held only by **chiasmata.** The diplotene stage may last for days or years, depending on the sex and organism (up to 45 years or so in female humans).

In females, the chromosomes are very active in transcription during diplotene, as the egg busily stores up materials for use during the first few divisions of embryonic development. In frogs and other animals in which levels of transcription are particularly elevated, the chromosomes adopt a special structure with very prominent loops and are known as **lampbrush chromosomes** (see Fig. 13–12). These loops are visible because the DNA is coated with huge numbers of nascent RNA transcripts and their associated proteins.

During **diakinesis,** which corresponds to prometaphase of meiosis I, homologous chromosomes once again shorten and condense. At metaphase I, the bivalents (pairs of homologous chromosomes) are aligned at the metaphase plate (see Fig. 48–1). Each of the homologues is oriented to one of the poles of the meiotic spindle. Homologues are held together by chiasmata. At the transition to anaphase I, chiasmata and cohesion between sister chromatids are resolved in order to allow segregation. After telophase I, there is no DNA replication, and cells enter directly in the second meiotic division, which is similar to mitosis. In the eggs of most female vertebrates, meiosis is arrested at metaphase II until fertilization.

The normal separation of chromosomes or chromatids is referred to as **disjunction** (disjoining). Mistakes in this separation are referred to as **nondisjunction.** Nondisjunction in meiosis I and II results in the

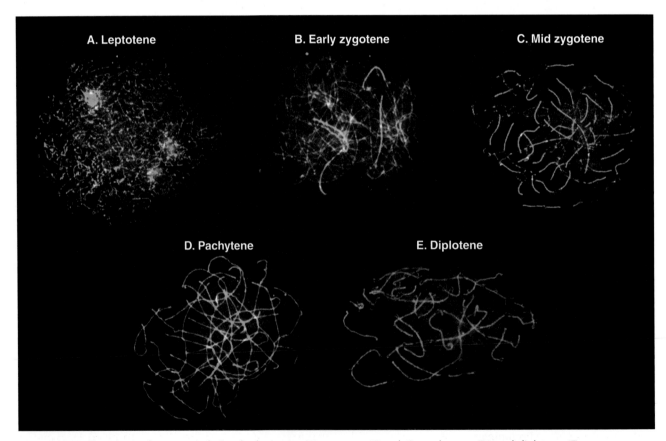

Figure 48-2 Chromosomal structures during the leptotene *(A)*, zygotene *(B* and *C)*, pachytene *(D)*, and diplotene *(E)* stages of meiotic prophase. Human oocyte synaptonemal complex has been stained with anti-Scp3 *(green)* and anti-centromere antibody *(red [A to D only])*, with DAPI staining of the DNA *(blue)*. (Courtesy of Charles Tease, Maj Hulten, and Geraldine Hartshorne, University of Warwick, Coventry, England.)

production of gametes with either too many or too few chromosomes, a condition known as **aneuploidy.**

Much of our knowledge of meiosis is based on studies from the budding yeast, *Saccharomyces cerevisiae.* Budding yeast has several key advantages for the study of meiosis. First, it is possible to induce a synchronous wave of meiosis in yeast cultures. This is key for biochemical analysis of meiosis. Second, the use of powerful genetic analysis has enabled an extensive study of the role of particular gene products in meiosis in vivo. Third, because yeast meiosis produces four equivalent spores, it is possible to examine all products of meiosis genetically and biochemically.

Pairing

Pairing describes the side-by-side alignment of homologues at a distance. Homologous chromosomes are paired in nonmeiotic cells in some organisms, such as the fruit fly *Drosophila* and budding yeast *S. cerevisiae,* but not in vertebrates. As mentioned earlier, pairing involves a process whereby homologous sequences somehow search for one another. In yeast, it appears that the entire genome is searched because even when a single gene is transposed onto a different chromosome, this gene can still find its homologous partner. In humans, small regions of transposed chromosomes can also be detected in the homology search. In certain organisms, such as *Caenorhabditis elegans* or *Drosophila* males, pairing can involve specialized DNA sequences; however, this does not generally appear to be the case.

Pairing is a very early event that starts during or before the leptotene phase, and it appears to be intimately involved with the onset of genetic recombination (Fig. 48–3). Genetic analysis in budding yeast reveals that mutants defective in the earliest stages of recombination are also defective in homologue pairing. It has been estimated that homologous chromosomes interact at about 190 sites per nucleus in budding yeast. This is similar to the number of meiotic recombination events (about 260) and suggests that sites of interaction may be involved in the initiation of recombination.

The mechanism for the global sequence scanning and subsequent homologue pairing is not yet known. One suggestion is that short regions of DNA become single-stranded (presumably as a result of interactions with specific proteins, such as Dmc1p; see section on recombination that follows) and then somehow "invade" double-stranded DNA molecules looking for matching sequences. Preliminary contacts are probably unstable, and the synergistic effect of numerous contacts might be required for stable pairing. It is likely that the recombination process somehow reinforces

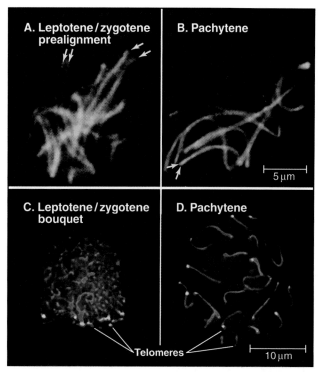

Figure 48-3 Chromosomal arrangements in meiotic prophase. *A* and *B,* Homologous chromosomes are aligned side by side before the synaptonemal complex forms. These yeast chromosomes were visualized using fusion of the protein Spo27 to green fluorescent protein. *A,* Early zygotene. Little synaptonemal complex is present, but homologous chromosomes are paired. *B,* Pachytene. All chromosomes are tightly synapsed. *C* and *D,* The bouquet arrangement of chromosomes in meiosis of the rat. *C,* Early zygotene nucleus showing clustered telomeres in the bouquet. *D,* Pachytene. Telomeres are no longer clustered. Telomeres are labeled red with an antibody to the protein RAP1; synaptonemal complex is labeled green with an antibody to Scp3. (*A* and *B,* Adapted from van Heemst D, James F, Poggeler S, et al: Spo76p is a conserved chromosome morphogenesis protein that links the mitotic and meiotic programs. *Cell* 98: 261–271, 1999. Copyright 1999, with permission from Elsevier Science. *C* and *D,* Adapted from Scherthan H, Jerratsch M, Li B, et al: Mammalian meiotic telomeres: Protein composition and redistribution in relation to nuclear pores. *Mol Biol Cell* 11: 4189–4203, 2000.)

this effect. However, homologues still pair in some systems lacking meiotic recombination (e.g., *Drosophila* recombination mutants like mei-W8), synaptonemal complex formation (asynaptic mutants in yeast), or both (e.g., in normal *Drosophila* males!).

Chromosomal *Ikebana:* The Bouquet Stage

In the transition from leptotene to zygotene, a special arrangement of chromosomes is observed in many organisms. Telomeres group together, attached to the inner nuclear membrane (see Fig. 48–3C). Chromosomes radiate from this point into the nucleus, spreading in a shape resembling a bouquet of flowers, hence the name "bouquet stage." The bouquet seems to be a nearly universal feature of this phase of meiosis, although there are relevant exceptions, as in *C. elegans* and *D. melanogaster*.

Formation of the bouquet starts in leptotene with the attachment of telomeres to the nuclear membrane. Later on, telomeres aggregate and form a plaque at the site of contact with the nuclear membrane. Ultrastructural analysis reveals that this attachment point is a continuation of the synaptonemal complex. Pairing requires microtubules, and the centrosome is frequently located in the cytoplasm next to the telomere plaque. In human spermatocytes and oocytes, cytoplasmic actin filaments connect telomeric attachments.

This very special chromosomal arrangement is thought either to facilitate the pairing of homologues or possibly to improve the chance of contact between homologous regions in synapsis. The bouquet is scattered at pachytene, with dispersal of the telomeres on the membrane, followed by centrosome separation. By diplotene, the telomeres have detached from the nuclear membrane.

Synapsis: Synaptonemal Complex Formation

Synapsis is the intimate association of homologous chromosomes mediated by the **synaptonemal complex.** Synapsis begins in zygotene and is complete throughout pachytene. The role of synapsis is not completely understood. It used to be thought that the synaptonemal complex was responsible for aligning the homologous chromosomes, and that only after this had been achieved would recombination occur. However, this is not the case. Homologue pairing clearly precedes synapsis, and pairing is intimately connected with the initiation of recombination. It now appears that the role of synapsis is to bring the recombination process efficiently to a close and to convert the sites where recombination has occurred into chiasmata that will hold homologous chromosomes paired until anaphase of meiosis I.

The overall architecture of the synaptonemal complex is highly conserved among different species. When mature, this structure looks roughly like railroad tracks with a third rail running down the center wherever homologues are fully paired (Figs. 48–4 and 48–5). The two outer rails are termed lateral elements, whereas the central rail is termed the central element. Thin transverse filaments lying perpendicular to the axial elements appear to connect the lateral elements to each other and to the central element.

Most of the chromosomal DNA extends outward from the synaptonemal complex as loops. No DNA

sequence has definitively been associated with the base of the loops in meiotic chromosomes, and it is not known if particular classes of sequences are associated with the synaptonemal complex. Loop length is quite constant within one species (e.g., about 20,000 bp in *S. cerevisiae*) but varies a lot among different species. In human females, the synaptonemal complex is roughly 50% longer than it is in males. A great many studies have revealed that the length of the synaptonemal complex is directly proportional to the frequency of meiotic recombination. In fact, human females undergo recombination at about twice the frequency of males.

Synaptonemal complex assembly starts in lepto-

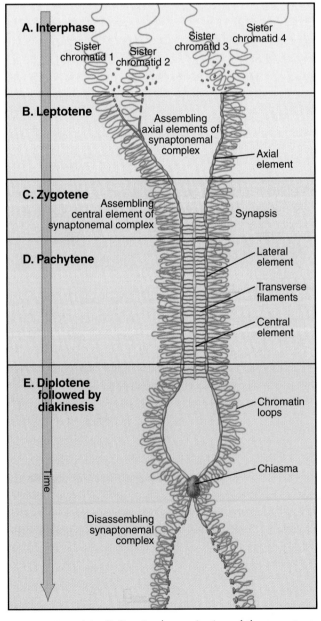

Figure 48–4 *A to E,* Structural organization of the synaptonemal complex during the various stages of meiotic prophase.

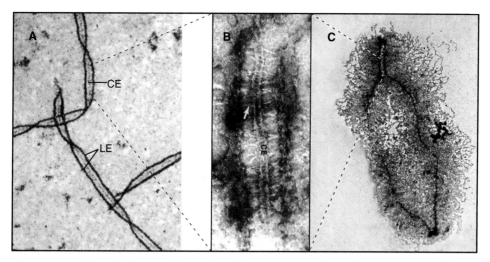

Figure 48–5 Selected electron micrographs of the synaptonemal complex. *A,* Low-magnification view of maize synaptonemal complexes stained with silver. The lateral (LE) and central elements (CE) are clearly seen. *B,* A negatively stained cricket synaptonemal complex following treatment with deoxyribonuclease (DNase). The central element (*CE*) and transverse filaments (*arrow*) are visible. *C,* A whole mount of zygotene chromosome of the silk moth. Cells in meiotic prophase were swollen and then lysed under gentle conditions with detergent. The chromosomes were then centrifuged onto thin carbon films so that they could be examined by electron microscopy. The synaptonemal complex is easily seen on this chromosome. Chromatin loops radiate outward, both from the unpaired axial elements and the paired lateral elements (where synapsis has occurred). (*A,* Adapted from Gillies CB: Electron microscopy of spread maize pachytene synaptonemal complexes. Chromosoma 83:575–591, 1981. *B,* Adapted from Solari AJ, Moses MJ: The structure of the central region in the synaptonemal complexes of hamster and cricket spermatocytes. J Cell Biol 56:145–152, 1973, by copyright permission of the Rockefeller University Press. *C,* From Rattner JB, Goldsmith M, Hamkalo BA: Chromatin organization during meiotic prophase of Bombyx mori. Chromosoma 79:215–224, 1980.)

tene with the appearance of axial elements along the length of each homologue (see Fig. 48–4). Normally, one axial element forms for each pair of sister chromatids, but sometimes splitting of each axial element is observed. Synapsis begins during zygotene as the axial elements align in parallel, leaving a gap of 900–1000 Å, and the central element forms between them. Synapsis begins at a number of sites along each pair of bivalents. By pachytene, a continuous synaptonemal complex is observed between homologous chromosomes.

It is important to emphasize that *synapsis*, the formation of the synaptonemal complex, is different from *pairing*, which describes the onset of an ordered genetic and physical interaction between homologous chromosomes. Although both processes are intimately related, several lines of evidence highlight differences between them. In yeast, mutants affecting synaptonemal complex formation do not affect pairing (i.e., homologous chromosomes pair but do not synapse). In natural polyploid organisms, like plants, there is more than one component genome, so there are more than two homologous chromosomes. When the component genomes are very different, homologues belonging to different components (called homeologues) can still pair with each other but do not synapse or recombine.

Pairing normally precedes synapsis, although in cases in which presynaptic homologue pairing has not occurred, a "zipper" effect from synaptonemal complex assembly can contribute to pairing.

The distribution of chiasmata along the arms of a chromosome is not random. An unknown mechanism ensures that a minimum spacing is maintained between them. Thus, one crossover event *interferes* with the occurrence of others in nearby regions of the chromosome. In a typical human spermatocyte with 23 pairs of homologues, about 50 chiasmata are observed. The larger chromosomes typically have four of them. The smallest chromosomes have one, and intermediate-sized chromosomes usually have two or three. One role of the synaptonemal complex appears to be establishment of this "crossover interference." The fission yeast *Schizosaccharomyces pombe* and the mold *Aspergillus nidulans* lack both synaptonemal complexes and crossover interference. Further evidence for a role of the synaptonemal complex in crossover interference is the observation that, in budding yeast *zip1* mutants, which lack synaptonemal complex, crossover interference is abolished. Presumably, the phenomenon of crossover interference has something to do with the processing of crossovers to turn them into mature chiasmata.

Synaptonemal Complex Components

Components of the synaptonemal complex have been identified through both genetic and biochemical approaches. Perhaps the best studied is the budding yeast protein Zip1p, which is found in mature synaptonemal complex, but not in the unpaired axial elements. Zip1p is predicted to have extensive regions of coiled-coil and is thought to assemble into a rod-shaped dimer. If the length of the Zip1p coiled-coil is altered, then synaptonemal complexes are produced in which the spacing between lateral elements is altered. This provides strong evidence that Zip1p is a key component of the transverse filaments in *S. cerevisiae* (Fig. 48–6).

In *zip1* mutants, the axial elements form, but homologous chromosomes are unable to synapse, and they pair only loosely. Recombination appears to be initiated but fails to be completed at about 10% of sites. As a result, the cells become arrested in pachytene (see later discussion of the pachytene checkpoint). Studies of this mutant show clearly that recombination can be initiated before chromosomes are tightly synapsed. In addition, they suggest that the role of the synaptonemal complex may be more in the proper termination of recombination than in chromosomal alignment.

In mammals, the protein Scp1 (called Syn1 in the hamster) is also localized in the transverse filaments. There is no sequence homology between Zip1p and Scp1/Syn1, but all of them share a common structure: a coiled-coil flanked by two globular domains. Scp1 is one of several identified cancer testis antigens. It is frequently expressed in human malignant diseases.

Several protein components of the axial/lateral elements have also been identified. In yeast, the Red1 protein is required for assembly of axial elements. Interestingly, in *red1* mutants, recombination is reduced (about three-fold) but not abolished. Mammalian Scp2 and Scp3 are components of the axial/lateral elements. After the synaptonemal complex starts to disappear in diplotene, Scp2 and Scp3 stay on the chromosomes. Scp2 only disappears totally after metaphase I, but Scp3 stays all along the chromosomes until anaphase I, and then only at the kinetochore until anaphase II. It has, therefore, been proposed to play a role in the special behavior of kinetochores during meiosis (see later section). Both proteins interact with members of the cohesin complex (see later discussion). Additionally, Scp3 interacts with Rad51p and Dmc1p, proteins involved in homologue recognition and the formation of recombination intermediates. Scp3-null mice do not form a synaptonemal complex, and chromosomes do not synapse. They are sterile owing to massive apoptosis in the gonads.

Recombination

Meiotic recombination in budding yeast and *C. elegans* initiates with cleavage of both strands of the DNA by a specialized enzyme called Spo11p (Box 48–2, Fig. 48–7A). Spo11p is a member of the class of enzymes called DNA topoisomerases (see Chapter 13). The reaction mechanism for these enzymes involves cleavage of one or both DNA strands (depending on the class of topoisomerase involved) in a reaction that produces a covalent linkage between a tyrosine on the enzyme and the cleaved phosphodiester backbone. This protein/DNA complex has been detected in yeast cells. Spo11-mediated double-strand breaks do not just occur at random in yeast; certain sites are preferred. Although the mechanism of site selection is not completely understood, it is known that, in addition to the DNA sequence of the chromosomes at that point, the formation of breaks is also influenced by the chromatin structure.

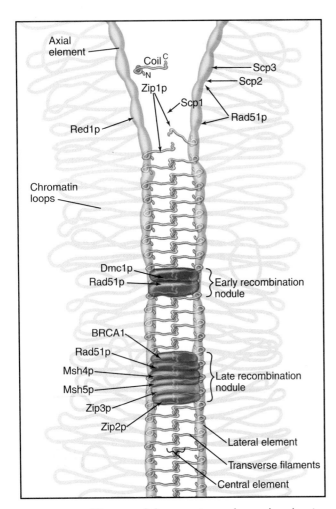

Figure 48-6 Diagram of the synaptonemal complex showing the locations of a number of well-characterized components.

box 48–2

BRIEF OVERVIEW OF GENETIC TERMINOLOGY

It is beyond the scope of this text to provide a comprehensive introduction to the field of genetics. However, to discuss genetic recombination and its role in meiosis, a number of terms used by geneticists should first be introduced (also see Box 5–1).

The **genotype** of an organism is the combination of genes that are present on the chromosomes of that organism. The **phenotype** is the physical manifestation of the action of these gene products (i.e., the appearance and macromolecular composition of the organism). In discussing recombination, scientists typically refer to the presence or absence of specific genetic markers. Each **genetic marker** is a particular DNA sequence in or around a gene that can be monitored by examining the phenotypes of the cells that carry it. A genetic marker might be the presence of a functional gene, a mutation with altered activity, or simply a polymorphism of DNA sequence that has no known functional consequence.

An organism that is **homozygous** for a particular genetic marker has the same sequence of that particular region of the DNA on both the maternal and paternal homologous chromosomes. A **heterozygous** organism has different forms of the genetic markers on the two homologous chromosomes. Although the physical events of genetic recombination can occur in both homozygotes and heterozygotes, they are most readily detected in the latter.

If two genetic markers are on different chromosomes, they will separate from one another in the anaphase of meiosis I 50% of the time as a result of the random distribution of chromosomes to the two spindle poles. If they are on the same chromosome, they will be *linked* to one another unless the chromosome undergoes a genetic recombination event between them. The greater the separation of two markers on one chromosome, the more likely it is for such an intervening recombination event to occur.

Two types of recombination events occur during meiosis (Fig. 48–7). The first of these—**gene conversion**—involves the *loss* of one or more genetic markers. This occurs by conversion of the DNA sequence on one chromosome into that on a second chromosome while keeping the second sequence intact. Thus, for a heterozygous trait A/a, gene conversion results in the production of a homozygous genotype A/A (or a/a). Gene conversion is thought to occur as the result of the invasion of a double helix by a region of DNA with complementary sequence, as shown in Figure 48–7.

The second type of recombination event—**crossing over**—involves the physical breakage and reunion of

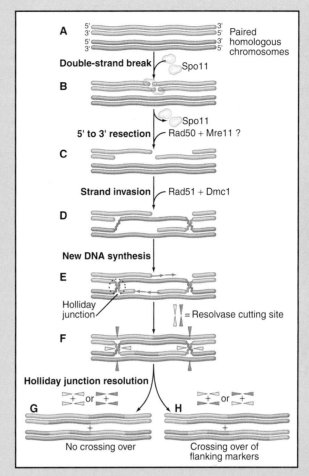

Figure 48–7 The events of recombination. Recombination occurs between homologues rather than sisters. *A,* Paired homologous chromosomes. *B,* Spo11 makes a double-strand break. *C,* Resection of the break. *D,* Strand invasion. *E,* New DNA synthesis fills the gaps. *F,* Sites of nuclease cutting as the Holliday junction is resolved. *G,* Symmetrical cutting gives no crossing over. *H,* Asymmetrical cutting gives crossing over. For further details, see text. (Reference: Paques F, Haber JE: Multiple pathways of recombination induced by double-strand breaks in *Saccharomyces cerevisiae.* Microbiol Mol Biol Rev 63:349–404, 1999.)

DNA strands on two different chromosomes. This is what most people think of when they think of recombination. In recombination by crossing over, the makeup of genetic markers remains constant; it is the linkage between different markers that changes.

In mice, as in yeast, the action of Spo11p and the generation of double-strand breaks are required for the normal pairing and synapsis of homologous chromosomes. In Spo11-null mice, recombination is not initiated and synapsis, if it occurs at all, is aberrant, often involving nonhomologous chromosomes (Fig. 48–8). In these mutant mice, spermatocytes die by apoptosis early in meiotic prophase, and oocytes die somewhat later. Interestingly, the nematode *C. elegans* and the fruit fly *D. melanogaster* do not require Spo11p-induced double-strand breaks for synapsis of homologous chromosomes.

The next stage of meiotic recombination in yeast involves the processing of the double-strand breaks. This is carried out by a $5' \rightarrow 3'$ exonuclease, which chews back one strand of the double helix (a process called resection), leaving single-stranded tails at the $3'$ end of the DNA molecules (see Fig. 48–7C). These tails can be detected in leptotene before synaptonemal complex formation. The exonuclease appears to be the product of two genes called *RAD50* and *MRE11*. These proteins are similar to two *Escherichia coli* proteins (SbcC and SbcD) that are well known to have exonuclease activity.

Following processing of the double-strand breaks, the single-stranded tails "invade" the homologus chromosome, displacing one DNA strand and base-pairing with the other. This produces branched intermediates known as **Holliday junctions** (see Fig. 48–7D and *E*). This happens in early pachytene and requires the products of the *RAD51* and *DMC1* genes. Double Holliday junctions persist throughout most of pachytene but are then converted to mature crossover and non-crossover recombination products.

Rad51p and Dmc1p are homologues of the *E. coli*

RecA protein. These enzymes polymerize into nucleo-protein filaments on DNA and use adenosine triphosphate (ATP) to catalyze homologous pairing and strand exchange reactions (i.e., to insert a single-stranded region of DNA into a double helix, displacing one of the two paired strands). Rad51p is required for cellular life and thus clearly has an essential function in addition to meiosis. This may be in the repair of DNA damage. In contrast, Dmc1p appears to be required only in meiosis, and mutants lacking the protein are defective in the pairing of homologues. Rad51p and Dmc1p are found in structures called **early recombination nodules** that appear along the axial elements during leptotene or early zygotene (see Fig. 48–6). Early nodules do not correspond with crossover sites but may have a role to play in the initiation of recombination, possibly serving as sites of double-strand break formation.

Crossover recombination products that are produced by cleavage of Holliday junctions during pachytene form structures that can be seen on the synaptonemal complex (see Fig. 48–7F). These structures are called **late recombination nodules.** Although the nodules are only seen by electron microscopy, it is widely assumed that foci seen along the synaptonemal complex in immunostaining experiments correspond to the nodules. One component of late nodules is Mlh1, a protein required for meiotic recombination in mammals (see Fig. 48–6). Although Rad51p and Dmc1p are largely dissociated from chromosomes in pachytene, some Rad51p is present in late nodules, where it co-localizes with BRCA1 (the human tumor suppressor protein mutated in certain types of breast cancer). Late nodules are converted into chiasmata during the diplotene stage. Chiasmata are thought to be specialized chromatin bridges between the homologues. They are held in place by chromosome arm cohesion that persists long after the synaptonemal complex has been disassembled and recombination intermediates have been resolved. Figure 48–9 shows the localization of several proteins involved in yeast synaptonemal complex structure and recombination.

A second system for segregating homologues in meiosis I has been found in fruit flies and budding yeast. This process, which has been called **distributive segregation,** functions on chromosomes that have *not* undergone genetic recombination. The distributive system senses chromosomal length, rather than sequence homology. Thus, a metacentric chromosome can undergo accurate distributive pairing and disjunction with *two* acrocentric chromosomes, provided that each corresponds roughly in length to one of the arms of the metacentric chromosome. The distributive segregation system can handle one or a few non-recombined chromosomes, but if there has been an overall breakdown in recombination, then massive nondisjunction

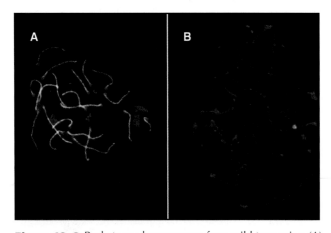

Figure 48–8 Pachytene chromosomes from wild-type mice (A) and mice in which the Spo11 gene has been disrupted (B). Pairing of homologous chromosomes is severely disrupted in the Spo11 mutant. (From Baudat F, Manova K, Yuen JP, et al: Chromosome synapsis defects and sexually dimorphic meiotic progression in mice lacking spo11. Mol Cell 6:989–998, 2000. Copyright 2000, with permission from Elsevier Science.)

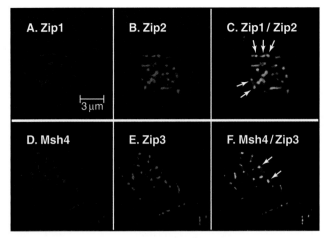

| A. Zip1 | B. Zip2 | C. Zip1 / Zip2 |
| D. Msh4 | E. Zip3 | F. Msh4 / Zip3 |

3 μm

Figure 48-9 Distribution of proteins involved in recombination in budding yeast meiotic chromosomes. *A to C,* Zip2 *(green)* binds at discrete sites along the synaptonemal complex, visible after staining with anti-Zip1 *(red). D to F,* Zip3 *(green),* which interacts with Zip2, co-localizes with the recombination enzyme Msh4 *(red)* at sites that correspond to late recombination nodules. In both cases, sites of co-localization appear yellow *(arrows).* (*A to C,* From Chua PR, Roeder GS: Zip2, a meiosis-specific protein required for the initiation of chromosome synapsis. Cell 93:349–359, 1998. Copyright 1998, with permission from Elsevier Science. *D to F,* From Agarwal S, Roeder GS: Zip3 provides a link between recombination enzymes and synaptonemal complex proteins. Cell 102:245–255, 2000. Copyright 2000, with permission from Elsevier Science.)

occurs. The mechanism of distributive segregation is unknown. One *Drosophila* mutant that affects the process is defective in a member of the kinesin family of molecular motor proteins (see Fig. 40–3). It is not known whether vertebrates have a functioning distributive segregation system.

Cohesion and Chromosomal Movements During Meiosis I

Chromosomes in mitosis achieve a dynamic alignment at the middle of the spindle as a result of a balance of forces. The two kinetochores of the sister chromatids are attached to opposite spindle poles, and mechanochemical motors located on the chromosomes actively pull each chromatid toward the pole that its kinetochore faces. This force does not produce any net poleward movement during metaphase because the two sister chromatids are held together until the onset of anaphase (see Fig. 47–7).

In meiosis I, paired homologues (called **bivalents**) are balanced at the metaphase plate. The structure of bivalents has two important differences from that of mitotic chromosomes. First, the kinetochore of each homologue is composed of the two kinetochores of the sister chromatids fused and acting as a single unit. The structure of the meiosis I kinetochore is most easily explained if the two kinetochores are each ro-

tated 90 degrees toward one another relative to their position on mitotic chromosomes (Fig. 48–10*A*). These sister kinetochores first visibly separate late in the first meiotic metaphase, when they move to opposite sides of the primary constriction. In yeast, this behavior requires the presence of a meiosis-specific kinetochore protein—monopolin—that associates with sister kinetochores from pachytene until anaphase of meiosis I. In some organisms, a strand of material visualized by a specialized silver-staining protocol connects the sister kinetochores. This physical connection is not broken in anaphase I, and sister centromeres are held together until anaphase II.

A second major difference between bivalents and mitotic chromosomes is in the force that resists the poleward pulling of the kinetochores and restrains the bivalent at the spindle midzone at metaphase. In meiosis I, this force arises from the adherence of homologues at chiasmata (Fig. 48–11; see also Fig. 48–10). Thus, recombination and chiasma formation are essential parts of the mechanism that guarantees the orderly segregation of homologous chromosomes in meiotic anaphase I. However, recombination alone is not sufficient to ensure the proper segregation of bivalents at meiosis I. This is shown most clearly by the *desynaptic* mutant of maize. In this mutant, homologous chromosomes synapse apparently normally and normal numbers of recombination events occur, producing chiasmata. However, these chiasmata frequently fall apart as the cells enter the first meiotic M phase. As a result, the homologues tend to segregate randomly in meiosis I. The underlying defect in the *desynaptic* mutation is not known, but the mutation behaves as expected for a defect in chromatid arm cohesion.

After premeiotic DNA replication, cohesion keeps sister chromatids together all along the arms. Once bivalents have oriented in the metaphase I spindle, chiasmata appear to be held in place by sister chromatid cohesion, which actually opposes homologue separation in the regions where exchange has occurred. At the onset of anaphase I, sister chromatid cohesion is released along the chromosome arms, allowing chiasmata to dissolve and homologous chromosomes to segregate to the spindle poles.

Sister chromatid cohesion at the centromeric regions is maintained until the onset of anaphase in meiosis II. This difference in the times at which sister cohesion is lost along the arms and in the centromeric region is essential for meiosis.

Work in yeasts, *Drosophila* and *Xenopus*, has identified a protein complex, the **cohesin complex**, required to hold sister chromatids together (see Fig. 47–14). In the budding yeast, two members of the cohesin complex disappear from chromosome arms during the first meiotic division but persist in the centromeres until the onset of anaphase II. One is Smc3p,

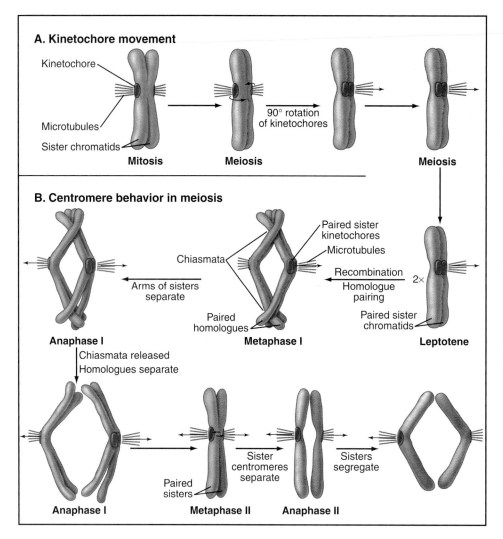

Figure 48-10 Chromosomal behavior during meiosis I and II. During meiosis I, sister chromatids are tightly paired along their lengths, kinetochore structure is altered, and homologues are held together at the metaphase plate by chiasmata. During anaphase I, loss of cohesion between the arms of sister chromatids releases the chiasmata and allows homologous chromosomes to segregate to opposite poles. During metaphase of meiosis II, sister chromatids are held together at their centromeres. Release of centromeric cohesion at meiosis II allows the sister chromatids to segregate to opposite spindle poles.

a cohesin subunit also required for mitosis. The other is **Rec8p,** a meiosis-specific cohesin subunit. Rec8 is the meiotic homologue of a protein called Scc1p, a key factor in the regulation of chromatid cohesion. Like Scc1p, Rec8 must be assembled onto the chromo-

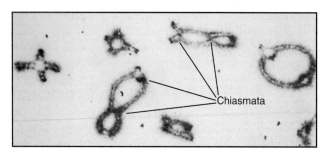

Figure 48-11 Bivalents at meiosis I metaphase are pulled toward the spindle poles by kinetochore-microtubule interactions but remain balanced at the metaphase plate because they are held together by chiasmata. These chromosomes are from a grasshopper. The chromosomes have been specifically stained with silver. (From Suja JA, de la Torre J, Gimenez-Abian JF, et al: Meiotic chromosome structure: Kinetochores and chromatid cores in standard and B chromosomes of Arcyptera fusca [Orthoptera] revealed by silver staining. Genome 34:19–27, 1991.)

some during the S phase preceding meiosis in order for it to regulate sister chromatid cohesion properly. If Rec8 is assembled on chromosomes after the premeiotic S phase, then sister chromatids separate prematurely in meiosis I. In mitosis, Scc1p is cleaved by a protease called **separase** at the onset of anaphase, and this cleavage is absolutely required for chromatid separation. In meiosis, Rec8p cleavage regulates chromatid separation in both meiosis I and meiosis II. In meiosis I, Rec8p is cleaved only along the chromosomal arms. This releases arm cohesion, permitting homologues to separate. However, Rec8p at centromeres remains intact. Cleavage of centromeric Rec8p at the onset of anaphase of meiosis II then releases the connection between centromeres and allows the sister chromatids to separate. The mechanism regulating the localized proteolysis of Rec8p in meiosis is not yet known.

Both Rec8p and Smc1p are found along chromosome cores containing axial elements or synaptonemal complexes. Analysis of mutants in these proteins has demonstrated that both are required for meiotic sister chromatid cohesion and axial element formation. This seems to establish a link between these two processes. Additionally, these proteins are necessary for recombination. In mammals, SMC1 and SMC3, two key members of the cohesin complex, have also been shown to interact with components of the synaptonemal complex lateral elements.

In addition to alterations in the organization of the chromosomes, spindle formation and structure differ between meiotic and mitotic cells. For example, meiotic spindles typically lack astral microtubules and may lack localized poles (perhaps because centrioles are often absent).

Behavior of the Sex Chromosomes in Meiosis

Of the 46 human chromosomes, the two **sex chromosomes** carry genes that define the sex of the individual. The other 22 pairs of chromosomes are called **autosomes.** The behavior of sex chromosomes and autosomes exhibits important differences during meiosis.

In particular, if genetic recombination is absolutely required to stabilize homologous chromosomes at the metaphase plate in meiosis I, then how is this accomplished for the X and Y chromosomes? The answer in most mammals is that the X and Y chromosomes have a short region of homologous sequence (about 2.6 million base pairs in humans) that does pair and undergo genetic recombination during meiosis. This is called the **pseudoautosomal region.** This region must undergo genetic recombination in every meiosis I cell if the X and Y chromosomes are subsequently to be partitioned correctly. Thus, the X and Y chromosomes act like short homologous chromosomes with large regions of unrelated DNA attached (Fig. 48–12).

The pairing between X and Y chromosomes in pachytene often extends beyond the pseudoautosomal region into the sex-specific portions of the chromosomes. However, this pairing never results in recombination. This confirms that pairing alone is not sufficient for recombination: homologous sequences must also be present. Regions of the X and Y chromosomes that do not pair in meiosis become highly condensed during late pachytene.

Cell Cycle Regulation of Meiotic Events

Meiosis employs the full set of functions that are required for the regulation of cell division in somatic cells (see Chapters 43 to 46). However, the peculiarities of the meiotic cell cycle require further mechanisms of regulation. One major difference between meiotic cells and somatic cells is that the meiotic chromosomes must undergo recombination and chiasma

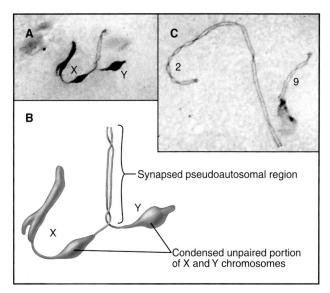

Figure 48-12 The sex chromosomes of a Chinese hamster at pachytene. *A* and *B,* The X and Y chromosomes are paired at the pseudoautosomal region. Elsewhere, the unpaired chromatin adopts a highly condensed morphology. *C,* Autosomes are completely synapsed and show a lesser degree of condensation. (From Dresser ME, Moses MJ: Synaptonemal complex karyotyping in spermatocytes of the Chinese hamster *(Cricetulus griseus).* IV. Light and electron microscopy of synapsis and nucleolar development by silver staining. Chromosoma 76:1–22, 1980.)

formation to segregate properly at the first meiotic division. It now appears that there is no mechanism to detect whether or not recombination has occurred in yeast. Yeast cells that are completely defective in recombination proceed through meiosis with normal timing but disastrous consequences; the chromosomes cannot align properly during meiosis I, and they assort randomly to the daughter cells. On the other hand, cells are able to detect the presence of stalled or abnormal recombination intermediates. Such intermediates accumulate if there are problems with the core recombination enzymes or if the assembly of the synaptonemal complex (required for the completion of recombination) is defective. When such problems are detected, cells arrest in the pachytene stage of meiotic prophase I. This pachytene checkpoint has been studied mainly in *S. cerevisiae,* but there is evidence that the mechanism is conserved. In mammals, germ cells that are arrested at the pachytene checkpoint owing to defects in recombination undergo apoptosis and are eliminated.

Studies in budding and fission yeasts have also revealed the existence of a DNA replication checkpoint in meiosis, involving the Rad proteins as well as the downstream kinase Chk2. If replication defects are detected, this checkpoint keeps Cdk1 activity levels low by maintaining phosphorylation in Tyr[15] and blocking entry into meiosis I (see Chapter 43).

Many of the proteins involved in mitotic checkpoints are present in meiotic cells. Proteins like ataxia telangiectasia–mutated (ATM) kinase, ataxia telangiectasia and Rad3 (ATR) protein kinase, Chk1, and the human homologue of *S. pombe* Rad1 (see Chapter 46) are associated with meiotic chromosomes in prophase, and it has been suggested that they could be involved in the meiotic checkpoint.

Suppression of DNA Replication Between Meiosis I and Meiosis II

One of the unique aspects of meiosis is that the process involves two M phases with no intervening S phase. Upon exit from meiosis I, Cdk1 kinase is reactivated immediately. This blocks assembly of prereplication complexes (see Chapter 45), thereby blocking DNA replication. Two pathways have been identified so far that contribute to reactivation of Cdk1. These pathways are not mutually exclusive and seem to be universally conserved.

The first pathway involves the down-regulation of translation of Wee1 protein kinase in meiosis. Wee1 is a mitotic inhibitor (see Fig. 43–7) that inactivates Cdk1 by phosphorylation at Tyr[15]. The absence of Wee1 in meiosis I was first observed in *Xenopus laevis* but seems to be a universally conserved way of reactivating Cdk1 without an S phase. Ectopic expression of Wee1 in mature *Xenopus* oocytes prevents reactivation of Cdk1 immediately after the meiosis I division. As a result, the oocytes re-enter interphase and replicate their DNA.

The second mechanism for differentiating meiosis from mitosis involves activation of a specialized mitogen-activated protein (MAP) kinase pathway by c-Mos, a meiotic-specific kinase. This pathway also activates Cdk1 and other unknown substrates, with profound effects on the meiotic cell cycle (see next section).

The Metaphase II Arrest and the MAPK Pathway

Oocytes of many vertebrates arrest in metaphase II of meiosis until they are fertilized. The activity responsible for this arrest was originally identified in *Xenopus laevis* and called **cytostatic factor** (CSF). CSF was discovered when cytoplasm from a *Xenopus laevis* egg (arrested in metaphase of meiosis II) was injected into one blastomere of a frog embryo at the two-cell stage. Once the injected blastomere entered mitosis, it became blocked at metaphase, just like the egg. Therefore, CSF is an activity that can even block somatic cells indefinitely at metaphase in mitosis. CSF activity appears in meiosis II and disappears after fertilization.

One active component of CSF is the *Xenopus* homologue of a well-known viral oncogene, *v-mos*, which was first identified as the transforming gene of

a cancer virus that causes solid tumors in mice (Moloney murine sarcoma virus). Using DNA hybridization, a cellular gene corresponding to *v-mos* was isolated from *Xenopus*. This gene is called **c-mos.** The *v-mos* gene is a mutant form of the cellular *c-mos* gene. *c-mos* is expressed only in oocytes and eggs, and not at all in somatic cells. Injection of either v-mos or c-Mos proteins into dividing blastomeres of early frog embryos arrested the cells at metaphase (Fig. 48–13). These experiments led to the proposal that c-Mos was CSF.

CSF arrest is known to be produced by the MAP kinase (MAPK) signal transduction pathway (see Fig. 29–5). Mos activates the pathway by phosphorylating MEK (MAPK-activating kinase), which then activates MAPK. MAPK then activates a downstream kinase called p90Rsk (see Fig. 48–13*D*). Introduction of constitutively active c-Mos or p90Rsk into *Xenopus* eggs is sufficient to induce CSF arrest. However, this version

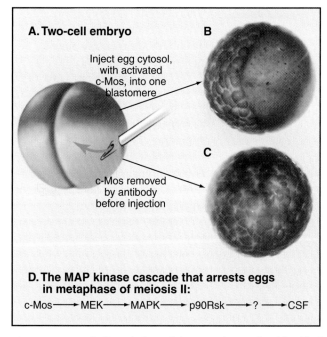

D. The MAP kinase cascade that arrests eggs in metaphase of meiosis II:

c-Mos ⟶ MEK ⟶ MAPK ⟶ p90Rsk ⟶ ? ⟶ CSF

Figure 48–13 *A*, Description of the experiment that identified c-Mos as an essential component of cytostatic factor (CSF) required for arrest of eggs in meiotic metaphase. One blastomere of a *Xenopus* embryo at the two-cell stage was injected with cytoplasm from a metaphase-arrested egg containing CSF activity. *B*, This blastomere (*right half of the embryo*) remained blocked in metaphase while the left blastomere divided many times. *C*, The same experiment was performed, but prior to injection, the c-Mos was removed from the egg cytoplasm by absorption with a specific antibody. Both the injected and uninjected blastomeres continued to divide normally. *D*, The MAP kinase pathway leading to metaphase II arrest in vertebrate eggs. (*B* and *C*, Micrographs courtesy of George Vande Woude, NCI, Frederick, MD; adapted from Sagata N, Watanabe N, Vande Woude GF, et al: The c-Mos proto-oncogene product is a cytostatic factor responsible for meiotic arrest in vertebrate eggs. Nature 342:512–518, 1989.)

of the pathway is not the whole story. P90Rsk can be depleted from a CSF-arrested extract, and the metaphase arrest is maintained. This means that there must be at least one unidentified step in the pathway beyond p90Rsk.

Regulation of *c-mos* is very important for meiosis; activation of this MAPK pathway is involved both in the metaphase II arrest caused by CSF and suppression of DNA replication between the two meiotic divisions. At the metaphase-anaphase transition that occurs upon fertilization of the egg, a transient increase in intracellular free Ca^{2+} apparently activates a protease of the calpain class that destroys c-Mos. Inactivation of c-Mos after meiosis, with subsequent inactivation of MAPK and p90Rsk, is required for entry into the first embryonic mitosis.

Timing of Meiosis in Humans

The fate of cells undergoing meiosis, as well as the timing of meiotic events, differs significantly between males and females.

Males produce about 100 million sperm a day in a process called spermatogenesis. This process continues throughout adult life. Spermatogenesis starts with the division of stem cells called **spermatogonia** and involves eight divisions prior to meiosis. These divisions are unusual in that cytokinesis is incomplete, and the cells remain connected by intercellular bridges. The process could produce up to 256 cells, but usually some cells die and others fail to divide, so that a more typical number is around 200 cells coming from the initial stem cell division. When these cells pass through meiosis (at which point they are referred to as spermatocytes) the final result is about 800 postmeiotic **spermatids.** Spermatids then undergo a complex program of differentiation, resulting in the production of the highly specialized **spermatozoa.** The entire process of spermatogenesis takes about 64 days, the bulk of which is spent in meiosis I. About 16 days are spent in pachytene, the longest stage of the meiosis I prophase. In contrast, only about 8 hours are spent in meiosis II.

In females, the ovary contains a total of about 100,000 primordial follicles, each with an oocyte that is arrested in the diplotene stage of meiosis at about the 12th to 16th week of fetal life. Following puberty, a small number of oocytes become activated and grow each month. One of these activated oocytes matures fully and is shed in response to a surge of luteinizing hormone. The others undergo programmed cell death and degenerate in a process known as atresia. As the oocyte is shed from the ovary, it completes meiosis I and becomes arrested at metaphase of meiosis II. It remains arrested at this stage until fertilization occurs.

In human females, only one mature egg is produced as a result of meiosis. All of the cell divisions are asymmetrical, with the other cells produced by the meiotic cleavages being very small and short-lived. These small cells are referred to as **polar bodies.** Note the marked contrast of these asymmetric meiotic divisions to those in the male, where each spermatocyte gives rise to four spermatozoa of equal size.

Meiotic Defects and Human Disease

Abnormalities in meiosis are surprisingly common but are not widely observed in the population because their consequences are extremely severe. In fact, meiotic abnormalities are a leading cause of fetal death, particularly during the first trimester of pregnancy in humans. The two major causes of problems are nondisjunction in the meiotic divisions and the generation of chromosomal rearrangements.

When chromosomes do not segregate properly in one or both meiotic divisions (nondisjunction), the products of meiosis do not have the normal haploid chromosomal complement. Gametes that have gained an entire set of chromosomes are referred to as **polyploid.** In human embryos, polyploidy is a common type of chromosomal abnormality, with triploidy (69 chromosomes) being the most common form. It is estimated that between 1% and 3% of all conceptions are triploids. Two thirds of these arise as a result of two sperm fertilizing one egg (nothing wrong with meiosis there!). In other cases, they come from a diploid gamete, the result of a defective meiotic segregation. The vast majority of triploid embryos do not survive to term.

Most chromosomal abnormalities in human embryos result from the loss or gain of one or more chromosomes. This condition is referred to as **aneuploidy.** In most cases, zygotes arising from aneuploid gametes do not produce viable embryos. Instead, they undergo fetal death. (Any fetal death is a spontaneous abortion, commonly called a miscarriage.) In one study of 10,000 conceptions, it was found that 15% of embryos were lost by spontaneous abortion. Of these, about half (8%) suffered from meiotic abnormalities. Just under 6% of conceptions had either trisomies or polyploidy of the autosomes; 96% of these spontaneously aborted. Loss of an X chromosome was found in 1.4% of the embryos, of which 99% spontaneously aborted. Much better tolerated were rare trisomies or polyploidy of the sex chromosomes (0.2% of conceptions); 80% of those affected survived. Table 48–1 describes these results in greater detail. Of the meiotic abnormalities affecting fetuses that survived to term, 20% were due to trisomy 21 (see later discussion) and

table 48–1

ANEUPLOIDY INVOLVING THE SEX CHROMOSOMES IN HUMANS

Karyotype	Frequency	Sex	Characteristics
47,XXY*	1/700	M	Klinefelter's syndrome; increased height; sterility, a proportion may have some learning difficulties
47,XYY	1/700	M	Increased height; generally fertile; typically with chromosomally normal offspring; a proportion may have some learning difficulties
47,XXX	1/1000	F	Increased height; generally fertile; typically with chromosomally normal offspring; a proportion have serious learning difficulties
45,X	1/10,000	F	Turner's syndrome; reduced height; infertility; normal intelligence; 99% of these embryos terminate as spontaneous abortions

*This number gives the total number of chromosomes, followed by the complement of sex chromosomes.
(From Thompson MW, McInnes RR, Willard HF: Genetics in Medicine, 5th ed. Philadelphia: WB Saunders, 1991, p. 215.)

30% were attributable to abnormal segregation of the sex chromosomes. It is likely that these figures underestimate the frequency of meiotic abnormalities and spontaneous abortion during very early pregnancy, as most fetuses lost in the first 4 to 6 weeks of gestation usually are not sent to the laboratory for karyotyping. Nonetheless, this study revealed that spontaneous abortion is an efficient protective mechanism for the elimination of chromosomal imbalances that arise from errors in meiosis.

The remaining chromosomal abnormalities of meiotic origin are structural rearrangements. These rearrangements most likely arise from chromosomal breakage followed by illegitimate recombination between nonhomologous chromosomes. A rearrangement that does not involve net gain or loss of chromosomal material is called a **balanced rearrangement.** Carriers of balanced rearrangements do not usually have problems except in reproduction. The reproductive difficulties are due to an increased production of gametes having chromosomal deletions and/or duplications because of difficulties in meiotic chromosomal synapsis and crossover. A fetus with an unbalanced rearrangement will usually undergo spontaneous abortion, but in some instances, such rearrangements result in a liveborn child with multiple malformations and mental retardation.

Meiotic errors involving a few of the autosomes can produce fetuses that survive to birth. Individuals trisomic for chromosome 21 (a condition commonly known as **Down syndrome**) have mental retardation and characteristic phenotypic features. Although these individuals may live to adulthood, they have a decreased life expectancy. A very few individuals who are trisomic for chromosomes 13 and 18 also survive to birth; however, they typically die shortly thereafter. Why do individuals with Down syndrome survive whereas others affected by aneuploidy do not? It may be that there are no genes whose dosage is critical for survival among the very small number (225) of genes on chromosome 21.

The frequency of certain types of aneuploidy, such as trisomy for chromosome 21, is strongly correlated with the age of the mother. Statistics indicate that only 0.04% of the children of mothers who are 20 years old have trisomy 21. This number rises dramatically with maternal age, so that nearly 5% of the conceptions in mothers 45 years old have trisomy 21 (Fig. 48–14). The reason for this dramatic increase is not known, although many suggestions have been

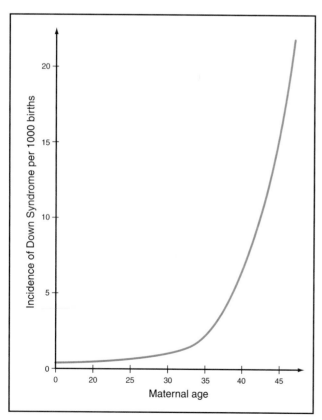

Figure 48–14 The relationship between maternal age and the incidence of Down syndrome.

proposed. Some believe that during the many years of arrest of oocytes in meiosis I diplotene, chiasmata joining homologous chromosomes gradually dissociate. Alternatively, there could be a tendency for the ovary to release the healthiest oocytes first; those that are trisomic for chromosome 21 may be released later in life. Interestingly, although the frequency of births of individuals with 47,XXX and 47,XXY chromosome complements (see Table 48–1 for explanation of nomenclature) also shows a correlation with maternal age, the frequency of occurrence of 45,X does not. This suggests that more than one mechanism may be responsible for the generation of aneuploid offspring.

Abnormalities in spermatogenesis also contribute to human aneuploidy. When sperm are examined, 2% to 5% are found to be aneuploid. It is known that about 7% of instances of trisomy 21 are of paternal origin. Meiotic abnormalities involving defects in crossing over and chiasma formation are also found in a significant percentage of infertile men who have decreased production of viable sperm.

▌ **Selected Readings**

Ellis N, Goodfellow PN: The mammalian pseudoautosomal region. Trends Genet 5:406, 1989.

Honigberg SM, McCarroll RM, Esposito RE: Regulatory mechanisms in meiosis. Curr Opin Cell Biol 5:219, 1993.

Loidl J: Coming to grips with a complex matter. A multidisciplinary approach to the synaptonemal complex. Chromosoma 100:289, 1991.

Miyazaki WY, Orr-Weaver TL: Sister-chromatid cohesion in mitosis and meiosis. Annu Rev Genet 28:167, 1994.

Rieder CL, Cole R: Chromatid cohesion during mitosis: Lessons from meiosis. J Cell Sci 112:2607, 1999.

Roeder GS: Meiotic chromosomes: It takes two to tango. Genes Dev 11:2600, 1997.

Roeder GS: Sex and the single cell: Meiosis in yeast. Proc Natl Acad Sci USA 92:10450, 1995.

Roeder GS, Bailis JM: The pachytene checkpoint. Trends Genet 16:395, 2000.

Sagata N: What does Mos do in oocytes and somatic cells? Bioessays 19:13, 1997.

Stoop-Myer C, Amon A: Meiosis: Rec8 is the reason for cohesion. Nature Cell Biol 1:E125, 1999.

West SC: Enzymes and molecular mechanisms of genetic recombination. Annu Rev Biochem 61:603, 1992.

Zickler D, Kleckner N: Meiotic chromosomes: Integrating structure and function. Annu Rev Genet 33:603, 1999.

chapter 49

PROGRAMMED CELL DEATH

The Necessity for Cell Death in Multicellular Organisms

The ability to undergo **programmed cell death** (Box 49–1) is a built-in latent capacity in virtually all cells of multicellular organisms. Cell death is extremely important in embryonic development, maintenance of tissue homeostasis, establishment of immune self-tolerance, killing by immune effector cells, and regulation of cell viability by hormones and growth factors. It has even been proposed to be the default program for all metazoan cells, and it is believed that cells remain healthy only as long as they receive survival signals from other cells. Abnormalities of the cell death program are important in a number of diseases, including cancer, Alzheimer's disease, and acquired immune deficiency syndrome (AIDS).

Classes of Cells That Undergo Programmed Cell Death

A variety of cells undergo programmed cell death. These can be separated into at least seven distinct classes (see examples in Fig. 49–1).

Harmful Cells

During molecular maturation of T-cell antigen receptors (see Chapters 29 and 30), immature T cells in the thymus (known as thymocytes) rearrange the genes encoding the receptor α and β chains. Many newly created receptors bind to foreign antigens, but others interact with self-antigens. Cells with receptors recognizing self-antigens are potentially harmful and are eliminated through programmed cell death. Interestingly, the drug cyclosporin A, which inhibits pro-

grammed cell death in thymocytes, can cause autoimmune disease.

Cells with damaged DNA tend to accumulate mutations, and they, too, are potentially harmful to the organism. DNA damage induces programmed cell death in many cell types.

Cells that harbor infectious agents, such as viruses, are also harmful to the organism. One mechanism to eliminate infected cells is through the action of cytotoxic T lymphocytes, which kill cells, in part, by inducing them to undergo programmed cell death.

Developmentally Defective Cells

To function properly, the T-cell receptor must recognize major histocompatibility complex (MHC) glycoproteins on other cells during antigen presentation (see Chapter 29). T lymphocytes whose T-cell receptors cannot interact with the spectrum of MHC glycoproteins expressed in a given individual are ineffective in the immune response. These cells die by apoptosis. Overall, defects in T-cell receptor assembly are extremely common, and up to 95% of immature T cells die by apoptosis without leaving the thymus.

Similar selection steps occur during the maturation of B lymphocytes (see Chapter 30), which is accomplished by a combination of gene rearrangements and facilitated mutagenesis. B lymphocytes expressing antibodies directed against self-antigens or producing antibodies whose affinity for antigen is below a critical threshold are eliminated through programmed cell death.

Excess Cells

The use of programmed cell death for quality control during development is not limited to the immune system, but is also extremely important during brain de-

767

box 49–1

KEY TERMS

Programmed Cell Death: An active cellular process that culminates in cell death. This may occur in response to developmental or environmental cues, or as a response to physiological damage detected by the cell's internal surveillance networks.

Necrosis (Accidental Cell Death): Cell death that results from irreversible injury to the cell. Cell membranes swell and become permeable. Lytic enzymes destroy the cellular contents, which then leak out into the intercellular space, leading to the mounting of an inflammatory response.

Apoptosis: One type of programmed cell death characterized by a particular pattern of morphologic changes. The name comes from the ancient Greek, referring to shedding of the petals from flowers or leaves from trees. Apoptosis is observed in all metazoans, including both plants and animals, but the genes encoding proteins involved in apoptosis have yet to be detected in single-celled organisms, such as yeasts.

Apoptotic death occurs in two phases. During the *latent phase*, the cell looks morphologically normal but is actively making preparations for death. The *execution phase* is characterized by a series of dramatic structural and biochemical changes that culminate in the fragmentation of the cell into membrane-enclosed *apoptotic bodies*. Activities that cause cells to undergo apoptosis are said to be *pro-apoptotic*. Activities that protect cells from apoptosis are said to be *anti-apoptotic*.

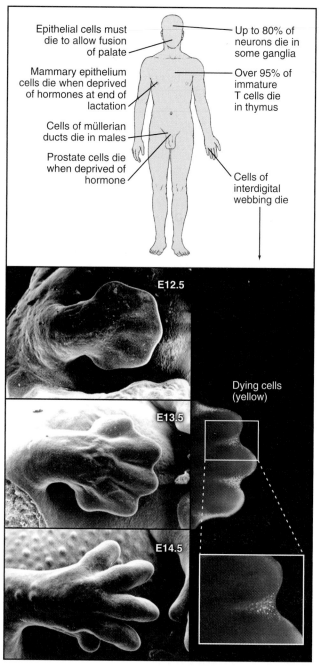

Figure 49–1 *Upper panel,* Types of cells that undergo programmed cell death. *Lower panel,* Programmed cell death in the embryonic mouse paw. At day 12.5 of development, the digits are fully connected by webbing. By day 13.5, the webbing has started to die, and by day 14.5, all of the webbing cells are gone. *Bottom right panel,* Nuclei of cells undergoing programmed cell death take up acridine orange, whereas cells of the surrounding healthy tissue do not. (Micrographs courtesy of William Wood and Paul Martin, Department of Anatomy and Developmental Biology, University College of London.)

velopment. Embryonic ganglia often have many more neurons than required to enervate their target muscles. Production of excess cells appears to be part of a strategy to ensure that a sufficient number of axons reach their targets. Excess neurons that do not make appropriate connections have no function and so are eliminated by programmed cell death. Up to 80% of neurons in certain developing ganglia die this way. The brain is the most seriously affected organ in mice lacking one of several essential death factors.

Unnecessary Cells

During development of many vertebrates, the digits of hands and feet are connected by a tissue webbing. Cells in this webbing serve no purpose in humans and are eliminated by programmed cell death.

The müllerian ducts develop into the female oviduct. In male embryos, progenitors of the müllerian ducts develop, even though they have no function. Programmed cell death eliminates the constituent cells of these embryonic ducts.

Obsolete Cells

The elimination of obsolete cells is most evident in organisms, such as insects and amphibians, that undergo metamorphosis during development. For example, programmed cell death initiated by a burst of thyroid hormone is responsible for resorption of the tadpole tail.

Mammals also use programmed cell death to eliminate obsolete tissues during embryogenesis. During craniofacial development, the hard palate develops from two lateral precursors, each covered in a protective layer of epithelial cells. As the two halves grow together at the midline of the nasopharynx, they remain separated by this covering of epithelium until, in response to a developmental cue, the epithelial cells at the midline undergo programmed cell death. Then the two halves of the palate can fuse. Failure of the epithelial cells to die at the appropriate time may interfere with the fusion of the palate.

Populations of cells that are fully functional may become obsolete as a result of physiological changes in the status of an organism. For example, in male mammals, certain accessory glands of the reproductive system are regulated by the levels of circulating male hormone. If hormone levels fall below a critical threshold, these organs, including the prostate, virtually disappear in a very brief time as their constituent cells undergo massive programmed death. Should levels of circulating androgens rise once again, the remaining prostatic stem cells proliferate and reconstruct the gland. A similar cycle of growth and involution is seen in the female in the mammary gland, which exhibits substantial differences in size and cellular composition in the lactating and nonlactating state. Interference with survival signaling by sex hormones is one important strategy commonly taken in the treatment of breast and prostate cancer.

Virus-Infected Cells

At least part of the loss of mature CD4$^+$ T helper cells (see Chapter 30) in persons infected with HIV-1 apparently results from programmed cell death. When exposed to agents that would normally stimulate cell proliferation, these cells instead undergo apoptosis. Paradoxically, it appears that many of these dying cells are not themselves infected with HIV.

Chemotherapeutic Killing of Cells

Exposure of cancer cells to many of the agents used in chemotherapy does not kill them outright. Instead, the cells die because the drugs cause intracellular damage that acts as a signal for the induction of apoptotic cell death.

■ Signals That Induce Programmed Cell Death

Cells undergo programmed death in response to both internal surveillance mechanisms and signals sent (or not sent) by other cells. Thus, some cells effectively

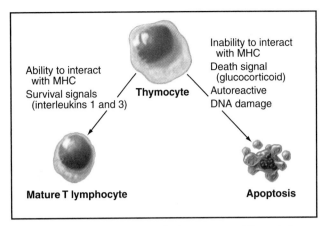

Figure 49-2 Examples of signals that promote differentiation or programmed cell death of a T lymphocyte in the thymus. Thymocytes that make functional T-cell receptors that do not recognize self-antigens mature, provided they receive survival signals, such as interleukin-1 and -3. Thymocytes undergo apoptosis if they produce defective T-cell receptor, recognize self-antigens, suffer DNA damage, or receive a death stimulus (glucocorticoid hormone). More than 95% of immature thymocytes die without leaving the thymus.

"volunteer" to die, whereas other cells are "nominated" for death by others (Fig. 49–2).

Cells that "volunteer" to die do so for a myriad of reasons. Two of the most widely studied death stimuli are DNA damage and inappropriate signals to proliferate. Examples of DNA damage that commonly trigger cell death are double-strand breaks induced by ionizing radiation and DNA breaks or other damage induced by chemotherapeutic agents. Cells that die in response to inappropriate signals to proliferate include those infected by certain viruses or overexpressing genes involved in cell proliferation (such as *c-myc* and *c-fos;* see Chapter 44). This ability to recognize an inappropriate stimulus to proliferate and respond to it by undergoing apoptosis may be an important defense against cancer.

Cells can be "nominated" for death by other cells in at least three ways. First, cells recognized as foreign (or harboring foreign pathogens) undergo programmed cell death when attacked by cytotoxic T lymphocytes. Second, cells may undergo programmed cell death if nurturing signals sent by other cells or the extracellular matrix are withheld. Survival signals include the lymphokines, such as interleukin-1 and -3, which are essential for survival of thymocytes; nerve growth factor, which is required for survival of many neurons; and extracellular matrix, which is required for survival of epithelial cells. Third, some cells respond to certain growth factors by undergoing programmed cell death. Examples include death of thymocytes in response to glucocorticoid hormones secreted by the adrenal glands, and the death of certain epithelial cells in response to transforming growth factor-β_1 (TGF-β_1).

The list of signals that cause cells to undergo programmed cell death is ever-increasing and bewilderingly complex. The complexity arises both from the number of different signals and from the diversity of cellular responses to a given signal. This diversity is illustrated by the following observations.

1. Certain cells die when hormonal levels rise (e.g., thymocytes in response to glucocorticoids), whereas others die as hormone levels decline (e.g., cells of the ventral prostate following castration).

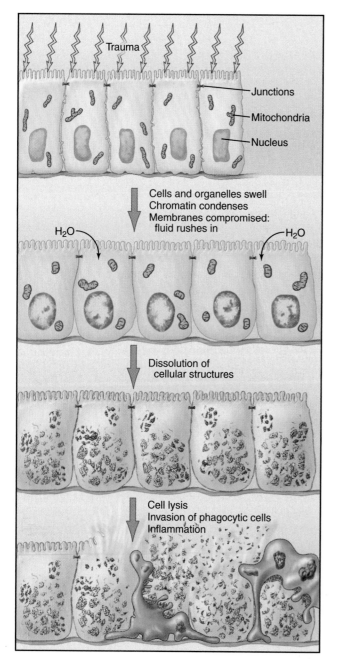

Figure 49–3 Necrosis is a result of injury to cells. Typically, groups of cells are affected. In most cases, necrotic cell death leads to an inflammatory response (red "angry" macrophages).

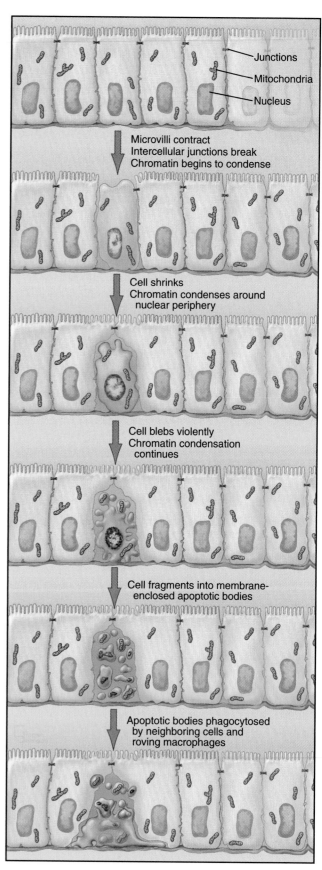

Figure 49–4 Apoptosis—active cellular suicide—typically affects single cells. Neighboring cells remain healthy. Apoptotic cell death usually does not lead to an inflammatory response.

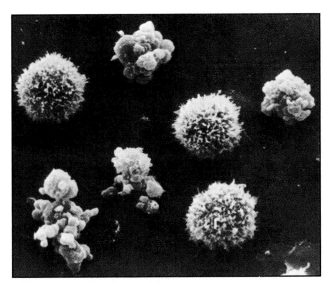

Figure 49-5 Scanning electron micrograph of intact and apoptotic mouse sarcoma cells. Intact cells are covered with microvilli, whereas apoptotic cells have numerous smooth blebs. These cells were stimulated to undergo apoptosis as a result of interference with RNA metabolism. (From Wyllie AH, Kerr JFR, Currie AR: Cell death: The significance of apoptosis. Int Rev Cytol 68:251–305, 1980.)

2. Inhibition of protein synthesis protects some cell types against programmed cell death, whereas in others, this inhibition leads directly to cell death.
3. Expression of the p53 tumor suppressor protein (see later section) in certain cell types leads to cell cycle arrest and promotes cell survival, whereas in others, it triggers programmed cell death.

In short, understanding and predicting the cellular life/death responses to the various stimuli that cells encounter may ultimately require an understanding of the complete web of individual and social interactions that are fundamental to the existence of complex metazoans.

Accidental Cell Death Versus Programmed Cell Death: Necrosis Versus Apoptosis

There are two primary pathways by which cells die. The path for accidental cell death is called **necrosis**. Accidental cell death occurs when cells receive a structural or chemical insult from which they cannot recover. Examples of such insults include ischemia (lack of oxygen), extremes of temperature, and physical trauma. The hallmark of necrosis is that cells die because they are *damaged*. In contrast, cells that die by programmed cell death commit suicide actively as the result of activation of a dedicated intracellular program. Often, they appear completely healthy prior to

committing suicide. For programmed cell death, the most commonly described pathway is **apoptosis**.

Necrosis corresponds to what most of us naively imagine cell death would be like: the cell falls apart and is digested by its own lytic enzymes (Fig. 49–3). Typically, loss of plasma membrane integrity is an early event in necrotic death. This allows water to rush into the dying cell, causing it to swell greatly so that the plasma and organelle membranes burst. As a result, the cell undergoes a generalized process of autodigestion and dissolution, culminating in the spilling of the cytoplasmic contents out into the surroundings. This, in turn, produces local inflammation, as phagocytic cells flock to the site, ingest the debris, and become activated (see Chapter 23). Because many agents that damage cells act over areas that are large compared to the size of a single cell, necrosis often involves large groups of neighboring cells.

In contrast to necrosis, apoptosis involves cell shrinkage, rather than cell swelling. Apoptosis is characterized by a reproducible pattern of structural alterations of both the nucleus and cytoplasm (Fig. 49–4). In order of appearance, these include (1) loss of microvilli and intercellular junctions (Fig. 49–5); (2) shrinkage of the cytoplasm; (3) dramatic changes in cytoplasmic motility with activation of a violent program of blebbing (Fig. 49–6); (4) loss of plasma mem-

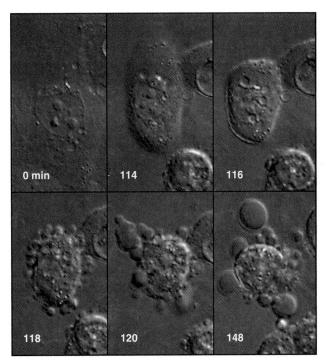

Figure 49-6 Apoptosis of a transformed pig kidney cell following exposure to etoposide, a drug used in cancer chemotherapy. The dramatic cytoplasmic blebbing results in the disassembly of the cell into membrane-enclosed vesicles. (Courtesy of L. M. Martins and K. Samejima, Wellcome Institute for Cell Biology, University of Edinburgh.)

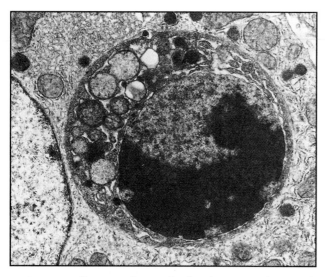

Figure 49-7 Electron micrograph of a phagocytosed apoptotic body containing a nuclear fragment. The nucleus of the epithelial cell that engulfed this apoptotic body is shown at left. In this case, apoptosis occurred during allograft rejection in a pig. (From Wyllie AH, Kerr JFR, Currie AR: Cell death: The significance of apoptosis. Int Rev Cytol 68:251–305, 1980.)

brane asymmetry, with the distribution of phosphatidyl serine being randomized so that it appears in the outer membrane leaflet; (5) changes in the organization of the cell nucleus, typically involving the hypercondensation of the chromatin and its collapse against the nuclear periphery; and (6) the "explosive" fragmentation of the cell into membrane-enclosed **apoptotic bodies** containing remnants of the nucleus, mitochondria, and other organelles. The plasma membrane retains its integrity throughout the entire process.

In tissues, apoptotic bodies are rapidly phagocytosed by surrounding cells (Fig. 49–7). Apoptosis can thus be considered to be the disassembly of the cell into "bite-sized" vesicles. Because these vesicles remain membrane bound, the cellular contents are never released into the environment. Furthermore, surface markers on apoptotic bodies suppress the activation of macrophages that ingest them. As a result, apoptotic death does not lead to an inflammatory response.

▌ Two Phases of Programmed Cell Death by Apoptosis

Apoptosis begins with a signal that can come from within the cell (e.g., detection of radiation-induced DNA breaks) or from without (e.g., a decrease in the level of an essential growth factor or hormone). This pro-apoptotic signal induces the cell to make a decision to commit suicide. By and large, the cellular decision-making process is not understood.

Initially, cells that are committed to undergo programmed cell death are in a **latent phase** of apoptosis (Fig. 49–8). Although embarked on a pathway of

gene expression (and/or other events) that leads to their inevitable death at some later time, while in the latent phase, these cells look essentially as normal and healthy as their neighbors. The duration of the latent phase of apoptosis is extremely variable, ranging from a few hours to several days. This is the case even for highly uniform populations of starting cells that are all at the same position in the cell cycle when the signal to die is given. The reason for this variability is not known.

Ultimately, the cells enter the **execution phase** of apoptosis, in which they undergo the dramatic morphologic and physiological changes described earlier. These changes are extremely rapid in comparison to the length of the latent phase and are typically completed within an hour or so. In contrast to the apparently diverse pattern of regulatory events that appears to characterize the latent phase in different cell types, the final execution phase of apoptosis appears to be much more conserved.

P53 and the Events of the Latent Phase

In some cell types, new protein synthesis must occur between the receipt of the signal triggering the death pathway and the onset of apoptotic execution. For example, thymocytes exposed to glucocorticoid hormones undergo apoptosis, reflecting the normal physiological pathway for regulating the population of the thymus by the adrenal gland. If, however, the thymocytes are cultured in the presence of a protein synthesis inhibitor, such as cycloheximide, following glucocorticoid exposure, they remain viable. Such observations give strong support to the notion of apoptosis as cellular suicide.

Protein synthesis during the latent phase of programmed cell death is not universally required. For example, cycloheximide actually induces programmed cell death in some cell types and has no effect on programmed cell death in other cells.

Little is known about the identity of the death-promoting proteins that are synthesized during the la-

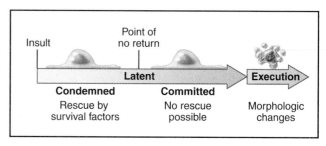

Figure 49-8 The two phases of apoptosis. Note that the latent phase can be subdivided into two stages: a *condemned* stage, during which the cell is proceeding on a pathway toward death but can still be rescued if it is exposed to anti-apoptotic activities, and a *committed* stage, beyond which rescue is impossible.

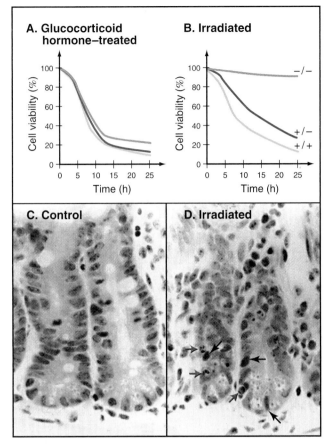

Figure 49-9 *A* and *B*, Time course of survival of thymocytes from three strains of mice after exposure to glucocorticoids (*A*) or irradiation (*B*). Cell death was due to apoptosis. The strains were as follows: *yellow,* wild-type mice; *red,* heterozygous mice having one good copy of the *p53* gene and one defective copy; *blue,* mice lacking a functional copy of the *p53* gene. Thymocytes lacking p53 are resistant to radiation-induced apoptosis but show normal induction of apoptosis following exposure to glucocorticoid hormone. *C* and *D,* Induction of p53 accumulation following radiation of the small intestine. *C,* Control sample. *D,* Irradiated sample. *Black arrows,* cells with increased levels of p53. *Red arrows,* apoptotic cells. (*A* and *B,* Reprinted with permission from Nature. From Lowe SW, Schmitt EM, Smith SW, et al: P53 is required for radiation-induced apoptosis in mouse thymocytes. Nature 362:847–849, 1993. Copyright 1993, Macmillan Magazines Limited. *C* and *D,* Courtesy of John Hickman, Molecular and Cellular Pharmacology Group, University of Manchester, England.)

tent phase of apoptosis. However, in many instances, genes up-regulated by the **p53** tumor suppressor protein are likely to be involved. P53 is involved in the regulation of cell cycle progression in response to DNA damage (see Chapter 46). When cells sense DNA damage induced by agents such as ionizing radiation, levels of p53 rise dramatically (Fig. 49-9). This p53 typically causes the cell to delay its entry into S phase until the damage has been repaired. P53 also is involved in triggering an apoptotic response in instances in which the damage is too severe to repair. The action of this tumor suppressor protein is very important in the body's defense against cancer. Nonfunc-

tional p53 genes are found in about 50% of all human cancers.

A direct connection between p53 and apoptosis was first noticed when the cloned p53 gene was introduced into a number of different cell types. In most cells, overexpression of p53 causes a cell cycle arrest at the G_1/S boundary. However, overexpression of cloned p53 in certain cancer-derived cell lines causes the cells to undergo apoptosis.

The role of p53 in apoptosis was confirmed when researchers constructed strains of transgenic mice lacking a functional p53 gene ("p53 knockout mice"). These mice develop normally but are extremely prone to cancer at a very young age. This rules out any absolute requirement for p53 in the programmed cell deaths that occur during embryogenesis in the mouse. Nonetheless, p53 is involved in apoptosis of certain mouse cells. Thymocytes isolated from p53 knockout mice are extremely resistant to the induction of apoptosis by ionizing radiation and other agents that cause DNA breaks (see Fig. 49-9C). However, p53 is not involved in all types of apoptosis, even in thymocytes. For example, thymocytes isolated from p53 knockout mice show normal induction of apoptosis following exposure to glucocorticoid hormone.

P53 appears to function as a transcriptional activator to promote apoptosis. P53 controls, among others, the well-studied death-promoting genes *Bax, Fas* (*CD95/APO*-1), and *APAF*-1 (see later sections). Other genes activated by p53, such as *PUMA* (p53 modulated upregulator of apoptosis), *Killer/*DR5, *Noxa,* etc., may also be involved in promoting cell death during the latent phase of apoptosis.

Not All Programmed Cell Death Occurs by Apoptosis

In recent years, the terms apoptosis and programmed cell death have come to be viewed as synonymous. This is incorrect. A number of well-documented examples exist of cells that undergo programmed cell death without exhibiting the dramatic structural changes that are the basis of the term apoptosis.

Programmed cell death of intersegmental muscles in the tobacco hawkmoth shortly after emergence of the adult from its cocoon differs in several ways from classical apoptosis. The chromatin does not condense, there is no detectable digestion of the DNA, and there is no obvious ruffling or "boiling" of the cytoplasm. Instead, there is a substantial induction of the polyubiquitin gene, which plays an important role in intracellular protein degradation (see Chapter 24). Induction of this gene is not detected during apoptosis in thymocytes. Thus, although these muscle cells unquestionably undergo programmed cell death, they apparently do not use the apoptosis pathway.

■ Genetic Analysis of Programmed Cell Death

Several key components involved in the apoptotic execution of mammalian cells were first identified in a genetic analysis of the tiny nematode worm, *Caenorhabditis elegans*. Because *C. elegans* is optically clear, it is possible to see every cell in a developing worm using differential interference contrast (Nomarski) optics. This has enabled investigators to develop a complete fate map for *C. elegans*: that is, one can choose any cell in an adult worm and tell its exact history all the way back to the fertilized egg. These studies have led to the surprising discovery that, of the 1090 somatic cells produced during embryogenesis of the *C. elegans* hermaphrodite, 131 undergo programmed cell death at reproducible locations and times. Thus, programmed cell death is one of the most common fates for newborn *C. elegans* cells.

Mutations in at least 14 *C. elegans* genes affect programmed cell death (Fig. 49–10). These may be divided into three classes: (1) genes that mark cells for subsequent programmed death; (2) genes involved in cell killing and its regulation; and (3) genes involved in the phagocytosis and subsequent processing of the cell corpses. These mutants are collectively known as ced (*cell death abnormal*) **mutants.**

The three most famous cell death genes are **ced-3, ced-4,** and **ced-9.** *Ced-3* and *ced-4* are required for cells to undergo programmed cell death. If either gene is inactivated, all cells throughout the organism that should die by programmed cell death are reprieved. These cells remain alive and are apparently functional. Interestingly, these worms have normal life spans. This suggests that programmed cell death may not be involved in the normal aging process, at least not in *C. elegans*. *Ced-9* is a regulator of *ced-3* and *ced-4*. In *ced-9* loss-of-function mutants, many cells die that should normally stay alive. This is deleterious for the organism, and *ced-9* mutants are not viable.

These genes all have mammalian counterparts (discussed more fully in the section that follows). Ced-3 is a member of a specialized family of cell death proteases called caspases (see later section). Ced-4 is a scaffolding protein that plays an essential role in the activation of caspases from their zymogen precursors. Its mammalian counterpart is **Apaf-1** (*a*poptotic *p*rotease-*a*ctivating *f*actor-1). Ced-9 is a member of the **Bcl-2** family of cell death regulators. In mammals, some Bcl-2 family members protect against cell death, whereas others actively promote cell death.

To date, eight genes involved in the phagocytosis and processing of the cell corpses have been characterized. Several are signaling proteins with roles in reorganizing the cytoskeleton to permit the cell to move toward and engulf its target. Another, the *nuc-1* gene, encodes the nuclease that digests the DNA of the dead cell. In the worm, digestion of the DNA occurs in lysosomes of cells that ingest the corpse. In mammals, this digestion occurs within the dying cell itself. The process of phagocytosis in apoptosis is surprisingly complex, probably involving both ligand-receptor interactions and directed cell motility.

■ Proteins Regulating Apoptosis

This and the next section list and briefly describe some of the major proteins that regulate apoptosis. The subsequent section describes two particular cell death pathways in some detail.

Bcl-2 Family

The *C. elegans ced-9* gene protects cells against programmed cell death. In *ced-9* mutants, many cells that should normally survive into the adulthood of the organism instead die during development. The human *Bcl-2* gene is at least partly functionally homologous to the *C. elegans ced-9* gene. Expression of human *Bcl-2* in developing *C. elegans ced-9* mutants reduced the level of programmed cell death. This ability of a human gene to protect cells of a nematode is good evidence that at least some of the fundamental mechanisms involved in programmed cell death have been conserved over great evolutionary distances.

Bcl-2 is only one member of a large family of

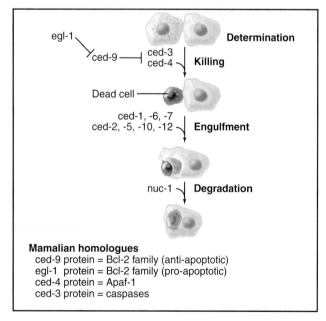

Mamalian homologues
ced-9 protein = Bcl-2 family (anti-apoptotic)
egl-1 protein = Bcl-2 family (pro-apoptotic)
ced-4 protein = Apaf-1
ced-3 protein = caspases

Figure 49–10 Genetic dissection of programmed cell death. The *ced* (cell death abnormal) mutants of the nematode worm *C. elegans* affect the killing, engulfment, and degradation stages of programmed cell death.

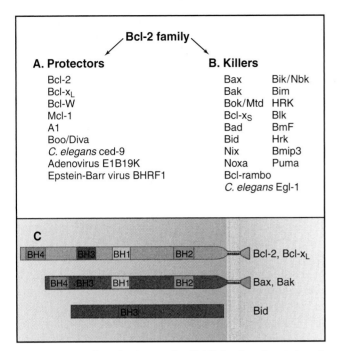

Figure 49–11 Introduction to the Bcl-2 family of proteins. *A*, Protectors. *B*, Killers. *C*, Bar diagrams of protein domain organization.

Bcl-x_L, and Bax can all form channels through artificial membranes. When reconstituted in vitro, these channels only allow the passage of small ions, and their importance for the regulation of apoptosis is not known.

Genetic experiments in mice have revealed several different functions for Bcl-2 family members. Mice born lacking Bcl-2 have deficiencies of the immune system that are best understood if one role of this protein in vivo is to render lymphocytes resistant to pro-apoptotic signals during immune system maturation. In contrast, loss of Bcl-x_L is lethal. Embryos die, apparently as a result of widespread cell death of central and peripheral neurons and hematopoietic cells of the liver. Loss of Bax (a pro-apoptotic family member) results, as expected, in insufficient deaths of T cells and B cells, resulting in hyperplasia of lymphoid tissues. Loss of Bax plus Bak renders cells highly resistant to apoptosis by the mitochondrial death pathway mediated by Bid (see subsequent discussion).

Bcl-2 Family Members and Cancer

A gene that prevents cells from dying poses a potential danger in multicellular organisms, in which rates

related proteins. Some family members protect cells from death (anti-apoptotic); others actively promote cell death (pro-apoptotic) (Fig. 49–11). Bcl-2 family members are defined by the presence of one to four blocks of conserved protein sequence called **BH domains** (*B*cl-2 *h*omology). Anti-apoptotic Bcl-2 family members typically have four of these domains. Pro-apoptotic family members may have three of these domains, although a number of these proteins have only the BH3 domain. The BH3 domain is thought to participate in protein-protein interactions that regulate cell death. For example, Bcl-2 protein forms a complex with a pro-apoptotic Bcl-2 family member called Bax. This complex formation can modulate the ability of Bcl-2 protein to protect cells against death stimuli.

Anti-apoptotic Bcl-2 family members protect cells against many cell death stimuli (Fig. 49–12), but how they do so remains controversial. *C. elegans* CED-9 and mammalian Bcl-x_L can both bind to the *C. elegans* CED-4 scaffolding protein and interfere with its activation of the CED-3 caspase (see later discussion). Thus, the proteins may directly block activation of the cell death pathway. Anti-apoptotic Bcl-2 family members also appear to block the mitochondrial pathway to cell death (see later section) by preventing the efflux of cytochrome *c* from mitochondria in response to death-promoting stimuli. How they might do this was suggested by the x-ray structure of anti-apoptotic protein Bcl-x_L, which revealed a surprising similarity to a number of bacterial, pore-forming proteins that was not expected from the amino acid sequence. In fact, Bcl-2,

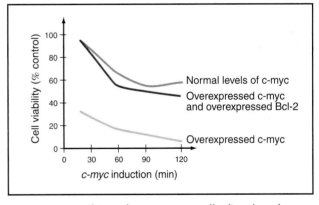

Figure 49–12 Chinese hamster ovary cells die when they are induced to express abnormally high levels of the c-myc protein, but simultaneous expression of the Bcl-2 protein rescues them from this effect. These cells contain many copies of the *c-myc* gene under control of a promoter that is activated when the cells are briefly exposed to high temperature (43°C for 90 minutes). The curves show the percentage of viable cells remaining at various times following the induction of *c-myc* expression. The *Bcl-2* gene was introduced into these cells on a plasmid molecule under the control of a viral promoter, which is always active. The upper curve represents the parental cell line lacking either the cloned *c-myc* or *Bcl-2* genes. (Note that about 40% of these cells die following the heat treatment used to induce *c-myc* expression.) The lower curve shows that the cells producing high levels of *c-myc* protein alone rapidly die by apoptosis. The middle curve shows that cells expressing both the c-myc and Bcl-2 proteins survive the treatment almost as well as the parental cells. (From Bissonnette RP, Echeverri F, Mahboubi A, et al: Apoptotic cell death induced by c-myc is inhibited by *bcl-2*. Nature 359:552–556, 1992.)

of cell proliferation and death must be balanced carefully. In fact, the name *Bcl-2* comes from the fact that this gene was isolated as the culprit responsible for certain types of B-cell lymphoma. These lymphomas arise when a chromosome translocation joins regions of chromosomes 14 and 18, moving the *Bcl-2* gene into the immunoglobulin heavy-chain gene cluster, a site of very active gene transcription in B cells. The elevated transcription of Bcl-2 is directly responsible for the cancerous phenotype in these patients, making Bcl-2 a cancer-promoting oncogene.

Unlike other oncogenes, *Bcl-2* overexpression does not cause cell proliferation. Instead, it disrupts the balance of regulation between life and death of the affected cells. Cells that overexpress Bcl-2 protein actually grow, if anything, more slowly than their counterparts that express normal levels of the protein. However, Bcl-2 overexpressers are highly resistant to many stimuli that normally promote cell death.

The gene encoding the pro-apoptotic Bcl-2 family member Bax is disrupted in one class of human colon cancers. Because Bax expression is induced by p53, which is also mutated in many colon cancers, it has been suggested that Bax may normally suppress tumors in the colon.

Certain viruses have acquired the ability to protect cells against apoptosis, which they use as part of their repertoire to overcome host defenses. For example, expression of the adenovirus *E1A* gene, which activates cellular programs leading to cell proliferation, typically causes cells to undergo apoptosis. This cellular response is mediated by p53, and adenovirus carries a second gene, *E1B*, that blocks the action of p53. Several other viruses also make polypeptides that inhibit apoptosis (see later discussion).

Proteins Involved in the Execution of Apoptosis

Caspases (cysteine aspartases) are specialized proteases that have cysteine at their active site and cleave on the C-terminal side of aspartate residues. Caspases inactivate cellular survival pathways and specifically activate other factors whose function is to promote cell death.

C. elegans has three major caspases, one of which (CED-3) is essential for cell death. In contrast, mammals have at least 14 caspase genes. Analysis based on sequence comparisons divides caspases into two major subfamilies. The caspase 1 subfamily encodes enzymes that process pro-interleukin-1β to yield mature interleukin-1β. Macrophages secrete this cytokine, which is involved in inflammation. In contrast, the caspase 3 subfamily of enzymes participates exclusively in apoptotic cell death.

All caspases are heterotetramers with two large and two small subunits associated into a compact, block-like molecule (Fig. 49–13). Like many proteases, caspases are synthesized as inactive zymogens consisting of an N-terminal prodomain, followed by domains encoding the large and small subunits. These domains are separated by aspartate residues, the cleavage target for caspases. Caspase maturation involves either autocatalytic processing of the zymogen (see later discussion) or cleavage of one zymogen by another active caspase. Caspase zymogens are apparently synthesized constitutively in all living cells.

The primary structure of the family of caspase zymogens involved in cell death reveals the presence of two classes of these enzymes (see Fig. 49–13). Caspase zymogens with long prodomains are known as **initiator caspases.** They are capable of autoactivation when complexed with the appropriate scaffolding factors (see later section) and, therefore, can initiate the apoptotic response. Sequences within the extended prodomains are involved in targeting the initiator caspase zymogens to the appropriate cellular locations and in interactions with scaffolding factors. The second class, **effector caspases,** have short prodomains. These enzymes are not capable of autoactivation under normal circumstances. Instead, they are

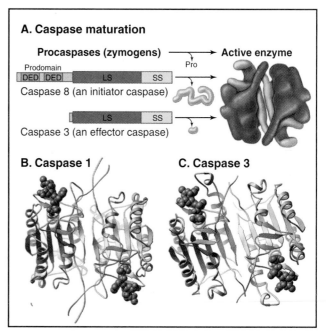

Figure 49–13 Summary figure describing the two classes of caspases. *A,* Initiator caspases have large prodomains that participate in subcellular targeting. Two procaspases come together to form the active enzyme *(right)*. *B* and *C,* Crystal structure of caspases 1 and 3. The catalytic residues come primarily from the large subunit *(blue)*. In the caspase 1–like enzymes (involved in the inflammatory response), the catalytic site is relatively open. In the caspase 3–like enzymes (involved in apoptosis), the small subunit *(yellow)* forms a "hood" that limits access to the active site.

KEEPING IT ALL STRAIGHT: THE KEY IS IN THE DOMAINS

There are so many different proteins involved in apoptosis that even experts have a difficult time keeping them all straight. However, an understanding of the general principles is much simplified if the following principle is kept in mind. Most proteins involved in apoptosis regulation are built from a relatively limited number of modules, many of which act as sites for protein-protein interactions. The following are the most important modules for apoptosis.

Bcl-2 family members are defined by the presence of short regions of conserved sequence, referred to as *BH domains* (Bcl-2 homology). One of these, the ~20 residue BH3 domain, found in all Bcl-2 family members, is thought to promote complex formation between Bcl-2 family members.

Caspase targeting and activation is regulated by three domains that, although they are not significantly related to one another at the level of amino acid sequence, all adopt a similar structure in solution. All are regions of ~80–90 residue that form a characteristic arrangement of six α-helix bundles.

1. The *death domain* (DD) is found in many proteins involved in signaling pathways related to cell death. These include cell death receptors, such as Fas (and others), and adapter molecules, such as FADD.
2. The *death effector domain* (DED) is found in adapters such as FADD, the prodomains of caspases 8 and 10, and in certain inhibitors of apoptosis.
3. The *caspase recruitment domain* (CARD) is found both in a number of adapter proteins involved in cell death, including CED-4 and Apaf-1, and in caspases 1, 2, and 9.

In general, these domains prefer to interact with themselves (i.e., DD-DD, DED-DED, and CARD-CARD). Such interactions are said to be homophilic. As a result, when a new apoptosis effector protein is cloned, it is possible to predict from an analysis of the sequence which of the known proteins it is likely to interact with.

proteins. **Adapter proteins** have multiple protein-protein interaction motifs and serve to link caspases to activated cell death receptors (see later section and Box 49–2). Somehow this binding orients the bound caspase zymogens in a favorable conformation so that they can cleave themselves, thereby releasing active caspases and starting the apoptotic cascade (see examples in later section).

Caspases are highly selective enzymes, cleaving a very small subset of cellular proteins found in both the nucleus and cytoplasm (Fig. 49–14). Although

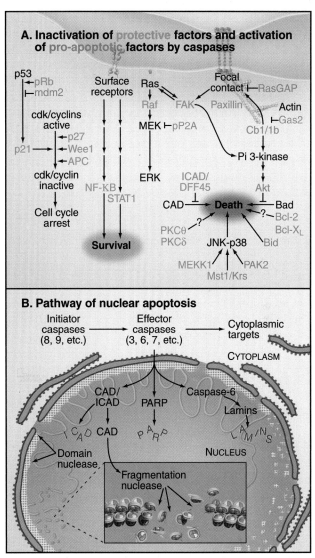

Figure 49–14 *A*, Some of the many proteins cleaved by caspases in apoptotic cell death. Proteins shown in green normally have a role in keeping the cell alive and are inactivated by caspases. Proteins shown in red are turned into active death-promoting factors as a result of caspase cleavage. Proteins shown in black are not cleaved and are included to show the pathways affected by cleavage. Caspases inactivate a number of pathways that promote cell survival, thereby strongly reinforcing the decision of the cell to die. *B*, Some of the roles of caspases in disassembly of the nucleus.

generally activated through processing by active initiator caspases.

Scaffolding proteins and **adapters** play an essential role in the activation of initiator caspases. The scaffolding proteins include both cell surface death receptors and the intracellular molecule **Apaf-1 (apoptotic protease activating factor 1)**. Upon receipt of a death stimulus, the relevant scaffolding protein forms an aggregate. This aggregate binds to initiator procaspases, either directly or through adapter

some of these targets are structural proteins, many others are involved in cellular signaling. For example, caspases cleave a number of protein kinases. Many kinases have autoregulatory domains that enable them to be switched on and off in response to physiological stimuli (see Fig. 27–4). In a number of cases, caspases cleave kinases so that regulatory domains are neatly removed, thereby producing constitutively active enzymes. Presumably, these unregulated kinases then activate factors that promote cell death. Caspases also cleave a number of proteins that normally function in the detection and repair of DNA damage.

In addition to the activities just described, caspases also act on a number of targets that directly promote cell death. The most obvious example of this is caspase activation of other caspases on the death cascade. Caspases also act on mitochondria, either directly or indirectly, to cause the release of factors that promote cell death. For example, caspases cleave the pro-apoptotic Bcl-2 family member Bid. Cleaved Bid then binds to mitochondria and promotes the release of cytochrome *c* (discussed in greater detail in a later section). Finally, caspase cleavage of an inhibitory chaperone is responsible for activation of the nuclease that ultimately destroys the chromosomal DNA of most cells undergoing apoptosis (see later discussion).

Natural Caspase Inhibitors

Several mammalian pox viruses make a serpin-like inhibitor of certain caspases called Crm1. (Serpins are special protease substrates that, upon cleavage, form a tight complex with the enzyme, functionally inactivating it.) Insect baculoviruses make two separate proteins—p35 and IAP—that inhibit apoptosis. The p35 protein is a broad-spectrum caspase inhibitor that may work by a serpin-like mechanism. IAP (inhibitor of apoptosis) proteins also block apoptosis, in some cases by inactivating caspases. Interestingly, several cellular homologues of the IAP proteins exist. Some of these apparently function as endogenous inhibitors of apoptosis.

CAD Nuclease and Its Chaperone ICAD

During apoptosis, the chromosomal DNA is cleaved by a nuclease (or nucleases) that acts in two stages. An initial cleavage of the chromosomes into fragments of roughly 50,000 base pairs is usually (but not always) followed by further cleavage of the DNA between nucleosomes, producing a characteristic "ladder" of DNA fragments with a periodicity of about 200 base pairs. This "ladder" is seen when the DNA is

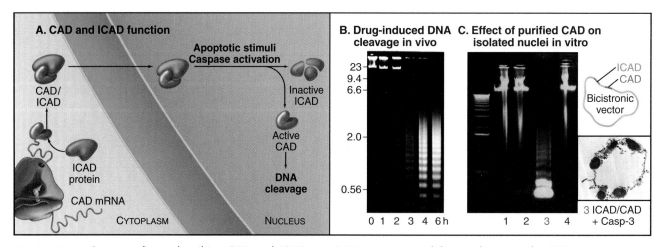

Figure 49–15 Summary figure describing CAD and ICAD. *A,* ICAD acts as an inhibitory chaperone for CAD, promoting folding of the protein on the ribosome and continuing as an inhibitor as CAD is stored in the nucleus. Cleavage of ICAD leads to CAD activation. *B,* Cleavage of the chromosomal DNA by CAD during chemotherapy-induced apoptosis of a leukemia cell line. DNA is separated according to size by electrophoresis on an agarose gel and stained with ethidium bromide. *C,* Cloned CAD and ICAD were expressed together in *E. coli* (the expression vector is diagrammed at the upper right) and incubated with nuclei. Only if ICAD was inactivated by cleavage with caspase 3 was active CAD released and able to degrade the nuclear DNA (lane 3). Other lanes: *Left,* DNA gel size markers; *Lanes 2 and 3,* nuclei incubated with buffer or caspase 3 alone, respectively; *Lane 4,* the same experiment as in lane 3 but performed using a mutant ICAD that could not be cleaved and inactivated by the caspase 3. This pure, activated CAD caused chromatin condensation and appearance of an apoptotic morphology in isolated cell nuclei. *Bottom right,* Electron micrograph of a thin section of one nucleus with condensed chromatin at the nuclear periphery. (*B,* From Kaufmann SH: Induction of endonucleolytic DNA cleavage in human acute myelogenous leukemia cells by etoposide, camptothecin, and other cytotoxic anticancer drugs: A cautionary note. Cancer Res 49: 5870–5878, 1989. *C,* Courtesy of K. Samejima, Wellcome Institute for Cell Biology, University of Edinburgh.)

isolated and subjected to gel electrophoresis. The responsible nuclease is called **CAD (caspase-activated DNase).** CAD is tightly regulated by *ICAD* **(inhibitor of CAD;** Fig. 49–15), a chaperone that must be present when CAD is being translated on the ribosome for CAD to fold into an active conformation. However, ICAD is also an inhibitor. CAD, when complexed with ICAD, is inactive as a nuclease. During apoptosis, ICAD is cleaved by caspases, and this releases active CAD nuclease. This elegant mechanism ensures that active CAD cannot be synthesized in the absence of its inhibitor. The complex of CAD and ICAD is also known as DFF (DNA fragmentation factor).

Two Pathways Leading to Cell Death

The Death Receptor Pathway

Cells express at least six different cell surface molecules that can function as death receptors. These receptors generally bind protein ligands that are expressed on the surface of other cells. Binding of its ligand by the receptor activates the receptor, turning on a pathway that can lead to cell death.

One well-characterized death receptor is called Fas (also known as Apo1 or CD95), a member of the tumor necrosis factor (TNF) receptor family (see Chapter 26). Fas is a type I membrane protein whose extracellular domain consists of 3 cysteine-rich domains (see Fig. 26–11, which shows the atomic structure of trimeric TNF receptor with bound ligand). Fas spends at least some of its time preassembled into a trimer. The cytoplasmic domain of Fas contains **death domain** of about 80 residues, which is shared by all of the so-called death receptors.

The ligand for the Fas receptor is a 40-kD intrinsic membrane protein called **Fas ligand.** This protein is present as a trimer on the surface of cells, including cytotoxic T lymphocytes, whose job, among others, is to rid the body of virally infected cells. When a cytotoxic T lymphocyte contacts a target cell, the Fas ligand on the lymphocyte surface binds to Fas on the target cell and initiates the death pathway (Fig. 49–16). Ligand binding somehow activates signaling from the intracellular death domain of Fas, possibly by stabilizing the trimer in the plane of the membrane (see Fig. 26–11). Bringing together three cytoplasmic death domains creates a binding site for an adapter protein called **FADD** (Fas-associated protein with a death domain). The Fas-FADD complex binds procaspase 8 through interactions with another type of motif called the **death effector domain,** present on both FADD and the prodomain of procaspase 8. On this molecular scaffold, procaspase 8 activates itself proteo-

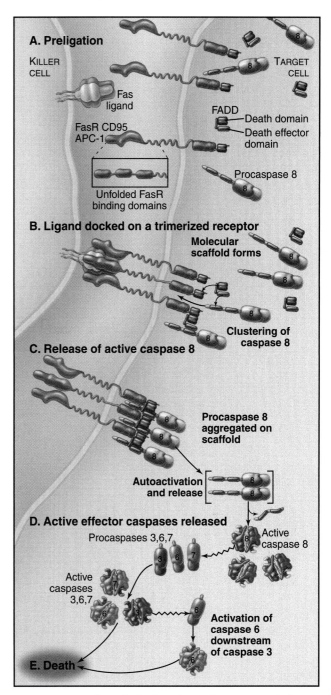

Figure 49-16 The cell death pathway downstream of the Fas cell death receptor. *A,* Preligation. *B,* Ligand docked on a trimerized receptor. *C,* Release of active caspase. *D,* Release of effector caspases. (See text for a description of the death pathway.)

lytically and triggers the death pathway as it activates downstream effector caspases. Interestingly, cells express a protein called FLIP that looks very much like a catalytically dead version of procaspase 8. This molecule is thought to compete with procaspase 8 for binding to FADD, thereby inhibiting the autoactivation

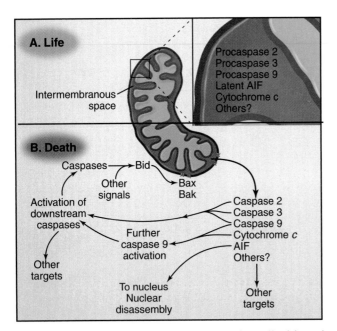

Figure 49-17 Mitochondria as integrators of a cell's life and death decisions. *A,* In healthy cells, a number of factors that promote apoptosis are stored in the intermembranous space of the mitochondria. *B,* In cells undergoing apoptosis, caspases trigger the pro-apoptotic Bcl-2 family members to induce the release of these death-promoting factors; this initiates an amplifying cycle that ultimately leads to cell death. *AIF,* apoptosis inducing factor.

of the caspase. The role of FLIP may be to dampen the Fas response locally to ensure that the cascade does not get activated by mistake.

Role of the Fas Death Receptor in Normal and Diseased Cells

Fas is emerging as an important factor in many cell death pathways. For example, Fas regulates the life span of activated tissue T and B lymphocytes. Normally, T cells die within a few hours of activation during an immune response. Activation initiates the expression of Fas ligand, which interacts with Fas already on the cell surface to trigger a death response. A similar mechanism (export of Fas and Fas ligand to the surface of the same cell) is responsible for some examples of p53-induced cell death and some, but not all, instances of cell death following exposure to chemotherapeutic agents.

Mouse mutants provide further evidence for an important role of the Fas system in immunoregulation. Mice lacking *Fas* (*lpr* mutation) or Fas ligand (*gld* mutation) accumulate excessive lymphocytes. In the appropriate genetic background, these mice tend to develop autoimmune disorders that, in some cases, resemble the human disease systemic lupus erythematosus. Evidence that Fas is involved in human systemic lupus erythematosus is still scant.

Expression of Fas ligand protects cells against im-

mune system cells that express Fas receptor. This is normally the case in immune-privileged tissues, like the lens of the eye and the testis, where it is desirable to avoid localized immune and inflammatory responses. Any immune effector cell that enters these tissues encounters Fas ligand and dies by apoptosis before it can act. Not surprisingly, certain tumor cells subvert this strategy as protection against the immune system. Melanoma cells expressing Fas ligand establish tumors particularly efficiently. Some tumor cells also defend themselves against immune surveillance with so-called **decoy receptors.** A secreted Fas decoy receptor blocks Fas ligand on cytotoxic cells. Other decoy receptors remain membrane bound but do not signal cell death because their intracellular domains lack functional death domains.

The Mitochondrial Pathway to Cell Death

Mitochondria are key players in an alternative pathway to cell death (Fig. 49–17). A variety of toxic insults trigger this pathway. Although the initial steps in this pathway are not yet known, in some cases, the apoptotic response is initiated when the death-promoting Bcl-2 family member Bid binds to mitochondria (Fig. 49–18). A process that requires either Bax or Bak opens a channel and releases the electron transport protein **cytochrome c** and other proteins from the intermembranous space into the cytoplasm. These mitochondrial proteins actively promote apoptotic cell death. In the cytoplasm, cytochrome *c* binds the scaffolding protein **Apaf-1,** a mammalian homologue of *C. elegans* CED-4 protein. This complex molecule interacts with caspases through an N-terminal **caspase recruitment domain.** Adjacent to this is the region of similarity to CED-4, which includes an adenosine triphosphatase (ATPase) domain. The C-terminal portion of Apaf-1 contains 12 WD-40 repeats, like those in β-subunits of trimeric G proteins (Chapter 27). This region of the molecule appears to act as a negative regulator of Apaf-1 function.

Binding of cytochrome *c* and deoxyadenosine triphosphate (dATP) removes the negative regulatory influence of the C-terminus of Apaf-1, thereby permitting binding and autoactivation of procaspase 9. This complex of Apaf-1, cytochrome *c,* caspase 9 (and possibly other subunits) is often referred to as the **apoptosome.** Active caspase 9 then cleaves procaspase 3, initiating the cell death cascade. This cascade can be further amplified in at least two ways. First, caspase 3 cleaves other effector caspases, directly amplifying the cascade. In addition, active caspases cleave Bid, which then binds much more efficiently to mitochondria, thereby releasing more mitochondrial factors, such as cytochrome *c,* and enhancing caspase 9 activation.

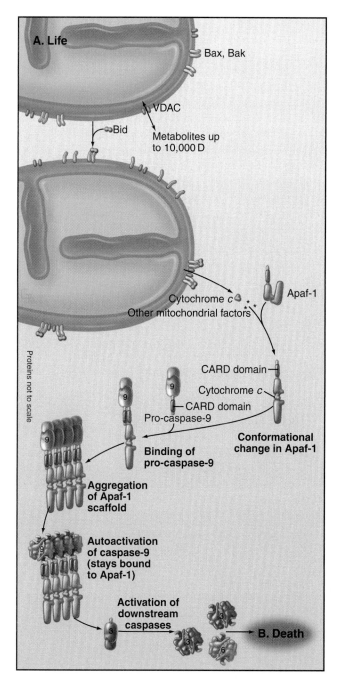

Figure 49-18 The mitochondrial cell death pathway from life (*A*) to death (*B*) (see text for description). There are a number of models for how the death-promoting factors, such as cytochrome *c,* are released by mitochondria. This figure shows only one of these in which Bax and Bak interact with the voltage-dependent anion channel (VDAC) and cause it to form a pore that releases cytochrome *c.* Released cytochrome *c* binds to Apaf-1, inducing a conformational change that, in turn, enables procaspase 9 to bind.

It was surprising to find that an essential protein like cytochrome *c* has a second function essential for death. Many studies support the Jekyll-and-Hyde–like nature of this protein in life and death.

Importance of Apoptosis in Human Disease

Apoptosis now accounts for a substantial percentage of all cell biology research. Why has this field so caught the scientific eye? There is no one reason, but one answer is the fact that apoptosis is a point of intersection between cell signaling pathways, cell structure, the cell cycle, and, of course, human disease. This chapter has mentioned the roles that aberrations in apoptosis play in the etiology of autoimmunity, AIDS, and cancer. Apoptosis is also emerging as a key factor in neurodegenerative diseases, such as Huntington's disease and Alzheimer's disease, as well as in myocardial infarction and stroke (Fig. 49–19). At a practical level, the realization that many successful chemotherapeutic agents act by inducing cancer cells to undergo apoptosis has meant that the search is now on for newer and better drugs that will elicit this response. An improved understanding of events during the latent phase of apoptosis may lead to the development of agents that will trigger an apoptotic response in tumor types that are currently resistant to chemotherapy. Conversely, the realization that a large fraction of the cell deaths in stroke are attributable to a wave of apoptosis that radiates outward from the original focus of ischemic death has led to the hunt for molecules that will prevent apoptosis during the critical period following the stroke or infarct. With such important practical problems to be solved, apop-

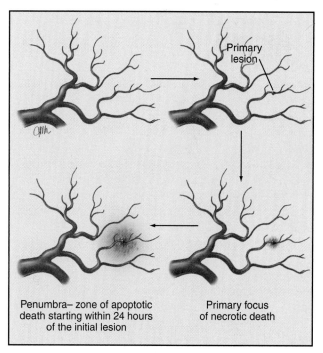

Figure 49-19 Secondary apoptotic death caused by oxygen deprivation in the penumbra greatly increases the size of the affected area of the brain in stroke.

tosis will continue to occupy a central position in cell biology research over the coming years.

▪ Selected Readings

Antonsson B, Martinou JC: The Bcl-2 protein family. Exp Cell Res 256:50–57, 2000.

Earnshaw WC, Martins LM, Kaufmann SH: Mammalian caspases: Structure, activation, substrates and functions during apoptosis. Annu Rev Biochem 68:383–424, 1999.

Kaufmann SH, Gores GJ: Apoptosis in cancer: Cause and cure. Bioessays 22:1007–1017, 2000.

Kaufmann SH, Hengartner MO: Programmed cell death: Alive and well in the new millennium. Trends Cell Biol 11:526–534, 2001.

Kelekar A, Thompson CB: Bcl-2-family proteins: The role of the BH3 domain in apoptosis. Trends Cell Biol 8:324–330, 1998.

Kroemer G, Reed JC: Mitochondrial control of cell death. Nature Med 6:513–519, 2000.

Meier P, Finch A, Evan G: Apoptosis in development. Nature 407:796–801, 2000.

Metzstein MM, Stanfield GM, Horvitz HR: Genetics of programmed cell death in *C. elegans:* Past, present and future. Trends Genet 14:410–416, 1998.

Nagata S: Apoptosis by death factor. Cell 88:355–365, 1997.

Raff MC: Social control on cell survival and cell death. Nature 356:397–400, 1992.

Rich T, Allen RL, Wyllie AH: Defying death after DNA damage. Nature 407:777–783, 2000.

Savill J, Fadok V: Corpse clearance defines the meaning of cell death. Nature 407:784–788, 2000.

Wyllie AH, Kerr JFR, Currie AR: Cell death: The significance of apoptosis. Int Rev Cytol 68:251–305, 1980.

INDEX

Note: Page numbers followed by b indicate boxed material; page numbers followed by f indicate figures; page numbers followed by t indicate tables.